WILLIAM F. MAAG LIBRARY
YOUNGSTOWN STATE UNIVERSITY

HANDBOOK OF PHYSIOLOGY

Section 11: Aging

HANDBOOK OF PHYSIOLOGY

A critical, comprehensive presentation of
physiological knowledge and concepts

Section 11: Aging

Edited by

EDWARD J. MASORO

Department of Physiology
The University of Texas Health Science Center

New York   Oxford
Published for the American Physiological Society
by Oxford University Press
1995

Oxford University Press

Oxford   New York   Toronto
Delhi Bombay Calcutta Madras Karachi
Kuala Lumpur Singapore Hong Kong Tokyo
Nairobi Dar es Salaam Cape Town
Melbourne Auckland Madrin

and associated companies in
Berlin Ibadan

Copyright © 1995 by the American Physiological Society

Published for the American Physiological Society by Oxford University Press, Inc.,
198 Madison Avenue, New York, New York 10016

Oxford is a registered trademark of Oxford University Press

All rights reserved. No part of this publication may be reproduced,
stored in a retrieval system, or transmitted, in any form or by any means,
electronic, mechanical, photocopying, recording, or otherwise,
without the prior permission of Oxford University Press.

Library of Congress Cataloging-in-Publication Data
Aging / edited by Edward J. Masoro.
p. cm.—(Handbook of physiology; section 11)
Includes bibliographical references and index.
ISBN 0-19-507722-9
1. Aging—Physiological aspects.   I. Masoro, Edward J.
II. American Physiological Society (1887–)
III. Series: Handbook of physiology (Bethesda, Md.); section 11.
[DNLM: 1. Aging—physiology.   QT 104 H236 1977 sect. 10]
QP6.H25   1977 sec.10   [QP86]   599'.01 s—dc20
[612.6'7]   DNLM/DLC   94-16

9 8 7 6 5 4 3 2 1

Printed in the United States of America
on acid-free paper

Preface

This Handbook, an up-to-date compendium of data on the physiology and the molecular aspects of biology of aging, provides the methodological and conceptual knowledge needed to carry out aging research successfully. I believe gerontologists, geriatricians, and biologists will find in these twenty-four chapters a source of unique and eminently useful information on aging in mammals with emphasis on human aging. Biologists who plan to initiate aging studies should find the book indispensable for avoiding pitfalls unique to gerontological research, pitfalls that have plagued the efforts of skilled biologists who are newcomers to gerontology.

Part I provides a broad overview of the current status of biological gerontology. The puzzle of why aging (senescence) occurs is examined. The concept of primary aging processes is considered; major views, both past and present, on the nature of these processes are assessed. The evolutionary theory of aging is presented as a framework for understanding why senescence occurs and as a guide for future studies in biological gerontology.

Methodological issues—the design and analysis of aging studies—are the focus of Part II, which includes discussions of the selection of human subjects and the use of animal models. There is also a chapter on the use of cells in culture as models of senescence.

Metabolic and molecular aspects of aging are discussed in Part III. A major theme is the influence of aging on bioenergetics, including the use of specific fuels (carbohydrates and fats) and the storage of energy (adipose tissue). This part should provide an invaluable source of basic information for gerontologists, geriatricians, and biomedical scientists concerned with those problems of the elderly related to obesity, glucose intolerance, type II diabetes, and atherosclerosis. Two of the chapters offer in-depth coverage of the molecular aspects of aging. These should provide gerontologists and physiologists with insights into mechanisms that underlie age-associated deterioration of the organism, including such diseases as rheumatoid arthritis, osteoarthritis, and cancer.

Part IV contains twelve chapters on age-related changes in the physiology of the organ systems and the integrated organism. Information here has been culled from widely dispersed physiological literature to offer a comprehensive and well-focused account of the physiology of aging in humans and other mammals.

Proposed modulators of senescence are discussed in Part V. Because such modulators can be important tools for the study of aging, this section should be of use to researchers in biological gerontology. Indeed, this is clearly illustrated by the wide use of the dietary restriction paradigm in experimental gerontology. This part should also provide those interested in developing interventions in human aging with a data base from which to develop approaches.

Topics not readily evident in the table of contents should be mentioned here. Chapter 15, on the endocrine system, is restricted to selected hormones, but almost all other hormones are covered extensively elsewhere: the pancreatic hormones (insulin and glucagon) in Chapters 7 and 24; the hormones influencing calcium metabolism and bone (parathyroid hormone, calcitonin, and 1,25 dihydroxy vitamin D) in Chapter 16; the thyroid hormone in Chapter 6; the adrenal medullary hormone in Chapter 7; melatonin in Chapter 23; and the gastrointestinal hormones in Chapter 20. Chapter 14 is the only chapter dedicated solely to the sense organs; it focuses on the methodological issues encountered in the study of age-related changes in sense organs and, in addition, provides an in-depth discussion of taste and smell. Information on other sense organs is presented in other chapters: vision, hearing, proprioception and vibratory sense in Chapter 12; macromolecular aspects of lens aging in Chapter 10; and cutaneous sense organs in Chapter 11. The autonomic nervous system is considered in Chapters 6, 7, 17, and 20, and skeletal muscle in Chapter 24. Temperature regulation is discussed in Chapter 6.

I am indebted to the following people for their critical analyses and constructive suggestions: Dr. William Adler, Dr. Steve Austad, Dr. Linda Bartoshuk, Dr. Bruce Baum, Dr. Rod Bronson, Dr. Neil Cherniack, Dr. John Cook, Dr. Vincent Cristofalo, Dr. J. Fred Dice, Dr. Murray Epstein, Dr. Barbara Gilchrest, Dr. Gary Grove, Dr. John Holloszy, Mr. Jeffrey House, Dr. John Johnson, Dr. Edward Lakatta, Mrs. Barbara Masoro, Dr. Michael Michelis, Dr. Richard Miller, Dr. Gregory Mundy, Dr. James Nelson, Dr. Thomas Norwood, Dr. Eric Poehlman, Dr. Gerald Reaven, Dr. Karen Reiser, Dr. Joseph Rogers, Dr. Robert Rosen, Dr. Lawrence Rubenstein, Dr. Robert Russell, Dr. Ilene Siegler, Dr. William Sonntag, and Dr. Richard Weindruch. To the extent to which their comments were followed, this book has been improved. I am also grateful to Ms. Susan Hannan of Oxford University Press who has overseen the copy-editing of this book with skill, patience, and tact. Finally, the invaluable help of Mrs. Kathleen Boehme in many different aspects of the preparation and processing of the manuscripts is gratefully acknowledged.

San Antonio, Texas   E. J. M
August 1, 1994

Contents

Contributors ix

I. OVERVIEW

1. **Aging: Current Concepts** 3
   Edward J. Masoro

II. METHODOLOGICAL ISSUES IN AGING RESEARCH

2. **Design and Analysis of Aging Studies** 25
   Paul T. Costa, Jr. and Robert R. McCrae

3. **Animal Models** 37
   Richard Weindruch

4. **Cell Culture as a Model** 53
   Vincent J. Cristofalo and Robert J. Pignolo

5. **Human Studies** 83
   Denis A. Evans

III. METABOLIC AND MOLECULAR ASPECTS OF AGING

6. **Energy Utilization** 95
   Roger J. M. McCarter

7. **Carbohydrate Metabolism** 119
   Jeffrey B. Halter

8. **Fat Metabolism and Adiposity** 147
   Dariush Elahi, Marianne McAloon Dyke, and Reubin Andres

9. **Gene Expression and Protein Degradation** 171
   Holly Van Remmen, Walter Ward, Robert V. Sabia, and Arlan Richardson

10. **Long-Lived Proteins: Extracellular Matrix (Collagens, Elastins, Proteoglycans) and Lens Crystallins** 235
    David R. Sell and Vincent M. Monnier

IV. ORGAN SYSTEM AND ORGANISMIC AGING

11. **Skin** 309
    Anjali Chuttani and Barbara A. Gilchrest

12. **Human Nervous System** 325
    Robert Katzman

13. **Maintenance and Regulation in Brain of Neurotransmission, Trophic Factors, and Immune Responses** 345
    Carl W. Cotman, Jennifer S. Kahle, and Andrew R. Korotzer

14. **Taste and Smell** 363
    Linda Bartoshuk and Valerie Duffy

15. **The Potential Role of Selected Endocrine Systems in Aging Processes** 377
    James F. Nelson

16. **Bone** 395
    Dike N. Kalu

17. **Cardiovascular System** 413
    Edward G. Lakatta

18. **Respiratory System** 475
    David Sparrow and Scott T. Weiss

19. **Renal and Urinary Tract Function** 485
    Robert D. Lindeman

20. **The Gastrointestinal Tract** 505
    Peter R. Holt

21. **Immune System** 555
    Richard A. Miller

22. **Loss of Integration and Resiliency with Age: A Dissipative Destruction** 591
    F. Eugene Yates and Laurel A. Benton

V. PROPOSED MODIFIERS OF AGING PROCESSES OR AGING PHENOTYPE

23. **Putative Interventions** 613
    Byung P. Yu

24. **Exercise** 633
    John O. Holloszy and Wendy M. Kohrt

    Index 667

Contributors

Reubin Andres, M.D.
Laboratory of Physiology
National Institute on Aging
National Institutes of Health and Division of Gerontology
University of Maryland & Baltimore VA Medical Center
Baltimore, Maryland

Linda Bartoshuk, Ph.D.
Department of Surgery, Section of Otolaryngology
Yale University School of Medicine
New Haven, Connecticut

Laurel A. Benton, M.D.
Department of Medicine
Medical Monitoring Unit
University of California at Los Angeles
Los Angeles, California

Anjali Chuttani, M.D.
Department of Surgery
Boston University School of Medicine
Boston, Massachusetts

Paul T. Costa, Jr., Ph.D.
Laboratory of Personality/Cognition
National Institute on Aging
National Institutes of Health
Baltimore, Maryland

Carl W. Cotman, Ph.D.
Department of Psychobiology
University of California, Irvine
Irvine, California

Vincent J. Cristofalo, Ph.D.
Center for Gerontological Research
Medical College of Pennsylvania
Philadelphia, Pennsylvania

Valerie Duffy, Ph.D.
School of Allied Health Professions
University of Connecticut
Storrs, Connecticut

Marianne McAloon Dyke, R.N., M.A.
Department of Medicine
Beth Israel Hospital
Boston, Massachusetts

Dariush Elahi, Ph.D.
Geriatric Service
University of Maryland at Baltimore
Baltimore, Maryland

Denis A. Evans, M.D.
Center for Research on Health and Aging
Rush-Presbyterian–St. Luke's Medical Center
Chicago, Illinois

Barbara A. Gilchrest, M.D.
Department of Dermatology
Boston University School of Medicine
Boston, Massachusetts

Jeffrey B. Halter, M.D.
Geriatrics Center and Institute of Gerontology
University of Michigan and VA Medical Center
Ann Arbor, Michigan

John O. Holloszy, M.D.
Department of Medicine
Washington University School of Medicine
St. Louis, Missouri

Peter R. Holt, M.D.
Department of Gastroenterology
St. Luke's-Roosevelt Hospital Center
New York, New York

Jennifer S. Kahle, Ph.D.
Department of Psychobiology
University of California, Irvine
Irvine, California

Dike N. Kalu, Ph.D.
Department of Physiology
University of Texas Health Science Center
San Antonio, Texas

Robert Katzman, M.D.
Department of Neuroscience
University of California, San Diego, School of Medicine
La Jolla, California

Wendy M. Kohrt, Ph.D.
Department of Medicine
Washington University School of Medicine
St. Louis, Missouri

Andrew R. Korotzer, Ph.D.
Department of Psychobiology
University of California, Irvine
Irvine, California

Edward G. Lakatta, M.D.
Laboratory of Cardiovascular Science
Gerontology Research Center
Baltimore, Maryland

Robert D. Lindeman, M.D.
VA Medical Center
Albuquerque, New Mexico

Roger J. M. McCarter, Ph.D.
Department of Physiology
The University of Texas Health Science Center
San Antonio, Texas

Robert R. McCrae, Ph.D.
Gerontology Research Center
National Institute on Aging
National Institutes of Health
Baltimore, Maryland

Edward J. Masoro, Ph.D. (Editor)
Department of Physiology
University of Texas Health Science Center
San Antonio, Texas

Richard A. Miller, M.D., Ph.D.
Institute of Gerontology
University of Michigan
Ann Arbor, Michigan

Vincent M. Monnier, M.D., Ph.D.
Institute of Pathology
Case Western Reserve University
Cleveland, Ohio

James F. Nelson, Ph.D.
Department of Physiology
University of Texas Health Science Center
San Antonio, Texas

Robert J. Pignolo, Ph.D.
Center for Gerontological Research
Medical College of Pennsylvania
Philadelphia, Pennsylvania

Arlan G. Richardson, Ph.D.
Department of Medicine
University of Texas Health Science Center
and the Geriatric Research, Education and Clinical Center
Audie L. Murphy Memorial Veteran's Hospital
San Antonio, Texas

Robert V. Sabia, M.S.
Department of Information Technology
University of Texas
San Antonio, Texas

David R. Sell, Ph.D.
Institute of Pathology
Case Western Reserve University
Cleveland, Ohio

David Sparrow, D.Sc.
Normative Aging Study
VA Outpatient Clinic
Boston, Massachusetts

Holly Van Remmen, Ph.D.
Department of Medicine
University of Texas Health Science Center
and the Geriatric Research, Education and Clinical Center
Audie L. Murphy Memorial Veteran's Hospital
San Antonio, Texas

Walter F. Ward, Ph.D.
Department of Physiology
University of Texas Health Science Center
San Antonio, Texas

Richard Weindruch, Ph.D.
Department of Medicine
University of Wisconsin
and VA—Geriatric Research, Education and Clinical Center
Madison, Wisconsin

Scott T. Weiss, M.D.
Channing Laboratory
Harvard Medical School
Boston, Massachusetts

F. Eugene Yates, M.D.
Department of Medicine
Medical Monitoring Unit
University of California at Los Angeles
Los Angeles, California

Byung P. Yu, Ph.D.
Department of Physiology
University of Texas Health Science Center
San Antonio, Texas

HANDBOOK OF PHYSIOLOGY

Section 11: Aging

I | OVERVIEW

1. Aging: current concepts

EDWARD J. MASORO | Department of Physiology, University of Texas Health Science Center, San Antonio, Texas

CHAPTER CONTENTS

Aging at the Population Level
    Life tables
    Survival curves
    Maximum life span
    Age-specific mortality rates
    Universality of aging
Aging at the Individual Level
Concept of Primary Aging Processes
    Classification of theories of aging
    Genetic programs akin to development and morphogenesis
    Homeostatic failure
        Generalized cellular homeostatic failure
        Failure in organismic homeostatic control systems
    Current status of the concept of primary aging processes
Evolutionary Biology of Aging
Manifestations of Aging Processes
    Age-associated disease processes
    Age-associated physiological changes
Summary and Conclusions

THE HUMAN AGING PHENOTYPE, the observable morphological and functional characteristics of aging, has been recognized for generations. Indeed, the phenotype was well described by Shakespeare in *As You Like It*:

> The sixth age shifts into lean and slipper'd pantaloon, with spectacles on nose and pouch on side, his youthful hose well sav'd, a world too wide, for his shrunk shank; and his big manly voice, turning again toward childish treble, pipes and whistles in his sound. Last scene of all, that ends this strange eventful history, is second childishness, and mere oblivion, sans teeth, sans eyes, sans taste, sans everything.

We can all see that similar age changes occur in other species, for example, our pets and farm animals. Little wonder that many people, including some biologists, think there is little to be learned about aging.

Any attempt to discuss aging in basic biological terms, however, quickly reveals that, for most species, the underlying mechanisms are not understood. This lack of knowledge makes it difficult to provide a generally acceptable definition of aging. Most gerontologists would probably accept the following definition as being free of errors of commission: *deteriorative changes with time during postmaturational life that underlie an increasing vulnerability to challenges, thereby decreasing the ability of the organism to survive*. Although many gerontologists undoubtedly would think that this definition suffers from important omissions, there would be much disagreement as to the nature of those omissions. Therefore, it should be viewed as a starting point for the discussion of aging.

If aging were broadly defined, it would refer to all time-related events that occur in the life of an organism, including those that are beneficial (such as developmental processes), those with neutral effects, and those of a deteriorative nature. The definition above refers only to the last category, and *senescence* would be a more correct term for this subset of aging. In common usage, however, the word *aging* refers to senescence (as in the name of the National Institute on Aging, the purpose of which is to study senescence). Therefore, in this chapter and in most of this book *aging* and *senescence* are used as synonyms, while specific terms are employed for other categories of aging (for example, *development*). Some chapters, however, use the term *aging* in the broad sense of all time-related events, and such usage is made clear (for example, see Chapter 2).

The fundamental issue to be explored in this book is the reason for the senescence of an organism that has developed into a complex structural and functional entity from a fertilized egg. The maintenance of such a complex system would appear to be a less formidable task than its development. Moreover, there is no a priori reason for the deterioration associated with senescence since biological organisms are thermodynamically open systems in which external energy sources can be drawn upon to repair damage. Nevertheless, in most species for which the database is adequate for a valid assessment of senescence, there is a stage of life at which deteriorative processes are not balanced by repair processes (that is, aging occurs), resulting in the deterioration of the organism, with death as the endpoint. The major goal of biological gerontology is to understand the biological mechanisms and causal chains underlying this deterioration.

AGING AT THE POPULATION LEVEL

The relationship between chronological age and population mortality characteristics has played and continues to play an important role in the field of gerontology. Such a role for mortality is somewhat surprising in that senescent processes need not be involved in the death of the organism. Nevertheless, proper analyses of mortality data have provided important gerontological insights.

Life Tables

Life tables are the source of data for mortality data analyses (108). They include the following columns of data as given in Table 1.1: age intervals (x), usually starting at birth and the length of the interval chosen by the tabulator (e.g., 0–1, 1–2, 2–3, etc. days for flies or years for humans); the number of individuals dying during the interval (d_x); the number of individuals alive at the beginning of the interval (l_x); the age-specific death rate (q_x) (i.e., the fraction of individuals alive at the start of the interval who die during that interval); the mean expectation of life (e_x) at the beginning of the age interval.

Survival Curves

Life tables are cumbersome and therefore not usually presented in published studies, even when sufficient data are available. Rather, survival curves are used in which the y axis denotes the percentage of the starting population alive (birth is usually the starting point) and the x axis denotes the chronological age of the population (98). Survival curves prepared by Fries and Crapo (38) for the population of the United States in 1910 and 1970 are shown in Figure 1.1. The point to be noted is that the curve in 1970 is more rectangular in shape than that in 1910; that is, a greater percentage of the population in 1970 lived to advanced ages than in 1910. Progressive rectangularization of the survival curve has occurred through the nineteenth and twentieth centuries

TABLE 1.1. *Life Table for 4,627 Male Houseflies* Musca domestica L. *(NAIDM Strain)*

x	d_x	l_x	1,000 q_x	e_x	x	d_x	l_x	1,000q_x	e_x
0–1	1.5	1000.0	1.5	16.88	30–31	8.4	49.1	171.1	5.11
1–2	2.8	998.5	2.8	15.90	31–32	5.6	40.6	137.9	5.07
2–3	3.7	995.7	3.7	14.94	32–33	6.7	35.0	191.4	4.80
3–4	2.8	992.0	2.8	14.00	33–34	4.3	28.3	151.9	4.82
4–5	2.6	989.2	2.6	13.04	34–35	5.0	24.0	208.3	4.59
5–6	5.6	986.6	5.7	12.07	35–36	3.0	19.0	157.9	4.66
6–7	8.6	981.0	8.8	11.14	36–37	2.6	16.0	162.5	4.44
7–8	14.0	972.3	14.4	10.23	37–38	1.5	13.4	111.9	4.21
8–9	19.5	958.3	20.3	9.37	38–39	2.4	11.9	201.7	3.67
9–10	48.0	938.8	51.1	8.56	39–40	2.6	9.5	273.7	3.47
10–11	46.5	890.9	52.2	7.99	40–41	2.8	6.9	405.8	3.59
11–12	57.5	844.4	68.1	7.40	41–42	1.1	4.1	268.3	4.71
12–13	94.9	786.9	120.6	6.91	42–43	0.6	3.0	200.0	5.23
13–14	69.8	692.0	100.9	6.79	43–44	0.2	2.4	83.3	5.42
14–15	77.8	622.2	125.0	6.49	44–45	0.2	2.2	90.9	4.86
15–16	64.2	544.4	117.9	6.35	45–46	0.4	1.9	210.5	4.53
16–17	62.0	480.2	129.1	6.13	46–47	0.4	1.5	266.7	4.60
17–18	61.8	418.2	147.8	5.96	47–48	0.0	1.1	0.0	5.09
18–19	52.7	356.4	147.9	5.91	48–49	0.0	1.1	0.0	4.09
19–20	49.9	303.7	164.3	5.85	49–50	0.4	1.1	363.6	3.09
20–21	41.7	253.7	164.4	5.90	50–51	0.2	0.6	333.3	4.17
21–22	31.8	212.0	150.0	5.97	51–52	0.0	0.4	0.0	5.00
22–23	28.1	180.2	155.9	5.93	52–53	0.0	0.4	0.0	4.00
23–24	22.9	152.2	150.5	5.93	53–54	0.2	0.4	500.0	3.00
24–25	16.6	129.2	128.5	5.90	54–55	0.0	0.2	0.0	4.50
25–26	14.0	112.6	124.3	5.69	55–56	0.0	0.2	0.0	3.50
26–27	14.9	98.6	151.1	5.43	56–57	0.0	0.2	0.0	2.50
27–28	18.8	83.6	165.1	5.32	57–58	0.0	0.2	0.0	1.50
28–29	12.3	69.8	176.2	5.27	58–59	0.2	0.2	1000.0	0.50
29–30	8.4	57.5	146.1	5.29					

From Rockstein and Lieberman (97); used with permission.

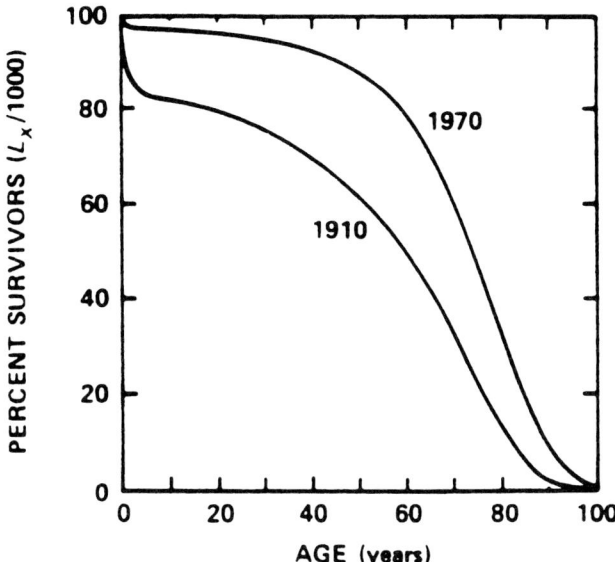

FIG. 1.1. Survival curves for United States population (men and women) in 1910 and 1970. [Reproduced from Fries and Crapo (38) with permission. Data for 1910 are from United States vital statistics reported in L. I. Dublin "The Possibility of Extending Human Life" in *The Harvey Lectures, 1922-1923*; data for 1970 are from Vital Statistics of the United States National Center for Health Statistics, 1970.]

in the United States and other developed nations. The major reason for this change in the shape of the survival curve is the increasing protection from premature death, including a marked reduction in the high rate of infant deaths. Social, economic, technological, and medical advances (sanitation engineering, nutrition, and immunization, for example) have protected the young from death caused by environmental hazards and infectious diseases.

Life expectancy of humans from birth and median length of life, which can be ascertained from survival curves, have increased throughout the course of the twentieth century. Assessment of those two parameters indicates that protection from premature death rather than changes in aging processes underlies the survival increases. Survival curves offer valuable information on the ability of the population to reach advanced ages and when appropriately analyzed, insights into aging processes.

Maximum Life Span

The information provided by survival curves that is most relevant to the study of aging is the maximum length of life (or the part of the survival curve approaching the maximum length of life). Indeed, the maximum length of life of a population has been viewed as an index of the rate of aging of the population. The reported maximum life spans of several species (37) are presented in Table 1.2. The maximum life spans of species have long been held to relate inversely to the rate of aging of the species. Finch et al. (37) and Promislow (90) have challenged the theoretical validity of using maximum life span as an index of the rate of aging. The basis of this challenge is discussed later, under *Age-Specific Mortality Rates*. In addition, Gavrilov and Gavrilova (40) have questioned the reliability of the recorded data on maximum life spans of species, pointing out that as the size of the population sample increases, so does the reported maximum life span. Therefore, one must conclude that the comparison of the human life span (based on a sample size of millions) with those of species maintained in zoos (based on very small sample sizes) is an unreliable index of the relative rate of aging, to say the least.

Moreover, the concept that a species has a genetically fixed life span has been questioned (12, 25). This challenge to conventional dogma is based on studies of the mortality characteristics of large populations of Mediterranean fruit flies and *Drosophila*. These studies will be considered later in this section in relation to the Gompertzian analysis of the rate of aging.

Age-Specific Mortality Rates

Age-specific mortality rates of humans (number of deaths per year per 1,000 individuals alive at the start of the year) relate to chronological age in the complex manner shown by the graphs prepared by Fries and Crapo (38) for the U.S. population in 1910 and 1970 (Figure 1.2). There is a high mortality rate at birth that falls until 10 years of age, when the probability of dying reaches a nadir. A marked increase in mortality rate during adolescence is associated primarily with accidental deaths. Starting at about age 30, an exponential increase in the age-specific mortality rate (note that the y axis of

TABLE 1.2. *Maximum Life Span of Common Mammalian Species**

Species	Maximum Life Span (years)
Laboratory mouse	4.5
Laboratory rat	5.5
Laboratory gerbil	3.8
Laboratory hamster	3
White-footed mouse	8
Domestic dog	20
Horse	46
Rhesus monkey	>35
Human	>110

*Data from Finch et al. (37); used with permission.

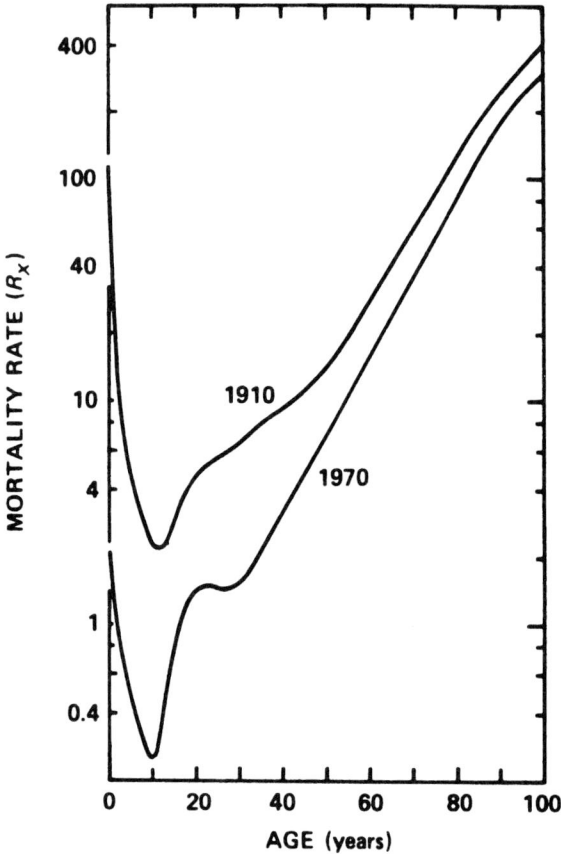

FIG. 1.2. The age-specific mortality rate (number of deaths per year per 1,000 individuals entering each age interval) is shown for year intervals from birth to 100 years for the United States population (men and women) in the years 1910 and 1970. [Reproduced from Fries and Crapo (38) with permission. Data for 1910 are from United States vital statistics reported in L. I. Dublin "The Possibility of Extending Human Life" in *The Harvey Lectures, 1922–1923*; data for 1970 are from Vital Statistics of the United States National Center for Health Statistics, 1970.]

Figure 1.2 is a log scale) begins and is sustained until 90 years of age, when the rate of increase in mortality rate decreases somewhat. It is the exponential increase that is important in gerontology. It should also be noted that, although the mortality rate in 1910 was greater than in 1970 at all ages, the slope of exponential increase was similar for the populations during both eras. Although the details of the relationship between age and age-specific mortality rate vary among species, an exponential increase over a considerable portion of the postmaturational period of life occurs with age in many species if they are maintained in an environment that protects them from premature death due to predators and other hazards (18). Finch (35) proposes that the exponential increase in age-specific mortality rate is evidence of senescence.

Many mathematical models have been proposed regarding the relationship between age-specific mortality rate and chronological age; those of Strehler and Mildvan (123), Sacher and Trucco (109), and Witten (136) are well-known examples and new models continue to be developed (50a). Finch (35) chose as a simple working model the Gompertz equation, which provides an adequate assessment of the postmaturational exponential increase in age-specific mortality rate with increasing age:

$$m(t) = Ae^{Gt}$$

where $m(t)$ is the age-specific mortality rate at age t (value of t calculated starting at the age of puberty); G is the exponential (Gompertz) mortality rate coefficient (i.e., the slope of the straight line component of the graphs in Figure 1.2) and is viewed as a quantitative index of the rate of aging; A is the age-independent mortality rate, which is usually estimated by extrapolation to $t = 0$, but which Finch calculates at puberty and calls the initial mortality rate (IMR); and e is the base of the natural logarithm.

The practical use of the Gompertz model is facilitated by calculating the mortality rate doubling time (MRDT), which relates to the Gompertz mortality rate coefficient as follows:

$$MRDT = \frac{\ln 2}{G}$$

The MRDT is inversely related to G but is a more natural expression than G because it relates directly to life span and is measured in the same units of time. Although recognizing the value of the Gompertz model in measuring actuarial senescence, Promislow (90) delineates the problems encountered in its use.

Data on the MRDT and the initial mortality rate (IMR) of common mammalian species (37) are presented in Table 1.3. Both the MRDT and the IMR vary among species. With the MRDT as a quantitative index of the rate of aging, the conclusion to be drawn is that rodents age much more rapidly than dogs or horses and that humans age more slowly than those two domestic species. Furthermore, based on the MRDT, the rate of aging of rhesus monkeys is, if anything, slower than that of humans, even though the maximum life span of humans is 110 years or so and that of rhesus monkeys only about 35 years. Finch et al. (37) concluded that the reason for this apparent paradox is that the IMR, which is not age-dependent, is much greater for rhesus monkeys than for humans. The IMR can be viewed as an index of vulnerability relating to both species and environmental characteristics. Thus, the use of maximum life span as an index of the rate of aging is clearly erroneous (90). One must view the interpretation of Finch

TABLE 1.3. *Initial Mortality Rate (IMR) and Mortality Rate Doubling Time (MRDT) of Common Mammalian Species**

Species	IMR deaths/yr/unit population	MRDT years
Laboratory mouse	0.03	0.27
Laboratory rat	0.002	0.3
Laboratory gerbil	0.1	0.9
Laboratory hamster	0.025	0.5
White-footed mouse	0.06	1.2
Domestic dog	0.02	3
Horse	0.0002	4
Rhesus monkey	0.02	15
Human	0.0002	8

*Data from Finch et al. (37); used with permission.

et al. cautiously, however, with regard to the rhesus monkey. Data on the IMR and the MRDT of rhesus monkeys are based on research colonies where there is a tendency to remove healthy young animals for research and to cull sickly old animals for tissues before they die. Such procedures distort both the IMR and the MRDT data. Indeed, Bowden and Williams (8) pointed out that available data on the longevity characteristics of nonhuman primate species must be viewed as tentative and that significant revision of these estimates is to be expected as further data become available.

The data in Table 1.4, which reflect the influence of environment on the IMR and the MRDT, are enlightening (35). Conditions ranging from a highly favorable environment, such as civilian life in the United States in 1980, to that of a prisoner of war of the Japanese in World War II markedly influence the IMR but have only a small effect on the MRDT. This indicates that while adverse environments strongly influence mortality rate, their influence on the rate of aging is less marked. That these findings relate not only to acute environmental events such as war but also to long-term unfavorable

TABLE 1.4. *IMR and MRDT of Various Human Populations**

Population	MRDT (years)	IMR (deaths/yr/unit population)
U.S. female, 1980	8.9	0.0002
Australian, 1944–45	8.2	0.0013
Australian prisoners of war (World War II)	7.7	0.0070
Dutch, 1945 (year in which German occupation ended)	7.8	0.0014
Dutch, 1946	7.6	0.0008

*Data from Finch (35); used with permission.

conditions is evident from the graphs in Figure 1.2, which show that the IMR in the U.S. population was much greater in 1910 than in 1970 but the MRDT was similar for both populations. Nevertheless, we know that environment can influence the rate of aging since dietary restriction in rats can increase the MRDT twofold (71).

It is well known that women live longer than men (50). However, analysis of the data of Gee and Veevers (41), graphically presented in Figure 1.3, indicate that the IMR is greater in men than in women, not that the MRDT is smaller. Thus it appears that the difference in longevity characteristics between men and women is not due to a difference in their rates of aging. Comfort (18) concluded that in most species females are longer-lived than males, though he also noted that there are a number of exceptions. The study of sex differences is not likely to be a promising approach to learning about mechanisms that influence the MRDT, but such knowledge may provide important information on the IMR and on aspects of the aging phenotype.

Two recent papers have questioned the use of the exponential increase in age-specific mortality rate as an operational index of the rate of aging. Carey et al. (12) studied more than one million Mediterranean fruit flies (*Ceratis capitata*) and showed that mortality rates do

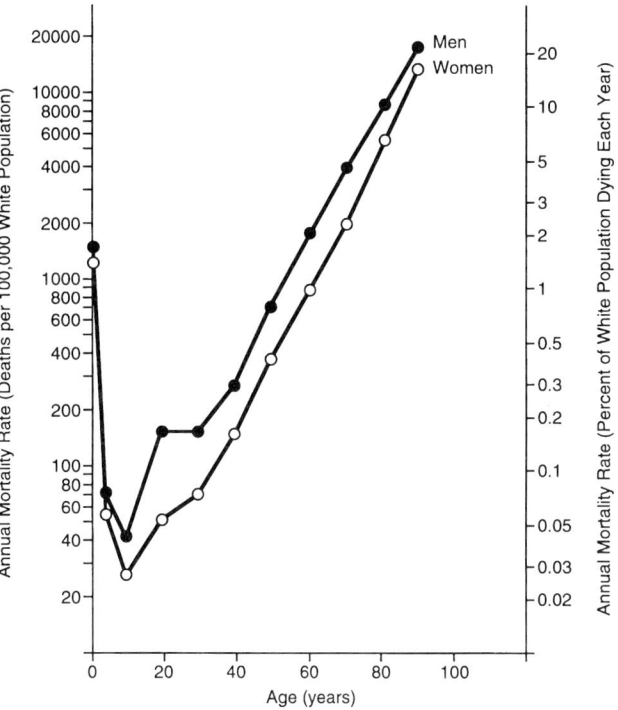

FIG. 1.3. The age-specific mortality rate (number of deaths per year per 100,000 white population) in females and males of the United States in 1976. [Reproduced from Hazzard (50) with permission.]

not increase monotonically with age. However, the researchers recognized that these findings may, in a sense, be artifactual because of the genetic heterogeneity of the population; as the population ages, individuals with genotypes conferring high rates of mortality are likely to die out, thereby transforming the population with advancing age into one consisting primarily of individuals with genotypes conferring low death rates. Curtsinger et al. (25) studied ten genotypes of *Drosophila melanogaster* (four inbred lines and six F_1 hybrids). The results of these studies also did not conform to a monotonic exponential increase in age-specific mortality rate with advancing age. In a single genotype, the mortality trajectory was best fit by a two-stage Gompertz model with no increase in age-specific mortality rate at ages greater than 30 days after emergence. These findings are not entirely new because, as is evident in Figure 1.2, human age-specific mortality rates in many instances do not continue to increase exponentially at very advanced ages. In addition, the studies of Carey et al. and Curtsinger et al. have been criticized on technical and/or theoretical grounds by Kowald and Kirkwood (58), Robine and Ritchie (95), Olshansky et al. (83), and Nusbaum et al. (82). Also, Brooks et al. (9a) found that age-specific mortality rates of inbred strains of the nematode *C. elegans* are in accord with the Gompertz model but as this chapter goes to press this conclusion is challenged (25a, 53a, 127a, 131a). However, deviations from the Gompertz model at least in some instances may be due to the genetic heterogeneity of the population. Indeed, Hirsch (50b) points out that it is likely that Gompertz functions cannot be extrapolated beyond 85 years of age in humans, and Vaupel and Carey (127) have formally addressed the issue of compositional changes in the population with regard to late life age-specific mortality rates. In my opinion, the fact that the Gompertz model does not accurately describe the age-specific mortality rates at advanced ages does not preclude its providing an approximate index of the rate of aging of a population when used appropriately.

Universality of Aging

Do all species experience senescence? There is no evidence that prokaryotes (bacteria) do (1). Bell (6) proposed that all multicellular organisms which have a germ line separate from a somatic line undergo senescence, whereas those without such a separation do not. Partridge and Barton (86) broadened this concept by stating that aging evolves in species in which there is a distinction between the parent organism and a smaller offspring. Moreover, Martinez and Levinton (66) report that asexual metazoans undergo senescence, and they propose that the evolution of somatic differentiation, not germ-line sequestration, is the necessary condition for the evolution of senescence.

The rate of senescence varies among species in a continuum from rapid to gradual to negligible (35). Moreover, in some species environmental variables apparently shift the rate of senescence from rapid to gradual or even toward negligible.

Rapid senescence refers to the abrupt onset of deterioration at some time after maturation, which results in a rapid exponential increase in mortality rate. Examples are short-lived invertebrates, such as rotifers, nematodes, and flies, with maximum life spans of less than a few months. Other examples of rapid senescence are semelparous species, such as annual plants, Pacific salmon, and marsupial mice, which die during or after the first period of reproduction. It should be noted, however, that not all gerontologists view the rapid deterioration following reproduction as senescence (56).

Gradual senescence refers to a slow, persistent progression of deterioration starting some time after maturation. An example is the exponential increase in human mortality rate shown in Figures 1.2 and 1.3. All placental mammals seem subject to gradual senescence, and it is this group of animals that most interests gerontologists because of the ultimate focus on human aging and the apparent similarity of the aging processes in placental mammals.

Examples of negligible senescence are seen in long-lived species in which clear evidence for a postmaturational increase in mortality rate has not been established. These include some species of anemones, clams, trees, fish, and reptiles. Whether these species age in the sense of undergoing senescence is difficult to say because conditions under which measurements are made may not be appropriate to obtain a clear-cut answer.

Indeed, although established for some species in the wild (89), senescence has not been documented for most species. This is the case not only for the long-lived species just discussed but also for many short-lived species. Because of predation, infection, and other environmental hazards, the accidental death rate is so high for many species (60) that most of the population do not live long enough to permit an evaluation of the occurrence of senescence.

AGING AT THE INDIVIDUAL LEVEL

Most gerontologists feel that chronological age is not a reliable index of the extent of senescence in an individual because the rate of aging varies considerably among individuals within a species. This thinking has led to the concept of biological age as distinct from chronological age (7). Although this concept is almost certainly a valid one, the means to measure biological age are thus far lacking. This does not reflect a lack of interest in the idea, however, for there has been much effort to develop methods of assessing the biological age of the individual.

Obviously, the exponential increase in the probability of dying, which is used as a measure of the rate of senescence of a population, cannot be applied to the individual. Therefore, the major thrust has been to develop biomarkers that will measure the biological age of the individual (5). The goal is to obtain easily executed, relatively noninvasive measurements which can serve as biomarkers of the rate of biological aging. The challenge is to validate one or more measurements as quantitative indices of biological age. This problem has not yet been resolved even with physiological measures, which would seem to be particularly useful for this purpose (68). Moreover, if there are several basic aging processes, no single biomarker is likely to be an index of all of them. To address this issue, attempts have been made to develop panels of biomarkers and mathematical models to assess total organismic aging. A major criterion of validity is the ability of the biomarker or panel of biomarkers to predict individual mortality risk with advancing age. Alas, Costa and McCrae (20) have shown that chronological age is a better predictor than any putative biomarker or panel. Practical and theoretical issues with regard to biomarkers of aging are discussed further in Chapters 2 and 22.

Validated measures of the rate of senescence in an individual are thus far lacking. The best that might be achieved with regard to the individual would be to assess the phenotype at various chronological ages. Unfortunately, the relationship of the phenotype to basic aging processes has not been defined at this stage of the development of biological gerontology. This issue is discussed further in Chapter 17 in relation to the heart.

CONCEPT OF PRIMARY AGING PROCESSES

Over the years much thought and effort have been expended in an attempt to understand the nature of the basic aging processes. Most biological gerontologists have long held that there are primary aging processes, and that much of the aging phenotype is secondary to these processes or that it constitutes further removed expressions of them. Twenty years ago, a single primary aging process was thought to be responsible for most of the aging phenotype (112). Although some gerontologists hold the view that the rate of aging is controlled by a yet to be identified central timer, others believe that there are several such processes (84). Moreover, the current view is that much of the aging phenotype may not involve deteriorations directly caused by aging processes (69). Rather, these may be compensatory responses (for example, cardiac hypertrophy) or nondeteriorative (for example, the graying of the hair) or secondary to chronic exposure to toxic environmental agents (for example, nervous system deterioration due to chronic exposure to carbon disulfide). Much research is now devoted to sorting out the various factors underlying the aging phenotype of an individual.

Twenty years ago, many biologists thought that primary aging processes were similar in all species, but there are now compelling reasons to believe that this is not likely (97, 100). The marked variation in the morphological and physiological manifestations of senescence among species strongly points to species differences in basic aging processes. Indeed, if aging is due to many different fundamental processes, the usefulness of the concept of primary aging processes must be called into question.

Classification of Theories of Aging

The many theories of aging proposed over the years have been aimed at identifying the nature of the primary aging process or processes. Their sheer number confounds, but many are closely interrelated. Moreover, since there may be many primary processes, particular theories need not be mutually exclusive. The challenge is to develop some order by classifying the theories in a logical fashion and identifying the interrelationships.

In fact, there have been many attempts to classify theories of aging; notable examples are those of Hart and Turturro (45), Hayflick (48), and Medvedev (74a). To date, however, the classifications have been less than satisfactory because many theories can be assigned to more than one of the classes. Therefore, a simple classification scheme, which avoids this problem and permits an orderly discussion of most extant theories of aging, is presented in Table 1.5.

One of two basic concepts underlies most theories of aging: *(1)* that aging is the result of genetic programs akin to those of development and morphogenesis or *(2)* that aging is due to evolutionarily nonadaptive homeostatic failures (that is, the inability of homeostasis to prevent deterioration of the living system). Direct evolutionarily adaptive selection for homeostatic failure is unlikely, and for that reason these are called "nonadaptive" theories of aging.

Genetic Programs Akin to Development and Morphogenesis

The appeal of theories of aging based on genetic programs akin to development and morphogenesis, such as the three examples listed in Table 1.5, relates to con-

TABLE 1.5. *Simple Scheme for Classifying Theories of Aging*

I. Genetic programs akin to development and morphogenesis
   Examples:
      Centralized clock theory of Kloeden et al. (57)
      Decreasing oxygen consumption hormone theory of Denckla (28)
      Codon-restriction theory of Strehler et al. (124)

II. Homeostatic failure
   A. Generalized cellular homeostatic failure
     Examples:
      Free radical theory of Harman (42)
      Free radical-glycation/Maillard reaction theory of Kristal and Yu (59)
      Somatic mutation theory of Szilard (125)
      Error castrophe theory of aging of Orgel (85)
   B. Failure in organismic homeostatic control systems
     Examples:
      Glucocortoid cascade hypothesis of Sapolsky et al. (111)
      Immunologic theory of aging of Walford (130)
      Neuroendocrine-immune theory of Fabris (32)

vincing evidence that genes play a major role in aging (21, 53, 72a). Often cited as evidence for such programed senescence is the fact that some adult insects are aphagic because of defective mouth parts and digestive organs (132). Because of these defects, the insects undergo rapid Gompertzian senescence. However, this does not mean that the senescence is genetically programmed in an evolutionarily adaptive sense akin to development. In this case, the failure to maintain digestive organs probably relates to the fact that *in the wild* it is not likely that these insects could have lived long enough for starvation to be a factor in evolutionary fitness. Thus there is no selection pressure to maintain these structures. Therefore, aging in these species is genetically programmed but not in a direct, evolutionarily adaptive sense akin to development. As discussed later, under EVOLUTIONARY BIOLOGY OF AGING, most modern evolutionary biologists interested in gerontology believe that senescence does not provide selective advantage and thus, unlike development, is not directly selected for (55).

Other lines of evidence cited in support of genetically programmed aging akin to development are the phenomena of apoptosis (programmed cell death) and proliferative arrest of normal diploid cells in culture. Multicellular organisms lose cells with advancing age (senescence), but a role for apoptosis in this loss has not been established. That apoptosis plays an important role in development is clear (91), and its importance in adults appears to relate to proliferative homeostasis. In the early 1960s, Hayflick and Moorhead (49) reported that human diploid fibroblasts in culture exhibit a limited number of cell divisions, a phenomenon that they suggested could serve as an in vitro model of senescence [see Chapter 4 as well as Cristofalo and Pignolo (24) and Martin (65) for a critical discussion of this model of aging]. It appears that a genetic program for inhibitors of DNA synthesis may underlie this limit in the number of cell divisions (88, 118). The relevance of limited in vitro cell proliferation to organismic aging remains to be established (100). Nonetheless, even if apoptosis and limited cell division are found to be intimately involved in the senescent deterioration of organisms, this does not mean that these deteriorative processes are genetically programmed in a fashion akin to development. A more likely scenario is that these postulated dysfunctions in apoptosis and cell division occur at ages too advanced for selection pressure to prevent them.

In summary, it is unlikely that aging is a continuation of developmental processes because, unlike development, it is not selected for as an evolutionarily adaptive process. This does not mean, however, that developmental processes cannot be closely linked to senescence. Developmental processes resulting in increased evolutionary fitness during early life might promote the deterioration of the organism at later ages (the concept of antagonistic pleiotropy is discussed later, under EVOLUTIONARY BIOLOGY OF AGING). Thus our attention is focused on theories proposing that senescence is a consequence of homeostatic failure. Although, such failure is probably genetically programmed, at least in some regard, it cannot be viewed as being akin to the evolutionarily adaptive genetic programs of development.

Homeostatic Failure

The organism's loss of highly regulated functioning as senescence progresses is a description of the aging phenotype. Indeed, "wear-and-tear" theories of aging were among the first offered (18). Early views of wear and tear focused on gross deterioration, for example, erosion of the teeth of herbivores (114), which results in senescence (that is, Gompertzian acceleration of mortality) due to inadequate nutrition, or damage to the wings of flies (96), which results in Gompertzian senescence because of reduced ability to obtain food or avoid predation. In recent years, the wear-and-tear concept has been extended to include cellular and molecular processes.

Initially, proponents of the wear-and-tear theories viewed aging as akin to the deterioration with time of inanimate objects (an all too familiar occurrence with automobiles). This view has been modified because living organisms are thermodynamically open systems, and thus there is no a priori reason why external energy cannot be utilized to maintain the organization of the organism. The fact is, however, that, at least in most species, the ability with age to use external energy to maintain complex structures and functions is not fully adequate; that is, repair processes fail to keep pace with some deteriorative processes. The nature of the homeostatic failure differs among species. Teeth are a good example. As we know, most herbivores cannot repair worn teeth. However, sea cows are able to do so (31). Thus, a fundamental issue in understanding the aging of a particular species is to learn why for some period during postmaturational life external energy can no longer be used to fully maintain the structural and functional properties of the organism (that is, inadequacy in one or more of the homeostatic systems occurs). Yates and Benton in Chapter 22 expand the concept of homeostasis to that of homeodynamics and develop the principle of homeodynamic senescence.

Generalized Cellular Homeostatic Failure. Since the early 1960s much emphasis has been placed on the concept of generalized cellular homeostatic failure, with the recognition that the rate of such failure (and probably its nature) may vary among species and cell types (29). The primary focus has been on the structure of macromolecules, with particular emphasis on nucleic acids and proteins and on such macromolecular assemblies as mitochondria and chromosomes. Before considering the mechanisms suggested as causes of this deterioration with age, it is informative to review the evidence regarding the extent to which deterioration occurs.

Chromosomal abnormalities, which include aneuploidy (extra or missing chromosomes) and structural abnormalities (chromosomal amplifications and breaks) increase with age (128). Whether these abnormalities cause aging or are a result of aging has not been established (113). Changes with age in DNA structure include increased frequency of single-strand breaks (81) and DNA cross-linking (126). There is a decline in methylation of DNA with age (135). Also, a loss of telomeric DNA sequences occurs with age (46), a finding that has been proposed by Wright and Shay (137) to underlie cellular senescence. Other than the fact that changes in DNA structure do occur with age, little can be said about the role of such changes in the aging processes (128). Although the limited available information does not indicate structural changes with age in mRNA, further work is needed in this area (27).

Aging does not increase the occurrence of proteins with altered primary structures (102). However, altered proteins do accumulate with age because of posttranslational modifications (39, 73, 120) that result from deamidation, proteolytic fragmentation, oxidation, nonenzymatic glycation, racemization, cross-linking, and conformational changes. These alterations could well be involved in the aging processes.

Mitochondrial structure deteriorates with age in some species and tissues (77). However, the role of this deterioration in aging is not established. Miquel and Fleming (78) proposed an oxygen-radical-mitochondrial injury theory of aging; further investigations by Miquel (76) and Wallace (131) have focused on the genomic instability of mitochondria and the occurrence with age of mitochondrial DNA deletions and other types of injury to the mitochondrial genome. Such age-associated changes have indeed been found (19, 47, 52, 54, 63, 64, 138). It has been theorized that with advanced age these alterations cause some cells to be unable to meet their need for bioenergy, rendering them nonfunctional (62, 80). Many investigators have reported that the number of mitochondria decreases with age, as does the cellular content of cytochrome oxidase (67). In many cellular membranes, fluidity also decreases with age, because of changes in phospholipid and cholesterol content, altered lipid structure, and altered protein-lipid interactions (94).

Many theories of aging address the causes and/or the consequences of age-associated alterations in the structure of macromolecules and macromolecular assemblies. One of the first was the "somatic mutation" theory (125), which postulated that aging is due to random "hits" that inactivate large chromosomal regions. This concept, developed from the large body of research done in the 1950s on the effects of radiation and radiation damage, was viewed as causal in the deterioration of cellular and organismic function with age. Related to this theory is the "intrinsic mutagenesis" theory of Burnet (10), who proposed that each species is endowed with a specific genetic constitution that has greater or lesser ability to regulate the fidelity of genetic material and its replication. The accumulation of mutations or errors, then, was viewed as the basis of aging. Cristofalo (22) points out that neither theory is supported by a substantial body of evidence. Moreover, the study of Clark and Rubin (16), showing a similar longevity of haploid and diploid wasps, provides strong evidence against the somatic mutation theory.

The "error catastrophe" theory of Orgel (85), which posits that aging is caused by macromolecular alterations, has been the subject of much study. According to this theory, if an error is made in the synthesis of a protein involved in the generation of genetic material or the protein-synthesizing apparatus, an error-containing protein would be produced, which would in turn cause further errors. In this way, the number of error-containing proteins would expand, resulting in an "error crisis" that would cause a marked deterioration in cellular function (that is, the functional deficits found in senescence). However, an essential requirement for the validity of this theory, the accumulation of proteins with altered primary structures, does not occur (102). Thus this provocative theory has been all but abandoned.

There are, however, changes in gene expression with age, some genes exhibiting decreased expression while others show increased expression (93). These changes could relate to alterations in DNA, intrinsic changes in transacting factors, or to changes in neural and endocrine regulators of gene expression, among other factors. Such changes in gene expression could well lead to homeostatic failure. Related to this concept is Cutler's theory of "dysdifferentiation" (26), which proposes that, with age, tissue-specific genes will lose their tissue specificity. Strong evidence supporting this theory has not appeared.

Many of the theories of generalized cellular homeostatic failure relate to the effects of fuel and fuel use. The view that fuel use may be involved in aging was first suggested by Rubner (105), who reported that the life span of domestic animal species correlated inversely with the metabolic rate per unit of body weight. Over the years, studies have both supported and disputed such a role for metabolic rate (67). It now appears that while metabolic rate may be a factor influencing the rate of aging, other factors can mask this action (72). One mechanism by which fuel use may influence aging processes is the generation of damaging reactive oxygen products such as hydrogen peroxide, superoxide, and hydroxyl radicals (11). This aspect of fuel use relates to the "free radical" theory, which was first proposed by Harman (42) and is again the focus of much study (119). Moreover, it is now known that reactive oxygen molecules are generated by biochemical reactions other than those involved in fuel use (121), thus broadening the scope of cellular functions that could cause free radical damage. Recent studies (2, 13, 92, 117, 140) have yielded findings in accord with the concept that oxidative damage plays a role in senescence. The available data do not establish a causal role for free radical or oxidative damage in senescence of most species (23, 101, 139), although the recent study of Sohal and Orr (85a), in which a transgenic *Drosophila melanogaster* model was used, provides strong evidence for such a role in that species.

Another potential for damage by fuel is the glycation reaction between reducing sugars and proteins or nucleic acids, and Cerami has proposed the "glycation" theory of aging (14). Through a series of reactions initiated by the Schiff base reaction, glycation results in advanced Maillard products (79), which cause protein cross-linking, nucleic acid–protein cross-linking, and other functional alterations of the macromolecules. As originally proposed, this theory addressed alterations in long-lived extracellular proteins, such as collagen, but it has since been expanded to include cellular macromolecules. Functional deficits suggested as attributable to glycation reactions range from changes in elastic properties to altered enzymatic functions to genomic changes. Kristal and Yu (59) proposed the "free radical–glycation/Maillard reaction" theory of aging, which embraces both the free radical and glycation theories, and also emphasizes the interaction of these biochemical processes.

The accumulation of macromolecular and supramolecular damage shows that the damage removal and repair mechanisms are not sufficient to counteract all injury. Indeed, the possible relationship between the rate of aging and DNA repair has been the subject of study (43, 44), but so far the information is not definitive (129). Whitehead and Grigliatti (133) provided evidence that the DNA repair system can play a role in the longevity of adult *Drosophila melanogaster*, but their findings do not establish a role for inadequate DNA repair in the normal aging of this species. Also, inadequate removal of damaged proteins by proteolysis may be another factor in the aging of cells; there is evidence that the rate of degradation of at least some proteins declines with age, usually accompanied by an equivalent reduction in rate of synthesis and thus a decreased rate of turnover (27).

This discussion has in no way exhausted the list of specific mechanisms that have been proposed and studied as causes for the disturbance of cellular homeostasis with increasing age. An in-depth coverage of the mechanisms just discussed as well as others which have been proposed to be involved in the disturbed cellular homeostasis underlying senescence is presented in Chapter 9. To date, clear evidence of a causal role in aging has not been established for any of the proposed mechanisms.

Failure in Organismic Homeostatic Control Systems. Another view of aging is that primary aging processes occur in specific cells that function in organismic homeostatic control systems (34). The change in the operation of a control system is viewed as the cause of the dysfunctions in many other cells; that is, these dysfunctions are considered secondary to disordered organismic homeostatic control function (36).

An example of a theory of aging based on this concept is the "glucocorticoid cascade" hypothesis of Sapolsky et al. (111). Basic to this theory is the presence in the hippocampus of neurons that contain a high density of glucocorticoid receptors and serve in the negative feedback control system regulating plasma glucocorticoid levels. Stress-induced increases in plasma glucocorticoid levels, which occur inevitably during daily life, are thought to down-regulate the hippocampal glucocorticoid receptors, resulting in periods of glucocorticoid hypersecretion. It is proposed that these periods of glucocorticoid hypersecretion, coupled with insults such as ischemia with advancing age, cause a loss of hippocampal neurons. As a consequence, there would be a feedforward cascade of sustained hyperadrenocorticism, with subsequent widespread deterioration (that is, senescence) resulting in such conditions as immunosuppression, osteoporosis, and impaired cognition. This provocative theory was based on research with the rat model; a subsequent study in rats has not provided support for this theory (107).

Many other theories based on disordered endocrine, neuroendocrine, and/or neural organismic regulatory systems have been proposed. These theories have implicated not only hormonal excesses but also hormonal deficits, such as the growth hormone deficit concept proposed by Rudman et al. (106).

A similar line of reasoning led Walford (130) to link age changes in the immune system to organismic aging in general. He theorized that age-associated immune system dysfunction contributes to a wide range of age-associated degenerative processes not usually considered immunological in origin. Fabris (32) recently proposed a complex theory of aging that linked the immune and neuroendocrine systems and their interactions to organismic aging.

Assessment of disordered neuroendocrine functions indicates that the factor underlying age change is not chronological time but rather events (for example, stress) occurring during the life of the animal (34). A further discussion of neuroendocrine function and aging is presented in Chapter 15.

A general discussion of the loss with age in the integration and stability of organisms is presented in Chapter 22. Lipsitz and Goldberger (64a) have proposed that a generalized loss in the complexity of organ system function is a basic characteristic of aging, a phenomenon for which they believe measurements can be developed based on chaos theory and the related concept of fractals.

Current Status of the Concept of Primary Aging Processes

Obviously, there has been no lack of theories concerning the nature of primary aging processes. Thus far, however, in the case of most species, strong evidence has not been provided in support of any of these theories. Although it is not difficult to show age changes, clear evidence of an age change as causal in the aging processes has yet to be established in most species. The reason for this lack of evidence may stem from the difficulty of establishing cause and effect when multiple processes are involved over an extended period. In fact, the question arises as to the very usefulness of the concept of primary aging processes if senescence does indeed result from many different primary processes and their interactions.

EVOLUTIONARY BIOLOGY OF AGING

Conceptual developments in the field of the evolutionary biology of aging may provide the framework needed for further advances in biological gerontology. Because aging reduces the genetic contribution of individuals to future generations, most evolutionary biologists believe that senescence results from a declining force of natural selection with age after sexual maturation (15); that is, the power of natural selection to favor advantageous alleles or to eliminate deleterious alleles declines with age after reproduction commences. This decline results from the high death rate at young ages in most species in the wild due to predation, infection, and other environmental hazards and consequently a marked decrease in the contribution to progeny with increasing postmaturational age.

Evolutionary biologists define aging (senescence) as a progressive decline in the age-specific fitness components of an organism due to internal physiological deterioration. The major aspects of fitness are age-specific fecundity and survival probability, which quantitatively determine fitness.

Most evolutionary biologists now view as unlikely the concept that aging is a positive force for selective advantage (that is, evolutionarily adaptive) by eliminating old individuals, thereby making resources available to their progeny, and by increasing the rate of succession of generations, thereby improving the chances for adaptation to changes in environment (56). This concept is based on *"group selection,"* which is nearly universally rejected by evolutionary biologists on logical grounds except in extraordinary cases. For example, group selection rather than individual selection can occur in the case of parasitic organisms not readily transmitted to another host. In such circumstances, a population of a parasitic species with a genotype conferring a low rate of reproduction may have selective advantage over a population of the same species with a high rate of reproduction, if this high rate of parasite reproduction kills the host. In contrast, under most circumstances, individuals with genotypes enabling the generation of the greatest number of viable progeny have selective advantage.

If senescence results from a declining force of natural selection, then the rate of aging should be markedly influenced by both environmental hazards (predation, starvation, infection, etc.) and the nature of the genetic trade-off between reproduction and subsequent survival; that is, current evolutionary theory predicts that aging should occur at slower rates in populations (or species) that have lower mortality rates due to lessened environmental hazards or higher fertility rates at older ages (100).

It is difficult to test this hypothesis in the laboratory.

However, Rose and his colleagues (51, 99) have reported studies with *D. melanogaster* showing that after 25 generations a stock developed by postponing culture reproduction evolved an increased longevity, a finding in accord with the hypothesis. Also, a study comparing bats with other mammals living in the wild (4) and a study of opossums living in different habitats (3) both support the concept that the lower the level of environmental hazard, the slower the rate of aging.

Two potential mechanisms have been proposed as the genetic basis of this evolutionary concept of aging (134a): antagonistic pleiotropy and accumulation of deleterious mutations expressed late in life.

Antagonistic pleiotropy, clearly and forcefully presented more than 35 years ago by Williams (134), is the proposition that some genes with beneficial effects at young ages have deleterious consequences at advanced ages. By this genetic mechanism, natural selection actively increases the rate of aging in the course of promoting overall (mean) fitness.

Mutation accumulation, first postulated by Medawar (74), is the proposition that if the effect of a detrimental gene mutation occurs only late in life, then the force of selection will be too weak to oppose its establishment and spread. According to this view, aging arises from an accumulation of late-acting deleterious mutations.

Draye et al. (31a) point out the difficulties encountered when attempting to obtain evidence establishing the occurrence of these genetic mechanisms. However, there is some experimental evidence supporting both antagonistic pleiotropy and the mutation accumulation mechanisms of aging. Quantitatively, the relative importance of each has yet to be defined (86). Moreover, other genetic mechanisms may exist.

Most theories of aging have focused on physiological causes. Evolutionary biologists recognize that physiological processes link the genetic mechanisms to senescence. As discussed earlier, under CONCEPT OF PRIMARY AGING PROCESSES, for most species the nature of this linkage is not known. The erosion of teeth in herbivores appears to be an instance where the nature of the linkage has been established (61). Another linkage between the evolutionary theory of aging and physiological processes is seen in the deleterious consequences of reproduction as a cause of rapid deterioration (viewed by many as senescence) in semelparous species, such as the Pacific salmon. One reason the nature of the linkages has not been identified for most species is the possibility that multiple physiological vehicles are involved, thereby complicating the identification of specific processes.

Current views on the evolutionary biology of aging can be summarized as follows: *(1)* all organisms that have a soma distinct from a germ line undergo senescence, *(2)* senescence results from the decline with age in the force of natural selection after reproduction commences, *(3)* possible genetic mechanisms of aging are the accumulation of deleterious late-acting genes and antagonistic pleiotropy, *(4)* the number of genes involved in the aging processes remains to be determined as do the genetic similarities and differences among and within species in regard to senescence, *(5)* the similarity in aging phenotypes among related species may result from a common ancestral species, *(6)* the apparent synchronization of age changes within a species may occur because senescence is the result of a decrease in the force of natural selection.

The evolutionary theory of aging provides a strong unifying base for gerontology. It should play an important guiding role in the future development of gerontology, for example, by *(1)* focusing on the possibility of diversity of aging mechanisms within species as well as among species, *(2)* providing a theoretical basis for the synchronization in some species of age-associated physiological deteriorations and of sources of mortality, *(3)* guiding the choice of animal models and the use of comparative biology for the study of aging, *(4)* providing a theoretical basis for a relationship between senescence and physiological adaptations of species to the environment, *(5)* bridging the dichotomy between the programed and stochastic concepts of aging, and *(6)* providing a theoretical basis for the antiaging action of dietary restriction.

Indeed, the evolutionary concept of aging has given rise to the provocative "disposable soma" theory proposed by Kirkwood (55). The tenet of this theory is that the basic function of an organism is to transform free energy from its environment into progeny. To do so, part of the energy must be used for somatic maintenance. The theory proposes that the force of selection results in apportioning energy between maintenance of the soma and reproduction so as to maximize evolutionary fitness. As a consequence, less energy is used for repair of the soma than is required for indefinite survival of the organism. It further proposes that the extent of the investment in somatic maintenance depends on ecological niche. A species with a high rate of mortality due to the environmental hazards of the niche in which it lives will invest little in maintenance of the soma, and the converse is the case for species living in a protected environment. This theory is attractive because it views aging caused by wear and tear not as a thermodynamic inevitability but rather as a balance struck between the use of energy for somatic maintenance and for reproduction.

MANIFESTATIONS OF AGING PROCESSES

With advancing age, organisms exhibit a spectrum of alterations in morphological and physiological characteristics. Many of these alterations may be deteriorations directly due to aging processes, while others may be compensatory responses, which if not appropriately regulated may also be deteriorative. In addition, some of these altered characteristics may not be the result of aging per se but may be caused by chronic exposure to toxic agents (chemical, biological, or other). A current challenge is that of determining which of the many characteristics of aged animals and people directly or indirectly relate to aging processes. Two general characteristics of aging organisms—age-associated disease processes and age-associated physiological changes—will be discussed in this regard.

Age-Associated Disease Processes

A procedure of subject selection that has been widely adopted in human studies of aging involves excluding persons with discernible disease. This is referred to by Rowe et al. (104) as "cleaning up" the physiological data. In animal studies of aging, there has also been a major effort to choose animals free of disease (70). Yet many diseases either occur only at advanced ages or are more prevalent among the aged; that is, they are age-associated disease processes. The conceptual basis for selecting subjects without disease is that by so doing "normal" aging can be studied (116). This concept requires further discussion.

In a thoughtful paper, Brody and Schneider (9) addressed the issue of the relationship between aging and age-associated diseases. They classified such diseases as *age-related* or *age-dependent* diseases. *Age-related* diseases were defined as those with an age pattern of occurrence in which the primary aging processes are not directly involved. *Age-dependent* diseases were defined as those in which the primary aging processes are involved in the pathogenesis. The problem then becomes one of deciding how to categorize a particular disease. The major criterion used by Brody and Schneider is the age pattern of the occurrence of morbidity or mortality due to the disease. If this pattern is similar to that of the age-specific death rate, the disease is classified as age-dependent, but if the pattern differs from that of the age-specific death rate, the disease is classified as age-related. According to their schema, following human diseases were classified as age-dependent: acute myocardial infarction, ischemic heart disease, cerebrovascular disease, type II diabetes, osteoporosis, Alzheimer's disease, and Parkinson's disease. The following were classified as age-related: multiple sclerosis, amyotrophic lateral sclerosis, gout, peptic ulcer, and most cancers, with the exception of prostatic cancer.

This attempt to relate age-associated diseases to aging processes is commendable. Because of our lack of knowledge of primary aging processes, however, it is difficult to assess its validity. Cancer is a case in point. Although the age pattern of the occurrence of and death from most cancers differs from the age-specific mortality rate, cancer is predominantly a disease of the aged (30, 87). Moreover, the occurrence of cancer involves equivalent periods of the life span in different species (110); for example, it occurs primarily between two and four years of age in rats and between 50 and 100 years of age in humans. Although this age association tends to implicate aging processes in the pathogenesis of cancer, there are other possible explanations. For the occurrence of cancer, multiple genetic alterations over an extended period of time are required (122). Mutations of both tumor-promoter and tumor-suppressor genes are believed to be involved (110). In the case of human colorectal cancer, Fearon and Vogelstein (33) have presented evidence that these cancers result from mutational activation of oncogenes coupled to mutational inactivation of suppressor genes and that four to five such mutations are involved. Clearly, time is required for this to occur. But are aging processes involved? The absolute time difference in the occurrence of cancers between humans and rats does not provide a clear answer: not only could the faster rate of aging in rats be a factor but also a faster mutation rate or a lower number of mutations required for the occurrence of cancer in rats could be implicated.

Although the question of a role for aging processes in carcinogenesis cannot be answered unequivocally at this time, Miller (75) points out that three processes (speciation, dietary restriction, and selective breeding) which influence the rate of aging have parallel effects on cancer incidence; he believes this is strong circumstantial evidence for a role of aging in cancer. Moreover, if the evolutionary theory of aging is correct, many age-associated diseases, including cancer, are to be expected as an inevitable component of senescence because of the declining force of natural selection with age.

Clearly, at this stage of knowledge, excluding age-associated disease as a part of "normal" aging is not warranted if normal is defined as "usual," which is the common usage. This is not to imply that studying aging in the absence of disease does not provide valuable information, but such studies should be called "aging in the absence of disease" rather than "normal aging."

Age-Associated Physiological Changes

Changes with age in physiological processes are obvious even from the casual observation of people and animals of different ages. Indeed, these changes are the major subject of this book. Many such changes in the physiological systems of humans were quantitatively evaluated some 30 to 40 years ago by Nathan Shock, whose results are graphically summarized in Figure 1.4 (115). These and many other studies have shown that with advancing age deterioration occurs in most physio-

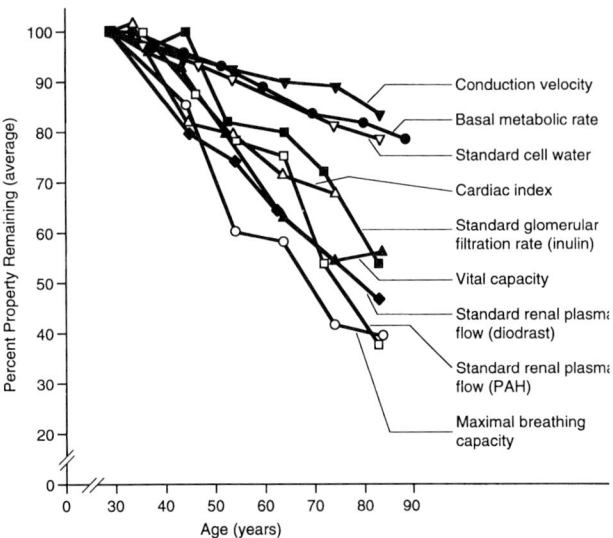

FIG. 1.4. Age changes in human physiological systems based on cross-sectional studies. [Figure prepared by Shock (115). Reproduced with permission.]

logical systems, although its extent varies from person to person.

The studies of Shock have been criticized because the extent to which disease influenced the findings was not evaluated. Indeed, knowledge of disease status permits the reductionist approach of assessing physiological performance in the presence and absence of a particular disease process, and such information is invaluable. Nevertheless, age-associated disease processes may be an integral part of aging and thus a major factor in senescent physiological deterioration in many individuals.

Another criticism is that the early physiological studies were cross-sectional; that is, subjects varying in age were studied at the same point in time. Each group born in a specific calendar time frame is called a *cohort*, and one problem with this design is that of cohort effects; that is, different cohorts have had different experiences. Cohort effects confound interpretation of findings in relation to aging. Another problem with the design is that of selective mortality; that is, only those who survive to a particular age can be studied, and the older the cohort, the smaller the percent of the original group still alive. Selective mortality also confounds interpretations of findings with regard to aging.

Longitudinal studies (measurements of the same subject over a long period of time) avoid those problems but have other drawbacks. These include the stability over time of the population being studied, alterations in measurement procedures due to changes in laboratory personnel and changes in assay methods and/or the instruments used for the assays, and the adaptation of subjects to the testing procedures. These issues have been seriously addressed but not entirely overcome. While many of the findings of early studies have now been confirmed qualitatively, quantitative differences have emerged, for example, in pulmonary vital capacity, cardiac output at rest, and basal metabolic rate. Further discussion of cross-sectional and longitudinal study designs can be found in Chapters 2 and 5, and in Part IV, Organ Systems and Organismic Aging.

The outstanding physiological differences between the young and the old are the reduced ability to meet challenges and the reduced capacity of the physiological systems. For example, elderly people show a decreased ability to maintain body temperature when challenged by hot or cold environments (17) and the running of the marathon takes longer, as reflected by the running times of the world record holders in each age range (38).

Rowe and Kahn (103) point out that even in the absence of discernible disease there is a heterogeneity with respect to many age-associated physiological changes that has largely been ignored as investigators have focused on the mean of the age group. They propose that for a given physiological function, the aging population without discernible disease be divided into a "usual" aging subgroup, exhibiting a level of physiological change with age similar to the mean, and a "successful" aging subgroup, exhibiting minimal change. They further propose that those who show little deterioration with age in a constellation of physiological functions be regarded as undergoing broadly "successful" aging in physiological terms. Rowe and Kahn conclude that the effects of the aging processes have been exaggerated and that the difference between "successful" and "usual" aging relates primarily to such extrinsic factors as diet, exercise, personal habits, and psychosocial influences. This view is provocative, but it is important to recognize that genetics is probably an important factor underlying the heterogeneity of the population undergoing "normal" aging, and there is also very likely a complex interaction between intrinsic aging processes and environmental factors. (For a discussion of this issue with regard to the skin, see Chapter 11.)

Indeed, marked deterioration of the physiological systems is evident in most people at advanced ages. Some of this deterioration is caused by disease and for this reason is often said not to be due to the aging processes. However, if most age-associated diseases are an integral part of senescence, as suggested by the evolutionary theory of aging, then dismissal of deterioration caused by disease as a part of the aging processes is not warranted. Similarly, environmental, life-style, and psychosocial characteristics can often have a negative long-term impact on the physiological systems, and this impact may be due to the actions of those characteristics on aging processes. The complex interactions of these many factors and the aging processes are far from being understood; until this understanding is achieved, it is at best premature and probably inappropriate to conclude that the effects of aging processes on the physiological systems have been exaggerated. Moreover, before age-related changes in physiological processes can be used as valid biomarkers of aging, these many issues must first be resolved.

SUMMARY AND CONCLUSIONS

Aging refers to the postmaturational deterioration of the organism, and the goal of biological gerontology is to understand the reasons for that deterioration. Population studies have yielded important information for gerontology: the data on age-specific mortality rates have been most useful, and the MRDT serves as an important index of the occurrence of aging and of its rate. It is likely that aging occurs in all species that have a soma separate from the germ line, but unequivocal proof of this view is lacking.

Aging is difficult to assess in the individual. While the concept of biological age as distinct from chronological age is almost certainly valid, it remains to be clearly established by measurement. As already stated, the development of biomarkers that serve as indices of the biological age of the individual has been vigorously pursued, but attempts to validate these biomarkers have so far been unsuccessful.

Gerontologists have long believed that there are primary aging processes and have expended much thought and research effort attempting to identify those processes. The many theories of aging proposed over the years were hypotheses about the nature of the primary processes. The theories can be divided into two categories: *(1)* genetic programs akin to development and morphogenesis and *(2)* homeostatic failure. On the basis of current views of the evolutionary biology of aging, it is not likely that theories in the first category have any validity. Despite the many ideas proposed and the effort devoted to their investigation, for most species the nature of the primary aging processes is not known. Indeed, the concept of primary aging processes is of value only if they are few in number. However, if in most species aging results from many different independent as well as interacting underlying processes, the concept of primary aging processes may not even be useful.

Conceptual developments in the evolutionary biology of aging may provide a unifying base for gerontology that can guide future research. Evolutionary biologists define aging as a persistent decline in age-specific fitness components due to internal physiological deterioration. They view the decline with age in the force of natural selection as the reason for senescence. The physiological processes involved in senescence may be many and may differ among species as well as within species.

Many diseases occur only at advanced ages or are more prevalent at advanced ages. In selecting human or animal subjects for the study of aging, great effort is made to exclude those with discernible disease, even though current knowledge does not reveal the extent of involvement of aging processes in age-associated diseases. Indeed, age-associated diseases would be predicted as likely to result from the decline in the force of natural selection with age. Thus, at this time, exclusion of age-associated disease as part of "normal" aging is not warranted. However, important information will continue to emerge from studies of aging in the absence of disease. Moreover, studies over the age range of young adulthood through middle age can be executed with most of the subjects free of the confounding problem of markedly debilitating diseases.

With advancing age, deterioration occurs in most physiological systems of humans and animals. The outstanding physiological differences between young and old are the reduced ability to meet challenges and the reduced functional capacity of the physiological systems. Even in the absence of discernible disease, there is a marked heterogeneity in age-associated physiological changes within a given population. Those individuals who show little age change in a particular physiological process are referred to as the "successful" aging group for that physiological process. Those who show little deterioration with age in a constellation of physiological functions are regarded as exhibiting broadly "successful" aging in physiological terms. Nevertheless, at a sufficiently advanced age, it appears that all people and animals will exhibit significant physiological deterioration.

REFERENCES

1. ARKING, R. *Biology of Aging Observation and Principles.* Englewood Cliffs, NJ: Prentice-Hall, 1991.
2. ARKING, R., S. BUCK, A. BERRIOS, S. DWYER, and G. T. BAKER. Elevated paraquat resistance can be used as a bioassay for longevity in a genetically based long-lived strain of *Drosophila*. *Dev. Genet.* 12: 362–370, 1991.
3. AUSTAD, S. N. Retarded senescence in an insular population of Virginia opossums (*Didelphis virginiana*). *J. Zool.* 229: 695–708, 1993.
4. AUSTAD, S. N., and K. E. FISCHER. Mammalian aging, metabolism and ecology: evidence from the bats and marsupials. *J. Gerontol.: Biol. Sci.* 46: B47–B53, 1991.
5. BAKER, G. T., III, and R. SPROTT. Biomarkers of aging. *Exp. Gerontol.* 23: 223–239, 1988.
6. BELL, G. Evolutionary and nonevolutionary theories of senescence. *Am. Naturalist* 124: 600–603, 1984.
7. BORKAN, G. A., and A. H. NORRIS. Assessment of biological age using a profile of physical parameters. *J. Gerontol.* 35: 177–184, 1980.

8. BOWDEN, D. M., and D. D. WILLIAMS. Aging. *Adv. Vet. Sci. Comp. Med.* 28: 305–341, 1984.
9. BRODY, J. A., and E. L. SCHNEIDER. Diseases and disorders of aging: a hypothesis. *J. Chron. Dis.* 39: 871–876, 1986.
9a. BROOKS, A., G. J. LITHGOW, and T. E. JOHNSON. Mortality rates in a genetically heterogeneous population of *Caenorhabditis elegans*. *Science* 263: 668–671, 1994.
10. BURNET, M. *Intrinsic Mutagenesis: A Genetic Approach for Aging*. New York: Wiley, 1974.
11. CADENAS, E. Biochemistry of oxygen toxicity. *Annu. Rev. Biochem.* 58: 79–110, 1989.
12. CAREY, J. R., P. LIEDO, D. OROZCO, and J. W. VAUPEL. Slowing of mortality rates at older ages in large medfly cohorts. *Science* 258: 457–461, 1992.
13. CARNEY, J. M., P. E. STARKE-REED, C. N. OLIVER, R. W. LANDRUM, M. S. CHENG, J. WU, and R. A. FLOYD. Reversal of age-related increase in brain protein oxidation, decrease in enzyme activity, and loss in temporal and spatial memory by chronic administration of the spin-trapping compound N-tert-butyl-α-phenylnitrone. *Proc. Natl. Acad. Sci. USA* 88: 3633–3636, 1991.
14. CERAMI, A. Hypothesis: glucose as a mediator of aging. *J. Am. Geriatr. Soc.* 33: 626–634, 1985.
15. CHARLESWORTH, B. *Evolution in Age-Structured Populations*. Cambridge: Cambridge University Press, 1980.
16. CLARK, A. M., and M. A. RUBIN. The modification by X-irradiation of the life span of haploids and diploids of the wasp, *Habrobracon* Sp. *Radiat. Res.* 15: 244–253, 1961.
17. COLLINS, K. J., and A. N. EXTON-SMITH. Thermal homeostasis in old age. *J. Am. Geriatr. Soc.* 31: 519–524, 1983.
18. COMFORT, A. *The Biology of Senescence* (3rd ed.), London: Elsevier, 1979.
19. CORTOPASSI, G. A., and N. ARNHEIM. Detection of a specific mitochondrial DNA deletion in tissue of older humans. *Nucleic Acids Res.* 18: 6927–6933, 1990.
20. COSTA, P. T., and R. R. MCCRAE. Concepts of functional or biological age. In: *Principles of Geriatric Medicine*, edited by R. Andres, E. L. Bierman, and W. R. Hazzard. New York: McGraw-Hill, 1984, p. 30–37.
21. COVELLI, V., D. MOUTON, V. DIMAJO, Y. BOUTHILLIES, C. BANGRAZI, J. MEVEL, S. REBESSI, G. DORIA, and G. BIOZZI. Inheritance of immune responsiveness, life span, and disease incidence in interline crosses of mice selected for high or low multispecific antibody production. *J. Immunol.* 142: 1224–1234, 1989.
22. CRISTOFALO, V. J. Overview of biological mechanism of aging. *Annu. Rev. Gerontol. Geriatr.* 10: 1–22, 1991.
23. CRISTOFALO, V. J., and R. G. ALLEN. Additional thoughts on free radicals and life span. *Aging: Clin. Exp. Res.* 5: 239–240, 1992.
24. CRISTOFALO, V. J., and R. J. PIGNOLO. Replicative senescence of human fibroblast-like cells in culture. *Physiol. Rev.* 73: 617–638, 1993.
25. CURTSINGER, J. W., H. H. FUKUI, D. R. TOWNSEND, and J. W. VAUPEL. Demography of genotypes: failure of the limited life-span paradigm in *Drosophila melanogaster*. *Science* 258: 461–463, 1992.
25a. CURTSINGER, J. W., H. H. FUKUI, L. XIU, A. KHAZAELI, and S. FLETCHER. Rates of mortality in populations of *Caenorhabditis elegans*. *Science* 266:826, 1994.
26. CUTLER, R. G. Dysdifferentiation and aging. In: *Molecular Biology of Aging: Gene Stability and Gene Expression*, edited by R. S. Sohal, L. Birnbaum, and R. G. Cutler. New York: Raven Press, 1985, p. 307–340.
27. DANNON, D. B., and N. J. HOLBROOK. Alterations in gene expression with aging. In: *Handbook of the Biology of Aging* (3rd ed.), edited by E. L. Schneider and J. W. Rowe. San Diego: Academic Press, 1990, p. 97–115.
28. DENCKLA, W. D. Role of pituitary and thyroid glands in the decline of minimal O_2 consumption with age. *J. Clin. Invest.* 53: 572–581, 1974.
29. DICE, J. F. Cellular and molecular mechanisms of aging. *Physiol. Rev.* 73: 149–159, 1993.
30. DIX, D. The role of aging in cancer incidence: an epidemiological study. *J. Gerontol.* 44: 10–18, 1989.
31. DOMNING, J. P. Marching teeth of the manatee. *Nat. Hist.* 92: 8–10, 1983.
31a. DRAYE, X., P. BULLENS, and F. A. LINTS. Geographic variations in life history strategies in *Drosophila melanogaster*. I Analysis of wild caught populations. *Exp. Gerontol.* 29: 205–222, 1994.
32. FABRIS, N. A neuroendocrine-immune theory of aging. *Int. J. Neurosci.* 51: 373–375, 1990.
33. FEARON, E. R., and B. A. VOGELSTEIN. Genetic model for colorectal tumorigenesis. *Cell* 61: 759–767, 1990.
34. FINCH, C. E. Neural and endocrine approaches to the resolution of time as a dependent variable in the aging processes in mammals. *Gerontologist* 28: 29–42, 1988.
35. FINCH, C. E. *Longevity, Senescence and the Genome*. Chicago: University of Chicago Press, 1990.
36. FINCH, C. E., and P. W. LANDFIELD. Neuroendocrine and autonomic functions in aging mammals. In: *Handbook of the Biology of Aging* (2nd ed.), edited by C. E. Finch and E. L. Schneider. New York: Van Nostrand Reinhold, 1985, p. 567–594.
37. FINCH, C. E., M. C. PIKE, and M. WITTEN. Slow mortality rate accelerations during aging in some animals approximate that of humans. *Science* 249: 902–905, 1990.
38. FRIES, J. F., and L. M. CRAPO. *Vitality and Aging*. San Francisco: W. H. Freeman, 1981.
39. GAFNI, A. Altered protein metabolism in aging. *Annu. Rev. Gerontol. Geriatr.* 10: 117–131, 1991.
40. GAVRILOV, L. A., and N. S. GAVRILOVA. *The Biology of Life Span: A Quantitative Approach*. Chur, Switzerland: Harwood Academic Publications, 1990.
41. GEE, E. M., and J. E. VEEVERS. Accelerating sex differential in mortality: an analysis of contributing factors. *Soc. Biol.* 30: 75–85, 1983.
42. HARMAN, D. Aging: a theory based on free radical and radiation biology. *J. Gerontol.* 11: 298–300, 1956.
43. HART, R. W., and F. B. DANIEL. Genetic stability in vitro and in vivo. *Adv. Pathobiol.* 7: 123–141, 1980.
44. HART, R. W., and R. B. SETLOW. Correlation between deoxyribonucleic acid excision repair and lifespan in a number of mammalian species. *Proc. Natl. Acad. Sci. USA* 71: 2169–2173, 1974.
45. HART, R. W., and A. TURTURRO. Theories of aging. In: *Review of Biological Research in Aging*, edited by M. Rothstein. New York: Alan R. Liss, 1985, vol. 1, p. 5–18.
46. HASTIE, N. D., M. DEMPSTER, M. G. DUNLOP, A. M. THOMPSON, D. K. GREEN, and R. C. ALLSHIRE. Telomere reduction in human colorectal carcinoma and with aging. *Nature* 346: 866–868, 1990.
47. HATTORI, K., M. TANAKA, S. SUGIYAMA, T. OBAYASHI, I. TAKAYUKI, T. SATAKE, Y. HANAKI, J. ASAI, M. NAGANO, and T. OZAWA. Age-dependent increase in deleted mitochondrial DNA in the human heart: possible contributing factor to presbycardia. *Am. Heart J.* 121: 1735–1742, 1991.
48. HAYFLICK, L. Theories of biological aging. *Exp. Gerontol.* 20: 145–159, 1985.
49. HAYFLICK, L., and P. S. MOORHEAD. The serial cultivation of human diploid cell strains. *Exp. Cell Res.* 25: 585–621, 1961.

50. HAZZARD, W. R. Biological basis of the sex differential in longevity. *J. Am. Geriatr. Soc.* 34: 455–471, 1986.
50a. HIRSCH, A. G., R. J. WILLIAMS, and P. MEHL. Kinetics of medfly mortality. *Exp. Gerontol.* 29: 197–204, 1994.
50b. HIRSCH, H. R. Can an improved environment cause maximum lifespan to decrease? Comments on lifespan criteria and longitudinal Gompertzian analysis. *Exp. Gerontol.* 29: 119–137, 1994.
51. HUTCHINSON, E. W., and M. R. ROSE. Quantitative genetic analysis of postponed aging in *Drosophila melanogaster*. In: *Genetic Effects in Aging II*, edited by D. E. Harrison. Caldwell, NJ: Telford Press, 1990, p. 66–87.
52. IKEBE, S., M. TANAKA, K. OHNO, W. SATO, K. HATORI, T. KONDO, Y. MIZUNO, and T. OZAWA. Increase of deleted mitochondrial DNA relative to normal DNA in Parkinsonian striatum by kinetic PCR analysis. *Biochem. Biophys. Res. Commun.* 172: 483–489, 1990.
53. JOHNSON, T. E. Increased life-span of age-1 mutants in *Caenorhabditis elegans* and lower Gompertz rate of aging. *Science* 249: 908–912, 1990.
53a. JOHNSON, T. E. Rates of mortality in populations of *Caenorhabditis elegans*. *Science* 266:828, 1994.
54. KADENBACH, B., and J. HÖCKER-MÜLLER. Mutations of mitochondrial DNA and human death. *Naturwissenschaften* 77: 221–225, 1990.
55. KIRKWOOD, T. B. L. The disposable soma theory of aging. In: *Genetic Effects on Aging II*, edited by D. E. Harrison. Caldwell, NJ: Telford Press, 1990, p. 9–19.
56. KIRKWOOD, T. B. L., and T. CREMER. Cytogerontology since 1881: a reappraisal of August Weismann and a review of modern progress. *Hum. Genet.* 60: 101–121, 1982.
57. KLOEDEN, P. E., R. RÖSSLER, and O. E. RÖSSLER. Does a centralized clock for ageing exist? *Gerontology* 36: 314–322, 1990.
58. KOWALD, A., and T. B. L. KIRKWOOD. Explaining fruit fly longevity. *Science* 260: 1664–1665, 1993.
59. KRISTAL, B. S., and B. P. YU. An emerging hypothesis: synergistic induction of aging by free radicals and Maillard reactions. *J. Gerontol.: Biol. Sci.* 47: B107–B114, 1992.
60. LACK, D. *The Natural Regulation of Animal Numbers*. Oxford: Clarendon Press, 1954.
61. LAWS, R. M. Dentition and ageing of the hippopotamus. *E. Afr. Wildlife J.* 6: 19–52, 1968.
62. LINNANE, A. W. Mitochondria and aging: the universality of bioenergetic disease. *Aging Clin. Exp. Res.* 4: 267–271, 1992.
63. LINNANE, A. W., A. BAUMER, R. J. MAXWELL, H. PRESTON, C. ZHANG, and S. MARZUKI. Mitochondrial gene mutation: the ageing process and degenerative disease. *Biochem. Int.* 22: 1067–1079, 1990.
64. LINNANE, A. W., S. MARZUKI, T. OZAWA, and M. TANAKA. Mitochondrial DNA mutations as a major contributor to aging and degenerative diseases. *Lancet* 1: 642–645, 1989.
64a. LIPSITZ, A., and A. L. GOLDBERGER. Loss of "complexity" and aging. Potential applications of fractals and chaos theory to senescence. *J. Am. Med. Assoc.* 267: 1806–1809, 1992.
65. MARTIN, G. M. Clonal attenuation: causes and consequences. *J. Gerontol.: Biol. Sci.* 48: B171–B172, 1993.
66. MARTINEZ, D. E., and J. S. LEVINTON. Asexual metazoans undergo senescence. *Proc. Natl. Acad. Sci. USA* 89: 9920–9923, 1992.
67. MASORO, E. J. Metabolism. In: *Handbook of the Biology of Aging* (2nd ed.), edited by C. E. Finch and E. L. Schneider. New York: Van Nostrand Reinhold, 1985, p. 540–563.
68. MASORO, E. J. Physiological system markers of aging. *Exp. Gerontol.* 23: 391–394, 1988.
69. MASORO, E. J. Biology of aging: facts, thoughts, and experimental approaches. *Lab. Invest.* 66: 500–510, 1991a.
70. MASORO, E. J. Use of rodents as models for the study of "normal aging": conceptual and practical issues. *Neurobiol. Aging* 12: 639–643, 1991b.
71. MASORO, E. J. The role of animal models in meeting the gerontologic challenge for the twenty-first century. *Gerontologist* 32: 627–633, 1992.
72. MASORO, E. J., and R. J. M. MCCARTER. Aging as a consequence of fuel utilization. *Aging: Clin. Exp. Res.* 3: 117–128, 1991.
72a. MCGUE, M., J. W. VAUPEL, N. HOLM, and B. HARVOLD. Longevity is moderately heritable in a sample of Danish twins born 1870–1880. *J. Gerontol.: Biol. Sci.* 48: B237–B244, 1993.
73. MCKERROW, J. Nonenzymatic post translational amino acid modifications in aging: a brief review. *Mech. Ageing Dev.* 10: 371–377, 1979.
74. MEDAWAR, P. B. *An Unsolved Problem of Biology*. London: H. K. Lewis, 1952.
74a. MEDVEDEV, Z. A. An attempt at a rational clarification of theories of aging. *Biol. Rev.* 65: 375–398, 1990.
75. MILLER, R. A. Gerontology as oncology. Research on aging as the key to the understanding of cancer. *Cancer* 68: 2496–2501, 1991.
76. MIQUEL, J. An update on the mitochondrial-DNA mutation hypothesis of cell aging. *Mutat. Res.* 275: 209–216, 1992.
77. MIQUEL, J. A., A. C. ECONOMOS, J. FLEMING, and J. E. JOHNSON, JR. Mitochondrial roles in cell aging. *Exp. Gerontol.* 15: 575–591, 1980.
78. MIQUEL, J., and J. E. FLEMING. A two step hypothesis on the mechanism of in vitro cell aging. Cell differentiation followed by intrinsic mitochondrial mutagenesis. *Exp. Gerontol.* 19: 31–36, 1984.
79. MONNIER, V. M. Nonenzymatic glycosylation, the Maillard reaction and the aging processes. *J. Gerontol.: Biol. Sci.* 45: B105–B111, 1990.
80. MÜLLER-HÖCKER, J. Mitochondria and ageing. *Brain Pathol.* 2: 148–158, 1992.
81. NAKANISHI, K., A. SHIMA, J. FUKUDA, and S. FUJITA. Age-associated increase of single-stranded regions in the DNA of mouse brain and liver cells. *Mech. Ageing Dev.* 10: 273–281, 1979.
81a. NESSE, R. M. Life table tests of evolutionary theories of aging. *Exp. Gerontol.* 23: 445–453, 1988.
82. NUSBAUM, T. J., J. L. GRAVES, L. D. MUELLER, and M. R. ROSE. Fruit fly aging and mortality. *Science* 260: 1567, 1993.
83. OLSHANSKY, S. J., B. A. CARNES, and C. K. CASSEL. Fruit fly aging and mortality. *Science* 260: 1565–1567, 1993.
84. OLSON, C. B. A review of why and how we age: a defense of multifactorial aging: *Mech. Ageing Dev.* 41: 1–28, 1987.
85. ORGEL, L. E. The maintenance of the accuracy of protein synthesis and its relevance to aging. *Proc. Natl. Acad. Sci. USA* 49: 512–517, 1963.
85a. ORR, W. C., and R. S. SOHAL. Extension of life span by overexpression of superoxide dismutase and catalase in *Drosophila melanogaster*. *Science* 263: 1128–1130, 1994.
86. PARTRIDGE, L., and N. H. BARTON. Optimality, mutation and the evolution of ageing. *Nature* 362: 305–311, 1993.
87. PITOT, H. C. Aging and cancer: some general thoughts. *J. Gerontol.: Biol. Sci.* (special issue) 44: 5–9, 1989.
88. PORTER, M. B., and J. R. SMITH. Role of endogenous proteins as negative growth modulators during in vitro cellular aging of human diploid fibroblasts. *Annu. Rev. Gerontol. Geriatr.* 10: 53–70, 1991.
89. PROMISLOW, D. E. L. Senescence in natural populations of mammals: a comparative study. *Evolution* 45: 1869–1887, 1991.

90. PROMISLOW, D. E. L. On size and survival: progress and pitfalls in the allometry of life span. *J. Gerontol.: Biol. Sci.* 48: B115–B123, 1993.
91. RAFF, M. C. Social controls on cell survival and cell death. *Nature* 356: 397–399, 1992.
92. REVEILLAUD, I., A. NIEDZWIECKI, K. G. BENSCFY, and J. E. FLEMING. Expression of bovine superoxide dismutase in *Drosophila melanogaster* augments resistance to oxidative stress. *Mol. Cell Biol.* 11: 632–640, 1991.
93. RICHARDSON, A., and I. SEMSEI. Effect of aging on translation and transcription. In: *Review of Biological Research in Aging*, edited by M. Rothstein. New York: Alan R. Liss, 1987, vol. 3, p. 467–483.
94. RIVNAY, B., S. BERGMAN, M. SHINITZKY, and A. GLOBERSON. Correlations between membrane viscosity, serum cholesterol, lymphocyte activation and aging in man. *Mech. Ageing Dev.* 12: 119–126, 1980.
95. ROBINE, J. M., and K. RITCHIE. Explaining fruit fly longevity. *Science* 260: 1665, 1993.
96. ROCKSTEIN, M. Biology of aging insects. In: *Topics in the Biology of Aging*, edited by P. L. Krohn. New York: John Wiley, 1966, p. 43–61.
97. ROCKSTEIN, M., and H. M. LIEBERMAN. A life table for the common housefly, *Musca domestica*. *Gerontologia* 3: 23–36, 1959.
98. ROCKSTEIN, M., J. CHESKY, and M. SUSSMAN. Comparative biology and evolution of aging. In: *Handbook of the Biology of Aging*, edited by C. E. Finch and L. Hayflick. New York: Van Nostrand Reinhold, 1977 p. 3–34.
99. ROSE, M. R. Laboratory evaluation of postponed senescence in *Drosophila melanogaster*. *Evolution* 38: 1004–1010, 1984.
100. ROSE, M. R. *Evolutionary Biology of Aging*. New York: Oxford University Press, 1991.
101. ROTH, G. S. Are free radicals causes or effects of aging? The entropy theory. *Aging: Clin. Exp. Res.* 5: 241–242, 1993.
102. ROTHSTEIN, M. Evidence for and against the error catastrophe hypothesis. In: *Modern Biological Theories of Aging*, edited by H. R. Warner, R. N. Butler, R. L. Sprott, and E. L. Schneider. New York: Raven Press, 1987, p. 139–154.
103. ROWE, J. W., and R. L. KAHN. Human aging: usual and successful. *Science* 237: 143–149, 1987.
104. ROWE, J. W., S. Y. WANG, and D. ELAHI. Design, conduct, and analysis of human aging research. In: *Handbook of the Biology of Aging* (3rd ed.), edited by E. L. Schneider and J. W. Rowe. San Diego: Academic Press, 1990, p. 63–71.
105. RUBNER, M. *Das Problem der Lebensdauer und Seine Beziehungen Zum Wachstum und Ernäbrung*. Munich: Oldenburg, 1908.
106. RUDMAN, D., A. G. FELLER, H. S. NAGRAJ, G. A. GERGANS, P. Y. LALITHA, A. F. GOLDBERG, R. A. SCHLENKER, L. COHN, I. W. RUDMAN, and D. E. MATTSON. Effects of human growth hormone in men over 60 years old. *N. Engl. J. Med.* 323: 1–6, 1990.
107. SABATINO, F., E. J. MASORO, C. A. MCMAHAN, and R. W. KUHN. Assessment of the role of the glucocorticoid system in the aging processes and in the action of food restriction. *J. Gerontol.: Biol. Sci.* 46: B171–B179, 1991.
108. SACHER, G. A. Life table modification and life prolongation. In: *Handbook of the Biology of Aging*, edited by C. E. Finch and L. Hayflick. New York: Van Nostrand Reinhold, 1977, p. 582–638.
109. SACHER, G. A., and E. TRUCCO. The stochastic theory of mortality. *Ann. N. Y. Acad. Sci.* 96: 985–1007, 1962.
110. SAGER, R. Tumor suppressor genes: the puzzle and the promise. *Science* 246: 1406–1412, 1989.
111. SAPOLSKY, R. M., L. C. KREY, and B. S. MCEWEN. The neuroendocrinology of stress and aging: the glucocorticoid cascade hypothesis. *Endocr. Rev.* 7: 284–301, 1986.
112. SCHNEIDER, E. L. Theories of aging, a perspective. In: *Modern Biological Theories of Aging* edited by H. R. Warner, R. N. Butler, R. L. Sprott, and E. L. Schneider. New York: Raven Press, 1987, p. 1–4.
113. SEN, S., G. TALUKDER, and A. SHARMA. Age-related alterations in human chromosome composition and DNA content in vitro during senescence. *Biol. Rev.* 62: 25–44, 1987.
114. SEVERINGHAUS, C. W. Tooth development and wear as criteria of age in white-tailed deer. *J. Wildlife Mgt.* 13: 195–216, 1949.
115. SHOCK, N. W. The science of gerontology. In: *Proceedings of Seminars 1959–61*, edited by E. C. Jeffers. Durham, NC: Council on Gerontology, Duke University Press, 1962.
116. SHOCK, N. W. (Editor) *Normal Human Aging: The Baltimore Longitudinal Study of Aging* (NIH Publ. No. 84–2450), Washington, D. C.: U.S. Government Printing Office, 1984.
117. SMITH, C. D., J. M. CARNEY, P. E. STARKE-REED, C. N. OLIVER, E. R. STADTMAN, and R. A. FLOYD. Excess brain protein oxidation and enzyme dysfunction in normal aging and in Alzheimer's disease. *Proc. Natl. Acad. Sci. USA* 88: 10540–10543, 1991.
118. SMITH, J. R. DNA synthesis inhibitors in cellular senescence. *J. Gerontol.: Biol. Sci.* 45: B32–B35, 1990.
119. SOHAL, R. S. The free radical hypothesis of aging: an appraisal of the current status. *Aging Clin. Exp. Res.* 5: 3–17, 1993.
120. STADTMAN, E. Protein modifications in aging. *J. Gerontol.: Biol. Sci.* 43: B112–B120, 1988.
121. STADTMAN, E. R. Protein oxidation and aging. *Science* 257: 1220–1224, 1992.
122. STANBRIDGE, E. J., and P. C. NOWELL. Origins of human cancer revisited. *Cell* 63: 867–874, 1990.
123. STREHLER, B. L., and A. S. MILDVAN. General theory of mortality and aging. *Science* 132: 14–21, 1960.
124. STREHLER, B., G. HIRSCH, D. GUSSECK, R. JOHNSON, and M. BICK. Codon-restriction theory of aging and development. *J. Theor. Biol.* 33: 429–474, 1971.
125. SZILARD, L. On the nature of the aging process. *Proc. Natl. Acad. Sci. USA* 45: 30–45, 1959.
126. TICE, R. R., and R. B. SETLOW. DNA repair and replication in aging organisms and cells. In: *Handbook of the Biology of Aging* (2nd ed.), edited by C. E. Finch and E. L. Schneider. New York: Van Nostrand Reinhold, 1985, p. 173–224.
127. VAUPEL, J. W., and J. R. CAREY. Compositional interpretations of medfly mortality. *Science* 260: 1666–1667, 1993.
127a. VAUPEL, J. W., T. E. JOHNSON, and G.J. LITHGOW. Rates of mortality in populations of *Caenorhabditis elegans*. *Science* 266:824, 1994.
128. VIJG, J. DNA sequence changes in aging: how frequent, how important? *Aging: Clin. Exp. Res.* 2: 105–123, 1990.
129. VIJG, J., and D. L. KNOOK. DNA repair in relation to aging processes. *J. Am. Geriatr. Soc.* 35: 532–541, 1987.
130. WALFORD, R. L. *The Immunologic Theory of Aging*. Copenhagen: Munksgaard, 1969.
131. WALLACE, D. C. Mitochondrial genetics: a paradigm for aging and degenerative diseases? *Science* 256: 628–632, 1992.
131a. WANG J.-L., H-G MÜLLER, W. B. CAPRA, and J. R. CAREY. Rates of mortality in populations of *Caenorhabditis elegans*. *Science* 266:827–828, 1994.
132. WEISMANN, A. Life and death. In: *Essays on Heredity and Kindred Biological Problems*, edited by E. B. Poulton, S. Schonland, and A. E. Shipley. Oxford: Clarendon Press, 1889, p. 1–66.

133. WHITEHEAD, I., and T. A. GRIGLIATTI. A correlation between DNA repair and longevity in adult *Drosophila melanogaster*. *J. Gerontol.: Biol. Sci.* 48: B124–B132, 1993.
134. WILLIAMS, G. C. Pleiotropy, natural selection, and the evolution of senescence. *Evolution* 11: 398–411, 1957.
134a. WILLIAMS, G. C., and R. M. NESSE. The dawn of Darwinian medicine. *Quart. Rev. Biol.* 66: 1–22, 1991.
135. WILSON, V. L., R. A. SMITH, S. MA, and R. G. CUTLER. Genomic 5-methyldeoxycytidine decrease with age. *J. Biol. Chem.* 262: 9948–9951, 1987.
136. WITTEN, M. A return to time, cells, systems, and aging: III Gompertzian models of biological aging and some possible roles for critical elements. *Mech. Ageing Dev.* 32: 141–177, 1985.
137. WRIGHT, W. E., and J. W. SHAY. Telomere positional effects and the regulation of cellular senescence. *Trends Genet.* 8: 193–197, 1992.
138. YEN, T.-C., J.-H. SU, K.-H. KING, and Y.-H. WEI. Aging-associated 5 kb deletion in human liver mitochondrial DNA. *Biochem. Biophys. Res. Commun.* 178: 124–131, 1991.
139. YU, B. P. Need the free radical theory of aging be linked to the metabolic rate theory? *Aging: Clin. Exp. Res.* 5: 243–244, 1993.
140. YU, B. P., D. W. LEE, C. G. MARLER, and J. H. CHOI. Mechanisms of food restriction: protection of cellular homeostasis. *Proc. Soc. Exp. Biol. Med.* 193: 13–22, 1990.

II | METHODOLOGICAL ISSUES IN AGING RESEARCH

2. Design and analysis of aging studies

PAUL T. COSTA, JR.
ROBERT R. McCRAE

Gerontology Research Center, National Institute on Aging, National Institutes of Health, Baltimore, Maryland

CHAPTER CONTENTS

Stability and Change in Mean Levels
    Cross-sectional designs
    Longitudinal designs
    Cross-sequential designs
    Demonstrating stability of mean levels
    Elaborations of the basic design
    Representativeness and attrition in longitudinal studies
    Screening for clinical conditions
Stability and Change in Individual Differences
    Potential problems in the measurement of rank-order stability
Advanced Topics in Design and Analysis of Aging Studies
    Changes in variance and in structure
    Biomarkers and functional age: flawed concepts
    Growth curves and age changes
    Survival analysis and the identification of risk factors
    Correlates of change
    Causal inferences from observational data
Some Considerations for the Design of Longitudinal Studies
    Combining cross-sectional and longitudinal designs
    Combining hypothesis-driven and exploratory research
    Creative exploitation of the data

MASORO HAS DEFINED AGING as the detrimental changes that occur in postmaturational life (see Chapter 1). Finch (30) has a broader view of aging which includes all kinds of time-related changes in organisms. We would suggest a still broader view, defining *aging* as what happens to an organism over time. This view encourages the study of stability as well as change. After all, it is as important to know which functions are preserved as it is to know which develop or deteriorate. An understanding of the mechanisms that underlie stability may suggest ways to alter the mechanisms of senescence.

In this chapter we will discuss some of the basic issues in designing studies and analyzing data to make reasonable inferences about maturational changes, nonmaturational changes, and stability over time. Our experience has been chiefly with the study of psychological variables in human aging, but the logic applies equally to studies of physiological variables and animals. We will discuss briefly some of the more sophisticated techniques for analyzing longitudinal data that have been developed by statisticians and methodologists, and we will conclude with some considerations for the design and implementation of multidisciplinary longitudinal studies.

STABILITY AND CHANGE IN MEAN LEVELS

The simplest question usually asked in studies of aging is, "Does x decline (or increase) with age?" Vital capacity and visual acuity decline with age; reaction time and vascular stiffness increase. These statements refer to populations, not individuals, and they are usually answered by an examination of mean levels in individuals of different ages. When different groups of individuals are measured at the same time, the design is *cross-sectional*; when the same individuals are measured at different ages, the design is *longitudinal*. Other designs are possible: different individuals can be measured at different times to control the effects of repeated measurement or to assess the effects of secular trends, such as the changing American diet.

Figure 2.1 summarizes some basic designs. In this example, three independent groups are examined—two with members born in 1930 and one with members born in 1950. A comparison of mean scores from Test A with scores from Test B is a longitudinal design; comparison of Test B and Test C scores with Test D scores is the familiar cross-sectional design. A comparison of Test A with Test C scores is called a *cross-sequential* analysis, and a comparison of Test A with Test D is a *time-sequential* analysis.

Cross-Sectional Designs

By far the most common design in aging research is cross-sectional. Organisms of different ages are compared in terms of a single parameter using analysis of variance. Cross-sectional designs are shortcuts that sometimes tell us what would happen if we had the time and patience to conduct longitudinal research. They are based on the premises that (*1*) the individuals compared are in fact comparable and (*2*) age changes in the future will mirror those of the past. In many cases these assumptions are plausible. Laboratory animals of a con-

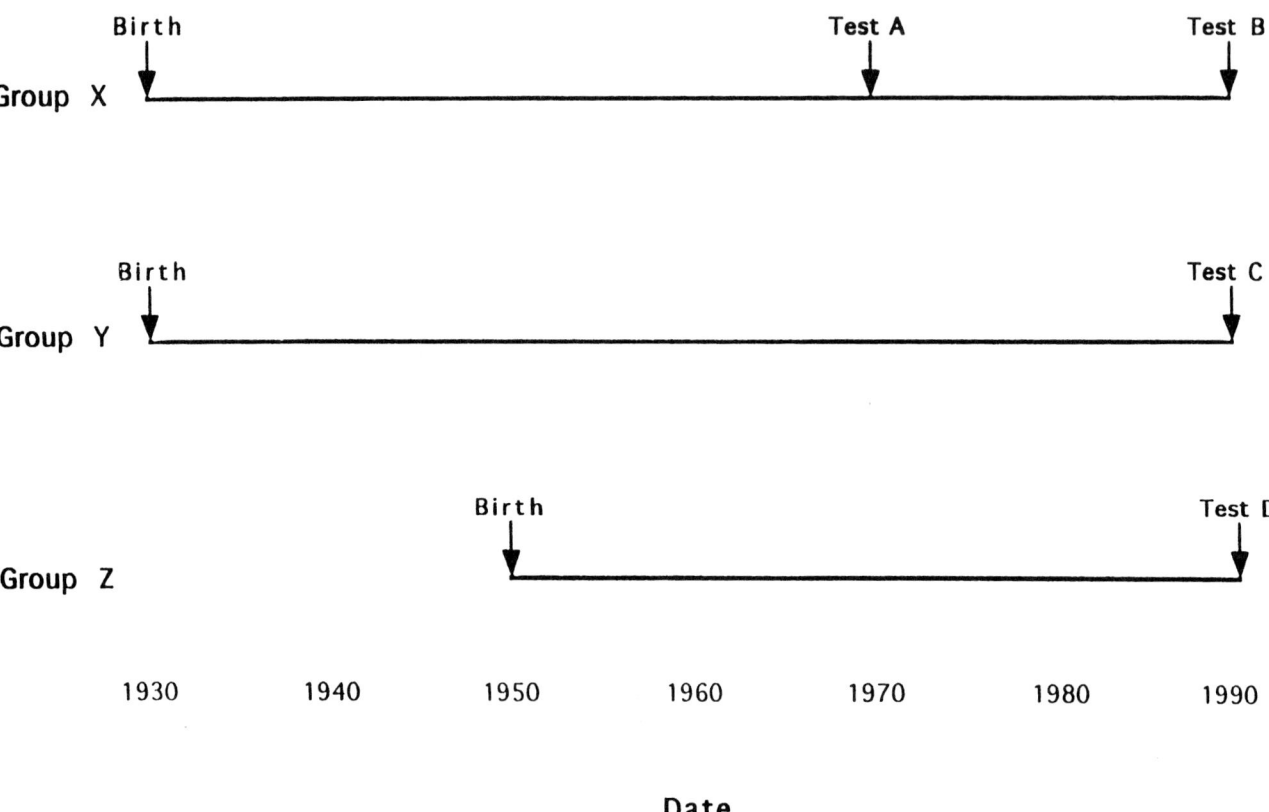

FIG. 2.1. Illustration of alternative designs for the examination of mean level stability or change.

stant strain raised in standard conditions are well suited to cross-sectional comparisons.

Human beings, by contrast, pose many challenges to the assumptions implicit in cross-sectional research. When college students are compared with nursing home residents, age differences are confounded with differences in education and health status. When 60-year-olds are compared with 90-year-olds, aging is confounded with selective mortality. It is certainly possible to conduct meaningful cross-sectional studies of human subjects, but a great deal of thought must be given to making the groups comparable for all relevant variables except age. A group of healthy college alumni in their 70s would make a better comparison group for college students than a group of nursing home residents. Where a strict case-control matching strategy is not feasible, potentially confounding variables can be measured and used as covariates.

These refinements of simple cross-sectional comparisons never resolve all potential problems. A college degree obtained in 1920 may not be fully comparable to the same degree obtained in 1990. Key covariates may be overlooked even by a careful researcher. And without the aid of a crystal ball, how can young subjects who are fated to die prematurely be screened out to match older subjects already selected for longevity? For reasons such as these, longitudinal studies have long been considered a necessity in studies of human aging.

Longitudinal Designs

In longitudinal designs change is measured directly in the same group of subjects. Each individual is his or her own control, so any differences between the first and second measurements cannot be attributed to effects of time and place of birth, early life experiences, or innate individual differences. If reliable and valid measures are used, the observed difference between Time 2 and Time 1 values on the variable in question are direct assessments of change.

But is change necessarily the result of aging? Clearly not. Any number of variables other than intrinsic aging processes may be the cause of observed changes. In particular, studies of human aging must take into account the effects of the particular historical era in which they are conducted. Helson (33) showed that women became more psychologically independent from college age to middle adulthood during the period from the 1960s to the 1990s. Their mothers, however, who matured in a more conservative era, did not show this effect. Physiological examples of such secular effects would be expected because of historical changes in diet and exercise, other life-style variables, and medical practice. The most dramatic example is the extension of the human life span in the twentieth century.

Advances in measurement technology can also complicate the interpretation of longitudinal data. When more sensitive diagnostic procedures are used, more instances of disease will be discovered even if the true prevalence of the disease has not changed. Longitudinal researchers must often choose between continuing standard but outdated instruments and introducing improved measures. When a new measure is introduced, it is often wise to allow a period of calibration in which both old and new measures are employed on the same subjects. A comparison of results allows an estimation of the effects attributable to measurement technology.

Another potential confound in longitudinal studies is the effect of measurement itself on subjects and their behavior. In cognitive testing, individuals typically perform a bit better on the second administration of a test. Without taking into account this practice effect, longitudinal studies of cognitive development may underestimate the magnitude of decline. The use of parallel forms—different versions of the test—is a partial solution, although the mere experience of taking a test tends to have some effect on future test performance. A familiar instance of measurement effects is seen in longitudinal studies of blood pressure, which typically show higher levels on the first measurement because the unfamiliar experience is stressful (35).

Cross-Sequential Designs

The most extreme example of a measurement effect is a study of animal aging that employs invasive measures that require that the animal be killed. Longitudinal measurement is impossible here, but there is an alternative to cross-sectional studies that may be useful in some cases—the cross-sequential design with independent samples (47). In this design, individuals born at the same time are compared at different times. A group of young animals might be randomly divided into two groups—one measured at Time 1, the other allowed to live until measurement at Time 2. The mean difference would estimate the changes over time in the full sample.

Cross-sequential designs are infrequently used, although they have many possible applications in aging research, particularly in humans. Suppose, for example, that a study of glucose tolerance had been conducted on a group of 40-year-olds in 1965. If the same measurements were taken on a comparable group of 70-year-olds in 1995, mean differences would estimate age changes. Thus, a quasi-longitudinal study can be conducted even when the original subjects can no longer be located. When the original subjects can be retested, cross-sequential designs that examine a supplemental sample at Time 2 form a valuable basis for replication. If effects seen in the longitudinal analysis are not found in the cross-sequential analysis, a practice effect may be suspected.

Like longitudinal designs, cross-sequential designs confound true aging changes with historical changes in the period of study. There are other designs (that is, time-sequential; see 47) that are intended to deconfound these, but they themselves are confounded in other ways. After a number of ingenious attempts, it has become clear that no research design and no method of analysis can unequivocally demonstrate the existence of aging effects (1, 17). Time of birth, age at measurement, and time of measurement are mathematically linked and can never be unconfounded. As a result, any effect that might be attributed to any one of those factors can be equally well explained by combinations of the other two.

This does not mean that research on aging is impossible. It does, however, mean that scientific judgment is needed in assessing the evidence. Every scientific explanation faces rival hypotheses, but some are more plausible than others. The most convincing evidence of true age effects comes from a replicated and reasonable pattern of evidence. If cross-sectional age differences point in the same direction as longitudinal changes, and if the latter are replicated by cross-sequential results, then aging may represent the most parsimonious explanation. If the results are consistent with theories of aging, so much the better.

Demonstrating Stability of Mean Levels

Not all variables show age changes, and the demonstration of stability may be as important as the discovery of change. This is particularly true in areas in which changes are expected. Age stereotypes suggest that older men and women are particularly prone to depression, but epidemiological and longitudinal studies dispute this (7, 25). Rodeheffer et al. (44) have shown no decline in cardiac output in healthy aging men, despite the increasing incidence of coronary heart disease in older men in general.

Demonstrating stability, however, is statistically problematic. When no significant differences are found, flaws in the design or limitations of sample size are plausible explanations, and it is difficult to publish null results in many professional journals. The use of careful controls and large samples can blunt these criticisms. In addition, it is useful to compute and report a confidence interval around the estimate of change (55) to show the estimated upper boundary for change. For example, after finding no consistent evidence of age changes in the scales of the NEO Personality Inventory, Costa and McCrae (21, p. 860) concluded that "if there are maturational changes in personality, they are likely to account for a change of less than one standard deviation during the full course of adult life."

Elaborations of the Basic Design

The discussion so far has concerned the simple case of young vs. old, or Time 1 vs. Time 2. In practice, most designs are more complex. Several different age groups may be examined in cross-sectional analyses, and several different time points may be measured in longitudinal designs. Many longitudinal studies (such as the Baltimore Longitudinal Study of Aging, or BLSA; 51) incorporate cross-sectional designs by following several different age cohorts simultaneously. These designs are capable of providing very detailed information. Age changes are rarely linear; different variables show age effects at different times, and they often show accelerated change in old age. Such patterns can only be detected by measuring the variable at several points in the life span.

One practical question in the design of longitudinal studies concerns the measurement interval. If the interval is too long, the true pattern of change may be missed; conversely, too frequent measurements are costly in terms of investigator expense and imposition on research subjects. Cross-sectional studies covering a wide age range can provide some guidance by suggesting the rates of change and the portions of the life span in which most change occurs. In effect, cross-sectional studies can be seen as a source of hypotheses about age changes to be tested in longitudinal designs.

In many studies the question concerns not simply the existence or extent of age-related changes, but the underlying mechanisms. These can be studied experimentally by manipulating environmental conditions or drug treatments; they can also be studied in quasi-experimental designs (11) by comparing age changes in different groups (for example, men and women, blacks and whites, smokers and nonsmokers). There are many analytical techniques that can be applied to such data. Significant Time X Condition interaction terms in repeated measures analyses of variance (38) indicate differential aging processes; in analyses of continuous data, rates of change can be estimated by regression analyses within condition, and differences between betas can be statistically tested (12).

Representativeness and Attrition in Longitudinal Studies

No study that relies on volunteers is likely to be truly representative of the general population, because people who decline to participate will probably be systematically different from the participants. This problem is compounded when long-term longitudinal studies are conducted: fewer people will commit themselves to such a study, and some attrition is bound to occur with the passage of time.

Different strategies have been adopted by the major longitudinal studies with regard to initial representativeness and potential attrition. The Berkeley Guidance Study (40) was designed to be fully representative of the community by recruiting every third baby born in Berkeley, California, during an 18-month interval. At the other extreme, the BLSA relied on a "snowball" technique in which the original, highly educated volunteers asked their friends and family members to join, and they in turn asked more people. The Normative Aging Study (6) selected participants on the basis of geographical and occupational stability to ensure minimum attrition.

The degree of importance of sample representativeness depends in part on the variables studied. BLSA participants have historically been quite unrepresentative with respect to education, but comparisons with a national sample showed that they were very similar with respect to major dimensions of personality (26), and the same conclusions about the stability of personality have been reached by researchers using representative (53) and nonrepresentative (21) samples. Goudy (31), in an analysis of the effects of attrition in a retirement study, concluded that attrition in longitudinal studies may be a less serious source of bias than is often suggested.

Certainly, concerns about representativeness should not discourage researchers from undertaking longitudinal studies. The effects of attrition can be examined by comparing those remaining in the study with dropouts on initial status; if the differences are small, then it is likely that the effects of attrition are minor. Similarly, separate analyses can be conducted in subsamples to test the potential effects of variables for which the sample is unrepresentative. The BLSA sample as a whole is much better educated than the general population, but there is still a range of education; if less-well-educated BLSA participants do not differ from better-educated participants in the rate of change of the variable of interest, then the sample as a whole probably does not differ from the general population.

Screening for Clinical Conditions

If the object of a study is to examine change in a variable due to aging per se, it would seem reasonable to exclude individuals in whom change might more plausibly be attributed to other causes, specifically disease. However, a number of diseases increase in frequency with age, and many normative age changes (such as increasing glucose intolerance) are indistinguishable from preclinical manifestations of certain diseases (such as diabetes). Thus, when elderly men and women with any disease are excluded from a study, the remaining sample is not so much normal as supernormal and thus is hardly representative of the population in general.

There is no universally satisfactory solution to this problem. It makes no sense to tally dental caries in people who have lost all their teeth, so they would have to be excluded from a study of age and tooth decay. There may also be some justification for excluding patients with coronary artery disease from a study of aging and pulmonary function, but there is probably no good a priori reason to exclude them from a study of aging and depth perception. Researchers must make reasonable exclusions, but they should not reflexively exclude subjects from a study of normal aging merely because they have a clinically significant disease.

In many cases, the wisest course is to analyze and report results with and without relevant clinical exclusions. The findings might be interpreted as estimates of the lower and upper bounds, respectively, of true aging effects.

STABILITY AND CHANGE IN INDIVIDUAL DIFFERENCES

All variables studied by gerontologists show individual differences to some degree. Individuals of the same age differ among themselves because of constitutional factors, life experiences, health status, and a host of other factors. These individual differences themselves may be highly variable (state-like) or relatively stable (trait-like). Body weight, for example, can show substantial fluctuations over the period of a decade, whereas height is more nearly constant; psychological well-being is less stable than personality traits like extraversion.

Stability in individual differences is usually expressed in terms of a correlation coefficient between scores at Time 1 and Time 2; the higher the correlation, the more predictable Time 2 standing is from Time 1 standing (see 37 for a fuller treatment). It should be noted that correlations are sensitive to the rank ordering of individuals but not to absolute levels. It is thus possible (and not uncommon) to find stability in rank ordering and change in mean levels for the same variable. Height decreases in old age with the settling of the vertebral column, but most tall people remain tall relative to their age peers.

Conversely, for some variables it is possible to find stability in mean levels with no stability in individual differences. This can occur if some people increase while others decrease on the variable. How happy or sad one is on a given day is likely to be a poor predictor of how happy one will be twenty years later, but the average mood of a group of people may be quite stable over that interval.

In fact, knowledge about stability or change in mean levels tells us nothing whatever about the stability of individual differences, and cross-sectional and cross-sequential studies, which are quite useful in identifying mean level changes, give no clues about rank-order stability. To know if an individual changes in comparison to age peers, we must have data from two different time periods on the same group of individuals. In the case of human beings, the retrospective study provides a shortcut: we ask the individuals how they were years ago and compare it to present standing. But retrospective studies are subject to many biases and lapses of memory (32, 57), and they are impossible in studies of animals. To answer questions about rank-order stability, longitudinal studies are indispensable.

Perhaps because longitudinal studies are relatively rare, gerontologists have paid less attention to the course of individual differences than to changes in mean levels. Even when longitudinal data are available, rank-order stability is often ignored. For example, Borkan and Norris (9) describe careful longitudinal analyses of fat distribution in adult males but neglect to report the stability of individual differences. The same is true of a study of serum cholesterol conducted by Hershcopf et al. (34).

One reason for this neglect may be the confusion of rank-order stability with reliability. When a test is administered twice over a two-week period, the correlation between the scores is usually (and correctly) interpreted as retest reliability, an indication of how well the test procedure yields reproducible results. The same correlation, however, between tests administered ten years apart has a very different interpretation, because it is influenced not only by properties of the test and conditions of test administration but also by changes in the underlying variable over the time interval. Reliability is always an important concern in measurement and doubly so in longitudinal studies where unreliability can vitiate both predictors and criteria. But a researcher who is confident that the methods being applied yield highly reproducible findings ought not to assume that retest correlations will be high if the retest interval is substantial. This is an empirical question of great interest and one of the chief reasons for conducting longitudinal studies.

Individual differences in many biological variables (for example, handedness, eye color, height) are very stable, and researchers sometimes assume that this is true of all biological variables, provided that they are reliably assessed. Studies of risk factors that assess predictors at a single point in time implicitly make this assumption, but it is a questionable assumption and one that is sometimes flatly incorrect. For example, hostility, as measured by the Cook-Medley Hostility Scale, has been associated with higher rates of coronary artery disease and death (5), and many researchers have assumed that chronic hostility over a period of many years contributes to the disease. Yet hostility scores in college students are only modestly predictive of hostility scores twenty years later ($r = 0.39$) (54). Perhaps stronger associations would be found if hostility were initially measured at a later age, when personality is fully developed (42); or perhaps what matters is some critical event that occurs during adolescence. In either case, it should be clear that relative standing on variables can change across the life span and that predictive associations cannot be understood fully without an appreciation of the stability or instability of individual differences. Longitudinal researchers should routinely report both short-term retest reliability and longitudinal stability of their variables.

For many biologists, individual differences are regarded merely as a source of error, to be minimized (if not eliminated) by breeding pure strains and maintaining a constant environment. Those who are interested in human aging, however, cannot avoid individual differences and should not disregard them. We know that personality traits are highly stable. The 40-year-old extravert is likely to become an 80-year-old extravert, still seeking many and varied social contacts, and that fact may be crucial in planning a successful retirement. How stable are individual differences in glucose tolerance, immune functioning, and muscle mass? Surely that knowledge would be useful in planning a healthy old age.

Potential Problems in the Measurement of Rank-Order Stability

Because stability coefficients can only be calculated from longitudinal data, the methodological problems uniquely posed by cross-sectional designs are moot. This does not mean that there are no potential problems in the measurement of rank-order stability. One issue is representativeness. Individuals who volunteer for and remain in a longitudinal study may systematically differ from others, not only in the mean level of a variable but also in its cross-time stability. For example, longitudinal participants may drop out of a study when their health declines, and the same declines in health may alter their standing on many variables of interest. Stability estimates from the remaining, healthy part of the sample may be exaggerated and therefore may not generalize well to the population as a whole.

In research using questionnaire data, estimates of stability may be inflated by consistencies in response style. In a study of 201 BLSA men retested on the Cornell Medical Index after intervals of 8–17 years, individual differences in the total number of physical symptoms reported were quite stable ($r = 0.72$) (19). While some people exaggerate their health complaints, others minimize them, and these tendencies are quite persistent over time. Therefore, the stability coefficient may reflect the stability of reporting style more than the stability of objective medical condition, and objective indicators or informant reports may provide a better estimate of the stability of medical symptoms.

Although stability coefficients may sometimes be spuriously inflated, they are almost always systematically attenuated by unreliability of measurement. The short-term reliability of an instrument sets an upper boundary to the observable long-term stability. The stability of the true scores—the retest correlations that would be obtained under conditions of perfect measurement—can be estimated by dividing the observed stability by the retest reliability coefficient. In a 24-year longitudinal study of personality, the observed retest correlation for friendliness was 0.65, and the scale's reliability was 0.84; the estimated true-score 24-year stability was therefore 0.78 (24).

ADVANCED TOPICS IN DESIGN AND ANALYSIS OF AGING STUDIES

The discussion so far has assumed that researchers are concerned with basic descriptive studies of aging: Does the variable increase or decrease as a result of aging processes? Do individuals have a characteristic level of the variable that they retain over time? There are, however, many more sophisticated questions that can be asked, and methodologists have continued to offer new designs and new methods of analysis (see 14, 48 for up-to-date reviews).

Changes in Variance and in Structure

Populations are characterized not only by their means but also by their variances. One of the early and enduring hypotheses of gerontological research has been the idea that variance increases with age, that is, that the range of individual differences becomes more pronounced with increasing age. It may be true as a general rule that health deteriorates with advancing age, but some older people preserve a remarkable level of functioning. As a result, there may be increased variance in standing on health-related variables.

The increasing variance hypothesis makes sense if we assume that most people begin in the normal range of a variable and that changes are due to disease processes that appear in different people at different times. For example, there is little variance in measures of mental status among 60-year-olds, because almost everyone is cognitively intact and receives a near-perfect score. As a few individuals develop dementing disorders, their scores decline and variance increases in the group.

However, it is by no means true that variance increases for all variables with age. Personality scores, for example, show constant variances across the adult life span (41). The variance hypothesis is useful as a reminder that there are important individual differences and that they are usually retained and sometimes increased with age: old people are not all alike. It is also, of course, advisable for any investigator to examine variances as a function of age. Not only is this information intrinsically of interest, it is also relevant to the choice of statistical techniques, which sometimes presuppose equal variances in the groups being compared.

Other questions can be asked about changes in the relations between variables. Two variables that are positively correlated in young individuals may be negatively correlated in older individuals. This possibility can be particularly important when a group of indicators are summed to form an index, on the assumption that they all reflect the same underlying process. Such an index developed on young people might be meaningless when applied to older people, because the indicators no longer have the same functional significance. This problem has been treated extensively in discussions of factorial invariance in psychological data (e.g., 28) and may arise in studies of aging physiology. In general, it is worthwhile to examine relations between variables within age groups as well as across them.

Biomarkers and Functional Age: Flawed Concepts

Researchers studying aging are often frustrated by the fact that they can neither manipulate nor hurry the chronological aging process. If one wishes to test whether a drug treatment or exercise regimen extends the life span, one normally has to wait until the organism dies a natural death. It would be convenient if some intermediate criterion were available which would predict life span and which could be studied over a shorter period of time. The search for such a criterion was one of the reasons that the idea of biomarkers and indices of functional or biological age became popular.

Although there are many variations, all these proposals suggest that the processes of aging can be traced in many different psychological and physiological functions. Differences in standing on age-related variables might be used to estimate the rate at which aging is progressing. A high rate of aging would imply early mortality; interventions which slowed the rate of aging would probably extend the life span.

Attractive as this proposition is, it has turned out to be unrealistic (2). The actual indices suggested have suffered from a variety of statistical confounds (16, 18). The gravest problems are found in cross-sectional studies that estimate rate of aging from relative standing on a set of functions. A 70-year-old man may have the same vital capacity as the average 40-year-old, from which it is (mistakenly) inferred that he has been aging slowly. This inference ignores the fact that there are initial individual differences that are confounded with any change due to aging; it also ignores errors of measurement.

In principle, longitudinal studies could determine the rate of change in a variety of functions, and some proposed indices of biological age would average these rates of change to determine the rate of aging. The basic flaw in this version is that there is no single "rate of aging" (20, 39). Different functions change over time at different rates and for different reasons, and none can be considered a marker of some basic process of aging.

This does not mean that there are no variables that predict mortality, such as cholesterol level, blood pressure, smoking status—we usually call them "risk factors." In many cases, these are legitimate intermediate criteria for intervention studies. If exercise reduces serum cholesterol levels, it may extend life, but it does so because it improves coronary artery functioning, not because it slows some mysterious "rate of aging."

Growth Curves and Age Changes

Once we know that a variable is in general higher (or lower) in older than in younger individuals, we may wish to become more specific. When in the life course does the decline begin? How rapidly does it progress? Is the decline linear or is it accelerated with increasing age (as in the case of visual memory measures; [3])? Such questions are simple elaborations of the issue of stability or change in mean levels and may be answered by a more fine-grained analysis of the same data. For example, a cross-sectional study of divergent thinking abilities (the hypothesized basis of creativity) showed increases to about age 40 and accelerated decline thereafter; longitudinal analyses confirmed this conclusion (43).

That study used curvilinear regression to model the data, but many other functions can also be used. For example, Bock (8) used logistic equations to describe growth in stature among children. Exponential growth might also occur, or cyclic fluctuations might be found. Fitting data to many different curves is relatively straigtforward for a competent statistician; the basic problem lies in collecting appropriate data. More complex curves require more data points, and the timing of data collection should be geared to the expected timing of changes. Complex models may prove less easy to replicate than simpler models; if so, the latter are to be preferred.

These designs consider normative age changes, that is, patterns of change that are common to all individuals. It is possible to compare age curves for different groups (for example, mortality curves for men and women); it is also of considerable interest to be able to predict age changes in individuals: cardiologists would surely like to know which of their patients have rapidly progressing arteriosclerosis; neurologists would like to predict the time course of dementing disorders for their individual patients and their patients' families.

Calculating individual regression slopes for longitudinal data points is one possibility, although the number of data points required for reliable estimates can be formidable (49). One contemporary approach uses hierarchical linear models (10) in which both group and individual changes are examined simultaneously. Such models can incorporate nonlinear as well as linear changes and can compare analyses done in subgroups.

Survival Analysis and the Identification of Risk Factors

The Duke Longitudinal Studies of Aging (52) are among the few in which all participants are followed until death. In most other studies, follow-up ends at an earlier point, and in any case, analyses of the data are usually conducted on an ongoing basis. This presents a problem for the study of risk factors, because at any given time, all the results are not in.

Epidemiologists often analyze such data using survival analysis (see 56 for a lucid presentation of the basic ideas). This approach considers how long individuals "survive" (remain healthy, etc.) under various conditions. For example, smokers and nonsmokers might be compared for mortality experience after 10 years. Even though most individuals, including most smokers, might still be alive, survival analysis could indicate whether 10-year mortality was higher for the smoking group. Like multiple regression, survival analysis can take into account different groups, covariates, and interaction terms (although the robustness of the findings may be questionable when complicated models are fit to a small number of cases). Modifications of the method can take into account different periods of surveillance that might result from late entry into the study or loss to follow-up.

Correlates of Change

Sometimes the topic of interest is not a qualitative endpoint but a quantitative change. Some people show rapid changes ("age rapidly"), whereas others show slower changes ("age slowly"). At first glance, it would appear that a useful way to understand these different rates of change would be to correlate change scores with external variables. For example, we might measure mental status at Time 1 and Time 2, subtract the first score from the second to estimate change, and correlate the change score with, say, vitamin intake.

This seemingly straightforward design has been the object of continuing controversy among methodologists (e.g., 27, 45), because measurement error at both times is confounded with true change. Residual scores, correcting for initial level, have sometimes been recommended as a more suitable measure of change than raw difference scores, but Rogosa (45) argues convincingly against this position as a general prescription.

If the error of measurement is small compared with the magnitude of true changes, then correlation of raw change scores will be meaningful; if the error of measurement is very large, or true change is very small, then no statistical adjustment is likely to make the data meaningful. As a prerequisite to analysis of change scores, some understanding of their reliability is needed.

One approach uses information from the longitudinal stability of the measure. If retest stability is very high—it approaches the short-term retest stability of the measure—and if variance is similar on both occasions, then there can be little individual difference in the rate of true change and the search for correlates is probably useless. Another approach is to gather data from more than two time points in order to assess the consistency of change in individuals. If person X changes twice as much as person Y on each of four occasions, it seems reasonable to conclude that person X really does have a higher rate of change. Rogosa and Willett (46) have suggested that individual growth curves, based on three or more observations, may be used to study correlates of change.

Asendorpf (4) has suggested another possibility. He recommends that the change scores be validated by using two different methods of measuring the variable of interest and calculating change scores for both. Only if the correlation is significant should one proceed to correlations with external variables. One advantage of this strategy is that it encourages researchers to build into their designs multiple measures of the constructs of interest, permitting internal validations of each measure and replications across the different measures.

The discussion so far has been predicted on the assumption that change scores in one variable are to be correlated with an external variable measured at one time. Researchers might also wish to correlate changes in one variable with changes in others. In principle, this approach is possible, but the difficulties of using a single change score are multiplied when two change scores are used. In particular, errors of measurement for the two change variables may be correlated, leading to spurious associations between change scores. This analytical approach is probably best avoided unless both rates of change are estimated from multiple observations.

Causal Inferences from Observational Data

One of the first lessons taught in courses on research methods is that it is hazardous to draw causal inferences from correlational data. The fact that, in a population with a wide age range, vital capacity is correlated with grip strength (36) does not necessarily mean that loss of vital capacity *causes* loss of grip strength. It is conceivable that loss of grip strength leads to reduced exercise and thus to lowered vital capacity. It is quite possible that some third, unmeasured variable or variables (such as exercise or intrinsic aging processes in the musculoskeletal system) produces both effects. It is also possible that the association is artifactual, a reflection of the fact that many body systems independently decline with age.

Some of these alternatives can be examined statistically in cross-sectional data. For example, we can use the technique of partial correlation to see if there is still some association between vital capacity and grip strength after we have controlled statistically for the effects of chronological age: if the partial correlation is nonsignificant, the most parsimonious explanation is that the association is an artifact of age distribution. Such designs eliminate some possibilities, but they are never definitive. We may have overlooked important confounding variables (gender, for instance), or we may not be able to measure adequately the variables we wish to control.

Experimental manipulation with random assignment to treatments is the preferred basis for making causal inferences, but chronological aging cannot be manipulated, and interventions are not always feasible. There are considerable data showing an association between the personality trait of antagonistic hostility and coronary artery disease (5), so reducing levels of antagonism might be expected to reduce coronary artery disease. Unfortunately, no one knows how to reduce antagonism. Other interventions (such as assigning individuals to smoking and nonsmoking groups) are unethical.

For these reasons, prospective longitudinal designs are often of great scientific value, particularly when the question is one of temporal priority. Causes precede effects. If decline in grip strength precedes decline in vital capacity, we know that loss of vital capacity cannot be the cause of loss of grip strength. Evidence that poor emotional and social adjustment precedes adolescent drug use (50) strengthens the argument that those adjustment difficulties are contributing causes.

Strengthens, however, is the operative word here, because longitudinal studies are subject to many of the same ambiguities as cross-sectional studies with regard to causal inference. Unmeasured third variables (or third variables measured at the wrong time; see 13) may still be the true causal agent. This is often overlooked in epidemiological studies, where the fact of a predictive association is often regarded as evidence of a causal relation.

Statisticians and methodologists are currently devoting a great deal of time to the design and analysis of longitudinal studies as the basis of causal inferences; Rogosa (45) provides a valuable reminder of the complexities involved. Just as no combination of cross-sectional, longitudinal, and sequential designs can prove the existence or absence of a maturational change, so no statistical manipulation can turn an observational design into an experimental design. Nevertheless, intelligent statistical analysis of longitudinal data can be very informative, particularly in ruling out some alternative hypotheses.

SOME CONSIDERATIONS FOR THE DESIGN OF LONGITUDINAL STUDIES

Full-scale longitudinal studies, in which large panels are studied frequently over a period of many years on a wide range of variables, are, predictably, rare. They are expensive to begin and maintain, and their pay-off is usually far in the future (sometimes to the benefit of a whole new generation of scientists). Yet longitudinal studies offer many unique research opportunities and, properly designed, are an extremely cost-effective way of conducting research. Any individual or group contemplating a longitudinal study should, of course, review in great detail the designs of previous studies (e.g., 51) to assess their strengths and limitations. Chapter 5 in this volume is also informative. In the following section we offer a few additional suggestions.

Combining Cross-Sectional and Longitudinal Designs

Several classic longitudinal studies have followed a single cohort over time (40). The strengths of this method include control over differences in time of birth and the ability to focus on a single age group and its shaping life experiences. But such pure longitudinal studies also have powerful limitations, including difficulty in generalizing to other cohorts and problems in separating aging from time of measurement effects.

An alternative approach is to follow a sample chosen from a wide age range. Longitudinal changes can be compared with cross-sectional age differences to strengthen conclusions about maturational changes and to assess generalizability across different generations. When the full age range is included in the sample, different topics can be pursued: while one scientist studies menopause, another can trace functional decline in old age. Finally, the availability of different age cohorts means that cross-sectional studies can be carried out at any time as a basis for new hypotheses to be tested longitudinally. Perhaps most compelling, the findings from these studies can be published years before longitudinal analyses are feasible.

Combining Hypothesis-Driven and Exploratory Research

In the early years of longitudinal studies, collecting almost any data was informative. Today, it would seem prudent to design studies first and foremost to test specific hypotheses about aging. These would provide a rationale for the study and would also guide decisions about age range, sample composition, and frequency of measurement. For example, if it is hypothesized that physical activity is a major determinant of rates of aging, then the sample should be selected to include a combination of sedentary, reasonably active, and highly active people. If changes in key variables are expected to be rapid, then the intervals between assessments must be kept short.

However, we have not reached the point in our understanding of the aging process where we can specify with any certainty all the key questions that remain to be answered. The appropriate hedge is to build into the study collection of a variety of data that permit explorations. These should include standard baseline measures that permit comparisons with other longitudinal studies and that cover a wide spectrum. For example, in the area of personality research, longitudinal studies should include measures of the five dimensions of personality traits that are currently thought to summarize most individual differences (23, 29). Basic physiological, psychological, and demographic information should routinely be included, and, wherever possible, blood samples and other body fluid and tissue samples should be collected and stored for future retrospective–prospective analyses.

In addition, however (and as time and resources allow), it is wise to include new and untried variables, solely to see what happens to them with age. Every advance in technology brings with it new variables that established longitudinal researchers wish they had been able to include in their studies years ago. No new study should be begun without a generous sampling of such state-of-the-art variables and measures.

Creative Exploitation of the Data

There are many ways to make longitudinal studies cost-effective. A follow-up study can convert a cross-sectional archive into a longitudinal study (15). Different longitudinal studies can be analyzed together to capitalize on differing samples. Mailed questionnaires can supplement or substitute for in-person visits.

However designed, any longitudinal study will ultimately generate a large archive of data. The best longitudinal investigator is not the one who patiently waits 20 years to test a focused hypothesis but the one who wrings the most possible information out of whatever data are available (22). Much of that information may not even relate to the study of aging but may speak to basic science or address a current research question with data that happen to be available.

Interdisciplinary collaborations, though sometimes made difficult by the different traditions of data analysis in different disciplines, offer intriguing possibilities: we know about relations between exercise and cardiovascular fitness, but what about relations between exercise and, say, dermatological status? Probably no one would fund a grant to find out, but if the data are available it would be a pity not to analyze them. The ultimate payoff from longitudinal studies is a fuller understanding of the aging process, but the costs of longitudinal research can be defrayed in part by good science of any description.

REFERENCES

1. ADAM, J. Sequential strategies and the separation of age, cohort, and time-of-measurement contributions to developmental data. *Psychol. Bull.* 85: 1309–1316, 1978.
2. ADELMAN, R. C. Biomarkers of aging. [Editorial] *Exp. Gerontol.* 22: 227–229, 1987.
3. ARENBERG, D. Differences and changes with age in the Benton Visual Retention Test. *J. Gerontol.* 33: 534–540, 1978.
4. ASENDORPF, J. B. Beyond stability: predicting inter-individual differences in intra-individual change. *Eur. J. Pers.* 6: 103–117, 1992.
5. BAREFOOT, J. C., W. G. DAHLSTROM, and R. B. WILLIAMS, JR. Hostility, CHD incidence and total mortality: a 25-year follow-up study of 255 physicians. *Psychosom. Med.* 45: 59–63, 1983.
6. BELL, B., C. L. ROSE, and A. DAMON. The Normative Aging Study: an interdisciplinary and longitudinal study of health and aging. *Int. J. Aging Hum. Dev.* 3: 5–17, 1972.
7. BLAZER, D. The epidemiology of depression in late life. *J. Geriatr. Psychiatry* 22: 35–52, 1989.
8. BOCK, R. D. Prediction of growth. In: *Best Methods for the Analysis of Change,* edited by L. M. Collins and J. L. Horn. Washington, DC: American Psychological Association, 1991, p 126–136.
9. BORKAN, G. A., and A. H. NORRIS. Fat redistribution and the changing body dimensions of the adult male. *Hum. Biol.* 49: 495–514, 1977.
10. BRYK, A. S., and S. W. RAUDENBUSH. *Hierarchical Linear Models: Applications and Data Analysis Methods.* Newbury Park, CA: Sage, 1992.
11. CAMPBELL, D. T., and J. C. STANLEY. *Experimental and Quasi-experimental Designs for Research.* Chicago: Rand McNally, 1963.
12. COHEN, J., and P. COHEN. *Applied Multiple Regression/Correlation Analysis for the Behavioral Sciences.* Hillsdale, NJ: Erlbaum, 1975.
13. COHEN, P. A. source of bias in longitudinal investigations of change. In: *Best Methods for the Analysis of Change,* edited by L. M. Collins and J. L. Horn. Washington, DC: American Psychological Association, 1991, p. 18–25.
14. COLLINS, L. M., and J. L. HORN (Editors) *Best Methods for the Analysis of Change.* Washington, DC: American Psychological Association, 1991.
15. CORNONI-HUNTLEY, J., H. E. BARBANO, J. A. BRODY, B. COHEN, J. J. FELDMAN, J. C. KLEINMAN, and J. MADANS. National Health

and Nutrition Examination I—Epidemiologic followup survey. *Public Health Rep.* 98: 245–251, 1983.
16. COSTA, P. T., JR., and R. R. MCCRAE. Functional age: a conceptual and empirical critique. In: *Second Conference on the Epidemiology of Aging* (NIH Publ. No. 80–969), edited by S. G. Haynes and M. Feinlieb. Washington, DC: U. S. Government Printing Office, 1980, p. 23–46.
17. COSTA, P. T., JR., and R. R. MCCRAE. An approach to the attribution of age, period, and cohort effects. *Psychol. Bull.* 92: 238–250, 1982.
18. COSTA, P. T., JR., and R. R. MCCRAE. Concepts of functional or biological age: a critical view. In: *Principles of Geriatric Medicine,* edited by R. Andres, E. Bierman, and W. Hazzard. New York: McGraw-Hill, 1985a, p. 30–37.
19. COSTA, P. T., JR., and R. R. MCCRAE. Hypochondriasis, neuroticism, and aging: when are somatic complaints unfounded? *Am. Psychol.* 40: 19–28, 1985b.
20. COSTA, P. T., JR., and R. R. MCCRAE. Measures and markers of biological aging: "a great clamoring . . . of fleeting significance." *Arch. Gerontol. Geriatr.* 7: 211–214, 1988a.
21. COSTA, P. T., JR., and R. R. MCCRAE. Personality in adulthood: a six-year longitudinal study of self-reports and spouse ratings on the NEO Personality Inventory. *J. Pers. Soc. Psychol.* 54: 853–863, 1988b.
22. COSTA, P. T., JR., and R. R. MCCRAE. Multiple uses for longitudinal personality data. *Eur. J. Pers.* 6: 85–102, 1992a.
23. COSTA, P. T., Jr., and R. R. MCCRAE. *The Revised NEO Personality Inventory (NEO-PI-R) and NEO Five-Factor Inventory (NEO-FFI) Professional Manual.* Odessa, FL: Psychological Assessment Resources, 1992b.
24. COSTA, P. T., JR, and R. R. MCCRAE. Trait psychology comes of age. In: *Nebraska Symposium on Motivation: Psychology and Aging,* edited by T. B. Sonderegger. Lincoln: University of Nebraska Press, 1992c, p. 169–204.
25. COSTA, P. T., JR., and R. R. MCCRAE. Depression as an enduring disposition. In: *Diagnosis and treatment of depression in late life: Results of the NIH Consensus Development Conference,* edited by B. D. Lebowitz, C. F. Reynolds, III, L. S. Schneider, and A. J. Friedhoff. Washington, DC: American Psychiatric Press, 1994, p. 155–167.
26. COSTA, P. T., Jr., R. R. MCCRAE, A. B. ZONDERMAN, H. E. BARBANO, B. LEBOWITZ, and D. M. LARSON. Cross-sectional studies of personality in a national sample: 2. Stability in neuroticism, extraversion, and openness. *Psychol. Aging* 1: 144–149, 1986.
27. CRONBACH, L. J., and L. FURBY. How should we measure "change"—or should we? *Psychol. Bull.* 74: 68–80, 1970.
28. CUNNINGHAM, W. R. Issues in factorial invariance. In: *Best Methods for the Analysis of Change,* edited by L. M. Collins and J. L. Horn. Washington, DC: American Psychological Association, 1991, p. 106–113.
29. DIGMAN, J. M. Personality structure: emergence of the five-factor model. *Annu. Rev. Psychol.* 41: 417–440, 1990.
30. FINCH, C. E. *Longevity, Senescence and the Genome.* Chicago: University of Chicago Press, 1990.
31. GOUDY, W. J. Effects of sample attrition and data analysis in the retirement history study. *Exp. Aging Res.* 11: 161–167, 1985.
32. HALVERSON, C. F., JR. Remembering your parents: reflections on the retrospective method. *J. Pers.* 56: 435–443, 1988.
33. HELSON, R. Comparing longitudinal studies of adult development: toward a paradigm of tension between stability and change. In: *Studying Lives Through Time,* edited by D. Funder, R. Parke, C. Tomlinson-Keasey, and R. Widaman. Washington, DC: American Psychological Association, 1993, p. 93–119.
34. HERSHCOPF, R. J., D. ELAHI, R. ANDRES, H. L. BALDWIN, G. W. RAIZES, D. D. SCHOCKEN, and J. D. TOBIN. Longitudinal changes in serum cholesterol in man: an epidemiologic search for an etiology. *J. Chronic Dis.* 35: 101–114, 1982.
35. KANNEL, W. B., and T. GORDON (Editors). *The Framingham Study: An Epidemiological Investigation of Cardiovascular Disease.* Washington, DC: Department of Health, Education, and Welfare, 1968–1974.
36. KANNEL, W. B., and H. HUBERT. Vital capacity as a biomarker of aging. In: *Biomarkers Conference.* Bethesda, MD: National Institute on Aging, 1982, p. 145–160.
37. KENNY, D. A., and D. T. CAMPBELL. On the measurement of stability in over-time data. *J. Pers.* 57: 445–481, 1989.
38. KEPPEL, G. *Design and Analysis: A Researcher's Handbook* (2nd ed.). Englewood Cliffs, NJ: Prentice-Hall, 1982.
39. LUDWIG, F. C., and M. E. SMOKE. The measurement of biological age. *Exp. Aging Res.* 6: 497–522, 1980.
40. MACFARLANE, J. W. Studies in child guidance. I. Methodology of data collection and organization. *Monogr. Soc. Res. Child Dev.* 3(No. 6, whole No. 19), 1938.
41. MCCRAE, R. R. Curiouser and curiouser! Modifications to a paradoxical theory of personality coherence. *Psychol. Inquiry* 4: 300–303, 1993.
42. MCCRAE, R. R., and P. T. COSTA, JR. *Personality in Adulthood.* New York: Guilford, 1990.
43. MCCRAE, R. R., D. ARENBERG, and P. T. COSTA, JR. Declines in divergent thinking with age: Cross-sectional, longitudinal, and cross-sequential analyses. *Psychol. Aging* 2: 130–137, 1987.
44. RODEHEFFER, R., G. GERSTENBLITH, L. C. BECKER, J. L. FLEG, M. L. WEISFELDT, and E. G. LAKATTA. Exercise cardiac output is maintained with advancing age in healthy human subjects: cardiac dilatation and increased stroke volume compensate for a diminished heart rate. *Circulation* 69: 203–213, 1984.
45. ROGOSA, D. Myths about longitudinal research. In: *Methodological Issues in Aging Research,* edited by K. W. Schaie, R. T. Campbell, W. Meredith, and S. C. Rawlings. New York: Springer, 1988, p. 171–209.
46. ROGOSA, D., and J. B. WILLET. Understanding correlates of change by modeling individual differences in growth. *Psychometrika* 50: 203–228, 1985.
47. SCHAIE, K. W. Quasi-experimental research designs in the psychology of aging. In: *Handbook of the Psychology of Aging* (1st ed.), edited by J. E. Birren and K. W. Schaie. New York: Van Nostrand Reinhold, 1977, p. 39–69.
48. SCHAIE, K. W., R. T. CAMPBELL, W. MEREDITH, and S. C. RAWLINGS (Editors) *Methodological Issues in Aging Research.* New York: Springer, 1988.
49. SCHLESSELMAN, J. J. Planning a longitudinal study. II. Frequency of measurement and study duration. *J. Chronic Dis.* 26: 561–570, 1973.
50. SHEDLER, J., and J. BLOCK. Adolescent drug use and psychological health: a longitudinal inquiry. *Am. Psychol.* 45: 612–630, 1990.
51. SHOCK, N. W., R. C. GREULICH, R. ANDRES, D. ARENBERG, P. T. COSTA, JR., E. G. LAKATTA, and J. D. TOBIN. *Normal Human Aging: The Baltimore Longitudinal Study of Aging* (NIH Publ. No. 84-2450). Washington, DC: National Institutes of Health, 1984.
52. SIEGLER, I. C. Psychological aspects of the Duke Longitudinal Studies. In: *Longitudinal Studies of Adult Psychological Development,* edited by K. W. Schaie. New York: Guilford, 1983, p. 136–190.
53. SIEGLER, I. C., L. K. GEORGE, and M. A. OKUN. Cross-sequential analysis of adult personality. *Dev. Psychol.* 15: 350–351, 1979.
54. SIEGLER, I. C., A. B. ZONDERMAN, J. C. BAREFOOT, R. B. WILLIAMS, JR., P. T. COSTA, JR., and R. R. MCCRAE. Predicting personality in adulthood from college MMPI scores: implications for follow-up studies in psychosomatic medicine. *Psychosom. Med.* 52: 644–652, 1990.

55. SUSSKIND, E. C., and E. W. HOWLAND. Measuring effect magnitudes in repeated measures ANOVA designs: implications for gerontological research. *J. Gerontol.* 35: 867–876, 1980.
56. WILLET, J. B., and J. D. SINGER. How long did it take? Using survival analysis in educational and psychological research. In: *Best Methods for the Analysis of Change,* edited by L. M. Collins and J. L. Horn. Washington, DC: American Psychological Association, 1991, p. 310–327.
57. WOODRUFF, D. S., and J. E. BIRREN. Age changes and cohort differences in personality. *Dev. Psychol.* 6: 252–259.

3. Animal models

RICHARD WEINDRUCH | Department of Medicine, University of Wisconsin and Veterans Administration—Geriatric Research Education and Clinical Center, Madison, Wisconsin

CHAPTER CONTENTS

Selection of an Appropriate Animal Model
    Animal models and the main ways of studying aging
    Defined longevity characteristics
    Awareness of late-life disease patterns
    Defined environmental conditions
        Diet
        Housing, husbandry, and microbial status
        Exercise
    Genetic characteristics
    Availability and cost
Patterns of Animal Use in Aging Studies
    Animal use in aging research, 1972–1992
    Overuse of the male Fischer 344 rat
Need for the Use of a Wide Spectrum of Models
    Lessons from nonmammals
    Rodents
    Carnivores
    Nonhuman primates
Summary and Conclusions

IN RESEARCH ON THE BIOLOGY OF AGING, although many investigators focus on the in vitro senescence of cell lines (see Chapter 4), the larger share of experiments use animal models to ask relevant questions about organisms at various ages. This chapter addresses the selection and use of animal models for the study of aging and provides investigators new to gerontology with key concepts such as the importance of using models with well-defined longevity characteristics and being keenly aware of the health status of the old animals being studied. In that process, common pitfalls that have made it difficult to interpret certain gerontological data are identified and discussed.

Because the main goal of most gerontologists is to learn from experiments how to improve the quality or increase the duration of human life, animals provide the investigator with a living model so that questions may be asked which cannot be asked of humans due to ethical, technical, economic, or other concerns. Not surprisingly, a great diversity of animals ranging in complexity from protozoans to nonhuman primates have been studied. Obviously, there is not a single best (or two best) animal model in which to study aging processes; instead, there is a diversity of possibilities from among which researchers need to make wise choices. Unfortunately, this great diversity has been underutilized in aging research, and a very large percentage (~75%) of studies on the biology of aging have used either mice or rats. As a result of this "rodent dominance" of the field and of my own experience, the emphasis here is on rodent models. It is, however, likely that much could be learned about basic aging processes in humans by studying animals other than rodents, and the development and use of a broad range of experimental models, is strongly encouraged.

Certain animal models have been used preferentially to study particular aspects of aging. Because mice are the preferred model in immunology, for example, they are used most often by immunogerontologists. For biochemical and physiological studies, rats are used more frequently than mice because of their greater size (and consequently higher tissue yields) and the ease of making physiological measurements. A third example concerns other simpler but genetically well-defined animals, such as *Drosophila melanogaster* and *Cenorhabditis elegans*, that provide elegant systems for investigating genetic influences on the rate of aging. These examples of preferential usage reflect a normal extension of the existing knowledge base. One might question whether important opportunities are being missed by the continued study of specific topics in the same models.

Several excellent reviews (for example, refs. 15, 20, 35, 36) have been published on animal models of aging. Table 3.1 provides an overview of these articles. Because of space limitations, no attempt is made here to review comprehensively either of the extent to which these many animal models are used in research or the advantages and shortcomings inherent in their use. Instead, the goal is to provide the readers with practical information about animal models that is complementary to published research and that will help them conduct and interpret biological research on aging. Areas of controversy are also addressed. Four main questions are considered in this chapter: *(1)* What are some of the critical elements that require careful consideration when selecting an animal model for aging studies? *(2)* In view

TABLE 3.1. *Recommended Review Articles on Animal Models for Aging Research*

Topic	Main Message	Reference
Models for genetic analysis of mechanisms of aging	Focuses on nonmammalian models and argues that genetic studies of aging are far too uncommon in organisms such as *C. elegans* and *D. melanogaster*, which are well suited for such analyses.	35
Mammalian models in aging research	A broad spectrum of animal models should be used to investigate the primary aging processes; however, there are several criteria (for example, known life table, free of infectious diseases, reasonably short life span, available at reasonable cost), which should be met for a model to be suitable for aging research.	11, 36
Alternative animal models for research on aging	There is great value to studying aging in diverse animal models. This summary of an NIA workshop discusses current knowledge about many species which have not been widely studied from the standpoint of aging but may provide important opportunities to facilitate the discovery of primary aging processes.	20, 32
New models to study the biology of senescence	"Species comparisons across many levels of biological organization involving the life histories of many species besides the usual few mammals, insects and nematodes importantly expand the view of mechanisms which limit life spans."	15

of the robust effects of dietary restriction on aging and diseases (see Chapter 23), should ad libitum feeding be abandoned as the standard way to feed animals? *(3)* What has the pattern of use of animal models been in aging research? *(4)* What are the advantages of using a wide variety of animal models in aging research?

SELECTION OF AN APPROPRIATE ANIMAL MODEL

The selection of a suitable animal model is clearly an important initial decision that powerfully shapes the course of the research being considered. Perhaps even more significant is the fact that such decisions can have very long-term ramifications for the investigator, who may continue to study a particular model for many years. Prominent examples of this include the work of Johnson on the genetic basis of longevity determination in the nematode *C. elegans* (27), Lints's studies of genetic and other aspects of aging in *D. melanogaster* (33), and the research on the influences of dietary restriction in male Fischer 344 rats carried out by Masoro and co-workers (39).

Animal Models and the Main Ways of Studying Aging

Several experimental approaches to the investigation of biological aging are possible. A listing of such approaches (Table 3.2) shows that animal models have been a component of much of the research that biogerontologists have pursued. The most common type of biological aging study involves the characterization of the influence of normal aging on measures thought of either as producing biosenescence or as being key consequences of aging processes. The design is most commonly cross-sectional, and animals of two ages (young vs. old), or preferably of more than two ages (young, middle-aged, old, and very old), are compared. Longitudinal studies are also done to characterize the influence of aging. (For a discussion of issues pertaining to experimental design, see Chapter 2.) As discussed later, under (Awareness of Late-Life Disease Patterns), studies of this and other types are commonly flawed by the investigators' failure to address a chronic concern in aging work: the health status of the older animals. Were the changes observed in the older animals a result of age or of a disease process associated with aging? The most meaningful comparisons in gerontology are those made among healthy animals varying in age.

Another significant type of aging study employs animals or data which have already been published on them and examines the basis of differences in longevity among species. In these studies, data are not typically gathered from animals differing in age. Sacher (46), employed this approach quite successfully, utilizing published data on 215 mammalian species for life span (L, in years), adult brain weight (E, in grams), adult body weight (S, in grams), specific metabolic rate (M, in watts/g body weight), deep body temperature (T_b, in

TABLE 3.2. *Ways to Explore the Biology of Aging Utilizing Experimental Animals*

Changes with normal aging in morphology, function, etc.

Causes of differences in longevity among species

Causes of differences in longevity within a species (for example, among congenic and transgenic strains, gender-associated)

Models of accelerated aging (for example, Senescence Accelerated Mouse, thymectomy, irradiation)

Models of decelerated aging (for example, dietary restriction, deprenyl treatment)

°C), and other parameters. He further analyzed these data and discovered that L was related to the other four variables as follows:

$$\log L = 0.62 \log E - 0.41 \log S - 0.52 \log M + 0.026T + 0.90$$

Sacher interpreted this to mean that species life span was related to two main factors. First, there is a cephalization factor (roughly related to the amount of body weight comprised of brain weight), which is positively related to L. Second, there is a metabolic factor such that species L is inversely related to M. Also described was a weaker and surprisingly positive correlation between L and T_b.

Although this interspecies approach can only provide correlative data, it has been constructively employed. A classic example is the study by Hart and Setlow (18), which demonstrated a positive correlation between DNA repair capacity in UV-irradiated fibroblasts and the life span of the species from which the cells were derived. Another example is Cutler's work (12) on the relationships between species life span and antioxidants.

A third type of aging study uncovers the sources of differences in longevity within a species. A good example of this approach is an investigation by Smith and Walford (49), which determined the longevity of mouse strains congenic at the main histocompatibility complex (known as the H-2 locus in mice). A total of 14 mouse strains were used in this experiment. Seven of these were congenic on the C57BL/10 background, four on the A strain background, and three on C3H. Many differences were observed in both average and maximum life span among the H-2 congenic strains within each of the three backgrounds. This study provided evidence that the main histocompatibility complex and genes linked thereto are some of the gene systems involved in controlling the rate of aging. This link has led to more recent studies to clarify the basis of these correlations.

A fourth way of studying aging uses animal models of accelerated aging. A main advantage of these models is that one can produce old animals in a shorter periods of time than usual and, therefore, generate life tables more quickly. An example of this is the Senescence Accelerated Mouse (SAM), the use of which as a gerontological model was reviewed by its discoverers (53). This strain has an average life span of only ~1 yr (that is <50% of the average life span of a moderately long-lived mouse strain). The SAM strain was derived as a genetic variant of the AKR/J strain. During sister–brother mating to maintain the inbred strain, investigators observed that certain litters showed features of accelerated aging (low activity, low glossiness of hair, skin coarseness, etc.). Importantly, whereas the parental strain is well known to develop thymic lymphoma at a very high incidence at an early age, SAM mice show only about a 15% incidence.

There are now many sublines of the SAM strain, each of which shows a different dominant pathology in late life. For example, the SAM-P/1 subline develops senile amyloid, SAM-P/3 shows degenerative joint disease, SAM-P/6 is a model for osteoporosis, SAM-P/8 shows overt deficits in learning and memory, and SAM-P/9 develops cataracts. The SAM strain is probably of greater gerontological interest than most of the many other short-lived rodent strains because SAM's late-life disease profile appears to be less dominated by a single lethal disorder than, for example, NZB mice (autoimmune hemolytic anemia), (NZB $\times$ NZW)F_1 (systemic lupus-like disease in females), MRL/lpr mice (lymphoproliferative disease), spontaneously hypertensive rat strains, and many others.

In addition to genetically determined models of accelerated aging, investigators have attempted to develop animals that age at an accelerated pace. One example of this approach is adult thymectomy in mice, which was done to test the importance of thymic involution in aging. The results showed that the adult-thymectomized mice had a shorter life span than controls (26), and that they showed accelerated aging of the immune system (43). Many other examples of models of accelerated aging (for example, irradiation, graft vs. host reaction, and various environmental stresses,) exist in the literature (and especially in the earlier gerontological literature), but these will not be discussed here (for a consideration of certain of these see ref. 55). Not surprisingly, the results of this work show that there are many ways to experimentally shorten life span, and some of these do mimic certain aspects of normal aging.

A fifth way of studying aging processes develops and applies interventions to establish animal models of decelerated aging. An example is the life span increase in *Drosophila* associated with the overexpression of genes encoding the antioxidant enzymes catalase and superoxide dismutase (42a). As covered in detail in Chapter 23, two other prominent examples are dietary restriction (a well-established example) and deprenyl treatment (which may have efficacy). Interestingly, dietary restriction increases maximum life span and retards aging processes in both long-lived and short-lived rodent models (60), including the SAM strain (53). An intervention such as dietary restriction provides the investigator with an in vivo model, (a live animal), in which to study the biology of decelerated aging. Most investigators of dietary restriction share the view that these studies help to clarify which aging processes are the most important. Other investigators examine the possibility of direct human applicability by testing the effects of dietary restriction on age-sensitive biological measures either in monkeys (24, 30) or in humans (57).

Further discussion of the use of nonhuman primate models in gerontology and of the monkey dietary restriction studies is provided later, under NEED FOR THE USE OF A WIDE SPECTRUM OF MODELS.

Defined Longevity Characteristics

Arguably the most fundamental requirement of any aging study that employs an animal model is to know, with a high level of confidence, the age of the subjects relative to the survival characteristics of the species. It is most desirable that such survival data have been generated for animals raised in environments resembling those used in the current research. A common problem is to consider the chronologically oldest group of animals in a study "old" when, biologically, they are not old. The data required to provide this information are known as a *life table*, from which survival curves for the animal model can be constructed (see discussion in Chapter 1). Although there are published reports from most areas of biogerontology that demonstrate the problem of inappropriately labeling animals "old", Walford's editorial "When Is a Mouse Old?" is a clear discussion of how this problem affects immunogerontology (56).

Numerous mouse and rat strains are available for use in gerontological studies. These can be arbitrarily subdivided into short-lived strains (that is, mean life spans ≤15 months) and long-lived strains (that is, mean life spans ≥25 months). An important consideration is whether aging is best studied in short-lived or long-lived strains of a species. Although there is not widespread agreement on this question, I believe that long-lived strains are superior models. This opinion is based on the fact that short-lived strains show their own very distinct and homogeneous pathology profiles, resulting in death at an age that can only be considered very young for the species. Although there are long-lived strains that show rather homogeneous and temporally compressed late-life disease patterns, these patterns typically are not as pronounced as those observed in the short-lived models. Finally, there is an intuitive appeal in studying aging in a strain that is a long-lived representative of the species.

To this end, in the late 1970s Roy Walford and I (62, 63) developed a long-lived mouse strain for use in aging studies, the (C3H.SW/Sn × C57BL10.RIII/Sn)F_1 hybrid. The intent was to develop a very healthy and long-lived mouse model for the study of aging and its modulation by dietary restriction. An F_1 hybrid was chosen because the existing literature clearly showed that they usually live signifcantly longer than their inbred parents. The selection of the parents for this F_1 hybrid was based on the results of the aforementioned longevity study of the influence of *H-2* type on the longevity of mice fed standard laboratory diets ad libitum (49). The female parent (C3H.SW/Sn) was the longest lived among four *H-2* congenic strains tested on the C3H background, with a tenth-decile life span of 34.7 months. The male parent (C57BL10.RIII/Sn) was the longest lived among nine *H-2* congenic strains tested on the C57LBL10 background and showed a tenth-decile life span of 39.2 months. Use of this C3B10F_1 hybrid in a dietary restriction study is illustrated below under "Should ad libitum feeding be abandoned . . ."

The longevity characteristics of several important and potentially worthwhile aging models are not well defined. For example, as Masoro (36) pointed out, the rabbit is often considered as a model for expanded use in aging research; however, reliable life-table data for rabbits are unavailable (11). As a result, we do not know when a rabbit is old. Another good example is the rhesus monkey. Although attempts have been made to evaluate life table–related measures for this species, to my knowledge good life-table data for acceptably large numbers of rhesus monkeys do not exist. Finch (16; Table 3.1) has estimated the initial mortality rate per yr for rhesus monkeys (0.02), the doubling time for the mortality rate (8 yr), and the maximum life span (>35 yr) (see also Table 1.3 of Chapter 1). Yet, as footnote 31 to Finch's table shows, these estimates are based on scattered data from several sources. Further, none of the data appear to be the result of a highly controlled longevity study in this species. As a result, generalizations about apparent differences in mortality characteristics between rhesus monkeys and humans may be premature.

Awareness of Late-Life Disease Patterns

One prerequisite to the conduct of meaningful aging research is a knowledge of the disease patterns of the organism under study and of any specific diseases present. This knowledge is essential for the evaluation of the health status of older animals. The investigator therefore needs to state clearly in any report what was done to evaluate the health status of the animals (assessment for the presence of pathogenic microorganisms, gross autopsy, histopathology, etc.) and what the results of that evaluation were. Also, if animals are excluded from further study because of the presence of disease, the criteria used for such exclusion need to be defined. By taking these steps, other investigators will know with some confidence whether the study involved healthy older animals or sick ones.

An unresolved issue of major importance in aging research is the extent to which aging processes and disease processes overlap. Some researchers argue that disease is not part of the aging process whereas other workers have more difficulty separating aging processes from disease processes. Although my thoughts on this issue have vacillated over the past 15 years, I currently believe that certain of the diseases of aging expressed by a given animal model are likely to be reflections of dominant aging processes in that genotype. As a result, awareness of a model's disease tendencies should only promote a better understanding of aging in that animal. For example, if a given animal model is especially prone to problems of glucose regulation prior to reaching old age, one might suspect that a large percentage of animals of this genotype will develop diabetes and show biochemical changes associated with high blood glucose when they become old. Likewise, age-associated changes that depend on the accumulation of glycated or glycooxidized molecules (31) would likely be more overt in such a model than in another animal model, which is instead highly prone to develop late-life cancers but not inclined to display alterations in glucoregulation.

Defined Environmental Conditions

The environmental conditions under which experimental animals are raised can powerfully influence gerontological investigations. The strongest influence on the rate of aging known in mammalian models is that exerted by diet and, specifically, the nonmalnutritional restriction of caloric intake (39, 60; see also Chapter 23). Other major factors relating to an animal's habitat involve housing and husbandry procedures, microbiological characterization, and level of physical activity. Selected aspects of these three types of environmental influence are discussed in the next section. Although most of this information directly concerns rodent models of aging, certain of the basic principles (for example, overfeeding shortens life span, health status must be carefully monitored, microbial status needs to be defined) have broader pertinence.

Diet

Types of diets used. Most gerontological studies in rodents have used either commercially available nonpurified diets or defined purified diets. There are two types of nonpurified diet: *open formula* (which has a defined, fixed composition) and *closed formula* (in which the manufacturer does not provide the exact composition). Purified diets differ from nonpurified diets in that they are made of refined proteins (casein is very commonly used), carbohydrates (sucrose, cornstarch), and fat (often corn oil), with added vitamin and mineral mixtures. A potential disadvantage of nonpurified diets is that they are more prone to contamination by nonnutritive substances than are the purified diets.

A 1977 American Institute of Nutrition (AIN) report (1) suggested that the AIN-76™ diet be the standard purified diet for rodent studies. The widespread use of a single diet is favorable if it facilitates the meaningful comparison of data but detrimental if it discourages attempts to improve diets. It is noteworthy that the AIN committee decided "that the diet should not contain quantities of vitamins and minerals highly in excess of the requirements for rats and mice as set forth by the Committee on Animal Nutrition, National Research Council" (42). Later, an AIN workshop resulted in recommendations for possible changes in the AIN-76 diet (44). The AIN rodent diet was again reformulated in 1993 (42a). Despite the obvious appeal of using a completely defined diet for many nutritional studies, to be accepted as an adequate standard for aging studies, the AIN-76 diet must be shown to yield maximum health spans and life spans as great as less defined or less widely used diets.

Should ad libitum feeding be abandoned as the standard way to feed animals in aging research? Since the 1930s it has been known that dietary restriction can profoundly extend survival in rodents (40). It also produces this outcome in many other animals, including rotifers, water fleas, and spiders (60). Results of studies carried out since the early 1970s show that rats and mice on dietary restriction stay biologically younger longer, as judged by evaluating several diverse age-sensitive measures. Most of the spontaneous neoplastic diseases of late life which afflict mice and rats are retarded by dietary restriction (61). The life span–extending and antiaging actions of dietary restriction have largely been studied in rodents, with restriction being initiated very early in life (~4–6 wk of age); however, similar outcomes occur when it is first imposed at 6 months (64) or 12 months (2, 59, 62) of age. Therefore, the actions of dietary restriction do not depend in any dominant way on tampering with processes that occur early in the life span.

The purpose here is not to review the dietary restriction paradigm but rather to illustrate the potent influence that the level of caloric intake exerts on longevity and disease patterns in rodent models. Figure 3.1 shows survival curves from a study (63) carried out on female mice from the C3B10F$_1$ hybrid strain. The life span of the mice increased with the severity of dietary restriction (Fig. 3.2). Comparing the mice fed 85 kcal/wk to those fed 40 kcal/wk (DR cohort), life span (average and tenth decile) was increased in the DR cohort by about 35%. The dominant pathology in C3B10F$_1$ hybrid mice is cancer, with lymphoma and hepatoma being the two most common neoplasms. The ability of dietary restriction to oppose the development of cancer is illustrated in Figure 3.3, which plots the survival curves for the mice fed either 85 or 40 kcal/wk, along with the age of death for mice that displayed a tumor at autopsy. Tumor incidence was 78% for the control group and 38% for mice on dietary restriction. Lymphoma was the

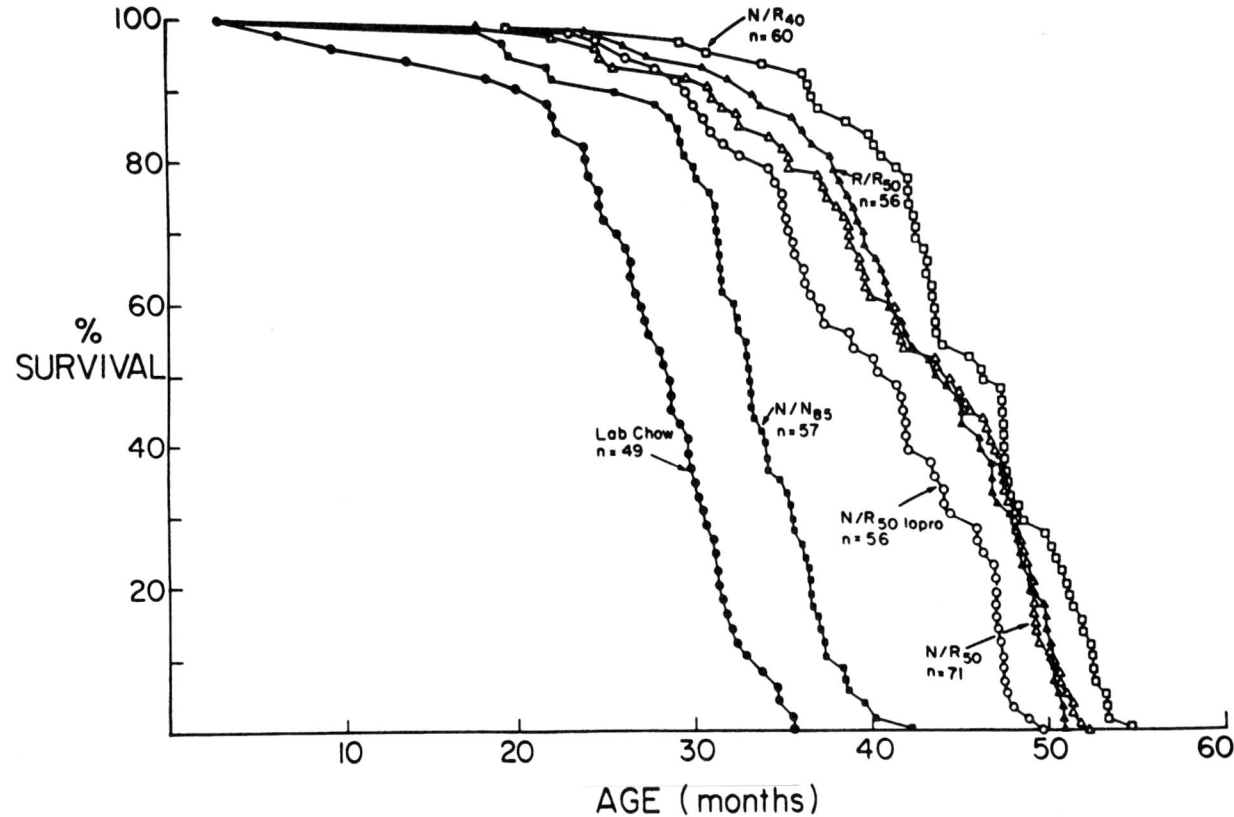

FIG. 3.1. Survival curves of female C3B10RF$_1$ mice fed ad libitum and restricted diets. Diet groups: Lab Chow (Purina Lab Chow^{RM}) ad libitum; N/N$_{85}$, normal caloric intake before weaning and thereafter 85 kcal/wk or ~25% less than ad libitum levels; N/R$_{50}$, fed normally before weaning, restricted postweaning to 50 kcal/wk; R/R$_{50}$, restricted in feeding level both before and after weaning; N/R$_{50lopro}$, restricted after weaning to 50 kcal/wk with a decrease with age in the protein content of the diet; N/R$_{40}$, restricted after weaning to 40 kcal/wk. Adult body weights for these groups averaged ~50 g for Lab Chow, ~35 g for N/N$_{85}$, and 20–25 g for the other four groups subjected to more severe dietary restriction. [From (63) with permission.]

most common neoplasm, found in 46% of control mice compared to 13% of mice on restricted diets. Average life spans for mice developing lymphoma in control and dietary restriction cohorts were 31 and 42 months, respectively. The next most common tumor was hepatoma, found in about 20% of mice from each diet cohort; however, mice from the group under dietary restriction bearing hepatoma lived an average of 44 months, 10 months longer than hepatoma-bearing controls. These data suggest that in mice the rate of aging (and disease development, as discussed below) is directly related to caloric intake.

There is another critically important point illustrated in Figure 3.3: Cancer was not found in any mouse from the diet-restricted cohort that died after 49 months of age. These very long-lived, apparently cancer-free mice totaled 18 in number (or 30% of the cohort under dietary restriction). It appears that dietary restriction creates a situation that prevents the occurrence of the usual pathologies that afflict aging animals, thereby providing an opportunity to study healthy animals at ages that otherwise would be unattainable. It is likely that any major insights into the causes of death in very old diet-restricted animals would produce important new understanding of basic aging processes that limit health and life spans. Intensive biological study of extremely old animals whose lives are greatly prolonged by dietary restriction should be encouraged.

These strong actions of dietary restriction have led some investigators to question the suitability of ad libitum feeding as the standard for feeding rodents in aging research (7, 36). Indeed, this issue extends beyond gerontology and is germane to a diverse set of very large long-term experiments, such as those conducted in toxicology and drug safety evaluations. Accordingly, researchers and policy makers in these latter disciplines have recently shown great interest in the dietary restriction paradigm as it applies to long-term evaluations of drug safety (18a, 21). This interest has been driven by very real concerns, such as the requirement that a drug

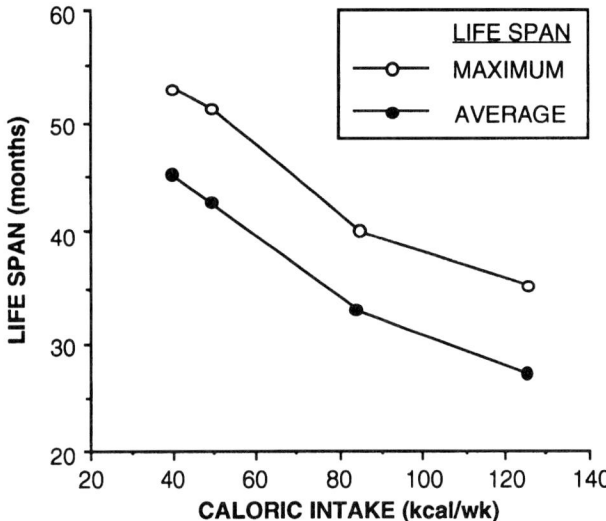

FIG. 3.2. Relationship between caloric intake and life span in female C3B10RF$_1$ mice. Dietary restriction was initiated at 3 wk of age. Four cohorts of mice (n = 49–71) were fed either 125, 85, 50 or 40 kcal/wk. Maximum life span is defined as the average of the cohort's longest-lived decile. [Adapted from (63) with permission.]

tion should provide the toxicologist with a "cleaner" animal model (that is, one with a lower background of diseases associated with lower caloric intakes) in which to evaluate the test substance. However, the use of dietary restriction in toxicology studies may so strongly oppose the development of induced tumors that levels may become low enough to cause problems with statistical power. With respect to aging research, it is my opinion that ad libitum feeding should be avoided, especially in models prone to obesity. The importance of studying healthy old animals cannot be overemphasized, and the appropriate restriction of caloric intake is one major step toward achieving that critical result in most of the commonly used rodent models. This is not to endorse the use of severe dietary restriction (for example, 50% of ad libitum intake) as a "normal" way to feed experimental animals; however, a regimen of 80% or so of the unrestricted intake level, which improves the long-term health of the animals under study, makes a great deal of sense.

Housing, Husbandry, and Microbial Status. Other critical environmental aspects of the aging animal model concern how the animals are housed, maintained, and monitored for the presence of infectious diseases. It is essential that aging studies be carried out in a well-defined environment. Further, a detailed description of

be tested for safety in laboratory rodents for a two-year period only to find that large numbers of the ad libitum–fed rats die before that time, irrespective of exposure to the compound under study. Also, use of dietary restric-

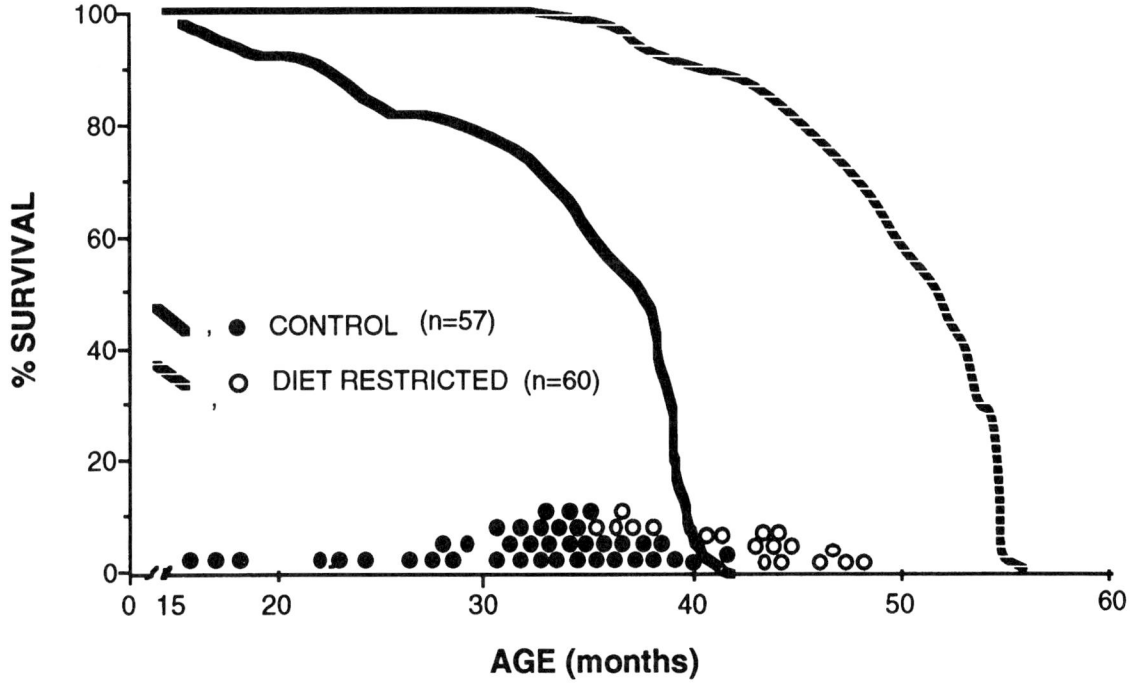

FIG. 3.3. Influence of dietary restriction started at 3 wk of age on life span and tumor incidence of female mice from the long-lived C3B10RF$_1$ hybrid strain. Survival curves are those for the 85 kcal/wk (control) and 40 kcal/wk (diet-restricted) cohorts shown in Figure 3.1. Circles show the age of death for tumor-bearing mice. [Adapted from (63) with permission.]

housing, husbandry, and the monitoring of microbial status is a critical component of publications describing studies of animals maintained for long periods of time. The widely accepted view is that rats and mice should be housed under specific-pathogen-free (SPF) conditions to minimize the risk of infectious diseases. The barrier utilized to oppose the entrance and spread of infectious agents in the colony may range in complexity from groups of many rooms to a filter hood on a single cage. This is not to say that it is impossible to have very long-lived and healthy rodent colonies using conventional (that is, nonbarrier) methods. An example is provided by the C3B10F$_1$ mice just described, which were raised in a conventional (but very clean) facility and displayed no evidence of infection over the 4.5 yr of study. What SPF conditions do provide is a means to reduce greatly the odds of developing a disastrous outbreak of infection in an aging colony. Kay (28) discusses the aftermath of such an occurrence involving Sendai virus infection of the animal facility at the Gerontology Research Center in 1976.

What is the influence of barrier housing on longevity? Does it extend life span and, if so, how do any such actions compare in size to those exerted by dietary restriction? These questions are perhaps best answered by the study of Snyder et al. (51), who used four groups of male Lobund-Wistar rats: *(1)* conventionally housed and fully fed (CV-F), *(2)* conventionally housed and on dietary restriction (CV-DR), *(3)* isolator housed germ-free and fully fed (GF-F), and *(4)* germ-free and on dietary restriction (GF-DR). The median length of life of ad libitum–fed CV and GF rats was quite similar (31 and 34 months, respectively). Dietary restriction increased the median life span of CV and GF rats to ~38 months. The maximum (tenth decile) life spans ranked GF-DR = 45 months, CV-DR = 44 months, GF-F = 39 months, and CV-F = 36 months. Interestingly, GF-F rats ate less than CV-F rats and weighed 6% less as adults. Therefore, any increases in longevity caused by the germ-free environment were very mild compared to those caused by dietary restriction affected only median life span, and may have resulted from a mild dietary restriction due to the germ-free status.

Four review articles resulting from the 1990 conference "Animal Models for Aging Research" provide especially useful and up-to-date information on housing, husbandry, and the evaluation of microbial status. Selected points from these reviews are summarized in the paragraphs that follow.

Clough (8) has reviewed and carefully tabulated the available published guidelines for the housing of rodents. The topics covered were ambient air temperature (optimal temperature 23° ± 3°C), relative humidity (optimal ~55%, but more data are needed on how levels of humidity influence survival of airborne pathogens), lighting levels (current levels may be too high for some animals), photoperiods, sound levels (50 dB), cage sizes, and ventilation rates (15 air changes/h probably sufficient). Of these factors, the author was most concerned about sound and concluded: "Current recommendations [are] all related to human ear function and are irrelevant to animal hearing. This factor is the one most likely to give rise to discomfort and lack of well-being in these species (rats and mice)."

As part of an extremely useful overview on the use of rodent models to study "normal" aging, Masoro (37) reviewed the influences of number of animals housed per cage, dark–light cycle, and ambient temperature on the longevity of mice and rats. Many studies have examined the effect of housing density on longevity, but results are quite variable. Shifting the dark–light cycle rendered no effect on longevity of mice in one study. As for temperature, it is known that rats housed at a range of 25°–30°C live longer than those housed at less than 10°C or at more than 30°C; however, data are lacking on the longevity of animals housed at different temperatures within the 10°–25°C range.

Two other articles discuss the need for a more standardized microbiological characterization of rodents for aging studies (48, 54). Both identify the main organisms of concern and provide protocols for monitoring the presence of those bacteria, viruses, and other microbes. Such microbiological characterization is now an essential part of maintaining a colony of aging rodents, and its importance cannot be overstated.

Exercise. The level of physical activity is still another important variable to consider in aging research. As detailed in Chapter 24 of this volume, the level of physical activity of rodents can influence survival patterns and other age-sensitive outcomes. In general, offering rodents the opportunity to exercise leads to increases in average life span but not maximum life span (22).

To determine the influence of dietary restriction on the rate of aging in nonhuman primates, our group is conducting studies in thirty male rhesus monkeys at the Wisconsin Regional Primate Research Center. We are also investigating normal aging in many animals of diverse ages (2–37 yr) not subjected to dietary manipulation. One concern is that animals be given adequate opportunity for physical activity. However, we have found it futile to provide older animals with an opportunity to exercise because they prefer a sedentary lifestyle. One could argue that this preference indicates that the nonhuman primate provides an excellent model for most human primates with respect to this behavioral characteristic.

Genetic Characteristics

Yet another basic factor influencing animal models of aging concerns genetic characteristics and quality control (14). From a genetic standpoint, there are various types of animals available. In rodents these range from outbred stocks to highly inbred strains. It is estimated that there are over 300 inbred strains of mice and 100 of rats available worldwide. In addition, there are F_1 hybrids, congenic, transgenic, recombinant inbred, and recombinant congenic strains. Festing (14) argues convincingly against the use of outbred stocks in gerontological research. He also argues that some form of genetic quality control must be maintained to document the authenticity of the strains under investigation. The conclusion was reached that newer quality control methods based on DNA restriction fragment length polymorphisms have many advantages over more traditional approaches and will likely dominate future testing.

A striking example of the potential difficulties connected with outbred strains is illustrated by the very popular Sprague-Dawley rat. Because the breeding stock used to produce Sprague-Dawley rats differs from supplier to supplier, there is often huge heterogeneity among what is reported for this strain. For example, in a dietary restriction study carried out by Berg and Simms (3), body weights for adult female Sprague-Dawley rats fed ad libitum averaged 280 g; however, these rats weighed less than the diet-restricted group (300 g) in the study of Merry and Holehan (41) for rats fed 50% of the ad libitum intake level. The vast differences in growth potentials of what are called "Sprague-Dawley rats" are discussed by Merry and Holehan (41).

Availability and Cost

It is possible to purchase old rats and mice from well-characterized strains at reasonable prices from the colonies subsidized by the National Institute on Aging (NIA). Sprott (52) summarizes the history of decisions made since the 1970s by administrators at the NIA in concert with outside experts in developing the NIA's very important animal model program. Eight genotypes of mouse (C57BL/6NNia, DBA/2NNia, CBA/CaNNia, BALB/cNNia, [C57BL/6NNia × C3H/NNia]F_1, [C57BL/6NNia × DBA/2NNia]F/i1, [BALB/cNNia × C57BL/6NNia]F_1, and Swiss Webster [outbred]) and three genotypes of rat (Fischer 344/NNia, Brown Norway/BiRijNia [Fischer 344/NNia × Brown Norway/BiRijNia]F_1 are now available (19). The survival characteristics of most of these models have been published (11), as have their age-specific pathologies (6). Animals from these strains are usually available at most ages over the life span.

A significant broadening of animal availability occurred in September 1993. Rats and mice of diverse ages fed either ad libitum or a restricted diet (40% < ad libitum intake from 14 wk of age) can now be purchased. These animals are raised at the huge SPF facility at the National Center for Toxicological Research in Jefferson, Arkansas). There are three rat genotypes and three mouse genotypes available.

Despite the reasonable costs of these old animals relative to the expense required to produce them, for most investigators with a new interest in gerontology, obtaining adequate numbers of old animals presents a serious financial obstacle. Unfortunately, today's peer review process typically demands having good pilot data if researchers are to attain a fundable ranking for longer-term inquiry, and this means that investigators often must procure and study old animals prior to having significant funding to do so. An increase of funds earmarked for animal purchase in pilot studies in gerontology is a major need, and one that is being met in part by an NIA program that makes limited numbers of old mice and rats available gratis to new investigators in gerontology for pilot experiments.

PATTERNS OF ANIMAL USE IN AGING STUDIES

In this section, patterns of animal usage in gerontology over the last 20 yr are analyzed. This analysis elucidates the obvious "rodentcentricity" of biogerontology. Not only are rodents the heavily favored model, but other obviously interesting rodent models have been all but ignored in favor of the standard laboratory rat (*Rattus norvegicus*) and laboratory mouse (*Mus musculus*) species. For example, the white-footed mouse (*Peromyscus* sp.) lives about twice as long as normal laboratory mice, yet *Peromyscus* has been little studied gerontologically (see ref. 47) with defined laboratory strains only now being established (Fig. 3.4) (50). As a result, the causes underlying the vastly different life-span potentials of these two types of mouse remain unclear. Further aggravating the situation is the fact that more and more workers have chosen to investigate one particular rat model (Fischer 344) such that a very large part of recent biogerontological research concerns one animal model.

Animal Use in Aging Research, 1972–1992

Although a diverse group of animals (other than humans) has been used in aging research since the early 1970s, the vast majority of work has involved mice and, increasingly, rats (Fig. 3.5). In the four journals surveyed, a total of 2,476 different animal usages was found. Of these, 1,877 (76%) were either rats or mice. Rats were used in 1,179 studies (48%), whereas mice were the subjects in 698 studies (28%). Only 599 studies (24%) involved neither rats nor mice. Figure 3.5 illustrates the upswing in the frequency of rat studies and the decline in the use of mice. Indeed, if present

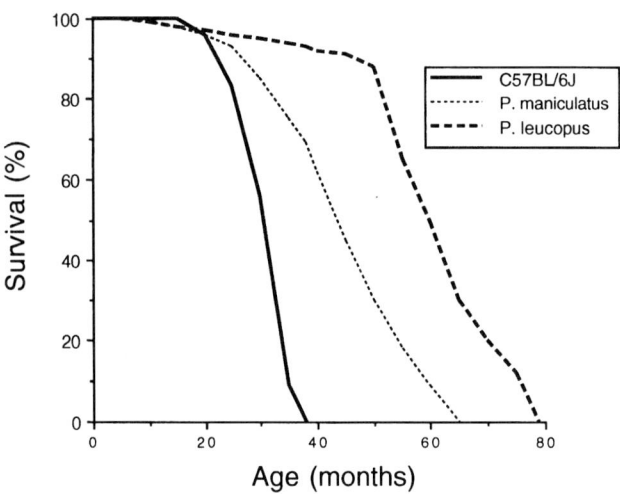

FIG. 3.4. Survival curves for two species of *Peromyscus* (the white-footed mouse) and one strain (C57BL/6J) of *Mus musculus* (the laboratory mouse) under laboratory conditions. [Redrawn from (50) with permission.]

trends continue, one could forecast that mice will no longer be used in aging research in the next century.

The overall frequency of use of the next most often studied organisms (after rats and mice) is illustrated in Figure 3.6. *Drosophila* holds a solid position as the third most frequently studied species in aging research, with 132 of the reports surveyed investigating this organism. A large gap then separates *Drosophila* from the next eight most frequently utilized animal types. Other organisms studied in the surveyed literature were dogs (24 reports), lizards (22 reports but none after 1984), cows (18 reports), other rodents [18 reports, with 11 on guinea pigs, three on *Peromyscus*, three on gerbils, and one describing *Mastomys* (an animal intermediate in size between rats and mice)], crustaceans (12 reports), mollusks (nine reports), frogs (seven reports), sheep (five reports), and an assortment of even lesser studied beasts.

In the four journals examined, it appears that an unfortunate trend toward even less frequent investigation of nonrodent models is ongoing (Fig. 3.5). For example, if one considers the period 1985–1992 (38% of the time period analyzed), only 119 investigations used animals other than rats and mice, accounting for only 21% of the nonrat/nonmouse studies. There may be a good reason for this trend because the year 1985 marked the time when Alex Comfort stepped down as Editor-in-Chief of *Experimental Gerontology*. It was an obvious by-product of Comfort's strong belief in the importance of studying aging in diverse models [see his classic text (10)] that this journal published the vast majority of nonrodent data.

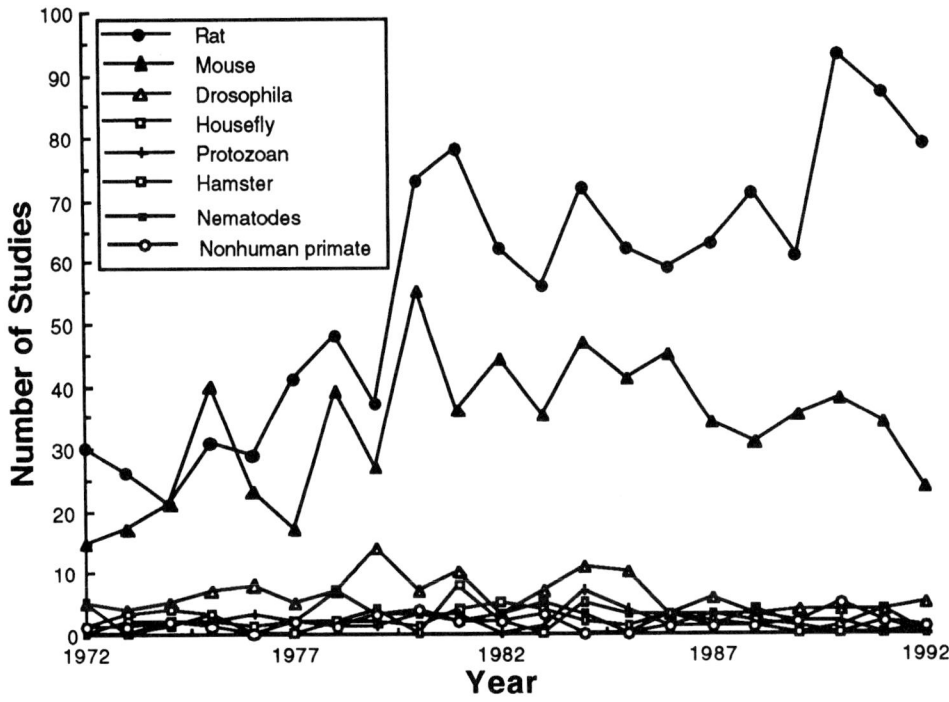

FIG. 3.5. Animal usage patterns in gerontology studies from 1972 to 1992. Data are derived from the animals studied in the reports published in four of the main biogerontology journals (*AGE*, *Experimental Gerontology*, *Journals of Gerontology*, and *Mechanisms of Aging and Development*). The figure shows only the most commonly used animals.

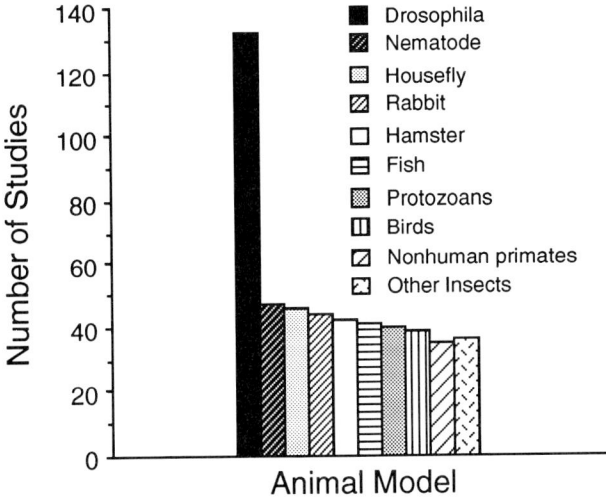

FIG. 3.6. Animals other than rats and mice used in gerontology studies from 1972 to 1992. Data are derived from the animals studied in the reports published in four of the main biogerontology journals (*AGE, Experimental Gerontology, Journals of Gerontology,* and *Mechanisms of Aging and Development*).

Overuse of the Male Fischer 344 Rat

The greater use of rats can correlated with the growing study of the male Fischer 344 (F344) strain. F344 rats were the subjects of 52 of the 95 reports (55%) involving rats which were published in the *Journals of Gerontology* from 1985 to 1992. This situation and its possible ramifications were the subject of editorial commentary in 1991 (58). It is important to underscore the fact that the problems are generic and not at all specific to male F344 rats. Some of the main points made follow.

The very wide use of the F344 rat as a gerontological model is due in large part to the NIA originally making this strain available to the research community. However, it should be noted that the NIA has made two other rat strains [Brown Norway (BN) and (F344 × BN)F_1] available, but, until recently, few investigators have used them (D. Hazzard, personal communication). It is clearly an unfavorable situation when such a large fraction of new knowledge on the biology of aging is confined to one rat strain. The extent to which the results from the many studies of aging F344 rats are generalizable to other aging organisms is a matter that must be confronted. Although a funding agency promoted the use of this particular animal model, the ultimate responsibility for this situation rests with investigators, who have largely disregarded the issue, possibly because they have been unaware of the limiting effects of using a single rat strain and also because of the difficulty in obtaining the resources needed to procure and maintain another less available genotype or multiple genotypes.

Another problem with using the male F344 strain lies in the failure of investigators to assess sufficiently the health/disease status of the animals. This issue was discussed earlier, under Awareness of Late-Life Disease Patterns, and the point was made that the investigator not only must be aware of the existence of disease processes but also must assess the consequences of the existing disease status on the study. That disease status of animal models is an issue for research is well illustrated by the male F344 model. Nephropathy of increasing severity with advancing age is a characteristic often found in male F344 rats (9). However, this easily recognized morphological lesion appears to be of little functional consequence until the lesions become severe, a condition rarely seen until advanced ages (34). Importantly, the possibility that nephropathy has interfered with the results of an aging study can be evaluated by combining histological and clinical chemistry evaluations. Another extremely common lesion found in male F344 rats, which occurs with increasing prevalence with advancing age, is testicular interstitial cell tumors. These lesions provide good reason to eliminate the use of F344 rats from reproductive aging research; however, they do not appear to cause problems that would significantly interfere with other research. These tumors neither metastasize nor do they appear to contribute to the death of the rat. However, like most rat or mouse strains with reasonably long average life spans (>2 yr), male F344 rats do have other neoplastic diseases that influence mortality and interfere with aging studies. Leukemia and pituitary adenoma are particular problems. The presence of such lesions must be known to the investigators and taken into account when interpreting the research.

The male F344 rat model also provides an unambiguous example of the importance of recognizing that environmental conditions can either retard or enhance disease processes. As a result, conditions should be sought which minimize the diseases of aging. In male F344 rats fed ad libitum a semipurified diet containing casein as the protein source, ~50% had severe nephropathy by 24 months and almost all by 27 months of age (34). However, when soy protein was substituted as the protein source in the diet of ad libitum–fed rats, almost none of the rats showed serious kidney lesions through 24 months and only ~30% displayed such lesions by 27 months of age (25). Finally, restricting food intake to 60% of that of the ad libitum–fed rats strongly prevented the occurrence of severe nephropathy even when the diet contained a high level (35%) of casein (38). Thus investigators in gerontology should monitor their rodent model for disease status and establish and utilize conditions that minimize the occurrence of disease.

In sum, gerontological studies must maximize the separation of the study of aging from that of diseases in a variety of animal models. The available literature strongly suggests that male F344 rats are overused and that inadequate attention is often given to the health status of old animals. The unfortunate result is a gerontological literature that often compares young healthy rats with old and possibly sick rats. This situation requires correction by encouraging investigators and reviewers to seriously concern themselves with the health/disease status of old animals. Further, the field will benefit by achieving a more balanced use of rat strains (which appears to be under way due to recent increased availability) and by adopting conditions that minimize and delay the occurrence of disease as standard operating procedure.

NEED FOR THE USE OF A WIDE SPECTRUM OF MODELS

Although much of this article has reflected the rat- and mouse-dominated nature of biogerontology, it is necessary to underscore again that exciting opportunities exist in less investigated animal models.

Lessons from Nonmammals

One need only spend a few hours (or a few months) reading Finch's book *Longevity, Senescence, and the Genome* (16) to appreciate the breadth of research possibilities currently being ignored in biogerontology (for a much briefer discussion, see ref. 15). In this book, the life histories of many eukaryotes are carefully considered to define what is known about the processes of biological senescence in these species. A great deal remains to be learned from a broad array of animals heretofore little studied from a gerontological perspective. In the meantime, studies on a few nonmammals, such as *C. elegans* (27) and *Drosophila* (45), which have long been investigated by small numbers of gerontologists, continue to provide important new insights largely dealing with the genetic basis of longevity.

Rodents

In view of the overuse of the F344 rat, it is highly appropriate to encourage the development of several genotypes suitable for aging research, that is, free of serious disease until advanced age, with no single disease being almost solely responsible for death. Candidates include Lobund-Wistar rats (50), the Wistar line used by Beauchene et al. (2), BN, and the F_1 hybrids made by mating F344 with BN rats. As stated, it is encouraging that the NIA has developed two of these models, and animals of diverse ages and subjected to dietary restriction are available. Therefore, the problem of lack of diversity in the rat studies is being corrected. However, investigators must not use animals from NIA-sponsored colonies with the belief that they are reagent-grade rats free of disease because of the NIA stamp of approval. Instead, the investigator should be fully aware of the age-related diseases expected for the genotype and must monitor the rats used in light of this.

As for mice, it is certain that transgenic and other genetically altered strains represent an important new type of animal resource. For example, the role that free radicals may play in aging processes is being productively explored using superoxide dismutase (SOD)–transgenic mice, which show elevated CuZn-SOD activities (2.0–3.5-fold higher in various brain regions) and increased resistance to certain paradigms of oxidative stress (23). This and many other newly created mouse strains are begging intensive gerontological application.

There are several other rodent models worthy of study. *Peromyscus* has already been mentioned as important to investigate so that the basis of its long life span relative to that of *Mus musculus* can be discerned. The usage and characteristics of other lesser used rodent models, such as hamsters, gerbils, guinea pigs, rabbits, and *Mastomys*, have been well reviewed elsewhere (11, 36).

Carnivores

The domestic dog (*Canis familiaris*) and cat (*Felis catus*) have been used in gerontological research to a limited extent. Young dogs and cats have been studied from a variety of biological standpoints. Cats have been much studied by neurophysiologists and dogs by a diverse group of biologists (with much investigation by physiologists). It appears that cats and dogs serve as good models for a number of diseases and late-life disorders which affect humans (reviewed in ref. 11). However, it does not appear that genetically well-defined strains of cat or dog have been used in aging studies (36).

An interesting, long-term study of 48 dogs (Labrador retrievers) fed either conventionally or subjected to dietary restriction (25% < ad libitum starting at 8 wk of age) is being conducted by investigators at Ralston-Purina Co. (St. Louis). Although the ultimate intent is to learn about the influence of dietary restriction on late-life health and longevity, this report describes effects on the incidence of hip dysplasia in these growing dogs (29). It was observed that fewer dogs on dietary restriction showed signs of hip dysplasia based on evaluations done at several ages up to 2 yr. These dogs were also studied for a number of measures of gerontological interest, including immune function, antioxidant enzyme activity, and glucoregulation (R. Kealy, personal communication).

Nonhuman Primates

Because of their close phylogenetic relationship to humans, there is a great appeal to the study of aging in nonhuman primates. However, because of issues of cost and the exceedingly limited availability of old nonhuman primates of known age and health status, the gerontological study of these animals has been very limited. Major gaps in knowledge exist even among the most commonly studied of the species, exemplified by the aforementioned lack of good life-table data for rhesus monkeys (*Macaca mulatta*). The fact remains that certain major age-related events occur only in primates (and not in other mammals). A prominent example is that true menstruation occurs only among certain primate species. Therefore, it makes great sense to study menopause in nonhuman primates (17), as was reported in 1979 in the first book on aging in nonhuman primates (4). Nearly all of that volume's thirty chapters report the influences of age on one or more of a diverse set of more than 250 behavioral, morphological and physiological outcomes in a collaborative study of a group of pigtail macaques (*Macaca nemestrina*). Yet, to have assembled a group of animals of sufficiently advanced age, it was necessary to include wild caught animals of uncertain age as subjects.

Davis and Leathers (13) edited a similar book, which describes a diversity of behavioral and pathological studies conducted by several research teams on 15 rhesus monkeys 4–31 yr of age when studied over the period 1952–1981. Analysis of age-related changes in sensory organ morphology was emphasized, but differences among age groups in brain and lung chemistry and endocrine gland morphology were also found. This is a reasonable source of data on aging in this species; however, the older monkeys in this study were subjected to radiation in their youth such that one must wonder how normal aging was studied in these animals. Also, there were only three monkeys in each of the five age groups studied.

Two other publications are very useful in that they contain a great deal of information on nonhuman primate models of aging. *Mammalian Models for Aging Research* (11) discusses the suitability and availability of the various species of nonhuman primates for different types of aging study from the standpoints of life span, body size, diet, nature of the menstrual cycle, and breeding record in captivity. The review also contains useful coverage of husbandry issues. Bowden and Williams (5) also provide a very useful review of aging in nonhuman primates, which emphasizes findings on reproductive, cognitive, neural, and visual aging.

Two studies with the goal of determining the influences of dietary restriction on the rate of aging in nonhuman primates address the same fundamental question, though they are quite different in many important aspects. The NIA study (24) is much the larger of the two and includes a total of 129 animals from two species (rhesus and squirrel monkeys), whereas the University of Wisconsin (UW) (30) study involves thirty male rhesus monkeys but is being expanded with the addition of 48 more animals. Other major differences involve diet composition and the method used to determine the level of dietary restriction.

The main findings of the first year of the NIA's study (24) showed that dietary restriction could safely be imposed in the monkeys, but they do not support the notion that a 30% dietary restriction was actually being imposed in all cohorts. This was especially true for the squirrel monkeys, where only minor effects on body weight gain were seen. As for the rhesus monkeys, body weight differences between animals under dietary restriction and controls were more clear-cut. Data were also reported for blood chemistry and hematological measures. Although some age-related changes were reported (for example, decreased levels of peripheral blood lymphocytes [PBL], decreased serum alkaline phosphatase activity, increased serum creatinine levels) influences of 1 yr of dietary restriction were generally not observed.

Our group has reported the experimental design, methodology, and findings from the UW study's first year (30). The main observations after 1 yr were that: (*1*) all monkeys appeared to be in excellent health; (*2*) average body weights for controls increased by 9%, while monkeys under dietary restriction did not gain weight; (*3*) monkeys on the restricted diet had less body fat than controls, whereas the amount of lean body mass was not significantly influenced by dietary restriction; and (*4*) diet did not overtly influence the other measures. These early data indicate that dietary restriction can be safely instituted in adult monkeys.

We are now seeing major effects of dietary restriction on age-sensitive biological outcomes. The monkeys on the restricted diet weigh about 30% less than the controls and have much less body fat and slightly reduced lean body mass. The monkeys on the restricted diet have reduced blood glucose and increased insulin sensitivity (29a) and reduced metabolic rate (Kemnitz et al, in preparation). These and other data suggest that dietary restriction in rhesus monkeys is capable of exerting strong effects on measures known to change with aging and/or thought to be involved in aging processes. More time and study are required to know whether the rate of aging is being altered in this important animal model.

SUMMARY AND CONCLUSIONS

A great diversity of animals, ranging in complexity from protozoans to nonhuman primates, have been studied from a gerontological standpoint. Clearly, certain animal models have been used preferentially to study particular aspects of aging (for example, mouse for immunology, rat for physiology, *C. elegans* and *Drosophila* for genetics). Unfortunately, despite the presence of so many possible animal models and the important new understandings that would likely come from their investigation, about 75% of biogerontological studies published in four major aging journals since the late 1960s have employed either mice or rats. Recent trends are disheartening as they indicate that the use of nonrodents continues to decline. Also, the use of the rat is increasing, while that of the mouse is declining. Aging research has seen an extremely heavy use of the male F344 rat, though this is being corrected as several new and suitable rodent models are now available.

To gain the most from gerontological studies, there is an absolute need for well-defined animal models, both at the genetic level and in the environment in which they live. A common and very serious problem has been investigators' lack of awareness of the late-life disease patterns of the animal model under study. The result in many studies is that the health status of the older animals is unknown and unreported. In this circumstance one does not know if healthy or sick older animals were studied. In short, knowledge of a model's disease patterns and an appropriate evaluation of health status based on these data maximizes the separation of the study of aging from that of late-life diseases. Also, adopting a slightly less than ad libitum food intake level as the control would provide a powerful way to facilitate the study of healthy old animals. This is just one of many areas of great opportunity concerning animal models for aging research.

This research is supported by the National Institute on Aging (RO1 AG10536 and PO1 AG11915), the American Cancer Society (CN-57), and the Wisconsin Regional Primate Research Center. The author sincerely appreciates the comments provided by Drs. Judd Aiken, Daniel Muller, and Thomas Pugh, as well as the assistance of Ms. Jocelyn Rang in the preparation of this manuscript.

REFERENCES

1. AMERICAN INSTITUTE OF NUTRITION. Committee on Standards for nutritional studies. Report of the American Institute of Nutrition ad hoc *J Nutr.* 107: 1340–1348, 1977.
2. BEAUCHENE, R. E., C. W. BALES, C. S. BRAGG, S. T. HAWKINS, and R. L. MASON. Effect of age on initiation of feed restriction on growth, body composition, and longevity of rats. *J. Gerontol.* 41: 13–19, 1986.
3. BERG, B. N., and H. S. SIMMS. Nutrition and longevity in the rat. III. Food restriction beyond 800 days. *J. Nutr.* 74: 23–32, 1961.
4. BOWDEN, D. M. (Ed). *Aging in Nonhuman Primates.* New York: Van Nostrand Reinhold, 1979.
5. BOWDEN, D. M., and D. D. WILLIAMS. Aging. In: *Advances in Veterinary Science and Comparative Medicine. Research on Nonhuman Primates,* edited by C. E. Cornelius and C. F. Simpson. Orlando, FL: Academic Press, 1984, vol. 28, p. 305–341.
6. BRONSON, R. T. Rate of occurrence of lesions in 20 inbred and hybrid genotypes of rats and mice sacrificed at 6 month intervals during the first years of life. In: *Genetic Effects on Aging II,* edited by D. E. Harrison. Caldwell, NJ: Telford Press, 1990, p. 279–358.
7. CHERKIN, A. Letter to the Editor. *Age* 2: 51, 1979.
8. CLOUGH, G. Suggested guidelines for the housing and husbandry of rodents for aging studies. *Neurobiol. Aging* 12: 653–658, 1991.
9. COLEMAN, G. L., S. W. BARTHOLD, G. W. OSBALDISTON, S. J. FOSTER, and A. M. JONAS. Pathological changes during aging in barrier-reared Fischer 344 rats. *J. Gerontol.* 32: 258–278, 1977.
10. COMFORT, A. *The Biology of Senescence* (3rd ed.), New York: Elsevier, 1979.
11. COMMITTEE ON ANIMAL MODELS FOR RESEARCH ON AGING. *Mammalian Models for Research on Aging.* Washington, DC: National Academy Press, 1981.
12. CUTLER, R. G. Antioxidants and longevity of mammalian species. In: *Molecular Biology of Aging,* edited by A. D. Woodhead, A. D. Blackett, and A. Hollaender. New York: Plenum Press, 1985, p. 13–73.
13. DAVIS, R. T., and C. W. LEATHERS (Eds). *Behavior and Pathology of Aging in Rhesus Monkeys.* New York: Alan R. Liss, 1985.
14. FESTING, M. F. W. Genetic quality control of laboratory animals used in aging studies. *Neurobiol. Aging* 12: 673–677, 1991.
15. FINCH, C. E. New models for new perspectives in the biology of senescence. *Neurobiol. Aging* 12: 625–634, 1991a.
16. FINCH, C. E. *Longevity, Senescence, and the Genome.* Chicago: University of Chicago Press, 1991b.
17. GRAHAM, C. E., O. R. KLING, and R. A. STEINER. Reproductive senescence in female nonhuman primates. In: *Aging in Nonhuman Primates,* edited by D. M. Bowden. New York: Van Nostrand Reinhold, 1979, p. 183–202.
18. HART, R. W., and R. B. SETLOW. Correlation between deoxyribonucleic acid excision-repair and lifespan in a number of mammalian species. *Proc. Natl. Acad. Sci. U.S.A.* 71: 2169–2173, 1974.
18a. HART, R. W., E. NEUMAN, R. ROBINSON. (eds.). *Dietary Restriction: Implications for the Design and Interpretation of Toxicity and Carcinogenicity Studies.* Berlin: Springer-Verlag, in press.
19. HAZZARD, D. G., R. T. BRONSON, G. E. MCCLEARN, and R. STRONG. Selection of an appropriate animal model to study aging processes with special emphasis on the use of rat strains. *J. Gerontol.* 47: B63–B64, 1992.
20. HAZZARD, D. G., H. R. WARNER, and C. E. FINCH. National Institute on Aging, NIH, workshop on alternative animal models for research on aging. *Exp. Gerontol.* 26: 411–439, 1991.
21. HENRY, C. J., D. B. CLAYSON, G. N. RAO, F. J. C. ROE, R. J. SCHEUPLEIN, and D. E. STEVENSON. Impact of dietary restriction on bioassays and recommendations for future research: panel discussion. In: *Biological Effects of Dietary Restriction,* edited by L. Fishbein. Berlin: Springer-Verlag, 1991, p. 321–336.
22. HOLLOSZY, J. O., and F. K. SMITH. Effects of exercise on longevity of rats. *Fed. Proc.* 46: 1850–1853, 1987.
23. HUANG, T.-T., E. J. CARLSON, S. A. LEADON, and C. J. EPSTEIN. Relationship of resistance to oxygen free radicals to CuZn-superoxide dismutase activity in transgenic, transfected, and trisomic cells. *FASEB J.* 6: 903–910, 1992.
24. INGRAM, D. K., R. G. CUTLER, R. WEINDRUCH, D. M. RENQUIST, J. J. KNAPKA, M. APRIL, C. T. BELCHER, M. A. CLARK, C. D. HATCHERSON, B. MARRIOTT, and G. S.ROTH. Dietary

restriction and aging: the initiation of a primate study. *J. Gerontol.* 45: B148–B163, 1990.
25. IWASAKI, K., C. A. GLEISER, E. J. MASORO, C. A. MCMAHAN, E. J. SEO, and B. P. YU. The influence of dietary protein source on longevity and age-related disease processes of Fischer rats. *J. Gerontol.* 43: B5–B12, 1988.
26. JEEJEEBHOY, H. F. Decreased longevity of mice following thymectomy in adult life. *Transplantation* 12: 525–526, 1971.
27. JOHNSON, T. E., D. B. FRIEDMAN, N. FOLTZ, P. A. FITZPATRIDK, and J. E. SHOEMAKER. Genetic variants and mutations of *Caenorhabditis elegans* provide tools for dissecting the aging processes. In: *Genetic Effects on Aging II*, edited by D. E. Harrison. Caldwell, NJ: Telford Press, 1990, p. 101–127.
28. KAY, M. M. B. Immunologic aging patterns: effect of parainfluenza type 1 virus infection on aging mice of eight strains and hybrids. In: *Genetic Effects on Aging*, edited by D. Bergsma and D. E. Harrison. New York: Alan R. Liss, 1978, p. 213–240.
29. KEALY, R. D., S. E. OLSSON, K. L. MONTI, D. F. LAWLER, D. N. BIERY, R. W. HELMS, G. LUST, and G. K. SMITH. Effects of limited food consumption on the incidence of hip dysplasia in growing dogs. *J. Am. Vet. Med. Assoc.* 201: 857–863, 1992.
29a. KEMNITZ, J. W., E. B. ROECKER, R. WEINDRUCH, D. F. ELSON, S. T. BAUM, and R. N. BERGMAN. Dietary restriction increases insulin sensitivity and lowers blood glucose in rhesus monkeys. *Am J Physiol* (Endocrinol. Metob. 29) 266: E540–E547, 1994.
30. KEMNITZ, J. W., R. WEINDRUCH, E. B. ROECKER, K. CRAWFORD, P. KAUFMAN, and W. B. ERSHLER. Dietary restriction of adult male rhesus monkeys: design, methodology, and preliminary findings from the first year of study. *J. Gerontol.* 48: B17–B27, 1993.
31. KRISTAL, B. S., and B. P. YU. An emerging hypothesis: synergistic induction of aging by free radicals and Maillard reactions. *J. Gerontol.* 47: B107–B114, 1992.
32. LINTS, F. A. (Ed). *Non-mammalian Models for Research on Aging. Interdisciplinary Topics in Gerontology.* 1985a, vol. 21, Basel: Karger, pp. 1–183.
33. LINTS, F. A. Insects. In: *Handbook of the Biology of Aging,* (2nd ed.), edited by C. E. Finch and E. L. Schneider. New York: Van Nostrand Reinhold, 1985b, p. 146–169.
34. MAEDA, H., C. A. GLEISER, E. J. MASORO, I. MURATA, C. A. MCMAHAN, and B. P. YU. Nutritional influences on aging of Fischer 344 male rats: II. Pathology. *J. Gerontol.* 40: 671–688, 1985.
35. MARTIN, G. M., and M. S. TURKER. Model systems for the genetic analysis of mechanisms of aging. *J. Gerontol.* 43: B33–B39, 1988.
36. MASORO, E. J. Animal models in aging research. In: *Handbook of the Biology of Aging,* (3rd ed), edited by E. L. Schneider and J. W. Rowe. San Diego: Academic Press, 1990, p. 72–94.
37. MASORO, E. J. Use of rodents as models for the study of "normal aging": conceptual and practical issues. *Neurobiol. Aging.* 12: 639–643, 1991.
38. MASORO, E. J., K. IWASAKI, C. A. GLEISER, C. A. MCMAHAN, E. SEO, and B. P. YU. Dietary modulation of the progression of nephropathy in aging rats: an evaluation of the importance of protein. *Am. J. Clin. Nutr.* 49: 1217–1227, 1989.
39. MASORO, E. J., I. SHIMOKAWA, and B. P. YU. Retardation of the aging processes in rats by food restriction. *Ann. N. Y. Acad. Sci.* 621: 337–352, 1991.
40. MCCAY, C. M., M. F. CROWELL, and L. A. MAYNARD. The effect of retarded growth on the length of the life span and on the ultimate body size. *J. Nutr.* 10: 63–79, 1935.
41. MERRY, B. J., and A. M. HOLEHAN. Onset of puberty and duration of fertility in rats fed a restricted diet. *J. Reprod. Fertil.* 57: 253–259, 1979.
42. National Research Council (NRC). Nutrient requirements of the mouse. In: *Nutrient Requirements of Laboratory Animals,* (3rd revised ed.), Washington DC: National Academy of Sciences, 1978, p. 38–53.
42a. ORR, W. C., and R. S. SOHAL. Extension of life-span by overexpression of superoxide dismutase and catalase in *Drosophila melanogaster. Science* 263: 1128–1130, 1994.
43. PACHCIARZ, J. A., and P. O. TEAGUE. Age-associated involution of cellular immune function. I. Accelerated decline of mitogen reactivity in spleen cells of adult thymectomized mice. *J. Immunol.* 116: 982–988, 1976.
44. REEVES, P. G. AIN-76 diet: should we change the formulation? *J. Nutr.* 119: 1081–1082, 1989.
44a. REEVES, P. G., F. H. NIELSEN, and G. C. FAHEY, JR. AIN-93 purified diets for laboratory rodents: Final report of the American Institute of Nutrition ad hoc Writing Committee on the Reformulation of the AIN-76A Rodent Diet. *J. Nutr.* 123: 1939–1951, 1993.
45. ROSE, M. R. Evolutionary genetics of aging in *Drosophila.* In: *Genetic Effects on Aging II,* edited by D. E. Harrison. Caldwell, NJ: Telford Press, 1990, p. 41–55.
46. SACHER, G. A. Evaluation of the entropy and information terms governing mammalian longevity. In: *Interdisciplinary Topics in Gerontology,* edited by R. G. Cutler. Basel: Karger, 1976, vol. 9, p. 69–82.
47. SACHER, G. A., and R. W. HART. Longevity, aging and comparative cellular and molecular biology of the house mouse, *Mus musculus,* and the white-footed mouse, *Peromyscus leucopus.* In: *Genetic Effects on Aging,* edited by D. Bergsma and D. E. Harrison. New York: Alan R. Liss, 1978, p. 71–96.
48. SEBESTENY, A. Necessity of a more standardized microbiological characterization of rodents for aging studies. *Neurobiol. Aging* 12: 663–668, 1991.
49. SMITH, G. S., and R. L. WALFORD. Influence of the main histocompatibility complex on aging in mice. *Nature* 270: 727–729, 1977.
50. SMITH, G. S., M. D. CREW, and R. L. WALFORD. *Peromyscus* as a gerontologic animal: aging and the MHC. In: *Genetic Effects on Aging II,* edited by D. E. Harrison. Caldwell, NJ: Telford Press, 1990, p. 457–472.
51. SNYDER, D. L., M. POLLARD, B. S. WOSTMANN, and P. LUCKERT. Life span, morphology, and pathology of diet- restricted germ-free and conventional Lobund-Wistar rats. *J. Gerontol.* 45: B52–B58, 1990.
52. SPROTT, R. L. Development of animal models of aging at the National Institute on Aging. *Neurobiol. Aging* 12: 635–638, 1991.
53. TAKEDA, T., M. HOSKAWA, and K. HIGUCHI. Senescence-accelerated mouse (SAM): a novel murine model of accelerated senescence. *J. Am. Geriatr. Soc.* 39: 911–919, 1991.
54. VAN DER LOGT, J. T. M. Necessity of a more standardized virological characterization of rodents for aging studies. *Neurobiol. Aging* 12: 669–672, 1991.
55. WALFORD, R. L. *The Immunologic Theory of Aging.* Copenhagen: Munksgaard, 1969.
56. WALFORD, R. L. When is a mouse old? *J. Immunol.* 117: 352–353, 1976.
57. WALFORD, R. L., S. B. HARRIS, and M. W. GUNION. The calorically restricted low-fat nutrient-dense diet in biosphere 2 significantly lowers blood glucose, total leukocyte count, cholesterol, and blood pressure in humans. *Proc. Natl. Acad. Sci. U. S. A.* 89: 11533–11537, 1992.
58. WEINDRUCH, R., and E. J. MASORO. Concerns about rodent models for aging research. *J. Gerontol.* 46: B87–B88, 1991.
59. WEINDRUCH, R., and R. L. WALFORD. Dietary restriction in mice beginning at one year of age: effects on lifespan and spontaneous cancer incidence. *Science* 215: 1415–1418, 1982.

60. WEINDRUCH, R., and R. L. WALFORD. *The Retardation of Aging and Disease by Dietary Restriction.* Springfield, IL: Thomas, 1988.
61. WEINDRUCH, R., D. ALBANES, D. and KRITCHEVSKY. The role of calories in carcinogenesis. In: *Hematology/Oncology Clinics of North America,* edited by D. W. Nixon. Philadelphia: Saunders, 1991, p. 79–89.
62. WEINDRUCH, R., S. R. S. GOTTESMAN, and R. L. WALFORD. Modification of age-related immune decline in mice dietarily restricted from or after midadulthood. *Proc. Natl. Acad. Sci. U. S. A.* 79: 898–902, 1982.
63. WEINDRUCH, R., R. L. WALFORD, S. FLIGIEL, and D. GUTHRIE. The retardation of aging in mice by dietary restriction: longevity, cancer, immunity and lifetime energy intake. *J. Nutr.* 116: 641–654, 1986.
64. YU, B. P., and E. J. MASORO, and C. A. MCMAHAN. Nutritional influences on aging of Fischer 344 rats. I. Physical, metabolic and longevity characteristics. *J. Gerontol.* 40: 657–670, 1985.

4. Cell culture as a model

VINCENT J. CRISTOFALO
ROBERT J. PIGNOLO

Center for Gerontological Research, Medical College of Pennsylvania, Philadelphia, Pennsylvania

CHAPTER CONTENTS

Historical Development of Cell Cultures for the Study of Aging
Relevance of In Vitro Cellular Senescence to In Vivo Aging
    Cell cultures as models
    Cellular mortality, cellular clocks, and death as an end point for aging
    Aging and evolution
    In vivo–in vitro parallel changes
Caveats in the Use of Cell Cultures as Models
Cellular and Molecular Markers of Senescence In Vitro and In Vivo
Mechanistic Studies of In Vitro Replicative Senescence
    Stochastic mechanisms
    Signal transduction pathways
    Genetic mechanisms
        Deterministic processes
        Genes isolated from selective libraries and monoclonal antibody pools
Summary and Conclusions

HISTORICAL DEVELOPMENT OF CELL CULTURES FOR THE STUDY OF AGING

IN METAZOA, after fertilization of the egg and initial cell divisions, the cells of the embryo differentiate into a germ cell lineage and a somatic cell lineage. The germ cell lineage is potentially immortal, in the sense that the complement of genes can be passed on indefinitely. The somatic cells, however, are destined for further differentiation and ultimately for aging and death. A question of major interest is whether biological aging is a cellular phenomenon or a result of failures in integrative function that occur at the supracellular level. Thus in addition to the organismic "clock(s)," which determines maximum life span potential, are there cellular clocks that can operate within the organism and independently outside the organism (in vitro) to determine cellular life span?

In vitro studies by Carrel and co-workers (27–30) initially suggested that individual cells, when separated from the organism, are potentially immortal in the same way that bacteria and most protozoa are considered immortal. However, it is now well established that populations of normal human diploid fibroblasts can proliferate in culture only for finite periods of time. Typically, after explanation there is a period of rapid proliferation during which the cultures can be subcultivated frequently. This period is followed by a time of declining proliferative capacity when the cells change size and morphology, become granular, and accumulate debris, until ultimately the culture is incapable of proliferation. The work of Swim and Parker (268), Hayflick and Moorhead (114), and others established the generality of this limited life span phenomenon. These authors described a variety of human tissues from fetal, neonatal, and adult individuals that were incapable of unlimited proliferation. A similar limitation on the growth of chick cells has been noted (90, 108). Beginning early in the 1960s, in a large number of laboratories throughout the world, this observation of limited proliferative life span has been made in both chick and human cells, as well as in cells from other mammalian species. The doubling capacities of various cultured populations are reproducible within relatively narrow limits. For example, about 60 population doublings occur in human embryonic fibroblasts, while embryonic chick fibroblasts have a replicative potential of about 25 doublings.

In addition to the studies of fibroblasts, a limited in vitro life span has been described in a variety of cell types, including glial cells (207), keratinocytes (219), vascular smooth muscle cells (15), lens cells (270), endothelial cells (171), and lymphocytes (274). These findings and those of Hayflick and co-workers (111, 114) do not support the notion that isolated animal cells are capable of unlimited proliferation in culture, as proposed by Carrel (27–30) and Ebeling (64, 65). Carrel's results have been criticized in detail by Hayflick (112, 113). However, Suda et al. (266) reported that mouse embryonic stem cells can be maintained in vitro for up to 250 cumulative doublings with no indication of crisis or transformation. These authors concluded that embryonic stem cells, before differentiation into somatic and germ cells, are immortal. In theory, their data are consistent with the general concept of immortality of the germ line. Nevertheless, most of the cell lines isolated either were pseudodiploid or ultimately became pseudodiploid. The essence of the report by Suda et al. is that an apparently (chromosomally) normal cell line can have an indefinite replicative life span, although this is not characteristic of all such cell lines derived from mice. Furthermore, no consideration was given to the possibility of cryptostructural chromosomal abnormalities that were undetected. Thus the question of whether cells are immortal before differentiation into somatic and germ lines remains controversial.

In this chapter we present a brief overview of the historical development of cellular gerontology, a discussion of the strengths and limitations of studying cell aging in vitro compared to cell aging in vivo and to organismic aging, as well as a discussion of findings from selected research. We believe the areas of research included in this chapter are driving the study of cellular gerontology. For additional perspectives, other reviews have been published by Hay (107), Cristofalo (39), Cristofalo and Stanulis-Praeger (45), Stanulis-Praeger (256), Macieira-Coelho (143), Norwood et al. (179), and Goldstein (78).

Initially, the inability of cell cultures to proliferate indefinitely was ascribed to such technical difficulties as inadequate nutrition, pH variation, toxic metabolic products, and microcontaminants. Hayflick and Moorhead (114) showed, however, that cell degeneration was unrelated, at least in any simple way, to any of these factors. When mixtures of young and old populations, distinguishable by karyotypic markers, were grown in the same pool of medium, the older population was lost after it had undergone a total of approximately 50 population doublings, while the younger population would continue to proliferate until the 50 or so doublings expected for this population had been completed. These results seem to rule out any direct effect of media composition, the presence of contaminating microorganisms, or toxic end products of metabolism. Loss of proliferative capacity cannot be related to depletion by serial dilution of some essential, nonreplicating, nonsynthesized metabolite, since the initial presence of 2^{50} (i.e., adequate for 50 population doublings) molecules of even the lightest element, hydrogen, would have a mass in excess of that of a single cell. However, we cannot formally rule out the gradual uncoupling of the synthesis of some essential metabolite from cell growth and division that would result in a gradual depletion through changes in the relative concentrations of various metabolites.

Hayflick and Moorhead concluded that the limited life span phenomenon could be programmed and/or that genetic damage may be accumulated, and they interpreted their observation as a cellular expression of senescence.

RELEVANCE OF IN VITRO CELLULAR SENESCENCE TO IN VIVO AGING

The suggestion that aging changes in vivo are reflected in various properties of tissue cultures has a long history. For example, it has been known since the early 1900s that age-associated changes in plasma can inhibit cell growth in vitro (30). In addition, the time elapsing prior to cell migration from explanted tissue fragments increases with increasing age (29, 30). These are both examples of the expression in vitro of aging in vivo. The studies of Hayflick and Moorhead (114), Hayflick (111), and many other workers (45) focused attention on the occurrence of senescence in vitro.

Studies of cells and tissues in culture have made enormous contributions to the understanding of the biology of growth, metabolism, reproduction, differentiation, and disease. For example, over 100 pathological conditions have been characterized by the use of predominantly fibroblast-like cell cultures established from affected donors (143). It is not surprising, then, that the use of cell culture models has been extended to include the study of aging. Although the use of cell cultures to study age-related phenomena began in the early 1920s, their use did not become generalized until the 1960s.

The use of cell cultures has the advantage of providing a defined and manipulable environment for a single cell type in which fundamental mechanisms associated with aging can be examined. It also has the disadvantage of separating the cell type under study from various control elements, including interactions with other cell types in the body.

In considering the relevance of aging in cell culture to aging in vivo, several assumptions must be made. First, we must assume that aging has a cellular basis. Since all processes in the organism are based in cells, this assumption seems reasonable. Second, cells in culture show deteriorative changes in structure and function that lead to a decline in homeostatic capability and an increased probability of dying (see Chapter 1). Thus the process observed during serial subcultivation of fibroblasts in culture *is* aging by the above criteria. The central issue is whether aging in vitro bears any relationship to aging of the whole organism, that is, whether studies carried out in cell culture have any relevance to aging in the individual.

One must bear in mind that little is known about the fundamental process of aging, or senescence. (Although the term *aging* is commonly used to refer to postmaturational processes which are deteriorative and lead to an increased vulnerability, the more correct term for this is *senescence*. *Aging* can refer to any time-related process. In this chapter, however, *senescence* and *aging* are used interchangeably.) Certainly, it is a complex phenomenon that may well have both environmental and intrinsically programmed components. Moreover, senescent changes involve different kinds of cells and tissues and thus may have various mechanisms for their occurrence. The aging of fixed postmitotic cells, such as neurons, may proceed by a different set of mechanisms than that of proliferating tissues, such as skin, the lining of the gut, and the blood-forming elements. Matrix macromolecules, such as collagen and elastin, represent an additional component with, presumably, their own parameters of senescent degeneration. Then, there are the potentially profound effects of interactions among these components during senescence.

Cell Cultures as Models

In vitro studies of aging have used two kinds of cell culture. The predominant kind are fetal- or neonatal-derived cultures, which when serially subcultured show aging changes, some of which parallel aging changes in vivo. The other related paradigm is that of cells derived from donors of different ages and studied after only one or a few subcultivations. In either case, attempts to relate changes in individual cells to organismic changes form the basis of a model for organismic change.

One source of confusion is the misunderstanding of how scientists use models and how the results of such studies can be extrapolated to what happens in the organism. The term *model* is used with several different meanings in biology. The various kinds have been discussed by Ransom (216). He defines a model as "a representation of structure." In biology there are two general kinds of modeling. One is based on analogy, which involves relating one process to another because there are clear similarities. For example, if one wishes to study fundamental aspects of flight in animals, one can study the wing action of bees, birds, and bats. Even though these are quite different organisms from the point of view of flight, each can serve as a model for the other. A second type of modeling is probably unique to biology, modeling by homology. Highly conserved genetic sequences provide an evolutionary history of biological processes that can be used to relate processes in one organism to the same processes in another. Modeling by homology must also lead to modeling by analogy. Thus, the rat is a model, by homology, for humans because most of the physiology of the rat, including the process of aging, is conserved evolutionarily. The rat is also a model of aging by analogy because there are point-by-point similarities between physiological processes in the rat and in the human.

Cells in culture are models for organismic aging at an entirely different level. Consider that cell types in vivo differ from one another primarily in that they express some different genes. They are models for one another by homology in that every human somatic cell has the same genetic information as every other cell from that individual. This situation holds for human somatic cells in culture as well. Cells in vitro are also potential models by analogy because changes in such features as cell size, shape, elements of metabolism, and cytoplasmic inclusions, among others, are similar to those occurring in vivo (see below). Prominent among these cellular alterations are changes in gene expression with in vitro age. Biological aging of organisms is also characterized by changes in gene expression.

However, the question of the role and/or relevance that aging in a particular model may have to aging of the organism as a whole may be unrelated to the usefulness of the model in studying the mechanisms that regulate the limitation of life span (42).

Cellular Mortality, Cellular Clocks, and Death as an End Point for Aging

The process of aging in human cell cultures probably reflects the presence of intracellular "clocks" that can operate in the absence of other higher order "clocks," such as those of the neuroendocrine system, and can be studied under controlled environmental conditions. Furthermore, since organs and tissues show changes with age in vivo, either the tissue and organ level changes are based in cellular changes that will then be reflected in culture or cells in a tissue are "immune" to aging and are thus immortal. The notion that normal cells are immortal in vivo or in vitro has never been established. To the contrary, it is well established that normal somatic cells, in vivo and in vitro, either undergo senescence or immortalize with the acquisition of some of the characteristics of tumor cells.

Three terms that must be carefully distinguished are *death, longevity,* and *aging*. In evaluating aging, death is the end point often used. Given that the increase in age-specific death rate is widely interpreted as a measure of aging rate, it is of little use in shedding light on the biological mechanisms responsible for the changes that occur. In fact, in considering the biological basis of the senescence process, death is a very poor end point, since the time and cause of death are subject to great variability. "Nonaccidental" death occurs when the failure of one or more physiological systems becomes incompatible with life. However, aging and age-related changes are occurring in other systems as well, although those changes may not limit life span. The biological basis underlying the regulation of such changes may be the same, even though the time course and end point may be different. The fact that the trajectory of senescence of a particular cell type is such as to be irrelevant to the limitation of the organismic life span does not preclude the potential relevance of the mechanism by which the senescent changes occur. Indeed, some replicating cell types have an aging trajectory that would accommodate a much longer organismic life span than is observed.

Given that the definition of organismic aging is at present amorphous and vague, it is very difficult to pinpoint the relationship between aging in vitro and in vivo. However, the following discussion examines how and why cell cultures can be exploited to understand the biology of aging.

Aging and Evolution

One apparent paradox in evaluating the relevance of aging in cell cultures to aging in vivo derives from the general premise that aging is nonadaptive; that is, it is not selected for in an evolutionary sense. Since the decline in proliferative activity exhibited by cell cultures appears to be deterministic (genetically regulated) and may have adaptive significance in suppressing uncontrolled proliferation, the argument can be made that cell senescence in vitro cannot be aging. The logic of this argument may be flawed. Although organismic aging may be nonadaptive and may result from the decline in the force of natural selection, that does not define the function or role of individual cell populations within the organism in this process. It seems that the forces that shape the evolutionary success of a species could very well include processes in which the senescence of a given cell population is adaptive for the evolutionary success of the organism but irrelevant to the organismic aging process. There are many examples in early development which fit this model. Similarly, one could argue that these *adaptive* changes in certain cell types, while important for the evolutionary success of the species, represent an example of antagonistic pleiotropy in which the mechanisms of senescence, once activated, continue to be expressed and thus lead to continued cellular deterioration beyond the time or stage when it is *useful*. A fundamental question, however, is whether studies on the aging and dynamics of cell populations in vitro can yield information about the mechanisms of aging in vivo. Perhaps, for example, studies with cell cultures will elucidate the mechanism(s) underlying the workings and limits of biological clocks, which determine the trajectory of deteriorative changes.

In Vivo–In Vitro Parallel Changes

It is probable that any direct relationship between in vivo and in vitro aging, as described for fibroblasts, involves cells that are capable of continued proliferation in vivo. It is known, for example, that after an initially high rate of cell doubling, the proliferation rate of some cell types in vivo gradually, but continually, slows down (132) (Some cells of the gastrointestinal system have an increased proliferative activity and would appear to be an exception [8].) Buetow (24) tabulated and reviewed the literature on age-associated changes in cellular proliferation rates in vivo. In general, there is a decline in mitotic activity in a wide variety of human and rodent tissues. Many of the studies of cell proliferation in vivo, however, fall short of elucidating the relative contribution of intrinsic vs. extrinsic factors (alterations in the extracellular matrix, for example). Thus, evaluation of various biochemical and morphological parameters of functional capacity that accompany the decline in proliferative capacity in vitro may be of considerable importance to understanding of the mechanisms of senescence and the control of cell proliferation in vivo. Another group of studies bearing on this point involves the serial transplantation of normal somatic tissues to new, young, inbred hosts each time the recipient approaches old age (3, 52, 55, 98–101, 125, 126, 212, 225, 242). In general, normal cells serially transplanted to inbred hosts seem to show a decline in proliferative capacity and probably cannot survive indefinitely. Also, Olsson and Ebbesen (182) found that mouse epidermis from old donors retained an increased susceptibility to carcinogens whether they were transplanted into young or old recipients.

Decreased antibody production by spleen cells (but not bone marrow cells) transplanted from old mice into young irradiated recipients suggests that senescence of immune-reactive cells in mice may be related to a change undergone by these cells when they migrate from bone marrow to spleen (70). Harrison and Doubleday (101), Harrison et al. (102), Ogden and Micklem (180), and Albright and Makinodan (3) found that proliferative capacity was reduced in spleen cells derived from old animals and transplanted into young irradiated hosts. The trauma of transplantation, however, cannot be ruled out absolutely as a contributing factor to proliferative decline.

Perhaps one of the strongest sources of support for the relationship of a limited life span in vitro to aging in situ springs from a variety of work that suggests a cumulative effect of in situ aging plus in vitro aging by showing a relationship between the age of the cell donor and the proliferative capacity of the cells derived from that donor (80, 111, 153). Martin et al. (153) showed a regression of approximately 0.20 cell doublings/year from ages 0–90 in a large number of subjects. The regression was highly significant ($p < 0.001$) even though the variance was large. An inverse relationship between replicative life span and donor age has also been rigorously demonstrated for skin fibroblasts derived from aged Fischer 344 rats (201).

An extensive study (233) of the in vitro growth of skin fibroblasts from old and young human donors showed a statistically significant decrease in the rate of fibroblast outgrowth, in vitro life span, cell population replication rate, and cell number at confluence of cultures derived from old donors when compared to parallel cultures from young donors. The differences between cells from young and old donors grown in vitro, while significant, were not as large as the differences found between early- and late-passage fetal lung (WI-38) fibroblasts.

In a subsequent study, Smith et al. (251) compared the clone size distribution of cultures derived from individuals of various ages. The population used was essentially the same as that used by Schneider and Mitsui (233) in the earlier study described above. Smith et al. found that cultures of fetal origin gave rise to the highest percentage of rapidly growing colonies, whereas cultures from old adults gave rise to the lowest percentage of large colonies. A comparable relationship between growth potential and donor age has been found for mouse aorta, media, and adventitia (151). A relationship between growth potential and maximal life span of the donor has also been found for several other species (77, 142, 152).

Similar in vivo–in vitro parallels have been found for human liver cells (133) and for epidermal cells (219) from young and old subjects. Decreased replicative capacity with increasing donor age has also been found for 17 lines of human arterial smooth muscle cells (15). An inverse relationship between replicative life span of human keratinocytes and donor age was reported by Willie et al. (287). Keratinocytes derived from neonates grew for approximately 50 population doublings, while those derived from adults were senescent after about 30 population doublings. In both cases, the cells became arrested in the G_1 phase of the cell cycle. In addition, an inverse relationship between proliferative response and differentiation suggests that these processes may be regulated in an integrated manner.

A finding by Ryan et al. (230) supported the concept that cell replicative life spans are genetically determined. They found that skin fibroblasts from three pairs of monozygotic twins showed no significant difference in replicative life span within each twin pair but did show such differences among pairs. In addition, Röhme (223) described the replicative life span for cells from a series of mammals of different life spans, and although some of these cell lines eventually underwent immortalization, the decline in replicative capacity was seen clearly (see, for example, Pignolo et al. [201]). Thus species maximum life span potential is expressed in fibroblast culture in terms of proliferative capacity.

Correlated with the above are findings that show age-related changes in cell physiology. For example, cell cultures derived from adult lung have lysosomal enzyme characteristics after only 12–14 passages that are similar to those of fetal cells after 35–50 passages (49), and adult skin cells show cell-cycle characteristics after only a few passages that are similar to those of degenerating fetal cell cultures (141, 145). Goldstein et al. (77) and Martin et al. (149, 153) showed that cells from patients with Hutchinson-Gilford syndrome or Werner syndrome, both of which are associated with progeroid syndromes, have a reduced proliferative capacity compared with control cells from normal donors of the same ages. Progeroid syndromes are generally defined by the premature appearance of characteristics of senescence. None of them can be considered a phenocopy of normal human aging, since all the characteristics of aging are not present. Thus, Martin (149) suggested that they be referred to as "segmental" progeroid syndromes because they approximate certain aspects of the aging process. The evidence for a limited replicative life span is much stronger for the case of Werner syndrome than it is for Hutchinson-Gilford syndrome (progeria or progeria of childhood). Other workers have reported decreased mitotic activity, DNA synthesis, and cloning efficiency for cells from affected subjects (54, 175). In addition, cells derived from diabetic individuals have a reduced ability to grow and survive in culture, as reflected in a reduced plating efficiency (80). These studies, however, are complicated by other factors (see Goldstein [82] for example). Another genetic disorder correlated with early onset of senescence as determined by in vitro studies is Down syndrome (149, 231). The work describing changes in the replication of Down syndrome cells is controversial (115).

The possibility exists that these relationships are indirect and that the cell culture system is simply a model to study the regulation of cell proliferation which, in turn, shows age-associated changes. Even then, however, it represents an important model for aging since the two principal age-associated diseases, cancer and atherosclerosis, represent failures in the regulation of cell proliferation. Martin and Sprague (150, 151) reviewed the contrasting properties of hyperplastoid cells (normal cells that proliferate and have a limited replicative life span in culture) and neoplastoid cells (cells that have abnormal properties including an indefinite life span in culture) in culture and have speculated on their use as model systems for the study of various proliferation-related pathologies.

In other studies, Macieira-Coelho and co-workers showed that interspecies differences in fibroblast replicative behavior in vitro parallel the differences in species life span and that vulnerability to immortalization in culture is related to species life span and to rate of neoplasia development in vivo (142). This correlative evidence remains to be completely explored.

It is of interest that Soukupova et al. (254), in studying the latent period in cell growth, showed that explants of tissues from young donors appeared to contain a large quantity of cells capable of migration and division, whereas the tissues of older donors behaved like mosaics of tissue regions with fewer cells, or perhaps no cells, capable of division. Their study did not distinguish between intrinsic changes in the cells and extrinsic factors, such as collagen accumulation, which may impede the migration of cells from explanted tissue.

In addition to the loss of division potential associated with in vitro and in vivo cell aging already described, many other significant alterations that occur with in vitro senescence also occur with senescence in vivo (Table 4–1). These changes include, but are not limited to, the diminution of steady-state *EPC-1* mRNA levels, the overexpression of collagenase and stromelysin, and a decrease in accumulation of a tissue inhibitor of metalloproteinases (TIMP-1). These and other alterations that occur with cellular aging in vitro and in vivo are described in detail later under CELLULAR AND MOLECULAR MARKERS.

Overall, it is clear that characteristic aging changes in vivo are expressed in cell culture. Detailed analysis of these changes shows that they have the same apparent trajectory as aging in vitro and appear tightly coupled to the capacity for cell proliferation.

CAVEATS IN THE USE OF CELL CULTURES AS MODELS

Several questions have been leveled at the use of cell cultures as a primary model system for the study of aging. For example, if the limited life span of cells studied in vitro is truly relevant to aging, then it should be characteristic of cultures derived from all vertebrate species. The senescence of cells in culture has been carefully documented for human (110, 111, 114) and avian (108) cell cultures, and for cultures derived from the marsupial *Potorous tridactylis* (243). However, a number of reports involving various rodent cell cultures (127, 196, 277, 292), cultures derived from marsupials (255), and cultures of marine fish cells (217) indicate that all these cells maintain their proliferative capacity for what seem to be indefinite periods without any major alteration in karyotype. However, when many of these cell cultures are followed carefully they show the period of declining proliferative capacity (senescence) prior to the development of indefinite proliferative capacity (286). For a series of cultures that transform, Röhme (223) described the declining proliferative capacity prior to the emergence of the transformed population. In addition, certain cultures derived from human lymphoid elements seem to retain the normal diploid karyotype and have an indefinite life span (134, 168). One can offer the explanation documented in some cases (213) that these are not truly normal diploid cells and that minor or even undetectable changes in karyotype could be imparting the properties of neoplastic growth, that is, indefinite proliferation, on the culture. The best documented example of immortalized cells that display apparently normal karyotypes but have undetectable or cryptic changes in karyotype that are causally related to transformation is in chronic myelogenous leukemia (CML). A small subset of CML-affected individuals do not exhibit the typical 9;22 translocation but do display the c-abl-bcr fusion transcript and protein characteristic of the disease (170). Thus molecular changes causally related to neoplastic transformations can occur in the absence of karyotypic changes. In addition, the possible role of viruses in long-term, apparently diploid lymphoid cells is exceedingly interesting. It would appear, for instance, that most long-term lymphoid cultures have the Epstein-Barr virus. The idea that some, but not all, long-term lymphoid cultures can be maintained with optimal concentrations of interleukin-2 (IL-2) remains controversial (9).

A second area of past controversy involved the interpretation of the data describing the population dynamics of diploid cultures. Initially, it was not clear whether the progressive decline in cell proliferation was due to a uniform increase in cell generation times in the culture or whether the culture was a heterogeneous population containing an increasing fraction of cells that were incapable of dividing, or both. A number of lines of evidence appeared to favor the latter alternative. For example, Merz and Ross (161) showed that in very low-density populations the percentage of cells undergoing division within a fixed time period decreased as a function of the number of subcultivations. The increase in the fraction of "nondividers" in the population was clearly an age-related phenomenon. It was not clear, however, whether

TABLE 4.1. *Parallel Changes with Cellular Aging In Vitro and In Vivo*

	Selected References
Decreased proliferative capacity	111, 153, 233
Decreased saturation density	41, 233
Increased ploidy	56, 72
Loss of migratory capacity	254
Decreased mitogenic response to serum/growth factors	205, 245
Increase in cell size	244, 265
Decrease in colony size distribution	251
Overexpression of collagenase	163, 253
Overexpression of stromelysin	162
Decreased response to calcium ion	211
Decreased expression of TIMP-1	162
Decreased expression of *EPC-1*	see text
Decreased expression of IGFBP-3	80a
Changes in cellular morphology	244, 265

the same pattern of cell division prevailed in mass culture populations.

Macieira-Coelho and co-workers (144–146) reported an increased heterogeneity in the length of the division cycle in late-passage cells, due principally to an increased G_1 period and to the fact that the fraction of cells included in DNA synthesis decreased as a function of culture age.

Shortly thereafter evidence was gathered that further supported this interpretation. For example, Cristofalo and Sharf (44) showed that for the human diploid cell lines WI-38 and WI-26 there is an exponentially decreasing fraction of the cell population that can incorporate [^{3}H]thymidine into DNA. This fraction is directly related to the proliferative capacity of the cell population. A time-related decline in the proportion of cells labeled with [^{3}H]thymidine has been reported for several other cell types, including adult skin fibroblasts (278). Senescent fibroblasts have a predominantly 2C (diploid) DNA content (295), with an increase in unlabeled cells showing a 4C DNA content representing G_1 tetraploids (293). Cells with higher ploidy numbers also appear in senescent populations (293).

The replicative potential of human fibroblast-like cells derived from the same origin and maintained under tightly controlled conditions in mass culture is reproducible to within a very narrow range of population doublings. This reproducibility is often taken to mean that the in vitro life span of cultures derived and serially cultivated in a similar manner is in some way programed. However, clonal populations of cells established from mass cultures of different in vitro ages display a bimodal distribution of replication capacities (148, 249, 250). The distribution of clones shifted to those displaying increasingly shorter life spans as the population from which the clones were derived aged, and the fastest growing clones, when subcloned, again exhibited a bimodal distribution with respect to replicative capacity. Interestingly, the longest-lived clones were always able to achieve the same number of population doublings as the mass cultures from which the clones were derived. Clones derived from aged donors also displayed shorter life spans with increasing donor age (251). Merz and Ross (161), Smith and Hayflick (249), and Smith and Whitney (250) examined the doubling potential of several hundred clones derived from fibroblast cultures. In all cases, there was a large variation in clone size and life span (doubling potential) among the clones isolated from a single mass culture.

Martin and Sprague (151) observed the growth kinetics and morphology of clones and subclones of diploid human skin cultures. Their studies also demonstrated extensive heterogeneity in the cultures. A similar observation was made by Pious et al. (204). Further information on the heterogeneity of diploid cell cultures comes from the work of Absher and co-workers (1, 2), whose investigations, using microcinematography to follow the interdivision times of clones from populations of various ages, revealed a gradual lengthening of average interdivision time with successive generations in all genealogies studied regardless of passage level. In addition, their studies showed that after the first two divisions there was a marked variation in the interdivision times of daughter cells derived from a single clone. Late-passage cells exhibited much greater variation; interdivision times of daughter cells in any clone appeared not to be related in any simple way to one another or to the interdivision time of the parent. Further support for the notion of heterogeneity in diploid cell cultures has come from the work of Bowman and colleagues (16, 159).

In general, then, the evidence appears very strong that the loss of proliferative capacity in diploid cell populations is a very well-regulated phenomenon in which substantial heterogeneity develops in the population, and that changes include both an increased generation time and the failure of an increasing fraction of the population to replicate at all. Cristofalo (39) suggested that fibroblast aging may follow a differentiation lineage model. Martin et al. (154) also suggested that the finite life span may represent a differentiation of cell types and that the process of diploid cell growth may have an in vivo counterpart in hyperplastic processes. Bayreuther et al. (12) interpreted this in vitro age-related heterogeneity as a series of differentiation events as well, and defined an 11-stage lineage sequence composed of distinct pre- and postmitotic cell types. However, work by Quinn et al. (214) provides evidence that clonal senescence and terminal differentiation of myogenic stem cells are separate processes. Interestingly, senescent WI-38 cells exhibit a loss of the enzyme cortisone reductase (7). Reduction of cortisone to cortisol is a differentiated function for lung fibroblasts associated with the production of surfactant in fetal lung alveolar cells. In this case, senescent fibroblasts lose a differentiated function, perhaps gaining one or more as yet undetermined functions in the process.

Another issue to be resolved is whether the limitation on the life span of diploid cells is the result of inhospitable environmental factors, such as accumulation of misinformation, mutation, or deficiencies in the medium or of a "program" that predetermines cell death, or both. The mixing experiments of Hayflick and Moorhead (114) mentioned above, in which karyotypically distinguishable young and old cells were allowed to proliferate in the same medium, showed that the young cells were able to achieve their entire growth potential in the same medium in which the old cells degenerated. They interpreted this finding as proof that the medium composition was adequate for all the cells. Yet the results showed that the medium was adequate for the growth of the young cells only for a limited period, and the findings indicated nothing at all about the requirements for prolonged growth of cells or for the growth of old cells.

Little, if anything, is known about differences in the nutritional requirements of young vs. old cultures or of young vs. old individuals, so evaluation of this point is, at present, impossible. It is possible to conclude, however, that the growth requirements of young and senescent cells, if different, would reflect physiological differences that arise with senescence.

Some laboratories have reported that various components of the cell culture medium can extend the life span of chick and human cells. For the most part, those components were not chemically defined, such as various combinations of sera from different species, embryo extract, serum albumin, and tryptose phosphate broth (107). In every case, however, growth ultimately declined in the same way, although somewhat later. Attempts to repeat the findings of Todaro and Green (275) using a partially purified preparation of serum albumin were unsuccessful in achieving an extension of replicative life span in WI-38 fibroblasts (V. J. Cristofalo and J. Horton, unpublished data, 1994). In a comparison of the capacity of different sera to promote cell adhesion and growth, Cooper and Goldstein (37) found that human serum curtails replicative life span in strains of human skin fibroblasts, both in terms of calendar time and in terms of cumulative population doublings.

Little or no data are available on the effect of chemically defined substances on the life span. Both Cristofalo (38) and Macieira-Coelho (140) showed that cortisone and hydrocortisone can extend the life span of human cell cultures; however, this is probably not a nutritional effect in the usual sense. Several other investigators (71, 88, 130, 164, 227, 246, 271) confirmed this increased proliferative activity for a variety of fibroblast-like cell types after treatment with hydrocortisone, cortisone, or other corticosteroids. With these hormones, just as in the cases cited above, replicative senescence is postponed but not eliminated.

These examples and others support the view that environmental factors can affect the life span of cells in culture (even that of the hardiest, permanently proliferating cell line if the environment becomes severe enough). This is an experimental fact. Of biological significance, however, is not whether environment can affect life span but rather whether in normal cells there is also a "program" underlying these environmental effects. In support of this possibility is the observation of many workers that cultures from a single stock, such as WI-38 cells, grown in different laboratories with various standard, commercially available media all show a similar number of generations before degeneration of the culture.

The capacity of genetic and humoral factors to modulate DNA synthetic capacity and life span of fibroblasts in culture suggests that senescent cells, even those that are derived from single cells, are composed of heterogeneous subpopulations in terms of their ability to respond to mitogenic stimulation. These subpopulations can be divided operationally into those that are *conditionally* arrested and those that are *irreversibly* arrested, depending on their ability to respond to exogenous factors and initiate DNA synthesis (Fig. 4.1). Senescent cells that are conditionally arrested may be manipulated by various treatments to undergo at least one additional round of DNA replication. Manipulations include the addition of phorbol 12-myristate 13-acetate (PMA) or hydrocortisone to culture medium (38, 58), the incubation of cells with plasma membranes derived from young or senescent preparations extracted under basic conditions (69), transient expression of an inducible *c-fos* construct (200), or Simian virus 40 (SV40) infection (83). For example, late-passage cultures containing an exogenously added murine *c-fos* gene under the control of the sheep metallothionein promoter can be induced to enter DNA synthesis. The percentage of [^{3}H]thymidine-labeled cells was as much as six-fold higher in induced cells as in uninduced controls, provided the senescent cells used were conditionally arrested. If irreversibly arrested cells were selected by extended serial passaging in culture or by treatment with bromodeoxyuridine, the effect of the introduced *c-fos* construct upon induction was lost (200). Similarly, treatment of senescent cells with plasma membranes was ineffective if irreversibly arrested cells were selected (69).

Senescent cells that are irreversibly arrested cannot respond to the above manipulations (except SV40 infection) by entering DNA synthesis. SV40 infection is unlike other genetic or humoral manipulations in that it can drive senescent cells into DNA synthesis even when the cells are exhaustively selected for a nondividing phenotype. Senescent cells selected in this way and manipulated to enter DNA synthesis do not go on to mitosis (see below, under Deterministic Processes).

There is strong evidence that both genetic and stochastic processes occur with senescence in culture (51). Genetic "triggering" events and subsequent or concomitant uncoupling of regulated processes are not mutually exclusive. Dysregulation may result because of programmed events, and then unregulated processes could contribute to the ultimate proliferative decline. Alternatively, programed events may result in the cessation of proliferation, which in turn increases the likelihood of unregulated, deteriorative processes and renders the cell more susceptible to environmental insults.

A related question is whether the in vitro life span of cultured diploid cells reflects a genetically determined number of population doublings or whether it is a func-

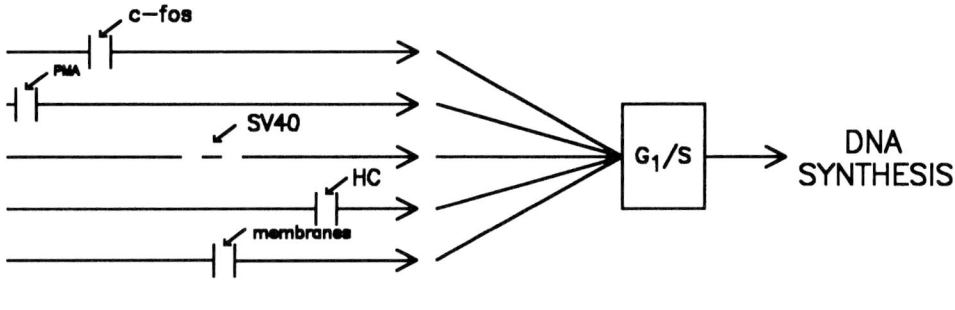

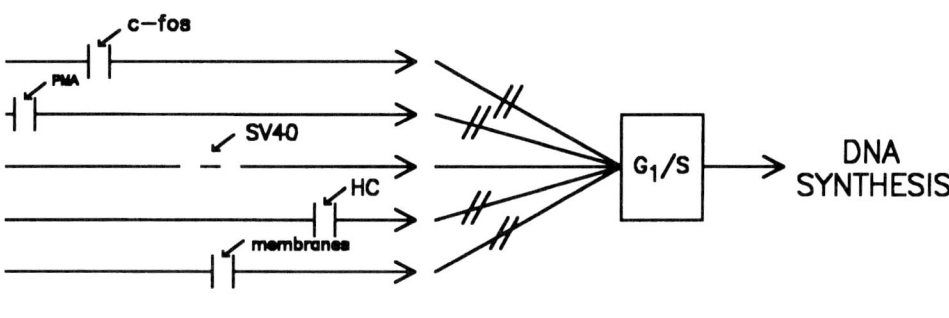

FIG. 4.1. Heterogeneity of senescent cells in culture. Multiple parallel pathways leading to DNA synthesis, one or more of which may be blocked in senescent cells (*ART*). These block(s) may be overcome in conditionally arrested cells by a variety of manipulations at putative target sites but not in irreversibly arrested cells, except by SV40 infection. *PMA*, phorbol 12-myristate 13-acetate; *HC*, hydrocortisone.

tion of time spent in culture. Initial evidence seemed to support the latter. For example, Hay and Strehler (108) and Weissman-Shomer and Fry (284) showed that chick cells subcultivated at high population densities went through fewer doublings than those at low population densities, but calendar life spans were essentially equivalent. Hay et al. (109) grew chick cells overlaid with agar to restrict divisions; upon subsequent cultivations, the culture died out at the same time as controls, irrespective of the number of divisions achieved. These workers concluded that the life span of cultured embryonic chick cells was a function of calendar time rather than of number of divisions undergone. Similarly, WI-38 diploid fetal lung fibroblasts subcultivated after 5 wk in stationary phase in medium containing 0.1% serum (v/v) were reported to have undergone fewer divisions than the continuously subcultivated controls, but all cultures reached phase III at the same point in calendar time (158).

In contrast to these findings, Dell'Orco et al. (57) maintained newborn human foreskin fibroblasts in a nondividing state in 0.5% serum for up to 177 days. When serum concentration was increased and the cells resumed division, they achieved approximately the same number of doublings as continuously proliferating controls, which became senescent after 32 doublings. Cultures that had been kept under maintenance conditions, however, lived a total of 287 days, while controls lived only 77 days. Dell'Orco's observations have been supported by Goldstein and Singal (79) who found that continually subcultivated clones and those maintained in stationary phase and then subcultured achieved about the same number of population doublings—56 and 53, respectively. However, a clear-cut extension of the calendar life span (75 days) was found for the cultures held in stationary phase. In addition, Harley and Goldstein (93) showed that, at any given time in circular outgrowths of human skin fibroblasts, mitotic cells at the circumference will have undergone more replications than cells located more centrally and are older. Similar findings supporting the view that replicative life span depends on cumulative population doublings have been presented by Mellgren (160) and Nielsen and Ryan (174) for chick embryo fibroblasts.

Other experiments (48) have shown that phase-out in young WI-38 cultures is determined primarily by population doublings. However, in old populations, events during the maintenance period could shorten life span to some degree.

It has also been reported that serial subcultivation of the human diploid fibroblast line from the Tokyo Metropolitan Institute of Gerontology (TIG-1) maintained in log phase resulted in cultures whose calendar life span was shortened but whose cumulative population doublings were increased when compared to cells serially cultivated by a 1:4 split (122). No morphological differences were noted between the two populations.

Angello et al. (6) showed that when fibroblasts were maintained in low serum at low densities, the cells lost replicative capacity. However, when fibroblasts were maintained in low serum at high densities, they did not lose replicative capacity.

To determine whether the frequency of subcultivation, that is, trypsin treatments, affected replicative life span, Hadley et al. (89) subcultivated cells at 1:10 and 1:1000 dilutions. The latter received fewer trypsin treatments and showed no increase in life span. In fact, a decrease in replicative life span was observed.

Taken together, the above findings indicate that chronological time appears to be significantly less important than division events in determining in vitro life span.

CELLULAR AND MOLECULAR MARKERS OF SENESCENCE IN VITRO AND IN VIVO

The steady loss of replicative potential is accompanied by a greater heterogeneity of cell sizes as well as a shift to much larger cell sizes (43, 87). Characteristic morphological alterations accompany the changes in cell size seen with senescence in culture (222). An increase in nuclear size (165), in nucleolar size (13, 14), and in the number of multinucleated cells (155) parallels the increase in cell size seen in slowly replicating or nonreplicating cultures. Prominent Golgi apparati, an evacuated endoplasmic reticulum, increased numbers of cytoplasmic microfilaments, vacuolated cytoplasm, and large lysosomal bodies have been observed in senescent human fibroblasts (20, 36, 135). Similar changes in cell size and morphology have been described for fibroblasts from aged donors (244, 265).

The increase in cell size exhibited by senescent cells in culture appears to be associated with their inability to utilize all of the growth surface available to them (87). Although larger cells are more likely to be nondividing in late-passage cultures—and there is a greater chance of finding enlarged cells in senescent cultures that have a reduced capacity to incorporate [³H]thymidine (166, 167)—large cells at any passage have reduced replicative capacities (5, 187).

Late-passage cultures display a reduced harvest density and a lowered saturation density at the plateau phase of growth (41, 146). At the end of their in vitro life span, substantial cell death occurs; however, a stable population emerges which can exist in a viable, although nonproliferative, state for many months (156). This stable population is capable of maintaining only an extremely low saturation density representing less than 5% of that achieved by early-passage cultures. The observed decrease in saturation densities most likely reflects an increased sensitivity to intercellular contact, since the forced contact of senescent cells, which is produced by overseeding, promotes the loss of cells from the culture until a density is achieved that is comparable to the density normally reached in the absence of such forced contact (203a). Thus, the original diploid cell life history formulation of Hayflick and Moorhead (114), which included a primary outgrowth phase, a period of vigorous growth, and a period of declining proliferation, must be amended to include a phase of cell death and the emergence of a long-lived postmitotic population (Fig. 4.2).

Whether alterations in the nature of cell contact among senescent cells can be attributed to changes at the level of extracellular matrix (ECM), to specific secretory proteins not connected with the ECM, or to membrane-associated molecules is unclear. Recent findings

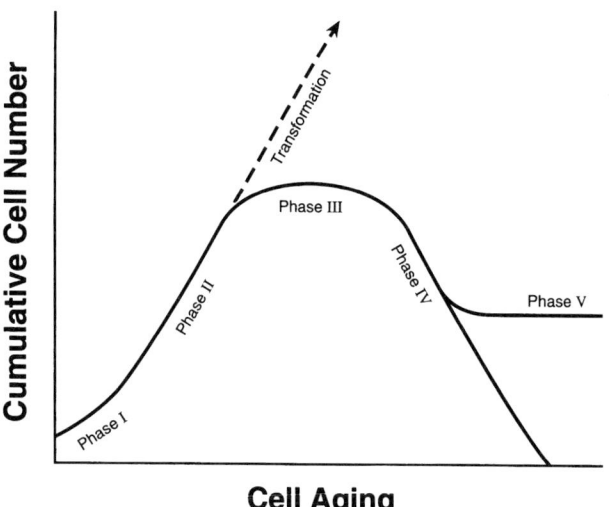

FIG. 4.2. Stages in the in vitro life history of normal human diploid fibroblasts. Phase I, outgrowth from explant; phase II, period of vigorous proliferation; phase III, decline in proliferative capacity; phase IV, cessation of proliferation and cell death; phase V, emergence of a stable, viable, but essentially nonproliferating cell population. *Dotted line* indicates the possibility, as a rare event, phase II cells may transform into an immortalized population acquiring an indefinite proliferation potential.

suggest that many proteins associated with the ECM are overexpressed in both senescent human fibroblasts and in fibroblasts from aged donors, as well as in fibroblasts from donors with progeroid syndromes (124, 147, 163, 172, 252, 253), including alpha 1 (I) procollagen, fibronectin, collagenase, and stromelysin. Fibronectin is also differentially expressed in late-passage fibroblasts in terms of the unmasking of antigenic determinants unique to senescence (208) and is correlated with increased cell size (129). The ECM, however, cannot exclusively account for the phenotypic changes that occur in late-passage cells. For example, when young fibroblasts are placed on ECM derived from senescent cells, they continue to proliferate with no apparent growth or morphological changes (V. J. Cristofalo and J. McIlhenney, unpublished data).

The differential expression of specific secretory proteins, such as IGF-I (65), IGF-I binding protein-3 (81), TIMP-1 (162), plasminogen activator inhibitor types 1 and 2 (128, 285, S. Goldstein, personal communication), and *EPC-1* (203), further demonstrates the complex changes that occur. Indirect evidence also indicates that alterations in membrane-associated molecules occur (69, 193, 258), since membrane preparations isolated from senescent cells (and quiescent young cells) can be inhibitory to cell proliferation when isolated under some conditions but stimulatory under other methods of extraction and preparation (see below under Deterministic Processes). In fact, membranes prepared from a variety of sources can be stimulatory depending on the method of extraction (69).

In general, as cells approach the end of their proliferative life span in vitro, the synthesis rate of macromolecules decreases, while the cellular content of macromolecules, except DNA, increases (Table 4.2). These observations are very reminiscent of the phenomenon of unbalanced growth in bacteria described over 30 years ago by Cohen and Barner (35). In senescent cells,

TABLE 4.2. *Cellular Changes with Senescence In Vitro*

Feature	Alteration	Selected References
Cell size	Increase	43, 87
Nuclear size	Increase	165
Saturation density	Decrease	41, 146
DNA content	No change	293, 295
RNA content	Increase	234
Protein content	Increase	47, 59
Glycogen content	Increase	222
Lipid content	Increase	47
Lysosome content	Increase	20, 36, 135
DNA synthesis rate	Decrease	44
RNA synthesis rate	Decrease	146, 235 206, 17
Protein synthesis rate	Decrease	45

it appears that DNA synthesis becomes uncoupled from other macromolecular syntheses and that there is a general dysregulation of coordinated processes.

As mentioned earlier (under CAVEATS IN THE USE OF CELL CULTURES . . .), studies by Yanishevsky et al. (295) have shown that most of the nondividing cells in senescent WI-38 populations have a 2C DNA content. This implies that the cells were arrested in the G_1 phase of the cell cycle. Also noted was an increase in unlabeled cells with a 4C DNA content. Subsequent studies of Yanishevsky and Carrano (293) indicated that these cells were G_1 tetraploids and not G_2 diploids. Thus senescent WI-38 cells remain essentially diploid to very near the end of their in vitro life span, when they exhibit structural chromosomal changes and increasing levels of tetraploidy and polyploidy.

Similar chromosomal alterations occur with in vivo cell aging (56, 72). At least one study has reported a small decrease in DNA content in human fibroblasts with in vitro age (232). It should be noted that there is an inherent bias in all of the studies designed to evaluate chromosomal changes with aging in vitro in that cytogenetic analyses can only be carried out with proliferating cells—that is, the least senescent cells in the aged culture.

Schneider and Shorr (234) reported the amount of all species of cellular RNA (ribosomal, transfer, and messenger) to be elevated in late-passage cultures, with the ratio of mRNA to total cellular RNA remaining constant in cells before and after senescence. Johnson et al. (121), however, showed that the ratio of mRNA to rRNA was about 30% lower in senescent cells than in young cells. Protein content also increases with increasing in vitro age (47). Since RNA and protein synthesis increase as cells progress from early to late G_1, it has been suggested (43, 234) that the uncoupling of cell growth from cell division, evidenced by increased cell-cycle times and/or the apparent late G_1 block in senescent cells, may result in the net accumulation of these and other macromolecules as well as increased cell size. Decreased protein turnover accompanied by, or as the result of, impaired protein degradation and removal machinery may account for an increase in protein content (59). Increased cell size (see the beginning of this section) and the related idea of continued growth in the absence of DNA synthesis and division may be the basis for the accumulation of RNA and protein as well as other macromolecules in senescent cells.

DNA, RNA, and protein synthetic rates decrease in late population doubling level cultures and may be related to the altered template activity in senescent cells. The loss of DNA synthetic capacity and arrest in late G_1 (see the final paragraphs of this section) would limit the absolute number of unique transcription events (and subsequently the number of potential translations) of those genes normally induced during S phase, G_2, and mitosis. Changes in chromatin structure with senescence could also result in a net decrease of transcription events due to an inaccessibility of local template regions. Ryan and Cristofalo (228), for example, showed an age-associated reduction in chromatin template activity in WI-38 cells that was consistent with a decrease in the number of net transcriptional events.

There is a marked reduction in the rate of RNA synthesis in senescent cells (146, 228, 235), and in transcription levels in response to serum stimulation (206). Bowman et al. (17), however, suggested that the in vitro age-related decline in RNA synthesis may be due almost entirely to the decreased synthesis of nucleolar RNA.

Although in vitro age-related decreases in protein synthesis have been reported (45), it is unclear if these changes have to do with impaired translational capacity, translational control, or mRNA template availability. Seshadri et al. (237a) has reported that early passage, quiescent and senescent fibroblasts synthesize protein at similar rates, and although the mRNAs encoding five ribosomal proteins (L5, P1, S3, S6, and S10) were equivalently expressed in senescent cells, there was a decline in mRNA for the ribosomal L7 protein.

Several lines of evidence support the concept that senescent cells are blocked in late G_1 near the G_1/S boundary in the cell cycle. The thymidine kinase activity in old, slowly proliferating cultures of WI-38 cells was found to be similar to that of young, rapidly dividing populations (40, 181). This apparent anomaly first raised the possibility that senescent cells retained the ability to phosphorylate thymidine and thus may be arrested in late G_1, since thymidine kinase is cell cycle–regulated and appears at the G_1/S boundary (40, 181). Subsequently, Olashaw et al. (181) found that thymidine triphosphate (TTP) synthesis is not impaired in senescent cells. The addition of serum to density-arrested populations of young and old cells induced TTP synthesis to a similar extent after 12 h in both populations. However, a far greater percentage of young cells subsequently initiated DNA synthesis as compared to old cells. Induction of thymidine kinase activity and TTP synthesis are cell cycle–dependent events that normally occur in late G_1, suggesting that senescent cells might be blocked in a state distinct from G_0 and with properties of late G_1.

Additional support for a late G_1 block comes from examining nuclear fluorescence following staining with quinacrine dihydrochloride (84). As serum-stimulated cells traverse G_1 and reach S, the staining pattern changes from bright and homogeneous to attenuated and segregated. The fluorescence pattern of senescent cells is typical of late G_1. Nucleolar association is also consistent with senescent cells arresting in late G_1 (V. J. Cristofalo, B. Martin, B. Razi, M. Anderson, and R. J. Pignolo, unpublished results).

Rittling et al. (221) examined the expression of 11 cell cycle–dependent genes in senescent WI-38 cells and compared the results to those obtained in young cells. Following serum stimulation of quiescent cultures, every gene studied was expressed at least qualitatively, in senescent cells at similar times and to roughly similar levels as those in young cells. This includes thymidine kinase, a gene maximally expressed at the G_1/S boundary. Chang and Chen (32), however, reported decreases in thymidine kinase mRNA levels and thymidine kinase activity in senescent IMR-90 fibroblasts. In the same study, Chang and Chen found similar steady-state mRNA levels for ornithine decarboxylase and c-myc in young and senescent cells, although a decreased activity for the former. These data strongly suggest that both young and senescent cells appear to respond to fresh mitogens by carrying out some of the same cell cycle processes in roughly the same time frame. However, the ability to complete the mitogen-initiated cascade of signal transduction pathways and to synthesize DNA is lost in senescent cells.

Seshadri and Campisi (237) reported findings similar to those reported by Rittling et al. (221) and Chang and Chen (32) with cell cycle–regulated genes, but they noted the inability of senescent cells to produce the transcript for c-fos at steady-state levels comparable to those found in young cells (see later under Signal Transduction Pathways). Detection of c-fos mRNA accumulation in senescent cells appears to be technique-sensitive and may vary with such things as cell culture conditions (58, 186, 241). Prior to serum stimulation, for example, senescent cells preincubated with PMA show enhanced c-fos expression (58). However, it seems clear that c-fos regulation is different in young and senescent cells. Stein et al. (264) showed that other growth-regulated genes expressed in G_1 such as cdc2 and cyc A, are repressed (see later under Signal Transduction Pathways). If senescent cells are irreversibly arrested in a unique state different from the normal cell-cycle stages, then it is not surprising that G_0/G_1 growth-regulated genes are repressed. However, the fact that some G_0/G_1 growth-regulated genes are not repressed in cells that fail to replicate suggests that only particular pathways are affected.

MECHANISTIC STUDIES OF IN VITRO REPLICATIVE SENESCENCE

Stochastic Mechanisms

Stochastic mechanisms for cellular senescence can generally be explained in one of three ways: the "somatic mutation" theory, the "error catastrope" theory, or the "free radical damage" theory (see Chapter 1). However, these are not mutually exclusive. More sophisticated versions of some of the above theories have emerged to explain certain shortcomings of the original versions, although many of the refinements have also been equivocal.

The classical somatic mutation theory as put forth by Szilard (269) proposed random mutational "hits" which accumulated and produced a level of damage incompatible with life. A mathematical re-evaluation of this theory with respect to the finite replicative life span of normal diploid fibroblasts still required a mutation rate at least two orders of magnitude greater than experimental estimates (116); further refinements have invoked mutational interactions (169), the activity of transposable elements (53), and epimutations such as changes in methylation status (68). The most convincing evidence to date suggests that enforced and accelerated random changes in DNA demethylation by 5-azacytidine in human diploid fibroblasts can reduce proliferative capacity, although not in direct proportion to the final methylation status obtained during normal in vitro aging (86).

Differences in DNA repair capacity (103, 185) and susceptibility to mutagenesis (236) have been suggested to be proportional to species life span and may represent evolutionary change. Hart et al. (105) have also observed that in two species that are similar to each other, *Mus musculus* and *Peromyscus leucopus*, but that have different life spans, the longer-lived species demonstrated greater excision repair of UV-induced damage. Reduced DNA repair capacity with age of cells in culture (18, 76, 104, 157, 184) and with in vivo age (131) has also been reported, although contradictory results have also appeared (19, 247). This area of inquiry remains controversial.

The error catastrophe theory (183) predicts that the accumulation of random defects in cellular proteins involved in transcription and translation would be autocatalytic in that error-containing proteins would produce more error-containing proteins, ultimately reaching a level incompatible with continued normal cell function. Although there have been conflicting reports of the accuracy of the protein synthetic machinery in senescent fibroblasts (137, 189), the introduction of random errors into proteins by feeding low levels of amino acid analogs had no effect on the proliferative life span of cells allowed to incorporate such analogs for extended periods (229).

The ability of senescent cells to remove altered or partially degraded proteins may be impaired, however, and the resulting accumulation of functionally defective proteins may thus ensue (59, 85).

In vitro age-associated changes in protein structure and function have been reported (117, 218, 226), and these alterations must be distinguished from the random introduction of errors if they are the result of a regulated series of senescence-specific events. Two examples of senescence-specific alterations in protein structure are the cleavage of immunoprecipitated epidermal growth factor (EGF)–receptor by a leupeptin-sensitive protease in detergent extracts from senescent, but not young, fibroblasts (26a) and the overexpression of the two-chain form of cathepsin B in senescent cells (60). The latter probably also results from senescence-specific protease activity.

The free radical damage theory, usually attributed to Harman (96, 97), proposes that free radicals that escape destruction by protective enzyme systems, such as superoxide dismutase, cause cumulative damage to important biological structures. Balin et al. performed extensive studies showing that low oxygen tension and alpha tocopherol do not extend the replication potential of WI-38 cells (10, 11). To date very few reports describing the relationship between free radical generation and proliferative life span of human diploid cells have been produced. One such study noted that manipulated increases in cellular glutathione by N-acetylcysteine resulted in an extension of replicative life span of TIG-1 human fibroblasts (118). This result suggests that cellular defense mechanisms directed against the toxic effects of oxygen radicals may influence proliferative life span directly or that glutathione may indirectly modulate proliferation through its roles in mitogenic stimulation, protein synthesis, or the reduction of ribonucleotides (118).

Allen and Balin (4) have found no significant differences in the levels of either the cupro-zinc or mangano forms of superoxide dismutase in skin fibroblast lines derived from postnatal donors ranging from 4 to 98 years of age. This finding indicates that if oxygen radical scavengers exert an influence on aging, in general, they probably influence proliferative capacity by secondary mechanisms rather than by destruction of free radicals per se.

Signal Transduction Pathways

A major approach to studying the regulation of cessation of replication in senescent cells has been to examine at various levels pathways that likely play significant roles in regulating cell proliferation and adaptive responses (Tables 4.3, 4.4).

Human diploid fibroblasts, at or near the beginning of their in vitro replicative life span, vigorously respond to serum or a defined combination of growth factors by DNA synthesis and mitosis. As these cells approach the end of their proliferative potential in culture they become increasingly refractory to mitogenic signals (46,

TABLE 4.3. *Changes in Steady-State mRNA Levels with Senesence**

Cell Cycle Position	Expressed Similarly in Senescent Cells	Overexpressed in Senescent Cells	Underexpressed in Senescent Cells
G_0		EF-1α, MnSOD mt ETS, PAI-1 LPC-1†, SAG IGF-BP3, PAI-2 Stromelysin Collagenase	EPC-1 EPC-A2 TIMP-1 IGF-I
G_1	JE-3 c-myc 4F1, c-jun 2F1, jun B p53, ODC TK, Calcyclin Calmodulin‡	LPC-1† Fibronectin IGF-BP3	c-fos cdc-2 PCNA§ IGF-I cycA cdK2 cdK4
Constitutive	β₂M, β-actin		HSP70, HSP90 pHE-7

*Changes in the expression of genes that are regulated, at least in part, by pre-DNA replicative mechanisms are shown. The expressions of some genes listed above have both pre- and post-DNA replicative components, but only the pre-DNA replicative components are shown, since changes in post-DNA replicative expression may be related to the failure of senescent cells to enter S phase. †Dysregulation: transcription uncoupled from translation. ‡Dysregulation. transcription uncoupled from cell cycle regulation. §Processing failure.
NOTE: Differences of twofold or less are not distinguished.

119, 197). A decreased mitogenic response to growth factors in vitro has also been observed for in vivo–aged cells (205, 245). The basis for this loss of responsiveness cannot be attributed to either dramatic reductions in the number of cell-surface growth-factor receptors or to the affinities with which these receptors bind ligands. In WI-38 cells, for example, both the number of receptors for EGF, platelet-derived growth factor (PDGF), and insulin-like growth factor (IGF-I) (per unit cell surface area) and receptor affinity for their ligands remain essentially unchanged with in vitro age (73, 198, 199). Interestingly, senescent WI-38 cells do not produce the mRNA or the protein for IGF-I (68a). The IGF-I receptor, however, is equivalently made in young and senescent WI-38 cells (236a).

Changes at the level of the growth-factor receptor, however, can be delineated upon examination of tyrosine kinase activity. The EGF receptor from detergent-solubilized, immunoprecipitated WI-38 senescent cell preparations loses its ability to autophosphorylate both in the presence and in the absence of EGF stimulation (26). This ability appears to be dependent upon the

TABLE 4.4. *Changes in Proteins with Senesence**

Cell Cycle Position	Expressed Similarly in Senescent Cells	Overexpressed in Senescent Cells	Underexpressed in Senescent Cells
G_0	Cytochrome oxidase	Statin Cathepsin B/2 chains Stromelysin Calmodulin† IGF-BP3 Collagenase	EPC-1 Stability of EGF-R phosphorylation‡ Cortisone reductase
G_1		Calmodulin† Cathepsin B/2 chains	ODCase EF-1α RB phosphorylation§ cdc-2 kinase
Constitutive			HSP70, HSP90 DNA pol.α

*Changes in the expression of genes that are regulated, at least in part, by pre-DNA replicative mechanisms are shown. The expressions of some genes listed above have both pre- and post-DNA replicative components, but only the pre-DNA replicative components are shown since changes in post-DNA replicative expression may be related to the failure of senescent cells to enter S phase. †Not cell cycle–regulated; overexpressed at all points in G_1. ‡Increased lability, thus decreased functional stability. §RB phosphorylation decreased. NOTE: Differences of twofold or less are not distinguished.

nature of the extraction used to isolate the EGF receptor from senescent cells, since the kinase activity remains intact when examined in situ (21, 34). These results suggest the existence of a more labile form of the EGF receptor or closely associated moiety in senescent cells. Recently, Carlin et al. (26a) showed that an altered form of the EGF receptor is present in detergent extracts from senescent cells, but not young cells. This altered form is the cleavage product of an endogenous, leupeptin-sensitive proteolytic activity present in senescent cells.

Fibroblasts respond to mitogens through the intracellular actions of secondary events, including phospholipid turnover, protein kinase C activation, and calcium mobilization. Alterations in postreceptor transduction pathways have been documented for arachidonic acid (AA) and prostaglandin (PG) metabolism from phospholipids in senescent cells (50). Substantial increases in both AA and the subsequent production of PGs can be seen in late-passage human fibroblasts (50, 173). Given the ability of exogenously added PG_{E2} to inhibit the proliferation of replication-competent cells, the above results indicate a possible role for PGs as regulators of negative growth control. Although the release of AA from membrane phospholipids is mediated by phospholipase A_2, whose activity appears to be intact in senescent WI-38 cells, phospholipid turnover by phospholipase $C_\gamma 1$ in senescent IMR-90 cells (an Institute for Medical Research cell line) is impaired (33).

Calcium ion (Ca^{2+}) is a potent modulator of cell proliferation for fibroblasts (210) and, in fact, can completely replace serum or growth factors as mitogens at supraphysiological concentrations (209). Both proliferatively senescent and in vivo–aged fibroblasts have a reduced ability to respond to extracellular calcium as measured by increases in saturation density (211). Young and senescent WI-38 fibroblasts have similar resting (quiescent) intracellular Ca^{2+} levels and exhibit similar changes in cytosolic Ca^{2+} fluxes following growth factor stimulation (22). Skin fibroblasts from aged donors have slightly reduced cytosolic-free Ca^{2+} levels (195) and slightly elevated amounts of bound Ca^{2+} (194). The mRNA of the calcium-binding/regulatory protein calmodulin is expressed similarly in young and senescent cells in terms of timing and steady-state levels; however, the protein as detected by radioimmunoassay is uncoupled from the cell cycle and exists in variable amounts in senescent WI-38 cells (22). Calmodulin-associated phosphodiesterase activity also appears to be diminished in late-passage cells (F. L. Cianciarulo and V. J. Cristofalo, manuscript in preparation). Thus an immunologically active, but functionally inactive, pool of calmodulin may be present in senescent cells.

Signal transduction pathways mediated by protein kinase A (PKA) or protein kinase C (PKC) are not altered in senescent cells owing simply to inadequate concentrations of these enzymes (15a). However, recent findings indicate that senescent cells have an impaired ability to translocate PKC to the cell membrane following mitogen stimulation (58). The association of PKC with the cell membrane is taken to be an indication of the fidelity of this signal transduction pathway, which seems not to be intact in senescent cells. Taken together, the above results suggest that late-passage fibroblasts are unresponsive to mitogenic stimulation, in part because of faulty or unregulated second-messenger systems.

As mentioned above, (see earlier under CELLULAR AND MOLECULAR MARKERS . . .) a number of early- and late-cell cycle–regulated genes are expressed in senescent WI-38 fibroblasts, including *c-myc*, *H-ras*, and thymidine kinase (221). The early-response gene *c-fos*, however, is repressed in late-passage cells (237) under certain conditions, and the ability of these cells to form active AP-1 complexes is also severely reduced (220). Moreover, there is a tendency toward Jun-Jun homodimers in senescent cells in contrast to the Fos-Jun heterodimers seen in young cells (220). The forced expression of an inducible *c-fos* construct by transient transfection of senescent cells results in as much as a sixfold increase in the number of cells capable of initiating DNA synthesis (200). In contrast to these findings, the induction of *c-fos* in senescent fibroblasts by microinjection of oncogenic *c-Ha-ras* protein was not sufficient for DNA synthesis (224). The diminished capacity of senescent cells to make *c-fos* in response to various manipulations, however, may be in part a function of the cell culture conditions used prior to induction of the gene (58, 186, 241), as mentioned earlier under CELLULAR AND MOLECULAR MARKERS. . . .

While the repression of *c-fos* transcription provides evidence for an early block in one or more pathways potentially required for DNA synthesis, later events may also be required. For example, the accumulation of mRNAs for cyclins A and B, as well as two of the D-type cyclins, is diminished in senescent fibroblasts (264, 289). The expression of two cyclin-dependent kinase genes, cdk2 and cdk4, is also diminished in senescent cells (2a, 138a). The retinoblastoma (RB) gene product fails to be phosphorylated in senescent cells (263), most likely because of the absence of the *cdc2* gene product and associated cyclins (264). This is particularly intriguing given that the RB gene product binds SV40 large T antigen and that large T antigen is capable of facilitating escape from senescence (238, 291). As mentioned below, T-antigen deletion mutants lacking either the RB- or p53-binding domains are unable to mediate escape from senescence (238). That unregulated antioncogenes may in some way prevent senescent cells from entering S phase is supported by studies in which antisense oligomers to RB and another antioncogene, p53, can extend the in vitro life span of human diploid fibroblasts by about one-third (91).

The hallmark of senescence in culture is the inability of cells to replicate their DNA. The formal possibility exists, then, that replicative enzymes themselves and/or replication-associated processes, such as control of DNA hierarchical structural orders, are reduced or altered. There is, for example, a direct relationship between the concentration of DNA polymerase alpha and the rate of entry into S phase (187), suggesting that the local availability of a replicative enzyme may be rate limiting. This observation is supported by the failure of senescent fibroblasts to complement a temperature-sensitive DNA polymerase alpha mutant (178). Similarly, senescent cells are unable to express the proliferating cell nuclear antigen (PCNA), the co-factor of DNA polymerase delta, presumably by a posttranscriptional block (31). In senescent cells the replication-dependent histones are also repressed, and a variant histone polyadenylated RNA is expressed uniquely (237). Although these findings suggest gross changes in the DNA synthetic machinery of senescent cells, the observation that SV40 can initiate an additional round of semiconservative DNA synthesis in old cells (83) indicates that this machinery is still intact.

The examples cited point to a progressive reduction in the ability of normal cells to respond to environmental signals (for example, mitogenic stimulation) with increasing in vitro age. Normal fibroblast-like cells also have a progressive reduction in their ability to respond adaptively to environmental stresses. Liu et al. (136) and Luce and Cristofalo (138) reported a reduction in heat shock gene expression in response to acute hyperthermic exposure and sodium arsenite. Interestingly, the preinduction of heat shock genes in senescent cells reduced their increased thermal lability in response to acute hyperthermia (138). In addition, the mRNA for the mangano form of superoxide dismutase is increased in senescent human fibroblasts, presumably in response to environmental stresses to which they are more susceptible (128; R. G. Allen, B. Keogh, and V. J. Cristofalo, unpublished results, 1994).

Genetic Mechanisms

Deterministic Processes. The nonproliferative phenotype of senescent cells in culture is dominant over normal proliferative cells and immortalized cells, but not over immortalized variants that have high levels of DNA polymerase alpha (DNA pol α) or those transformed by DNA tumor viruses. Evidence supporting these observations comes from cell fusion studies in which senescent cells were fused to their young counterparts or to various immortalized cells (177, 188, 190, 259, 261). In each case, the replication-competent nucleus within each heterokaryon was observed for its ability to synthesize DNA in the presence of the senescent cell nucleus. For those fusions in which the replication-competent nucleus was inhibited, it was necessary for the cycling parental cell to be in early to mid-G_1 or in G_2. Ongoing DNA synthesis was not affected by the presence of the senescent cell nucleus (294). Quiescent, early-passage fibroblasts can replace senescent cells in these heterokaryon experiments with similar results (260, 262). In fusion studies using immortalized variants containing high levels of DNA pol α or cells transformed with DNA tumor viruses, senescent cells were not able to inhibit the replication-competent nucleus, and the senescent nucleus itself was then able to synthesize DNA (188, 261). Although HeLa cells can "rescue" senescent cell DNA synthesis, it has not been rigorously proved that they are immortalized by viral genes. Furthermore, Pendergrass et al. (188) showed that even young normal diploid fibroblasts, if they have sufficiently high concentrations of DNA pol α, can rescue up to 30% of senescent cells.

Experiments on the ability of transformed cell lines to complement recessive defects responsible for an immortalized phenotype reportedly identified at least four complementation groups (191, 192). In these experiments, the fusion of two immortalized cell lines would yield hybrids exhibiting either indefinite cell division (indicating the same genetic defect) or finite cell division (indicating different genetic defects). The former would then be assigned to the same complementation group, the latter to different groups. These results suggest that there is a limited number of genes or sets of genes that may be responsible for escape from senescence. The interpretation of these results has recently become more difficult given the reports that fusions of infinite life span cells of different complementation groups failed to exhibit finite life spans (230a) and that the fusion of cells within the same complementation group resulted in hybrids with limited life spans (285a, 63b). For example, Ryan et al. (230a) has shown that 52 of 53 fusions of indefinite life span cell lines failed to yield finite life span hybrids. As discussed later in this section, "escape" from senescence may not be regulated by the same steps that regulate senescence. However, these results further demonstrate the recessive nature of cellular immortality.

There are numerous reports documenting the presence of inhibitors of DNA synthesis in senescent cells, although the nature of these inhibitors is poorly understood and whether any of them play a causal role in senescence is unclear. In the heterokaryon studies already mentioned, when cycloheximide was included in the cell culture medium, no inhibition of DNA synthesis was observed in the young cells. This suggested that an inhibitor, presumably a protein, was produced by senescent cells that inhibited DNA synthesis in both members of the heterokaryon (25, 63). Senescent cell–derived cytoplasts can mimic the effect of intact senescent cells in fusion studies similar to those described above (63). In other experiments, inhibitory activity can be demonstrated using preparations of senescent cell membranes or membrane preparations of young cells made quiescent by a variety of methods (193, 258). The inhibitory activity present in senescent cell membranes is sensitive to the nature of the extraction used in the preparation of the membranes. As mentioned earlier under CELLULAR AND MOLECULAR MARKERS . . . , preparation of membranes under neutral or acidic conditions preserves the inhibitory activity, while basic conditions actually make senescent cell membranes stimulatory (69).

The idea that senescent cells actively make an inhibitor of DNA synthesis is further supported by the observation that poly A^+ RNA derived from senescent fibroblasts, when microinjected into proliferation-competent cells, can inhibit their entry into DNA synthesis (139). Poly A^+ RNA prepared from quiescent, early-passage fibroblasts showed a similar effect, although at a greater concentration. Presumably, cells of all ages make both stimulators and inhibitors of DNA synthesis. If the ratio of these substances in in vitro–aged cells changes, so too must their phenotype. A question of major interest, then, is whether inhibitors shown to be overexpressed in senescence represent merely a quantitative difference in inhibitors present throughout the life span or, alternatively, whether senescence is marked by a different spectrum of molecules unrelated to the inhibitors of DNA synthesis (and proliferation) present in normal young cells.

As already mentioned, as senescent cells reach an "irreversibly" arrested condition they attain a state distinct from either the G_0 phase that young cells achieve or any other definable state within the cell cycle (51). The pattern of gene expression exhibited by senescent cells, under conditions that would define the quiescent state in early-passage cells, is different from that of a functional G_0 state. The fact that late-passage cells can express some of the gene characteristics of the G_1/S boundary suggests an "abortive attempt" to initiate DNA synthesis and arrest in a unique state (Fig. 4.3).

Young cells can be made to resemble senescent cells, in terms of increased size and reduced proliferative capacity, under conditions of low density and low serum concentration (6). This finding suggests that an uncoupling of growth from DNA synthesis occurs with extended time in low serum. A functional "low serum" state may also occur in senescent cells as a consequence of signal transduction failures, resulting in a similar kind of uncoupling. Alternatively, a late G_1 block could prevent DNA synthesis without hindering cell growth and could also result in the uncoupling of growth from proliferation. If cells must complete S phase, G_2 events, and mitosis in order to return to G_0 from late G_1, then the inability to return to G_0 may gradually destroy the normal coordination of cell growth with cell division.

It is attractive to think that both young and senescent human diploid fibroblasts make related or identical inhibitors of DNA synthesis, one or more of which may lose tight regulatory control in late-passage cells and send them into proliferative decline. However, the evidence suggesting that senescent and quiescent young cells share a common inhibitor(s) of DNA synthesis is indirect and may occur because these cell types display a nongrowth phenotype rather than as an indication of a causal relationship between quiescence and senescence. The balance of both negative and positive modulating factors likely plays a critical role in the onset and progression of replicative arrest.

Although cells that escape from senescence to achieve an unlimited division potential are, by definition, immortal, it is not clear if the mechanism(s) by which immortality is achieved is related in any direct way to the mechanism(s) involved in senescence; that is, immortality is not simply a direct reversal of senescence. The genes activated or inactivated as a requirement for immortality may not be the same as those that regulate senescence as it occurs in normal cells.

Similarly, those chromosomes that have been reported to cause immortalized cells to acquire a senescent phenotype may not carry genes that play a direct role in senescence as it normally occurs. If such genes are replaced, as was accomplished in the microcell fusion studies described at the end of this section, finite life spans are achieved for the recipients, suggesting that proliferative controls have been restored. It is unclear, however, if the same controls that, when disrupted, mediate escape from senescence are also responsible for senescence to occur as a programmed event after an undetermined number of population doublings.

The DNA-containing SV40 can transform normal human diploid fibroblast (HDF) cultures and confer onto them an indefinite proliferative potential (120, 276). Transformation of cells by SV40 requires integration of at least part of the viral genome, and this process occurs more efficiently in dividing cells. Infection of cells by SV40 results in a prolongation or increase in replicative life span followed by a dramatic decline in proliferative capacity or *crisis*. The relationship between senescence and crisis is unclear, although Stein has suggested similarities between in vitro–aged and precrisis cells (257). As a rare event, SV40-infected cells that survive crisis may acquire the potential for indefinite pro-

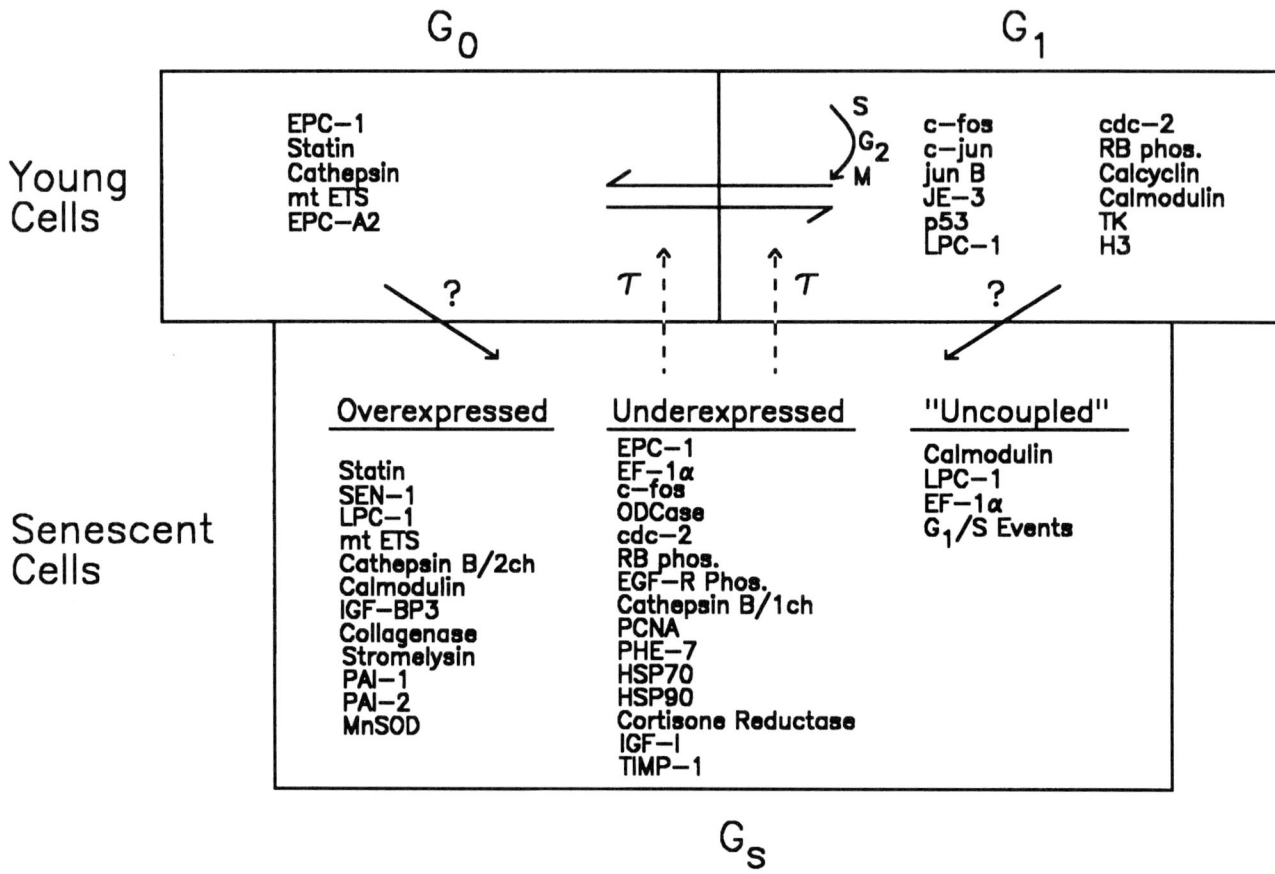

FIG. 4.3. Representation of growth states available to young and senescent fibroblasts and the molecular markers that define each state. G_s, senescence-specific growth state; τ, putative transitional pathways by which conditionally arrested cells may re-enter cell cycle; ?, pathways by which young cells become senescent by an unknown mechanism(s).

liferation. Nondividing senescent cells are refractory to transformation. Infection of senescent cells by SV40, however, does result in the re-initiation of an additional round of DNA synthesis (83), although the ability of senescent cells to divide is not restored.

Evidence that the cessation of proliferation may be a programmed phenomenon has been provided by studies that characterized the reversible escape from cellular senescence using SV40 large T antigen as mediator of this transition (215, 291). The SV40 large T antigen can promote escape from senescence through a two-step process. The continued expression of large T antigen allows cells to undergo significantly more population doublings and thus postpones the onset of the senescent phenotype relative to cultures not expressing large T antigen (*mortality 1,* M1). The continued expression of large T antigen is required for cells to suppress the onset of senescence initially and throughout the period of extended life span, its removal resulting in the rapid decline in replicative capacity (291). Cells in which SV40 large T antigen has been de-induced (repressed) and subsequently re-induced show what might be interpreted as a reversibly senescent phenotype. These de-induced cells display characteristic senescent morphology and express molecular markers associated with senescence (239). Although large T antigen is capable of extending the in vitro life span of cells that constitutively express it, ultimately these cells also become proliferatively senescent. This stage has been described as the *mortality 2* (M2) stage of senescence (240, 291). At an extremely low frequency, immortalization-competent SV40 large T antigen–transfected fibroblast clones can overcome M2 and transform into permanent cell lines (240). The inactivation of M2 loci may occur via genetic instability, resulting in mutation or aneuploidy, and may likely be caused by SV40 large T antigen itself. The presence of both RB protein–binding activity [adenovirus E1A or human papillomavirus (HPV) E7] and p53 protein–binding activity (adenovirus E1B or HPV E6) can permit cells to override the M1 mechanism, but neither binding activity alone is capable of replacing SV40 large T antigen (238, 240). Similarly, a mutant SV40 T antigen defective in p53 binding or an SV40 T antigen mutant defective in RB binding cannot independently bypass the M1 mechanism (238, 240). These findings, however, do not define a discrete mechanism, since RB- and p53-binding activities are not completely understood and SV40 large T antigen is a multifunctional molecule with additional, potentially unknown interactions.

The fact that SV40 large T antigen can override the M1 mechanism does not unequivocally indicate that RB- and p53-binding activities are regulating cellular senescence. The SV40 large T antigen may be acting so late in G_1 as to bypass any upstream senescence-specific regulatory events and, in effect, may be inactivating the normal functions of RB and p53 as antioncogenes in order to form a continuous loop between DNA synthesis and cell division until M2 is reached. This idea assumes that changes in the functions of RB and p53 with in vitro aging are not causative events but rather, downstream or secondary effects of senescence.

An interesting event that coincides with the loss of DNA synthetic capacity in fibroblasts aged in vitro is the shortening of telomeres (94). This finding has suggested the hypothesis that with the shortening of telomeres is an associated loss of genetic information at or near the ends of chromosomes which is responsible for replicative decline. It also provides an attractive model for the way in which cells might "count" divisions. This hypothesis further suggests that there is a loss of telomerase activity in normal human fibroblasts (92, 95), which is preserved or restored in cells that have obtained an immortalized phenotype. This hypothesis, does not, however, adequately explain the rapid cessation of division by reversibly senescent SV40 large T antigen–transformed fibroblasts when T antigen is de-induced or the continued proliferation of these cells when T antigen is re-induced. Neither the time required for a putative loss of telomerase activity in the former case nor the re-acquisition of genetic material initially lost during senescence in the latter case is consistent with this hypothesis. To explain such inconsistencies, Wright and Shay (290) proposed that senescence could be regulated by essential genes near the ends of chromosomes, not as the result of a physical loss of genetic material at these regions (although this would also occur), but by the activation or inactivation of telomeric sequences by changes in adjacent local chromatin condensation. This formulation could also explain the heterogeneity seen in the proliferative potential of clones derived from mass cultures at different in vitro ages if heterochromatic regions of telomeric DNA were in a dynamic state whose probability of encroaching upon critical regulatory genes increased with shortening telomere length. Alternatively, shortened telomere length may be an effect of senescence rather than a primary cause or characteristic of senescence in mammalian cells only. D'Mello and Jazwinski (61), for example, found no change in telomere length during the aging of *Saccharomyces cerevisiae*.

Some of the most compelling evidence in support of a genetic basis for cellular senescence has been the finding that the introduction of particular chromosomes into immortalized cells causes them to acquire a senescent phenotype. The search for chromosomes carrying senescence-inducing genes has relied on the cytogenetic comparison of hybrids between immortal and normal human diploid fibroblasts for the loss of specific chromosomes and the concomitant potential for unlimited division potential, usually defined as >100 population doublings. Thus far, these studies have implicated human chromosomes 1 and 4 as putative sites for senescence-related genes. These studies have also indicated that senescence-related genes may be limited to a small number of chromosomes and, although functionally redundant, are sufficient to cause a senescent phenotype only in immortalized cells belonging to a specific subgroup (see above under Deterministic Processes).

The evidence that human chromosome 1 is involved in cellular senescence came from cell fusion studies between MRC-5 normal human fetal lung fibroblasts and an immortal Syrian hamster cell line (267). A karyotypic analysis of hybrid clones that displayed indefinite division potential revealed that human chromosome 1 was not present. Further, the transfer of a single copy of human chromosome 1 into the immortal hamster cell line by microcell fusion resulted in the appearance of characteristic cellular markers of senescence, including enlarged and irregular morphology, cessation of proliferation, and failure to initiate DNA synthesis as measured by the incorporation of [^{3}H]thymidine into nuclei.

That genes involved in cellular senescence may reside on human chromosome 4 is strongly indicated by the karyotypic analysis of hybrids between a human fibrosarcoma cell line and normal human fibroblasts (176). The introduction of human chromosome 4 into representative immortal cell lines of different complementation groups, based on indefinite division potential and analogous recessive defects (see above under Deterministic Processes), also supports this conclusion. The introduction of human chromosome 4 caused a reversal of the immortal phenotype displayed by a single complementation group represented by two carcinoma-derived cell lines and a glioblastoma. The human chromosome 4 had no effect on any of the cell lines representing the other complementation groups (176).

The introduction of a normal Chinese hamster X chromosome into a nickel-transformed Chinese hamster cell line with an Xq chromosome deletion has also been reported to induce the cessation of proliferation in these previously immortal cells (123). Although the efficacy of the Chinese hamster X chromosome to confer a senescent phenotype was severely reduced when contributed by later-passage donor cells, this reduction was reversed by treatment of the donor cell line with 5-azacytidine. This suggests that a senescence gene or genes may be regulated by DNA methylation.

The greatest drawbacks to interpreting these findings are the failure of some clones containing introduced chromosomes to exhibit the cessation of division and the inability to adequately control for gene dosage effects occurring either at the level of chromosome copy number or unregulated gene expression.

Genes Isolated from Selective Libraries and Monoclonal Antibody Pools.

The list of molecular markers of senescence in culture has dramatically increased as a result of examining genes isolated from selective libraries and monoclonal antibody (MAb) pools. The first attempts at constructing cDNA libraries from young and senescent cell populations and screening by plus/minus hybridization uncovered both a cDNA-encoding fibronectin (124) and a cDNA-containing homology to elongation factor I alpha (74, 75), the transcripts of which were found to be overexpressed in senescent cells. A novel sequence, SAG (senescence-associated gene), has recently been isolated by this method (288), and its expression, although not cell cycle–regulated, increases in parallel with in vitro age. Analysis of DNA sequencing information revealed that SAG contains a putative DNA-binding domain and thus may serve a functional role as a regulatory protein.

Using similar techniques, but with starting material from Werner's syndrome fibroblasts, a total of 18 differentially expressed genes were found to have preferentially higher steady-state mRNA levels in Werner's syndrome fibroblasts as compared to normal fibroblasts (172). Nine of these genes were identified as known sequences, six coding for secreted proteins associated with the extracellular matrix. Of the nine unknown genes, seven included repetitive short nuclear elements. Moreover, five of the nine known genes were also found to be overexpressed in in vitro–aged fibroblasts. It is particularly interesting to note the overexpression of the gene for IGF binding-protein-3 (81), given its variable role in regulating IGF-I–stimulated DNA synthesis and WS3-10, an unknown gene that shows the greatest similarity to *Drosophila* MP20 and chicken SM22, two muscle proteins of unknown function (272, 273). In addition, the amount of IGFBP3 in medium conditioned by fibroblasts increased with the age of the donor from which the cells were derived (80a).

The sensitivity with which differentially expressed genes can be isolated from cDNA libraries depends, in large part, on techniques used for the enrichment of unique or favored sequences. For example, screening of G_0 subtracted cDNA libraries from young and senescent WI-38 fibroblasts has uncovered at least 11 differentially expressed genes (62). Both random screening and screening using subtractive probes were used to isolate cDNA copies of genes which were predominantly expressed in either early or late population doubling level (PDL) cells. Genes expressed predominantly in young cells included *EPC-1* (early PDL cDNA-1), a G_0-specific marker in young fibroblasts identical to the pigmented epithelial-derived differentiation factor (PEDF) and related to a family of serine protease inhibitors (203), and *EPC-A2*, a human homolog of the transcription factor *twist*. Mitochondrial genes encoding cytochrome b and subunit 4 of NADH CoQ reductase, as well as *LPC-1* (late PDL cDNA-1), were more abundantly expressed in late-passage fibroblasts (62). *LPC-1*, whose expression in senescent cells is uncoupled from the cell cycle but is strictly regulated in young cells (202), has recently been identified as a marker protein (p63) of the ER-Golgi intermediate compartment (106) related to a swine cardiogenic shock protein (23). These sequences provide the first direct molecular evidence that in vitro–aged fibroblasts may exist in a growth state distinct from the G_0 state of early PDL cells. In addition, the diminished capacity of skin fibroblasts from aged donors to accumulate the *EPC-1* transcript has been shown (R. J. Pignolo, R. G. Allen, M. O. Rotenberg, and V. J. Cristofalo, unpublished data, 1994). In this study, steady-state *EPC-1* mRNA levels were evaluated in 27 skin fibroblast cell lines from donors ranging in age from 12 fetal weeks to 94 years. All cell lines analyzed had normal karyotypes and had completed less than 60% of their in vitro replicative life span.

The above studies have taken the approach that an analysis of differentially expressed genes will reveal changes that may, in part, play a causal role in senescence or, at the very least, help define a molecular phenotype of the senescent cell. Implicit in this approach is the hypothesis that senescence is a multifactorial process requiring the balance and interaction of both positive and negative regulatory factors.

In contrast to this strategy, other investigators have searched for genes that specifically inhibit entry into DNA synthesis. The most promising work has employed a functional assay for the isolation of relevant sequences. This isolation of genes by expression phenotype scores the ability of full-length cDNAs, transfected or microinjected into young cells, to inhibit DNA synthesis. Three clones, coined "SDI" clones (senescent cell–derived inhibition of DNA synthesis), promote such a phenotype (248, 176a). Two of the three have roughly equivalent transcript levels in young and senescent cells, and a third, SDI-1, has elevated levels in late-passage cells or in early-passage cells made quiescent by long-term serum deprivation. SDI-1 has recently been identified as an inhibitor of multiple G_1 cyclin-cdk (cyclin-dependent kinase) complexes, shown to be inducible by p53, and alternatively called Cip 1, Waf 1,

Pic 1, or p21 (173a, 154a, 119a). The overexpression of this variously known protein has been implicated in the growth arrest of HDF cells, National Institutes of Health 3T3 cells, several tumor lines, as well as the radiation-induced G_1 arrest of normal fibroblasts (119a, 176a, 63a). Thus far, no senescence-specific inhibitor of DNA synthesis has been found.

Another approach has exploited the use of MAbs to recognize epitopes of gene products uniquely or predominantly expressed as cells age in vitro. The best examples of such MAbs are those that recognize determinants on statin (279–282) and terminin (283), a nonproliferating-cell-specific nuclear protein and a senescence-specific fragment derived from a larger protein found in young cells, respectively. Statin is related to a family of genes sharing homology with elongation factor I alpha. Terminin is the result of an age-related post-translational modification/proteolysis. MAb technology has also been used to identify epitopes unique to senescence that map to fibronectin (208).

The budding yeast *Saccharomyces cerevisiae* has been used as a model system for cellular senescence, exhibiting characteristic biomarkers of in vitro aging, including finite cell division, increased cell size, and increased generation time (67). Six clones isolated from a yeast genomic DNA library showed differential expression as a function of age (66). It will be interesting to examine the role of human homologs to these clones should they exist.

SUMMARY AND CONCLUSIONS

The life history of fibroblast and fibroblast-like cells includes an initial stage of outgrowth and establishment in culture, a period of vigorous proliferation (which has a variable length depending on such factors as the tissue of origin and the age of the donor, among others), a period of declining proliferative vigor (which includes substantial cell death), and finally the emergence of an (apparently) long-lived population unable to proliferate in response to growth factors. During the phase of declining proliferative vigor, the cells acquire characteristics, some of which are similar to the characteristics of cells in older individuals. Eventually, the culture completely loses proliferative capacity. A comparable life history has been described for glial cells, keratinocytes, vascular smooth muscle cells, endothelial cells, and lymphocytes, suggesting that this life history is characteristic of those cell types that, in vivo, retain the capacity for proliferation throughout the life span.

Numerous studies have shown a correlation between the age of the tissue donor and the replicative life span of the cells in culture. In addition, for a small sample of species, there is a direct correlation between fibroblast replicative life span in vitro and maximum life span potential of the species.

The period in the life history usually referred to as the "senescent phase" is probably more complicated than was originally thought, since studies with life span modulators suggest that there is a "conditionally" senescent state from which cells can be "rescued" for one or more additional rounds of DNA synthesis. Finally, the cells enter an "obligatory" arrested state in which only SV40 infection can reverse the block to DNA synthesis but not the block to mitosis.

The modern era of aging research in tissue culture commenced in the 1960s. The inception of the field really began with the recognition by Hayflick and Moorhead (114) that the phenomenon of senescence in vitro paralleled, in some of its characteristics, cell aging in vivo and thus provided a model in which to study the cellular mechanisms underlying senescence under controlled environmental conditions.

Research in this area began with a detailed characterization and comparison of young vs. senescent cell morphology and physiology. These studies provided the basis for a wide variety of subsequent studies that addressed possible mechanisms underlying cell senescence. These included studies on DNA repair, protein synthetic errors, chromatin structure and function, and mechanisms for modulating replicative life span. Many of the alterations accompanying senescence in vitro have also been demonstrated to occur in vivo.

There have been two major directions of research in this area. The first began with studies of cell-cycle kinetics, which evolved into studies of differential responses to growth factors, signal transduction mechanisms, and differential gene expression. The results show that as cells in culture age there is an increase in cell-cycle time, due primarily to an increase in the G_1 phase. Cells are arrested in senescence primarily with a 2C DNA content, suggesting a block in the pre-DNA synthetic phase.

Young cells that are serum/growth factor–starved respond to the addition of fresh serum (growth factors) by traversing G_0/G_1, synthesizing DNA, and dividing. Senescent cells handled in precisely the same way bind and metabolize (at least partially) growth factors and carry out many of the reactions of G_0/G_1, but do not synthesize DNA. Two noteworthy differences in the cascade of reactions that follow growth factor addition to senescent cells are an altered regulation and attenuated expression of the early response gene *c-fos* and a substantial reduction in the ability to translocate PKC to the cell membrane. The significance of either of these changes is not understood at this time.

Other studies in this same vein took advantage of SV40/T antigen as a probe of the mechanisms of proliferative arrest. The evidence seems strong that overcoming senescence involves overcoming two different blocks: M1, a block to DNA synthesis, and M2, a block to post-DNA synthetic events.

In parallel with these studies, a second approach through genetic analysis has been used. Studies began with the observation that in heterokaryons senescence was dominant, which suggested that an inhibitor was expressed in senescent cells that prevented them from replicating. Later studies, in which preparations of senescent (and quiescent young) cell mRNA were microinjected into young cells, suggested that senescence was controlled by negative regulators. The next major thrust in the evolution of these studies was based on the search for differentially expressed genes, especially the putative antiproliferative gene(s) that may be characteristic of senescence. These studies were performed using various methodologies, including the construction of selective libraries. To date, although several antiproliferative genes have been identified, these have all been associated with nongrowing cells, whether nongrowth is the result of contact inhibition or serum deprivation in young or senescent cells. In contrast, at least one gene, *EPC-1*, has been shown to be expressed in young, serum-starved or contact-inhibited (quiescent) cells but not in senescent cells treated in the same way. The correlation between the expression of these genes and aging in vivo, with few exceptions (*EPC-1*, for example), remains to be established.

As a result of this research, several overriding concepts have emerged. *(1)* There is no clear evidence that the process by which normal cells regulate proliferation through the expression of proliferation suppressors has anything directly to do with the process by which senescence is regulated. *(2)* The senescent state is not merely a case of irreversible quiescence, except in a very limited operational sense. Senescent cells appear to be in a unique state that is not identical to any of the defined segments of the cell replication cycle. Senescence is characterized by a general loss of integrative function, resulting in cellular dysfunction that leads either to cell death or to acquisition of a strikingly different phenotype that is irreversibly postreplicative. Perhaps senescence in this postreplicative cell type is a process by which cell populations are prevented from unlimited proliferation and thus would have an adaptive value in vivo. *(3)* Specific genes that are differentially expressed in senescent cells may be regulators of the process or, alternatively, may be the downstream effects of a higher order change that then results in a new but dysfunctional phenotype. Thus far, there is no information that sheds further light on these options.

REFERENCES

1. ABSHER, P. M., and R. G. ABSHER. Clonal variation and aging of diploid fibroblasts. *Exp. Cell Res.* 103: 247–255, 1976.
2. ABSHER, P. M., R. G. ABSHER, and W. D. BARNES. Genealogies of clones of diploid fibroblasts. Cinemicrophotographic observations of cell division patterns in relation to population age. *Exp. Cell Res.* 88: 95–104, 1974.
2a. AFSHARI, C. A., P. J. VOJTA, L. A. ANNAB, P. A. FUTREAL, T. B. WILLARD, and J. C. BARRETT. Investigation of the role of G_1/S cell cycle mediators in cellular senescence. *Exp. Cell Res.* 209: 231–237, 1993.
3. ALBRIGHT, J., W., and T. MAKINODAN. Decline in the growth potential of spleen-colonizing bone marrow stem cells of long-lived aging mice. *J. Exp. Med.* 144: 1204–1213, 1976.
4. ALLEN, R. G., and A. K. BALIN. Developmental changes in the superoxide dismutase activity of human skin fibroblasts are maintained in vitro and are not caused by oxygen. *J. Clin. Invest.* 82: 731–734, 1988.
5. ANGELLO, J. C., W. R. PENDERGRASS, T. H. NORWOOD, and J. PROTHERO. Proliferative potential of human fibroblasts: an inverse dependence on cell size. *J. Cell. Physiol.* 132: 125–130, 1987.
6. ANGELLO, J. C., W. R. PENDERGRASS, T. H. NORWOOD, and J. PROTHERO. Cell enlargement: one possible mechanism underlying cellular senescence. *J. Cell. Physiol.* 140: 288–294, 1989.
7. ARONSON, J. F., J. W. MCCLASKEY, and V. J. CRISTOFALO. Human fetal lung fibroblasts: observations on origin and stability in culture. *Mech. Ageing Dev.* 21: 229–244, 1983.
8. ATILLASOY, E., and P. R. HOLT. Gastrointestinal proliferation and aging. *J. Gerontol.* 48: B43–B49, 1993.
9. AUNE, T. M., and S. L. POGUE. Generation and characterization of continuous lines of $CD8^+$ suppressor T lymphocytes. *J. Immunol.* 142: 3731–3739, 1989.
10. BALIN, A. K., D. B. P. GOODMAN, H. RASMUSSEN, and V. J. CRISTOFALO. The effect of oxygen tension on the growth and metabolism of WI-38 cells. *J. Cell. Physiol.* 89: 235–250, 1976.
11. BALIN, A. K., D. B. P. GOODMAN, H., RASMUSSEN, and V. J. CRISTOFALO. The effect of oxygen and vitamin E on the life span of human diploid cells in vitro. *J. Cell Biol.* 74: 58–67, 1977.
12. BAYREUTHER, K., P. I. FRANCZ, J. GOGOL, M. MAIER, and H. G. MEINRATH. Differentiation of primary and secondary fibroblasts in cell culture systems. *Mutat. Res.* 256: 233–242, 1991.
13. BEMILLER, P. M., and L. H. LEE. Nucleolar changes in senescing WI-38 cells. *Mech. Ageing Dev.* 8: 417–427, 1976.
14. BEMILLER, P. M., and J. E. MILLER. Cytological changes in senescing WI-38 cells: a statistical analysis. *Mech. Ageing Dev.* 10: 1–15, 1979.
15. BIERMAN, E. L. The effect of donor age on the in vitro lifespan of cultured human arterial smooth-muscle cells. *In Vitro Cell. Dev. Biol.* 14: 951–955, 1978.
15a. BLUMENTHAL, E. J., A. C. K. MILLER, G. H. STEIN, and A. M. MALKINSON. Serine/threonine protein kinases and calcium-dependent protease in senescent IMR-90 fibroblasts. *Mech. Ageing Dev.* 72: 13–24, 1993.
16. BOWMAN, P. D., and C. W. DANIEL. Aging of human fibroblasts in vitro: surface features and behavior of aging WI-38 cells. *Mech. Ageing Dev.* 4: 147–158, 1975.
17. BOWMAN, P. D., R. L. MEEK, and C. W. DANIEL. Decreased synthesis of nucleolar RNA in aging human cells in vitro. *Exp. Cell Res.* 101: 434–437, 1976a.
18. BOWMAN, P. D., R. L. MEEK, and C. W. DANIEL. Decreased unscheduled DNA synthesis in nondividing aged WI-38 cells. *Mech. Ageing Dev.* 5: 251–257, 1976b.
19. BRADLEY, M. O., L. C. ERICKSON, and T. W. KOHN. Normal DNA strand rejoining and absence of DNA crosslinking in progeroid and aging human cells. *Mutat. Res.* 37: 279–292, 1976.

20. BRANDES, D., D. G. MURPHY, E. B. ANTON, and S. BARNARD. Ultrastructural and cytochemical changes in cultured human lung cells. *J. Ultrastruct. Res.* 39: 465–483, 1972.
21. BROOKS, K. M., P. D. PHILLIPS, C. R. CARLIN, B. KNOWLES, and V. J. CRISTOFALO. EGF-dependent phosphorylation of the EGF receptor in plasma membranes isolated from young and senescent WI-38 cells. *J. Cell. Physiol.* 133: 523–531, 1987.
22. BROOKS-FREDERICH, K. M., F. L. CIANCIARULO, S. M. RITTLING, and V. J. CRISTOFALO. Cell cycle dependent regulation of Ca^{++} in young and senescent WI-38 cells. *Exp. Cell Res.* 205: 412–415, 1993.
23. BUCHMAN, T. G., D. E. CABIN, S. VICKERS, C. S. DEUTSCHMAN, E. DELGADO, M. M. SUSSMAN, and G. B. BULKLEY. Molecular biology of circulatory shock. Part II. Expression of four groups of hepatic genes is enhanced after resuscitation from cardiogenic shock. *Surgery* 108: 559–566, 1990.
24. BUETOW, D. E. Cell numbers vs. age in mammalian tissues and organs. In: *CRC Handbook of Cell Biology of Aging*, edited by V. J. Cristofalo. Boca Raton, FL: CRC Press, 1985, p. 1–115.
25. BURMER, G. C., C. J. ZEIGLER, and T. H. NORWOOD. Evidence for endogenous polypeptide-mediated inhibition of cell-cycle transit in human diploid cells. *J. Cell Biol.* 94: 187–192, 1982.
26. CARLIN, C. R., P. D. PHILLIPS, B. B. KNOWLES, and V. J. CRISTOFALO. Diminished in vitro tyrosine kinase activity of the EGF receptor of senescent human fibroblasts. *Nature* 306: 617–620, 1983.
26a. CARLIN, C. R., P. D. PHILLIPS, K. M. BROOKS-FREDERICK, S. MILLER, B. B. KNOWLES, and V. J. CRISTOFALO. Cleavage of the EGF receptor by an endogenous leupeptin-sensitive protease active in detergent extracts of senescent but not young human diploid fibroblasts. *J. Cell. Physiol.* 160: 427–434, 1994.
27. CARREL, A., and M. T. BURROWS. Cultivation of adult tissues and organs outside of the body. *JAMA* 55: 1379–1381, 1910a.
28. CARREL, A., and M. T. BURROWS. Cultivation of sarcoma outside of the body. *JAMA* 55: 1554, 1910b.
29. CARREL, A., and M. T. BURROWS. On the physiochemical regulation of the growth of tissues. *J. Exp. Med.* 13: 562–570, 1911.
30. CARREL, A., and A. H. EBLING. Age and multiplication of fibroblasts. *J. Exp. Med.* 34: 599–623, 1921.
31. CHANG, C., P. D. PHILLIPS, K. E. LIPSON, V. J. CRISTOFALO, and R. BASERGA. Senescent human fibroblasts have a post-transcriptional block in the expression of the proliferating cell nuclear antigen. *J. Biol. Chem.* 266: 8663–8666, 1991.
32. CHANG, Z.-F., and K. Y. CHEN. Regulation of ornithine decarboxylase and other cell cycle-regulated genes during senescence of IMR-90 human diploid fibroblasts. *J. Biol. Chem.* 263: 11431–11435, 1988.
33. CHOUDHURY, G. G., V. L. SYLVIA, and A. Y. SAKAGUCHI. Decline of signal transduction by phospholipase $C_{\gamma}1$ in IMR-90 human diploid fibroblasts at high population doubling levels. *FEBS Lett.* 293: 211–214, 1991.
34. CHUA, C. C., D. E. GEIMAN, and R. L. LADDA. Receptor for epidermal growth factor retains normal structure and function in aging cells. *Mech. Ageing Dev.* 34: 35–55, 1986.
35. COHEN, S. C., and H. D. BARNER. Studies on unbalanced growth in *Escherichia coli*. *Biochemistry* 40: 885–893, 1954.
36. COMINGS, D. E., and T. A. OKADA. Electron microscopy of human fibroblasts in tissue culture during logarithmic and confluent stages of growth. *Exp. Cell Res.* 61: 295–301, 1970.
37. COOPER, J. T., and S. GOLDSTEIN. Comparative studies on human skin fibroblasts: life span and lipid metabolism in medium containing fetal bovine or human serum. *In Vitro Cell. Dev. Biol.* 13: 473–476, 1977.
38. CRISTOFALO, V. J. Metabolic aspects of aging in diploid human cells. In: *Aging in Cell and Tissue Culture*, edited by E. Holeckova and V. J. Cristofalo. New York: Plenum Press, 1970, p. 83–119.
39. CRISTOFALO, V. J. Animal cell cultures as a model system for the study of aging. In: *Advances in Gerontological Research*, edited by B. L. Strehler. New York: Academic Press, 1972, vol. 4, p. 45–79.
40. CRISTOFALO, V. J. Cellular senescence: factors modulating cell proliferation in vitro. In: *INSERM*, edited by F. Bourliere, Y. Courtois, A. Macieira-Coelho and L. Robert. Paris: INSERM, 1973, vol. 27, p. 65–92.
41. CRISTOFALO, V. J. Cellular biomarkers of aging. *Exp. Gerontol.* 23: 297–305, 1988.
42. CRISTOFALO, V. J. On models and the study of senescence: reflections on the state of biogerontology and a farewell. *J. Gerontol.* 46: B207–B208, 1991.
43. CRISTOFALO, V. J., and D. KRITCHEVSKY. Cell size and nucleic acid content in the human diploid cell line WI-38 during aging. *Med. Exp. Int. J. Exp. Med.* 19: 313–320, 1969.
44. CRISTOFALO, V. J., and B. B. SHARF. Cellular senescence and DNA synthesis: thymidine incorporation as a measure of population age in human diploid cells. *Exp. Cell Res.* 76: 419–427, 1973.
45. CRISTOFALO, V. J., and B. M. STANULIS-PRAEGER. Cellular senescence in vitro. In: *Advances in Cell Culture*, edited by K. Mararmorosch. New York: Academic Press 1982, vol. 2, p. 1–67.
46. CRISTOFALO, V. J., D. L. DOGGETT, K. M. BROOKS-FREDERICH, and P. D. PHILLIPS. Growth factors as probes of cell aging. *Exp. Gerontol.* 24: 367–374, 1989.
47. CRISTOFALO, V. J., B. V. HOWARD, and D. KRITCHEVSKY. The biochemistry of human cells in culture. In: *Research Progress in Organic, Biological, and Medicinal Chemistry*, edited by U. Gallo and L. Santamaria. Amsterdam: North-Holland Publishing Company, 1970, vol. 2, p. 95–146.
48. CRISTOFALO, V. J., R. PALAZZO, and R. L. CHARPENTIER. Limited lifespan of human fibroblasts in vitro: metabolic time or replications? In: *Neural Regulatory Mechanisms During Aging*, edited by R. C. Adelman, J. Roberts, G. T. Baker, S. I. Baskin and V. J. Cristofalo. New York: Alan R. Liss, 1980, p. 203–206.
49. CRISTOFALO, V. J., N. PARRIS, and D. KRITCHEVSKY. Enzyme activity during the growth and aging of human cells in vitro. *J. Cell. Physiol.* 69: 263–272, 1967.
50. CRISTOFALO, V. J., P. D. PHILLIPS, T. SORGER, and G. GERHARD. Alterations in the responsiveness of senescent cells to growth factors. *J. Gerontol.* 44: 55–62, 1989.
51. CRISTOFALO, V. J., R. J. PIGNOLO, and M. O. ROTENBERG. Molecular changes with in vitro cellular senescence. In: *Aging and Cellular Defense Mechanisms*, edited by C. Franceschi, G. Crepaldi, V. J. Cristofalo, and J. Vijg. New York: The New York Academy of Sciences, 1992, vol. 663, p. 187–194.
52. CUDKOWICZ, G., A. C. UPTON, G. M. SHEARER, and W. L. HUGHES. Lymphocyte contact and proliferative capacity of serially transplanted mouse bone marrow. *Nature* 201: 165–167, 1964.
53. CUMMINGS, D. J. Mitochrondrial DNA in *Podospora anserina*: a molecular approach to cellular senescence. *Monogr. Dev. Biol.* 17: 254–266, 1984.
54. DANES, B. S. Progeria: a cell culture study on aging. *J. Clin. Invest.* 50: 2000–2003, 1971.
55. DANIEL, C. W., K. B. DEOHME, J. T. YOUNG, P. B. BLAIR, and L. J. FAULKIN. The in vivo lifespan of normal and preneoplastic mouse mammary glands: a serial transplantation study. *Proc. Natl. Acad. Sci. USA* 61: 52–60, 1968.

56. DEKNUDT, G., and A. LEONARD. Aging and radiosensitivity of human somatic chromosomes. *Exp. Gerontol.* 12: 237–240, 1977.
57. DELL'ORCO, R. T., G. B. MERTENS, and P. F. KRUSE, JR. Doubling potential and calender time of human diploid cells in culture. *Exp. Cell Res.* 84: 363–366, 1974.
58. DE TATA, V., A. PTASZNIK, and V. J. CRISTOFALO. Effects of the tumor promoting agent phorbol 12-myristate 13-acetate (PMA) on the proliferation of young and senescent WI-38 human diploid fibroblasts. *Exp. Cell Res.* 205: 261–269, 1993.
59. DICE, J. F. Altered intracellular protein degradation in aging: a possible cause of proliferative arrest. *Exp. Gerontol.* 24: 451–459, 1989.
60. DI PAOLO, B. R., R. J. PIGNOLO, and V. J. CRISTOFALO. Overexpression of the two-chain form of cathepsin B in senescent WI-38 cells. *Exp. Cell Res.* 201: 500–505, 1992.
61. D'MELLO, N. P., and S. M. JAZWINSKI. Telomere length constancy during aging of *Saccharomyces cerevisiae*. *J. Bacteriol.* 173: 6709–6713, 1991.
62. DOGGETT, D. L., M. O. ROTENBERG, R. J. PIGNOLO, P. D. PHILLIPS, and V. J. CRISTOFALO. Differential gene expression between young and senescent quiescent WI-38 cells. *Mech. Ageing Dev.* 65: 239–255, 1992.
63. DRESCHER-LINCOLN, C. K., and J. R. SMITH. Inhibition of DNA synthesis in senescent-proliferating human cybrids is mediated by endogenous proteins. *Exp. Cell Res.* 153: 208–217, 1984.
63a. DULIC, V., W. K. KAUFMANN, S. J. WILSON, T. D. TISTY, E. LEES, J. W. HARPER, S. J. ELLEDGE, and S. I. REED. p53-Dependent inhibition of cyclin-dependent kinase activities in human fibroblasts during radiation-induced G1 arrest. *Cell* 76: 1013–1023, 1994.
63b. DUNCAN, E. L., N. J. WHITAKER, E. L. MOY, and R. R. REDDEL. Assignment of SV40-immortalized cells to more than one complementation group for immortalization. *Exp. Cell Res.* 205: 337–344, 1993.
64. EBELING, A. H. The permanent life of connective tissue outside of the organism. *J. Exp. Med.* 17: 273–285, 1913.
65. EBELING, A. H. Measurement of the growth of tissues in vitro. *J. Exp. Med.* 34: 231–243, 1921.
66. EGILMEZ, N. K., J. B. CHEN, and S. M. JAZWINSKI. Specific alterations in transcript prevalence during the yeast lifespan. *J. Biol. Chem.* 264: 14312–14317, 1989.
67. EGILMEZ, N. K., J. B. CHEN, and S. M. JAZWINSKI. Preparation and partial characterization of old yeast cells. *J. Gerontol.* 45: B9–B17, 1990.
68. FAIRWEATHER, S., M. FOX, and B. P. MARGISON. The in vitro lifespan of MRC-5 cells is shortened by 5-azacytidine-induced demethylation. *Exp. Cell Res.* 168: 153–159, 1987.
68a. FERBER, A., C. D. CHANG, C. SELL, A. PTASZNIK, V. J. CRISTOFALO, H. OZER, D. LEROITH, and R. BASERGA. Failure of senescent human fibroblasts to express the IGF-I gene. *J. Biol. Chem.* 268: 17883–17888, 1993.
69. FREDERICH, K. M., P. D. PHILLIPS, and V. J. CRISTOFALO. Stimulation of DNA synthesis in senescent human cells following incubation with plasma membranes. *Exp. Cell Res.* 202: 386–390, 1992.
70. FRIEDMAN, D., and A. GLOBERSON. Immune reactivity during aging. II. Analysis of the cellular mechanisms involved in the deficient antibody response in old mice. *Mech. Ageing Dev.* 7: 299–307, 1978.
71. FULDER, S. J. The growth of cultured human fibroblasts treated with hydrocortisone and extracts of the medicinal plant *Panax ginseng*. *Exp. Gerontol.* 12: 125–131, 1977.
72. GALLOWAY, S. M., and K. E. BUCKTON. Aneuploidy and aging: chromosome studies on a random sample of the population using G-banding. *Cytogenet. Cell Genet.* 20: 78–95, 1978.
73. GERHARD, G. S., P. D. PHILLIPS, and V. J. CRISTOFALO. EGF- and PDGF-stimulated phosphorylation in young and senescent WI-38 cells. *Exp. Cell Res.* 193: 87–92, 1991.
74. GIORDANO, T., and D. N. FOSTER. Identification of a highly abundant cDNA isolated from senescent WI-38 cells. *Exp. Cell Res.* 185: 399–406, 1989.
75. GIORDANO, T., D. KLEINSEK, and D. N. FOSTER. Increase in abundance of a transcript hybridizing to elongation factor I alpha during cellular senescence and quiescence. *Exp. Gerontol.* 24: 501–513, 1989.
76. GOLDSTEIN, S. The role of DNA repair in aging of cultured fibroblasts from xeroderma pigmentosum and normals. *Proc. Soc. Exp. Biol. Med.* 137: 730–734, 1971.
77. GOLDSTEIN, S. Senescence. In: *Endocrinology*, edited by L. J. Degroot, G. F. Cahill, Jr., W. D. Odell, L. Martini, J. T. Potts, Jr., D. H. Nelson, E. Steinberger, and A. I. Winegrad. New York: Grune and Stratton, 1979, vol. 3, p. 2001–2028.
78. GOLDSTEIN, S. Replicative senescence: the human fibroblast comes of age. *Science* 249: 1129–1133, 1990.
79. GOLDSTEIN, S., and D. P. SINGAL. Senescence of cultured human fibroblasts: mitotic vs. metabolic time. *Exp. Cell Res.* 88: 359–364, 1974.
80. GOLDSTEIN, S., J. W. LITTLEFIELD, and J. S. SOELDNER. Diabetes mellitus and aging: diminished plating efficiency of cultured human fibroblasts. *Proc. Natl. Acad. Sci. USA* 64: 155–160, 1969.
80a. GOLDSTEIN, S., E. J. MOERMAN, and R. C. BAXTER. Accumulation of insulin-like growth factor binding protein-3 in conditioned medium of human fibroblasts increases with chronologic age of donor and senescence in vitro. *J. Cell. Physiol.* 156: 294–302, 1993.
81. GOLDSTEIN, S., E. J. MOERMAN, R. A. JONES, and R. C. BAXTER. Insulin-like growth factor binding protein 3 accumulates to high levels in culture medium of senescent and quiescent human fibroblasts. *Proc. Natl. Acad. Sci. USA* 88: 9680–9684, 1991.
82. GOLDSTEIN, S., E. J. MOERMAN, J. S. SOELDNER, R. E. GLEASON, and D. M. BARNETT. Chronologic and physiologic age affect replicative life-span of fibroblasts from diabetic, prediabetic, and normal donors. *Science* 199: 781–782, 1978.
83. GORMAN, S. D., and V. J. CRISTOFALO. Reinitiation of cellular DNA synthesis in BrdU-selected nondividing senescent cells by simian virus 40 infection. *J. Cell. Physiol.* 125: 122–126, 1985.
84. GORMAN, S. D., and V. J. CRISTOFALO. Analysis of the G_1 arrest position of senescent WI-38 cells by quinacrine dihydrochloride nuclear fluorescence-evidence for a late G_1 arrest. *Exp. Cell Res.* 167: 87–94, 1986.
85. GRACY, R. W., K. U. YUKSEL, M. L. CHAPMAN, J. K. CINI, M. JAHANI, H. S. LU, B. ORAY, and J. M. TALENT. Impaired protein degradation may account for the accumulation of "abnormal" proteins in aging cells. In: *Modern Aging Research, Modification of Proteins During Aging*, edited by R. C. Adelman and E. E. Dekker. New York: Alan R. Liss, 1985, vol. 7, p. 1–18.
86. GRAY, M. D., S. A. JESCH, and G. H. STEIN. 5-Azacytidine-induced demethylation of DNA to senescent level does not block proliferation of human fibroblasts. *J. Cell. Physiol.* 149: 477–484, 1991.
87. GREENBERG, S. B., G. L. GROVE, and V. J. CRISTOFALO. Cell size in aging monolayer cultures. *In Vitro Cell. Dev. Biol.* 13: 297–300, 1977.
88. GROVE, G. L., and V. J. CRISTOFALO. Characterization of the cell cycle of cultured human diploid cells: effects of aging and hydrocortisone. *J. Cell. Physiol.* 90: 415–422, 1977.

89. HADLEY, E. C., E. D. KRESS, and V. J. CRISTOFALO. Trypsinization frequency and loss of proliferative capacity in WI-38 cells. *J. Gerontol.* 34: 170–176, 1979.
90. HAFF, R. F., and H. E. SWIM. Serial propagation of 3 strains of rabbit fibroblasts: their susceptibility to infection with vaccinia virus. *Proc. Soc. Exp. Biol. Med.* 93: 200–204, 1956.
91. HARA, E., H. TSURUI, A. SHINOZAKI, S. NAKADA, and K. ODA. Cooperative effect of antisense-Rb and antisense-p53 oligomers on the extension of lifespan in human diploid fibroblasts, TIG-1. *Biochem. Biophys. Res. Commun.* 179: 528–534, 1991.
92. HARLEY, C. B. Telomere loss: mitotic clock or genetic time bomb? *Mutat. Res.* 256: 271–282, 1991.
93. HARLEY, C. B., and S. GOLDSTEIN. Cultured human fibroblasts: distribution of cell generations and a critical limit. *J. Cell. Physiol.* 97: 509–516, 1978.
94. HARLEY, C. B., A. B. FUTCHER, and C. W. GREIDER. Telomeres shorten during aging of human fibroblasts. *Nature* 345: 458–460, 1990.
95. HARLEY, C. B., H. VAZIRI, C. M. COUNTER, and R. C. ALLSOPP. The telomere hypothesis of cellular aging. *Exp. Gerontol.* 27: 375–382, 1992.
96. HARMAN, D. Aging: a theory based on free radical and radiation chemistry. *J. Gerontol.* 11: 298–300, 1956.
97. HARMAN, D. The free radical theory of aging. In: *Modern Biological Theories of Aging,* edited by H. R. Warner, R. N. Butler, R. L. Sprott, and E. L. Schneider. New York: Raven Press, 1987, p. 81–87.
98. HARRISON, D. E. Normal function of transplanted mouse erythrocyte precursors for 21 months beyond donor life spans. *Nature New Biol.* 237: 220–222, 1972.
99. HARRISON, D. E. Normal production of erythrocytes by mouse marrow continuous for 73 months. *Proc. Natl. Acad. Sci. USA* 70: 3184–3188, 1973.
100. HARRISON, D. E. Normal function of transplated marrow cell lines from aged mice. *J. Gerontol.* 30: 279–285, 1975.
101. HARRISON, D. E., and J. W. DOUBLEDAY. Normal function of immunologic stem cells from aged mice. *J. Immunol.* 114: 1314–1317, 1975.
102. HARRISON, D. E., C. M. ASTLE, and J. W. DOUBLEDAY. Cell lines from old immunodeficient donors give normal reponses in young recipients. *J. Immunol.* 118: 1223–1227, 1977.
103. HART, R. W., and R. B. SETLOW. Correlation between deoxyribonucleic acid excision-repair and lifespan in a number of mammalian species. *Proc. Natl. Acad. Sci. USA* 71: 2169–2173, 1974.
104. HART, R. W., and R. B. SETLOW. DNA repair in late-passage human cells. *Mech. Ageing Dev.* 5: 67–77, 1976.
105. HART, R. W., G. A. SACHER, and T. L. HOSKINS. DNA repair in a short- and a long-lived rodent species. *J. Gerontol.* 34: 808–817, 1979.
106. HAURI, H.-P., and A. SCHWEIZER. The endoplasmic reticulum-Golgi intermediate compartment. *Curr. Opin. Cell Biol.* 4: 600–608, 1992.
107. HAY, R. J. Cell strain senescence in vitro: cell culture anomaly or an expression of a fundamental inability of normal cells to survive and proliferate. In: *Aging in Cell and Tissue Culture,* edited by E. Holeckova and V. J. Cristofalo. New York: Plenum Press, 1970, p. 7–24.
108. HAY, R. J., and B. L. STREHLER. The limited growth span of cell strains isolated from the chick embryo. *Exp. Gerontol.* 2: 123–135, 1967.
109. HAY, R. J., R. A. MENZIES, H. P. MORGAN, and B. L. STREHLER. The division potential of cells in continuous growth as compared to cells subcultivated after maintenance in stationary phase. *Exp. Gerontol.* 3: 35–44, 1968.
110. HAYAKAWA, M. Progressive changes of the growth characteristics of the human diploid cells in serial cultivation in vitro. *Tohoku J. Exp. Med.* 98: 171–179, 1969.
111. HAYFLICK, L. The limited in vitro lifetime of human diploid cell strains. *Exp. Cell Res.* 37: 614–636, 1965.
112. HAYFLICK, L. Aging under glass. *Exp. Gerontol.* 5: 291–303, 1970.
113. HAYFLICK, L. The cellular basis for biological aging. In: *Handbook of the Biology of Aging,* edited by C. E. Finch and L. Hayflick. New York: Van Nostrand Reinhold Company, 1977, p. 159–179.
114. HAYFLICK, L., and P. S. MOORHEAD. The serial cultivation of human diploid cell strains. *Exp. Cell Res.* 25: 585–621, 1961.
115. HOEHN, H., M. SIMPSON, E. M. BRYANT, P. S. RABINOVITCH, D. SALK, and G. M. MARTIN. Effects of chromosome constitution on growth and longevity of human skin fibroblast cultures. *Am. J. Med. Genet.* 7: 141–154, 1980.
116. HOLLIDAY, R., and T. B. L. KIRKWOOD. Predictions of the somatic mutation and mortilization theories of cellular ageing are contrary to experimental observations. *J. Theor. Biol.* 93: 627–642, 1981.
117. HOLLIDAY, R., and G. M. TARRANT. Altered enzymes in aging human fibroblasts. *Nature* 238: 26–30, 1972.
118. HONDA, S., and M. MATSUO. Relationship between the cellular glutathione level and in vitro life span of human diploid fibroblasts. *Exp. Gerontol.* 23: 81–86, 1988.
119. HOSOKAWA, M., P. D. PHILLIPS, and V. J. CRISTOFALO. The effect of dexamethasone on epidermal growth factor binding and stimulation of proliferation in young and senescent WI-38 cells. *Exp. Cell Res.* 164: 408–414, 1986.
119a. HUNTER, T. Braking the cycle. *Cell* 75: 839–841, 1993.
120. JENSEN, F., H. KOPROWSKI, and J. A. PONTEN. Rapid transformation of human fibroblast cultures by simian virus 40. *Proc. Natl. Acad. Sci. USA* 50: 343–348, 1963.
121. JOHNSON, L. F., H. T. ABELSON, S. PENMAN, and H. GREEN. The relative amounts of the cytoplasmic RNA species in normal, transformed, and senescent cultured cell lines. *J. Cell. Physiol.* 90: 465–470, 1976.
122. KAJI, K., and M. MATSUO. A low density inoculation method for the serial subcultivation of human diploid fibroblasts: an efficient model for the study of cellular ageing. *Mech. Ageing Dev.* 13: 219–225, 1980.
123. KLEIN, C. B., K. CONWAY, X. W. WANG, R. K. BHAMRA, X. LIN, M. D. COHEN, L. ANNAB, J. C. BARRETT, and M. COSTA. Senescence of nickel-transformed cells by an X chromosome: possible epigenetic control. *Science* 251: 796–799, 1991.
124. KLEINSEK, D. A. Selection of mRNAs expressed during cellular senescence in vitro. *Age* 12: 55–60, 1989.
125. KROHN, P. L. Heterochronic transplantation in the study of ageing. In: *Proceedings of the Royal Society, Review Lectures on Senescence, Series B,* London: The Royal Society, 1962a, vol. 157, p. 128–147.
126. KROHN, P. L. Transplantation and aging. In: *Topics of the Biology of Aging,* edited by P. L. Krohn. New York: J. Wiley, 1962b, p. 125–148.
127. KROOTH, R. S., M. W. SHAW, and B. K. CAMPBELL. A persistent strain of diploid fibroblasts. *J. Natl. Cancer Inst.* 32: 1031–1040, 1964.
128. KUMAR, S., A. J. MILLIS, and C. BAGLIONI. Expression of interleukin 1-inducible genes and production of interleukin 1 by aging human fibroblasts. *Proc. Natl. Acad. Sci. USA* 89: 4683–4687, 1992.
129. KUMAZAKI, T., R. S. ROBETORYE, S. C. ROBERTORYE, and J. R. SMITH. Fibronectin expression increases during in vitro cellular senescence: correlation with increased cell area. *Exp. Cell Res.* 195: 13–19, 1991.

130. LAISHES, B. A., and G. M. WILLIAMS. Conditions affecting primary cell cultures of functional adult rat hepatocytes. II. Dexamethasone enhanced longevity and maintenance of morphology. *In Vitro Cell. Dev. Biol.* 12: 821–832, 1976.
131. LAMPIDIS, T. J., and G. E. SCHRAIBERGER. Age-related loss of DNA repair synthesis in isolated rat myocardial cells. *Exp. Cell Res.* 96: 412–416, 1975.
132. LEBLOND, C. P. Classification of cell populations on the basis of their proliferative behavior. *Natl. Cancer Inst. Monogr.* 14: 119–145, 1964.
133. LE GUILLY, Y., M. SIMON, P. LENOIR, and M. BOUREL. Long term culture of human adult liver cells: morphological changes related to in vitro senescence and effect of donor's age on growth potential. *Gerontologia* 19: 303–313, 1973.
134. LEVY, J. A., M. VIROLAINEN, and V. DEFENDI. Human lymphoblastoid lines from lymph node and spleen. *Cancer Lett.* 22: 517–524, 1968.
135. LIPETZ, J., and V. J. CRISTOFALO. Ultrastructural changes accompanying the aging of human diploid cells in culture. *J. Ultrastruct. Res.* 39: 43–56, 1972.
136. LIU, A. Y. C., H. S. CHOI, Y. K. LEE, and K. Y. CHEN. Molecular events involved in transcriptional activation of heat shock genes become progressively refractory to heat stimulation during aging of human diploid fibroblasts. *J. Cell. Physiol.* 149: 560–566, 1991.
137. LUCE, M. C., and C. L. BUNN. Decreased accuracy of protein synthesis in extracts from aging human diploid fibroblasts. *Exp. Gerontol.* 24: 113–125, 1989.
138. LUCE, M. C., and V. J. CRISTOFALO. Reduction in heat shock gene expression correlates with increased thermosensitivity in senescent human fibroblasts. *Exp. Cell Res.* 202: 9–16, 1992.
138a. LUCIBELLO, F. C., A. SEWING, S. BRUSSELBACH, C. BURGER, and R. MULLER. Deregulation of cyclins D1 and E and suppression of cdk2 and cdk4 in senescent human fibroblasts. *J. Cell Sci.* 105: 123–133, 1993.
139. LUMPKIN, C. K. J., J. K. MCCLUNG, O. M. PEREIRA-SMITH, and J. R. SMITH. Existence of high abundance antiproliferative mRNAs in senescent human diploid fibroblasts. *Science* 232: 393–395, 1986.
140. MACIEIRA-COELHO, A. Action of cortisone on human fibroblasts in vitro. *Experientia* 22: 390–391, 1966.
141. MACIEIRA-COELHO, A. The decreased growth potential in vitro of human fibroblasts of adult origin. In: *Aging in Cell and Tissue Culture,* edited by E. Holeckova and V. J. Cristofalo. New York: Plenum Press, 1970, p. 83–119.
142. MACIEIRA-COELHO, A. Metabolism of aging cells in culture. *Gerontology* 22: 3–8, 1976.
143. MACIEIRA-COELHO, A. *Biology of Normal Proliferating Cells In Vitro. Relevance for In Vivo Aging.* Basel: Karger, 1988.
144. MACIEIRA-COELHO, A., and L. BERUMEN. The cell cycle during growth inhibition of human embryonic fibroblasts in vitro. *Proc. Soc. Exp. Biol. Med.* 144: 43–47, 1973.
145. MACIEIRA-COELHO, A., and J. PONTEN. Analogy in growth between late passage human embryonic and early passage human adult fibroblasts. *J. Cell Biol.* 43: 374–377, 1969.
146. MACIEIRA-COELHO, A., J. PONTEN, and L. PHILLIPSON. The division cycle and RNA synthesis in diploid human cells at different passage levels in vitro. *Exp. Cell Res.* 42: 673–684, 1966.
147. MANN, D. M., P. J. MCKEOWN-LONGO, and A. J. MILLIS. Binding of soluble fibronectin and its subsequent incorporation into the extracellular matrix by early and late passage human skin fibroblasts. *J. Biol. Chem.* 263: 2756–2760, 1988.
148. MARTIN, G. M. Cellular aging: clonal senescence. *Am. J. Pathol.* 89: 484–511, 1977.
149. MARTIN, G. M. Genetic syndromes in man with potential relevance to pathobiology of aging. In: *Genetic Effects on Aging,* edited by D. Bergsma and D. E. Harrison. New York: Alan R. Liss, 1978, p. 5–39.
150. MARTIN, G. M., and C. A. SPRAGUE. Clonal senescence and atherosclerosis. *Lancet* 2: 1370–1371, 1972.
151. MARTIN, G. M., and C. A. SPRAGUE. Symposium on in vitro studies related to atherogenesis. Life histories of hyperplastoid cell lines from aorta and skin. *Exp. Mol. Pathol.* 18: 125–141, 1973.
152. MARTIN, G. M., C. E. OGBURN, and C. A. SPRAGUE. Effects of age on cell division capacity. In: *Aging: A Challenge to Science and Society,* edited by D. Danon, N. W. Shock and M. Marois. Oxford: Oxford University Press, 1981, vol. 1, p. 124–135.
153. MARTIN, G. M., C. A. SPRAGUE, and C. J. EPSTEIN. Replicative lifespan of cultivated human cells. Effects of donor age, tissue, and genotype. *Lab. Invest.* 23: 86–92, 1970.
154. MARTIN, G. M., C. A. SPRAGUE, T. H. NORWOOD, and W. R. PENDERGRASS. Clonal selection, attenuation and differentiation in an in vitro model of hyperplasia. *Am. J. Pathol.* 74: 137–154, 1974.
154a. MARX, J. How p53 suppresses cell growth. *Science* 262: 1644–1645, 1993.
155. MATSUMURA, T. Multinucleation and polyploidization of aging human cells in culture. *Adv. Exp. Med. Biol.* 129: 31–38, 1980.
156. MATSUMURA, T., Z. ZERRUDO, and L. HAYFLICK. Senescent human diploid cells in culture: survival, DNA synthesis and morphology. *J. Gerontol.* 34: 328–334, 1979.
157. MATTERN, M. R., and P. A. CERUTTI. Age-dependent excision repair of damaged thymine from gamma-irradiated DNA by isolated nuclei from human fibroblasts. *Nature* 254: 450–452, 1975.
158. MCHALE, J. S., M. L. MOUTON, and J. MCHALE. Limited culture lifespan of human diploid cells as a function of metabolic time instead of division potential. *Exp. Gerontol.* 6: 89–93, 1970.
159. MEEK, R. L., P. D. BOWMAN, and C. W. DANIEL. Establishment of mouse embryo cells in vitro. *Exp. Cell Res.* 107: 277–284, 1977.
160. MELLGREN, J. Effects of the number of cell divisions and of added isologous nucleic acids on aging of normal human fibroblasts in vitro. *Pathol. Eur.* 10: 215–219, 1975.
161. MERZ, G. S., and J. D. ROSS. Viability of human diploid cells as a function of in vitro age. *J. Cell. Physiol.* 74: 219–221, 1969.
162. MILLIS, A. J., M. HOYLE, H. M. MCCUE, and H. MARTINI. Differential expression of metalloproteinase and tissue inhibitor of metalloproteinase genes in aged human fibroblasts. *Exp. Cell Res.* 201: 373–379, 1992.
163. MILLIS, A. J., J. SOTTILE, M. HOYLE, D. M. MANN, and V. DIEMER. Collagenase production by early and late passage cultures of human fibroblasts. *Exp. Gerontol.* 24: 559–575, 1989.
164. MILO, G. E., and B. C. CASTRO. Conditions for transformation of human fibroblast cells: an overview. *Cancer Lett.* 31: 1–13, 1986.
165. MITSUI, Y., and E. L. SCHNEIDER. Increased nuclear sizes in senescent human diploid fibroblast cultures. *Exp. Cell Res.* 100: 147–152, 1976a.
166. MITSUI, Y., and E. L. SCHNEIDER. Relationship between cell replication and volume in senescent human diploid fibroblasts. *Mech. Ageing Dev.* 5: 45–56, 1976b.
167. MITSUI, Y., J. R. SMITH, and E. L. SCHNEIDER. Equivalent proliferation potential of different size classes of human diploid fibroblasts. *J. Gerontol.* 36: 416–419, 1981.
168. MOORE, G. E., and W. F. MCLIMANS. The life span of the

cultured normal cell: concepts derived from studies of human lymphoblasts. *J. Theor. Biol.* 20: 217–226, 1968.
169. MORLEY, A. A. Is ageing the result of dominant or co-dominant mutations? *J. Theor. Biol.* 98: 469–474, 1982.
170. MORRIS, C. M., A. E. REEVE, P. H. FITZGERALD, P. E. HOLLINGS, M. E. J. BEARD, and D. C. HEATON. Genomic diversity correlates with clinical variation in Ph-negative chronic myeloid leukaemia. *Nature* 320: 281–283, 1986.
171. MUELLER, S. N., E. M. ROSEN, and E. M. LEVINE. Cellular senescence in a cloned strain of bovine fetal aortic endothelial cells. *Science* 207: 889–891, 1980.
172. MURANO, S., R. THWEATT, R. J. SHMOOKLER-REIS, R. A. JONES, E. J. MOERMAN, and S. GOLDSTEIN. Diverse gene sequences are overexpressed in Werner syndrome fibroblasts undergoing premature replicative senescence. *Mol. Cell. Biol.* 11: 3905–3914, 1991.
173. MURATO, S.-I., Y. MITSUI, and M. KAWAMURA. Effect of in vitro aging on 6-ketoprostaglandin $F_{1\alpha}$-producing activity in cultured human diploid lung fibroblasts. *Biochim. Biophys. Acta* 574: 351–355, 1979.
173a. NASMYTH, K., and T. HUNT. Dams and sluices. *Nature* 366: 634–635, 1993.
174. NIELSEN, P. J., and J. M. RYAN. Cumulative population doublings as the determinant of chick cell lifespan in vitro. *J. Cell. Physiol.* 107: 371–378, 1981.
175. NIENHAUS, A. J., B. DE JONG, L. P. TEN KATE, and F. H. OSWALD. Fibroblast culture in Werner's syndrome. *Humangenetik* 13: 244–246, 1971.
176. NING, Y., J. C. WEBER, A. M. KILLARY, D. H. LEDBETTER, J. R. SMITH, and O. M. PEREIRA-SMITH. Genetic analysis of indefinite division in human cells: evidence for a cell senescence-related gene(s) on human chromosome 4. *Proc. Natl. Acad. Sci. USA* 88: 5635–5639, 1991.
176a. NODA, A., Y. NING, S. F. VENABLE, O. M. PEREIRA-SMITH, and J. R. SMITH. Cloning of senescent cell derived inhibitors of DNA synthesis using an expression screen. *Exp. Cell Res.* 211: 90–98, 1994.
177. NORWOOD, T. H., W. R. PENDERGRASS, C. A. SPRAGUE, and G. M. MARTIN. Dominance of the senescent phenotype in heterokaryons between replicative and post-replicative human fibroblast-like cells. *Proc. Natl. Acad. Sci. USA* 71: 2231–2235, 1974.
178. NORWOOD, T. H., A. SAULEWICZ, F. HANAOKA, and W. R. PENDERGRASS. Failure by senescent fibroblasts to complement a DNA polymerase α mutant (Abstract). *Ann. Meet. Geroniol. Soc. Am.* 44th San Francisco CA 1991, p. 354. Published in *The Gerontologist* by the Gerontological Society of America (GSA).
179. NORWOOD, T. H., J. R. SMITH, and G. H. STEIN. Aging at the cellular level: the human fibroblastlike cell model. In: *Handbook of the Biology of Aging*, edited by E. L. Schneider and J. W. Rowe. San Diego: Academic Press, 1990, p. 131–154.
180. OGDEN, D. A., and H. S. MICKLEM. The fate of serially transplanted bone marrow cell populations from young and old donors. *Transplantation* 22: 287–293, 1976.
181. OLASHAW, N. E., E. D. KRESS, and V. J. CRISTOFALO. Thymidine triphosphate synthesis in senescent WI38 cells. Relationship to loss of replicative capacity. *Exp. Cell Res.* 149: 547–554, 1983.
182. OLSSON, L., and P. EBBESEN. Aging decreases the activity of epidermal G_1 and G_2 inhibitors in mouse skin independent of grafting on old or young recipients. *Exp. Gerontol.* 12: 59–62, 1977.
183. ORGEL, L. E. The maintenance of the accuracy of protein synthesis and its relevance to aging. *Proc. Natl. Acad. Sci. USA* 49: 517–521, 1963.

184. PAINTER, R. B., J. M. CLARKSON, and B. R. YOUNG. Ultraviolet-induced repair replication in aging diploid human cells (WI-38). *Radiat. Res.* 56: 560–564, 1973.
185. PAPPENHOLZ, V. Correlation between DNA repair of embryonic fibroblasts and different life span of 3 inbred mouse strains. *Mech. Ageing Dev.* 7: 131–150, 1978.
186. PAULSSON, Y., M. BYWATER, S. PFEIFER-OHLSSON, R. OHLSSON, S. NILSSON, C. H. HELDIN, B. WESTERMARK, and C. BETSHOLTZ. Growth factors induce early pre-replicative changes in senescent human fibroblasts. *EMBO J.* 5: 2157–2162, 1986.
187. PENDERGRASS, W. R., J. C. ANGELLO, M. D. KIRSCHNER, and T. H. NORWOOD. The relationship between the rate of entry into S phase, concentration of DNA polymerase alpha, and cell volume in human diploid fibroblast-like monokaryon cells. *Exp. Cell Res.* 192: 418–425, 1991a.
188. PENDERGRASS, W. R., J. C. ANGELLO, A. C. SAULEWICZ, and T. H. NORWOOD. DNA polymerase alpha and the regulation of entry into S phase in heterokaryons. *Exp. Cell Res.* 192: 426–432, 1991b.
189. PENDERGRASS, W. R., G. M. MARTIN, and P. BORNSTEIN. Evidence contrary to the protein error hypothesis for in vitro senescence. *J. Cell. Physiol.* 87: 3–13, 1976.
190. PEREIRA-SMITH, O. M., and J. R. SMITH. Phenotype of low proliferative potential is dominant in hybrids of normal human fibroblasts. *Somatic Cell Mol. Genet.* 8: 731–742, 1982.
191. PEREIRA-SMITH, O. M., and J. R. SMITH. Evidence for the recessive nature of cellular immortality. *Science* 221: 964–966, 1983.
192. PEREIRA-SMITH, O. M., and J. R. SMITH. Genetic analysis of indefinite division in human cells: identification of four complementation groups. *Proc. Natl. Acad. Sci. USA* 85: 6042–6046, 1988.
193. PEREIRA-SMITH, O. M., S. F. FISHER, and J. R. SMITH. Senescent and quiescent cell inhibitors of DNA synthesis. Membrane-associated proteins. *Exp. Cell Res.* 160: 297–306, 1985.
194. PETERSON, C., and J. E. GOLDMAN. Alterations in calcium content and biochemical processes in cultured skin fibroblasts from aged and Alzheimer donors. *Proc. Natl. Acad. Sci. USA* 83: 2758–2762, 1986.
195. PETERSON, C., R. R. RATAN, M. L. SHELANSKI, and J. E. GOLDMAN. Cytosolic free calcium and cell spreading decrease in fibroblasts from aged and Alzheimer donors. *Proc. Natl. Acad. Sci. USA* 83: 7999–8001, 1986.
196. PETURSSON, G., J. G. COUGHLIN, and C. MEYLAN. Long-term cultivation of diploid rat cells. *Exp. Cell Res.* 33: 60–67, 1964.
197. PHILLIPS, P. D., K. KAJI, and V. J. CRISTOFALO. Progressive loss of the response of senescing WI-38 cells to platelet-derived growth factor, epidermal growth factor, insulin, transferrin, and dexamethasone. *J. Gerontol.* 39: 11–17, 1984.
198. PHILLIPS, P. D., E. KUHNLE, and V. J. CRISTOFALO. [^{125}I] EGF binding ability is stable throughout the replicative life span of WI-38 cells. *J. Cell. Physiol.* 114: 311–316, 1983.
199. PHILLIPS, P. D., R. J. PIGNOLO, and V. J. CRISTOFALO. Insulin-like growth factor-I: specific binding to high and low affinity sites and mitogenic action throughout the life span of WI-38 cells. *J. Cell. Physiol.* 133: 135–143, 1987.
200. PHILLIPS, P. D., R. J. PIGNOLO, K. NISHIKURA, and V. J. CRISTOFALO. Renewed DNA synthesis in senescent WI-38 cells by expression of an inducible chimeric c-fos construct. *J. Cell. Physiol.* 151: 206–212, 1992.
201. PIGNOLO, R. J., E. J. MASORO, W. W. NICHOLS, C. I. BRADT, and V. J. CRISTOFALO. Skin fibroblasts from Fischer 344 rats undergo similar changes in replicative life span but not immortalization with caloric restriction of donors. *Exp. Cell Res.* 201: 16–22, 1992.
202. PIGNOLO, R. J., M. O. ROTENBERG, and V. J. CRISTOFALO.

Differential expression of a novel cell cycle-regulated transcript in late population doubling level WI-38 cells (Abstract). *Ann. Meet. Gerontol. Soc. Am. 44th San Francisco CA 1991*, p. 74. published in *The Gerontologist* by Gerontological Society of America (GSA).

203. PIGNOLO, R. J., M. O. ROTENBERG, and V. J. CRISTOFALO. Senescent WI-38 cells fail to express EPC-1, a gene induced in young cells upon entry into the G$_o$ state. *J. Biol. Chem.* 268: 8949–8957, 1993.

203a. PIGNOLO, R. J., M. O. ROTENBERG, and V. J. CRISTOFALO. Alterations in contact and density-dependent arrest state in senescent WI-38 cells. *In Vitro Cell. Dev. Biol.* 30: 471–476, 1994.

204. PIOUS, D. A., R. N. HAMBURGER, and S. E. MILLS. Clonal growth of primary human cell cultures. *Exp. Cell Res.* 33: 495–507, 1964.

205. PLISKO, A., and B. A. GILCHREST. Growth factor responsiveness of cultured human fibroblasts declines with age. *J. Gerontol.* 38: 513–518, 1983.

206. POCHRON, S. F., A. R. O'MEARA, and M. J. KURTZ. Control of transcription in aging WI-38 cells stimulated by serum to divide. *Exp. Cell Res.* 116: 63–74, 1978.

207. PONTEN, J. Aging properties of glia. In: *INSERM*, edited by F. Bourliere, Y. Courtois, A. Macieira-Coelho and L. Robert. Paris: INSERM, 1973, vol. 27, p. 53–64.

208. PORTER, M. B., O. M. PEREIRA-SMITH, and J. R. SMITH. Novel monoclonal antibodies identify antigenic determinants unique to cellular senescence. *J. Cell. Physiol.* 142: 425–433, 1990.

209. PRAEGER, F. C., and V. J. CRISTOFALO. The growth of WI-38 cells in a serum-free, growth factor-free, medium with elevated calcium concentrations. *In Vitro Cell. Dev. Biol.* 22: 355–359, 1986a.

210. PRAEGER, F. C., and V. J. CRISTOFALO. Modulation of WI-38 cell proliferation by elevated levels of CaCl$_2$. *J. Cell. Physiol.* 129: 27–35, 1986b.

211. PRAEGER, F. C., and B. A. GILCHREST. Influence of increased extracellular calcium concentration and donor age on density-dependent growth inhibition of human fibroblasts. *Proc. Soc. Exp. Biol. Med.* 182: 315–321, 1986.

212. PRICE, G. B., and T. MAKINODAN. Immunologic deficiencies in senescence. II. Characterization of extrinsic deficiencies. *J. Immunol.* 108: 413–417, 1972.

213. PUCK, T. T., C. A. WALDREN, and J. H. TJIO. Some data bearing on the long term growth of mammalian cells. In: *Symposium on Topics in the Biology of Aging*, edited by P. L. Krohn. New York: J. Wiley, 1966, p. 101–123.

214. QUINN, L. S., T. H. NORWOOD, and M. NAMEROFF. Myogenic stem cell commitment probability remains constant as a function of organismal and mitotic age. *J. Cell. Physiol.* 134: 324–336, 1988.

215. RADNA, R. L., Y. CATON, K. K. JHA, P. KAPLAN, G. LI, F. TRAGONOS, and H. L. OZER. Immortalization of origin-defective simian virus 40 tsA-transformed human fibroblasts is temperature dependent. *Mol. Cell. Biol.* 9: 3093–3096, 1989.

216. RANSOM, R. *Computers and Embryos: Models in Developmental Biology*. New York: J. Wiley, 1981.

217. REGAN, J. D., M. M. SIGEL, W. H. LEE, K. A. LLAMAS, and A. R. BEASLEY. Chromosomal alterations in marine fish cells in vitro. *Can. J. Genet. Cytol.* 10: 448–453, 1968.

218. REZNICK, A. Z., A. DOVRAT, L. ROSENFELDER, S. SHUPUND, and D. GERSHON. Defective enzyme molecules in cells of aging animals are partially denatured, totally inactive, normal degradation intermediates. In: *Modern Aging Research, Modification of Proteins During Aging*, edited by R. C. Adelman and E. E. Dekker. New York: Alan R. Liss, 1985, vol. 7, p. 69–81.

219. RHEINWALD, J. G., and H. GREEN. Serial cultivation of strains of human epidermal keratinocytes: the formation of keratinizing colonies from single cells. *Cell* 6: 331–334, 1975.

220. RIABOWOL, K., J. SCHIFF, and M. Z. GILMAN. Transcription factor AP-1 activity is required for initiation of DNA synthesis and is lost during cellular aging. *Proc. Natl. Acad. Sci. USA* 89: 157–161, 1992.

221. RITTLING, S. R., K. M. BROOKS, V. J. CRISTOFALO, and R. BASERGA. Expression of cell cycle-dependent genes in young and senescent WI-38 fibroblasts. *Proc. Natl. Acad. Sci. USA* 83: 3316–3320, 1986.

222. ROBBINS, E., E. M. LEVINE, and H. EAGLE. Morphological changes accompanying senescence of cultured human diploid cells. *J. Exp. Med.* 131: 1211–1222, 1970.

223. RÖHME, D. Evidence for a relationship between longevity of mammalian species and life-spans of normal fibroblasts in vitro and erythrocytes in vivo. *Proc. Natl. Acad. Sci. USA* 78: 5009–5013, 1981.

224. ROSE, D. W., G. MCCABE, J. R. FERAMISCO, and M. ADLER. Expression of c-fos and AP-1 activity in senescent human fibroblasts is not sufficient for DNA synthesis. *J. Cell. Biol.* 119: 1405–1411, 1992.

225. ROSENDAAL, M., G. S. HODGSON, and T. R. BRADLEY. Haemopoietic stem cells are organised for use on the basis of their generation age. *Nature* 264: 68–69, 1976.

226. ROTHSTEIN, M. The alteration of enzymes in aging. In: *Modern Aging Research, Modification of Proteins During Aging*, edited by R. C. Adelman and E. E. Dekker. New York: Alan R. Liss, 1985, vol. 7, p. 53–67.

227. ROWE, D. W., B. J. STARMAN, W. Y. FUJIMOTO, and R. H. WILLIAMS. Differences in growth response to hydrocortisone and ascorbic acid by human diploid fibroblasts. *In Vitro Cell. Dev. Biol.* 13: 824–830, 1977.

228. RYAN, J. M., and V. J. CRISTOFALO. Chromatin template activity during aging in WI-38 cells. *Exp. Cell Res.* 90: 456–458, 1975.

229. RYAN, J. M., G. DUDA, and V. J. CRISTOFALO. Error accumulation and aging in human diploid cells. *J. Gerontol.* 29: 616–621, 1974.

230. RYAN, J. M., D. G. OSTROW, X. O. BREAKEFIELD, E. S. GERSHON, and L. UPCHURCH. A comparison of the proliferative and replication lifespan kinetics of cell cultures derived from monozygotic twins. *In Vitro Cell. Dev. Biol.* 17: 20–27, 1981.

230a. RYAN, P. A., V. M. MAHER, and J. J. MCCORMICK. Failure of infinite life span human cells from different immortality complementation groups to yield finite life span hybrids. *J. Cell. Physiol.* 159: 151–160, 1994.

231. SCHNEIDER, E. L., and C. J. EPSTEIN. Replication rate and lifespan of cultured fibroblasts in Down's syndrome. *Proc. Soc. Exp. Biol. Med.* 141: 1092–1094, 1972.

232. SCHNEIDER, E. L., and B. J. FOWLKES. Measurement of DNA content and cell volume in senescent human fibroblasts utilizing flow multiparameter single cell analysis. *Exp. Cell Res.* 98: 298–302, 1976.

233. SCHNEIDER, E. L., and Y. MITSUI. The relationship between in vitro cellular aging and in vivo human age. *Proc. Natl. Acad. Sci. USA* 73: 3584–3588, 1976.

234. SCHNEIDER, E. L., and S. S. SHORR. Alteration in cellular RNAs during the in vitro lifespan of cultured human diploid fibroblasts. *Cell* 6: 179–184, 1975.

235. SCHNEIDER, E. L., Y. MITSUI, R. TICE, S. S. SHORR, and K. BRAUNSCHWEIGER. Alteration in cellular RNAs during the in vitro lifespan of cultured human diploid fibroblasts. II. Synthesis and processing of RNA. *Mech. Ageing Dev.* 4: 449–458, 1975.

236. SCHWARTZ, A. G. Correlation between species life span and capacity to activate 7,12-dimethylbenz(a)anthracene to a form mutagenic to a mammalian cell. *Exp. Cell Res.* 94: 445–447, 1975.

236a. SELL, C., A. PTASZNIK, C. D. CHANG, J. SWANTEK, V. J. CRISTOFALO, and R. BASERGA. IGF-I receptor levels and the proliferation of young and senescent human fibroblasts. *Biochem. Biophys. Res. Commun.* 194: 259–265, 1993.

237. SESHADRI, T., and J. CAMPISI. Repression of c-fos transcription and an altered genetic program in senescent human fibroblasts. *Science* 247: 205–209, 1990.

237a. SESHADRI, T., J. A. UZMAN, J. OSHIMA, and J. CAMPISI. Identification of a transcript that is down-regulated in senescent human fibroblasts. *J. Biol. Chem.* 268: 18474–18480, 1993.

238. SHAY, J. W., O. M. PEREIRA-SMITH, and W. E. WRIGHT. A role for both RB and p53 in the regulation of human cellular senescence. *Exp. Cell Res.* 196: 33–39, 1991.

239. SHAY, J. W., M. D. WEST, and W. E. WRIGHT. Re-expression of senescent markers in deinduced reversibly immortalized cells. *Exp. Gerontol.* 27: 477–492, 1992.

240. SHAY, J. W., W. R. WRIGHT, and H. WERBIN. Defining the molecular mechanisms of human cell immortalization. *Biochim. Biophys. Acta* 1072: 1–7, 1991.

241. SHIGEOKA, H., and H. C. YANG. Early kinase C dependent events in aging human diploid fibroblasts. *Mech. Ageing Dev.* 55: 49–59, 1990.

242. SIMINOVITCH, L., J. E. TILL, and E. A. MCCULLOCH. Decline in colony-forming ability of marrow cells subjected to serial transplantation into irradiated mice. *J. Cell. Physiol.* 64: 23–31, 1964.

243. SIMONS, J. W. J. W. A theoretical and experimental approach to the relationship between cell variability and aging in vitro. In: *Aging in Cell and Tissue Culture,* edited by E. Holeckova and V. J. Cristofalo. New York: Plenum Press, 1970, p. 25–39.

244. SIMONS, J. W. I. M., and C. VAN DEN BROEK. Comparison of ageing in vitro and ageing in vivo by means of size analysis using a Coulter counter. *Gerontologia* 16: 340–351, 1970.

245. SLAYBACK, J. R. B., L. W. Y. CHEUNG, and R. P. GEGER. Comparative effects of human platelet growth factor on the growth and morphology of human fetal and adult diploid fibroblasts. *Exp. Cell Res.* 110: 462–466, 1977.

246. SMITH, B. T., J. S. TORDAY, and C. J. P. GIROUD. The growth promoting effect of cortisol in human fetal lung cells. *Steroids* 22: 515–524, 1973.

247. SMITH, C. A., and P. C. HANAWALT. Repair replication in cultured normal and transformed human fibroblasts. *Biochim. Biophys. Acta* 447: 121–132, 1976.

248. SMITH, J. R. Inhibitors of DNA synthesis derived from senescent human diploid fibroblasts. *Exp. Gerontol.* 27: 409–412, 1992.

249. SMITH, J. R., and L. HAYFLICK. Variation in the life-span of clones derived from human diploid cell strains. *J. Cell Biol.* 62: 48–53, 1974.

250. SMITH, J. R., and R. G. WHITNEY. Intraclonal variation in proliferative potential of human diploid fibroblasts: stochastic mechanism for cellular aging. *Science* 207: 82–84, 1980.

251. SMITH, J. R., O. PEREIRA-SMITH, and E. L. SCHNEIDER. Colony size distribution as a measure of in vivo and in vitro aging. *Proc. Natl. Acad. Sci. USA* 75: 1353–1356, 1978.

252. SOTTILE, J., M. HOYLE, and A. J. MILLIS. Differential response of early and late passage fibroblasts to collagenase stimulatory factor in conditioned media. *Coll. Relat. Res.* 8: 361–374, 1988.

253. SOTTILE, J., D. M. MANN, V. DIEMER, and A. J. MILLIS. Regulation of collagenase and collagenase mRNA production in early- and late-passage human diploid fibroblasts. *J. Cell. Physiol.* 138: 281–290, 1989.

254. SOUKUPOVA, M., E. HOLECKOVA, and P. HNEVKOVSKY. Changes of the latent period of explanted tissues during ontogenesis. In: *Aging in Cell and Tissue Culture,* edited by E. Holeckova and V. J. Cristofalo. New York: Plenum Press, 1970, p. 41–56.

255. STANLEY, J., D. PYE, and A. MACGREGOR. Comparison of doubling numbers attained by cultured animal cells with life span of species. *Nature* 255: 158–159, 1975.

256. STANULIS-PRAEGER, B. M. Cellular senescence revisited: a review. *Mech. Ageing Dev.* 38: 1–48, 1987.

257. STEIN, G. H. SV40-transformed human fibroblasts: evidence for cellular aging in precrisis cells. *J. Cell. Physiol.* 125: 36–44, 1985.

258. STEIN, G. H., and L. ATKINS. Membrane-associated inhibitor of DNA synthesis in senescent human diploid fibroblasts: characterization and comparison to quiescent cell inhibitor. *Proc. Natl. Acad. Sci. USA* 83: 9030–9034, 1986.

259. STEIN, G. H., and R. M. YANISHEVSKY. Entry into S phase is inhibited in two immortal cell lines fused to senescent human diploid cells. *Exp. Cell Res.* 120: 155–165, 1979.

260. STEIN, G. H., and R. M. YANISHEVSKY. Quiescent human diploid cells can inhibit entry into S phase in replicative nuclei in heterodikaryons. *Proc. Natl. Acad. Sci. USA* 78: 3025–3029, 1981.

261. STEIN, G. H., R. M. YANISHEVSKY, L. GORDON, and M. BEESON. Carcinogen-transformed human cells are inhibited from entry into S phase by fusion to senescent cells but cells transformed by DNA tumor viruses overcome the inhibition. *Proc. Natl. Acad. Sci. USA* 79: 5287–5291, 1982.

262. STEIN, G. H., L. ATKINS, M. BEESON, and L. GORDON. Quiescent human diploid fibroblasts: common mechanism for inhibition of DNA replication in density-inhibited and serum-deprived cells. *Exp. Cell Res.* 162: 255–260, 1986.

263. STEIN, G. H., M. BEESON, and L. GORDON. Failure to phosphorylate retinoblastoma gene product in senescent human fibroblasts. *Science* 249: 666–669, 1990.

264. STEIN, G. H., L. F. DRULLINGER, R. S. ROBETORYE, O. M. PEREIRA-SMITH, and J. R. SMITH. Senescent cells fail to express cdc2, cyc A, and cycB in response to mitogen stimulation. *Proc. Natl. Acad. Sci. USA* 88: 11012–11016, 1991.

265. STEINHAGEN, M. Effect of donor age on clonal differentiation of human skin fibroblasts in vitro. *Gerontology* 31: 27–38, 1985.

266. SUDA, Y., M. SUZUKI, Y. IKAWA, and S. AIZAWA. Mouse embryonic stem cells exhibit indefinite proliferative potential. *J. Cell. Physiol.* 33: 197–201, 1987.

267. SUGAWARA, O., M. OSHIMURA, M. KOI, L. A. ANNAB, and J. C. BARRETT. Induction of cellular senescence in immortalized cells by human chromosome 1. *Science* 247: 707–710, 1990.

268. SWIM, H. E., and R. F. PARKER. Culture characteristics of human fibroblasts propagated serially. *Am. J. Hyg.* 66: 235, 1957.

269. SZILARD, L. On the nature of the aging process. *Proc. Natl. Acad. Sci. USA* 45: 30–45, 1959.

270. TASSIN, J., E. MALAISE, and Y. COURTOIS. Human lens cells have an in vitro proliferative capacity inversely proportional to the donor age. *Exp. Cell Res.* 123: 388–392, 1979.

271. THRASH, C. R., and D. D. CUNNINGHAM. Stimulation of division of density-inhibited fibroblasts by glucocorticoids. *Nature* 242: 399–401, 1973.

272. THWEATT, R., C. K. LUMPKIN, and S. GOLDSTEIN. A novel gene encoding a smooth muscle protein is overexpressed in senescent

human fibroblasts. *Biochem. Biophys. Res. Commun.* 187: 1–7, 1992.
273. THWEATT, R., S. MURANO, R. D. FLEISCHMANN, and S. GOLDSTEIN. Isolation and characterization of gene sequences overexpressed in Werner syndrome fibroblasts during premature replicative senescence. *Exp. Gerontol.* 27: 433–440, 1992.
274. TICE, R. R., E. L. SCHNEIDER, D. KRAM, and P. THORNE. Cytokinetic analysis of impaired proliferative response of peripheral lymphocytes from aged humans to phytohemagglutinin. *J. Exp. Med.* 149: 1029–1041, 1979.
275. TODARO, G. J., and H. GREEN. Serum albumin supplemented medium for long-term cultivation of mammalian fibroblast strains. *Proc. Soc. Exp. Biol. Med.* 116: 688–692, 1964.
276. TODARO, G. J., S. R. WOLMAN, and H. GREEN. Rapid transformation of human fibroblasts with low growth potential into established cell lines by SV40. *J. Cell. Physiol.* 62: 257–265, 1963.
277. VALENTI, C., and E. A. FRIEDMAN. Long-term cultivation of diploid rabbit skin cells. *Tex. Rep. Biol. Med.* 26: 363–380, 1968.
278. VINCENT, R. A., and P. C. HUANG. The proportion of cells labeled with tritiated thymidine as a function of population doubling level in cultures of fetal, adult, mutant, and tumor origin. *Exp. Cell Res.* 102: 31–42, 1976.
279. WANG, E. A 57,000-mol-wt. protein uniquely present in nonproliferating cells and senescent human fibroblasts. *J. Cell Biol.* 100: 545–551, 1985a.
280. WANG, E. Rapid disappearance of statin, a nonproliferating and senescent-cell specific protein, upon reentering the process of cell cycling. *J. Cell Biol.* 101: 1695–1701, 1985b.
281. WANG, E. Statin, a non-proliferation-specific protein, is associated with the nuclear envelope and is heterogeneously distributed in cells leaving quiescent state. *J. Cell. Physiol.* 140: 418–426, 1989.
282. WANG, E., and S. L. LIN. Disappearance of statin, a protein marker for nonproliferating and senescent cells, following serum-stimulated cell-cycle entry. *Exp. Cell Res.* 167: 135–143, 1986.
283. WANG, E., and G. TOMASZEWSKI. Granular presence of terminin is the marker to distinguish between the senescent and quiescent states. *J. Cell. Physiol.* 147: 514–522, 1991.
284. WEISSMAN-SHOMER, P., and M. FRY. Chick embryo fibroblast senescence in vitro: pattern of cell division and life span as a function of cell density. *Mech. Ageing Dev.* 4: 159–166, 1975.
285. WEST, M. D., W. E. WRIGHT, and J. W. SHAY. Transcriptional mechanisms regulating the over-expression of plasminogen activator inhibitor-1 in senescent fibroblasts (Abstract). *Ann. Meet. Gerontol. Soc. Am. 44th San Francisco CA 1991*, p. 314. published in The Gerontologist by the Gerontological Society of America (GSA).
285a. WHITAKER, N. J., E. L. KIDSTON, and R. R. REDDEL. Finite life span of hybrids formed by fusion of different simian virus 40–immortalized human cell lines. *J. Virol.* 66: 1202–1206, 1992.
286. WILLIAMS, J. R., and K. L. DEARFIELD. Nonhuman fibroblast-like cells in culture. In: *CRC Handbook of Cell Biology of Aging*, edited by V. J. Cristofalo. Boca Raton, FL: CRC Press, 1985, p. 433–451.
287. WILLIE, J. J., N. R. PITTELKOW, G. D. SHIPLEY, and R. E. SCOTT. Integrated control of growth and differentiation of normal human prokeratinocytes cultured in serum-free medium: clonal analyses, growth kinetics and cell cycle studies. *J. Cell. Physiol.* 121: 31–44, 1984.
288. WISTROM, C., and B. VILLEPONTEAU. Cloning and expression of SAG: a novel marker of cellular senescence. *Exp. Cell Res.* 199: 355–362, 1992.
289. WON, K.-A., Y. XIONG, D. BEACH, and M. Z. GILMAN. Growth-regulated expression of D-type cyclin genes in human diploid fibroblasts. *Proc. Natl. Acad. Sci. USA* 89: 9910–9914, 1992.
290. WRIGHT, W. E., and J. W. SHAY. Telomere positional effects and the regulation of cellular senescence. *Trends Genet.* 8: 193–197, 1992.
291. WRIGHT, W. E., O. M. PEREIRA-SMITH, and J. W. SHAY. Reversible cellular senescence: implications for immortalization of normal human diploid cells. *Mol. Cell. Biol.* 9: 3088–3092, 1989.
292. YAFFE, D. Retention of differentiation potentialities during prolonged cultivation of myogenic cells. *Proc. Natl. Acad. Sci. USA* 61: 477–483, 1968.
293. YANISHEVSKY, R., and A. V. CARRANO. Prematurely condensed chromosomes of dividing and non-dividing cells in aging human cell cultures. *Exp. Cell Res.* 90: 169–174, 1975.
294. YANISHEVSKY, R. M., and G. H. STEIN. Ongoing DNA synthesis continues in young human diploid cells (HDC) fused to senescent HDC, but entry into S phase is inhibited. *Exp. Cell Res.* 126: 469–472, 1980.
295. YANISHEVSKY, R., M. L. MENDELSOHN, B. H. MAYALL, and V. J. CRISTOFALO. Proliferative capacity and DNA content of aging human diploid cells in culture: a cytophotometric and autoradiographic analysis. *J. Cell. Physiol.* 84: 165–170, 1974.

5. Human studies

DENIS A. EVANS | *Center for Research on Health and Aging, Rush-Presbyterian-St. Luke's Medical Center, Chicago, Illinois*

CHAPTER CONTENTS

Approaching the Study of Human Aging—Advantages of Longitudinal Studies
Study Populations and the Role of Epidemiological Studies
    Large-scale population-based studies
    Investigating common conditions of multifactorial origin
Measuring Health and Disease among Older Persons
    Function and disease
    Measurement issues
      Measurement of physical function
      Measurement of cognitive function
Practical Considerations in Conducting Studies among Older Persons
    Obtaining and maintaining study participation
    Other practical considerations

THE PURPOSE OF A WELL-DESIGNED RESEARCH STUDY is to answer a question, so in designing any study, the essential first step is to specify the question of interest. Previous chapters have dealt with general design considerations in aging research (Chapters 1 and 2) and with design issues in studying aging in animal models (Chapter 3) and in cell culture systems (Chapter 4). This chapter focuses on studies of humans, with emphasis on the special requirements of studies that involve older persons.

Many considerations enter into designing a study, including the nature of the question, available resources for conducting the study, and the experience and knowledge of the investigators. Attempts at conducting studies in which the question is vague or poorly considered usually end in failure. Having specified the question of interest with as much precision as possible, the investigator must choose an approach or study design that will provide the most accurate answer. In contrast to in vitro animal studies, most human studies are observational rather than experimental or interventional; the major exceptions are randomized trials of experimental therapies. A number of basic observational study designs with many possible variations and combinations of features have evolved to address research questions.

Stated most directly, most questions related to aging involve considerations of change. Deciding how to approach such questions requires at least a basic understanding of the value and difficulties of longitudinal study designs, because the essence of aging is change over time. Longitudinal study designs that directly consider change often have distinct advantages over other approaches, and for this reason they will be emphasized here. Although many of the same principles apply to a study's design regardless of its size, in this chapter the emphasis is on large-scale studies. Many of the relevant human studies are large-scale, and the issues peculiar to these studies are not covered in detail elsewhere in this volume.

APPROACHING THE STUDY OF HUMAN AGING—ADVANTAGES OF LONGITUDINAL STUDIES

In general, longitudinal study designs (see Chapter 1) are powerful tools for investigating scientific questions. Their usefulness is especially important in studying aging because aging is fundamentally a process of change in individual organisms, and longitudinal approaches permit direct measurement of change in individuals. Study designs that approach aging without measuring change are necessarily indirect, at least to some degree. Longitudinal studies have other well-recognized general applications as well. For example the relationships of variables to one another in time can be understood clearly from longitudinal studies, which is especially important if the study is concerned with whether one variable may have a causal relation with another. The meaning of an association is often clarified if it can be determined which variable arose first. For example, does an observed association between a measure of depression and a measure of poor physical health reflect the impact of depression on physical health or vice versa? One can make a plausible argument for either path, or both; knowing the relation between these variables in time is essential to understanding how they might affect one another.

Longitudinal studies also permit uniform measurement of the predictors (risk factors) prior to any distortion by the outcome (disease). The presence of a disease often alters behavior; for example, a person may well change eating, smoking, or alcohol consumption habits after a heart attack. If one wants to explore the relation of such health-related habits to the risk of having a heart attack, it is well to measure them before the heart attack occurs.

To achieve these advantages, longitudinal studies must be conducted with rigorous attention to methodological detail. In this regard they are substantially more challenging than cross-sectional studies because they require data collection at multiple times and because the validity of their results depends strongly on attaining high rates of participation at each of these measurement points.

Much of our current knowledge of human aging does not come from longitudinal studies but from studies in which the variables of interest are measured at the same time. These are often referred to as "cross-sectional" studies. Because such studies do not directly measure change, it is necessary to infer from single-point measurements what happens as a person ages. To study the effect of age on another variable of interest in a cross-sectional study, we typically tabulate values of this variable for persons of different ages. From this tabulation, we draw inferences about how this variable behaves as persons become older. The underlying concept of interest is change in this variable with age for each person. In cross-sectional studies, however, we cannot directly measure change with age for each person. Instead, we are comparing the variable of interest for groups of different persons, who, among their many other differences, happen also to be of different ages, and, from this comparison, we indirectly infer the behavior of this variable with age. Practically, this inference from cross-sectional data is subject to substantial errors arising from the many differences (other than age) that characterize the persons making up the different age groups. One major source of such differences is frequently labeled "cohort effects." In this usage, a cohort is understood to be a group of persons who remain together and can be followed as a group over time. Each of us can be regarded as belonging to a birth cohort (28) of persons born in a particular year or other time period, who then, in a sense, age together. A second source of error is selective (nonrandom) removal of persons from a population, typically removal by death or institutionalization of the sickest persons.

These sources of error may be illustrated by considering an imaginary cross-sectional study conducted in 1990 of cognitive and physical functions among persons 65–90 years of age. To estimate the effect of age on cognition, we might divide the participants into 5-year age groups and compare performance on tests of cognitive function across those groups. With regard to cohort effects, those comprising the 65–70-year-old group were born from 1920–1925 and those in the 85–90-year-old group were born from 1900–1905. Thus, these two groups are from different birth cohorts that have been exposed to different life experiences, such as a different average level of educational attainment and different types of occupations. These life experiences may modify cognitive test performance and the effects of cohort differences may be mistakenly attributed to the difference in age between groups. In studies of cognition, the use of cross-sectional data, ignoring cohort differences, has tended to overestimate decline in cognitive function with age (41, 42).

Selective removal from the population due to death or institutionalization might also distort our ability to make inferences regarding aging from this imaginary cross-sectional study. If we regard the question of interest as estimating changes in physical or cognitive function with age for the entire population and not merely for its healthy members, then such selective losses may lead to underestimation of these changes. Persons with cognitive or physical impairment are, on average, at higher risk either of death or of entering nursing homes (1, 6, 21). Those who have died, of course, cannot participate, and those in nursing homes may be difficult to identify and enroll in studies. Cross-sectional data, selectively omitting these persons, will underestimate loss of physical and cognitive function, because only older persons who have avoided death or institutionalization will be enrolled. In longitudinal studies, in contrast, a cohort of persons can be followed with sequential measurement of physical and cognitive function.

Our discussions have necessarily taken a very general view of longitudinal studies, emphasizing only the essential elements of multiple measurements over time for a defined group of individuals. This ignores the great range of additional complexity in this area with respect to both longitudinal study designs and to methods of analysis. Only a few additional points with basic practical implications will be briefly noted here. In designing longitudinal studies, one immediate practical consideration is whether one is dealing with variables that are best thought of as being either present or absent, that is, as dichotomies or, alternatively, as continuous variables. A second basic decision is how many times variables will be measured. A longitudinal study requires that variables be measured on the same individuals at at least two time points, but there are strong advantages to multiple measures in many situations (36). Many investigations of risk factors and disease are typically thought of as examining dichotomous variables at two time points. An individual may be thought of as exposed or unexposed to the risk factor of interest and as developing or not developing the disease under investigation. An initial contact defines the study cohort, eliminating persons with prevalent cases of the disease of interest, and permits uniform measurement of the risk factors of interest in the cohort prior to the overt onset of incident disease. After a period of time, usually a few years, a second contact allows the detection of incident disease that developed in this interval.

In more complex longitudinal studies, sequential measurements of the variables of interest are made at multiple time points and a wide range of analytical approaches are possible (7, 10, 19, 27, 32, 37, 39). It is important to keep measurement of the variables at each time as similar as possible and to use measures with low random variation (high reliability) between repeated determinations so as to maximize the ability to measure real change in the variables of interest. Because of the number and complexity of analytical approaches possible with sequentially collected data, it is essential to have the advice of a statistician knowledgeable in this area at the time the study is designed, as well as during analyses.

STUDY POPULATIONS AND THE ROLE OF EPIDEMIOLOGICAL STUDIES

Investigators conducting research relevant to older persons have a wide range of choices in selecting the persons they will ask to participate in studies. The most frequent approach is to select what are sometimes called "samples of convenience"; the major reasons for selecting potential participants are ease of access by the investigators and the anticipated willingness of these persons to volunteer for the study. This approach typically leads to enrollment of persons from special groups, such as older persons attending a clinic or members of a senior citizen's club or even acquaintances of the investigators. If older persons are to be compared to younger persons, the younger people may be selected from groups, such as college students, that are very different from those from which the older people are selected. Investigations in these special groups have made large contributions to our understanding of aging, and they remain an appropriate and reasonable way to approach many issues. Studies carried out in samples of convenience also have some large intrinsic limitations, however.

Large-Scale Population-Based Studies

Persons in special groups may differ greatly from older persons in the general population. Often, volunteers from special groups are of higher socioeconomic status and in better health than persons of similar age in the general population. If persons of different ages are selected from different special groups, any comparisons will reflect not only the age differences but also any other differences in the characteristics and compositions of these special groups. Awareness of these limitations has led to increasing emphasis on conducting studies in defined populations, for example, all persons residing in a specified geographic area.

The techniques for large-scale population studies of common chronic diseases have been highly developed in epidemiology, a discipline that has been defined as "the study of the distribution and determinants of health-related states or events in defined populations" (28). Therefore, at least to some extent, such population studies may appear to be the province of the epidemiologist. This appearance, however, is misleading; the value of a truly multidisciplinary approach in these studies cannot be overestimated. Typically, such studies require close collaboration among persons from such diverse disciplines as epidemiology, biostatistics, the medical and basic science fields most directly concerned with the substantive matters of interest, and the social sciences. Nonetheless, epidemiological research has made large contributions to understanding the causes and prevention of such conditions as coronary heart disease, hypertension, lung cancer, and chronic obstructive lung disease. To a large degree, the study of the health problems of older persons overlaps with the study of these common conditions. Thus an understanding of the health of older persons demands effective ways of studying common chronic conditions and of utilizing the special knowledge and techniques of epidemiology.

One difficulty with studies limited to samples of convenience is that the descriptive data from these samples are often of limited interest. For example, the prevalence or incidence of Alzheimer's disease in a clinical population is probably only of local administrative interest; estimates from a geographically defined community are of much greater interest because they may accurately reflect prevalence or incidence in the general population. A still larger reason for emphasizing studies in defined populations over those carried out in samples of convenience is the relevance of population-based studies to understanding the etiology and prevention of chronic diseases of multifactorial origin and other common health conditions. Such studies are playing an increasingly important role in aging research because the burden of ill health resulting from common chronic diseases or other health conditions is very large among older persons and has focused attention on the need to prevent or modify disease and disability in this age group.

Investigating Common Conditions of Multifactorial Origin

One feature of many common chronic diseases is that their occurrence is not explained by any one factor or by a simple combination of factors. Coronary heart disease does not arise from cigarette smoking alone, from elevated blood pressure alone, or from elevated serum cholesterol alone. Rather, each of these (together with many other factors, a number of which are unknown) makes a contribution to the occurrence of the disease, and changing any factor potentially alters the occurrence of the disease. Thus each may be considered a risk factor for coronary heart disease, and identification of potentially reversible risk factors opens avenues for disease prevention. Multiple risk factor models of disease occurrence may well be applicable to understanding the occurrence and prevention of many common chronic problems of older persons, and greater understanding of the techniques of study design and analysis widely used in epidemiological research is likely to contribute substantially to advances in aging. This is especially likely to be true for longitudinal studies, both because of their general advantages in understanding the relation between possible causal factors and the occurrence of disease and because of the special relevance of longitudinal studies to understanding aging (see earlier under APPROACHING THE STUDY OF HUMAN AGING . . .).

One strong advantage of studying defined populations in investigating risk factors for common chronic conditions is that, at least for some diseases, they provide assurance that those persons identified as having a disease are truly comparable with those identified as not having that disease. An alternative approach is the case-control study that uses the medical care system to identify cases of a disease (for example, persons hospitalized with the illness) and then compares these cases to controls selected from the general population. Such case-control studies have proved useful in identifying risk factors for many illnesses (29) and have the additional advantage of being typically much less expensive than cohort studies. The approach of comparing cases identified through the medical care system with population controls has substantial potential for bias, however, if the cases identified through receipt of medical care differ systematically in important ways from all the cases in the general population. For example, if persons with the disease of interest are more likely to come to medical attention if they are also of higher socioeconomic status, then factors associated with high socioeconomic status may appear to be artifactually associated with the disease. This disadvantage may be especially relevant to etiological studies of common chronic problems in older persons; chronic diseases and other health problems are common in the older age groups, and, for at least some of these illnesses, only a fraction of persons with the condition may have it detected and recorded during the routine delivery of medical care.

Case-control studies of Alzheimer's disease offer a practical example of this situation. Some case-control studies (15, 47) that used the existing medical care system to identify cases but selected control subjects from population samples have found an inverse relation between cigarette smoking and risk of Alzheimer's disease. However, Alzheimer's disease is one of the common illnesses of older persons for which the fraction of disease that comes to medical attention is unknown and may be small. The possibility of bias according to characteristics reflecting access to medical care, including higher socioeconomic status (18), makes the results of these case-control studies difficult to interpret. The prevalence of cigarette smoking is substantially higher among persons from lower socioeconomic strata (20, 45), and this bias may account, at least in part, for the lower prevalence of smokers among cases. It is noteworthy that the one study (43) reporting a positive association between smoking and Alzheimer's disease used cases identified through a U.S. Veterans Administration facility, a hospital likely to have a large number of smokers among its patients. Much closer comparability between persons with the condition and unaffected persons can usually be achieved in studies of defined populations with ascertainment of disease independent of existing systems of medical care. The study design in the defined population can be either a longitudinal cohort study in which persons initially free of the condition of interest are followed for its occurrence over a defined period of time or a case-control study in which both affected and unaffected persons are randomly selected from the same defined population.

MEASURING HEALTH AND DISEASE AMONG OLDER PERSONS

Function and Disease

To some extent, we are accustomed to thinking of health as the absence of defined diseases. As researchers, then, we sometimes translate our overall goal of understanding and improving the health of older persons into one of understanding the mechanisms, treatment, and prevention of these diseases. This concept of health and aging is too narrow, however. It ignores the need to understand fundamental mechanisms of aging, an area treated in much more detail in other chapters. It also does not take into account that the absence of specified diseases does not fully define health, nor does their presence fully define poor health. The most telling criticism of definitions of health limited to the presence or absence of disease is that they ignore function, and, in the last few decades, the advantages of broader definitions of health emphasizing function have received increasing recognition (17, 44).

Both traditional, disease-specific and broader functional definitions of health have value in conceptualizing and conducting research among older persons. It is likely, in fact, that one key to making substantial progress in understanding common chronic problems of older persons will be increased knowledge of how these two concepts of health are related. A major advantage of functional definitions of health is that they may more closely reflect the aspects of health that are most important to older persons themselves because they represent what a person is able to actually do. A second advantage is that estimates of a person's function, either by that person or by an observer, appear to be good predictors of need for and utilization of health care and social services (5). In contrast, a major reason for using disease-based concepts of health is that most of our current thinking about causation and prevention is based on specific diseases. For example, we do analyses relating risk factors to coronary heart disease and implement major public health campaigns to assist in its prevention. It is reasonably assumed that successful efforts at reducing or preventing such diseases will result in substantial increases in health and function.

Measurement Issues

For many specific disease conditions, including the various manifestations of coronary heart disease (38), chronic obstructive lung disease (8), hypertension (3), Alzheimer's disease (31), and stroke (14, 48), formal criteria have been established and are usually suitable for use among older persons. No attempt will be made to review these criteria here. Measures of function among older persons are less clearly understood, however, and will be reviewed briefly. More comprehensive reviews (24, 46) are also available for the interested reader.

A person's function can be subdivided into many aspects, and each of these can be assessed in many different ways. The most basic conceptual division relevant to older persons, typically, is between physical and cognitive functions. In terms of assessment methods, measurement by open-ended, unspecified questions is usually distinguished from batteries of structured questions or other items with specified response categories. Within structured methods, report of function by either the subject or by a proxy respondent is separated from direct performance testing of function in which the subject is asked to carry out a defined task and performance is measured by a trained observer. For research purposes, defined, structured measurement techniques are strongly preferred because they reduce observer bias and permit combining results from multiple subjects in a meaningful fashion. Cognitive function in research studies is usually assessed by direct performance testing with measures ranging from brief batteries requiring only a few moments to administer to extensive arrays of neuropsychological performance tests. Physical function is assessed for research purposes in both ways. The most frequently used measures employ reporting by the subject or a proxy, but direct performance testing of physical function has become increasingly common as a research tool. Each of these approaches has both advantages and disadvantages so that the choice of the optimal measurement technique for a particular study usually depends on the purpose and design of that study.

Measurement of Physical Function A large number of measures of physical function have been extensively used to assess older persons in research studies. Most of these are report measures, and most also measure cognitive as well as physical functions. It is often difficult to be certain to what degree impairment measured by report may reflect impaired physical function and to what degree it may reflect impaired cognition. Most of the commonly used scales were developed to assess intensity of need for medical care services, especially among persons receiving institutional long-term care, but they are currently used for a much wider range of study purposes. These measures consist of questions asking whether the person carries out (or has the capacity to carry out) certain activities, such as walking across a small room, eating a meal, or walking up a flight of stairs. Among the more frequently used report measures are the Activities of Daily Living Scale developed by Katz and Akpom (25), the Older Americans Research and Service Center Measure (11), the Barthel Index (30), the Functional Health Scale developed by Rosow and Breslau (40), and the items used by Nagi (34).

These report measures have some important advantages. They provide a global assessment of function, can readily be administered by trained, nonmedical personnel, require little time, and can be administered either to the subject directly or to a proxy respondent, so that persons with severe impairment are not selectively excluded from assessment. Furthermore, impairment as measured by several of these scales has been shown to predict utilization of medical care services; thus impairment appears to reflect conventional ideas of poor health. One major disadvantage is lack of precision as to the source of impairment. While impairment on most of the items of these self-report or proxy-report scales reflects physical impairment, and the scales can, in general, be thought of as measures of physical functioning, possible confusion between physical and cognitive impairment is frequent. For example, inability to feed oneself might reflect either impaired function of one's hands or arms or impaired cognitive function. A second disadvantage is that differing reports of impairment on these scales may reflect differences in the ways people report impairment as well as actual differences in function. For example, most studies have shown that older women report more impaired physical function than do men. Is this difference due to actual greater prevalence of physical impairment among women or to a possible difference in the ways women and men report impairments?

An alternate method of evaluating physical function in older persons is by directly testing ability to perform specified tasks (16, 22). Either certain aspects of the performance can be recorded for analysis or an overall impression of ability to perform the task can be recorded by a trained observer. There has been much less experience with these measures in large-scale studies than there has been with the report measures described above. Because they have several advantages over report measures that are valuable in some situations, however, experience with direct performance testing of physical function is expanding rapidly. Direct performance testing of physical function is usually much more tightly focused on some particular aspect of function than are report measures. For example, one performance test used among older persons is the ability to rise from a chair without assistance from others or without using one's arms ("chair stands"). One way of administering and scoring this task is to record the amount of time required for a person to rise from a chair in this fashion five times. Because the information from direct performance testing is more tightly focused, it has the potential to provide greater insight into the reason for a person's impairment and into possible ways of modifying or preventing the impairment. This potentially very important advantage is responsible for much of the recent interest in direct performance testing. Direct performance testing of physical function also has disadvantages, however. One is that its emphasis on focused information is balanced by the lack of a global summary of overall function. While it is possible that an impression of global function might be gained from a comprehensive battery of performance tests, this approach has not been widely attempted and would probably require much more time than would the global impression provided by brief report measures. Another disadvantage is that proxy information cannot be used. Because performance testing requires direct participation by the subject, persons unable (typically because of cognitive impairment or severe physical illness) or unwilling to undergo testing are selectively excluded. Practically, this means that there is at least some tendency to exclude persons with the highest levels of impairment. Finally, direct performance testing is usually more complex and expensive to administer than are report measures of physical function; it requires more highly trained personnel and typically takes more time.

Measurements of physical function by report and by direct performance testing are not directly opposed. Rather, they are best seen as two alternatives that can be complementary, depending on the goals of individual studies. Many studies can make use of both approaches, with report of function providing a general assessment of function that is especially valuable in describing the participants and performance testing providing a detailed assessment of areas of special interest and importance.

Most existing studies of physical function of older persons have been either purely descriptive in approach or have used physical function as an independent variable, that is, these studies have sought to investigate the effects of impaired function on other variables of interest, such as use of health care services. More recently, there has been stronger emphasis on studies using impaired physical function as a dependent variable; that is, the purpose of the study is to identify other factors that are associated with or predict either good or impaired function. A major reason for this shift in study goals is an emphasis on identifying potentially reversible risk factors for decline in physical function. To at least some extent, the emphasis has changed from a goal of understanding the impact of poor function on the need for or utilization of services to a goal of preventing impairment and disability among older persons.

Measurement of Cognitive Function. Cognitive function is usually measured by direct performance testing rather than by report of the subject or a surrogate. A wide and complex variety of performance tests of various aspects of cognition have been used in aging research, and no attempt to comprehensively evaluate these measures will be made here. Several brief measures intended to provide a global assessment of an older person's cognitive abilities have been used extensively in research. Perhaps the two most widely used of these brief tests are the mental status questionnaire and its variants and the Mini-Mental State Examination. The mental status questionnaire was developed by Kahn et al. (23). A number of modified versions have been developed; the most widely used is the Short Portable Mental Status Questionnaire developed by Pfeiffer (35) and used in the Older Americans Resources and Services Program. This consists of ten brief questions that assess orientation and stock of current information. They include such questions as "What is today's date?" and "Who is the current president?" The measure requires little time to administer but does not assess many aspects of cognition and is not highly sensitive.

The Mini-Mental State Examination was developed by Folstein et al. (13). It includes some brief orientation items very similar to those used in the mental status questionnaire but, in addition, it attempts to very briefly assess some other aspects of cognitive function, such as memory and language. It has been very widely used in studies of Alzheimer's disease as an index of disease severity. Both the mental status questionnaire and the

Mini-Mental State Examination were originally used among hospitalized persons, but both have since been used in a number of large population-based studies (2, 9, 33, 35, 49). These measures or other very brief tests can provide a rapid global assessment of cognition that is extremely useful in large-scale studies of older persons. More detailed studies of cognitive function usually rely on structured batteries of performance tests of various aspects of cognition with tests chosen to emphasize those aspects of greatest importance to the particular study.

PRACTICAL CONSIDERATIONS IN CONDUCTING STUDIES AMONG OLDER PERSONS

Obtaining and Maintaining Study Participation

High rates of participation are usually necessary for valid study results, and researchers typically put great effort into obtaining such participation. Methods for doing so among older persons are similar to those used in younger age groups, but some areas deserve special emphasis. In many ways, it is useful to regard the process of attaining full participation as one of identifying and removing the barriers between potential participants and the study. Some of these barriers are unique to individual studies, but others can be anticipated to occur frequently in most studies of older persons. Perhaps the most frequent barrier to participation is failure to provide sufficient information for potential participants to decide if they wish to be part of the study. Investigators typically make conscientious efforts to inform potential participants about the research, but people considering participation frequently have questions or concerns that have not occurred to the investigators. In asking people to participate in a study, it is essential to encourage their questions; *listen* to these questions and respond directly to the issues *they* raise. Presentations or brochures that seem to give all the information relevant to the investigators may leave unanswered concerns in the minds of potential participants. If these issues are not sought and answered, the usual consequence is nonparticipation.

A second barrier is the burden of the study for the participants (for example, any potential discomfort or embarrassment, length of the interview or other data-gathering process). This burden is likely to be carefully considered by older persons in deciding whether to participate in a study, and experienced investigators are often appropriately sensitive to the issue. Minimizing participant burden is essential to achieving high rates of participation. One aspect of participant burden that is sometimes neglected, however, is the participants' views of the balance between this burden and the likely value of the study. Like most people, potential participants have little enthusiasm for activities that they regard as wasted time. As emphasized above, however, their criteria for judging a study may be substantially different from those of the investigators, but it is on the basis of their criteria that they will decide whether or not to participate. Therefore, careful efforts to put the reasons for conducting the study in ways that participants will find meaningful and willingness to discuss the value of the study with potential participants individually will often enhance participation. Occasionally, investigators have the view that older persons have large amounts of empty time and that it is, therefore, not necessary to consider scheduling or duration of study visits carefully. This view that older persons' time is somehow not as important as that of others is not widely shared by older persons themselves; instead, they may find it condescending and a barrier to participation.

In reducing the burden of study participation for older persons, it is often useful to consider bringing the study directly to the homes of the participants or, if this is not possible, to a location near their homes. Surveys of older persons typically identify transportation as a substantial unmet need (4). Studies that require older persons to provide their own transportation to inconvenient sites will frequently have difficulty securing adequate participation. In addition, physical and cognitive impairment become much more frequent with increasing age (9). If one wishes to have participation in a study open to persons with the full range of functions seen among older persons, it is necessary to take special care to be sure access is provided to those with impairments. In practical terms, this may mean carrying out study measurements in participants' homes or at least making special arrangements to transport older persons with impairments to the study center. In one recent community-based study (12) of Alzheimer's disease, for example, the evaluations by a neurologist and other clinical specialists were carried out in a neighborhood health center centrally located in a geographically defined community only a few square miles in area, but it was still necessary to perform 28% of the evaluations in participants' homes to achieve adequate participation. Older persons with impairments often have family members who care deeply about them. For successful participation, it is necessary to be able to explain the study clearly and carefully to these family members as well as to the participants themselves.

Maintaining participation over an extended period of time, often several years, is especially relevant to aging research because of the importance of longitudinal studies to this field. High rates of follow-up participation are essential to the validity of longitudinal study results. The most effective designs in this regard usually limit data collection at each follow-up contact to the information that is essential for answering the questions of major interest to the study. Adding nonessential data collection to follow-up visits sometimes appears attractive and cost-effective but may actually involve substantial risk for the study. The decision to do this should be made very cautiously because the increased participant burden resulting from additional data collection may lower participation, thus risking the ability of the study to test its central hypotheses. Another means of enhancing the validity of longitudinal studies while reducing respondent burden at follow-up is to use existing, regularly collected data sets for follow-up information. This requires that the existing data set be of high quality and suitable to the needs of the study, that there is a means of linking the study data with the existing data set, and that appropriate informed consent for access to the data set be obtained from each participant at the beginning of the study. If these requirements are met, however, this approach has the advantage of avoiding selective nonresponse while lowering participant burden. A practical example is the use of Medicare claims files maintained by the Health Care Finance Administration to provide information on utilization of hospital services by older persons participating in a study for which such utilization is an outcome of interest.

Other Practical Considerations

Time required for data collection is often longer in studies of older persons than for otherwise comparable studies of persons from younger age groups; budgets and planning should reflect this. Preparations to allow access to the study for those with impairments (see above) can require a great deal of time, but there are very likely other reasons for the greater time requirement as well. Many older persons appear to weigh carefully over a period of time whether or not to participate, so that multiple contacts may be needed to explain a study and arrange for participation. Some older persons appear to carefully consider study questions and respond more slowly than do younger participants.

Use of proxy respondents (that is, obtaining the answers to questions about a subject from an informant instead of directly from the subject) is an important but difficult issue in conducting research among older persons. In some situations (for example, a study limited to persons with moderate or severe dementia) the most reasonable approach may be to obtain all questionnaire responses from informants under the assumption that the presence of dementia will prevent the subjects from supplying accurate information directly. A more frequently encountered problem pertains to studies that enroll persons of varying physical and cognitive abilities. If one chooses not to have proxy respondents for some subjects, then there will be a strong tendency to eliminate from participation those with severe cognitive and physical impairment. This problem is especially severe for longitudinal studies because many common outcomes of interest (for example, development of a disease of interest or utilization of medical care services) may well be strongly associated with development of impairment. Therefore, exclusion of proxy respondents will lead to biased measurement of the outcome that may well be severe enough to threaten the validity of the study results. Nevertheless, the decision to use proxy respondents for some but not all subjects also poses difficulties. For some information, reports from proxy respondents are likely to differ from reports directly from participants. Because the distribution of proxy respondents will be nonrandom and related to the presence of severe physical or cognitive impairment, there is a possibility of biased measurement that might affect study results. Longitudinal studies with sequential measurements present a challenge in this regard because there is the possibility that observed changes may reflect a change from direct response to proxy response as well as an actual change in the variable of interest. The approach to using proxy response must vary according to the needs of each study, but perhaps the most frequent approach is to use proxy respondents for some subjects but to limit this use to situations in which the alternative would be to have data unavailable for that particular subject at that measurement point. Proxy responses should be labeled so that they can be distinguished from direct participant responses in data analyses. Implementation of this approach usually requires that authorization from a supervisor be obtained before study personnel obtain information from a proxy respondent so as to avoid overuse of proxies.

Finally, it is difficult to overestimate the value of pretesting questions, protocols, and procedures among older persons as similar as possible to the eventual participants before the use of these materials in the actual study (26). With pretesting, unanticipated problems that would have had serious effects on the study may be recognized and corrected. This is especially important for questions and procedures that have been successfully used in younger age groups but for which experience among older persons is limited.

REFERENCES

1. ABRAMSON, J. H., R. GOFIN, and E. PERITZ. Risk markers for mortality among elderly men—a community study in Jerusalem. *J. Chronic Dis.* 35: 565–572, 1982.
2. ALBERT, M. S., L. A. SMITH, P. A. SCHERR, J. O. TAYLOR, D. A. EVANS, and H. H. FUNKENSTEIN. Use of brief cognitive tests to identify individuals in the community with clinically-diagnosed Alzheimer's disease. *Int. J. Neurosci.* 57: 167–178, 1991.

3. AMERICAN HEART ASSOCIATION. *Recommendations for Human Blood Pressure Determination by Sphygmomanometers.* Dallas: American Heart Association, 1980.
4. BRANCH, L. G., and A. M. JETTE. The Framingham Disability Study: I. Social disability among the aging. *Am. J. Public Health* 71: 1202–1210, 1981.
5. BRANCH, L. G., and A. M. JETTE. A prospective study of long-term care institutionalization among the aged. *Am. J. Public Health* 72: 1373–1379, 1982.
6. CAMPBELL, A. J., C. DIEP, J. REINKEN, and L. MCCOSH. Factors predicting mortality in a total population sample of the elderly. *J. Epidemiol. Community Health* 39: 337–342, 1985.
7. CLAYTON, D. The analysis of event history data: a review of progress and outstanding problems. *Stat. Med.* 7: 819–841, 1988.
8. COMMITTEE ON STANDARDS FOR EPIDEMIOLOGIC SURVEYS IN CHRONIC RESPIRATORY DISEASE OF THE AMERICAN THORACIC SOCIETY. *Standards for Epidemiologic Surveys in Chronic Respiratory Disease.* New York: National Tuberculosis and Respiratory Disease Association, 1969.
9. CORNONI-HUNTLEY, J., D. B. BROCK, A. M., OSTFELD, J. O. TAYLOR, and R. B. WALLACE, (Eds). *Established Populations for Epidemiologic Studies of the Elderly Resource Data Book.* Washington, DC: US Government Printing Office, 1986.
10. COX, D. R. Regression models and life tables. *J. R. Stat. Soc., B.* 34: 187–220, 1972.
11. DUKE UNIVERSITY CENTER FOR THE STUDY OF AGING AND HUMAN DEVELOPMENT. *Multidimensional Functional Assessment: The OARS Methodology.* Durham, N.C.: Duke University, Press 1978.
12. EVANS, D. A., H. H. FUNKENSTEIN, M. S. ALBERT, P. A. SCHERR, N.R. COOK, M. J. CHOWN, L. E. HEBERT, C. H. HENNEKENS, and J. O. TAYLOR. Prevalence of Alzheimer's disease in a community population higher than previously reported. *JAMA* 262: 2251–2256, 1989.
13. FOLSTEIN, M. F., S. E. FOLSTEIN, P. R. MCHUGH. "Mini-mental state" a practical method for grading the cognitive state of patients for the clinician. *J. Psychiatr. Res.* 12: 189–198, 1975.
14. FOULKES, M. A., P. A. WOLF, T. R. PRICE, J. P. MOHR, and D. B. HIER. The Stroke Data Bank: design, methods and baseline characteristics. *Stroke* 19: 547–554, 1988.
15. GRAVES, A. B., C. M. VAN DUIJN, V. CHANDRA, L. FRATIGLIONI, A. HEYMAN, A. F. JORM, E. KOKMEN, K. KONDO, J. A. MORTIMER, W. A. ROCCA, S. L. SHALAT, H. SOLINEN, and A. HOFMAN. Alcohol and tobacco consumption as risk factors for Alzheimer's disease: a collaborative re-analysis of case-control studies. *Int. J. Epidemiol.* 20(suppl. 2): S48–S57, 1991.
16. GURALNIK, J. M., L. G. BRANCH, S. R. CUMMINGS, and J. D. CURB. Physical performance measures in aging research. *J. Gerontol.* 44: M141–M146, 1989.
17. HABER, L. D. Identifying the disabled: concepts and methods in the measurement of disability. *Soc. Secur. Bull.* 30: 17–35, 1967.
18. HEYMAN, A., W. E. WILKINSON, J. A. STAFFORD, M. J. HELMS, A. H. SIGMON, and T. WEINBERG. Alzheimer's disease: a study of epidemiological aspects. *Ann. Neurol.* 15: 335–341, 1984.
19. HUI, S., and J. BERGER. Empirical Bayes estimation of rates in longitudinal studies. *J. Am. Stat. Assoc.* 78: 753–760, 1983.
20. JACOBSEN, B. K., and D. S. THELLE. Risk factors for coronary heart disease and level of education: the Tromsø Heart Study. *Am. J. Epidemiol.* 127: 923–932, 1988.
21. JAGGER, C. and M. CLARKE. Mortality risks in the elderly; five-year follow-up of a total population. *Int. J. Epidemiol.* 17: 111–114, 1988.
22. JETTE, A. M., and L. G. BRANCH. Impairment and disability in the aged. *J. Chronic Dis.* 38: 59–65, 1985.
23. KAHN, R. L., A. I. GOLDFARB, M. POLLACK, and A. PECK. Brief objective measures for the determination of mental status in the aged. *Am. J. Psychiatry* 117: 326–328, 1960.
24. KANE, R. A., and R. L. KANE. *Assessing the Elderly: A Practical Guide to Measurement.* Lexington, MA: D. C. Heath, 1981.
25. KATZ, S., and C. A. AKPOM. A measure of primary sociobiological functions. *Int. J. Health Serv.* 6: 493–508, 1976.
26. KOHOUT, F. J. The pragmatics of survey field work among the elderly. In: *The Epidemiologic Study of the Elderly*, edited by R. B. Wallace and R. F. Woolson. New York: Oxford University Press, 1992, p. 91–119.
27. LAIRD, N., and J. WARE. Random-effects models for longitudinal data. *Biometrics* 38: 963–974, 1982.
28. LAST, J. M. (Ed). *A Dictionary of Epidemiology.* 2nd ed. New York: Oxford University Press, 1988.
29. MACMAHON, B., and T. F. PUGH. *Epidemiology Principles and Methods.* Boston: Little, Brown, 1970.
30. MAHONEY, F. I., and D. W. BARTHEL. Functional evaluation: the Barthel Index. *Rehabilitation* 14: 61–65, 1965.
31. MCKHANN, G., D. DRACHMANN, M. FOLSTEIN, R. KATZMAN, D. PRICE, and E. M. STADLAN. Clinical diagnosis of Alzheimer's disease. Report of the NINCDS-ADRDA Work Group under the auspices of Department of Health and Human Services Task Force on Alzheimer's Disease. *Neurology* 34: 939–944, 1984.
32. MUENZ, L. R., and L. V. RUBINSTEIN. Markov models for covariate dependence of binary sequences. *Biometrics* 41: 91–101, 1985.
33. MYERS, J. K., M. M. WEISSMAN, G. L. TISCHLER, C. E. HOLZER, III, P. L. LEAF, H. ORVASCHEL, J. C. ANTHONY, J. H. BOYD, J. D. BURKE, M. KRAMER, and R. STOLTZMAN, R. Six-month prevalence of psychiatric disorders in three communities 1980 to 1982. *Arch. Gen. Psychiatry* 41: 959–967, 1984.
34. NAGI, S. Z. An epidemiology of disability among adults in the United States. *Milbank Q.* 54: 439–468, 1976.
35. PFEIFFER, E. A short portable mental status questionnaire for the assessment of organic brain deficit in elderly patients. *J. Am. Geriatr. Soc.* 23: 433–441, 1975.
36. ROGOSA, D. Myths about longitudinal research. In: *Methodological Issues in Aging Research* edited by K. W. Schaie, R. T. Campbell, W. Meredith, and S. C. Rawlings. New York: Springer-Verlag, 1990, p. 171–209.
37. ROGOSA, D. R., and J. B. WILLETT. Understanding correlates of change by modeling individual differences in growth. *Psychometrika* 50: 203–228, 1985.
38. ROSE, G. A., H. BLACKBURN, R. F. GILLUM, and R. J. PRINEAS. *Cardiovascular Survey Methods.* (2nd ed.), Geneva: World Health Organization, 1982.
39. ROSNER, B. The analysis of longitudinal data in epidemiologic studies. *J. Chronic Dis.* 1979; 32: 163–173.
40. ROSOW, I., and N. BRESLAU. A Guttman health scale for the aged. *J. Gerontol.* 21: 556–559, 1966.
41. SCHAIE, K. W. The Seattle Longitudinal Study: a 21-year exploration of psychometric intelligence in adulthood. In: *Longitudinal Studies of Adult Psychological Development*, edited by K. W. Schaie. New York: Guilford, 1983, p. 64–135.
42. SCHAIE, K. W., and C. R. STROTHER. A cross-sequential study of age changes in cognitive behavior. *Psychol. Bull.* 70: 671–680, 1968.
43. SHALAT, S. L., B. SELTZER, C. PIDCOCK, and E. L. BAKER, JR. Risk factors for Alzheimer's disease: a case-control study. *Neurology* 37: 1630–1633, 1987.
44. SHANAS, E. Measuring the home health needs of the elderly in five countries. *J. Gerontol.* 26: 37–40, 1971.
45. SHEA, S, A. D. STEIN, C. E. BASCH, R. LANTIGUA, C. MAYLAHN, D. S. STROGATZ, and L. NOVICK. Independent associations of educational attainment and ethnicity with behavioral risk factors

for cardiovascular disease. *Am. J. Epidemiol.* 134: 567–582, 1991.
46. SPECTOR, W. D. Functional disability scales. In: *Quality of Life Assessments in Clinical Trials,* edited by B. Spilker. New York: Raven Press, 1990, p. 115–129.
47. VAN DUIJN, C. M., and A. HOFMAN. Relation between nicotine intake and Alzheimer's disease. *Br. Med. J.* 302: 1491–1494, 1991.
48. WHO TASK FORCE ON STROKE AND OTHER CEREBROVASCULAR DISORDERS. Recommendations on stroke prevention, diagnosis and therapy. *Stroke* 20: 1407–1431, 1989.
49. YU, E. S., W. T. LIU, P. LEVY, M. Y. ZHANG, R. KATZMAN, C. T. LUNG, S. C. WONG, Z. Y. WANG, and G. Y. QU. Cognitive impairment among elderly adults in Shanghai, China. *J. Gerontol.* 44: S97–S106, 1989.

III METABOLIC AND MOLECULAR ASPECTS OF AGING

6. Energy utilization

ROGER J. M. McCARTER | Department of Physiology, The University of Texas Health Science Center, San Antonio, Texas

CHAPTER CONTENTS

Energy Metabolism and Body Composition
Tissue Mass and Tissue Metabolism
Mitochondrial Content and Mitochondrial Metabolism
Whole-Body Metabolic Rate
    Twenty-four-hour energy expenditure
    Components of 24-hour energy expenditure
        Basal metabolic rate
        Physical activity
        Diet-induced thermogenesis
    Efficiency and energy utilization
Factors Modulating Metabolic Rate
    Temperature
    Neuroendocrine factors
    Dietary restriction
Metabolic Rate of Poikilotherms as a Function of Age
Energy Metabolism and Theories of Aging
    Rate of living theory
    Free radical theory
Conclusions

AGING AND ENERGY METABOLISM are linked in many ways. Theories of aging often assign energy metabolism a central role; it is widely believed that metabolic rate varies with age and that energy metabolism is implicated in problems and diseases of old age.

Historically, the interaction between aging and energy metabolism has been described in terms of intensity of metabolism or metabolic rate per unit of metabolic mass. This focus was established by the pioneering experiments of Rubner (162), which indicated an inverse relationship between longevity and metabolic rate. As elaborated by Pearl, this implied that "duration of life varies inversely with the rate of living" (147), and the concept received wide acceptance. Subsequent studies in a variety of species produced both supporting and opposing data. Current views on the interaction of aging and energy metabolism include metabolic rate but stress the importance of by-products of metabolism, such as free radicals, and the potentially damaging effects of metabolic fuels, such as glucose, in determining the rate of aging. It follows from "rate of living"–type theories that life is terminated by decreased availability of cellular energy. The idea that cells lose the ability to generate adenosine triphosphate (ATP) with time is supported by studies of DNA mutation in mitochondria of yeast and other fungi (143). These studies have been extended to mammalian tissues (106). They suggest that random mutations of mitochondrial DNA (mtDNA) accumulate with time and lead to both disease and the loss of ability to transform energy for maintenance of cellular integrity. Different rates of aging of tissues might then be a consequence of different rates of accumulation of mitochondrial damage. Despite the large volume of work in this area, however, it remains unclear whether the "fire of life" (96) burns less brightly with advanced age or whether the increased rate of living of small animals is a consequence of increased intensity of tissue metabolism or altered distribution of active tissues. A key factor in dealing with these issues is that body composition varies with age and species. The choice of an appropriate basis for comparing different species and ages thus becomes important. Since altered body composition may play a role in problems of advanced age, metabolic factors regulating the balance between energy input and output also affect the use of energy in old age.

The purpose of this chapter is to examine the interaction between energy metabolism and aging. Does the intensity of metabolism vary with age? If so, what factors are responsible for this? Is metabolic rate a key factor or do other aspects of energy metabolism provide a link between energy use and rate of aging? To address these issues, data obtained from humans and laboratory animals are discussed. Factors modulating metabolic rate are examined in relation to their variability with age, and the impact of such data on theories of aging is assessed. Under usual living conditions more than 90% of the energy utilized by cells is obtained from oxidative metabolism (19). Anaerobic pathways are utilized for acute energy generation, as in skeletal muscle fibers during brief, intense bouts of physical activity. This chapter, however, will focus on energy generation from oxidative metabolism because (1) lifetime energy metabolism is derived mainly from oxidative processes and (2) by-products of oxidative metabolism, such as free radicals, are implicated in mechanisms of aging. Several reviews provide additional information in this area (117, 152, 211).

ENERGY METABOLISM AND BODY COMPOSITION

There is a large disparity in the metabolic activity of different tissues, so tissue size in relation to total body mass is an important factor in determining whole-body energy utilization. Adipose tissue has the lowest rate of metabolism, so the simplest view of body composition is a two-component model in which body mass is divided into fat mass and fat-free mass (FFM) compartments. Measurements of energy metabolism are then related to the activity of the FFM. FFM can be estimated by measuring the lean body mass (LBM; the difference between total body mass and mass of adipose tissue) using a variety of techniques. Methods involve anthropometric measures of skin-fold thickness, densitometry, bioelectric impedance, and body water determination using total body ^{40}K (50, 66). Each of these measures provides a different value of LBM, and values can differ by as much as 30% (13). Figure 6.1 illustrates the variation of LBM with age as determined by three different techniques (densitometry, total body water, fat-soluble gases) in men and women. On average, the LBM declines in adulthood by about 0.3% per year in men and 0.2% per year in women. Much of the decline in LBM is thought to be a consequence of decreased muscle mass (160, 198). It should be noted that decline in LBM with age is not always found. For example, in Fischer 344 rats LBM increases over most of the life span. As shown in Figure 6.2, LBM increases with age in these rats and only the longest-lived rats, maintained under barrier conditions and fed ad libitum, exhibit a decrease in LBM during the final 10% of the life span.

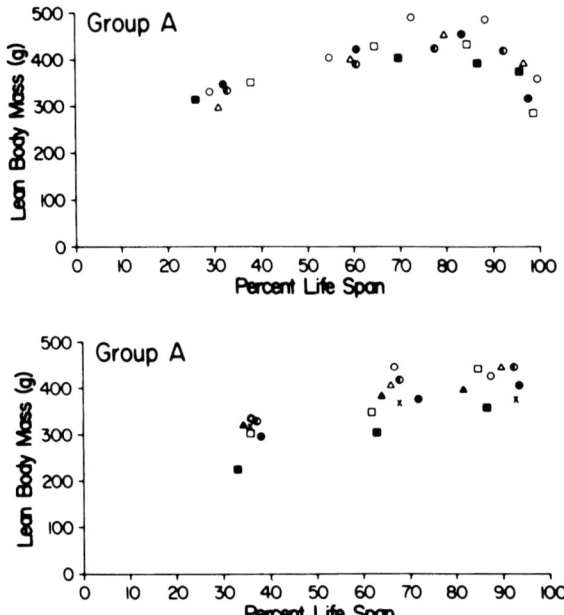

FIG. 6.2. Changes in lean body mass (LBM) during the life span of Fischer 344 rats. Longitudinal study in which similar symbols refer to repeated measures of same rat. *Group A* refers to rats fed ad libitum. *Upper panel* shows data derived from six longest-lived rats, *lower panel* from eight shortest-lived rats, from a colony of 115 rats. Reproduced from Yu et al. (214) with permission.

Not only does the amount of LBM change with age but its composition is also age-related. Table 6.1 shows the ratio of extracellular water (ECW) to intracellular water (ICW) in adult men and women. This ratio increases with age and, since data show constancy of

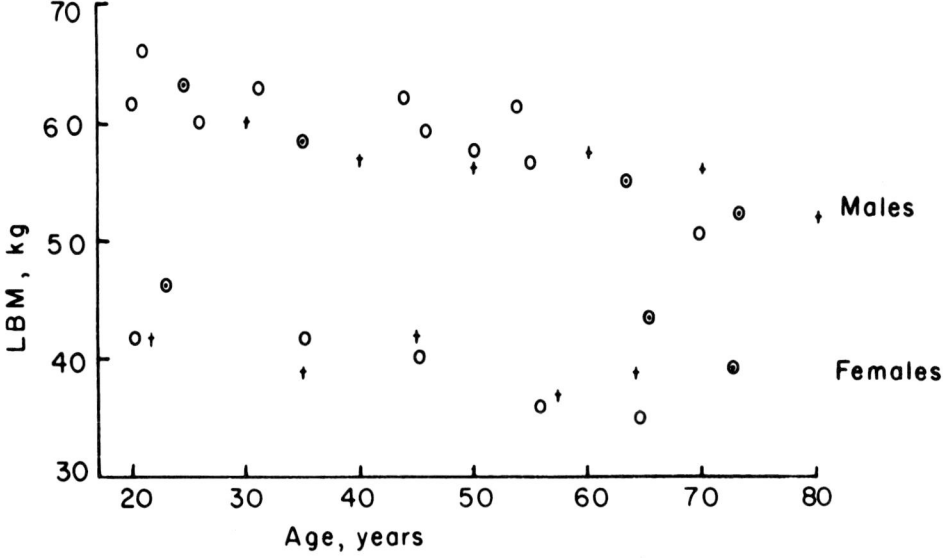

FIG. 6.1. Variation of lean body mass (LBM) with age in males and females. Cross-sectional data obtained using techniques of densitometry (○), total body water (+) and fat-soluble gases (⊙). Reproduced from Forbes (63) with permission.

TABLE 6.1. *Changes in Body Composition with Age*

	%Fat		ECW/ICW	
Age (yr)	Male	Female	Male	Female
25	20	30	0.735	0.889
45	24	33	0.806	0.960
65	28	36	0.893	1.043
85	32	40	1.083	1.143

ECW = extracellular water; ICW = intracellular water. Based on data obtained in cross-sectional studies [from Brozeck, 1965 (21)].

ECW with age (21), the increasing ratio is indicative of decreased ICW in older individuals. Table 6.1 also shows the well-known increase in adiposity with age. Longitudinal measurements of fat mass in Fischer 344 rats as a function of life span are shown in Figure 6.3. These changes follow a pattern similar to that of LBM with age, as demonstrated in Figure 6.2, although results are more variable. Variability of fat mass with age also appears to be a principal contributor to fluctuations of total body mass in humans, since longitudinal studies indicate only small variation in LBM with age (63).

Uncertainties regarding the precise nature of change in amount and composition of LBM or FFM limit the ability to interpret changes in energy utilization and energy balance with age. It should be particularly noted that the techniques used for routine determination of LBM or FFM have not been validated in the elderly; that is, comparisons of results for elderly humans using the various methods of obtaining LBM (50) are needed.

TISSUE MASS AND TISSUE METABOLISM

Skeletal muscle and adipose tissue are major components of total body mass: 40% and 21%, respectively, in "reference" adult men and 29% and 33%, respectively, in "reference" adult women (180). However, the metabolic rate per unit mass of these tissues is small in comparison with that of internal organs, such as brain, liver, heart, and kidneys. Therefore, the mass of internal

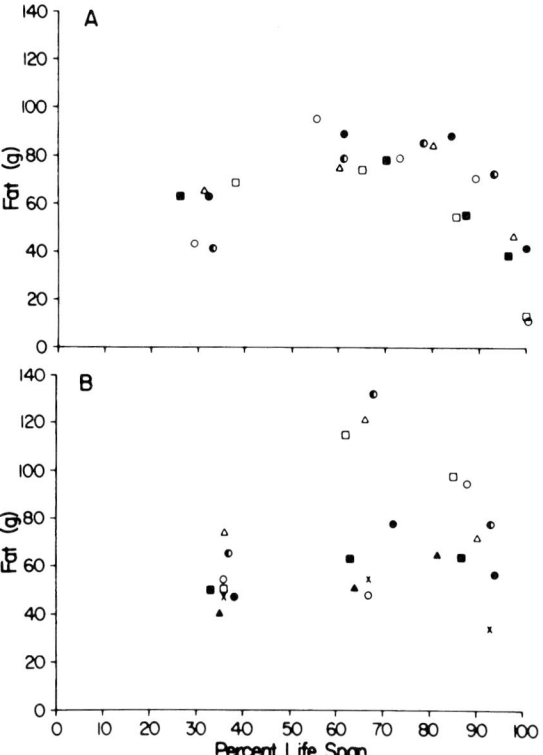

FIG. 6.3. Changes in fat mass over the life span of Fischer 344 rats. Longitudinal measurements in which similar symbols refer to repeated measures of the same rat. *Panel A* shows data derived from six longest-lived rats. *Panel B* shows data from eight shortest-lived rats. Reproduced from Bertrand et al. (132) with permission.

organs and their variation with age may exert a major effect on energy metabolism and energy balance. For example, the high metabolic rate per unit mass of infants is due in large part to the size of the brain in relation to total body mass (51). Table 6.2 shows data obtained in cross-sectional measurements in humans. Brain mass remains a relatively constant fraction of body mass during adulthood, whereas liver and kidney decrease and heart mass increases in relation to body mass. The summed masses of brain, liver, kidneys, and heart appear to remain constant through the seventh decade of life, whereas muscle mass decreases in relation

TABLE 6.2. *Organ Mass as a Percentage of Body Mass in Relation to Age in Humans*

Age years	Brain	Liver	Kidneys	Heart	Summed Organs	Muscle
31–40	2.2	2.48	0.46	0.54	5.7	41.8
41–50	2.3	2.56	0.45	0.58	5.9	40.2
51–60	2.4	2.42	0.47	0.56	5.9	—
61–70	2.7	2.14	0.41	0.63	5.9	33.9
>70	2.3	2.03	0.41	0.60	5.3	27.0

From Elia, 1991b (51) based on original data of Korenchevsky, 1961 (97).

TABLE 6.3. *Organ Mass as a Percentage of Body Mass for Different Adult Mammals*

Species	Brain	Liver	Kidneys	Heart	Summed Organs
Elephant	0.09	0.09	0.02	0.03	0.23
Steer	0.07	0.71	0.14	0.33	1.25
Horse	0.11	1.11	0.27	0.71	2.20
Sheep	0.20	1.85	0.31	0.54	2.90
Dog	0.75	4.20	0.70	0.85	6.50
Monkey	0.93	2.44	0.47	0.51	4.35
Guinea Pig	0.59	3.38	0.70	0.29	4.96
Rat	0.80	4.80	0.84	0.38	6.82

From data of Brody, 1945 (17).

to body mass with age. Table 6.3 shows relative organ masses in a variety of adult mammalian species, excluding humans. While there is considerable variability (e.g., 215) in general the masses of brain, kidneys, and heart are less than 1% of body mass, while liver can constitute more than 4% of body mass. In contrast, brain mass is about 2.5% and liver 2.5% of body mass in humans (Table 6.2). Data in Table 6.3 demonstrate that in large animals the summed masses of metabolically active tissues tend to be a small fraction of total body mass, whereas in small animals the active tissues are a larger fraction of total body mass. In addition to differences in organ:body mass ratios, changes in the composition of tissues have been found, as a function of both species and age. For example, rat brains may have a smaller proportion of glial cells with low metabolic activity than that found in the human brain (178), but there is an increased amount of metabolically inactive connective tissue with age in skeletal muscle (121). Also, bone density (and hence body density) decreases with age and is a function of ethnic origin (45, 63, 151, 197). These changes in tissue composition must be taken into account when estimating LBM. For example, changes in body density as a consequence of altered bone density might be interpreted as altered adiposity in hydrometric measurements of LBM. Knowledge of altered composition is therefore important for interpreting changes in metabolic rate. Differences in whole-body metabolic rate with age may be a consequence of altered metabolic rate per unit mass of the cells of older individuals. There are, however, at least two other possibilities to account for such changes: (1) altered tissue composition, as discussed above, and (2) altered contribution of different tissues to total body mass. Whole-body metabolic rate will decrease with age without any change in rate of individual tissues if those tissues having a lower rate of metabolism constitute an increasing fraction of total mass with age. In agreement with this concept, the data of Holliday (80) suggest that metabolic rate per unit mass of internal organs remains remarkably constant during growth and development in humans, at a time when organ mass:body mass ratios and whole-body metabolic rate change rapidly. Few data are available concerning organ metabolic rate over the life span, and there exists a clear need for such information. In adult men and women, data (51) indicate tissue metabolic rates as follows (kcal/kg organ mass/24 h): liver, 200; brain, 240; heart, 440; kidneys, 440; skeletal muscle, 13; adipose tissue, 4.5; other tissues such as bone, skin, intestines, etc. (obtained by difference), 12. These values demonstrate that resting skeletal muscle has a rate of metabolism three times higher than that of adipose tissue. However, adipose tissue, skeletal muscle, and the miscellaneous tissues represent essentially a different class in terms of metabolic activity when compared with heart, liver, kidneys, and brain. Indeed, even taking into account differences in mass of these tissues, liver and brain are estimated to account for more than 40% of the metabolic energy expenditure of adult men under resting conditions, with skeletal muscle providing 22% and adipose tissue 4% of the total (51). Given these differences in metabolic activity, it is not surprising that variation of whole-body metabolic rate over the life span depends greatly on how data are normalized, regardless of changes in intrinsic activity of the tissues. This is illustrated in Figure 6.4, using values of basal metabolic rate (BMR) obtained in humans (51). The characteristic rapid decline in BMR with development is demonstrated (solid circles) when metabolic rate is expressed in terms of body surface area or body mass. However, little variation with age is seen when metabolic rate is normalized to the summed mass of brain, liver, kidneys, and heart. The data of Korenchevsky (97) show decline in the contribution of liver, kidneys, and muscle and increase in adipose tissue as a fraction of total mass with advancing age in humans. Such changes in tissue distribution would be expected to result in lower whole-body metabolic rate independent of altered intensity of cellular metabolism. Several studies have measured the metabolic rates of organs in vitro rather than in situ, as discussed above. The pioneering work of Krebs (98) established conditions in vitro for maximal metabolic activity of isolated tissues and also demonstrated the large variability of results obtained with

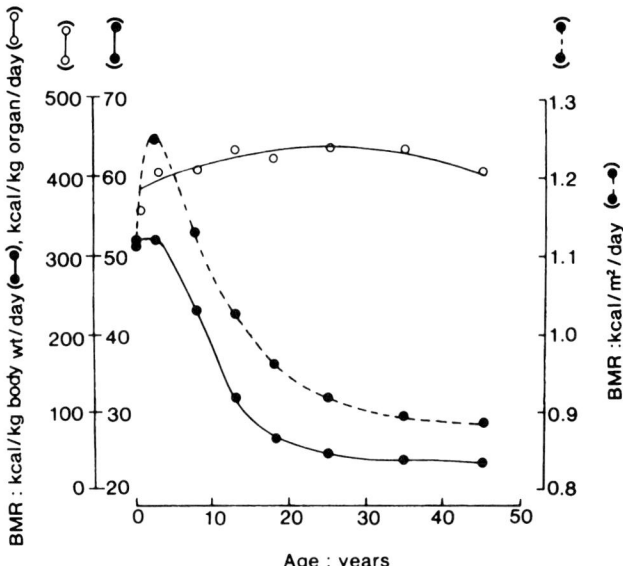

FIG. 6.4. Changes of basal metabolic rate (BMR) with age expressed in terms of body weight (*solid circles, solid line*), surface area (*solid circles, dashed line*), and summed weight of vital organs (*open circles*). Reproduced from Elia (51) with permission.

different media and under different conditions. Such studies of homogenates or tissue slices suggest decreased metabolic rate with age (7, 148, 157). However, conflicting results have also been obtained (40, 203). It is not clear how these data relate to metabolic rates in vivo since such results depend greatly upon incubation conditions (40, 51).

MITOCHONDRIAL CONTENT AND MITOCHONDRIAL METABOLISM

Given the uncertainties involved in relative mass and composition of active tissues, a more direct approach to comparing the metabolic activities of individuals or animals may be to compare mitochondrial content. These cellular organelles are the sites of ATP generation by oxidative metabolism, and they are uniquely sensitive to genetic damage: mtDNA is in close proximity to sites of reactive free radical generation and is not protected by the histones associated with nuclear DNA. Also, repair of damaged mtDNA is carried out with much less fidelity than exists for nuclear DNA (20, 30). Accumulation of altered mtDNA with time might therefore compromise energy transduction and lead to a breakdown of cell function. The surface area of mitochondrial membrane per unit of tissue volume may therefore be a useful index of metabolic activity. The work of Else and Hulbert (52–54) suggests such a basis for comparison. These authors used a comparative approach to demonstrate that the greater rates of energy metabolism of homeotherms vs. poikilotherms (at similar body mass and temperature) are associated with differences in mitochondrial volume density and mitochondrial membrane surface area (MMSA). Similarly, differences in metabolic rates of developing and mature animals, including humans, are associated with differences in MMSA. Organs such as heart, liver, brain, and kidneys develop oxidative metabolic capacity at different rates, and differences in MMSA are consistent with measured differences in energy metabolism of these tissues (84).

It might be expected, therefore, that during senescence there is organ-specific loss of capacity for energy metabolism associated with decreased MMSA. Few studies have been done in this area. Available literature suggests decreased mitochondrial volume density of liver, brain, and heart in rats (24, 77), but studies in vitro indicate no change in capacity for oxidative energy metabolism in liver of Fischer 344 rats of 10–30 months of age (163). Further studies are needed to determine tissue-specific MMSA, its correlation with organ energy metabolism, and the implications of such changes for whole-body energy metabolism.

While the work of Hulbert et al. (84) suggests a correlation between MMSA and metabolic rate, it should be noted that mitochondrial density is variable, depending on cellular activity and environmental conditions. So, for example, endurance exercise leads to increased mitochondrial density in skeletal muscle, an adaptation in line with the above concept. However, adaptation to the hypoxia of high altitude can also lead to increased mitochondrial density independent of altered metabolic rate (18, 144). Such plasticity of mitochondrial density suggests that caution should be exercised in inferring elevated rates of metabolism in vivo on the basis of increased MMSA.

WHOLE-BODY METABOLIC RATE

Many different measures of intensity of metabolism have been used for comparing members of different species or members of a given species who differ in size, age, and health. The most common measurement in humans is the BMR. In this procedure, oxygen consumption and carbon dioxide production of subjects are measured for brief time periods (usually less than 1 h) following overnight bed rest and a 12–14 h fast, with subjects resting quietly in a thermoneutral environment and having no physical activity until after the test. Results are usually normalized to body surface area. The BMR is not a measure of the lowest rate of metabolism, since metabolic rate during sleep is lower, but does provide a standardized set of conditions for comparing metabolism in different individuals and in the same individual with age. Measurement of BMR in other species is not possible because of the constraints involved. BMR also does not provide a measure of metabolic rate encountered under usual living conditions. For practical and theoretical reasons, the resting metabolic rate (RMR) is often determined as the metabolic rate encountered under resting conditions in a thermoneutral environment without the requirement of bed rest and overnight fast. In animal studies the RMR is estimated as the lowest metabolic rate encountered when animals are awake but not physically active, after several hours of acclimation to the measuring chamber (204).

For evaluating interactions between energy metabolism and aging, the most appropriate measure is the daily energy expenditure, or metabolic rate measured over 24 h. At best, this measurement is carried out under conditions that approximate usual living. This can be reasonably achieved by traditional methods of indirect calorimetry in studies of laboratory rodents (123). In humans and larger laboratory animals the recent availability of the "double-labeled (D_2 ^{18}O) water" technology has made it possible to obtain estimates of metabolic rate averaged over several days of measurement (211). This technology provides measures of total metabolism during several days of usual living. In combination with indirect calorimetry, diet, and body composition analysis, the method enables estimates of changes in whole-body metabolism as well as identification of factors responsible for these changes. Such studies in humans are under way, but results are not yet available (211).

Twenty-Four-Hour Energy Expenditure

There is general agreement that total daily energy expenditure (24EE) can be resolved into three major components: BMR, diet-induced thermogenesis (DIT), and physical activity. As illustrated in Figure 6.5, BMR is the largest of these components (60%–75%), with physical activity and DIT providing an additional 20%–40%. "Other" refers to energy metabolism induced by behavior (such as smoking cigarettes) or in response to the environment (such as the thermoregulatory response to cold). Variation of 24EE with age has been estimated from studies of daily caloric intake (130) and by indirect calorimetry in humans (200) and laboratory rodents (123).

Variation of total daily caloric intake with age was measured by McGandy et al. (130) in a cross-sectional study of 252 healthy adult men ranging in age from 20 to 99 yr. In addition, these authors measured basal oxygen consumption and estimated energy expenditure associated with a wide variety of usual physical activities. Their conclusion was that total, basal, and total

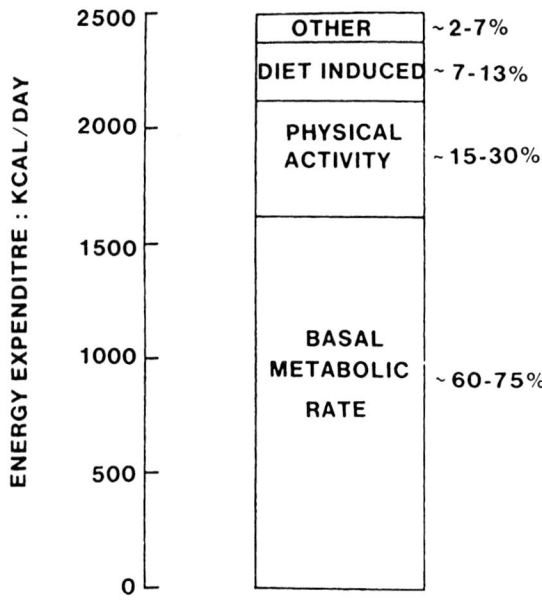

FIG. 6.5. Components of 24EE. Reproduced from Elia (50) with permission.

basal energy expenditure decrease with age in healthy individuals. Elahi et al. (49) found similar decreased caloric intake with age in a longitudinal study of adult men. Vaughan et al. (200) employed a large respiratory chamber and indirect calorimetry to study 24EE in 102 caucasian men and women aged 18–85 yr. Subjects were able to move freely during the 24-h measurement but had limited opportunity for physical activity. Despite similar levels of physical activity, total energy intake (8041 ± 1231 vs. 9029 ± 1206 kJ/day) and total energy expenditure (7815 ± 1193 vs. 9008 ± 1,473 kJ/day) were significantly lower in older (71 ± 6 yr) than younger (24 ± 4 yr) men and women. There was no significant difference in net energy balance (intake−expenditure) between the two groups. Expressed as a function of FFM, the daily energy expenditure of these two groups is shown in Figure 6.6. Interestingly, results for both groups were related by the same regression equation; that is, age was not a major determinant of 24EE as a function of FFM. In contrast to these studies in humans, McCarter and Palmer (123) found variable 24EE with age in male specific-pathogen-free Fischer 344 rats fed ad libitum or fed a life-prolonging restricted diet (60% of ad libitum intake). These results are shown in Figure 6.7 and were obtained under the usual living conditions of these laboratory rodents.

In summary, available literature is limited but indicates no consistent variation of 24EE with age in mammals. Changes of 24EE appear to be strongly correlated with body mass and composition rather than with age, although off-setting age-related changes in components of 24EE are possible and should be considered.

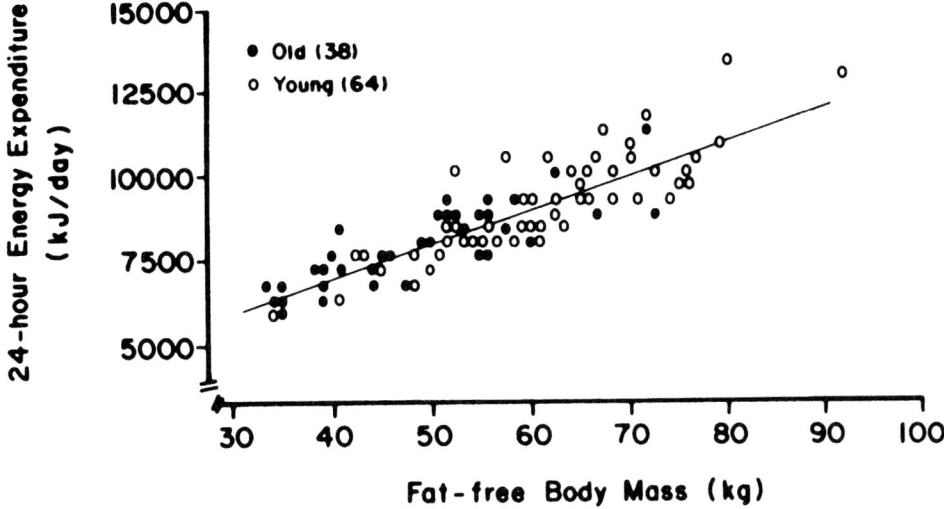

FIG. 6.6. Total daily energy expenditure of young (24 ± 4 yr, *open circles*) and old (71 ± 6 yr, *solid circles*) men and women as a function of FFM. Reproduced from Vaughan et al. (200) with permission.

Components of 24-Hour Energy Expenditure

Basal Metabolic Rate. By far the major component of 24EE is the BMR (Fig. 6.5). BMR and the related RMR have been extensively studied in humans. Almost all studies show decreased energy expenditure with age, both in cross-sectional and in longitudinal measurements (for review, see 152). However, there is controversy regarding the meaning of these data. The controversy is related to changes in body composition with age and the normalization procedures used to determine BMR or RMR. As already pointed out, BMR traditionally has been obtained by expressing metabolic rate per unit of body surface, with surface area estimated from measurements of body characteristics (usually height and mass). This concept originated with Sarrus and Rameaux (168), was validated by the experiments of Rubner (161), and then achieved wide acceptance after publication of large-scale trials involving measurement of more than 8,000 subjects (15). Although surface area continues to be used for expression of BMR, there are strong reservations regarding this normalization procedure (9), and standards based simply on height and mass have gained acceptance (50).

In parallel with these anthropometric measures, another set of standards developed. The research of Krogh (101) demonstrated that the resting metabolism of different species is related by a power function of body mass (W), such that $RMR = aW^n$, where a and n are constants. Kleiber (95) later showed the value of n to be approximately 0.74 for adult mammals (rather than the value of 0.67 expected for a surface area relation), leading to the concept of *metabolic mass* for normalization of whole-body metabolic rate, that is, metabolic mass = $W^{0.74}$ or $W^{3/4}$ as often used. Recent debate has focused on the value of this exponent (79), but the underlying biological basis of the relationship remains unknown. Other studies, directed at the origin of differences in metabolic rate between men and women, led to the concept of LBM or FFM as other means of normalizing MR (145, 206). Data such as those of Figure 6.6 (199) strongly indicate that much of the variance in metabolic rate, measured over 24 h as BMR or RMR, can be explained as a consequence of

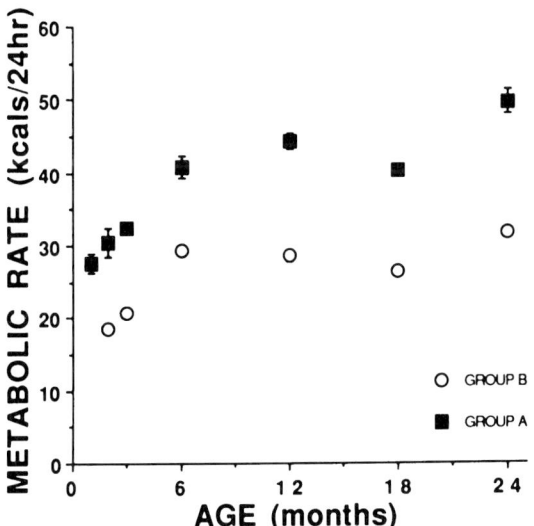

FIG. 6.7. Total daily energy expenditure of male Fischer 344 rats under usual living conditions. Metabolic rate measured from 6 wk to 24 months of age. *Solid squares*, rats fed ad libitum; *open circles*, rats fed 60% ad libitum. Reproduced from McCarter and Palmer (123) with permission.

differences in FFM. For example, differences in metabolic rate of men and women or of large and small individuals are minimized when metabolic rate is related to FFM (34, 35, 200). This method also has a biological basis in the well-known low metabolic rate of adipose tissue in comparison with other major tissues. Subtraction of adipose tissue or fat mass from body mass, therefore, provides a measure of metabolically active mass, which can be used to normalize metabolic rates of different individuals. There are of course problems related to this approach also. The first of these is that tissue components of FFM (liver, brain, kidneys, intestines, muscle, etc.) are not homogeneous in their metabolic activities (see TISSUE MASS AND TISSUE METABOLISM). The second is that the metabolic rate of adipose tissue is low but not negligible (about 4.5 kcal/kg/day). Taking these factors into account, equations derived by several authors relating metabolic rate to FFM can be evaluated. These equations have been summarized by Elia (50, Table 10) as being of two general types:

$$MR = K_1 + K_2 FFM \qquad (1)$$

$$MR = K_1 + K_2 FFM + K_3 FM \qquad (2)$$

where K_1, K_2, and K_3 are constants FM = fat mass. As is readily apparent from equations (1) and (2), the common means of expressing intensity of metabolism as MR/FFM will yield the constant K_2, provided K_1/FFM and/or $K_3 FM/FFM$ are negligible. This will be best approximated when FFM is large and/or K_1, K_3, and FM are small. These equations explain the frequent observation that MR/FFM decreases with increasing size. For example, using Equation (1), FFM of small individuals or animals is small and K_1/FFM may be a large fraction of the total. When FFM increases, the relative contribution of K_1/FFM to MR/FFM decreases. The apparently greater MR/FFM of smaller individuals than larger ones is then seen as a consequence of the relatively larger contribution of K_1/FFM to total metabolism. While such equations provide adequate descriptions of experimental data for intraspecific comparisons, they suffer from the absence of a clear biological basis, as noted for the power function ($MR = aW^n$) used for interspecific comparison of metabolic rates. However, the equations do provide results consistent with changes in body composition known to occur with aging. For example, Tzankoff and Norris in cross-sectional (198) and longitudinal studies (199) measured BMR and urine creatinine (as a measure of muscle mass) in volunteers. They concluded that decreased muscle mass with age could account for the entire observed age-related decrease in BMR. In line with this effect of muscle metabolism on BMR, the more recent experiments of Zurlo et al. (216) demonstrated in healthy male and female subjects that deviations of BMR from predicted values were correlated with differences in forearm skeletal muscle content.

In addition to the relationship between loss of muscle mass and decrease in metabolic rate with age, there exist a number of reports in which metabolic rate has been found to decrease with age independent of changes in FFM. For example, Morgan and York (133) found lower RMR in elderly subjects than in young subjects, despite similar values of FFM for both groups. Also, Fukagawa et al. (66) and Vaughan et al. (200) found decreased RMR and BMR, respectively, in old vs. young individuals independent of differences in FFM. These data suggest decreased MR/FFM with age, possibly as a consequence of decreased cellular energy metabolism or altered tissue composition. Also, as noted earlier, there is loss of FFM with advancing age in humans, and individuals with lower FFM exhibit a relatively higher value of MR/FFM. It is possible, therefore, that earlier reports of unchanged BMR with age are a consequence of overestimation of metabolic rate in elderly subjects due to normalization of MR to FFM, without taking into account contributions of the constants K_1 and K_3 as described earlier. Indeed, the work of several authors (35, 135) suggests decline of BMR with age independent of altered FFM as follows:

$$BMR = 601.2 + 21.0\ FFM - 2.6\ age$$

$$BMR = 441 + 21.9\ FFM - 2.4\ age$$

Whether such age-related decline in BMR is due to decreased rate of cellular energy metabolism or to altered composition of lean mass or of individual tissues is not known at this time. It should be pointed out that other work indicates that BMR is influenced also by genetic background and physical activity (16, 76, 150), in addition to the factors listed above. Since physical activity declines with age, possible effects of regular exercise on BMR are of particular interest. Despite the large volume of literature in this area and extensive research in humans and experimental animals, this issue remains unresolved, with evidence found for either no effect on BMR or increased BMR as a consequence of exercise training (188, 195, 196). Poehlman and Horton (152) have suggested that the different findings may be due in part to differences in the intensity of training, with only those individuals undergoing high levels of physical activity exhibiting increased BMR or RMR.

In summary, results of the very large number of studies in this area show that there is not a major decrease in basal or resting energy metabolism with age. However, future studies directed toward resolving age-related changes in BMR must take into account a formidable array of variables.

In comparison, there are relatively few reports of variation of RMR with age in laboratory animals. RMR has been reported to increase, decrease, or remain constant with age in rats (10, 42, 83). In addition, McCarter and Palmer (123) measured changes in resting metabolism over the life span of barrier-maintained Fischer 344 rats. RMR decreased from 3 to 18 months of age in these rats and then increased from 18 to 24 months of age. Similar trends were found when metabolic rate was expressed in terms of FFM or in terms of different power functions of body mass ($W^{0.75}$ or $W^{0.67}$). These results followed a trend similar to that seen with age in studies of the minimal oxygen consumption (MOC) as defined by Denckla (44). The MOC was defined to establish a standardized set of conditions for measuring basal metabolism in laboratory animals. Measurements by Denckla (44) in female Zivic-Miller rats and by McCarter et al. (124) in male Fischer 344 rats showed significant decline in MOC from 6 to 18 months of age with metabolic rate expressed per 100 g of FFM. However, since MOC is measured with rats under stage III anesthesia, the relevance of MOC data to aging processes is not clear.

Physical Activity. The contribution of physical activity to 24EE is large and variable (15%–30% of 24EE, see Fig. 6.5). The results of Ravussin et al. (156) show that much of the variation of 24EE between individuals is a consequence of differences in spontaneous activity, regardless of differences in body size. This component of 24EE includes energy expended in vigorous exercise as well as in the activities of usual daily living. This contribution also includes longer-lasting metabolic effects, which persist at the end of physical activity. Given the difficulty of assessing increased metabolic rate of exercise under usual living conditions, there are no studies to date that directly address the age-related variation of this component of 24EE. Such results will come from experiments using the doubly labeled water technique, in combination with direct measurements of BMR. However, there is a well-documented decrease in physical activity with age across phylogenetic lines. In humans there is a decrease with age in time devoted to active leisure activities and also a decrease with age in the intensity of those activities (33, 179). In laboratory rodents there is decreased spontaneous movement around cages (213) as well as decreased voluntary wheel running (82) with age. Decreased physical activity with age will lead to decrease in 24EE. In addition, decreased duration and intensity of exercise would be expected to result in altered body composition, that is, increased FM and decreased FFM with age, and thus a decrease in BMR and a further decrease in 24EE.

Diet-Induced Thermogenesis. A relatively minor contributor (~10%) to 24EE, DIT has two important components: an "obligatory" component, the thermic effect of food (TEF), and a "facultative" component related to activation of the sympathetic nervous system (SNS) and to activity of various metabolic cycles. TEF is a consequence of energy expended in digestion, absorption, and processing of ingested nutrients. The magnitude of TEF is a function of the size and composition of the meal, the frequency of meals (190), and the particular metabolic processing involved (89). Typically, the energy cost of carbohydrate processing is about 8% of ingested energy, fat 3%, and protein about 25% (60). Young (211) has pointed out that there is no information from long-term studies of the effects of age on TEF. Available evidence suggests that TEF is reduced in older vs. younger individuals following a test meal (133, 175). However, differences in TEF with age are small and probably are not a major factor in age-related variation of 24EE (211). Although large numbers of earlier studies produced equivocal results, later experiments demonstrated that TEF is lower in obese individuals than in lean individuals (37). Also, exercise potentiates TEF in lean subjects but not in obese subjects (151). Decreased physical activity and increased adiposity with age might therefore lessen the capacity of TEF to modulate whole-body energy balance. Altered physical activity and adiposity with age would result in a positive feedback, with more ingested energy stored as fat in the long term even if these effects are small on a 24-h basis. More studies are warranted to characterize age-related variations in TEF, especially using a longitudinal design. Current studies have been reviewed by Poehlman and Horton (152), but this active area of research is in a state of flux. In particular, it should be noted that James (86) and Jequier (88) have advocated a change in terminology, namely that TEF should be used to describe all of the responses that collectively result in increased energy expenditure following a meal. These authors propose that DIT be used to describe long-term effects of over- and undernutrition and that PPT (post-prandial thermogenesis) be used to describe the metabolic responses measured immediately following ingestion of food. If these definitions are adopted, then both PPT and DIT would involve obligatory and facultative components, and TEF would, presumably, incorporate all metabolic responses measured in PPT and DIT.

The facultative component of DIT dissipates about 3% of ingested food energy and is a function of SNS activity and metabolic cycle activity (61). There is much evidence for altered responsiveness and activity of the SNS with age (152). In general, levels of plasma norepinephrine, the major postganglionic neurotransmitter of the SNS, increase with age, suggesting increased sympathetic tone (174). Results of Poehlman et al. (154) suggest no difference with age in the clearance of norepinephrine and show that physically active older men exhibit an increased rate of appearance of plasma norepinephrine in comparison with younger or inactive older individuals. Schwartz et al. (174) demonstrated lower DIT in elderly individuals and less of an increase in plasma norepinephrine in response to a meal, suggesting blunted responsiveness of the SNS with age. Although contradictory results have been obtained, it appears that levels of physical activity and degree of adiposity may modulate the relationship between DIT and SNS activity with age (152). Rothwell (158) has pointed out the association between DIT, SNS activity, and the activity of particular metabolic cycles. Adaptive thermogenesis may be linked to altered protein and triglyceride turnover, Cori cycle activity, ion pumping (such as Na^+/K^+-ATPase), uncoupling of oxidative phosphorylation in brown adipose tissue (BAT), and substrate cycling (in futile cycles and/or ATP-generating cycles, such as glycolysis). Thermogenesis in BAT is a major component of adaptive energy metabolism in small animals. In adult humans the quantitative significance of this tissue is doubtful, although functional BAT has been found in individuals up to 80 yr of age (104). It seems likely that skeletal muscle plays a role in facultative thermogenesis in humans. Results of Astrup et al. (3) and Emorine et al. (55) indicate increased thermogenesis in skeletal muscle following carbohydrate feeding, and this may be mediated via beta-2 and beta-3 adrenergic receptors. There are no reports to date regarding age-related variations in this aspect of skeletal muscle metabolism. There is also little information regarding changes with age in the activities of the many metabolic cycles listed above, with the exception of protein turnover, which is known to decrease with age in humans and laboratory animals (see Chapter 9). Protein turnover is estimated to account for about 14% of the BMR in adult humans (51, Table 5), but maintenance of Na^+/K^+ gradients across cell membranes may be a major contributor (about 30% of the BMR; 71). Of particular interest are the so-called futile cycles, which dissipate ATP with no other net change in the organism (60). Examples are fructose-1,6-diphosphate hydrolysis by fructose diphosphatase and resynthesis by phosphofructokinase; interconversion of glucose and glucose-6-phosphate; breakdown and resynthesis of triglycerides involving both liver and adipose tissue; and breakdown and resynthesis of phosphoenolpyruvate. Current estimates are that such cycles play a minor role in thermogenesis (210). However, the age-related role of this seemingly energetically wasteful metabolism, together with that of "proton slippage" in mitochondrial oxidative phosphorylation, remains to be established. If there is an increase with age in energy dissipation (that is, increased utilization of energy in pathways not directly related to maintenance of cellular homeostasis), these metabolic cycles would be likely candidates for investigation.

Young (211) has identified the need for studies of long-term energy balance in humans and laboratory animals. Preliminary results from his laboratory suggest that both overfeeding and underfeeding for a period of 3 wk result in similar thermogenic responses to food in young and old individuals. On the basis of current information, therefore, it appears that, as in the case of BMR, age-related variation in DIT is small. However, given the large number of factors influencing the thermogenic response to food, and in particular the involvement of the SNS in this response, further research is needed to establish the precise role of this component of 24EE in aging.

Efficiency and Energy Utilization

The existence of "futile" cycles and the dissipation of proton gradients across inner mitochondrial membranes without coupled synthesis of ATP (proton slippage) suggests that the fraction of nutrient energy resulting in net ATP synthesis may be variable. Variable metabolic efficiency has been invoked as an explanation of the anti-aging action of dietary restriction and is implicit in wear-and-tear theories of aging (207). Masoro and McCarter (116) pointed out that "metabolic efficiency" may not be a useful concept in the context of aging processes. This is because of problems of definition and the difficulty of assigning "useful" and "wasteful" roles to particular metabolic activities or pathways. In line with this view, Flatt (60) suggests that metabolic efficiency has been a "conceptual trap rather than a tool" in studies of obesity. Flatt emphasizes that there are at least nine possible definitions of metabolic efficiency (Table 6.4). When considering the amount of physical work performed in relation to change in whole-body metabolic rate, metabolic efficiency can be determined relatively unambiguously (definition 2 of Table 6.4) and is about 25%. Even here, though, the method of measurement (mass-bearing vs. non-mass-bearing activity) will determine the outcome. In the case of carcass energy deposition as a fraction of total food energy input (definition 4 of Table 6.4), efficiency increases as energy input exceeds maintenance requirements. In this case, subtracting energy of maintenance from total energy intake (definition 5) has theoretical appeal but is difficult to establish in practice. In humans metabolic efficiency is most often utilized in comparisons of TEF; that is, TEFs in different individuals are compared as a fraction of their respective RMRs. RMR is in turn related to FFM, but since RMR is not directly proportional to FFM (as described earlier under Basal Metabolic Rate), comparisons between individuals of differing FFMs involve errors associated with normalization of RMR to FFM. The metabolic efficiency of nutrient storage (definition 6) can be calculated on the basis of

TABLE 6.4. *Possible Definitions of Metabolic Efficiency*

1. η_{work}	=	Work produced / Energy intake	Depends primarily on amount of physical activity performed
2. $\eta_{\Delta work}$	=	ΔWork produced / ΔMetabolic rate	Reproducible under well-defined conditions
3. $\eta_{coupling}$	=	Mechanical work produced / High-energy bond energy utilized	About 40%
4. η_{gross}	=	Energy retained / Energy intake	Depends primarily on intake/expenditure ratio; important in judging feed efficiency during meat production; negative when intake < expenditure
5. η_{net}	=	Energy retained / Energy intake above maintenance requirement	Similar in principle to Eq. 2 but difficult to assess with accuracy (particularly when intake is not substantially greater than expenditure) because maintenance requirements cannot be reliably established
6. $\eta_{storage}$	=	Cost of nutrient absorption and storage / ΔEnergy expenditure	Somewhat variable; depends primarily on importance of catecholamine (SNS)- mediated stimulation of metabolism relative to obligatory storage costs (i.e., ATP needed for synthesis of glycogen, protein, and adipose tissue triglycerides)
7. $\eta_{oxygen\ phosphatase}$	=	Energy recovered in high-energy bonds of ATP / Heat of combustion of substrate oxidized	Depends primarily on P:O ratio; reaches 67% for P:O ratio of 3 (because some proton leakage across the mitochondrial membrane always occurs, the P:O ratio can be substantially less than 3 at low rates of substrate oxidation)
8. $\eta_{metabolism}$	=	ATP replaced / ATP generated	Depends on metabolic costs incurred for substrate handling (i.e., ATP expenditure for transport, activation, substrate cycles)
9. $\eta_{ATPproduct}$	=	ATP replaced / ATP generated	Depends on metabolic costs incurred for substrate handling (i.e., ATP expenditure for transport, activation, substrate cycles)

From Flatt (60), reproduced by permission.

composition of the diet and a cost of ATP replacement of 20–22 kcal/mol. Flatt (60) suggests that metabolic efficiency may be most usefully expressed in terms of net yield of ATP (definitions 7–9). Because of differences in TEF, for example, net yields of ATP are 90%, 75%, and 55% for meals consisting entirely of fat, carbohydrate, or protein, respectively.

An alternative approach to this issue is to consider the change of energy output required to perform a given amount of work. This index is termed "economy" (57), and there is an evolving literature documenting effects of age on the economy of energy utilization. For example, a given speed of walking requires higher net energy expenditure in the elderly than in young adults (146). The basis of this decreased economy of movement with age is not clear, but it is apparently not a consequence of decreased physical activity with advanced age (114).

Under conditions of usual living, problems of energy balance are determined more by food intake than by energy expenditure (211). Intake is rarely fixed and will be adjusted to offset increased energy expenditure (60). The composition of ingested food is a major factor in energy balance. Ingested carbohydrate increases oxidation of carbohydrate and inhibits oxidation of fat, whereas ingested fat does not promote oxidation of carbohydrate or fat (1, 61, 173). Hence the composition of energy intake as well as the amount of food will influence metabolic cycles and energy expenditure. Understanding variation with age in energy substrate utilization must therefore precede attempts to invoke changes in metabolic efficiency as a factor in aging processes.

FACTORS MODULATING METABOLIC RATE

Temperature

Rates of the biochemical reactions that collectively make up whole-body metabolism are accelerated by increased temperature and slowed by decreased temperature. This effect occurs provided the change in temperature does not alter the chemical characteristics of the reactants and the enzymes catalyzing the reactions, such as by denaturing proteins or by changing the affinity of reactive sites. In general, the dependence of reaction rate on temperature follows the Arrhenius equation

$$\ln k_{T_2}/k_{T_1} = \frac{E\alpha(T_2 - T_1)}{RT_1T_2}$$

Where k_{T_1} and k_{T_2} are reaction rate constants at absolute temperatures T_1 and T_2, $E\alpha$ is the activation energy of reaction, assumed independent of temperature; and R is the universal gas constant. The ratio of the rate constants (k_{T_2}/k_{T_1}) when $T_2 - T_1 = 10°C$ is the Q_{10}. For many but not all biological reactions Q_{10} ranges between 2 and 3, that is, increase in temperature of 10°C results in a doubling to a tripling of reaction rate, or, in general, decrease in temperature of 10°C would be expected to lower metabolic rate to *1/2* or *1/3* of the initial value (209). Such effects would be expected in poikilothermic animals whose body temperature is a function of ambient temperature. In homeothermic animals, temperature is regulated about a "set point" (73). Fluctuations about this point because of inability to dissipate or conserve heat or resetting of the reference point (as in fever) would also lead to altered metabolic rate. In humans, body temperature is tightly regulated so that optimal rates of metabolic reactions are maintained. The regulation of core body temperature involves modulation of whole-body metabolic rate and control of heat dissipation. Ability to regulate body temperature and to adapt to different thermal environments declines with age (31). However, the extent of decline is highly variable, depending on health, fitness, intake of medications, and behavior, such as consumption of alcohol or smoking cigarettes (111). Individuals 65 yr and older have a thirty-five-fold higher risk than younger people of developing heat stroke or hyperthermia (core temperature $\geq$ 106°F); they also have increased vulnerability to hypothermia (core temperature $\leq$ 95°F). Vulnerability increases in part because of decreased perception of body temperature with age (32), but effector mechanisms may also be impaired (111).

In a hot environment and/or following strenuous exercise the primary mechanisms of heat dissipation in humans are increased skin blood flow and increased rate of sweating. Although earlier reports suggest unaltered skin vasodilation with age (75), more recent studies show decreased ability to redistribute blood flow from core to periphery in the elderly (91). This diminished response of skin blood flow to heat challenge may be related to structural changes in the skin vasculature (92), impaired vasoconstriction of blood vessels of the viscera, and increased threshold for sweating (167). The interesting study of Inoue et al. (85) demonstrates the importance of anatomical location: rates of sweating of the skin of the back were not age-related, but sweating of the skin of the thigh was always lower in elderly (60–71 yr) than in young (20–25 yr) male subjects. Level of physical activity plays a major role; Buono et al. (23) and Tankersley et al. (193) found no difference in sweat rates when young and old individuals of similar V_{O_2max} were compared. Indeed, several investigators have suggested that decline with age in V_{O_2max} (rather than decline of heat loss response per se) is related to decreased ability to dissipate heat (for example, 38), probably via altered sensitivity of the sweating response (135).

Response to cold challenge is also diminished with age. In addition to decrease in BMR and physical activity, there is reduced shivering and impaired sympathetic vasoconstrictor response with age. There is considerable variability between subjects in these responses, however. For example, Khan et al. (94) found that some but not all healthy elderly men and women (average age 68 yr) had diminished reflex sympathetic vasoconstrictor response to cold challenge in comparison with that of young men and women (average age 26 yr). In contrast to the age-related decrease in heat dissipation response, the decrease in adaptation to cold is not a function of physical fitness, but is related to adiposity (22). The variability in response of the elderly to cold may also be a consequence of different degrees of impairment of the SNS, and similar effects have been noted in diabetics (176). The ability to raise body temperature in response to pyrogens, that is, generation of fever, is also blunted with age (137). Since elevation of body temperature in response to bacterial infection is important for survival, this loss of responsiveness constitutes a significant risk factor for the elderly (170). Induction of fever is mediated by endogenously released cytokines. Release of interleukin 1, the endogenous pyrogen for which most information is available, appears to be unchanged with age (90). This suggests that peripheral rather than central factors may be involved in the diminished febrile response. In addition to the above factors, many elderly people are compromised in their ability to regulate body temperature because of frequent use of medications. Anticholinergic, antiadrenergic, or diuretic drugs, as well as antidepressants and monoamine oxidase inhibitors, will result in blunted response to thermal challenge, in addition to decreased responsiveness with age. The result is often an individual with poikilothermic rather than homeothermic characteristics (41). Such loss of ability to conserve or dissipate heat will in turn increase or decrease whole-body metabolic rate, in a positive feedback, with potentially life-threatening consequences.

Evidence also indicates altered thermoregulatory capability of laboratory rodents with age (6, 99, 191). Few studies have investigated the response to heat challenge in old vs. young animals, but available data suggest that, in contrast to humans, older rats have enhanced responsiveness, that is, decreased rate of heat storage in response to heat stress. The results of Kregel et al. (99) in male Fischer 344 rats show decreased rate of rise of core temperature during acute heating of old (24 months) vs. mature (12 months) rats. As found in humans, however, repeated exposure to heat stress results in more rapid heat storage and increased core temperature following heat challenge (99). The response to cold has been extensively investigated in laboratory rodents, in part because of interest in the ability of small animals to increase metabolic rate by nonshivering thermogenesis (NST). NST is a consequence of the uncoupling of oxidative phosphorylation in mitochondria of BAT. Thus in laboratory rodents temperature regulation in cold environments involves heat conservation by redistribution of blood flow and increased generation of heat from shivering thermogenesis as well as nonshivering thermogenesis. Foster and Frydman (64, 65) have estimated that during acute exposure to cold 25% of total oxygen consumption is due to BAT thermogenesis. Following acclimation to cold, however, NST in BAT accounts for 42% of thermogenesis in response to cold. The age-related decline in thermoregulatory ability of rodents is, however, extremely variable, depending on strain, sex, and level of physical activity (126, 127, 129). In particular, 23-month-old female Fischer 344 rats were able to maintain core temperature during cold challenge (6 h at 6°C), whereas male Fischer 344 rats of similar age exhibited decreased core temperature (−1.8°C) under the same conditions. Both sexes had similar increases in oxygen consumption during cold exposure, implying diminished ability to conserve heat in elderly male, but not female, rats. Surprisingly, BAT mass and GDP (guanosine 5′-diphosphate) binding (an index of BAT activity) decreased significantly with age in male rats but not in female rats (126). The results of McDonald et al. (128) are a striking demonstration of the protective effect of exercise in maintaining age-related ability to meet a cold challenge. Male Fischer 344 rats, 12 and 24 months of age, were subjected to 60 min of treadmill running (20 m/min on 0% grade) 5 days per week for 6 months. When faced with a cold challenge (6 h at 6°C), elderly control, sedentary rats exhibited a large decrease in core temperature (36.3–31.2°C), whereas in elderly exercised rats core temperature decreased by a much smaller amount (36.4–35.3°C). No significant differences were found in BAT mass per unit body mass or in GDP binding to mitochondria isolated from BAT. The authors concluded that decreased capacity for shivering thermogenesis due to decline in physical activity may be an important component of the age-related decline in thermoregulatory capability in rats. Later results of this research group indicate that the availability of carbohydrate as a fuel for the muscular activity of shivering thermogenesis is not a limiting factor in this age-related decrement (103).

In contrast to these studies of acute cold challenge, Holloszy and Smith (81) subjected adult (6-month-old) male Long-Evans rats to chronic intermittent cold exposure (4 h per day, 5 days per wk in water at 23°C until 32 months of age). Experimental rats ate 44% more food than controls and had significantly lower body masses, indicating significantly elevated daily metabolic rates. Despite repeated cold challenge and much higher rates of metabolism, life expectancy of experimental rats was not less than that of control rats.

Results in mice suggest the existence of an age limit for benefits of exercise. Talan and Ingram (192) compared responses to cold in control and exercised C57BL/6J mice (3 wk of forced treadmill or voluntary wheel running) using mice 28–30 months of age. Thirty-six percent of the exercised mice died, and the survivors exhibited no improvement in thermoregulatory response with repeated testing. In contrast, control, sedentary mice had increased tolerance to cold challenge with repeated testing. Also, the results of Tatelman and Talan (194) suggest that aged mice are less tolerant to cold because they produce less heat in response to cold challenge, perhaps due to decreased activation of NST and BAT. Laboratory animals also exhibit decreased febrile response with age (29, 59, 138), and this diminished response has been extensively investigated in rats. Elderly male (170) and female (169) rats have delayed onset of response and decreased magnitude of temperature change in comparison with young and adult rats following intraperitoneal inoculations with *Escherichia coli*. Age-related attenuation is associated with decreased heat output by BAT, rather than skeletal muscle, since endotoxin infection decreases muscle blood flow but increases perfusion of BAT (87). The results of Scarpace et al. (171) demonstrate that there is less capacity for thermogenesis in old rats, a consequence of decreased mitochondrial content as well as fewer available GDP binding sites in these animals. In addition, Scarpace et al. (172) showed diminished activation of BAT in old rats because of decreased numbers of β-adrenergic receptors and reduced activation of adenylate cyclase in the BAT of these animals.

Despite impressive advances in understanding mechanisms of heat production, much remains to be done. In particular, animal models should be employed in which health status and level of physical activity are identified with age. Unresolved issues include alterations with age in the sensing of body temperature, activity of the SNS, and responsiveness of peripheral tissues.

Neuroendocrine Factors

Nervous and hormonal systems play major roles in modulating metabolic rate via control of skeletal muscle and fuel mobilization. Age-related variations in carbohydrate metabolism and exercise are considered elsewhere (see Chapters 7 and 21). We will focus on age-related effects of thyroid hormone and the SNS, since these neuroendocrine systems are widely believed to directly modulate metabolic rate.

Boothby and Sandiford (14) popularized the use of BMR in the identification of thyroid disorders in humans, with deviations from normal values of BMR being categorized as a result of hypo- or hyperthyroid conditions. However, no clear relationship has been found between plasma levels of thyroid hormones and metabolic rate in euthyroid individuals (208). Moreover, while the turnover of thyroxine (T_4) decreases significantly with age in humans, it is not clear whether aging affects plasma levels of T_4 and T_3 (tri-iodothyronine, the metabolically active form of the hormone) (72, 141). In a recent study of 300 male subjects aged 17–78 yr Poehlman et al. (153) found that RMR was only weakly correlated with fasting levels of total and free T_3. FFM and $V_{O_{2max}}$ were major determinants of decreased RMR with age, and there was an inverse correlation between plasma T_3 (total and free) and age. On the basis of earlier studies Perlmutter and Riggs (149) suggested that decline with age in thyroid hormone metabolism is due mainly to decreased peripheral turnover of the hormone. This possibility and others have been investigated in animal studies. However, the studies also exhibit no clear effects of age. Plasma T_3 and T_4 levels have been found to be unchanged, decreased, or increased with age (62, 78, 205). The conversion of T_4 to T_3 is accomplished by 5'-deiodinases. Activity of these enzymes has been found to decrease (46) or to be unchanged (67) with age. No data are available on age-related variability of metabolic clearance of T_3 or on changes in concentration of plasma proteins (such as transthyretin), to which most of the plasma T_4 and T_3 are bound. There are also few studies regarding tissue responsiveness to T_4 or T_3 with age. Denckla (44) found decreased responsiveness with age of whole-body metabolic rate to exogenous T_3 in anesthetized female Zivic-Miller rats. In contrast, McCarter et al. (124) found increased sensitivity with age of MOC to exogenous T_3 in male Fischer 344 rats 6–18 months of age. T_3-induced malic enzyme and its mRNA decrease with age in tissues of laboratory rodents (132), suggesting decreased responsiveness of peripheral tissues to thyroid hormone with age. In summary, although variable results have been reported, the available literature suggests decreased influence of thyroid hormone on metabolic rate with age, probably as a consequence of peripheral factors rather than an age-related decline in output of the thyroid gland. Several issues remain unresolved; in particular, the role of thyroid hormone in modulating MR is not clear, despite the widely held perception of a direct influence of thyroid hormone on rate of metabolism.

Nevertheless, SNS activity is known to directly affect MR. As discussed earlier under Diet-Induced Thermogenesis, SNS activity is a major link in the facultative component of dietary thermogenesis. This occurs via activation of BAT in small animals and skeletal muscle and/or vital organ metabolism in humans (3, 167, 172). In addition, the results of Saad et al. (164) demonstrate a direct effect of SNS activity on 24EE and on RMR in adult Caucasians (but not in Pima Indians). These studies involved measurements of 24EE, 24-h urinary norepinephrine excretion, RMR, and metabolic rate following propranolol infusion (to block β-adrenergic receptors). Given these links between SNS activity and metabolic rate it is important to establish age-related variation in SNS activity. This activity, or sympathetic *tone*, is estimated from plasma concentrations of norepinephrine, by infusion of labeled norepinephrine to assess turnover rates. A majority of the many studies conducted in this area (reviewed in 152) indicate increased appearance of plasma norepinephrine in the elderly, but the increase in sympathetic tone with age may be a consequence of changes in body composition and level of physical activity. Studies of laboratory animals indicate that in addition to increased plasma norepinephrine with age there is a decline in content of norepinephrine of most, but not all, organs with age (58, 201). Such observations have been interpreted to indicate that activity of the SNS increases with age and that aging may be associated with a hyperadrenergic state, characterized by increased basal and increased stress-induced sympathetic activity (159). Metabolic consequences of these age-related changes in SNS activity are not yet well defined. However, the results of Odio and Brodish (140) demonstrate decreased capacity of old (22 months) male Fischer 344 rats to mobilize metabolic fuels (glucose and free fatty acids) in response to acute stress (electric shock of the foot) compared to adult (6 months) control rats.

Dietary Restriction

Studies in humans and various animals over the past century have demonstrated unequivocally that restriction of food intake leads to a decrease in metabolic rate per unit mass. Indeed, Garrow (68) has stated; "there is no investigator who has looked for this effect and failed to find it." Studies have been conducted in a wide variety of species, including several different strains of rodent, sheep, cattle, and humans, ranging in age from preadolescence to adulthood and using caloric restrictions of 10–50% of ad libitum intake (131, 207). The effect of calorie restriction on metabolic rate, therefore, appears to be a fundamental response of metabolism to reduced energy input, independent of age, species, and precise level of restriction. Most of these studies involved measurement of BMR and restriction of food for relatively short time periods: less than 6 months in the case of humans (131) and 2 months for rodents (207, Table 4.18. The more recent work of McCarter and McGee (122) shows that not only BMR but also 24EE declines following reduction of food intake in weanling Fischer 344 rats. However, the decrease in metabolic rate is a transient phenomenon: within 6 wk lean mass adjusted to the decreased input of calories so that 24EE per unit lean mass was the same in control and restricted rats. BMR exhibited a longer transient period but was not significantly different from control after 18 wk of restriction. These results were extended by McCarter et al (125) and McCarter and Palmer (123), who demonstrated that metabolic rate per unit lean mass of rats fed a restricted diet was not less than that of rats fed ad libitum over most of the life span. Similar results were demonstrated by Duffy et al. (47), who measured RMR and 24EE in 18-month-old Fischer 344 rats restricted to 60% of ad libitum intake from 6 wk of age. The response of whole-body metabolism when dietary restriction is initiated in adulthood has not been characterized. Work by Gonzalez-Pacheco et al. (70) suggests that a longer transient period is associated with metabolic adaptation to such restriction of food in adult rats. These authors found that BMR and 24EE remained depressed 6 wk after initiation of 40% dietary restriction in 6-month-old Fischer 344 rats. A longer time of adaptation of body mass to reduced food input in adulthood is also indicated by the results of Yu et al. (213). These authors restricted the food intake of 6-month-old rats by 40% and found that body mass required several months to adapt to the decreased food intake. The food consumption per unit mass of these rats remained depressed for at least 6 months following initiation of restriction (213, Figs. 2, 7). In contrast, Masoro et al. (118) demonstrated that in weanling rats food consumption per unit body mass was the same in restricted and control animals within 4 wk of the start of the restricted diet. Results of chronic starvation in humans also support the concept of metabolic adaptation to long-term restriction of food intake; that is, individuals subjected to long-term deprivation of food exhibit values of BMR within the normal range (8, 202). In contrast, the impressive studies of Benedict et al. (11) and Keys et al. (93) demonstrate that when moderate to severe dietary restriction is initiated for relatively short durations (less than 6 months) in adult humans, there is a decrease in BMR not accounted for by a corresponding decrease in metabolic mass.

The results of chronic dietary restriction have conceptual importance for current theories of aging since it has been suggested that reduction of metabolic rate is the mechanism by which dietary restriction retards aging processes (165). It is important to emphasize, therefore, that under the precise experimental conditions that lead to retardation of aging processes in laboratory rodents, there was no reduction of metabolic rate per unit metabolic mass over most of the life span (47, 123). Recent challenges (70, 113) to this concept should therefore be viewed within the broader context of the metabolic effects of dietary restriction in general and will be discussed further in the final section of this chapter.

METABOLIC RATE OF POIKILOTHERMS AS A FUNCTION OF AGE

Many studies have investigated metabolic rate of poikilothermic animals, both vertebrate and invertebrate. In general, these demonstrate a similar reciprocal relationship between body mass and metabolic rate per unit mass as discussed for mammals (12). The studies of Hulbert and colleagues (52, 84) indicate that homeotherms have far greater capacity for aerobic metabolism than poikilotherms of the same body mass and temperature. This difference in oxidative capacity is similar to measured differences in RMR (12) and is correlated with the greater volume density of mitochondria, surface area of mitochondrial membranes, and oxidative enzyme activity of homeotherms (84). As noted by Masoro (115), insufficient data are available regarding the life span of poikilotherms to establish clearly whether or not the low intensity of their metabolism is correlated with increased life span. A particular problem identified by Sohal and Allen (183) is that the concept of a species-specific life span may not strictly apply to poikilotherms, given the large number of environmental factors that influence life span. Because of the conveniently small size and short life span of insects, large numbers of studies designed to probe mechanisms of aging have been conducted with them, especially flies of different strains. Comparison of results of most of these studies is not possible because of the variable conditions employed (108). Also, in most studies metabolic rate was found to vary with age, depending on environmental temperature. Figure 6.8 demonstrates variation of oxygen consumption with age of male milkweed bugs housed at three different ambient temperatures. Note that metabolic rate increases, decreases, or remains constant with age depending on temperature (120). The impressive study of Arking et al. (2) demonstrates that oxygen consumption of different strains of *Drosophila melanogaster* decreases with age at high ambient temperatures ($\geq 25°C$) but remains relatively constant with age at lower ambient temperature (18°C). Although changes in metabolic rate with age are usually interpreted as altered intensity of cellular metabolism, none of the possibly confounding changes in body and tissue composition described earlier for mammals has been established in these animals.

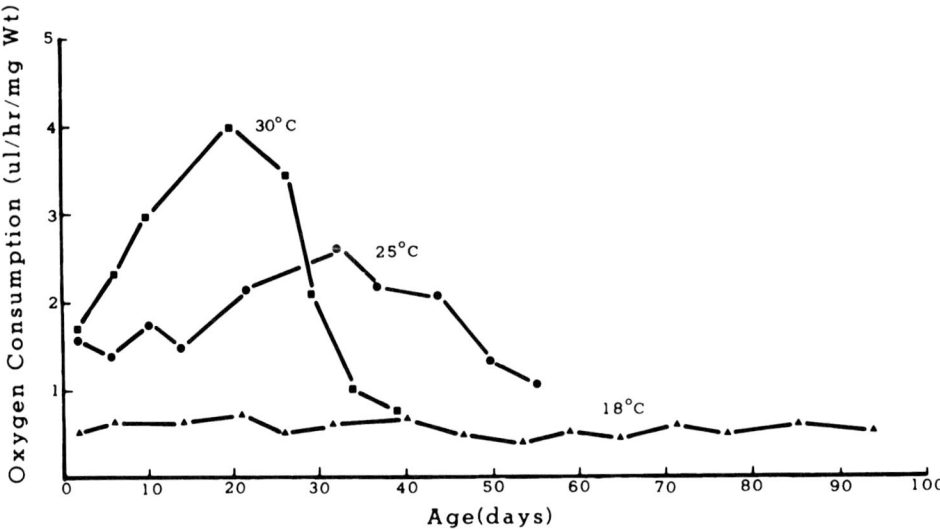

FIG. 6.8. Oxygen consumption of male milkweed bugs with age and at different ambient temperatures. Reproduced from McArthur and Sohal (120) with permission.

Changes with age of cellular pathways of energy metabolism in insects have been reviewed by Lints (107). Although much of the earlier literature documents decline in the structural integrity of mitochondria, together with decreased oxidative and glycolytic enzyme activity, recent studies indicate no change in levels of high-energy phosphates or activity of enzymes related to energy metabolism, provided appropriate substrates are supplied during measurement in vitro. Lints (107) suggests that compromised functional ability of these animals may be associated with altered permeability of mitochondrial membranes, leading to inadequate supply of substrate, rather than reduced capacity of mitochondria to generate ATP. As is the case in homeotherms, the nature and origins of change in metabolic rate per unit body mass with age in poikilotherms thus remain uncertain.

ENERGY METABOLISM AND THEORIES OF AGING

Rate of Living Theory

The concept that life span is linked to metabolic rate has a long and controversial history. Controversy centers on which definition of the link between metabolism and aging is assumed. There is evidence both in support of and against different versions, but collectively such theories are grouped under the description of Pearl (147) as the "rate of living" theory of aging. The theories have as their starting point the assumption that with the passage of time there is an accumulation of damage in proportion to the absolute magnitude of metabolism (162) or the consumption of a vital substance whose exhaustion limits life (147). Life span is thus determined by the rate at which these processes occur, and this in turn is determined by metabolic rate. So convinced was Rubner of the importance of these ideas that he suggested they might represent the "unity of a great law" (162). To this day the metabolic rate link is considered a possible mechanism of aging (112, 181, 182) in spite of an impressive array of contrary evidence (4, 5, 56, 81, 108).

A brief historical perspective will outline the basis of the controversy. Rubner (162) found that oxygen consumption per unit body mass over the adult life span was approximately the same (about 200 kcal/g/life span) in five different species of domestic animal despite a sixfold difference in life span. The suggestion that there might exist a finite lifetime metabolic potential gained support from experiments with fruit flies. Loeb and Northrop (109) reported that life span of *D. melanogaster* decreased as ambient temperature was raised from 10°C to 30°C. Since these insects are poikilotherms, the implication of these data was that increased temperature resulted in increased metabolic rate and so decreased longevity. Similar results were obtained by Pearl (147) using flies and cantaloupe seedlings and were incorporated into his "rate of living" theory of aging. Dramatic support was also provided by McArthur and Baillie (119). These authors found that life span decreased by 77% when brine shrimp (*(Daphnia)* were raised at 28°C vs. 8°C, but the total number of heartbeats per lifetime was similar at both temperatures. Many subsequent experiments were conducted using changes in temperature or physical activity as means of altering metabolic rate in a variety of poikilothermic animals. As Sohal and Allen (183) pointed out, few investigators actually measured rate of metabolism as a function of life span in these experiments, and the work of Newell (136) shows little change of metabolic rate with altered temperature in several different invertebrates. Despite the large number of reports in this area, there remains no consensus that increased rate of metabolism shortens life span in poikilothermic animals. However, as discussed by Sohal (183) and Lints (108), altered metabolic rate frequently has been found to modulate life span. Variable effects of altered metabolic rate may thus be interpreted in terms of genetically different abilities of organisms to respond to increased generation of toxic substances or increased rates of exhaustion of vital substances.

In mammals an inverse relationship has been shown to exist between metabolic rate per unit mass and life span in a number of different species (36) (Fig. 6.9). The graphs in Figure 6.9 are generated using estimates of metabolic rate and life span, and there appear to be identifiable hyperbolas for different mammalian species. It should be noted that hyperbolas approach their limiting values asymptotically. Therefore, at low metabolic rates small variability in metabolic rate may be associated with large differences in life span (Figure 6.9). Conversely, for animals of short life span, small differences in longevity may be associated with large differences in metabolic rate per unit mass. In this way, a twofold difference in the life spans of chimpanzees and humans may be associated with closely related values of metabolic rate per unit mass (48). These results show that in general mammals of high metabolic rate per unit mass have a shorter life expectancy than those of low metabolic rate per unit mass. It is tempting, therefore, to conclude that there exists a direct link between metabolic rate and rate of aging, but such a conclusion would be premature. The recent work of Austad and Fischer (5) suggests a different explanation. These authors point out that a large number of exceptions to predictions of the rate of living theory exist, particularly in the case of marsupials and bats. They found that lifetime energy expenditures among 164 mammalian species ranged from 39 to 1,102 kcal/g/life span, in contrast to the limited values suggested by Rubner (162) and Cutler (36).

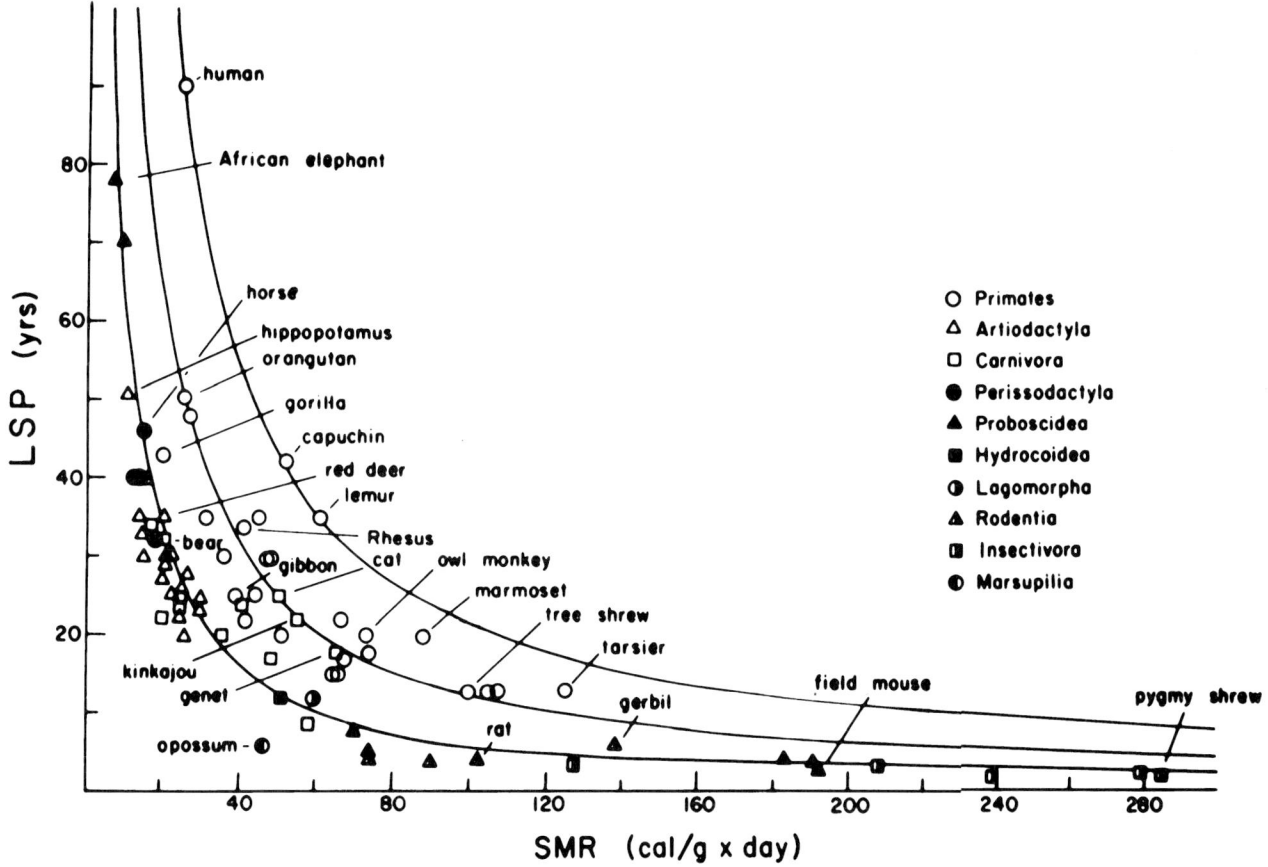

FIG. 6.9. Life span of selected mammals as a function of metabolic rate. *LSP*, life span potential, measured as life span in years for 90% mortality; *SMR*, specific metabolic rate, measured as basal metabolism in calories per gram body weight per day. Reproduced from Cutler (36) with permission.

Noting that there also exists an inverse relationship between body size and metabolic rate, Austad and Fischer (5) suggest that increased longevity may be a consequence of the survival value of increased body size, rather than decreased metabolic rate. Using this rationale, the long life expectancies of birds and bats, despite very high metabolic rates per unit mass, are a consequence of the survival value of their life-styles and are not related to metabolic rate. Similarly, the increased longevity of larger animals is a consequence of reduced environmental vulnerability rather than decreased metabolic rate per unit mass. Given the large number of conflicting results and the controversy in this literature, these suggestions offer an alternative explanation that certainly merits study (4).

A further test of the rate of living theory involves the search for mechanisms by which dietary restriction retards aging processes. Sacher (165) suggested that dietary restriction prolongs life as a consequence of its action in decreasing metabolic rate. Reduction of metabolic rate per unit mass in response to reduced food intake is one of the most well-established effects in nutritional physiology (68). The mechanism of action of dietary restriction suggested by Sacher (165) thus gained wide acceptance (207) and continues to be advanced as a viable possibility (70, 112). However, there is considerable evidence against this view. Masoro et al. (118) found that the food intake (calories/g body mass) of male Fischer 344 rats fed ad libitum or fed a life-prolonging restricted diet was the same over most of the life span. Since restricted rats lived about 40% longer, they consumed far more calories over their life span than rats fed ad libitum. McCarter and McGee (122) measured metabolic rate per unit body mass of restricted and ad libitum–fed rats under usual living conditions. They found that the decrease in metabolic rate following initiation of dietary restriction (as found by others) was a transient phenomenon; that is, metabolic rate of weanling rats adjusted to reduced food intake so that by 6 months of age both BMR and 24EE were similar in restricted and ad libitum–fed rats. These results were confirmed by Duffy et al. (47), who measured BMR and 24EE in 18-month-old Fischer 344 rats fed ad libitum or fed the restricted diet from 6 wk of age. Finally, McCarter and Palmer (123) found no difference in 24EE over the life span of ad libitum–fed and restricted rats. The important conclusion of all of these experiments is that when metabolic rate was assessed under conditions known to retard aging processes in Fischer 344 rats no differences were found between metabolic rates of rats fed ad libitum and those fed the restricted diet; that is, reduced metabolic rate is not an essential component of the life-prolonging action of dietary restriction. It is possible that metabolic rate is indeed decreased in key tissues of restricted rats, and this in turn signals a change of physiological status and decreased rate of aging (112). However, such key tissues have yet to be identified and such a limited effect on specific tissues would not serve as confirmation of the rate of living theory of aging.

On the basis of available information it thus seems unlikely that metabolic rate per se is a major determinant of the rate of aging. The large databases currently available (e.g. 5) provide too many exceptions to a simple and direct link between life span and metabolic rate as suggested by Rubner (162) and Pearl (147). However, the vigorous debate that attended the rate of living theory led to the formulation of other ways in which energy use might be linked to aging. These ideas relate to the cumulative effects of toxic by-products of energy metabolism, as exemplified by the "free radical" theory of aging (74), or to the toxic effects of the presence of circulating fuels, as in the "glycation theory" of aging (28). Since the latter is described in Chapter 7, a brief assessment will be given only of the former.

Free Radical Theory

Aerobic metabolism enables organisms to rapidly generate large amounts of metabolic energy from ingested nutrients. The obvious competitive advantage of this form of energy transduction carries with it a penalty: the oxygen required for combustion may also undergo a sequence of univalent reductions producing highly reactive and potentially damaging free radicals. Molecules produced in these reactions contain unpaired electrons and so are capable of combining with neighboring molecules and altering their function. For example, the electron transport processes involved in the mitochondrial generation of ATP also yield small numbers of $\dot{O}_{2-}$, H_2O_2, and $\dot{O}H$, which are capable of inducing damage in cellular organelles (26). H_2O_2 is also generated by peroxisome metabolism (134), and H_2O_2 and $\dot{O}_{2-}$ are generated in the course of site-specific protein oxidation (186). The biological significance of reactive oxygen species was recognized by Gerschman et al. (69) and was incorporated into a free radical theory of aging by Harman (74). Given the constant production and widespread cellular distribution of these compounds, the ability of organisms to limit their production, to defend against their presence, and to repair damage created by them seems a promising basis for aging processes. Cells do indeed possess extensive arrays of mechanisms to protect themselves against these substances. These include low molecular mass free radical scavengers, such as α-tocopherol, β-carotene, and ascorbate, and enzymes that destroy reactive oxygen species, such as superoxide dismutase (SOD), catalase, and glutathione peroxidase. Despite these defenses, however, oxidative damage of proteins, lipids, and DNA is known to occur in vivo (39). However, cellular damage may be removed or repaired by other systems, such as proteases and DNA repair mechanisms (43).

Evidence that free radical damage plays a role in aging has been recently reviewed by Sohal (182). The conclusion of this extensive review is that, in spite of the huge volume of work in the area, available evidence does not eliminate or positively implicate free radical damage as a component of aging processes. Several striking points are clear, however. (*1*) The rate of generation of reactive oxygen molecules is not positively correlated with rates of mitochondrial oxygen consumption. For example, H_2O_2 generation is highest under conditions of relatively low rates of oxygen consumption (110). (2) At least in *Drosophila,* antioxidant defenses are in excess of levels necessary to cope with usual physiological fluxes of reactive oxygen radicals (142, 177). Also, with age there is no generalized decline in antioxidant defense, and longevity is not correlated with overall levels of these defenses. (3) The balance between the rate of generation of reactive oxygen molecules and the rate of their destruction may be best indicated by rates of production of alkanes, such as *n*-pentane and ethane, as measured in exhaled air. These compounds are thought to be a measure of the level of lipid peroxidation in vivo. Age-related increase of these compounds in exhaled air has been found in both rodents and flies (166, 184), but more information is needed to establish clearly if such increases reflect increased accumulation of free radical damage with age. (*4*) Age-related damage attributable to reactive oxygen radicals, as measured by accumulation of lipofuscin, lipid peroxides, protein carbonyls, and compromised respiratory activity of mitochondria, appears modest at this stage. There is insufficient evidence to demonstrate that such damage plays a role in aging processes. Because of these factors Sohal (182) designates these ideas the "free radical hypothesis" (rather than theory) of aging, in acknowledgment of the absence at present of a firm base of experimental support. However, there is emerging awareness of the importance of free radical damage in age-associated diseases, such as atherosclerosis (187), cancer (189), and diabetes (139). Also, evidence shows that there are age-related increases in oxidatively modified proteins (185), DNA (27), and lipids (25, 102) and that life-prolonging dietary restriction reduces the extent of lipid peroxidation and increases levels of antioxidant defense (212, 105). Given the well-recognized multifactorial nature of aging processes, it seems likely that reactive oxidative radicals do indeed play a role in the degenerative aspects characteristic of aging. Hypotheses linking free radical damage and glycation reactions to aging are also emerging (100). Oxidative energy metabolism thus forms a framework for the constant generation of molecules not only essential to life (such as ATP) but which also destroy cellular organization (such as $\dot{O}H$). Existing evidence shows that rate of production of the latter is not correlated with rate of production of the former; that is, free radical damage is not a function of the rate of living but accumulates as a function of the duration of life.

CONCLUSIONS

Answers to questions raised at the beginning of this chapter can now be attempted. Does the intensity of metabolism vary with age and if so, what factors are responsible for this? From the foregoing discussion it is apparent that age is not an important determinant of metabolic rate. Changes in body composition and tissue composition, however, will affect whole-body metabolic rate by altering the contribution of tissues of differing rates of metabolism. Body composition is determined by long-term energy balance, and this is thought to be most influenced by the amount and composition of energy intake. It remains uncertain if the metabolic rate of individual tissues changes significantly with age, that is, if there is a decline in cellular metabolic activity with age and what factors may be responsible for this. Since there is a one hundredfold range in metabolic rate of individual tissues (from adipose to cardiac and renal tissues), it is not surprising that traditional methods of normalizing metabolic rate to such a heterogeneous mixture of tissues have provided controversial results. Data show that FFM is the major determinant of 24EE and that significant age-related variation occurs mostly as a consequence of decreased skeletal muscle mass. More information is needed on metabolic rates of specific tissues in vivo, on the size and composition of these tissues with age, and on mitochondrial density and function with age.

Is metabolic rate a key factor or do other aspects of energy metabolism provide the link between energy use and aging? Despite long-standing popular support and some experimental basis, the concept that metabolic rate is linked directly to aging processes is not supported by most current studies. There is some evidence that energy metabolism plays a role in aging processes; however, this evidence implicates components of the metabolic system, such as oxygen, fuels, and by-products of metabolism, rather than rate of metabolism, as factors contributing to the degeneration characteristic of old age.

REFERENCES

1. ACHESON, K. J., Y. SCHUTZ, T. BESSARD, K. ANANTHARAM, J. P. FLATT, and E. JEQUIER. Glycogen storage capacity and de

novo lipogenesis during massive carbohydrate overfeeding in man. *Am. J. Clin. Nutr.* 48: 240–247, 1988.
2. ARKING, R., S. BUCK, R. A. WELLS, and R. PRETZLAFF. Metabolic rates in genetically based long-lived strains of *Drosophila*. *Exp. Gerontol.* 23: 59–76, 1988.
3. ASTRUP, A. L., L. SIMONSEN, J. BULLOW, J. MADSEN, and N. J. CHRISTENSEN. Epinephrine mediates facultative, carbohydrate-induced thermogenesis in human skeletal muscle. *Am. J. Physiol.* 257: E340–E345, 1989.
4. AUSTAD, S. N. Testing the rate-of-living theory of longevity. *Gerontol. News.* 8: 4, 1991.
5. AUSTAD, S. N., and K. E. FISCHER. Mammalian aging, metabolism and ecology: evidence from the bats and marsupials. *J. Gerontol.* 46: B47–B53, 1991.
6. BALMAGIYA, T., and S. J. ROSOVSKY. Age-related changes in thermoregulation in male albino rats. *Exp. Gerontol.* 18: 199–210, 1983.
7. BARROWS, C. H., L. M. ROEDER, and J. A. FALZONE. Effect of age on the activities of enzymes and the concentration of nucleic acids in the tissues of female wild rats. *J. Gerontol.* 17: 144–147, 1962.
8. BEATTIE, J., and P. H. HERBERT. The estimation of metabolic rate in the starvation state. *Br. J. Nutr.* 1: 185–191, 1947.
9. BENEDICT, F. G. *Vital Energetics. A Study in Comparative Basal Metabolism*. Washington, DC: Carnegie Institute of Washington, Publication 503, 1938, p. 1–215.
10. BENEDICT, F. G., and G. MACLEOD. The heat production of the albino rat. II. Influence of environmental temperature, age and sex; comparison with basal metabolism in man. *J. Nutr.* 1: 381–395, 1929.
11. BENEDICT, F. G., W. R. MILES, P. ROTH, and M. SMITH. *Human Vitality and Efficiency under Prolonged Restricted Diet*. Washington DC: Carnegie Institute of Washington, Publication 280, 1919, p. 1–701.
12. BENNETT, A. J. Activity metabolism of the lower vertebrates. *Ann. Rev. Physiol.* 400: 447–469, 1978.
13. BERNSTEIN, R. S., J. C. THORNTON, and M. U. YOUNG. Prediction of resting metabolic rate in obese patients. *Am. J. Clin. Nutr.* 37: 595–602, 1983.
13a. BERTRAND, H. A., F. T. LYND, E. J. MASORO, and B. P. YU. Changes in adipose mass and cellularity through the adult life of rats fed ad libitum or a life-prolonging restricted diet. *J. Gerontol.* 35: 827–835, 1980.
14. BOOTHBY, W., and I. SANDIFORD. Normal values for standard metabolism. *Am. J. Physiol.* 90: 290–291, 1929.
15. BOOTHBY, W. M., and I. SANDIFORD. Summary of the basal metabolism data on 8614 subjects with special reference to the normal standards for the estimation of the basal metabolism rate. *J. Biochem.* 54: 783–803, 1922.
16. BOUCHARD, C., A. TREMBLAY, A. NADEAU, J. P. DESPRÉS, G. THERIAULT, M. R. BOULAY, G. LORTIE, C. LEBLANC and G. FOURNIER. Genetic effect in resting and exercise metabolic rates. *Metabolism* 38: 364–370, 1989.
17. BRODY, S. *Bioenergetics and Growth*. New York: Reinhold, 1945, 972 p.
18. BROOKS, G. A., and T. D. FAHEY. *Exercise Physiology*. New York: John Wiley and Sons, 1984, 726 p.
19. BROWN, A. C. Energy metabolism. In: *Physiology and Biophysics*, vol. 3, edited by T. C. Ruch and H. D. Patton. Philadelphia: W. B. Saunders, 1973, p. 85–104.
20. BROWN, W. M., M. GEORGE, and A. C. WILSON. Rapid evolution of animal mitochondrial DNA. *Proc. Natl. Acad. Sci. USA* 76: 1976–1971, 1979.
21. BROZEK, J. *Human Body Composition*. London: Pergamon Press, 1965, 311 p.
22. BUDD, G. M., J. R. BROTHERHOOD, A. L. HENDRIC, and G. E. JEFFERY. Effects of fitness, fatness and age on men's responses to whole body cooling in air. *J. Appl. Physiol.* 71: 2387–2393, 1991.
23. BUONO, M. J., B. K. MCKENZIE, and F. W. KASCH. Effects of ageing and physical training on the peripheral sweat production of human eccrine sweat gland. *Age Ageing* 20: 439–441, 1991.
24. BURNS, E. M., T. W. KRUCKERBERG, L. E. COMERFORD, and M. T. MUSCHMANN. Thinning of capillary walls and declining numbers of endothelial mitochondria in the cerebral cortex. *J. Gerontol.* 34: 642, 1979.
25. CAND, F., and J. VERDITTI. Superoxide dismutase, glutathione peroxidase, catalase and lipid peroxidation in the major organs of the aging rat. *Free Radic. Biol. Med.* 7: 59–63, 1989.
26. CARDENAS, E. Biochemistry of oxygen toxicity. *Ann. Rev. Biochem.* 58: 79–110, 1989.
27. CATHCART, R., E. SCHWIERS, R. L. SALU, and B. N. AMES. Thymine glycol and thymidine glycol in human and rat urine: a possible assay for oxidative DNA damage. *Proc. Natl. Acad. Sci. USA* 81: 5633–5637, 1984.
28. CERAMI, A. Hypothesis: glucose as a mediator of aging. *J. Am. Geriatr. Soc.* 33: 626–634, 1985.
29. CLARK, S. M., J. T. GEAN, and J. M. LIPTON. Reduced febrile responses to peripheral and central administration of pyrogen in aged squirrel monkeys. *Neurobiol. Aging* 1: 175–180, 1980.
30. CLAYTON, D. A. Replication of animal mitochondrial DNA. *Cell* 28: 693–705, 1982.
31. COLLINS, K. J., and A. N. EXTONNM-SMITH. Thermal homeostasis in old age. *J. Am. Geriatr. Soc.* 31: 519–524, 1983.
32. COLLINS, K. J., and A. N. EXTON-SMITH. Urban hypothermia preferred temperature and thermal perception in old age. *Br. Med. J.* 282: 175–177, 1981.
33. CUNNINGHAM, D., H. MONTOYE, H. METZNER, and J. KELLER. Active leisure time activities as related to age among males in a total population. *J. Gerontol.* 23: 551–556, 1968.
34. CUNNINGHAM, J. J. A re-analysis of the factors influencing basal metabolic rate in normal adults. *Am. J. Clin. Nutr.* 33: 2372–2374, 1980.
35. CUNNINGHAM, J. J. Body composition and resting metabolic rate: the myth of feminine metabolism. *Am. J. Clin. Nutr.* 36: 721–726, 1982.
36. CUTLER, R. Anti-oxidants, aging and longevity. In: *Free Radicals in Biology 6*, edited by W. A. Pryor. Orlando: Academic Press, 1984, p. 381.
37. D'ALESSIO, D. A., E. C. KAVLE, M. A. MOZZOLI, K. J. SMALLEY, M. POLANSKY, Z. V. KENDRICK, L. R. OWEN, M. C. BUSHMAN, G. BOWDEN, and O. E. OWEN. Thermic effect of food in lean and obese men. *J. Clin. Invest.* 81: 1781–1789, 1988.
38. DAVIES, C. T. M. Thermoregulation during exercise in relation to sex and age. *Eur. J. Appl. Physiol.* 42: 71–79, 1979.
39. DAVIES, K. J. A. Intracellular proteolytic systems may function as secondary anti-oxidant defenses. An hypothesis. *Free Radic. Biol. Med.* 2: 155–173, 1986.
40. DAVIES, M. On body size and tissue respiration. *J. Cell. Comp. Physiol.* 57: 135–147, 1961.
41. DAVIS, B. B., and T. V. ZENSER. Biological changes in thermoregulation in the elderly. In: *Homeostatic Function and Aging*, edited by B. B. Davis and W. G. Wood. New York: Raven Press, 1985, p. 137–166.
42. DAVIS, J. E. The effect of advancing age on the oxygen consumption of rats. *Am. J. Physiol.* 119: 28–33, 1937.
43. DEEMPLE, B., and J. HALBROOK. Inducible repair of oxidative DNA damage in *Escherichia coli*. *Nature (Lond.)* 304: 466–468, 1983.
44. DENCKLA, W. D. Role of pituitary and thyroid glands in the decline of minimal O_2 consumption with age. *J. Clin. Invest.* 53: 572–581, 1974.

45. DETENBECK, L. C., and J. JOWSEY. Normal aging in the bone of the adult dog. *Clin. Orthop.* 65: 76–80, 1969.
46. DONDA, A., and T. LAMARCHAND-BERAUD. Aging alters the activity of 5′-deiodinase in the adenohypophysis, thyroid gland and liver of the male rat. *Endocrinology* 124: 1305–1309, 1989.
47. DUFFY, P. H., R. J. FEUERS, J. A. LEAKEY, K. NAKAMURA, A. TURTURRO, and R. W. HART. Effect of chronic caloric restriction on physiological variables related to energy metabolism in the male Fischer 344 rat. *Mech. Ageing Dev.* 48: 117–133, 1989.
48. ECONOMOS, A. C. Beyond rate of living. *Gerontology* 27: 258–265, 1981.
49. ELAHI, V. K., D. ELAHI, R. ANDRES, J. D. TOBIN, M. G. BUTLER, and A. H. NORRIS. A longitudinal study of nutritional intake in men. *J. Gerontol.* 38: 162–180, 1983.
50. ELIA, M. Energy expenditure in the whole body. In: *Energy Metabolism,* edited by J. M. Kinney and H. N. Tucker. New York: Raven Press, 1991a, p. 19–59.
51. ELIA, M. Organ and tissue contribution to metabolic rate. In: *Energy Metabolism,* edited by J. M. Kinney and H. N. Tucker. New York: Raven Press, 1991b, p. 61–79.
52. ELSE, P. L., and A. J. HULBERT. Comparison of the "mammal machine" and the "reptile machine": energy production. *Am. J. Physiol.* 240: R3–R9, 1981.
53. ELSE, P. L., and A. J. HULBERT. An allometric comparison of the mitochondria of mammalian and reptilian tissues: the implications for the evolution of endothermy. *J. Comp. Physiol. [B]* 156: 3–11, 1985a.
54. ELSE, P. L., and A. J. HULBERT. Mammals: an allometric study of metabolism at tissue and mitochondrial level. *Am. J. Physiol.* 248: R415–R421, 1985b.
55. EMORINE, L. J., S. MARULLO, M. BRIEND-SUTREN, G. PATEY, K. TATE, C. DELAVIER-KLUTCHKO, and A. D. STROSBERG. Molecular characterization of the human β-3 adrenergic receptor. *Science* 245: 1118–1121, 1989.
56. ENESCO, H. E., A. MCTAVISH, and R. GARBERI. Spontaneous activity level and lifespan in rotifers: lack of support for the rate of living theory. *Gerontology* 36: 256–261, 1990.
57. ENOKA, R. M. *Neuromechanical Basis of Kinesiology* (2nd ed), Human Kinetics, (In press).
58. FELTON, S. Y., D. L. BELLINGER, T. J. COLLIER, P. D. COLEMAN, and D. L. FELTON. Decreased sympathetic innervation of spleen in aged Fischer 344 rats. *Neurobiol. Aging* 8: 159–165, 1987.
59. FERGUSON, A. V., W. L. VEALE, and K. E. COOPER. Age-related differences in the febrile response of the New Zealand white rabbit to endotoxin. *Can. J. Physiol. Pharmacol.* 59: 613–614, 1981.
60. FLATT, J. P. Energy costs of ATP synthesis. In: *Energy Metabolism: Tissue Determinants and Cellular Corollaries,* edited by J. M. Kinney and H. N. Tucker. New York: Raven Press, 1992, p. 319–343.
61. FLATT, J. P., E. RAVUSSIN, K. J. ACHESON, and E. JEQUIER. Effects of dietary fat on post-prandial substrate oxidation and carbohydrate and fat balances. *J. Clin. Invest.* 76: 1019–1024, 1985.
62. FLORINI, J. R., and J. F. REGAN. Age-related changes in hormone secretion and action. *Rev. Biol. Res. Aging* 2: 227–250, 1985.
63. FORBES, G. B. *Human Body Composition.* New York: Springer-Verlag, 1986, 341 p.
64. FOSTER, D. O., and M. L. FRYDMAN. Tissue distribution of cold-induced thermogenesis in conscious warm or cold-acclimated rats re-evaluated from changes in tissue blood flow: the dominant role of brown adipose tissue in the replacement of shivering by non-shivering thermogenesis. *Can. J. Physiol. Pharmacol.* 57: 257–270, 1978a.
65. FOSTER, D. O., and M. L. FRYDMAN. Non-shivering thermogenesis in the rat II. *Can. J. Physiol. Pharmacol.* 56: 110–122, 1978b.
66. FUKAGAWA, N. K., L. G. BANDANI, and J. B. YOUNG. Effect of age on body composition and resting metabolic rate. *Am. J. Physiol.* 259: E233–E238, 1990.
67. GAMBERT, S. R. Effect of age on the conversion of thyroxine (T_4) to 3,5,3′ tri-iodothyronine (T_3) by liver homogenate from fed and fasted Sprague-Dawley rats. *Age* 5: 88–91, 1982.
68. GARROW, J. S. *Energy Balance and Obesity in Man.* Oxford: Elsevier/North Holland, 1978, 195 p.
69. GERSCHMAN, R., D. L. GILBERT, S. W. NYE, P. DWYER, and W. O. FENN. Oxygen poisoning and X-irradiation: a mechanism in common. *Science* 19: 623–629, 1954.
70. GONZALES-PACHECO, D. M., W. C. BUSS, K. M. KOEHLER, W. F. WOODSIDE, and S. S. ALPERT. Energy restriction reduces metabolic rate in adult male Fischer-344 rats. *J. Nutr.* 123: 90–97, 1993.
71. GRANDE, F., and A. KEYS. Body weight, body composition and calorie status. In: *Modern Nutrition in Health and Disease,* edited by R. S. Goodhart and M. S. Shils. Philadelphia: Lea-Febiger, 1980, p. 3–34.
72. GREGERMAN, R. I. The age-related alteration of thyroid function and thyroid hormone metabolism in man. In: *Endocrines and Aging,* edited by L. Gitman. Springfield, IL: Charles C. Thomas, 1964, p. 161–173.
73. HARDY, J. D. Physiology of temperature regulation. *Physiol. Rev.* 41: 521–606, 1961.
74. HARMAN, D. Aging: a theory based on free radical and radiation chemistry. *J. Gerontol.* 11: 298–300, 1956.
75. HELLON, R. F., and A. R. LIND. The influence of age on peripheral vasodilation in a hot environment. *J. Physiol. (Lond.)* 141: 262–272, 1958.
76. HENRI, C. J. K., and D. G. REES. Basal metabolic rate and race. In: *Comparative Nutrition,* edited by K. Blaxten, and I. Macdonald. Paris: John Libbey, 1988, p. 149–161.
77. HERBENER, G. H. A morphometric study of age-dependent changes in the mitochondrial populations of mouse liver and heart. *J. Gerontol.* 31: 8–16, 1976.
78. HERLIHY, J. T., C. STACY, and H. BERTRAND. Effect of age and diet on the serum thyroid hormone levels in Fischer 344 rats. *Gerontologist* 30: A109, 1990.
79. HEUSNER, A. Body size and energy metabolism. *Ann. Rev. Nutr.* 5: 267–293, 1985.
80. HOLLIDAY, M. A. Metabolic rate and organ size during growth from infancy to maturity and during late gestation and early infancy. *Paediatrics* 47: 169–177, 1971.
81. HOLLOSZY, J. O., and K. SMITH. Longevity of cold-exposed rats: a re-evaluation of the "rate of living theory." *J. Appl. Physiol.* 61: 1656–1660, 1986.
82. HOLLOSZY, J. O., E. K. SMITH, M. VINING, and S. ADAMS. Effect of voluntary exercise on longevity of rats. *J. Appl. Physiol.* 59: 826–831, 1985.
83. HORST, K. L. O., L. B. MENDEL, and F. G. BENEDICT. The influence of previous diet, growth and age upon the basal metabolism of the rat. *J. Nutr.* 8: 139–162, 1934.
84. HULBERT, A. J., W. MANTAJ, and P. A. JANSSENS. Development of mammalian endothermic metabolism: quantitative changes in tissue mitochondria. *Am. J. Physiol.* 261: R561–R568, 1991.
85. INOUE, Y., M. NAKAO, T. ARAKI, and H. MURAKAMI. Regional differences in the sweating responses of older and younger men. *J. Appl. Physiol.* 71: 2453–2459, 1991.
86. JAMES, W. P. T. From SDA to DOT to TEF. In: *Energy Metabolism: Tissue Determinants and Cellular Corollaries,* edited by J. M. Kinney and H. N. Tucker. New York: Raven Press, 1992, p. 163–183.
87. JEPSON, M. M., D. J. MILLWARD, M. J. ROTHWELL, and M. J.

STOCK. Involvement of sympathetic nervous system and brown fat in endotoxin-induced fever in rats. *Am. J. Physiol.* 255: E617–E620, 1988.
88. JEQUIER, E. Discussion. In: *Energy Metabolism: Tissue Determinants and Cellular Corollaries,* edited by J. M. Kinney and H. N. Tucker. New York: Raven Press, 1992, p. 183–186.
89. JEQUIER, E., and Y. SCHUTZ. Energy expenditure in obesity and diabetes. *Diabetes Metab. Rev.* 4: 583–593, 1988.
90. JONES, P. G., C. A. KAUFFMAN, A. G. BERGMAN, C. M. HAYES, M. J. KLUEGER, and J. G. CANNON. Production of leukocytic pyrogen by monocytes from elderly persons. *Gerontology* 30: 182–187, 1984.
91. KENNEY, W. L. Control of heat-induced cutaneous vasodilation in relation to age. *Eur. J. Appl. Physiol.* 57: 120–125, 1988.
92. KENNEY, W. L., and J. JOHNSON. Control of skin blood flow during exercise. *Med. Sci. Sports Exerc.* 24: 303–312, 1992.
93. KEYS, A., J. BROZEK, A. HANSCHEL, O. MICKELSON, and H. L. TAYLOR. *The Biology of Human Starvation.* Minneapolis: University of Minnesota Press, 1950, 385 p.
94. KHAN, F., V. A. SPENCE, and J. J. F. BELCH. Cutaneous vascular responses and thermoregulation in relation to age. *Clin. Sci.* 82: 521–528, 1992.
95. KLEIBER, M. Body size and metabolism. *Hilgardia* 6: 315–353, 1932.
96. KLEIBER, M. *The Fire of Life.* New York: Krieger Publishing Co., 1975.
97. KORENCHEVSKY, V. *Physiological and Pathological Aging.* Basel: Karger Press, 1961, p. 38–47.
98. KREBS, H. A. Body size and tissue respiration. *Biochim. Biophys. Acta* 4: 249–269, 1950.
99. KREGEL, K. C., C. M. TIPTON, and D. R. SEALS. Thermal adjustments to nonexertional heat stress in mature and senescent Fischer 344 rats. *J. Appl. Physiol.* 68: 1337–1342, 1990.
100. KRISTAL, B., and B. P. YU. An emerging hypothesis: synergistic induction of aging by free radicals and maillard reactions. *J. Gerontol.* 47: B107–B114, 1992.
101. KROGH, A. *The Respiratory Exchange of Animals and Man.* London: Longmans Green, 1916.
102. LAGANIERE, S., and B. P. YU. Anti-lipoperoxidation action of food restriction. *Biochem. Biophys. Res. Commun.* 145: 1185–1191, 1987.
103. LARKIN, L., B. A. HOROWITZ, and R. B. MCDONALD. Effect of cold on serum substrate and glycogen concentration in young and old Fischer 344 rats. *Exp. Gerontol.* 27: 179–190, 1992.
104. LEAN, M. E. J., W. P. T. JAMES, G. JENNINGS, and P. TRAYHURN. Brown adipose tissue uncoupling protein content in human infants, children and adults. *Clin. Sci.* 71: 291–297, 1986.
105. LEE, D. W., and B. P. YU. Modulation of free radicals and superoxide dismutase by age and dietary restriction. *Aging* 2: 357–362, 1990.
106. LINNANE, A. W. Mitochondria and aging: the universality of bioenergetic disease. *Aging* 4: 267–271, 1992.
107. LINTS, F. A. Insects. In: *Handbook of the Biology of Aging* (2nd ed.), edited by C. E. Finch and E. L. Schneider. New York: Van Nostrand Reinhold Company, 1985, p. 146–169.
108. LINTS, F. A. The rate of living theory revisited. *Gerontology* 35: 36–57, 1989.
109. LOEB, J., and J. H. NORTHROP. On the influence of food and temperature on the duration of life. *J. Biol. Chem.* 32: 103–121, 1917.
110. LOSCHEN, G., L. FLOHE, and P. CHANCE. Respiratory chain linked H_2O_2 production in pigeon heart mitochondria. *FEBS Lett.* 18: 261–264, 1971.
111. LYBARGER, J. A., and E. H. KILBOURNE. Hyperthermia and hypothermia in the elderly: an epidemiologic review. In: *Homeostatic Function and Aging,* edited by B. B. Davis and W. G. Wood. New York: Raven Press, 1985, p. 149–156.
112. LYNN, W. S., and J. C. WALLWORK. Does food restriction retard aging by reducing metabolic rate? *J. Nutr.* 122: 1917–1918, 1992.
113. LYNN, W. S., J. C. WALLWORK, and D. H. COPPENHAVER. Overnutrition, uncontrolled organ growth and apoptosis. *J. Appl. Nutr.* 44: 3–15, 1992.
114. MARTIN, P. E., D. E. ROTHSTEIN, and D. D. LARISH. Effects of age and physical activity status on the speed-aerobic demand relationship of walking. *J. Appl. Physiol.* 73: 200–206, 1992.
115. MASORO, E. J. Metabolism. In: *Handbook of the Biology of Aging* (2nd ed.), edited by C. E. Finch and E. L. Schneider. New York: Van Nostrand Reinhold Company, 1985, p. 540–563.
116. MASORO, E. J., and R. J. M. MCCARTER. Dietary restriction as a probe of mechanisms of senescence. *Ann. Rev. Gerontol. Geriatr.* 10: 183–197, 1990.
117. MASORO, E. J., and R. MCCARTER. Aging as a consequence of fuel utilization. *Aging* 3: 117–128, 1991.
118. MASORO, E. J., B. P. YU and H. BERTRAND. Action of food restriction in delaying the aging processes. *Proc. Natl. Acad. Sci. USA* 79: 4239–4241, 1982.
119. MCARTHUR, J. W., and W. H. T. BAILLIE. Metabolic activity and duration of life. II. Metabolic rates and their relation to longevity in *Daphnia magna. J. Exp. Zool.* 53: 243–286, 1929.
120. MCARTHUR, M. C., and R. S. SOHAL. Relationship between metabolic rate, aging, lipid peroxidation and fluorescent age pigment in milkweed bug, *Oncopeltus fasciatus* (Hemiptera). *J. Gerontol.* 37: 268–274, 1982.
121. MCCARTER, R., and J. MCGEE. Influence of nutrition and aging on the composition and function of rat skeletal muscle. *J. Gerontol.* 42: 432–441, 1987.
122. MCCARTER, R. J., and J. R. MCGEE. Transient reduction of metabolic rate by food restriction. *Am. J. Physiol.* E175–E179, 1989.
123. MCCARTER, R. J., and J. PALMER. Energy metabolism and aging: a lifelong study in Fischer 344 rats. *Am. J. Physiol.* 263: E448–E452, 1992.
124. MCCARTER, R., J. T. HERLIHY, and J. M. MCGEE. Metabolic rate and aging: effects of food restriction and thyroid hormone on minimal oxygen consumption in rats. *Aging* 1: 71–76, 1989.
125. MCCARTER, R., E. J. MASORO, and B. P. YU. Does food restriction retard aging by reducing the metabolic rate? *Am. J. Physiol.* 248: E488–E490, 1985.
126. MCDONALD, R. B., C. DAY, K. CARLSON, J. S. STERN, and B. A. HORWITZ. Effect of age and gender on thermoregulation. *Am. J. Physiol.* 257: R700–R704, 1989b.
127. MCDONALD, R. B., B. A. HORWITZ, J. S. HAMILTON, and J. S. STERN. Cold- and norepinephrine-induced thermogenesis in younger and older Fischer 344 rats. *Am. J. Physiol.* 254: R457–R462, 1988a.
128. MCDONALD, R. B., B. A. HORWITZ, and J. S. STERN. Cold-induced thermoregulation in younger and older Fischer 344 rats following exercise training. *Am. J. Physiol.* 254: R908–R916, 1988b.
129. MCDONALD, R. B., J. S. STERN, and B. A. HORWITZ. Thermogenic responses of younger and older rats to cold exposure: comparison of two strains. *J. Gerontol.* 44: B37–B42, 1989a.
130. MCGANDY, R. B., C. H. BARROWS, JR., A. SPANIA, A. MEREDITH, J. L. STONE, and A. H. NORRIS. Nutrient intake and energy expenditure in men of different ages. *J. Gerontol.* 21: 581–587, 1966.
131. MITCHELL, H. H. *Comparative Nutrition of Man and Domestic Animals.* New York: Academic Press, 1962, 90 p.
132. MOORADIAN, A. D., L. DEEBAJ, and N. C. W. WONG. Age-related alterations in the response of hepatic lipogenic enzymes

to altered thyroid states in the rat. *J. Endocrinol.* 128: 79–84, 1991.
133. MORGAN, J. B., and D. A. YORK. Thermic effect of feeding in relation to energy balance in elderly men. *Ann. Nutr. Metab.* 27: 71–77, 1983.
134. MOSER, H. W. Peroxisomal diseases. *Adv. Pediatr.* 36: 1–38, 1989.
135. NADEL, E. R., K. B. PANDOLF, M. F. ROBERTS, and J. A. J. STOLWIJK. Mechanisms of thermal acclimation to exercise and heat. *J. Appl. Physiol.* 37: 515–520, 1974.
136. NEWELL, R. C. The effect of temperature fluctuations on the metabolism of intertidal invertebrates. *Am. Zool.* 9: 293–307, 1969.
137. NORMAN, D. C., D. GRAHN, and T. T. YOSHIKAWA. Fever and aging. *J. Am. Geriatr. Soc.* 33: 859–863, 1985.
138. NORMAN, D. C., R. H. YAMAMURA, and T. T. YOSHIKAWA. Fever response in old and young mice after injection of interleukin-1. *J. Gerontol.* 43: M80–M85, 1988.
139. OBERLEY, L. W. Free radicals and diabetes. *Free Rad. Biol. Med.* 5: 113–124, 1988.
140. ODIO, M. R., and A. BRODISH. Effects of age on metabolic responses to acute and chronic stress. *Am. J. Physiol.* 254: E617–E624, 1988.
141. OLSEN, T., P. LAWBERG, and J. WEEKE. Low serum tri-iodothyronine and high serum reverse-tri-iodothyronine in old age: an effect of disease not age. *J. Clin. Endocrinol. Metab.* 47: 1111–1115, 1978.
142. ORR, W., and R. S. SOHAL. The effects of catalase gene expression on lifespan and resistance to oxidative stress in transgenic. *Drosophila melanogaster. Arch. Biochem. Biophys.* 297: 35–41, 1992.
143. OSIEWACZ, H. D., and H. HERMANNS. The role of mitochondrial DNA rearrangements in aging and human diseases. *Aging* 4: 273–286, 1992.
144. OU, L. C., and S. M. TENNEY. Properties of mitochondria from hearts of cattle acclimatized to high altitude. *Respir. Physiol.* 8: 151–159, 1970.
145. OWEN, O. E., E. KARLE, and R. S. OWEN. A reappraisal of the caloric requirements of healthy women. *Am. J. Clin. Nutr.* 44: 1–19, 1986.
146. PEARCE, M. E., D. A. CUNNINGHAM, A. P. DONNER, P. A. RECHNITZER, G. M. FULLERTON, and J. H. HOWARD. Energy cost of treadmill and floor walking at self-selected paces. *J. Appl. Physiol.* 52: 115–119, 1983.
147. PEARL, R. *The Rate of Living.* New York: Alfred Knopf, 1928, 185 p.
148. PENG, M., Y. PENG, and F. CHEN. Age-dependent changes in the oxygen consumption of the cerebral cortex, hypothalamus, hippocampus and amygdaloid in rats. *J. Gerontol.* 32: 517–522, 1977.
149. PERLMUTTER, M., and D. S. RIGGS. Thyroid collection of radioactive iodide and serum protein-bound iodine concentration in senescence, in hypothyroidism and in hypopituitarism. *J. Clin. Endocrinol.* 9: 430–439, 1949.
150. PI-SUNYER, F. X. Discussion. In: *Energy Metabolism*, edited by J. M. Kinney and H. N. Tucker. New York: Raven Press, 1992, p. 60.
151. PI-SUNYER, F. X., and K. R. SEGAL. Relationship of diet and exercise. In: *Energy Metabolism: Tissue Determinants and Cellular Corollaries*, edited by J. M. Kinney and H. N. Tucker. New York: Raven Press, 1992, p. 187–209.
152. POEHLMAN, E., and E. S. HORTON. Regulation of energy expenditure in aging humans. *Ann. Rev. Nutr.* 10: 255–275, 1990.
153. POEHLMAN, E. T., E. M. BERKE, J. R. JOSEPH, A. W. GARDNER, S. M. KATZMAN-ROOKS, and M. I. GORAN. Influence of aerobic capacity, body composition and thyroid hormones on the age-related decline in resting metabolic rate. *Metabolism* 41: 915–921, 1992.
154. POEHLMAN, E. T., T. MCAULIFFE, and E. DANFORTH, JR. Effects of age and level of physical activity on plasma norepinephrine kinetics. *Am. J. Physiol.* 258: E256–E262, 1990.
155. RAVUSSIN, E., and C. BOGARDUS. Relationship of genetics, age and physical fitness to daily energy expenditure. *Am. J. Clin. Nutr.* 49: 968–975, 1989.
156. RAVUSSIN, E., S. LILLIOJA, T. E. ANDERSON, L. CHRISTIN, and C. BOGARDUS. Determinants of 24-hour energy expenditure in man. *J. Clin. Invest.* 78: 1568–1578, 1986.
157. ROSS, M. H., and J. O. ELY. Age-related changes in respiration of sliced liver of the rat. *J. Franklin Inst.* 258: 63–66, 1954.
158. ROTHWELL, N. *Hypothalamus and Thermogenesis in Energy Metabolism: Tissue Determinants and Cellular Corollaries*, edited by J. M. Kinney and H. N. Tucker. New York: Raven Press, 1992, p. 229–246.
159. ROWE, J. W., and B. R. TROEN. Sympathetic nervous system and aging in man. *Endocr. Rev.* 1: 167–179, 1980.
160. ROWE, J. W., R. ANDRES, J. D. TOBIN, A. H. NORRIS, and N. W. SHOCK. The effect of age on creatinine clearance in men: a cross-sectional and longitudinal study. *J. Gerontol.* 31: 155–163, 1976.
161. RUBNER, M. Über den Einfluss der Korpergrosse auf Stoff- und Kraft-wechsel. *Zh. Obshch. Biol.* 19: 535–562, 1883.
162. RUBNER, M. *Das problem der Lebensdauer und seine Beziehungen zum Wachstum under Ehrnarung.* Munich: Oldenburg 1908, 204 p.
163. RUMSEY, W. L., Z. V. KENDRICK, and J. W. STARNES. Bioenergetics in the aging Fischer 344 rat: effects of exercise and food restriction. *Exp. Gerontol.* 22: 271, 1987.
164. SAAD, M. F., S. A. ALGER, F. ZURLO, J. B. YOUNG, C. BOGARDUS, and E. RAVUSSIN. Ethnic differences in the sympathetically-mediated energy expenditure. *Am. J. Physiol.* 261: E789–E794, 1991.
165. SACHER, G. A. Life table modification and life prolongation. In: *Handbook of the Biology of Aging*, edited by C. Finch and L. Hayflick. New York: Van Nootrand Reinhold, 1977, p. 582–638.
166. SAGAI, M., and T. ISHINOSE. Age-related changes in lipid peroxidation as measured by ethane, ethylene, butane and pentane in respired gases of rats. *Life Sci.* 27: 731–738, 1980.
167. SAGAWA, S., K. SHIRAKI, M. K. YOUSEF, and K. MIKI. Sweating and cardiovascular responses of aged men to heat exposure. *J. Gerontol.* 43: M1–M8, 1988.
168. SARRUS, F., and J. F. RAMEAUX. Rapport sur un memoire adresse à l'Academic royale de medicine. *Bull. Acad. Natl. Med. (Paris)* 3: 1094–1100, 1838.
169. SCARPACE, P. J., B. S. BENDER, and S. E. BORST. The febrile response to *E. coli* peritonitis is impaired in senescent rats. *Gerontologist* 30: 215A, 1990.
170. SCARPACE, P. J., M. MATHENY, B. S. BENDER, and S. E. BORST. Impaired febrile response with age: role of thermogenesis in brown adipose tissue. *Proc. Soc. Exp. Biol. Med.* 200: 353–358, 1992a.
171. SCARPACE, P. J., M. MATHENY, and S. E. BORST. Thermogenesis and GDP binding with age in response to the novel agonist CGP-12177A. *Am. J. Physiol.* 262: E185–E190, 1992b.
172. SCARPACE, P. J., A. D. MOORADIAN, and J. E. MORLEY. Age-associated decrease in beta-adrenergic receptors and adenylate cyclase activity in rat brown adipose tissue. *J. Gerontol.* 43: B65–B70, 1988.
173. SCHUTZ, Y., J. P. FLATT, and E. JEQUIER. Failure of dietary fat intake to promote fat oxidation: a factor favoring the development of obesity. *Am. J. Clin. Nutr.* 50: 307–314, 1989.
174. SCHWARTZ, R. S., L. F. JAEGER, and R. C. VEITH. The impor-

tance of body composition to the increase in plasma norepinephrine appearance rate in elderly men. *J. Gerontol.* 42: 546–551, 1987.
175. SCHWARTZ, R. S., L. F. JAEGER, and R. VEITH. The thermic effect of feeding in older men: the importance of the sympathetic nervous system. *Metabolism* 39: 733–737, 1990.
176. SCOTT, A. R., I. A. MACDONALD, T. BENNET, and R. B. TATTERSAL. Abnormal thermoregulation in diabetic autonomic neuropathy. *Diabetes* 37: 961–968, 1988.
177. SETO, N. O. L., S. HAYASHI, and G. M. TENER. Overexpression of Cu-Zn superoxide dismutase in *Drosophila* does not affect lifespan. *Proc. Natl. Acad. Sci. USA* 87: 4270–4274, 1990.
178. SIESJO, B. K., and B. NILSSON. A method of determining blood flow and oxygen consumption in the rat brain. *Acta Physiol. Scand.* 96: 72–82, 1976.
179. SKINNER, J. S. *Age and Performance in Limiting Factors of Physical Performance*, edited by J. Keul. Stuttgart: Georg Thieme, 1973, p. 271–282.
180. SNYDER, W. S., M. J. COOK, E. S. NASSET, L. R. KARHAUSEN, G. P. HOWELLS, and I. H. TIPTON. *Report of the task group on reference man. International Commission on Radiological Protection, No. 23.* Oxford: Pergamon Press, 1975, p. 1–40.
181. SOHAL, R. S. The rate of living theory: a contemporary interpretation. In: *Insect Aging*, edited by K. G. Collatz and R. S. Sohal. Berlin: Springer-Verlag, 1986, p. 23–44.
182. SOHAL, R. S. The free radical hypothesis of aging. An appraisal of the current status. *Aging Clin. Exp. Res.* 5: 3–17, 1993.
183. SOHAL, R. S., and R. G. ALLEN. Relationship between oxygen metabolism, aging and development. *Adv. Free Rad. Biol. Med.* 2: 117–160, 1986.
184. SOHAL, R. S., A. MULLER, B. KOLETZKO, and H. SIES. Effect of age and ambient temperature on n-pentane production in adult housefly *Musca domestica. Mech. Ageing Dev.* 29: 317–326, 1985.
185. STADTMAN, E. R. Protein oxidation and aging. *Science* 257: 1220–1224, 1992.
186. STADTMAN, E., and C. N. OLIVER. Metal-catalyzed oxidation of proteins: physiological consequences. *J. Biol. Chem.* 266: 2005–2008, 1991.
187. STEINBERG, D. Antioxidants and atherosclerosis. *Circulation* 84: 1420–1425, 1991.
188. STEINHAUS, A. H. Studies in the physiology of exercise. I. Exercise and basal metabolism in dogs. *Am. J. Physiol.* 88: 658–677, 1928.
189. SUN, Y. Free radicals, antioxidant enzymes, and carcinogenesis. *Free Rad. Biol. Med.* 8: 583–599, 1990.
190. TAI, M. M., P. CASTILLO, and F. X. PI-SUNYER. Meal size and frequency: effect on the thermic effect of food. *Am. J. Clin. Nutr.* 54: 783–787, 1991.
191. TALAN, M. Body temperature of C57BL/6J mice with age. *Exp. Gerontol.* 19: 25–29, 1984.
192. TALAN, M. I., and D. K. INGRAM. Effects of voluntary and forced exercise on thermoregulation and survival in aged C57BL/6J mice. *Mech. Ageing Dev.* 36: 269–279, 1986.
193. TANKERSLEY, C. G., J. SMOLANDER, W. L. KENNEY, and S. M. FORTNEY. Sweating and skin blood flow during exercise: effects of age and maximum oxygen uptake. *J. Appl. Physiol.* 71: 236–242, 1991.
194. TATELMAN, H. M., and M. I. TALAN. Metabolic heat production during repeated cold stress in adult and aged male C57BL/6J mice. *J. Gerontol.* 45: B215–B219, 1990.
195. TERJUNG, R. L., and C. M. TIPTON. Exercise training and oxygen consumption. *Int. Z. Angew Physiol.* 28: 269–272, 1970.
196. TREMBLAY, A., E. FONTAINE, and A. NADEAU. Contribution of post-exercise increment in glucose storage to variations in glucose-induced thermogenesis in endurance athletes. *Can. J. Physiol. Pharmacol.* 63: 1165–1169, 1985.
197. TROTTER, M., G. F. BROMAN, and R. R. PETERSON. Density of bones of white and negro skeletons. *J. Bone Joint Surg.* 42A: 50–58, 1960.
198. TZANKOFF, S. P., and A. H. NORRIS. Effect of muscle mass decrease on age-related BMR changes. *J. Appl. Physiol.* 43: 1001–1006, 1977.
199. TZANKOFF, S. P. and A. H. NORRIS. Longitudinal changes in basal metabolism in man. *J. Appl. Physiol.* 45: 536–539, 1978.
200. VAUGHAN, L., F. ZURLO, and E. RAVUSSIN. Aging and energy expenditure. *Am. J. Clin. Nutr.* 53: 821–825, 1991.
201. VEGA, J. A., A. RICCI, and F. AMENTA. Age-dependent changes of the sympathetic innervation of the rat kidney. *Mech. Ageing Dev.* 54: 185–196, 1990.
202. VENKATACHALAM, P. Basal metabolism in nutritional edema. *Metabolism* 2: 128–141, 1954.
203. VON BERTALANFFY, L., and W. J. PIROZYNSKI. Tissue respiration and body size. *Science* 113: 559–600, 1951.
204. VONLANTHEN, M., R. J. MCCARTER, and D. CASTO. Metabolic effects of aminophylline in weanling rats. *Am. J. Physiol.* 258: R193–R197, 1990.
205. WARTOFSKY, L., and K. D. BURMAN. Alterations in thyroid function in patients with systemic illness: the "euthyroid sick syndrome." *Endocr. Rev.* 3: 164–217, 1982.
206. WEBB, P. Energy expenditure and fat free mass in men and women. *Am. J. Clin. Nutr.* 34: 1816–1826, 1981.
207. WEINDRUCH, R., and R. L. WALFORD. *The Retardation of Aging and Disease by Dietary Restriction.* Springfield, IL: A. H. Thomas, 1988.
208. WELLE, S., and K. S. NAIR. Relationship of resting metabolic rate to body composition and protein turnover. *Am. J. Physiol.* 258: E990–E998, 1990.
209. WILLIAMS, V. R., W. L. MATTICE, and H. B. WILLIAMS. *Basic Physical Chemistry for the Life Sciences.* San Francisco: Freeman and Co., 1978, p. 323–330.
210. WOLFE, R. R. The role of triglyceride-fatty acid cycling and glucose cycling in thermogenesis and amplification of net substrate flux in human subjects. In: *Hormones and Nutrition in Obesity and Cachexia*, edited by J. Muller, E. Danforth, A. G. Burger, and U. Siedentopp. Berlin: Springer-Verlag, 1990, p. 20–40.
211. YOUNG, V. R. Energy requirements in the elderly. *Nutr. Rev.* 50: 95–101, 1992.
212. YOUNGMAN, L. D., J. Y. PARK, and B. N. AMES. Protein oxidation associated with aging is reduced by dietary restriction on protein or calories. *Proc. Natl. Acad. Sci. USA* 89: 9112–9116, 1992.
213. YU, B. P., E. J. MASORO, and C. A. MCMAHAN. Nutritional influences on aging of Fischer 344 rats: I. Physical, metabolic, and longevity characteristics. *J. Gerontol.* 40: 657–670, 1985.
214. YU, B. P., E. J. MASORO, I. MURATA, H. B. BERTRAND, and F. T. LYND. Lifespan study of SPF Fischer 344 male rats fed ad libitum or restricted diets: longevity, growth, lean body mass and disease. *J. Gerontol.* 37: 130–141, 1982.
215. YU, B. P., G. WONG, H. LEE, H. A. BERTRAND, and E. J. MASORO. Age changes in hepatic metabolic characteristics and their modulation by dietary manipulation. *Mech. Ageing Dev.* 24: 67–81, 1984.
216. ZURLO, F., K. LARSON, C. BOGARDUS, and E. RAVUSSIN. Skeletal muscle metabolism is a major determinant of resting energy expenditure. *J. Clin. Invest.* 86: 1423–1427, 1990.

7. Carbohydrate metabolism

JEFFREY B. HALTER | *Geriatrics Center and Institute of Gerontology, University of Michigan, and VA Medical Center, Ann Arbor, Michigan*

CHAPTER CONTENTS

Epidemiology of Age-Related Changes of Carbohydrate Metabolism
Mechanisms for Age-Related Changes of Carbohydrate Metabolism
    Normal regulation of glucose metabolism
    Effects of aging
        Insulin secretion
        Insulin action
        Insulin-independent glucose uptake
        Glucose transport
        Effects of other hormones
    Confounding factors
        Adiposity
        Physical activity
        Dietary factors
        Hypertension
        Drugs
Diabetes Mellitus
    Mechanisms for development of non-insulin-dependent diabetes mellitus
    Metabolic consequences of diabetes mellitus
    Long-term consequences of diabetes mellitus

DIMINISHED HOMEOSTATIC CONTROL OF CARBOHYDRATE METABOLISM is a common characteristic of aging, particularly in humans, which is most apparent following challenge with a carbohydrate load, when the return to baseline of circulating glucose levels is delayed. Since glucose is the predominant form of carbohydrate used as fuel by cells, the terms "carbohydrate metabolism" and "glucose metabolism" will be used interchangeably in this chapter. When diminished homeostatic glucose regulation becomes sufficiently severe, circulating glucose levels following glucose ingestion may become very high and postabsorptive fasting glucose levels may become elevated to the extent that criteria for the diagnosis of diabetes mellitus are met. Many factors associated with aging probably contribute to age-related alterations of glucose metabolism and the high prevalence of diabetes mellitus among the elderly. This chapter will review the epidemiology of these age-related changes of glucose metabolism, the aging effects on physiological variables that are important to glucose homeostasis, the age-associated conditions that may contribute to impaired glucose tolerance, and the mechanisms that may lead to overt diabetes mellitus and its subsequent adverse effects.

EPIDEMIOLOGY OF AGE-RELATED CHANGES OF CARBOHYDRATE METABOLISM

The most standardized method used to evaluate glucose homeostasis in population-based epidemiological studies is the oral glucose tolerance test (OGTT). In this procedure, glucose levels in plasma are measured before and after ingestion of a standard oral load of dextrose (usually 75 g although the amount sometimes varies). An alternative approach is to measure the fall of glucose levels following intravenous (I.V.) glucose administration (IVGTT). Many cross-sectional studies have demonstrated that healthy older adults have higher glucose levels during OGTT and slower glucose disappearance during IVGTT than do young healthy subjects (see 6, 38 for reviews). The results from one such study are illustrated in Figure 7.1. Diagnostic criteria for various categories of impaired glucose tolerance have been developed, based at least in part on the risk for developing diabetes-related complications or further deterioration of glucose metabolism. The most widely used of these criteria, developed by the National Diabetes Data Group, are summarized in Table 7.1 (143). Similar criteria have been developed by the World Health Organization (222). Some studies of diabetes epidemiology have used a blood sample obtained 2 h after a glucose challenge or 2 h after a meal to provide a marker for abnormality. Advantages of the OGTT include simplicity of the protocol and its widespread use and standardization. Disadvantages of the OGTT include the relatively unphysiological nature of the challenge (few individuals ingest 75 g of pure sugar at one time during normal life) and the variability of OGTT results on repeated measurement in an individual (6, 103, 120).

Given these limitations, however, the OGTT has provided much information on incidence and prevalence

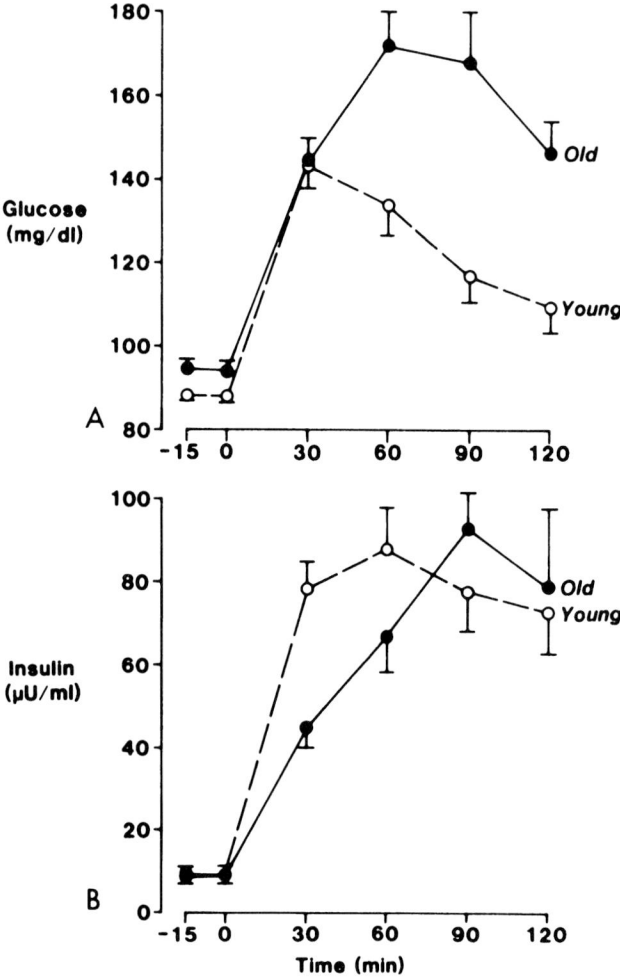

FIG. 7.1. Plasma glucose (upper) and insulin (lower) levels before and following oral ingestion of 100 g of glucose in healthy old (n = 18) and young (n = 18) subjects matched for relative body weight and socioeconomic group. Subjects were eating an ad libitum diet that included approximately 10% fewer total calories and 15% fewer carbohydrate calories in the old subjects. [From Chen et al. (31) with permission.]

rates for diabetes mellitus and impaired glucose tolerance. There is a high prevalence rate of both diabetes mellitus and impaired glucose tolerance among older humans in many ethnically diverse populations (3, 37, 58, 79, 80, 139, 211, 223, 225). Data from the National Health and Nutrition Examination Survey conducted by the National Center for Health Statistics from 1976 to 1980 indicate that nearly 10% of Americans 65–74 yr old had previously diagnosed diabetes mellitus and that an equal number were found to have undiagnosed diabetes mellitus by OGTT (80). An additional group of nearly 25% of the elderly population met criteria for impaired glucose tolerance. Not only does the prevalence of diabetes mellitus increase with age but also the incidence rate of new cases increases in people over the age of 65 yr to between 0.5% and 1% per year compared to <0.2% per year in individuals aged 25–44 yr. A simultaneous analysis of the incidence, prevalence, and mortality in the United States has indicated an increase of approximately 5% per year in the number of people with diabetes mellitus, most of whom are among the elderly population (82).

Diminished glucose tolerance has also been observed in animal models of aging. However, the data are more limited than findings in humans, and results are somewhat more variable (38). Assessment of glucose tolerance status is a substantially greater challenge in an experimental animal model because the methodology has not been standardized nearly to the extent that it has been in humans. Because of effects of stress hormones on glucose homeostasis, ideal studies would require indwelling catheters in trained animals. Previous studies have not done this and have sometimes not included a wide enough age range to separate changes of senescence from changes related to early development. Naturally occurring diabetes mellitus has been reported in Rhesus monkeys with onset in mid-to-late life and many metabolic characteristics that are similar to age-related human non-insulin-dependent diabetes mellitus (NIDDM) (20, 78).

TABLE 7.1 *Diagnostic Criteria for Diabetes Mellitus*

Category	Fasting Plasma Glucose	Oral OGTT*		
		1 h	2 h	3 h
Diabetes mellitus†	≥ 140 mg/dl (2 occasions)			
	< 140 mg/dl	≥ 200 mg/dl‡	≥ 200 mg/dl	
	Random hyperglycemia plus classic diabetes symptoms			
Impaired glucose tolerance	< 140 mg/dl	≥ 200 mg/dl‡	140–200 mg/dl	

*Criteria are based on 75-g glucose load, except for gestational diabetes for which 100 g is used. All values are venous plasma glucose.
†Patients meeting any one of the three criteria have diabetes mellitus.   ‡One value ≥ 200 mg/dl at 30, 60, or 90 min meets the criterion.

MECHANISMS FOR AGE-RELATED CHANGES OF CARBOHYDRATE METABOLISM

Maintenance of carbohydrate homeostasis is a complex process involving multiple regulatory systems and hormones. Aging and age-associated factors could potentially influence many of the systems involved in glucose homeostasis. Studies using radioisotopically labeled glucose or a combined I.V. and oral glucose clamp protocol have been used to compare aspects of glucose kinetics following oral glucose ingestion in normal old and young people (89, 176, 209). These studies suggest that glucose intolerance occurs in older people despite delayed absorption of oral glucose and delayed posthepatic glucose delivery. Greater hyperglycemia in the old results from delayed suppression of hepatic glucose output and decreased rate of peripheral glucose uptake following oral glucose ingestion. The hormone mechanisms contributing to age-related changes of glucose metabolism have been studied by many investigators. A brief discussion of normal control of glucose homeostasis follows, providing a framework from which to discuss observed effects of aging.

Normal Regulation of Glucose Metabolism

Carbohydrate metabolism in the postabsorptive fasting condition is tightly regulated by a feedback control system in which the circulating glucose level is the primary regulatory signal. A simplified version of this feedback control system is provided in Figure 7.2. Insulin and glucagon, secreted by the pancreatic β-cells and α-cells, respectively, are the two primary hormones involved in this feedback control system. Glucose is a direct stimulus for insulin secretion and also modulates the stimulatory effect of other endocrine, neural, and metabolic signals. Glucose also inhibits glucagon secretion either directly or via a paracrine effect of locally released insulin. Insulin and glucagon levels in turn regulate the liver, which is the primary organ of endogenous glucose production and thus the primary source of circulating glucose in the fasted state (42).

Approximately 80% of glucose utilization in the fasted state occurs independently of insulin availability (11, 42). The brain accounts for most of this insulin-independent glucose uptake, which becomes maximal at near normal fasting glucose levels. Glucose uptake by insulin-dependent tissues, primarily muscle, accounts for only a small percentage of overall glucose utilization in the fasted state. Recent work characterizing the molecular mechanisms for glucose transport has helped to clarify the differential specificity for glucose uptake as it relates to insulin availability by different tissues (14, 91). The predominant types of glucose transporters found on brain cell membranes (Glut 1 and Glut 3) are not affected by insulin. Maximum glucose uptake by the brain occurs at near normal fasting circulating glucose levels. In contrast, the primary type of glucose transporter in muscle and fat cells (Glut 4) is regulated by insulin. Insulin administration causes translocation of intracellular Glut 4 molecules to the surface membrane, where glucose uptake is enhanced dramatically (91, 92). Insulin is also important to maintain production of Glut 4 molecules by fat and muscle cells. Thus glucose levels are maintained during fasting by a relatively greater secretion of glucagon over insulin, favoring hepatic glucose production and minimizing glucose utilization by insulin-dependent tissues such as muscle and fat.

Following meal ingestion, a complex series of events ensues which minimizes the perturbation of glucose levels while maximizing the body's ability to store fuel (42). The rise in glucose levels accompanying meal ingestion provides a direct stimulus to insulin secretion. This rise in glucose also potentiates neural, endocrine, and metabolic signals that increase in association with ingestion of a meal to further enhance insulin secretion (45, 77, 163). At the same time, the combination of hyperglycemia and increased insulin secretion suppresses glucagon production, thus shifting the liver from an organ of glucose production to an organ of net glucose uptake and storage (17). While brain glucose uptake remains relatively unchanged, there is a substantial increase of insulin-mediated glucose utilization by muscle and fat tissue.

Several aspects of this complex regulatory system merit additional consideration. Assessment of rates of insulin secretion in vivo is complicated by the substantial liver extraction of insulin from portal vein blood. Thus, although variation of hepatic extraction of insulin

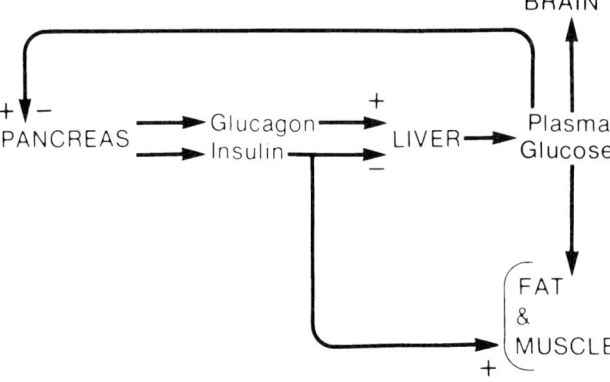

FIG. 7.2. Model illustrating key features of the feedback control system for regulation of steady-state plasma glucose levels. A key feature of this system is that changes of hormone secretion or hormone sensitivity will be modulated to minimize change in the glucose concentration and to maintain peripheral glucose utilization. [From Pfeifer et al. (159) with permission.]

does not appear to be regulated physiologically under most conditions, peripheral insulin levels provide only an indirect measure of pancreatic hormone secretion. The problem of hepatic extraction of insulin in vivo has been addressed in part by studying the circulating levels and kinetics of C-peptide (162), the amino acid–connecting peptide that is cleaved in the final stage of conversion of proinsulin to insulin and is co-secreted with insulin. Since C-peptide is not removed or metabolized by the liver, understanding its secretion rate and kinetics can allow direct estimation of insulin secretion rates in vivo. Another characteristic of this system, as for many other physiological endocrine/metabolic systems, is that glucose and insulin levels and secretion rates are not constant but vary over time, with a pulsatile pattern that is independent of meal ingestion (105, 196). Pulsatile variation of glucose levels under these circumstances is directly linked to pulsatile secretion of insulin (200).

Because of the feedback nature of the glucose regulatory system, it is extraordinarily difficult to interpret measures of insulin secretion or glucose metabolism in experimental protocols in which the feedback loop is operative. For example, when glucose levels are allowed to vary during OGTT, the insulin secretion response is a complex function of the change of glucose over time. As insulin is secreted and glucose levels fall, there is less of a stimulus for insulin secretion. One approach to studying the complexity of this feedback control system in more detail in vivo involves breaking the feedback loop by controlling one or more aspects of the system. Thus glucose clamp procedures have been developed to prevent the circulating glucose levels from changing during a protocol in which insulin secretion is changing over time (7, 40). Similarly, since glucose uptake by tissues will increase with increasing glucose level, interpretation of studies of glucose metabolism can be enhanced by maintenance of a constant glucose level in the environment.

Another characteristic of the feedback control system for control of glucose homeostasis involves the linkage between peripheral insulin action and insulin secretion. To the extent that there is resistance to insulin action to enhance glucose utilization in peripheral tissues, as occurs frequently in simple obesity, glucose levels will tend to be higher at a given insulin level, particularly following a challenge. However, the higher glucose level provides a greater stimulus to the pancreatic β-cell, resulting in greater secretion of insulin. Thus conditions associated with insulin resistance are characterized by hyperinsulinemia when there is normal pancreatic beta cell function to compensate for the insulin resistance. In fact, even further adaptation to insulin resistance may occur, resulting in enhanced β-cell sensitivity to glucose and greater insulin output for a given glucose challenge (12, 13). Again, this has been most clearly demonstrated in people with simple obesity. Such adaptation provides a mechanism for maintenance of relatively normal glucose levels and glucose tolerance in many people with simple obesity and insulin resistance.

Effects of Aging

Insulin Secretion. Many studies have been carried out to assess the effects of aging on insulin secretion in experimental animals and humans. While these studies taken together indicate that aging is associated with subtle impairments of insulin secretion, there is considerable variability among the findings (1). This variability is probably due to many factors, including the relatively small magnitude of the age effect, the use of a wide range of measures of pancreatic β-cell function of varying degrees of sensitivity, the use of different animal models, and the presence of multiple potential confounding factors in human studies.

Animal studies. Diminished portal vein insulin responses to glucose challenge have been observed with aging in male Sprague-Dawley rats (1). More specifically, this decrease is most apparent in the later phase of the multiphasic insulin secretory response to glucose challenge. Studies of insulin secretion from perfused pancreatic islets and perfused whole pancreas suggest a decline in insulin output with age (1, 101, 168, 188, 219). However, the magnitude of this age effect appears to vary according to the size and distribution of pancreatic islets (1, 165). This age effect appears to be most apparent when small islets are studied, which is the predominant type of islet in younger animals. Interpretation of some of these studies is hampered by the relatively limited age range of the animals studied. The observed decreases of insulin secretion occur between 2–4 months and 12 months, with little further decline at greater age. The use of Sprague-Dawley rats in these studies presents a problem because age-related obesity is prominent among these animals and so is a potential confounding factor. In fact, a number of age-related changes of insulin secretion have been modified by dietary and physical activity interventions in these animals (167).

Other work, using the Fischer 344 rat, has included a much wider age range to more clearly emphasize the effects of senescence (24, 44, 185, 197). Age-related obesity is substantially less of a problem in this animal model. These studies have also provided evidence for decreased insulin secretion by perfused isolated islets (44, 185). Although an age-related decline of insulin secretion has not been apparent in studies of whole perfused pancreas (185, 197), a study of the whole pancreas may miss aging changes in the number or size of islets. The age-related decline of insulin secretion is most clear when insulin secretion is expressed as a rate per β-cell (168). A further complication is that the age effect on insulin secretion in isolated islets may be limited primarily to male rats, as such an effect was not demonstrable in female rats in one study (185). Limited work has been done in aging mice and has not revealed consistent age changes.

A number of possible mechanisms for age-related changes in pancreatic β-cell function have been explored. Glucose transport into β-cells and subsequent oxidation via the enzyme glucokinase appear to be the primary signaling mechanisms for glucose-mediated insulin secretion (119). Studies of glucose oxidation by β-cells have yielded conflicting results, with some studies suggesting decreased glucose oxidation with aging (188) and others reporting an age-related increase of glucose oxidation (24, 185). Again, differences in experimental model and type and distribution of islet studied may contribute to the observed variability. Studies of more distal steps in insulin secretion have provided evidence that islets from aged animals demonstrate diminished margination of insulin secretion vesicles at the plasma membrane in response to glucose stimulation (44, 67). Other work has emphasized decreased production of cyclic adenosine monophosphate (cyclic AMP) via the adenyl cyclase system, a second-messenger system for regulation of insulin secretion, as a factor contributing to an age-related decline of insulin secretion (113). The effects of other islet hormones within the pancreatic islets on insulin secretion have also been considered. In particular, evidence has been presented for enhanced sensitivity of pancreatic β-cells to inhibition by somatostatin with aging (27).

Isolated islets have also been used to characterize the effects of aging on measures of insulin biosynthesis and on the secretion of newly synthesized vs. preformed insulin in response to glucose challenge. No age effect on levels of insulin messenger RNA has been observed (219). Aging has a greater effect on secretion of preformed insulin than on newly synthesized insulin, although both pools appear to be affected (64, 219). Proinsulin synthesis is also reduced as a function of age during high glucose stimulation (64, 219). These findings suggest multiple age-related alterations in the signal transduction and biosynthetic pathways leading to insulin secretion.

Human studies. Although substantial data exist on levels of insulin in the fasting state and during OGTT or following a meal, these data are extremely difficult to interpret because of their lack of sensitivity and specificity as quantitative measures of pancreatic β-cell function. A delayed insulin response during OGTT has been observed in some studies (see Fig. 7.1). Overall, the OGTT data suggest that gross impairment of pancreatic β-cell function is not characteristic of normal human aging (31, 57, 116, 166). Use of an I.V. injection of glucose as a challenge to the pancreatic β-cell has provided clear evidence for impaired pancreatic β-cell function in diabetic patients with fasting hyperglycemia (159, 163). However in nondiabetic individuals, the acute insulin secretory response to an I.V. glucose bolus is highly variable and has not provided evidence of an age-related impairment (29, 50, 156). The development of the hyperglycemic glucose clamp technique to provide a constant hyperglycemic stimulus by varying the exogenous glucose infusion rate over time has provided a useful approach to quantifying some aspects of pancreatic β-cell function (7). However, initial studies using this approach demonstrated little, if any, decrement in insulin secretory responses as a function of age (7, 40). The hyperglycemic clamp procedure has also been combined with oral glucose ingestion to assess the contribution of enteric mediators, such as gastric inhibitory polypeptide (GIP), to β-cell function in human aging (45). This study suggested a possible decreased β-cell sensitivity to GIP with age.

Another approach to providing better delineation of pancreatic β-cell function in humans is the use of C-peptide measurements in combination with the assessment of C-peptide kinetics to allow quantitative estimation of insulin secretory rates (162). When this approach has been applied to the study of insulin secretory responses of aging humans to meal ingestion or during a glucose infusion protocol designed to closely match circulating glucose levels, no age difference in absolute insulin secretion rate was observed (72). However, as illustrated in Figure 7.3, this study did suggest a diminished relative insulin secretory response in the older subjects. In contrast, others have found evidence for a diminished insulin secretory rate with age based on estimates of pancreatic insulin secretion during a prolonged I.V. glucose tolerance test protocol (29, 153). Another approach that has helped to identify age-related pancreatic β-cell functional deficits is to quantitate the potentiating effect of glucose on insulin secretory responses to a non-glucose stimulus, such as the amino acid arginine (29, 95).

One of the factors that may have limited interpretation of previous studies based solely on peripheral insulin levels is that there is evidence from a number of different laboratories for a small but consistent decrease in insulin clearance with age in humans (54, 121, 127, 172). Thus comparable circulating insulin levels in old and young subjects in the presence of diminished insulin clearance in the old subjects might suggest that the insulin secretory rate is actually somewhat decreased among the elderly.

Another problem in the interpretation of studies of pancreatic β-cell function in aging has to do with the potential confounding effect of coexistent insulin resistance in elderly people. The operation of the normal

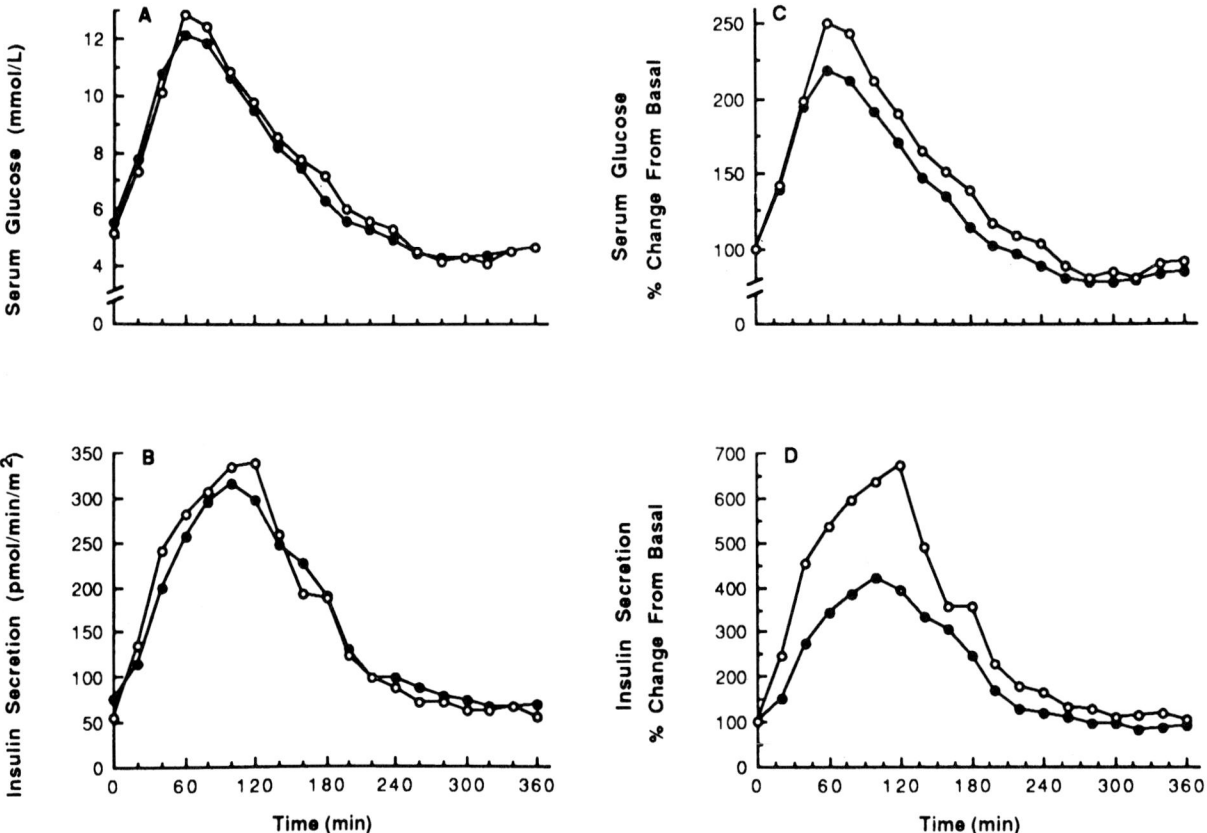

FIG. 7.3. Comparison of serum glucose levels and insulin secretion rates estimated by analysis of C-peptide kinetics in elderly (*solid circle*, n = 10) and young (*open circle*, n = 6) healthy subjects. Studies were carried out during a stepped I.V. glucose infusion designed to match circulating glucose levels between groups and to achieve levels similar to those during an OGTT. While no differences were observed in absolute insulin secretion rates between groups, the elderly group had a lower relative increase of insulin secretion. [From Gumbiner et al. (72) with permission.]

physiological feedback control mechanism for regulation of glucose homeostasis should result in hyperinsulinemia to compensate for the presence of insulin resistance if pancreatic β-cell function is completely normal. Thus the finding of similar pancreatic β-cell responses to glucose challenge in old and young subjects may, in fact, represent a relative impairment among the old, if the old subjects are also insulin resistant. When a group of older people was selected for study because they had a quantitative measure of insulin action similar to that of healthy young subjects, a more clear delineation of diminished pancreatic β-cell function was possible (95), as illustrated in Figure 7.4.

Future studies may be able to characterize subtle age-related impairments of pancreatic β-cell function even further. The pulsatile nature of endogenous insulin secretion and its relationship to fluctuations of circulating glucose levels can provide sensitive measures of normal glucose–pancreatic islet interaction (200). Disruption of this interaction has been demonstrated in subjects with impaired glucose tolerance compared to normal individuals (150) and in studies of apparently unaffected family members of patients with familial NIDDM (151). In fact, recent work has demonstrated that such an approach can help to identify subtle defects of insulin secretion in individuals who have the genetic marker for familial maturity onset diabetes of youth (MODY) but who do not yet demonstrate any impairment of glucose tolerance and who have apparently unaffected insulin secretory responses to a traditional I.V. glucose challenge (81). The application of such sensitive testing approaches may help to further characterize and quantitate the potential age changes in pancreatic β-cell function in humans.

Insulin Action. Many studies have provided evidence for resistance to the metabolic effects of insulin in aging animals and humans (see 38 for review). However, the interpretation of these findings is an ongoing challenge. One of the problems is that many factors can influence the metabolic effects of insulin. Thus the challenge is to sort out which of the findings with regard to insulin

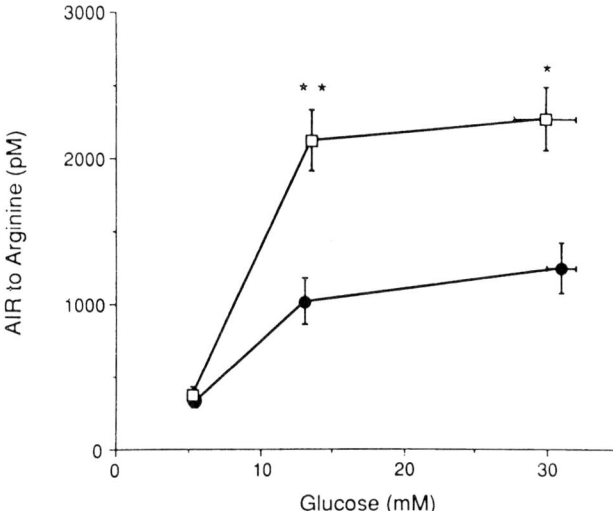

FIG. 7.4. Comparison of the acute insulin response (AIR) to a 5-g I.V. arginine bolus as a function of the plasma glucose level in exercise-trained older subjects (*solid circle*, n = 14) and exercise-trained younger subjects (*open square*, n = 11). Short-term glucose infusions were used to achieve elevated circulating glucose levels in subjects. *$P < 0.01$, **$P < 0.005$ for comparison of AIRs at similar glucose levels between old and young subjects. Both subject groups had similar sensitivities to insulin as measured during a frequently sampled IVGTT protocol. [From Kahn et al. (95) with permission.]

action in aging are secondary to other concomitants of aging. Another challenge in this area is the relative non-specificity of the term *insulin resistance*. There is no specific quantitative unit of insulin action. Rather, insulin action is assessed in relative terms by the measurement of an effect of insulin (such as glucose uptake) in a specific experimental situation or tissue site in comparison to similar measurements made under other experimental circumstances or in another set of animals or human subjects. Because insulin has many different metabolic effects, measurements can either provide an overall summary of them (for example, total body glucose metabolism in vivo) or emphasize a very specific effect (for example, translocation of Glut 4 transporters to the surface membrane of fat cells). A more detailed discussion of the potential interaction of specific variables with aging in the determination of sensitivity to insulin is provided later, under Confounding Factors.

Animal studies. Studies of aspects of insulin action in animal models of aging have been designed to establish the presence of insulin resistance, to define the contribution of external or environmental factors that may contribute to insulin resistance, and to establish cellular mechanisms that may explain resistance to insulin action. Much of the early evidence of age effects on insulin-mediated glucose metabolism in muscle and fat tissue is a result of changes in early life development. In particular, most studies have been done in Wistar and Sprague-Dawley rats, which rapidly become obese as they get older. Thus it has been particularly difficult to separate effects of obesity from aging in the development of insulin resistance. Studies in whole animals, perfused hind limbs, or isolated skeletal muscle have identified diminished glucose utilization in response to insulin as one overall marker of diminished insulin action across the life span (9, 66, 140, 169). Using a hyperinsulinemic euglycemic clamp approach, shifts to the right of the dose–response curves for both stimulation of glucose uptake and inhibition of hepatic glucose production as a function of insulin level have been demonstrated with increasing age for male Wistar rats (144). While these effects appear to be a continuous function of age, the largest effects occur in early life, with little further decline in insulin-stimulated glucose utilization between 4–6 month-old rats and older rats.

One mechanism that may contribute to age-related insulin resistance is a decline in insulin binding to cell surface membrane receptors. Diminished insulin binding and receptor number occur in early development in both fat and muscle cells, with little further change in insulin receptor number as a function of further aging (9, 144, 149). Thus changes in insulin receptor number and binding to the cell surface do not appear to be sufficient to explain the further decrease in insulin-mediated glucose uptake or the suppression of glucose production observed in experimental animals in later life. These findings suggest that there is a postreceptor component to the age-related impairment of insulin action under these circumstances.

One of the events that occurs in association with insulin stimulation of cellular metabolism is the activation of tyrosine kinase present in the cytoplasmic portion of the insulin receptor (93). This may be an important step in insulin-mediated signal transduction in terms of activating phosphorylase pathways. The study of skeletal muscle cell response to insulin has provided evidence for diminished insulin-mediated tyrosine kinase activity. A progressive decline has been observed during the life span of the male Wistar rat (102), and lower insulin-mediated tyrosine kinase activity has been observed in muscle from 24-month-old female Fischer 344 rats than in 2-month-old rats (9). The findings in Wistar rats contrast with results from liver tissue, in which no such age effect was observed. A decline in insulin-mediated autophosphorylation of the tyrosine kinase domain of the insulin receptor was also observed (9, 102), but only during early life development in the Wistar rats. Thus the observed life span–related decline in insulin receptor-mediated tyrosine kinase activity does not appear to be explained by diminished autophosphorylation of the tyrosine kinase domain of the insulin receptor itself.

Insulin's interaction with cell membrane receptors results in the internalization of the insulin receptor complex, which may be another important component of the cell signaling mechanism. Following this internalization, receptors are recycled to the cell surface. Studies using fat cells of male Sprague-Dawley rats have demonstrated a decrease of insulin receptor recycling between the ages of 2 and 12 months, an effect that was unrelated to any decrease in insulin receptor binding (210). However, this finding has not been extended to older rats.

Insulin is also an important regulator of fat-cell lipolysis. A diminished antipolytic effect of insulin has been demonstrated in adipocytes from aging Wistar rats (177). This effect appears to be dependent on the modulating influence of adenosine, as it is most apparent in the presence of a low concentration of an adenosine agonist. Similar to findings with insulin action in terms of glucose metabolism, this effect is most apparent when cells from very young animals are compared to cells from animals in early maturation, with little further decline in insulin's antipolytic action with further aging of the animal to senescence.

Human studies. Studies of insulin action in humans have emphasized comparisons between young, middle-aged, and old people. The hyperinsulinemic euglycemic clamp procedure has been employed to help delineate age-related changes in glucose metabolism in humans (40). A combination of this method with tritiated glucose infusion permits quantitative estimation of hepatic glucose production, thereby allowing more accurate assessment of the total glucose disposal rate. Studies using multiple infusion rates of insulin can characterize the dose–response relationship between insulin level and glucose utilization or suppression of hepatic glucose production. Such studies provide little evidence for an age-related impairment of insulin-mediated suppression of hepatic glucose production in humans (52, 124). However, there is substantial agreement among several different laboratories that insulin-mediated total glucose disposal declines with age (40, 52, 164, 182), as illustrated in Figure 7.5. Disadvantages of the glucose clamp technique include the relatively cumbersome nature of the procedure and, more importantly, the requirement of establishing substantially elevated circulating insulin levels during testing. Thus results of these studies include findings at circulating insulin levels that are rarely achieved under normal physiological circumstances. These studies have indicated that aging is associated with a shift to the right in the dose–response curve for insulin effects on glucose utilization, since glucose utilization at maximally stimulating insulin levels appears to be relatively unaffected (52, 182). Such findings are most compatible with a decrease in insulin action beyond the level of the insulin receptor.

Another approach to the assessment of insulin action in vivo has been to use glucose infusions of varying rates to match glucose levels over time and to directly assess

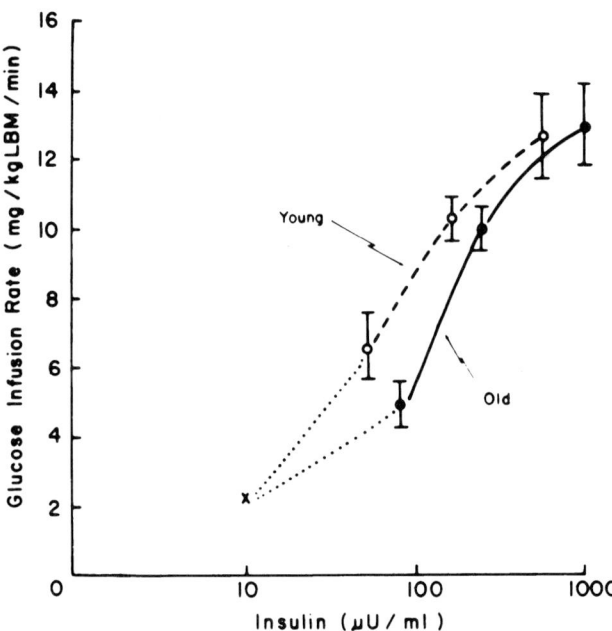

FIG. 7.5. Comparison of dose–response curves for insulin levels achieved during a euglycemic clamp protocol vs. glucose infusion rate needed to maintain euglycemia in healthy, nonobese young (n = 17) and old (n = 10) subjects. Experimental data extrapolated to known basal hepatic glucose production rates for young and old subjects. Glucose infusion rates were similar in young and old at the highest insulin level tested but significantly lower in the old at the low insulin infusion rate. [From Rowe et al. (182) with permission.]

forearm glucose uptake under these conditions. Such studies have also demonstrated diminished glucose utilization under conditions of comparable circulating glucose and insulin levels in old compared to young subjects (88).

Efforts to assess insulin action at more physiological insulin levels have focused on computer modeling to define parameters of insulin action based on the interaction between insulin and glucose levels during perturbation. The best established and validated method involves the use of an I.V. bolus injection of glucose alone or followed by an I.V. infusion of the sulfonylurea agent tolbutamide, with frequent blood sampling over 3 h for measurement of insulin and glucose levels (17). This method of data analysis identifies key parameters that allow close fitting of the observed data by the experimental model, which is based on known aspects of insulin–glucose physiology. This modeling approach estimates a quantitative parameter of insulin action (S_I), which has been extensively validated in animal and human studies, including direct comparison to measures of insulin action during a hyperinsulinemic glucose clamp protocol (17). Using this frequently sampled IVGTT approach, diminished sensitivity to insulin has been demonstrated in aging humans (29, 202). A more comprehensive analysis of several different modeling approaches to assessment of insulin action in a large cohort of healthy men has provided additional evidence for an age-related decline in tissue sensitivity to insulin (217).

The hyperinsulinemic glucose clamp approach has been used to assess other aspects of insulin action in human aging. The suppressive effect of insulin on circulating amino acid levels, as well as its antiproteolytic effect, appeared to be unaffected by age in such studies (61). Similarly, insulin-mediated suppression of lipolysis, as reflected by circulating free fatty acid levels, and insulin suppression of circulating glucagon levels have been observed to be similar in old and young subjects (124, 164). One possible limitation of these studies is that relatively high circulating insulin levels were required. Thus possible age differences in sensitivity to these effects at lower insulin levels have not been excluded. A combination of the euglycemic insulin clamp technique to measure glucose metabolism with indirect calorimetry to quantitate substrate oxidation and energy production can allow separate estimation of oxidative and nonoxidative components to alterations of glucose metabolism in conditions of insulin resistance. Such studies suggest that the age-related decline in glucose disposal in men is associated with a substantial decline in nonoxidative glucose metabolism but not with oxidative glucose metabolism (56). Interestingly, these age effects in men were not observed in women. Since other studies demonstrating age-related insulin resistance in humans have been limited to males, further work on more heterogeneous populations is clearly important.

Muscle is the most important site for insulin-mediated glucose disposal in quantitative terms. However, lack of accessibility of muscle tissue has hampered specific studies of insulin action on muscle tissue in humans. Fat cells are more readily available and have been investigated with regard to mechanisms of age-related changes in insulin action. Studies of insulin binding to adipocytes have yielded varying results, with some finding no age difference in insulin binding (52) and others suggesting an age-related decrease (22, 115, 155). Studies of insulin binding in monocytes have not identified an age-related decline (52, 88, 182). Insulin-mediated glucose transport has also been studied in adipocytes from humans. A decline in maximal glucose transport as measured by 3-O-methylglucose uptake was observed in cells from elderly men, but there was no effect on the glucose level for half-maximal transport (53). These findings are consistent with in vivo observations in the same subjects of comparably decreased glucose uptake over a range of glucose levels studied, despite constant insulin levels (55). Overall, these findings suggest a reduction of glucose transport capacity in fat cells from elderly people as opposed to a reduction in the function of glucose transport units. Studies of the effects of age on human adipose cell Glut 4 transporters and their regulation by insulin have not yet been reported.

Insulin-Independent Glucose Uptake. Diminished glucose uptake by peripheral tissues or following a challenge, as in age-related glucose intolerance, could be due in part to diminished delivery of insulin to tissues as a result of decreased insulin secretion or to diminished insulin action at peripheral tissues. However, there is evidence that a component of glucose uptake from the circulation occurs independently of insulin. Thus it is possible that an age-related impairment in this component of glucose uptake could contribute to impaired glucose tolerance with aging. One approach to the assessment of glucose utilization that depends more on glucose level than on insulin is to study the effect of changing glucose levels on glucose utilization when insulin is held constant, as during a hyperinsulinemic glucose clamp protocol. However, it is difficult to separate completely effects of glucose on glucose utilization and glucose–insulin interaction when insulin levels are high. Another approach has been to use somatostatin to suppress endogenous insulin secretion and then to measure glucose utilization during maintenance of a constant glucose level in the circulation. In one study using this approach, glucose utilization was lower in old subjects than in young subjects when glucose levels were maintained at approximately normal fasting levels. However, when glucose levels were raised to approximately 11 mM, glucose utilization rates were similar in both young and old (123). These findings suggest that, at least at some physiological glucose levels, non-insulin-mediated glucose uptake is reduced in elderly people.

Another approach to this issue has emerged from the kinetic modeling studies using the IVGTT protocol. Insulin-independent glucose utilization mediated by changes of glucose level, defined as glucose effectiveness (S_G), is one of the components of the physiological model. A solution to the model requires estimation of the parameter S_G, which is the fractional rate of glucose uptake during the IVGTT protocol. S_G is independent of insulin levels, or dependent only upon the initial fasting insulin level, and has been validated as a measure of glucose effectiveness by studies in experimental animals (2, 17). S_G is reduced in patients with NIDDM. Studies in humans have shown no difference in values for S_G in old persons and young persons (29, 202). However, as described in more detail below, epinephrine causes a greater fall in S_G in old subjects than in young subjects, which may contribute to the enhanced hyperglycemic effect of epinephrine in human aging (136).

Glucose Transport. Enhanced understanding of the molecular biology of glucose transport has allowed direct quantitative measurement of glucose transport molecules in cell membranes. The availability of such measurements has allowed direct testing of the possibility that changes of glucose transporter expression may contribute to diminished cellular glucose uptake in aging. Initial reports demonstrated reduced amounts of Glut 4 protein in membranes of both fat cells and gastrocnemius muscle when comparing 1–2-month-old Wistar or Sprague-Dawley rats with either 12- or 20-month-old animals (48, 84, 111). This decrease appears specific for the Glut 4 transporter because measurements of Glut 1 transporter protein showed no difference between groups (48). Assessment of Glut 4 messenger RNA suggested that the decrease in Glut 4 protein is a result of decreased biosynthesis (111). Decreased Glut 4 protein content in fat cells from older animals occurred both in the plasma membrane fraction and in the low-density microsome fraction. There was markedly less translocation of Glut 4 protein from the intracellular microsome fraction to the plasma membrane fraction upon exposure to insulin (48). The findings are compatible with observed decreases of cellular uptake of 3-O-methylglucose or 2-deoxyglucose as markers of cellular glucose transport activity (48, 71, 111).

A decrease of Glut 4 protein in muscle has also been observed in male Fischer 344 rats across the age range of 3–24 months (97), but this effect was most apparent in exercised, trained animals, with only very small changes observed in sedentary rats with age (9, 97). However, in a study of glucose uptake and Glut 4 protein in several muscles from Long-Evans rats of varying age, age-related decreases in both glucose uptake and Glut 4 protein were apparent when comparing 2- and 10-month-old animals, with no further decline in 25-month-old animals (71). These findings, illustrated in Figure 7.6, are most consistent with other work in experimental animals demonstrating changes in insulin action and glucose uptake primarily when comparing very young rats with mature rats but less so when comparing aged animals with mature animals. Thus these findings overall are most compatible with a change in insulin sensitivity and glucose metabolism with growth and development in experimental animals rather than as an effect of senescence.

Effects of Other Hormones. Many hormones interact with glucose metabolism in vivo and could contribute to age-related changes in this system. In particular, hormones released during stressful illness, including glucagon, catecholamines, growth hormone, and glucocorticoids, affect glucose metabolism by increasing circulating glucose levels. Glucagon secretion does not appear to be significantly influenced by aging in humans either in the fasting state or following amino acid stim-

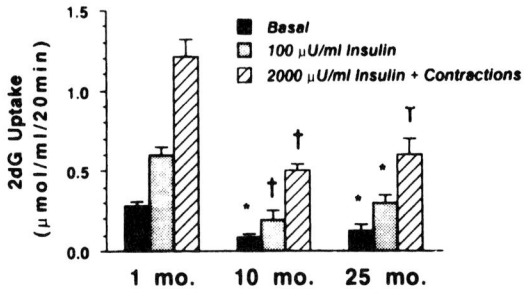

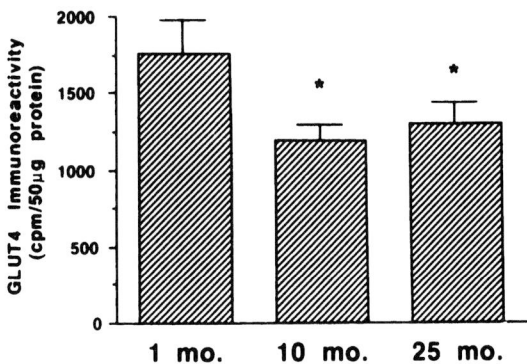

FIG. 7.6. *Top:* Comparison of glucose transport activities, as measured by uptake of 2 deoxyglucose (2dG), in epitrochlearis muscle from female Long-Evans rats of varying age. *$P < 0.01$, and †$P < 0.001$ vs. muscles from 1-month old rats. Values are mean ± standard error for five to eight muscles per group, except for basal uptake in 1-month-old rats where n = 14. *Bottom:* Glut 4 immunoreactive protein content compared in homogenates of epitrochlearis muscle from rats of varying age. Values are mean ± standard error for nine to ten muscles per group. * $P < 0.05$ vs. muscles from 1-month- old rats. [From Gulve et al. (71) with permission.]

ulation (16, 46, 195). Glucagon suppression by insulin also appears to be unaffected by age (124). However, older subjects have been reported to have greater hyperglycemic and hepatic glucose production responses to glucagon infusion, suggesting enhanced hepatic sensitivity to glucagon in these subjects (195).

Growth hormone secretion declines rather than increases with age and so cannot be directly implicated in age-related glucose intolerance. Consistent with the decline of growth hormone secretion in the elderly, particularly during the night, is the observation of the lack of an early morning rise of glucose levels, thought by some to be mediated by nocturnal growth hormone secretion. This "dawn" phenomenon of rising glucose level in the early morning has been described in normal humans but appears to be absent in the elderly (122, 178). Given the potential adverse effects on glucose metabolism of high levels of growth hormone, the current interest in the use of growth hormone to cause anabolic effects in elderly people should be accompanied by studies of the susceptibility of such individuals to growth hormone–mediated hyperglycemia. Initial trials with human growth hormone administration have demonstrated small effects on fasting and postchallenge glucose levels (19, 96, 117, 184).

Regulation of glucocorticoid production appears to be relatively normal in experimental animals and humans with aging (43, 192, 216). There has been some suggestion of subtle increases in corticosteroid levels at certain times of the day with aging, but these seem unlikely to be of significance in terms of glucose homeostasis. There is little information about the sensitivity of elderly animals or people to the hyperglycemic effects of glucocorticoids.

Catecholamines can have potent effects on glucose regulation by multiple mechanisms. Catecholamines interfere with insulin-mediated glucose disposal and stimulate hepatic glucose production, both primarily by β-adrenergic receptor mechanisms, and inhibit insulin secretion by an α_2-adrenergic mechanism (76). Plasma norepinephrine levels and norepinephrine release are consistently increased in aging humans (112, 205) and in aged animals when measured under carefully controlled experimental conditions to minimize the confounding effects of experimental stress (98). However, the role of endogenous sympathetic nervous system activity in age-related glucose intolerance remains uncertain. Improvement of glucose tolerance in elderly humans by dietary intervention occurs without any effect on circulating norepinephrine levels (30). In addition, age-related insulin resistance is poorly correlated with the degree of elevation of norepinephrine levels (202). Furthermore, short-term suppression of sympathetic nervous system activity does not result in any consistent improvement in insulin action in older individuals (201).

The sensitivity of elderly people to metabolic effects of catecholamines has also been studied. This issue is of particular relevance since a number of studies have demonstrated age-related decreases in nonmetabolic effects of catecholamines, both β-adrenergic (132, 189) and α-adrenergic (203, 204). No reduction in the insulin secretory response to the β-adrenergic agonist isoproterenol was observed in healthy older people despite the presence of diminished cardiac β-adrenergic responsiveness in these individuals (137). Thus the age-related decrease in adrenergic responsiveness may not apply to metabolic effects of catecholamines.

Epinephrine infusions have been used to study age interactions on insulin secretion and insulin action. The IVGTT procedure was used to allow estimation of both the insulin secretion response to glucose and quantitative measures of sensitivity to insulin (136). As illustrated in Figure 7.7, comparisons were made between young and old subjects who had virtually identical plasma glucose responses to the IVGTT protocol in the absence of epinephrine infusion. During infusion of a dose of epinephrine that achieved circulating epinephrine levels comparable to those achieved during physiological stress, significantly greater hyperglycemia was observed in the older subject group, indicating enhanced overall sensitivity to the hyperglycemic effects of epinephrine. However, the dose–response relationship for epinephrine inhibition of the insulin secretion response to I.V. glucose is identical between old and young subjects. Furthermore, old and young subjects were equally sensitive to the effects of epinephrine on diminishing tissue sensitivity to insulin. The primary difference was greater suppression in the old subjects of glucose effectiveness (S_G), the effect of glucose level on fractional glucose removal rate, as illustrated in Figure 7.8. Thus, while sympathetic nervous system activity and catecholamine release do not appear to be important in age-related changes of glucose metabolism in the normal resting state, enhanced sensitivity to metabolic effects of catecholamines may contribute to greater hyperglycemia under stressful situations. In this regard, an enhanced hyperglycemic response to experimental stress has been reported in aged rats (145).

Confounding Factors

A major challenge in the interpretation of age differences in measures of glucose metabolism is that glucose metabolism is sensitive to a wide range of influences. Thus it may be very difficult to specifically define effects of aging that are independent of other such influences. As summarized in Figure 7.9, it is likely that there are primary changes of pancreatic β-cell function and possibly changes of insulin action with aging that contribute to age-related changes of glucose metabolism. It is also likely that there are specific genetic factors that influence the expression of glucose intolerance with aging, although such genetic factors have not yet been defined. Several studies have attempted to control for the other variables that may affect glucose metabolism. Although there are exceptions, these studies suggest that there is a residual decline in glucose tolerance with age in both men and women but that this age effect is relatively modest in magnitude. The following discussion addresses a number of the specific confounding factors that can influence glucose metabolism.

Adiposity. Increased adiposity is a major factor that contributes to age-related alterations of glucose metabolism, particularly decreased insulin action. Both total adiposity and adipose mass distribution in humans appear to be important, with central distribution of body fat being particularly associated with metabolic

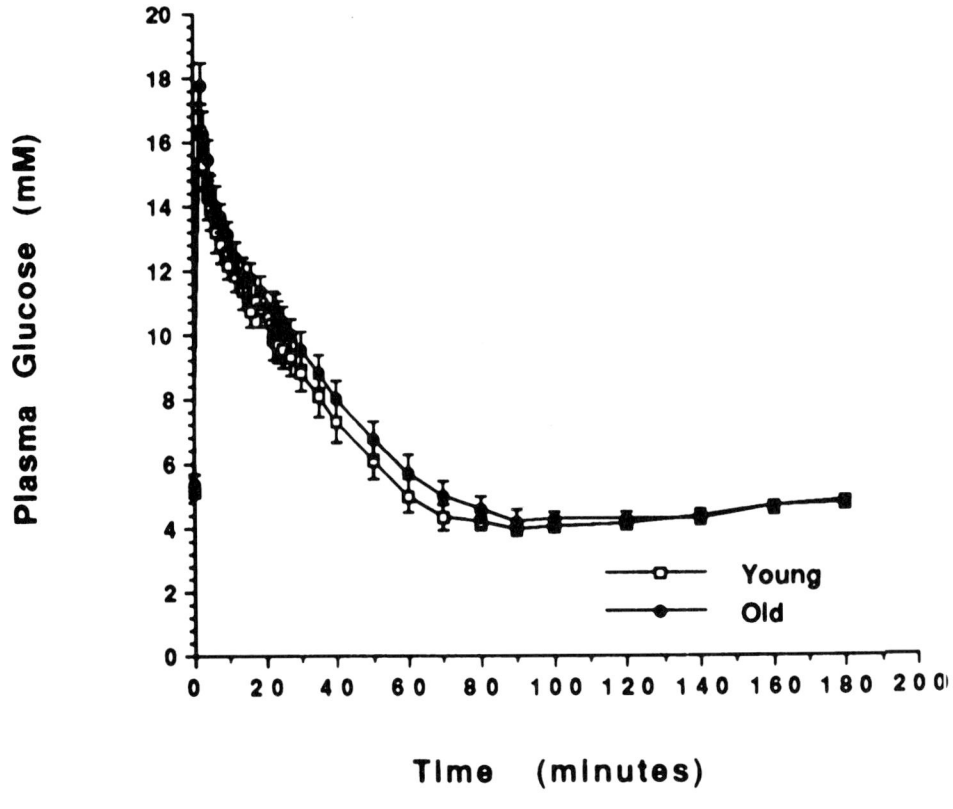
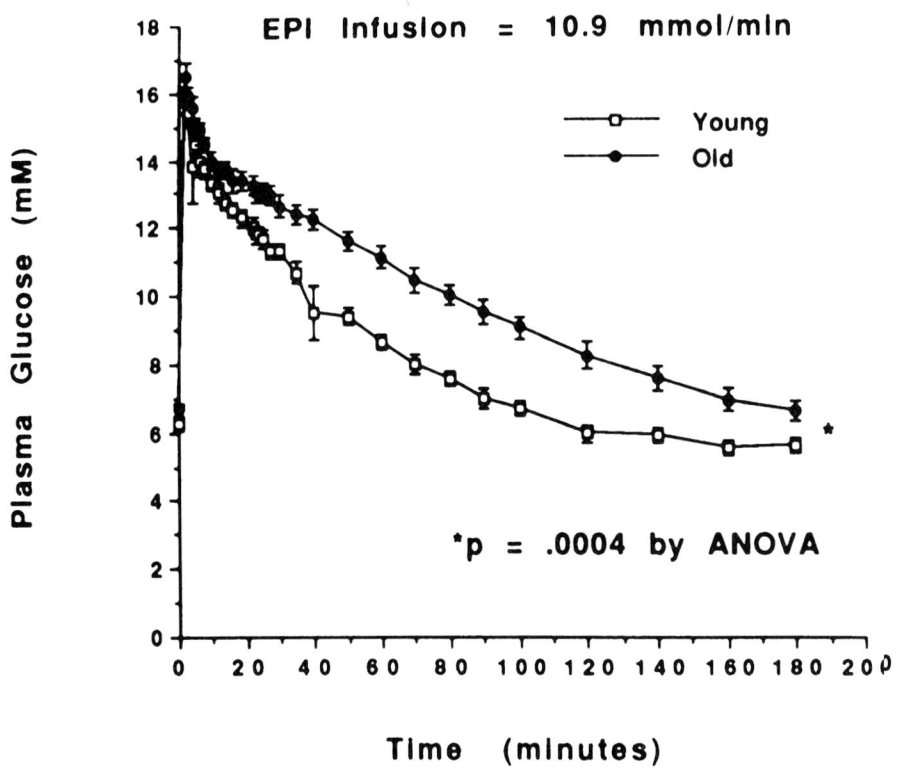

FIG. 7.7. Comparison of plasma glucose levels during an I.V. glucose tolerance test in healthy young (n = 7) and old (n = 7) subjects. *Upper panel:* IVGTT results in the absence of infusion of epinephrine (EPI). *Lower panel:* The slower decline of glucose levels in the old subject group during EPI infusion. Circulating EPI levels were comparable in both subject groups during EPI infusion. [From Morrow et al. (136) with permission.]

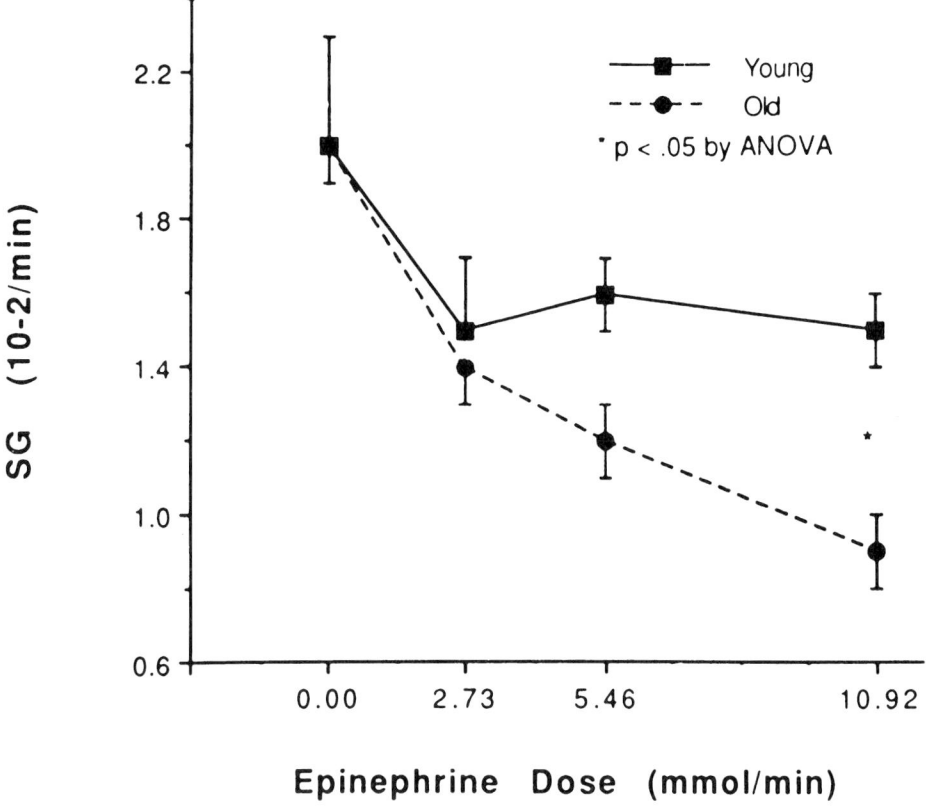

FIG. 7.8. Comparison of effects of increasing doses of epinephrine in healthy young (n = 7) and old (n = 7) subjects. S_G is a measure of glucose effectiveness obtained from minimal model analysis of IVGTT results. Epinephrine infusion reduced S_G values in both subject groups. This effect was greater in the old than the young. [From Morrow et al. (136) with permission.]

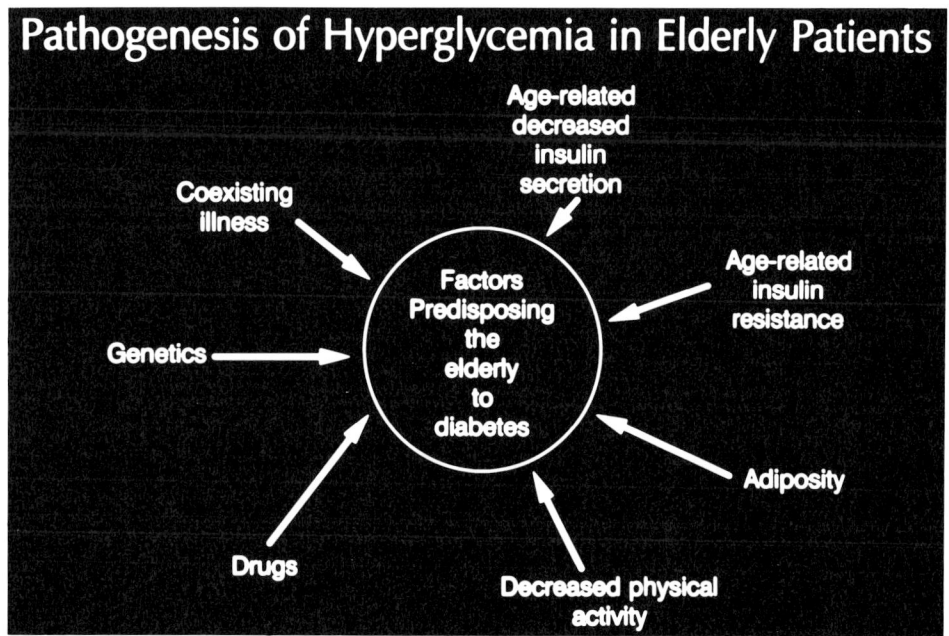

FIG. 7.9. Summary of factors which may contribute to the high rate of diabetes mellitus and impaired glucose tolerance among elderly people. [From Halter (75) with permission.]

abnormalities (21, 25, 33, 34, 100). Several studies in humans have attempted to control for the influence of adiposity by including a large sample size and multiple measurements of various aspects of body fat mass and distribution to control for age group differences statistically. Although these studies are not in full agreement, they suggest that there is a persistent effect of age on both glucose tolerance and insulin action that is independent of body fat mass and distribution in humans (25, 126, 166, 193). However, there is heterogeneity among the elderly population. Older people who meet the criteria for normal glucose tolerance have less adiposity, particularly central adiposity, and do not have a detectable decrease of insulin sensitivity (34, 100, 154).

Studies in experimental animals have been more problematic. Measures of insulin action and glucose transport as a function of age in fat cells have been substantially confounded by the concomitant increase of fat cell mass and fat cell size observed with age. Many of the age-related metabolic alterations in studies of fat cells have occurred during the phase of rapid increase of body size in early development and are associated directly with increased fat cell size. In fact, age-related changes of glucose metabolism have been reported to be entirely explained by variation of fat cell size (107). Studies of the Fischer 344 rat have been least affected by this problem, since this strain usually does not increase its body weight dramatically between maturity and late life. Measurements of insulin action and glucose metabolism in other tissues, such as skeletal muscle, may be less directly influenced by fat cell mass. However, it is possible that insulin resistance secondary to adiposity could indirectly affect muscle tissue as well.

The potential confounding effect of obesity on measures of pancreatic β-cell function and insulin secretion with aging is that obesity-related pancreatic β-cell adaptation and hyperinsulinemia may mask underlying age-related defects of β-cell function. Thus it is unlikely that observed impairments of β-cell function with age can be explained by coexisting adiposity.

Physical Activity. Diminished physical activity or bed rest in humans is associated with impaired glucose tolerance and insulin resistance. Conversely, exercise training improves glucose tolerance and enhances tissue sensitivity to insulin. Thus aging-associated decreased mobility and diminished physical activity may be important confounding factors in age-related changes of glucose homeostasis. There is limited information about the effects of exercise training on age-related changes of glucose metabolism in experimental animals. Exercise training improves insulin action in Sprague-Dawley rats between the ages of 12 and 16 months, but this effect could not be separated from the decreased adiposity associated with exercise training (130). Exercise training has been reported to increase glucose transport activity and the content of Glut 4, but not of Glut 1, in skeletal muscles of young rats (68). In one study the Glut 4 content of skeletal muscle increased more in 12-month-old Sprague-Dawley rats than in younger rats (49). In contrast, exercise training of Fischer 344 rats appears to be less effective in increasing skeletal muscle Glut 4 content. In fact, in this animal model, the age-related decrease of Glut 4 content was more apparent in exercise-trained animals than in sedentary animals (97). Differences in the animal model studied, the ages of the animals, and the duration and type of exercise training, as well as other differences of the specific experimental protocol may have contributed to these apparently discrepant findings.

There is substantially more information about the effects of exercise training on glucose tolerance and insulin action in aging humans. However, studies have been limited thus far to effects of aerobic exercise, with little investigation of strength training. In addition, most studies of exercise-training effects on metabolic function have been carried out in men. Healthy older men with greater degrees of physical fitness, usually assessed by measurement of maximal oxygen uptake during exercise, have better glucose tolerance and less evidence of insulin resistance than less active older men (85, 126, 190, 218). More physically fit elderly men also tend to have less body fat and less central adiposity. While some glucose intolerance appears to persist with age even when controlling for these factors, the age-related change is modest (126, 218). When insulin action was assessed with a glucose clamp protocol in healthy older men, degree of physical fitness and central adiposity were the most important predictors of insulin resistance, and age was not an independent predictor (126). Physically fit older men have also been reported to have higher levels of muscle Glut 4 (86).

Exercise training without concomitant weight reduction has had little effect on overall oral glucose tolerance in elderly men. However, a significant improvement in insulin action, measured either with a glucose clamp protocol or by computer modeling of IVGTT results, has been demonstrated in older men following exercise training (94, 208), as illustrated in Figure. 7.10. The reduction of insulin resistance accompanying exercise training under these circumstances is associated with diminished pancreatic β- cell sensitivity to stimulation (94), as would be expected from the physiology of the feedback control system affecting glucose and insulin. This compensatory effect may explain why the improvement of insulin action associated with exercise training does not affect overall glucose tolerance.

Dietary Factors. Dietary factors, particularly carbohydrate intake, are known to influence glucose tolerance.

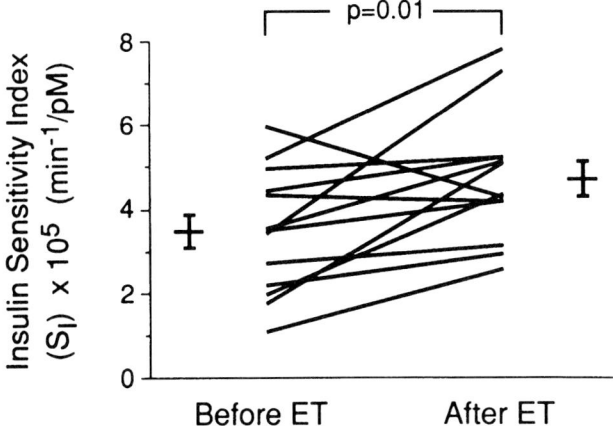

FIG. 7.10. Effect of a 6-month program of exercise training (ET) on insulin sensitivity in 13 older subjects. Insulin sensitivity was determined from minimal model analysis of frequently sampled IVGTT. [From Kahn et al. (94) with permission.]

In fact, standard instructions for carrying out an OGTT include a minimum dietary carbohydrate intake to minimize the acute effects of restricted carbohydrate intake on impairing glucose tolerance (143). Some studies have suggested that the total caloric intake of older adults may be relatively low and that carbohydrate intake in particular may be less compared to younger individuals (31, 160). Thus it is possible that impaired glucose tolerance in aging may be due in part to diminished dietary carbohydrate intake. Conversely, excessive intake of calories leading to obesity is an important contributing factor to insulin resistance and impaired glucose tolerance in an older adult population. Indeed, caloric restriction of experimental animals is associated with reduced body weight and less age-related impairment of insulin action (169). Circulating glucose levels and insulin levels are lower in lifelong diet-restricted rats and monkeys as well (35, 118).

Studies in humans have addressed the effects of short-term alteration of dietary carbohydrate intake on aspects of age-related changes in glucose metabolism. Healthy elderly people demonstrate improved glucose tolerance, enhanced tissue sensitivity to insulin, and improved pancreatic β-cell function when placed on an 85% carbohydrate diet for 3–5 days compared to an ad libitum diet (30). When old and young subjects were studied on comparable carbohydrate diet regimens, age differences in glucose tolerance, insulin secretion, and insulin action were reduced but still persisted (30, 31). Thus dietary carbohydrate intake is an additional factor that can contribute to age-related changes of glucose metabolism.

Hypertension. There is a growing body of evidence that some groups of people with essential hypertension have associated insulin resistance and glucose intolerance (51, 129, 170). Given the high prevalence rate of hypertension among the elderly, blood pressure may be an important variable when studying age-related glucose intolerance. Among the population of elderly people in Rancho Bernardo, California, increased blood pressure is associated with impaired glucose tolerance, or NIDDM, independently of the coexistence of obesity or use the of antihypertensive medications (174). However, the degree of association between insulin resistance or hyperinsulinemia and hypertension has varied considerably in different studies, perhaps related to the degree of obesity in the populations (73). The association between insulin resistance, glucose intolerance, and hypertension is strong in some Caucasian populations but does not appear to be present among other races or ethnic groups (187). Even in the predominantly Caucasian population of the Baltimore Longitudinal Study of Aging, little if any relationship between hyperinsulinemia and blood pressure was found after adjusting for other confounding variables (138). Similarly, insulin resistance is found in some animal models of hypertension, but not in others (60, 224).

The mechanism for the association of increasing blood pressure and insulin resistance is not known. One hypothesis is that hyperinsulinemia associated with insulin resistance causes hypertension by direct effects on the cardiovascular system such as stimulation of arterial smooth muscle proliferation (199) or effects on Ca^{2+} transport in vascular smooth muscle cells (224). Alternatively, it has been suggested that insulin resistance and hyperinsulinemia affect the cardiovascular system indirectly by activation of the sympathetic nervous system (36, 104). Administration of insulin, although at near pharmacological doses, can lead to increased sympathetic nerve activity and release of catecholamines (109, 183) and in addition may enhance vascular sensitivity to endogenous catecholamines (63). However, in short-term experiments, insulin administration increases sympathetic nervous system activity by causing vasodilation leading to a reflex increase of sympathetic activity and catecholamine release (5, 83). Thus one would have to postulate that longer-term exposure to elevated insulin levels has different cardiovascular effects from the antihypertensive effects of short-term insulin administration.

As discussed previously, there is evidence for increased sympathetic nervous system activity in human aging as well as insulin resistance and glucose intolerance. However, careful analysis of these factors in a population of otherwise healthy men and women has indicated that blood pressure and degree of adiposity are the best predictors of declining insulin action (202). Neither age nor circulating norepinephrine levels contribute independently to the age-related decrease of

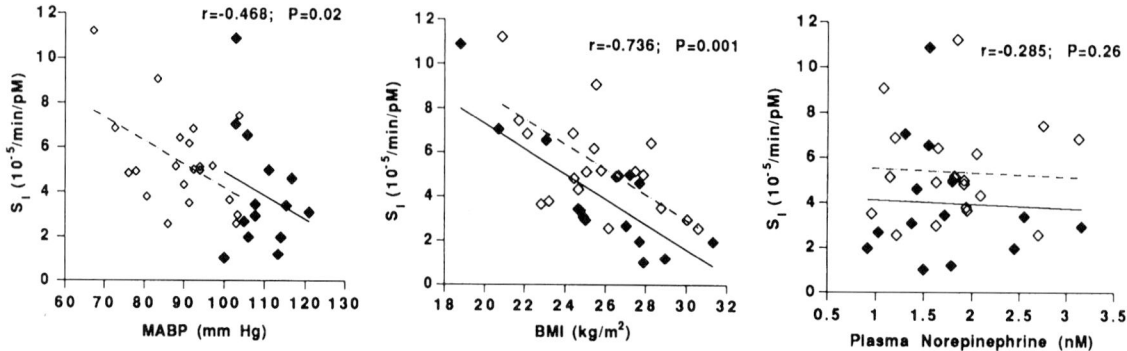

FIG. 7.11. Regression analysis of tissue sensitivity to insulin (S_I) in relation to mean arterial blood pressure (MABP), body mass index (BMI), and plasma norepinephrine level for healthy normotensive and hypertensive subjects aged 38–78 yr, adjusted for co-factor of blood pressure group. *Dashed line* is the regression line for normotensive subjects; *solid line,* for hypertensive subjects. In both groups, S_I was inversely related to blood pressure and BMI but not to plasma norepinephrine. [From Supiano et al. (201) with permission.]

insulin action. Similarly, among a group of older people, including those with mild hypertension, there was a close association between blood pressure and degree of adiposity as predictors of sensitivity to insulin but no relationship to norepinephrine levels (201), as illustrated in Figure 7.11. Furthermore, when sympathetic nervous system activity was suppressed during 10 days of treatment with the antihypertensive agent guanadrel, no improvement of sensitivity to insulin was observed.

An alternative hypothesis for the association between hypertension and insulin resistance is the adverse long-term effect on small blood vessels of exposure to hypertension (90). The loss of function of such small blood vessels could result in impaired delivery of glucose to tissues and thus diminished insulin-mediated glucose utilization. Thus this hypothesis postulates that insulin resistance is secondary to underlying long-term hypertension. The lack of association of insulin resistance with hypertension in some animal models and some human populations argues against this hypothesis, although it is possible that other genetic or physiological regulatory factors may prevent the development of insulin resistance under these circumstances.

Drugs. A number of pharmacological agents in common use have known effects on glucose metabolism. Since older adults commonly use pharmacological agents, any interpretation of alterations of glucose metabolism in such individuals must take into account the drugs they are using. Table 7.2 includes a list of drugs known to affect glucose metabolism. Because of the association of hypertension with insulin resistance and glucose intolerance, effects of antihypertensive agents on glucose metabolism have been of particular interest (87). Whereas none of the drug effects on glucose metabolism seem to be of large magnitude, a variety of effects have been documented (114). Hydrochlorothiazide causes insulin resistance, while the angiotensin-converting enzyme inhibitor captopril appears to enhance insulin sensitivity (167). The sympatholytic agent guanadrel has no consistent effect on insulin action (201). The α_2-adrenergic agonist clonidine diminishes glucose tolerance by α_2-adrenergic inhibition of insulin secretion (125).

DIABETES MELLITUS

The most common form of diabetes mellitus in older adults is NIDDM, or type II diabetes mellitus. NIDDM is a syndrome characterized by hyperglycemia, meeting the criteria indicated in Table 7.1. Other features of this

TABLE 7.2. *Drugs That May Cause Hyperglycemia*

Antihypertensives
  Diuretics
  β-adrenergic blockers
  α_2-adrenergic agonists
  ? Ca^{2+} channel blockers
Antiinflammatory agents
  Glucocorticoids
  Nonsteroidal antiinflammatory drugs
Stimulants
  Adrenergic agonists
  Nicotine
  Caffeine
Others
  Sex steroids (estrogen/progesterone)
  Phenytoin
  Pentamidine
  Nicotinic acid

syndrome include increased adiposity, hypertension, and disorders of lipid metabolism. Age of onset is usually relatively late in life, with the highest incidence rate among people over the age of 65 yr. There appears to be a strong genetic component to this condition. The prevalence of NIDDM among certain families is as high as 50%, and there is a very high concordance rate for NIDDM among identical twins, approaching 100% (10, 206). NIDDM probably develops in a progressive manner, with a period of impaired glucose tolerance preceding the development of overt NIDDM. However, only limited longitudinal data are available to affirm this hypothesis (146). People who meet the criteria for impaired glucose tolerance have a substantially increased risk of developing overt NIDDM, although this risk is only 1%–5% per year. Because of the relative nonspecificity of the OGTT and its variability within an individual, it is not an ideal marker to follow for the development of NIDDM. More specific predictive markers would be of great value to enhance understanding of the pathophysiology of this condition.

Mechanisms for Development of Non-Insulin-Dependent Diabetes Mellitus

Many studies have demonstrated that patients with NIDDM have substantial impairment of pancreatic β-cell function (see 163 for review) and diminished sensitivity to the metabolic effects of insulin (see 170 for review). However, there continues to be debate about which of these events is primary. Epidemiological studies of several different populations, including family members of patients with NIDDM, suggest that hyperinsulinemia and insulin resistance predict the subsequent development of NIDDM (74, 110, 194, 221). In other studies, subtle impairments of both pancreatic β-cell function and insulin action have been demonstrated in family members of patients with NIDDM (47, 151, 186) and in women who have had gestational diabetes (220), a condition that reverts to normal glucose tolerance following delivery but is a predictor of subsequent development of NIDDM.

In fact, it is likely that NIDDM is a heterogeneous disorder that ultimately may be shown to have many different genetic causes. Some of these causes may primarily involve defects in insulin action, whereas for others impairments of pancreatic β-cell function may be primary. Relatively rare individuals and families have been described with disorders of glucose metabolism secondary to defined abnormalities of the cellular insulin receptor, although these syndromes do not have phenotypic characteristics typical of NIDDM (207).

At least two genetic markers have now been identified with the development of MODY, an NIDDM syndrome that is an autosomal disorder appearing relatively early in life. One group of families with this disorder has genetic mutations of the glucokinase gene located on chromosome 7 (59). Glucokinase is the key glucose-metabolizing enzyme located in the pancreatic B cell which is responsible for generating the initial signal for glucose-mediated insulin secretion (119, 157). A genetic marker has been identified on chromosome 20 in another large kindred with this syndrome (15). Although the specific gene has not yet been identified, individuals who carry the genetic marker but do not yet have diabetes have a demonstrable impairment of insulin secretion but no measurable defect of insulin action (81). Study of the polymorphism of a repeat segment of the glucokinase gene has identified an allele associated with the presence of NIDDM in African Americans (32). Figure 7.12 illustrates the interaction of this marker with the age at onset of NIDDM in this population. Thus in these types of NIDDM, genetic factors associated with impaired pancreatic β-cell function appear to be the cause.

A hypothetical scheme illustrating key events in the development of NIDDM as a function of the interaction between insulin resistance and impaired insulin secretion is shown in Figure 7.13. In this scheme, factors such as aging, obesity, hypertension, and diminished physical activity, which are associated with insulin resistance, will tend to cause mild hyperglycemia. Hyperglycemia feeds back to provide ongoing stimulation to pancreatic β-cell function. When pancreatic β-cell function is normal, there is adaptation to the factors contributing to insulin resistance resulting in hyperinsulinemia and maintenance of normal glucose levels. However, in individuals who have a defect of pancreatic β-cell function, there is a maladaptive response with further deterioration of function and impaired insulin secretion, which worsens the hyperglycemia. Chronic hyperglycemia in turn appears to be a contributing factor to both impaired β-cell function and insulin resistance (108, 179–181), thus setting up a vicious cycle in which hyperglycemia is the net outcome. One possible mechanism for an effect of chronic hyperglycemia to impair pancreatic β-cell function is down-regulation of the β-cell glucose transporter Glut 2 (212). Such down-regulation could decrease the amount of glucose available for β-cell metabolism and the generation of signals for insulin secretion.

Metabolic Consequences of Diabetes Mellitus

Chronic, mild hyperglycemia may have few direct effects on overall body function. However, as hyperglycemia worsens, a series of events can ensue that may have devastating consequences, ultimately resulting in death. Marked hyperglycemia can cause an osmotic diuresis with loss of salt and water leading to volume

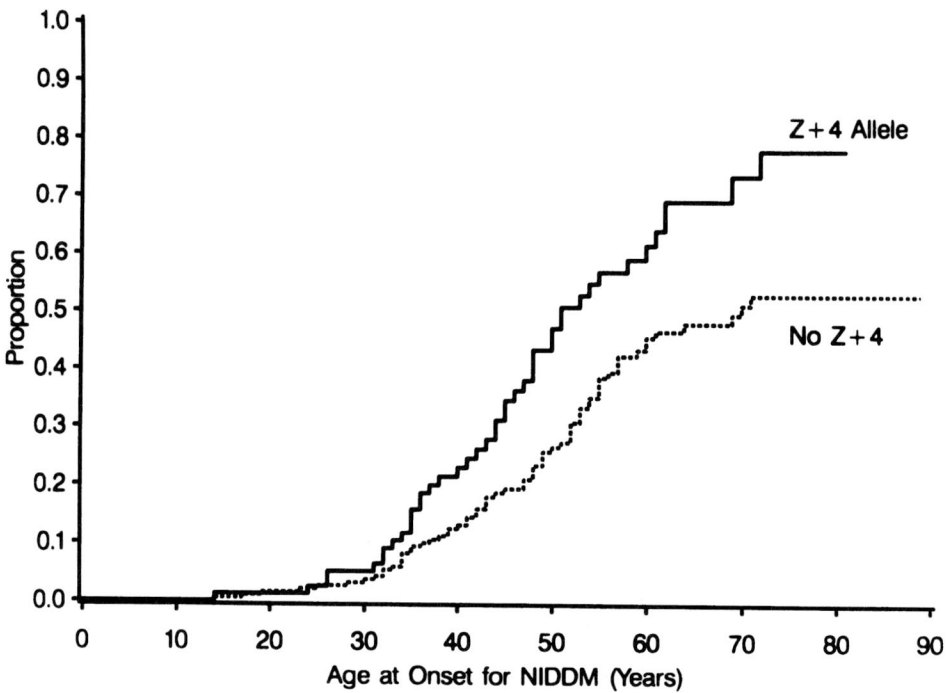

FIG. 7.12. Prevalence of NIDDM by age of onset among a group of 112 African Americans with or without the Z + 4 glucokinase allele (log-survival test, $P = 0.0014$). [From Chiu et al. (32) with permission.]

depletion, activation of stress hormones, and greater hyperglycemia. If volume depletion is not corrected, renal perfusion is compromised and the ability to excrete excess glucose is markedly diminished. This can lead to gross elevation of glucose levels and hyperosmolarity, leading to coma and even death. This syndrome of very poor diabetes control is termed *hyperosmolar non-ketotic coma* and is particularly prevalent in elderly individuals (135).

This condition appears to be an extreme example of stress hyperglycemia, because it is usually associated with a major stressful illness. As illustrated in Figure 7.14, people with NIDDM are more sensitive to the hyperglycemic effect of epinephrine than nondiabetic controls (152). Thus individuals with relatively stable,

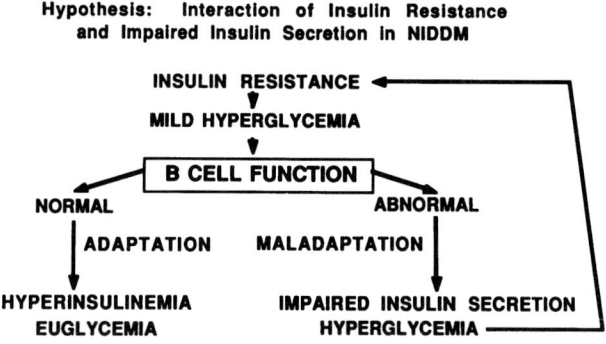

FIG. 7.13. Theoretical model describing the feedback effect of insulin resistance in individuals with normal pancreatic β-cell function, resulting in maintenance of euglycemia. In contrast, individuals with impaired pancreatic β-cell function are unable to adapt to insulin resistance, resulting in a vicious cycle in which hyperglycemia develops and leads to further deterioration of β-cell function and more severe insulin resistance.

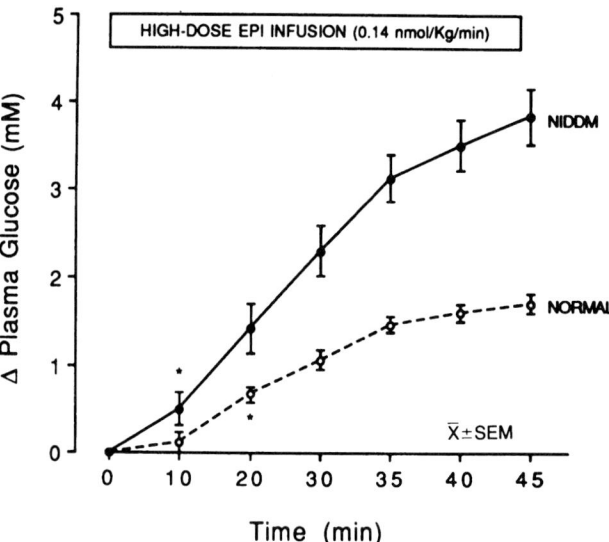

FIG. 7.14. Comparison of the increase from baseline of plasma glucose levels during infusion of epinephrine (EPI) in patients with NIDDM (n = 9) and normal subjects (n = 20). In addition to having a greater overall hyperglycemic response, the first significant increase of plasma glucose (*) occurred earlier in the NIDDM patients. [From Ortiz-Alonso et al. (152) with permission.]

moderate hyperglycemia may be at particular risk for metabolic decompensation when stress hormones are released during an acute illness. Normal individuals adapt to epinephrine-induced hyperglycemia by augmenting β-cell function to overcome the inhibitory effects of catecholamines on β-cells. However, pancreatic β-cell function is already severely impaired in people with NIDDM, and these individuals are not able to compensate for the further inhibitory effects of epinephrine.

Even moderate hyperglycemia may have a variety of adverse long-term effects on body function. Diminished cellular replicative capacity in vitro has been described in patients with diabetes mellitus (8, 65, 133, 215). Although this finding is somewhat variable and its long-term significance unclear, it is one factor to be considered as a possible explanation for an apparent acceleration of the aging process in people with diabetes.

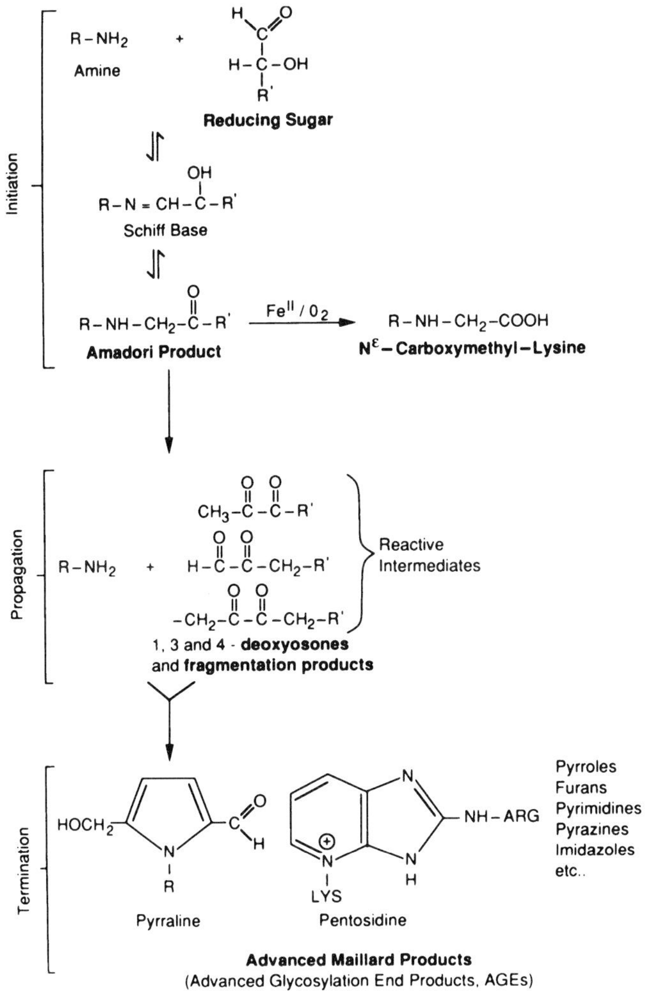

There has been substantial interest in the adverse effects of long-term exposure to elevated glucose levels on a number of important structural and functional proteins. Glucose can interact with proteins nonenzymatically to cause glycosylation. Accumulation of glycosylated proteins has been postulated to be a contributing factor to many aspects of aging (28, 131). Glycosylation of hemoglobin, for example, alters hemoglobin's physical structure and functional characteristics. The degree of glycosylation reflects the exposure of hemoglobin to glucose during the life span of the red blood cells in vivo. Measurement of glycosylated hemoglobin has been used clinically to assess overall glycemia during several weeks prior to the blood sample. In nondiabetic people, the glycosylated hemoglobin level increases with age (69), providing evidence that the age-related decrease of glucose tolerance in humans represents sufficient hyperglycemia over time to influence hemoglobin glycosylation. Similarly, an increase of protein glycosylation has been observed in some tissues of aging rats (147, 148).

Glycosylated proteins may undergo subsequent additional molecular rearrangements to form what have been described as advanced glycosylation end-products (23, 28, 131), as illustrated in Figure 7.15. One such product is pyrraline, which accumulates in tissues of diabetic humans and experimental animals and has been found in a number of tissues that are sites for long-term diabetes complications (128). Another product, pentosidine, has been identified from human collagen and is derived from pentose metabolism. As illustrated in Figure 7.16, collagen pentosidine increases as a function of

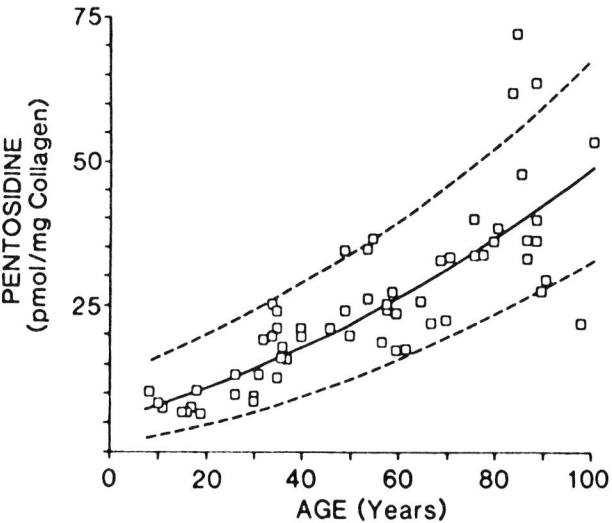

FIG. 7.15. General scheme for the process of nonenzymatic glycosylation and subsequent formation of advanced glycosylation end-products resulting from the Maillard reaction. [From Monnier (131) with permission.]

FIG. 7.16. Relationship between age and level of pentosidine in collagen among nondiabetic subjects from whom skin samples were obtained at autopsy. The regression line for this relationship and 95% confidence interval are shown ($y = 0.002 x^2 + 0.214x + 5.69$, $r = 0.86$). [From Sell and Monnier (191) with permission.]

age in nondiabetic individuals (191). Pentosidine accumulation appears to be greatest in some individuals with diabetes and associated end-stage renal disease. Because of the cross-linked nature of the proteins affected by these reactions, they have been postulated to contribute to a number of long-term diabetes complications by trapping proteins nonspecifically at the tissue level. Receptors for advanced glycosylation end-products have been identified in macrophages and monocytes. Stimulation of these receptors results in release of cytokines, including interleukin 1 and tumor necrosis factor, which in turn can promote growth responses in cells (214). Recent evidence suggests that such stimulation can also induce production of insulin-like growth factor 1, which could contribute to proliferation of mesenchymal cells (99).

Long-Term Consequences of Diabetes Mellitus

Regardless of its possible mechanism, diabetes mellitus is associated with a wide range of adverse long-term complications. Elderly people with NIDDM are at increased risk for the development of these complications (26, 70, 141, 142), as summarized in Table 7.3. In particular, the risk for cardiovascular disease, including heart attack and stroke, is greater in elderly people with diabetes and contributes to the significant morbidity and increased mortality associated with this condition. Accelerated development of atherosclerosis in this setting appears to result from the interaction of chronic hyperglycemia with multiple other risk factors associated with diabetes, including altered lipid metabolism, hypertension, obesity, and insulin resistance (18, 41, 106, 171). Increased risk for cardiovascular disease is also associated with impaired glucose tolerance, in the absence of overt diabetes mellitus (62, 198). High rates of amputation related to peripheral vascular disease in combination with peripheral neuropathy contribute to diminished quality of life among elderly people with diabetes. Risks of end-stage renal disease and retinal abnormalities leading to loss of vision are also increased in this population. Diabetic neuropathy is common in this population (70), but the epidemiology is not yet sufficiently defined to establish the degree of increased risk. Older people with diabetes mellitus appear to have subtle impairments of cognitive function, not explained by coexistent cerebrovascular disease (134, 158, 173, 213).

Although these risks are well established, there is no clear evidence that treatment of hyperglycemia lowers the risk for these complications among people with NIDDM. Because of the difficulty in measuring the rates of these complications and the long period of time it takes for them to develop, this issue has been difficult to investigate. However, recent data from the Diabetes Control and Complications Trial (DCCT) and the Stockholm Diabetes Intervention Study, trials of intensive diabetes management of young people with insulin-dependent diabetes, have provided clear evidence for a beneficial effect of achieving near-normal glucose levels (39, 175). While these findings cannot be directly extrapolated to older adults with NIDDM, they provide further evidence for the adverse long-term effects of chronic hyperglycemia. Indeed, based on the findings of the DCCT and the body of work linking hyperglycemia with metabolic and structural alterations in tissues subject to diabetes complications, the American Diabetes Association has concluded that achievement of euglycemia should be a treatment goal for all patients with diabetes mellitus (4). It is hoped that future work will provide clear treatment guidelines to minimize the substantial risks for long-term complications among the large population of older adults who have diabetes mellitus.

TABLE 7.3. *Important Long-Term Complications of Diabetes in the Elderly and Their Relative Risk**

Complication	Relative Risk
Macrovascular disease	
Coronary heart disease	2
Stroke	2
Amputation	10
Capillary microangiopathy	
Retinopathy–macular edema	1.4†
Renal disease	2
Neuropathy	?

*Risk compared to people of the same age who do not have diabetes [see Carter Center (26)]. †Relative risk for blindness.

REFERENCES

1. ADELMAN, R. Secretion of insulin during aging. *J. Am. Geriatr. Soc.* 37: 983–990, 1989
2. ADER, M., G. PACINI, Y. J. YANG, and R. N. BERGMAN. Importance of glucose per se to intravenous glucose tolerance. *Diabetes* 34: 1092–1103, 1985.
3. AGNER, E., B. THORSTEINSSON, and M. ERIKSEN. Impaired glucose tolerance and diabetes mellitus in elderly subjects. *Diabetes Care* 5: 600–604, 1982.
4. American Diabetes Association. Position statement: implications of the Diabetes Control and Complications Trial. *Diabetes* 42: 1555–1558, 1993.
5. ANDERSON, E. A., R. P. HOFFMAN, T. W. BALON, C. A. SINKEY, and A. L. MARK. Hyperinsulinemia produces both sympathetic neural activation and vasodilation in normal humans. *J. Clin. Invest.* 87: 2246–2252, 1991.
6. ANDRES, R. Aging and diabetes. *Med. Clin. North Am.* 55: 835–846, 1971.
7. ANDRES, R. and J. D. TOBIN. Aging and the disposition of glucose. *Adv. Exp. Med. Biol.* 61: 239–249, 1975.
8. ARCHER, F. J. and R. KAYE. Aging of diabetic and nondiabetic

skin fibroblasts in vitro: life span and sequential growth curves. *J. Gerontol.: Med. Sci.* 44: M93–M99, 1989.
9. BARNARD, R. J., LAWANI, L. O. MARTIN, D. A. YOUNGREN, J. F., SINGH, R. and S. H. SCHECK. Effects of maturation and aging on the skeletal muscle glucose transport system. *Am. J. Physiol.* 262 (*Endocrinol. Metab.* 25): E619–E626, 1992.
10. BARNETT, A. H., C. EFF, R. D. LESLIE, and D. A. PYKE. Diabetes in identical twins: a study of 200 pairs. *Diabetologia* 20: 87–93, 1981.
11. BARON, A. D., G. BRECHTEL, P. WALLACE, and S. V. EDELMAN. Rates and tissue sites of non-insulin- and insulin-mediated glucose uptake in humans. *Am. J. Physiol.* 255 (*Endocrinol. Metab.* 18): E769–E774, 1988.
12. BEARD, J. C., J. B. HALTER, J. D. BEST, M. A. PFEIFER, and D. PORTE, JR. Dexamethasone-induced insulin resistance enhances B cell responsiveness to glucose level in normal men. *Am. J. Physiol.* 247 (*Endocrinol. Metabl.* 10): E592–E596, 1984.
13. BEARD, J. C., W. K. WARD, J. B. WALLUM, and D. PORTE, JR. Relationship of islet function to insulin action in human obesity. *J. Clin. Endocrinol. Metab.* 65: 59–64, 1987.
14. BELL, G. I., Molecular defects in diabetes mellitus. *Diabetes* 40: 413–422, 1991.
15. BELL, G. I., K. S. XIANG, M. V. NEWMAN, S. WU, L. G. WRIGHT, S. S. FAJANS, R. S. SPIELMAN, and N. J. COX. Gene for non-insulin-dependent diabetes mellitus (maturity-onset diabetes of the young subtype) is linked to DNA polymorphism on human chromosome 20q. *Proc. Natl. Acad. Sci. U.S.A.* 88: 1484–1488, 1991.
16. BERGER, D., R. C. CROWTHER, J. C. FLOYD, S. PEK, and S. S. FAJANS. Effect of age on fasting plasma levels of pancreatic hormones in man. *J. Clin. Endocrinol. Metab.* 47: 1183–1189, 1978.
17. BERGMAN, R. N. Lilly lecture 1989. Toward physiological understanding of glucose tolerance. Minimal-model approach. *Diabetes* 38: 1512–1527, 1989.
18. BIERMAN, E. Atherogenesis in diabetes. *Arterioscler. Thromb.* 12: 647, 1992.
19. BINNERTS, A., J. H. P. WILSON, and S. W. J. LAMBERTS. The effects of human growth hormone administration in elderly adults with recent weight loss. *J. Clin. Endocrinol. Metab.* 67: 1312–1316, 1988.
20. BODKIN, M. L., METZGER, B. L. and B. C. HANSEN. Hepatic glucose production and insulin sensitivity preceding diabetes in monkeys. *Am. J. Physiol.* 256 (*Endocrinol. Metab.* 19): E676–E681, 1989.
21. BOLINDER, J., H. LITHELL, E. SKARFORS, and P. ARNER. Effects of obesity, hyperinsulinemia and glucose intolerance on insulin action in adipose tissue of sixty-year-old men. *Diabetes* 35: 282–290, 1986.
22. BOLINDER, J., J. OSTMAN, and P. ARNER. Influence of aging on insulin receptor binding and metabolic effects of insulin on human adipose tissue. *Diabetes* 32: 959–964, 1983.
23. BROWNLEE, M., A. CERAMI, and H. VLASSARA. Advanced glycosylation endproducts in tissue and the biochemical basis of diabetic complications. *N. Engl. J. Med.* 318: 1315–1321, 1988.
24. BURCH, P. T., D. K. BERNER, A. LEONTIRE, A. VOGIN, B. M. MATSCHINSKY, and F. M. MATSCHINSKY. Metabolic adaption of pancreatic islet tissue in aging rats. *J. Gerontol.* 39: 2–6, 1984.
25. BUSBY, M. J., M. F. BELLANTONI, J. D. TOBIN, D. C. MULLER, S. D. KAFONEK, M. R. BLACKMAN, and R. ANDRES. Glucose tolerance in women: the effects of age, body composition, and sex hormones. *J. Am. Geriatr. Soc.* 40: 497–502, 1992.
26. Carter Center of Emory University. Closing the gap: the problem of diabetes mellitus in the United States. *Diabetes Care* 8: 391–406, 1985.
27. CASAD, R. C., JR. and R. C. ADELMAN. Aging enhances inhibitory action of somatostatin in rat pancreas. *Endocrinology* 130: 2420–2422, 1992.
28. CERAMI, A. Glucose as a mediator of aging. *J. Am. Geriatr. Soc.* 33: 626–634, 1985.
29. CHEN, M., R. N. BERGMAN, G. PACINI, and D. PORTE, JR. Pathogenesis of age-related glucose intolerance in man: insulin resistance and decreased β-cell function. *J. Clin. Endocrinol. Metab.* 60: 13–20, 1985.
30. CHEN, M., J. B. HALTER, and D. PORTE, JR. Plasma catecholamines, dietary carbohydrate, and glucose intolerance: a comparison beteween young and old men. *J. Clin. Endocrinol. Metab.* 62: 1193–1198, 1986.
31. CHEN, M., J. B. HALTER, and D. PORTE, JR. The role of dietary carbohydrate in the decreased glucose tolerance of the elderly. *J. Am. Geriatr. Soc.* 35: 417–424, 1987.
32. CHIU, K. C., M. A. PROVINCE, and M. A. PERMUTT. Glucokinase gene is genetic marker for NIDDM in American blacks. *Diabetes* 41: 843–849, 1992.
33. COON, P. J., E. BLEECKER, D. DRINKWATER, D. MEYERS, and A. P. GOLDBERG. Effects of body composition and exercise capacity on glucose tolerance, insulin, and lipoprotein lipids in healthy older men: a cross-section and longitudinal intervention study. *Metabolism* 38: 1201–1209, 1989.
34. COON, P. J., E. M. ROGUS, D. DRINKWATER, D. C. MULLER, and A. P. GOLDBERG. Role of body fat distribution in the decline in insulin sensitivity and glucose tolerance with age. *J. Clin. Endocrinol. Metab.* 75: 1125–1132, 1992.
35. CUTLER, R. G. B. J. DAVIS, D. K. INGRAM, and G. S. ROTH. Plasma concentration of glucose, insulin, and percent glycosylated hemoglobin are unaltered by food restriction in rhesus and squirrel monkeys. *J. Gerontol. Biol. Sci.* 47: B9–B12, 1992.
36. DALY, P. A., and L. LANDSBERG. Hypertension in obesity and NIDDM. Role of insulin and sympathetic nervous system. *Diabetes Care* 14: 240–248, 1991.
37. DAMSGAARD, E. M. O. K. FABER, A. FROLAND, A. GREEN, M. HAUGE, N. V. HOLM, and S. IVERSEN. Prevalence of fasting hyperglycemia and known non-insulin-dependent diabetes mellitus classified by plasma C- peptide: Fredericia survey of subjects 60–74 yr. old. *Diabetes Care* 10: 26–32, 1987.
38. DAVIDSON, M. B. The effect of aging on carbohydrate metabolism: a review of the English literature and a practical approach to the diagnosis of diabetes mellitus in the elderly. *Metabolism* 28: 688–705, 1979.
39. DCCT Research Group. Outcomes of the diabetes control and complications trial (DCCT). *N. Engl. J. Med.* 329: 977–986, 1993.
40. DEFRONZO, R. A. Glucose intolerance and aging: evidence for tissue insensitivity to insulin. *Diabetes* 28: 1095–1101, 1979.
41. DEFRONZO, R. A. and E. FERRANNINI. Insulin resistance. A multifaceted syndrome responsible for NIDDM, obesity, hypertension, dyslipidemia, and atherosclerotic cardiovascular disease. *Diabetes Care* 14: 173–194, 1991.
42. DINNEEN, S., J. GERICH, and R. RIZZA. Carbohydrate metabolism in non-insulin-dependent diabetes mellitus. *N. Engl. J. Med.* 327: 707–713, 1992.
43. DODT, C., J. DITTMANN, J. HRUBY, E. SPÄTH-SCHWALBE, J. BORN, R. SCHÜTTLER, and H. L. FEHM. Different regulation of adrenocorticotropin and cortisol secretion in young, mentally healthy elderly and patients with senile dementia of Alzheimer's type. *J. Clin. Endocrinol. Metab.* 72: 272–276, 1991.
44. DRAZNIN, B., J. P. STEINBERG, and K. E. SUSSMAN. The nature of insulin secretory defect in aging rats. *Diabetes* 34: 1168–1173, 1985.
45. ELAHI, D., D. K. ANDERSEN, D. C. MULLER, J. D. TOBIN, J. C. BROWN, and R. ANDRES. The enteric enhancement of glucose-

stimulated insulin release: the role of GIP in aging, obesity, and non-insulin-dependent diabetes mellitus. *Diabetes* 33: 950–957, 1984.

46. ELAHI, D., D. C. MULLER, S. P. TZANKOFF, R. ANDRES, and J. D. TOBIN. Effect of age and obesity on fasting levels of glucose, insulin, glucagon, and growth hormone in man. *J. Gerontol.* 37: 385–391, 1982.

47. ERIKSSON, J., A. FRANSSILA-KALLUNKI, A. EKSTRAND, C. SALORANTA, E. WIDEN, C. SCHALIN, and L. GROOP. Early metabolic defects in persons at increased risk for non-insulin-dependent diabetes mellitus. *N. Engl. J. Med.* 321: 337–343, 1989.

48. EZAKI, O., N. FUKUDA, and H. ITAKURA. Role of two types of glucose transporters in enlarged adipocytes from aged obese rats. *Diabetes* 39: 1543–1549, 1990.

49. EZAKI, O., M. HIGUCHI, H. NAKATSUKA, K. KAWANAKA, and H. ITAKURA. Exercise training increases glucose transporter content in skeletal muscles more efficiently from aged obese rats than young lean rats. *Diabetes* 41: 920–926, 1992.

50. FELDMAN, J. M., and J. W. PLONK. Effect of age on intravenous glucose tolerance and insulin secretion. *J. Am. Geriatr. Soc.* 24: 1–3, 1976.

51. FERRANNINI, E., G. BUZZIGOLI, R. BONADONNA, M. A. GIORICO, M. OLEGGINI, L. GRAZIADEI, R. PEDRINELLI, L. BRANDI, and S. BEVILACQUA. Insulin resistance in essential hypertension. *N. Engl. J. Med.* 317: 350–357, 1987.

52. FINK, R. I., O. G. KOLTERMAN, J. GRIFFIN, and J. M. OLEFSKY. Mechanisms of insulin resistance in aging. *J. Clin. Invest.* 71: 1523–1535, 1983.

53. FINK, R. I., O. G. KOLTERMAN, M. KAO, and J. M. OLEFSKY. The role of the glucose transport system in the postreceptor defect in insulin action associated with human aging. *J. Clin. Endocrinol. Metab.* 58: 721–725, 1984.

54. FINK, R. I., R. R. REVERS, O. G. KOLTERMAN, and J. M. OLEFSKY. The metabolic clearance of insulin and the feedback inhibition of insulin secretion are altered with aging. *Diabetes* 34: 275–280, 1985.

55. FINK, R. I., P. WALLACE, and J. M. OLEFSKY. Effects of aging on glucose-mediated glucose disposal and glucose transport. *J. Clin. Invest.* 77: 2034–2041, 1986.

56. FRANSSILA-KALLUNKI, A, C. SCHALIN-JANTTI, and L. GROOP. Effect of gender on insulin resistance associated with aging. *Am. J. Physiol.* 263 (*Endocrinol. Metab.* 26): E780–E785, 1992.

57. FRENCH, L. R., F. C. GOETZ, A. M. MARTINEZ, J. R. BOEN, S. A. BUSHHOUSE, and J. M. SPRAFKA. Association between stimulated plasma C-peptide and age: the Wadena City health study. *J. Am. Geriatr. Soc.* 40: 309–315, 1992.

58. FRENCH, L. R., J. R. BOEN, A. M. MARTINEZ, S. A. BUSHHOUSE, J. M. SPRAFKA, and F. C. GOETZ. Population-based study of impaired glucose tolerance and type II diabetes in Wadena, Minnesota. *Diabetes* 39: 1131–1137, 1990.

59. FROGUEL, P., H. ZOUALI, N. VIONNET, G. VELHO, M. VAXILLAIRE, F. SUN, S. LESAGE, M. STOFFEL, J. TAKEDA, P. PASSA, A. PERMUTT, J. S. BECKMANN, G. I. BELL, and D. COHEN. Familial hyperglycemia due to mutations in glucokinase. *N. Engl. J. Med.* 328: 397–702, 1993.

60. FRONTONI, S., L. OHMAN, J. R. HAYWOOD, R. A. DEFRONZO, and L. ROSSETTI. In vivo insulin action in genetic models of hypertension. *Am. J. Physiol.* 262 (*Endocrinol. Metab.* 25): E191–E196, 1992.

61. FUKAGAWA, N. K., K. L. MINAKER, V. R. YOUNG, D. E. MATTHEWS, D. M. BIER, and J. W. ROWE. Leucine metabolism in aging humans: effect of insulin and substrate availability. *Am. J. Physiol.* 256 (*Endocrinol. Metab.* 19): E288–E294, 1989.

62. FULLER, J., M. J. SHIPLEY, G. ROSE, R. J. JARRETT, and H. KEEN. Coronary heart disease risk and impaired glucose tolerance: the Whitehall study. *Lancet* 1: 1373–1376, 1980.

63. GANS, R. O. B., H. J. G. BILO, W. W. A. V. MAARSCHALKERWEERD, R. J. HEINE, J. P. NAUTA, and A. J. M. DONKER. Exogenous insulin augments in healthy volunteers the cardiovascular reactivity to noradrenaline but not to angiotensin II. *J. Clin. Invest.* 88: 512–518, 1991.

64. GOLD, G., G. M. REAVEN, and E. P. REAVEN. Effect of age on proinsulin and insulin secretory patterns in isolated rat islets. *Diabetes* 30: 77–82, 1981.

65. GOLDSTEIN, S., R. J. MOERMAN, J. S. SOELDNER, R. E. GLEASON, and D. M. BARNETT. Chronologic and physiologic age affect replicative life-span of fibroblasts from diabetic, pre-diabetic and normal donors. *Science* 199: 781–782, 1978.

66. GOODMAN, M. N., S. M. DLUZ, M. A. MCELANEY, E. BELUR, and N. B. RUDERMAN. Glucose uptake and insulin sensitivity in rat muscle: changes during 3–96 weeks of age. *Am. J. Physiol.* 244 (*Endocrinol. Metab.* 7): E93–E100, 1983.

67. GOODMAN, M., J. W. LEITNER, K. E. SUSSMAN, and B. DRAZNIN. Insulin secretion in aging: studies with sequential gating of secretion vesicle margination and lysis. *Endocrinology* 119: 827–832, 1986.

68. GOODYEAR, L. J., M. F. HIRSHMAN, P. M. VALYOU, and E. S. HORTON. Glucose transporter number, function, and subcellular distribution in rat skeletal muscle after exercise training. *Diabetes* 41: 1091–1099, 1992.

69. GRAF, R., J. B. HALTER, and D. PORTE, JR. Glycosylated hemoglobin in normal subjects and maturity-onset diabetics. Evidence for a saturable system in man. *Diabetes* 27: 834–839, 1978.

70. GREENE, D. R. Acute and chronic complications of diabetes mellitus in older patients. *Am. J. Med.* 80(suppl. C): 39, 1986.

71. GULVE, E. A., E. J. HENRIKSEN, K. J. RODNICK, J. H. YOUN, and J. O. HOLLOSZY. Glucose transporters and glucose transport in skeletal muscles of 1- to 25-mo-old rats. *Am. J. Physiol.* 264 (*Endocrinol. Metab.* 27): E319–E327, 1993.

72. GUMBINER, B., K. S. POLONSKY, W. F. BELTZ, P. WALLACE, G. BRECHTEL, and R. I. FINK. Effects of aging on insulin secretion. *Diabetes* 38: 1549–1556, 1989.

73. HAFFNER, S. M. Editorial: Insulin and blood pressure: fact or fantasy? *J. Clin. Endocrinol. Metab.* 76: 541–543, 1993.

74. HAFFNER, S. M., M. P. STERN, H. P., HAZUDA, B. D. MITCHELL, and J. K. PATTERSON. Increased insulin concentrations in nondiabetic offspring of diabetic parents. *N. Engl. J. Med.* 319: 1297–1301, 1988.

75. HALTER, J. B. *Diabetes Update: Elderly Patients with Non-Insulin Dependent Diabetes Mellitus.* The Upjohn Company, Kalamazoo, MI: 1990.

76. HALTER, JB, J. C. BEARD, and D. PORTE, JR. Islet function and stress hyperglycemia: plasma glucose and epinephrine interaction. *Am. J. Physiol.* 247 (*Endocrinol. Metab.* 10): E47–E52, 1984.

77. HALTER, J. B., R. J. GRAF, and D. PORTE, JR. Potentiation of insulin secretory responses by plasma glucose levels in man: evidence that hyperglycemia in diabetes compensates for impaired glucose potentiation. *J. Clin. Endocrinol. Metab.* 48: 946–954, 1979.

78. HANSEN, B. C., and N. L. BODKIN. Heterogeneity of insulin responses: phases in the continuum leading to non-insulin-dependent diabetes mellitus. *Diabetologia* 29: 713–719, 1986.

79. HARRIS, M. I. Impaired glucose tolerance in the U.S. population. *Diabetes Care* 12: 464–474, 1989.

80. HARRIS, M. I., W. C. HADDEN, W. C. KNOWLER, and P. H. BENNETT. Prevalence of diabetes and impaired glucose tolerance and plasma glucose levels in U.S. population aged 30–74 yr. *Diabetes* 36: 523–534, 1987.

81. HERMAN, W. H., S. S. FAJANS, F. J. ORTIZ, M. J. SMITH, J. STURIS, G. I. BELL, K. S. POLONSKY, and J. B. HALTER. Abnormal insulin secretion, not insulin resistance, is the genetic or

primary defect of MODY in the RW pedigree. *Diabetes* 43: 40–46, 1994.

82. HERMAN, W. H., P. SINNOCK, E. BRENNER, J. L. BRIMBERRY, D. LANGFORD, A. NAKASHIMA, S. J. SEPE, S. M. TEUTSCH, and R. S. MAZZE. An epidemiologic model for diabetes mellitus: incidence, prevalence, and mortality. *Diabetes Care* 7: 367–371, 1984.

83. HILSTED, J., N. J. CHRISTENSEN, and S. LARSON. Effect of catecholamines and insulin on plasma volume and intravascular mass of albumin in man. *Clin. Sci.* 77: 149–155, 1989.

84. HISSIN, P. J., J. E. FOLEY, L. J. WARDZALA, E. KARNIELI, I. A. SIMPSON, L. B. SALANS, and S. W. CUSHMAN. Mechanism of insulin-resistant glucose transport activity in the enlarged adipose cell of the aged, obese rat. Relative depletion of intracellular glucose transport systems. *J. Clin. Invest.* 70: 780–790, 1982.

85. HOLLENBECK, C. B., W. HASKELL, M. ROSENTHAL, and G. M. REAVEN. Effect of habitual physical activity on regulation of insulin-stimulated glucose disposal in older males. *J. Am. Geriatr. Soc.* 33: 273–277, 1984.

86. HOUMARD, J. A., P. C. EGAN, P. D. NEUFER, J. E. FRIEDMAN, W. S. WHEELER, R. G. ISRAEL, and G. L. DOHM. Elevated skeletal muscle glucose transporter levels in exercise-trained middle-aged men. *Am. J. Physiol.* 261 (*Endocrinol. Metab.* 24): E437–E443, 1991.

87. HOUSTON, M.C. The effects of antihypertensive drugs on glucose intolerance in hypertensive nondiabetics and diabetics. *Am. Heart J.* 115: 640, 1988.

88. JACKSON, R. A., P. M. BLIX, J. A. MATTHEWS, J. B. HAMLING, B. M. DIN, D. C. BROWN, J. BELIN, J. A. H. RUBENSTEIN, and J. D. N. NABARRO. Influences of ageing on glucose homeostasis. *J. Clin. Endocrinol. Metab.* 55: 840–848, 1982.

89. JACKSON, R. A., M. I. HAWA, R. D. ROSHANIA, B. M. SIM, L. DISILVIO, and J. B. JASPAN. Influence of aging on hepatic and peripheral glucose metabolism in humans. *Diabetes* 36: 119–129, 1988.

90. JULIUS, S., T. GUDBRANDSSON, K. JAMERSON, S. T. SHAHAB, and O. ANDERSSON. The hemodynamic link between insulin resistance and hypertension. *J. Hypertens.* 9: 983–986, 1991.

91. KAHN, B. B. Facilitative glucose transporters: regulatory mechanisms and dysregulation in diabetes. *J. Clin. Invest.* 89: 1367–1374, 1992.

92. KAHN, B. B., and J. S. FLIER. Regulation of glucose-transporter gene expression in vitro and in vivo. *Diabetes Care* 13: 548–564, 1990.

93. KAHN, C. R., and M. F. WHITE. The insulin receptor and the molecular mechanism of insulin action. *J. Clin. Invest.* 82: 1151–1156, 1988.

94. KAHN, S. E., V. G. LARSON, J. C. BEARD, K. C. CAIN, G. W. FELLINGHAM, R. S. SCHWARTZ, R. C. VEITH, J. R. STRATTON, M. D. CERQUEIRA, and I. B. ABRASS. Effect of exercise on insulin action, glucose tolerance, and insulin secretion in aging. *Am. J. Physiol.* 258 (*Endocrinol. Metab.* 21): E937–E943, 1990.

95. KAHN, S. E., V. G. LARSON, R. S. SCHWARTZ, J. C. BEARD, K. C. CAIN, G. W. FELLINGHAM, J. R. STRATTON, M. D. CERQUEIRA, and I. B. ABRASS. Exercise training delineates the importance of B-cell dysfunction to the glucose intolerance of human aging. *J. Clin. Endocrinol. Metab.* 74: 1336–1342, 1992.

96. KAISER, F. E., A. J. SILVER, and J. E. MORLEY. The effect of recombinant human growth hormone on malnourished older individuals. *J. Am. Geriatr. Soc.* 39: 235–240, 1991.

97. KERN, M., P. L. DOLAN, R. S. MAZZEO, J. A. WELLS, and G. L. DOHM. Effect of aging and exercise on GLUT-4 glucose transporters in muscle. *Am. J. Physiol.* 263 (*Endocrinol. Metab.* 26): E362–E367, 1992.

98. KIRITSY-ROY, J. A., J. B. HALTER, S. M. GORDON, M. J. SMITH, and L. C. TERRY. Role of the central nervous system in hemodynamic and sympathoadrenal responses to cocaine in rats. *J. Pharmacol. Exp. Ther.* 255: 154–160, 1990.

99. KIRSTEIN, M., C. ASTON, R. HINTZ, and H. VLASSARA. Receptor-specific induction of insulin-like growth factor I in human monocytes by advanced glycosylation end product-modified proteins. *J. Clin. Invest.* 90: 439–446, 1992.

100. KOHRT, W. M., J. P. KIRWAN, M. A. STATEN, R. E. BOUREY, D. S. KING, and J. O. HOLLOSZY. Insulin resistance in aging is related to abdominal obesity. *Diabetes* 42: 273–281, 1993.

101. KOMATSU, M., N. YOKOKAWA, Y. NAGASAWA, I. KOMIYA, T. AIZAWA, N. TAKASU, and T. YAMADA. Gradual delay in glucose-induced first phase insulin secretion by the pancreatic islets of 7 week-, 6 month-, and 1 year-old rats. *J. Gerontol.: Biol. Sci.* 46: B59–B64, 1991.

102. KONO, S., H. KUZUYA, M. OKAMOTO, H. NISHIMURA, A. KOSAKI, T. KAKEHI, M. OKAMOTO, G. INOUE, I. MAEDA, and H. IMURA. Changes in insulin receptor kinase with aging in rat skeletal muscle and liver. *Am. J. Physiol.* 259 (*Endocrinol. Metab.* 22): E27–E35, 1990.

103. KOSAKA, K., Y. MIZUNO, and T. KUZUYA. Reproducibility of the oral glucose tolerance test and the rice-meal test in mild diabetics. *Diabetes* 15: 901–904, 1966.

104. LANDSBERG, L. Diet, obesity and hypertension: an hypothesis involving insulin, the sympathetic nervous system, and adaptive thermogenesis. *Q. J. Med.* 61: 1081–1090, 1986.

105. LANG, D. A., D. R. MATTHEWS, J. PETO, and R. C. TURNER. Cyclic oscillations of basal plasma glucose and insulin concentrations in human beings. *N. Engl. J. Med.* 301: 1023–1027, 1979.

106. LARSSON, B., K. SVARDSUDD, L. WELIN, L. WILHELMSEN, P. BJORNTORP, and G. TIBBLIN. Abdominal adipose tissue distribution, obesity and risk of cardiovascular disease and death: 13 year follow-up of participants in the study of men born in 1913. *Br. Med. J.* 288: 1401–1404, 1984.

107. LAWRENCE, J. C., JR., J. COLVIN, G. D. CARTEE, and J. O. HOLLOSZY. Effects of aging and exercise on insulin action in rat adipocytes are correlated with changes in fat cell volume. *J. Gerontol. Bio. Sci.* 44: B88–B92, 1989.

108. LEAHY, J. L., H. E. COOPER, D. A. DEAL, D. A., and G. C. WEIR. Chronic hyperglycemia is associated with impaired glucose indluence on insulin secretion: a study of normal rats using chronic in vivo glucose infusions. *J. Clin. Invest.* 77: 908–915, 1986.

109. LEMBO, G., R. NAPOLI, B. CAPALDO, G. RENDINA, G., IACCARINO, M. VOLPE, B. TRIMARCO, and L. SACCÀ. Abnormal sympathetic overactivity evoked by insulin in the skeletal muscle of patients with essential hypertension. *J. Clin. Invest.* 90: 24–29, 1992.

110. LILLIOJA, S., D. M. MOTT, B. V. HOWARD, P. H. BENNETT, H. YKI-JARVINEN, D. FREYMOND, B. L. NYOMBA, F. ZURLO, B. SWINBURN, and C. BOGARDUS. Impaired glucose tolerance as a disorder of insulin action. Longitudinal and cross-sectional studies in Pima Indians. *N. Engl. J. Med.* 318: 1217–1225, 1988.

111. LIN, J.-L., T. ASANO, Y. SHIBASAKI, K. TSUKUDA, H. KATAGIRI, H., ISHIHARA, H., TAKAKU, and Y. OKA. Altered expression of glucose transporter isoforms with aging in rats—selective decrease in GluT4 in the fat tissue and skeletal muscle. *Diabetologia* 34: 477–482, 1991.

112. LINARES, O. A., and J. B. HALTER. Sympathochromaffin system activity in the elderly. *J. Am. Geriatr. Soc.* 35: 448–453, 1987.

113. LIPSON, L. G., V. A. BOBRYCKI, M. J. BUSH, G. E. TIETJEN, and A. YOON. Insulin release in aging: studies on adenylate cyclase, phosphodiesterase, and protein kinase in isolated islets of langerhans of the rat. *Endocrinology* 108: 620–624, 1981.

114. LITHELL, H. O. L. Effect of antihypertensive drugs on insulin, glucose, and lipid metabolism. *Diabetes Care* 14: 203–209, 1991.
115. LONNROTH, P., and U. SMITH. Aging enhances the insulin resistance in obesity through both receptor and postreceptor alterations. *J. Clin. Endocrinol. Metab.* 62: 433–437, 1986.
116. MANEATIS, T., R. CONDIE, and G. REAVEN. Effect of age on plasma glucose and insulin responses to a test mixed meal. *J. Am. Geriatr. Soc.* 30: 178–182, 1982.
117. MARCUS, R., G. BUTTERFIELD, L. HOLLOWAY, L. GILLILAND, D. J. BAYLINK, R. L. HINTZ, and B. M. SHERMAN. Effects of short term administration of recombinant human growth hormone to elderly people. *J. Clin. Endocrinol. Metab.* 70: 519–527, 1990.
118. MASORO, E. J., R. J. M. MCCARTER, M. S. KATZ, and C. A. MCMAHAN. Dietary restriction alters characteristics of glucose fuel use. *J. Gerontol.: Biol. Sci.* 47: B202–B208, 1992.
119. MATSCHINSKY, F. M. Glucokinase as glucose sensor and metabolic signal generator in pancreatic β-cells and hepatocytes. *Diabetes* 39: 647–652, 1990.
120. MCDONALD, G. W., G. F. FISHER, and C. BURNHAM. Reproducibility of the oral glucose tolerance test. *Diabetes* 14: 473–480, 1965.
121. MCGUIRE, E. A., J. D. TOBIN, M. BERMAN, and R. ANDRES. Kinetics of native insulin in diabetic, obese, and aged men. *Diabetes* 28: 110–120, 1979.
122. MENEILLY, G. S., D. ELAHI, K. L. MINAKER, K. L., and J. W. ROWE. The dawn phenomenon does not occur in normal elderly subjects. *J. Clin. Endocrinol. Metab.* 63: 292–296, 1986.
123. MENEILLY, G. S., D. ELAHI, K. L. MINAKER, A. L. SCLATER, and J. W. ROWE. Impairment of noninsulin-mediated glucose disposal in the elderly. *J. Clin. Endocrinol. Metab.* 63: 566–571, 1989.
124. MENEILLY, G. S., K. L. MINAKER, D. ELAHI, and J. W. ROWE. Insulin action in aging man: evidence for tissue-specific differences at low physiologic insulin levels. *J. Gerontol.* 42: 196–201, 1987.
125. METZ, S. A., J. B. HALTER, and R. P. ROBERTSON. Induction of defective insulin secretion and impaired glucose tolerance by clonidine: selective stimulation of metabolic alpha-adrenergic pathways. *Diabetes* 27: 554–562, 1978.
126. MEYERS, D. A., A. P. GOLDBERG, M. L. BLEECKER, P. J. COON, D. T., DRINKWATER, and E. R. BLEECKER. Relationship of obesity and physical fitness to cardiopulmonary and metabolic function in healthy older men. *J. Gerontol.: Med. Sci.* 46: M57–M65, 1991.
127. MINAKER, K. L., J. W. ROWE, R. TONINO, and J. A. PALLOTTA. Influence of age on clearance of insulin in man. *Diabetes* 31: 851–855, 1982.
128. MIYATA, S., and V. MONNIER. Immunohistochemical detection of advanced glycosylation end products in diabetic tissues using monoclonal antibody to pyrraline. *J. Clin. Invest.* 89: 1102–1112, 1992.
129. MODAN, M., H. HALKIN, S. ALMOG, A. LUSKY, A. ESHKOL, M. SHEFI, A. SHITRIT, and Z. FUCHS. Hyperinsulinemia: a link between hypertension obesity and glucose intolerance. *J. Clin. Invest.* 75: 809–817, 1985.
130. MONDON, C. E., C. SIMS, C. B. DOLKAS, E. P. REAVEN, and G. M. REAVEN. The effect of exercise training on insulin resistance in sedentary year old rats. *J. Gerontol.* 41: 605–610, 1986.
131. MONNIER, V. M. Nonenzymatic glycosylation, the Maillard reaction and the aging process. *J. Gerontol.: Biol. Sci.* 45: B105–B111, 1990.
132. MONTAMAT, S. C. and A. O. DAVIES. Physiological response to isoproterenol and coupling of beta-adrenergic receptors in young and elderly human subjects. *J. Gerontol. Med. Sci.* 44: M100–105, 1989.
133. MOORADIAN, A. D. Tissue specificity of premature aging in diabetes mellitus: the role of cellular replicative capacity. *J. Am. Geriatr. Soc.* 36: 831–839, 1988.
134. MOORADIAN, A. D., K. PERRYMAN, J. FITTEN, G. D. KAVONIAN, and J. E. MORLEY. Cortical function in elderly non-insulin dependent diabetic patients. Behavioral and electrophysiologic studies. *Arch. Intern. Med.* 148: 2369–2372, 1988.
135. MORROW, L. A., W. H. HERMAN, and J. B. HALTER. Diabetes mellitus. In: *Oxford Textbook of Geriatric Medicine*, edited by J. G. Evans and T. F. Williams. Oxford: Oxford University Press, 1992, p. 131–140.
136. MORROW, L. A., G. S. MORGANROTH, W. H. HERMAN, R. N. BERGMAN, and J. B. HALTER. Effects of epinephrine on insulin secretion and action in humans. Interaction with aging. *Diabetes* 42: 307–315, 1993.
137. MORROW, L. A., S. G. ROSEN, and J. B. HALTER. Beta-adrenergic regulation of insulin secretion in the elderly: evidence of heterogeneity of beta-adrenergic responsiveness. *J. Gerontol.: Med. Sci.* 46: M108–M113, 1991.
138. MULLER, D. C., D. ELAHI, R. E. PRATLEY, J. D. TOBIN, and R. ANDRES. An epidemiological test of the hyperinsulinemia-hypertension hypothesis. *J. Clin. Endocrinol. Metab.* 76: 544–548, 1993.
139. MYKKANEN, L., M. LAAKSO, M. UUNSITUPA, and K. PYORALA. Prevalence of diabetes and impaired glucose tolerance in elderly subjects and their association with obesity and family history of diabetes. *Diabetes Care* 13: 1099–1105, 1990.
140. NARIMIYA, M., S. AZHAR, C. B. DOLKAS, C. E. MONDON, C. SIMS, D. W. WRIGHT, and G. M. REAVEN. Insulin resistance in older rats. *Am. J. Physiol.* 246 (*Endocrinol. Metab.* 9): E397–E404, 1984.
141. NATHAN, D. M., D. E. SINGER, J. E. GODINE, C. HODGSON HARRINGTON, and L. C. PERLMUTER. Retinopathy in older type II diabetics. Association with glucose control. *Diabetes* 35: 797–801, 1986.
142. NATHAN, D. M., D. E. SINGER, J. E. GODINE, and L. C. PERLMUTER. Non-insulin-dependent diabetes in older patients: complications and risk factors. *Am. J. Med.* 81: 837–842, 1986.
143. National Diabetes Data Group. Classification and diagnosis of diabetes mellitus and other categories of glucose intolerance. *Diabetes* 28: 1039–1057, 1979.
144. NISHIMURA, H., H. KUZUYA, M. OKAMOTO, Y. YOSHIMASA, K. YAMADA, T. IDA, T. KAKEHI, and H. IMURA. Change of insulin action with aging in conscious rats determined by euglycemic clamp. *Am. J. Physiol.* 254 (*Endocrinol. Metab.* 17): E92–98, 1988.
145. ODIO, M. R., and A. BRODISH. Effects of age on metabolic responses to acute and chronic stress. *Am. J. Physiol.* 254 (*Endocrinol. Metab.* 17): E617–E624, 1988.
146. OHLSON, L. O., B. LARSSON, P. BJORNTORP, H. ERIKSSON, K. SVARDSUDD, L. WELIN, G. TIBBLIN, and L. WILHELMSEN. Risk factors for type 2 (non-insulin-dependent) diabetes mellitus: thirteen and one-half years of follow-up of the participants in a study of Swedish men born in 1913. *Diabetologia* 31: 798–805, 1988.
147. OIMOMI, M., Y. KITAMURA, S. NISHIMOTO, S. MATSUMOTO, H. HATANAKA, and S. BABA. Age-related acceleration of glycation of tissue proteins in rats. *J. Gerontol.* 41: 695–698, 1986.
148. OIMOMI, M., Y. MAEDA, F. HATA, Y. KITAMURA, S. MATSUMOTO, H. HATANAKA, and S. BABA. A study of the age-related acceleration of glycation of tissue proteins in rats. *J. Gerontol.: Biol. Sci.* 43: B98–B101, 1988.
149. OLEFSKY, J. M., and G. M. REAVEN. Effects of age and obesity

on insulin binding to isolated adipocytes. *Endocrinology* 96: 1486–1498, 1975.
150. O'MEARA, N. M., J. STURIS, E. VAN CAUTER, and K. S. POLONSKY. Lack of control by glucose of ultradian insulin secretory oscillations in impaired glucose tolerance and in NIDDM. *J. Clin. Invest.* (in press), 92: 262–271, 1993.
151. O'RAHILLY, S., R. C. TURNER, and D. R. MATTHEWS. Impaired pulsatile secretion of insulin in relatives of patients with non-insulin-dependent diabetes. *N. Engl. J. Med.* 318: 1225–1230, 1988.
152. ORTIZ-ALONSO, F. J., W. H. HERMAN, D. L. ZOBEL, T. J. PERRY, M. J. SMITH, and J. B. HALTER. Effect of epinephrine on pancreatic B-cell and A-cell function in patients with non-insulin dependent diabetes mellitus. *Diabetes* 40: 1194–1202, 1991.
153. PACINI, G., F. BECCARO, A. VALERIO, R. NOSADINI, and G. CREPALDI. Reduced beta-cell secretion and insulin hepatic extraction in health elderly subjects. *J. Am. Geriatr. Soc.* 38: 1283–1289, 1990.
154. PACINI, G., A. VALERIO, F. BECCARO, R. NOSADINI, C. COBELLI, and G. CREPALDI. Insulin sensitivity and beta-cell responsivity are not decreased in elderly subjects with normal OGTT. *J. Am. Geriatr. Soc.* 36: 317–323, 1988.
155. PAGANO, G., M. CASSADER, A. DIANA, E. PISU, C. BOZZO, F. FERRERO, and G. LENTI. Insulin resistance in the aged: the role of the peripheral insulin receptors. *Metabolism* 30: 46–49, 1981.
156. PALMER, J. P., and J. W. ENSINCK. Acute-phase insulin secretion and glucose tolerance in young and aged normal men and diabetic patients. *J. Clin. Endocrinol. Metab.* 41: 498–503, 1975.
157. PERMUTT, M. A., K. C. CHIU, and Y. TANIZAWA. Glucokinase and NIDDM: a candidate gene that paid off. *Diabetes* 41: 1367–1372, 1992.
158. PERLMUTTER, L. C., M. K. HAKAMI, C. HODGSON-HARRINGTON, J. GINSBERG, J. KATZ, D. E. SINGER, and D. M. NATHAN. Decreased cognitive function in aging non-insulin-dependent diabetic patients. *Am. J. Med.* 77: 1043–1048, 1984.
159. PFEIFER, M. A., J. B. HALTER, and D. PORTE, JR. Insulin secretion in diabetes mellitus. *Am. J. Med.* 70: 579–588, 1981.
160. POEHLMAN, E. T., T. L. MCAULIFFE, D. R. VAN HOUTEN, and E. DANFORTH. Influence of age and endurance training on metabolic rate and hormones in healthy men. *Am. J. Physiol.* 259 (*Endocrinol. Metab.* 22): E66–E72, 1990.
161. POLLARE, T., H. LITHELL, and C. BERNE. A comparison of the effects of hydrochlorthiazide and captopril on glucose and lipid metabolism in patients with hypertension. *N. Engl. J. Med.* 321: 868–873, 1989.
162. POLONSKY, K. S., J. LICINIO-PALXAO, B. D. GIVEN, W. PUGH, P. RUE, J. GALLOWAY, T. KARRISON, and B. FRANK. Use of biosynthetic human C-peptide in the measurement of insulin secretion rates in normal volunteers and type I diabetic patients. *J. Clin. Invest.* 77: 98–105, 1986.
163. PORTE, D., JR. β-cells in type II diabetes mellitus. *Diabetes* 40: 166–180, 1991.
164. RATZMANN, K. P., S. WITT, P. HEINKE, and B. SCHULZ. The effect of ageing on insulin sensitivity and insulin secretion in non-obese healthy subjects. *Acta Endocrinol.* 100: 543–549, 1982.
165. REAVEN, E. P., and G. M. REAVEN. Structure and function changes in the endocrine pancreas of aging rats with reference to the modulating effects of exercise and caloric restriction. *J. Clin. Invest.* 68: 75–84, 1981.
166. REAVEN, G. M., N. CHEN, C. HOLLENBECK, and Y.-D. I. CHEN. Effect of age on glucose tolerance and glucose uptake in healthy individuals. *J. Am. Geriatr. Soc.* 37: 735–740, 1989.
167. REAVEN, E., D. CURRY, J. MOORE, and G. REAVEN. Effect of age and environmental factors on insulin release from the perfused pancreas of the rat. *J. Clin. Invest.* 71: 345–350, 1983.
168. REAVEN, E. P., G. GOLD, and G. M. REAVEN. Effect of age on glucose-stimulated insulin release by the b-cell of the rat. *J. Clin. Invest.* 64: 591–599, 1979.
169. REAVEN, E., D. WRIGHT, C. E. MONDON, R. SOLOMON, H. HO, and G. M. REAVEN. Effect of age and diet on insulin secretion and insulin action in the rat. *Diabetes* 32: 175–180, 1983.
170. REAVEN, G. M. Role of insulin resistance in human disease. *Diabetes* 37: 1595–1607, 1988.
171. REAVEN, G. M. Insulin resistance, hyperinsulinemia, hypertriglyceridemia, and hypertension. Parallels between human disease and rodent models. *Diabetes Care* 14: 195–202, 1991.
172. REAVEN, G. M., M. S. GREENFIELD, C. E. MONDON, M. ROSENTHAL, D. WRIGHT, and E. P. REAVEN. Does insulin removal rate from plasma decline with age? *Diabetes* 31: 670–673, 1982.
173. REAVEN, G. M., L. W. THOMPSON, D. NAHUM, and E. HASKINS. Relationship between hyperglycemia and cognitive function in older NIDDM patients. *Diabetes Care* 13: 16–21, 1990.
174. REAVEN, P. D., E. L. BARRETT-CONNOR, and D. K. BROWNER. Abnormal glucose tolerance and hypertension. *Diabetes Care* 13: 119–125, 1990.
175. REICHARD, P., B-Y. NILSSON, and U. ROSENQVIST. The effect of long-term intensified insulin treatment on the development of microvascular complications of diabetes mellitus. *N. Engl. J. Med.* 329: 304–309, 1993.
176. ROBERT, J.-J., J. C. CUMMINS, R. R. WOLFE, M. DURKOT, D. E. MATTHEWS, X. H. ZHAO, D. M. BIER, and V. R. YOUNG. Quantitative aspects of glucose production and metabolism in health elderly subjects. *Diabetes* 31: 203–211, 1982.
177. ROLBAND, G. C., E. D. FURTH, J. M. STADDON, E. M. ROGUS, and A. P. GOLDBERG. Effects of age and adenosine in the modulation of insulin action on rat adipocyte metabolism. *J. Gerontol.: Biol. Sci.* 45: B174–B178, 1990.
178. ROSENTHAL, M., and G. M. ARGOUD. Absence of the dawn glucose rise in nondiabetic men compared by age. *J. Gerontol.: Med. Sci.* 4: M57–M61, 1989.
179. ROSSETTI, L., A. GIACCARI, and R. A. DEFRONZO. Glucose toxicity. *Diabetes Care* 13: 610–630, 1990.
180. ROSSETTI, L., G. I. SHULMAN, W. ZAWALICH, and R. A. DEFRONZO. Effect of chronic hyperglycemia on in vivo insulin secretion in partially pancreatectomized rats. *J. Clin. Invest.* 80: 1037–1044, 1987.
181. ROSSETTI, L., D. SMITH, G. I. SHULMAN, D. PAPACHRISTOU, and R. A. DEFRONZO. Correction of hyperglycemia with phlorizin normalizes tissue sensitivity to insulin in diabetic rats. *J. Clin. Invest.* 79: 1510–1515, 1987.
182. ROWE, J. W., K. L. MINAKER, J. A. PALLOTTA, and J. S. FLIER. Characterization of the insulin resistance of aging. *J. Clin. Invest.* 71: 1581–1587, 1983.
183. ROWE, J. W., J. B. YOUNG, K. L. MINAKER, A. L. STEVENS, J. PALLOTTA, and L. LANDSBERG. Effect of insulin and glucose infusions on sympathetic nervous system activity in normal man. *Diabetes* 30: 219–225, 1981.
184. RUDMAN, D., A. G. FELLER, H. S. NAGRAJ, G. A. GERGANS, P. Y. LALITHA, A. F. GOLDBERG, R. A. SCHLENKER, L. COHN, I. W. RUDMAN, and D. E. MATTSON. Effects of human growth hormone in men over 60 years old. *N. Engl. J. Med.* 323: 1–6, 1990.
185. RUHE, R. C., D. L. CURRY, S. HERRMANN, and R. B. MCDONALD. Age and gender effects on insulin secretion and glucose sensitivity of the endocrine pancreas. *Am. J. Physiol.* 262 (*Regulatory Integrative Comp. Physiol.* 31): R671–R676, 1992.
186. SAAD, M. F., W. C. KNOWLER, D. J. PETTITT, R. G. NELSON, D. M. MOTT, and P. H. BENNETT. The natural history of impaired

glucose tolerance in the Pima Indians. *N. Engl. J. Med.* 319: 1500–1506, 1988.

187. SAAD, M. F., S. LILLIOJA, B. L. NYOMBA, C. CASTILLO, R. FERRARO, M. DEGREGORIO, E. RAVUSSIN, W. C. KNOWLER, P. H. BENNETT, B. V. HOWARD, and C. BOGARDUS. Racial differences in the relation between blood pressure and insulin resistance. *N. Engl. J. Med.* 324: 733–739, 1991.

188. SARTIN, J. L., M. CHAUDHURI, S. FARINA, and R. C. ADELMAN. Regulation of insulin secretion by glucose during aging. *J. Gerontol.* 41: 30–35, 1986.

189. SCARPACE, P. J. Decreased receptor activation with age. Can it be explained by desensitization? *J. Am. Geriatr. Soc.* 36: 1067–1071, 1988.

190. SEALS, D. R., J. M. HAGBERG, W. K. ALLEN, B. F. HURLEY, G. P. DALSKY, A. A. EHSANI, and J. O. HOLLOSZY. Glucose tolerance in young and older athletes and sedentary men. *J. Appl. Physiol.: Respir. Environ. Exercise Physiol.* 56: 1521–1525, 1984.

191. SELL, D. R., and V. M. MONNIER. End-stage renal disease and diabetes catalyze the formation of a pentose-derived crosslink from aging human collagen. *J. Clin. Invest.* 85: 380–384, 1990.

192. SHERMAN, B., C. WYSHAM, and B. PFOHL. Age-related changes in the circadian rhythm of plasma cortisol in man. *J. Clin. Endocrinol. Metab.* 61: 439–443, 1985.

193. SHIMOKATA, H., D. C. MULLER, J. L. FLEG, J. SORKIN, A. W. ZIEMBA, and R. ANDRES. Age as independent determinant of glucose tolerance. *Diabetes* 40: 44–51, 1991.

194. SICREE, R. A., P. Z. SIMMET, H. O. M. KING, and J. S. COVENTRY. Plasma insulin response among Nauruans. Prediction of deterioration in glucose tolerance over 6 years. *Diabetes* 36: 179–186, 1987.

195. SIMONSON, D. D., and R. A. DEFRONZO. Glucagon physiology and aging: evidence for enhanced hapatic sensitivity. *Diabetologia* 25: 1–7, 1983.

196. STAGNER, J. I., E. SAMOLS, and G. C. WEIR. Sustained oscillations of insulin, glucagon and somatostatin from the isolated canine pancreas during exposure to a constant glucose concentration. *J. Clin. Invest.* 65: 939–942, 1980.

197. STARNES, J. W., E. CHEONG, and F. M. MATSCHINSKY. Hormone secretion by isolated perfused pancreas of aging Fischer 344 rats. *Am. J. Physiol.* 260 (*Endocrinol. Metab.* 23): E59–E66, 1991.

198. STERN, M. P., and S. M. HAFFNER. Body fat distribution and hyperinsulinemia as risk factors for diabetes and cardiovascular disease. *Arteriosclerosis* 6: 123, 1986.

199. STOUT, R. W. Insulin as a mitogenic factor: role in the pathogenesis of cardiovascular disease. *Am. J. Med.* 90(suppl. 2A): 62S–65S, 1991.

200. STURIS, J., E. VAN CAUTER, J. D. BLACKMAN, and K. S. POLONSKY. Entrainment of pulsatile insulin secretion by oscillatory glucose infusion. *J. Clin. Invest.* 87: 439–445, 1991.

201. SUPIANO, M. A., R. V. HOGIKYAN, L. A. MORROW, F. J. ORTIZ-ALONSO, W. H. HERMAN, R. N. BERGMAN, and J. B. HALTER. Hypertension and insulin resistance: role of sympathetic nervous system activity. *Am. J. Physiol.* 262 (*Endocrinol. Metab.* 25): E935–E942, 1992.

202. SUPIANO, M. A., R. V. HOGIKYAN, L. A. MORROW, F. J. ORTIZNM-ALONSO, W. H. HERMAN, A. T. GALECKI, and J. B. HALTER. Aging and insulin resistance: role of blood pressure and sympathetic nervous system activity. *J. Gerontol.: Med. Sci.* 48: M237–M243, 1993.

203. SUPIANO, M. A., R. V. HOGIKYAN, A. M. STOLTZ, N. ORSTAN, and J. B. HALTER. Regulation of venous alpha- adrenergic responses in older humans. *Am. J. Physiol.* 260 (*Endocrinol. Metab.* 23): E599–E607, 1991.

204. SUPIANO, M. A., O. A. LINARES, J. B. HALTER, K. M. RENO, and S. G. ROSEN. Functional uncoupling of the platelet alpha$_2$-adrenergic receptor adenylate cyclase complex in the elderly. *J. Clin. Endocrinol. Metab.* 64: 1160–1164, 1987.

205. SUPIANO, M. A., O. A. LINARES, M. J. SMITH, and J. B. HALTER. Age-related differences in norepinephrine kinetics: effect of posture and sodium-restricted diet. *Am. J. Physiol.* 259 (*Endocrinol. Metab.* 22): E422–E431, 1990.

206. TATTERSALL, R. B., and D. A. PYKE. Diabetes in identical twins. *Lancet* 2: 1120, 1972.

207. TAYLOR, S. I. Lessons from patients with mutations in the insulin-receptor gene. *Diabetes* 41: 1473–1490, 1992.

208. TONINO, R. P. Effect of physical training on the insulin resistance of aging. *Am. J. Physiol.* 256 (*Endocrinol. Metab.* 19): E352–E356, 1989.

209. TONINO, R. P., K. L. MINAKER, and J. W. ROWE. Effect of age on systemic delivery of oral glucose in men. *Diabetes Care* 12: 394–398, 1989.

210. TRISCHITTA, V., and G. M. REAVEN. Evidence of a defect in insulin-receptor recycling in adipocytes from older rats. *Am. J. Physiol.* 254 (*Endocrinol. Metab.* 17): E39–E44, 1988.

211. TUOMILEHTO, J., A. NISSINEN, S.-L. KIVELA, J. PEKKANEN, E. KAARSALO, E. WOLF, A. ARO, S. PUNSAR, and M. J. KARVONEN. Prevalence of diabetes mellitus in elderly men aged 65 to 84 years in eastern and western Finland. *Diabetologia* 29: 611–615, 1986.

212. UNGER, R. H. Diabetic hyperglycemia: link to impaired glucose transport in pancreatic β-cells. *Science* 251: 1200–1205, 1991.

213. U'REN, R. C., M. C. RIDDLE, M. D. LEZAK, and M. BENNINGTON-DAVIS. The mental efficiency of the elderly person with type II diabetes mellitus. *J. Am. Geriatr. Soc.* 38: 505–510, 1990.

214. VLASSARA, H., M. BROWNLEE, K. R. MANOGUE, C. A. DINARELLO, and A. PASAGIAN. Cachectin/TNF and IL-1 induced by glucose-modified proteins: role in normal tissue remodeling. *Science* 240: 1546–1548, 1988.

215. VRACKO, R., and B. H. MCFARLAND. Lifespans of diabetic and non-diabetic fibroblasts in vitro: results of replicative determinations. *Exp. Cell Res.* 129: 345–350, 1980.

216. WALTMAN, C., M. R. BLACKMAN, G. P. CHROUSOS, C. RIEMANN, and S. M. HARMAN. Spontaneous and glucocorticoid-inhibited adrenocorticotropic hormone and cortisol secretion are similar in healthy young and old men. *J. Clin. Endocrinol. Metab.* 73: 495–502, 1991.

217. WALTON, C., I. F. GODSLAND, A. J. PROUDLER, C. FELTON, and V. WYNN. Evaluation of four mathematical models of glucose and insulin dynamics with analysis of effects of age and obesity. *Am. J. Physiol.* 262 (*Endocrinol. Metab.* 25): E755–E762, 1992.

218. WANG, J. T., L. T. HO, K. T. TANG, L. M. WANG, Y.-D. I. CHEN, and G. M. REAVEN. Effect of habitual physical activity on age-related glucose intolerance. *J. Am. Geriatr. Soc.* 37: 203–209, 1989.

219. WANG, S. Y., P. A. HALBAN, and J. W. ROWE. Effects of aging on insulin synthesis and secretion: differential effects on preproinsulin messenger RNA levels, proinsulin biosynthesis, and secretion of newly made and preformed insulin in the rat. *J. Clin. Invest.* 81: 176–184, 1988.

220. WARD, W. K., C. L. W. JOHNSTON, J. C. BEARD, T. J. BENEDETTI, J. B. HALTER, and D. PORTE, JR. Insulin resistance and impaired insulin secretion in subjects with histories of gestational diabetes mellitus. *Diabetes* 34: 861–869, 1985.

221. WARRAM, J. H., B. C. MARTIN, A. S. KROLEWSKI, J. S. SOELDNER, and C. R. KAHN. Slow glucose removal rate and hyperinsulinemia precede the development of type II diabetes in the offspring of diabetic patients. *Ann. Intern. Med.* 113: 909–915, 1990.

222. World Health Organization. *WHO Expert Committee on Diabetes Mellitus: Second Report.* Geneva: World Health Organization, Tech. Rep. Ser., no 646, 1980.
223. WINGARD, D. L., P. SINSHEIMER, E. L. BARRETT-CONNOR, and J. B. MCPHILLIPS. Community-based study of prevalence of NIDDM in older adults. *Diabetes Care* 13(suppl. 2): 3–8, 1990.
224. ZEMEL, M. B., J. D. PEULER, J. R. SOWERS, and L. SIMPSON. Hypertension in insulin-resistant Zucker obese rats is independent of sympathetic neural support. *Am. J. Physiol.* 262 (*Endocrinol. Metab.* 25): E368–E371, 1992.
225. ZIMMET, P., and S. WHITEHOUSE. The effect of age on glucose tolerance: studies in a Micronesian population with a high prevalence of diabetes. *Diabetes* 28: 617–623, 1979.

8. Aging, fat metabolism, and adiposity

DARIUSH ELAHI | *Laboratory of Physiology, National Institute on Aging, National Institutes of Health, and Division of Gerontology, University of Maryland & Baltimore VA Medical Center, Baltimore, Maryland*

MARIANNE McALOON DYKE | *Department of Medicine, Beth Israel Hospital, Boston, Massachusetts, and Division of Gerontology, University of Maryland & Baltimore VA Medical Center, Baltimore, Maryland*

REUBIN ANDRES | *Laboratory of Physiology, National Institute on Aging, National Institutes of Health, and Division of Gerontology, University of Maryland & Baltimore VA Medical Center, Baltimore, Maryland*

CHAPTER CONTENTS

Fat Mass
    Direct methods of measuring fat mass
    Indirect methods of measuring fat mass
        Height-weight tables
        Total body density
        Skin-fold measurements
        Isotope dilution
        Total body potassium
        In vivo neutron-activation analysis
        Dual photon absorptiometry
        Bioelectrical impedance analysis
    Measurement of body fat distribution
        Anthropometric measurements
        Computerized tomography and magnetic resonance
    Recommendation on fat mass measurements
Adiposity and Age-Associated Diseases
    Glucose intolerance
    Obesity
    Serum lipoproteins and atherosclerosis

DIFFERENCES IN BODY WEIGHT AND HEIGHT in men and women during aging have been the focus of several population studies in North America. In the United States, the Health Examination Survey (HES, 1960–1962) was a nationwide survey with a probability sample of 7,710 community-dwelling civilians 18–70 years of age. Its successors, the National Health and Nutrition Examination Survey (NHANES) I and II (1, 99), were conducted from 1971 to 1974 and from 1976 to 1980. NHANES I and II included probability samples of more than 20,000 community-dwelling civilians 18–74 years old. The Framingham Heart Study and 4.2 million policies of the life insurance companies also provided time trends in body weight during aging. The Framingham Study began in 1948 with a cohort of 5,209 men and women between the ages of 30 and 62 yr (30). These individuals were recalled and examined every 2 yr thereafter. Policies from 25 insurance companies were pooled and reported in great detail in book form as the *Build Study 1979* (29). Such large-scale, long-term epidemiological studies show trends for the general population.

In order to use height and weight data to assess overweight or severely overweight subjects, it has become internationally accepted to combine these measurements into a single value, the body mass index (BMI), also called the Quetelet Index. It is intuitively obvious that taller individuals will weigh more than shorter individuals when both groups are equally obese or equally lean. This weight is "corrected" for height by comparing wt/ht^2 since it has been shown that weight tends to vary as the square of height in many populations. BMI is generally expressed as kg/m^2.

The BMI is distributed in populations with skewness toward high values. Thus there are no obvious rules along the distribution axis to define such cutpoints as the upper and lower limits of normal weight-for-height or the range of BMIs that should be designated "overweight" or "severe overweight." Yet there are important reasons for designating BMI ranges that can be so classified. Such ranges or cutpoints are needed to compare the prevalence of overweight or severe overweight among populations, to give public health advice regarding healthy weights, and to provide goals for care-givers to follow with patients.

The arbitrary nature of any proposed standards based solely on population distributions must be understood. The limitation of these standards can be accepted in view of the uses to which they are put, as noted above. Alternative methods of arriving at definitions of the obese state will be discussed below. The most widely used standards for defining overweight and severe overweight have come from NHANES II (99). Cutpoints were derived from data on men and women in the 20–29-yr-old range. Sex-specific BMIs between the 85th

TABLE 8.1. *BMI of 20–29-Year-Old Subjects*

	85th Centile	95th Centile
Men	27.8	31.1
Women	27.3	32.3

and 95th centiles were defined as "overweight" and BMIs above the 95th centile were defined as "severe overweight." Thus 15% of men and women in their twenties were defined as being above normal weight, and of these, 5% were defined as severely overweight. The BMIs for these cutpoints are shown in Table 8.1.

In NHANES II, the percentage of overweight and severely overweight Americans in each decade of age up to 65–74 yr reflects the increase in body weight during the adult years of life, at least until the onset of old age, as shown in Table 8.2.

The data show that between the ages of 25 and 55 yr, overweight increases in both white and black men and then decreases in both groups from age 55 to age 74 yr. However, between the ages of 35 and 55 yr there is a greater prevalence of overweight in blacks. In white women, the prevalence of overweight increases from age 25 to age 65 yr and then stabilizes. In black women, the prevalence of overweight is much higher than in white women and increases from 30% for the decade 25–34 yr to 60% for the decade 45–54 yr, double that of white women in the same age group. In general, comparisons of HES, NHANES I, and NHANES II show that the prevalence of overweight is increasing in the United States (Fig. 8.1). It should be noted that these data were collected from a noninstitutionalized population and certainly are not representative of the aged population in nursing homes or other long-term care facilities.

Overweight has also been commonly characterized as the weight-for-height that is 20% over that recommended by the Metropolitan Life Insurance Co. Tables (1). It needs only to be noted here that the percentage of overweight individuals in the U.S. population will be only slightly larger than percentages computed by the use of NHANES II distributions. The mean BMIs of the midpoint of the medium frame for men and women of average height (69–70 in for men and 64–65 in for women) in the 1983 Metropolitan Tables (1), when corrected by height of shoes and weight of indoor clothes (1 in and 5 lb for men; 1 in and 3 lb for women), are 22.4 kg/m² for both men and women. Increasing this value by 20% gives a BMI cutpoint for overweight of 26.9, a value close to the 85th centile cutpoints of 27.8 for men and 27.3 for women.

The current cycle of NHANES data collection (1988–1994) is still in progress. Preliminary results of the first half of this cycle (1988–1991) show a surprisingly large increase of approximately 8% in overweight and severe overweight in men and women in the U.S. population since the NHANES II data. Body weight is clearly much more difficult to control than other risk factors, such as cigarette smoking, dietary change, and blood pressure control.

The prevalence of morbid conditions increases in the obese state. Hypertension, dyslipoproteinemia, and diabetes are more common in overweight individuals than in nonoverweight individuals. In the NHANES, hypertension was defined as systolic blood pressure of 160 mm Hg or higher and diastolic blood pressure of 95 mm Hg or higher. The relative risk of hypertension in adults aged 20–75 yr is threefold higher in overweight than in nonoverweight individuals. Between the ages of 20 and 44 yr and 45 and 75 yr, the relative risk of hypertension in overweight individuals is 5.6 times and 1.9 times higher than in nonoverweight adults, respectively. White overweight men and women have a greater risk of hypertension than blacks. Economic status does not appear to influence the relative risk of hypertension.

The relative risk of hypercholesterolemia (defined as

TABLE 8.2. *NHANES II (1976–80): Percentage of Overweight and Severely Overweight Persons 20–74 Yr of Age by Race, Sex, and Age**

	Men				Women			
	White		Black		White		Black	
Age	Overweight	Severely Overweight	Overweight	Severely Overweight	Overweight	Severely Overweight	Overweight	Severely Overweight
20–24	12.7	4.3	5.5	4.2	9.6	3.4	23.7	4.9
25–34	20.9	6.7	17.5	6.5	17.9	7.5	33.5	16.9
35–44	28.2	8.3	40.9	17.1	24.8	10.3	40.8	26.3
45–54	30.5	10.7	41.4	12.0	29.9	12.2	61.2	21.9
55–64	28.6	8.7	26.0	12.8	34.8	13.5	59.4	23.3
65–74	25.8	8.4	26.4	10.4	36.5	12.2	60.8	26.1

*Overweight = sex-specific BMI ≥ 85% of examinees 20–29 yr of age, excluding pregnant women. Severely Overweight = sex-specific BMI ≥ 95% of examinees 20–29 yr of age, excluding pregnant women.

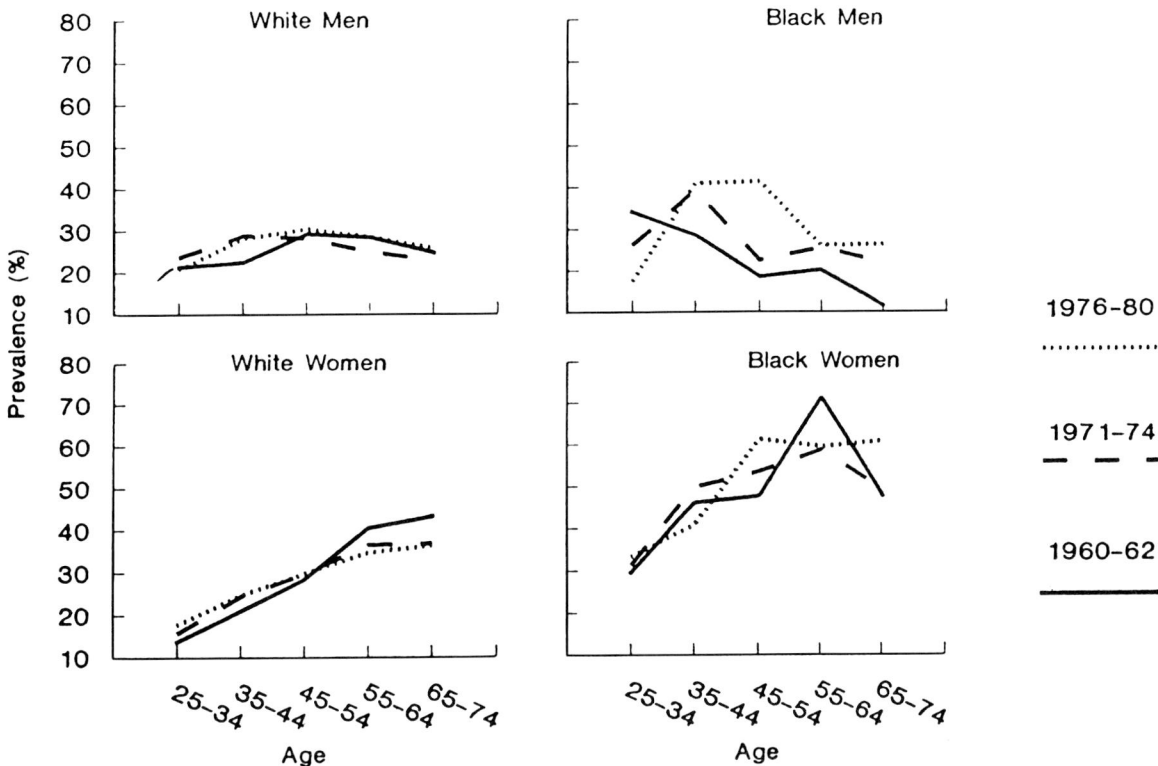

FIG. 8.1. Prevalence of overweight, United States, 1960–1980. Source: Division of Health Examination Statistics, National Center for Health Statistics, Washington, D.C.

a level of 250 mg/dl or higher) in adults aged 20–25 yr is 1.5 times higher in overweight vs. nonoverweight individuals. Between the ages of 20 and 44 yr, the relative risk is 2.1 times higher in overweight vs. nonoverweight adults. In the age range 45–75 yr, overweight is not associated with increased risk of hypercholesterolemia. The risk is higher in overweight black men compared to overweight white men, white women, and black women. Overweight men with low socioeconomic status have an increased risk compared to the other groups. In overweight women, race or socioeconomic status are not associated with an increased risk of hypercholesterolemia.

Compared to white men, the prevalence of diabetes in adults aged 20–75 yr is 30, 70, and 100% higher in white women, black men, and black women, respectively. Diabetes is more prevalent in blacks than in Caucasians. The prevalence in blacks aged 65–74 years is 26% compared to 18% among Caucasians in the same age group. The relative risk of diabetes in adults aged 20–75 yr is threefold higher in overweight vs. nonoverweight individuals. Between the ages of 20 and 44 yr and 45 and 74 yr, the relative risk is 3.8 and 2.1 times higher in overweight than in nonoverweight adults, respectively.

The health implications of overweight and obesity, as reviewed from the above data, generally support a higher relative risk in the aged. It is possible for an individual such as a master athlete (for example, a basketball player or a weight lifter) to be overweight and not obese. However, two individuals with the same height and weight cannot be distinguished as obese or muscular from calculation of their BMIs. To assess the health implications of obesity, a method is required to distinguish overweight from obesity. This is most relevant in the aged since total body weight begins to decrease but percent fat does not. Furthermore, it has recently become evident that in obesity the pattern of body fat distribution may have health implications. Thus in addition to the quantity of fat in the body, the location of fat plays a dominant role in determining whether obesity will be benign or malignant in its influence on the risk factor being examined. This is best exemplified in the development of diabetes and hypertension.

The fat mass of the body, its location, and its tissue plane (subcutaneous vs. deep) can be estimated using a variety of techniques. Measurement of body composition is difficult, and none of the methods can be regarded as ideal. The techniques currently employed have both advantages and disadvantages. The most consistent, reliable method, currently the "gold standard," is the determination of density by underwater weighing. The natural history of body mass (body composition) with age is generally derived from cross-sectional data, there being few longitudinal data, but reliable cross-sectional data are not available for the elderly population (above 75 yr of age).

FAT MASS

Aging is associated with alterations in body composition, namely an increase in adipose tissue mass with a concomitant decrease in fat-free mass (FFM) or lean tissue. Major changes in body composition occur with redistribution of body fat mass and body cell mass without a concomitant alteration in body weight. This is exemplified by comparing a young group with an average age of 30 yr (mean body weight 73.4 kg) to an older group with an average age of 70 yr (mean body weight 73.8 kg). In the young group, fat comprised 18.3% of weight in contrast to the older group with 26.3% (85). The increase in relative fatness is compounded by the fact that, in general, aging is also associated with weight gain and, therefore, an even greater increase in absolute fat mass. Furthermore, the regional distribution of fat mass is altered with age. Desirable techniques allow the assessment of both obesity and its regional distribution. In this review, methods for assessing body composition will be discussed, with emphasis on their use for the study of aging. The prevalence of obesity and its health implications as a function of age will also be addressed.

Body composition can be measured using direct or indirect methods. The only direct method of measurement is anatomical (that is, dissection of cadavers). Commonly employed indirect methods are subjective (i.e., based on one's impression or rule of thumb) or estimate the amount of fat tissue using anthropometric assessment. The anthropometric methods routinely utilized are height and weight; total body density; skin-fold thickness measurements; isotope dilution measurements; total body potassium determinations; dual photon absorptiometry; bioelectrical impedance analysis; girth, depth, breadth, and length measurements; X-ray computerized tomography and magnetic resonance imaging. In addition, specialized centers have neutron activation (neutron irradiation) instruments and whole-body gamma-ray counting systems where prompt-gamma-neutron activation analysis (PGNA), delayed gamma-neutron activation analysis (DGNA), and inelastic neutron scattering (INS) can be performed. With the latter devices, it is possible to measure total body nitrogen, calcium, phosphorous, sodium, chloride, and carbon. The procedures, however, are prohibitively expensive, have a total radiation exposure of approximately 3.0 mSV, and require approximately 120 min to complete.

Most indirect measurements of total body fat are based on compositional differences between the estimated weight of lean and fat tissues. Since fat is void of water and potassium with a density of approximately 0.9 g/cm^3, measurement of total body water, potassium, and total body density can be used to estimate FFM. It should be noted that a subtle difference exists between FFM and lean body mass. FFM represents the total body weight minus the estimated mass of fat. Excluded in the estimated mass of fat are the soluble fat component, that is, the ether-soluble fraction, of the adipose tissue and fat stored in nonadipose tissue sites. Thus the water and protein fractions of adipose tissue are included in FFM. Lean body mass equals total body weight minus weight of adipose tissue, which includes the weight of water and the protein fractions of adipose tissue.

Direct Methods of Measuring Fat Mass

Since 1940, 34 adult dissections have been performed in subjects ranging in age from 35 to 94 yr (31, 48–50, 96, 133, 134). These data are supplemented by the reports of nineteenth-century anatomists who weighed many tissues. Although the nineteenth-century anatomists completed approximately 25 dissections, data on only 10 cadavers have been reported. The cadavers ranged in age from 21 to 45 yr (see 31, Table 1). The nineteenth-century data are incomplete with respect to adipose and nonadipose tissue mass.

The most extensive investigation is the Brussels Cadaver Study conducted by Clarys and co-workers (31). To gain experience with their techniques, they initially dissected two cadavers. They then conducted 25 additional dissections in 12 males and 13 females, who ranged in age from 55 to 94 yr and none of whom were emaciated or had any physical abnormalities. There were 12 embalmed and 13 nonembalmed cadavers. To minimize evaporative losses, nonembalmed dissection and weighing were completed within 24 h of death. The purpose of the study was to provide normative weight data on tissues and organs and to compare indirect methods of anthropometric estimation of body composition to actual direct measurement. Indirect assessment included anthropometric measurements, nhotography, underwater weighing, and soft-tissue radiographs. The results of the 25 dissections are presented in Tables 8.3 and 8.4. In females, 40% of total body weight was adipose tissue compared to 28% in males. The term *adipose tissue–free weight* (ATFW), which represents the total body weight minus the weight of all dissectible adipose tissue, may be preferable to the term *lean body weight* (31). When expressed as ATFW,

TABLE 8.3. *Description of Subjects, Brussels Cadaver Analysis Study, Vrije Universiteit, Brussels*

				Description of Subjects						Gross Tissue Weights (kg)				
Sex	Group	Subject	Age (yr)	Cause of Death	Supine Length	Estimated Stature*	Weight at Receipt	Weight at Dissection	Skin	Adipose	Muscle	Bone	Undifferentiated Tissues
Male	Embalmed	3	73	Heart disease	157.1	156.2	—	52.8	2.56	17.3	17.3	7.4	8.4
		5	78	Heart disease	163.8	162.8	—	70.4	3.8	20.6	26.9	8.9	10.2
		6	78	Respiratory insuff	168.0	167.0	69.9	71.5	4.7	17.8	26.3	11.7	10.9
		9	70	Natural	160.1	159.2	52.4	58.5	3.3	18.0	20.1	7.9	9.2
		10	83	Natural	168.5	167.5	46.4	51.7	3.3	12.1	17.9	9.8	8.6
		13	72	Carcinoma	166.8	165.8	60.7	65.1	3.7	16.9	25.7	9.6	9.1
	Mean		76		164.0	163.1	57.3	61.7	3.6	17.1	22.4	9.2	9.4
	SD		5		4.6	4.6	10.2	8.6	0.7	2.8	4.4	1.6	1.0
Male	Unembalmed	17	65	Heart disease	167.1	166.1	54.8	54.8	3.2	9.7	23.3	8.8	9.7
		20	59	Heart disease	174.2	173.2	76.8	76.8	4.3	20.8	31.2	10.1	10.4
		23	81	Natural	177.9	176.9	61.0	61.0	2.7	17.0	21.8	8.7	10.8
		25	73	Heart disease	173.0	172.0	85.1	85.1	4.6	25.7	34.8	10.3	9.7
		26	73	Heart disease	164.6	163.6	57.7	57.7	2.9	25.3	15.8	7.3	6.3
		27	55	Suicide	187.6	186.5	88.9	88.9	5.5	20.8	40.4	11.1	11.1
	Mean		68		174.1	173.0	70.7	70.7	3.9	19.9	27.9	9.4	9.7
	SD		10		8.2	8.2	14.8	14.8	1.1	5.9	9.2	1.4	1.8
Mean			72		169.1	168.1	65.4	66.2	3.7	18.5	25.1	9.3	9.5
SD			8		8.2	8.2	14.3	12.5	0.9	4.6	7.4	1.4	1.4
Female	Embalmed	4	83	Carcinoma	149.2	148.3	—	61.6	4.1	25.3	16.9	7.0	8.3
		7	94	Heart disease	152.4	151.5	44.3	49.1	2.9	16.0	15.4	7.7	7.1
		8	79	Heart disease	158.0	157.1	45.2	48.3	3.2	14.4	16.0	7.4	7.4
		11	84	Unknown	158.7	157.8	68.8	75.4	3.7	35.6	18.6	8.0	9.5
		12	69	Carcinoma	169.6	168.6	61.4	62.9	3.9	18.0	20.3	10.0	10.8
		14	70	Accident	161.2	160.2	60.4	63.4	3.6	26.9	18.8	7.3	6.8
	Mean		80		158.2	157.2	56.0	60.1	3.6	22.7	17.6	7.9	8.3
	SD		9		7.1	7.1	10.8	10.2	0.5	8.1	1.9	1.1	1.6
	Unembalmed	15	79	Heart disease	160.7	159.7	58.9	58.9	3.1	21.6	18.3	7.7	8.1
		18	83	Heart disease	173.3	172.3	74.2	74.2	3.3	40.1	14.3	8.8	7.7
		19	82	Renal insuff	162.6	161.7	48.2	48.2	2.5	18.6	13.3	7.4	6.3
		21	77	Heart disease	152.2	151.3	71.6	71.6	3.5	28.0	23.4	7.6	9.1
		22	68	Natural	154.5	153.6	69.0	69.0	3.4	32.0	19.3	6.7	7.6
		24	86	Leukemia	157.4	156.5	61.2	61.2	3.6	29.3	14.6	7.7	6.0
		28	82	Heart disease	164.4	163.5	68.8	68.8	3.1	29.3	21.7	7.3	7.5
	Mean		80		160.8	159.8	64.6	64.6	3.2	28.4	17.8	7.6	7.5
	SD		6		7.1	7.0	9.0	9.0	0.3	7.0	3.9	0.6	1.1
Mean			80		159.6	158.6	61.0	62.5	3.4	25.8	17.8	7.7	7.9
SD			7		6.9	6.9	10.3	9.4	0.4	7.8	3.0	0.8	1.3
Total Mean			76		164.1	163.2	63.0	64.3	3.5	22.3	21.3	8.5	8.7
SD			9		8.9	8.8	12.2	10.9	0.7	7.3	6.6	1.4	1.6

*Estimated stature = supine length × 0.993 + 0.095 ± 0.815 cm.

Reprinted from Clarys, J. P., A. D. Martin, D. T. Drinkwater. Gross tissue weights in the human body cadaver dissection. *Human Biology*, 56, 1984, by permission of the Wayne State University Press.

TABLE 8.4. Gross Tissue Weights in the Adult Human Body as a Percent of Body Weight and Adipose Tissue–Free Weight (ATFW), Brussels Cadaver Analysis Study, Vrije Universiteit Brussels

Sex	Group	Subject	Weight (kg)	Tissue Weights as % of Body Weight						ATFW (kg)	Tissue Weights as % of ATFW				
				Skin (%)	Adipose (%)	Muscle (%)	Bone (%)	Undifferentiated Tissue (%)	Total (%)		Skin (%)	Muscle (%)	Bone (%)	Undifferentiated Tissue (%)	Total (%)
Male	Embalmed	3	52.8	4.7	32.7	32.7	13.9	15.9	100.0	35.5	7.0	48.6	20.7	23.7	100.0
		5	70.4	5.4	29.2	38.2	12.7	14.5	100.0	49.8	7.6	54.0	17.9	20.5	100.0
		6	71.5	6.6	24.9	36.8	16.4	15.3	100.0	53.7	8.8	49.0	21.9	20.4	100.0
		9	58.5	5.6	30.8	34.4	13.5	15.8	100.0	40.5	8.1	49.7	19.5	22.8	100.0
		10	51.7	6.4	23.4	34.7	19.0	16.6	100.0	39.6	8.3	45.3	24.8	21.6	100.0
		13	65.1	5.7	25.9	39.5	14.8	14.0	100.0	48.2	7.8	53.4	20.0	18.9	100.0
	Mean		61.7	5.7	27.8	63.1	15.0	15.3		44.6	7.9	50.0	20.8	21.3	
	SD		8.6	0.7	3.6	2.6	2.3	1.0		7.0	0.6	3.3	2.3	1.8	
	Unembalmed	17	54.8	5.9	17.8	42.5	16.1	17.7	100.0	45.1	7.2	51.7	19.6	21.5	100.0
		20	76.8	5.6	27.1	40.6	13.1	13.5	100.0	56.0	7.7	55.8	18.0	18.5	100.0
		23	61.0	4.4	27.8	35.7	14.3	17.7	100.0	44.0	6.1	49.5	19.8	24.6	100.0
		25	85.1	5.4	30.1	40.9	12.1	11.4	100.0	59.4	7.8	58.6	17.4	16.3	100.0
		26	57.7	5.1	43.9	27.4	12.7	10.9	100.0	32.4	9.1	48.8	22.7	19.4	100.0
		27	88.9	6.1	23.4	45.5	12.5	12.5	100.0	68.1	8.0	59.4	16.3	16.3	100.0
			70.7	5.4	28.4	38.8	13.5	14.0	100.0	50.8	7.6	54.0	19.0	19.5	100.0
	Mean		70.7	5.4	28.4	38.8	13.5	14.0		50.8	7.6	54.0	19.0	19.5	
	SD		14.8	0.6	8.8	6.4	1.5	3.0		12.8	1.0	4.6	2.3	3.2	
Mean			66.2	5.6	28.1	37.4	14.3	14.6		47.7	7.8	52.0	19.9	20.4	
SD			12.5	0.6	6.4	4.9	2.0	2.3		10.4	0.8	4.3	2.4	2.6	
Female	Unembalmed	4	61.6	6.7	41.1	27.4	11.3	13.5	100.0	36.3	11.4	46.5	19.3	22.9	100.0
		7	49.1	5.9	32.6	31.3	15.6	14.6	100.0	33.1	8.7	46.5	23.2	21.6	100.0
		8	48.3	6.6	29.8	33.0	15.3	15.2	100.0	33.9	9.4	47.1	21.8	21.7	100.0
		11	75.4	4.9	47.2	24.6	10.7	12.6	100.0	39.8	9.3	46.7	20.2	23.9	100.0
		12	62.9	6.2	28.6	32.3	15.8	17.1	100.0	44.9	8.6	45.2	22.2	24.0	100.0
		14	63.4	5.6	42.5	29.6	11.6	10.7	100.0	36.5	9.7	51.5	20.1	18.7	100.0
	Mean		60.1	6.0	37.0	29.7	13.4	14.0	100.0	37.4	9.5	47.2	21.1	22.1	100.0
	SD		10.2	0.7	7.7	3.2	2.4	2.2		4.4	1.0	2.2	1.5	2.0	
	Unembalmed	15	58.9	5.2	36.7	31.1	13.1	13.8	100.0	37.3	8.2	49.2	20.8	21.8	100.0
		18	74.2	4.4	54.1	19.3	11.8	10.4	100.0	34.1	9.7	41.9	25.7	22.7	100.0
		19	48.2	5.3	38.7	27.6	15.4	13.1	100.0	29.6	8.6	45.0	25.1	21.3	100.0
		21	71.6	4.9	39.0	32.7	10.6	12.8	100.0	43.6	8.0	53.6	17.4	21.0	100.0
		22	69.0	4.9	46.3	28.0	9.7	11.0	100.0	37.0	9.2	52.2	18.1	20.4	100.0
		24	61.2	5.8	47.9	23.9	12.6	9.8	100.0	31.9	11.2	45.8	24.3	18.7	100.0
		28	68.8	4.5	42.6	31.5	10.5	10.8	100.0	39.5	7.9	54.8	18.4	18.9	100.0
	Mean		64.6	5.0	43.6	27.7	12.0	11.7		36.1	9.0	48.9	21.4	20.7	
	SD		9.0	0.5	6.2	4.8	1.9	1.5		4.7	1.2	4.9	3.6	1.5	
Mean			62.5	5.5	40.5	28.6	12.6	12.7		36.7	9.1	48.1	21.3	21.3	
SD			9.4	0.7	7.4	4.1	2.2	2.2		4.4	1.1	3.8	2.7	1.8	
Total Mean			64.3	5.5	34.6	32.9	13.4	13.6		42.0	8.5	50.0	20.6	20.9	
SD			10.9	0.7	9.3	6.3	2.2	2.4		9.5	1.2	4.4	2.6	2.3	

Reprinted from Clarys, J. P., A. D. Martin, D. T. Drinkwater. Gross tissue weights in the human body cadaver dissection. *Human Biology*, 56, 1984, by permission of the Wayne State University Press.

48% of weight was muscle in females compared to 52% in males. In females, 21% of ATFW was bone compared to 20% in males. Although this series represents the best available data on direct measurement of adipose tissue, it should be noted that the cadavers averaged 76 yr of age and would generally be considered to be obese; therefore, the results may not be applicable to younger subjects.

The Brussels study provided both tissue mass measurements and anthropometric measurements in the same cadavers. The investigators reported a validated equation for the estimation of muscle mass in male subjects (93). Total muscle mass (TMM, g) can be accurately predicted (SEE = 1.53 kg, r^2 = 0.97) by measuring stature ($STAT$, cm), thigh circumference (CTG, cm, midway between inguinal crease and midpoint of patella), corrected for the front thigh skin-fold thickness, forearm circumference (FG, cm, at maximum girth), and calf circumference (CCG, cm, at maximum girth), corrected for medial calf skin-fold thickness:

$$TMM = STAT(0.0533\ CTG^2 + 0.0987\ FG^2 + 0.0331\ CCG^2) - 2,445$$

This equation is the only cadaver-validated equation and is probably the best anthropometric estimate of total skeletal muscle mass. It should be noted that this equation was derived from data in men only, who ranged in age from 55 to 83 yr. Undoubtedly, age-related decline in muscle mass had occurred in these subjects, and caution should be used in applying the equation to younger subjects.

Indirect Methods of Measuring Fat Mass

Height–Weight Tables. Body weight is the easiest and certainly the most commonly used determinant of obesity and can be measured accurately. Height is another simple, easily obtained measurement. The basis for defining normal weight (sometimes referred to as optimal, ideal, desirable, or recommended) largely stems from actuarial data collected at various time intervals during this century. In general, the mortality experiences of 25 insurance companies have been pooled and reported in great detail. The data collected from 1935 to 1953 were reported in 1959 and the data collected from 1954 to 1972 in 1980. From analyses of these data sets, the Metropolitan Life Insurance Co. published tables of optimal weight ranges based on actuarial mortality data as a function of height. The recommendations were gender-specific, and three sets of overlapping weight ranges for each of three body frames (small, medium, and large) were provided for heights of 4′10″ to 6′ in women and 5′2″ to 6′4″ in men. Neither of the tables (1959 or 1983) included age as a variable. Thus weights in the 1959 table were recommended for ages 25 yr and up and in the 1983 table for ages 25–59 yr. The most commonly employed standards for optimal weight are the 1959 "Desirable Weight" table (11) and the 1983 "Height–Weight" table (12). These tables are updates of similarly formulated Metropolitan Life Insurance "ideal weight" tables of 1942 for women (9) and 1943 for men (10). The rationale behind the construction of the 1942 and 1943 tables was not provided.

The "optimal" weight tables, derived from combined mortality experiences of the insured population in North America, may not be appropriate for the general population for several reasons. The major criticisms are that the insured subjects are not representative of the general population and that height and weight are not the best estimates of optimal weight. Furthermore, the possible impact of cigarette smoking on optimal weight was not evaluated. The designation of three body frame sizes was not based on measurements from the insured population, revealing further inadequacies of the tables. The optimal weight range for any individual can vary from 6 to 26 lb, depending on which height and frame are chosen. In addition, depending on the version of the table used (1959 or 1983), optimal weight for two individuals of equal stature can differ considerably; recommended weights in the later table are higher than in the earlier table.

In recent years a different standard of relative obesity has been used more frequently. As previously mentioned, the relationship of relative obesity to height and weight was described in 1842 by M. A. Quetelet (107) and is known as the Quetelet Index, or BMI. This standard does not rely on any table, which is advantageous. A range of 20–27 kg/m^2 for women and 20–25 kg/m^2 for men is frequently recommended as the standard of normality for body weight (16). This recommendation is based on the widely used, generally accepted rule that individuals studied in clinical research are classified as nonobese if their "obesity index" is between 90% and 120% of the recommended weight. Obesity index is computed as the subject's weight divided by his or her "desirable" weight (mid-weight of the medium frame in the 1959 Metropolitan Table). It is important to realize that obesity index, as calculated from the 1959 table, and BMI are linearly related. BMI, computed from the mid-weight of the medium frame divided by height squared (kg/m^2) in the 1959 Metropolitan Desirable Weight Table, is remarkably constant and averages 20.7 kg/m^2 for women and 22 kg/m^2 for men, with coefficients of variation of only 1.1% and 1.2%, respectively. However, since the height and weight measurements of the tables include shoes and clothing, a correction should be made. It is recommended that 2 in and 5 lb be subtracted for women and 1 in and 7 lb be subtracted for men. Thus the corrected BMIs average 21.2 and 21.6 kg/m^2 for women and men, respectively.

The controversy in the recommendation of optimal weight has not been resolved. Between 1973 and 1992, four NIH-sponsored conferences on obesity were held (13, 26, 27, 51). The recommendations from the Consensus Development Conference on Health Implications of Obesity, held in February 1985 did not show a clear preference for either the 1959 or the 1983 version of weight standards. The tables were recognized as being deficient because age was not included as a variable, but no age recommendations were offered. The 1992 consensus conference still recognized this deficiency but did not resolve the issue (13).

Andres et al. have examined mortality rates by gender as a function of body mass and age (8). The database comprised the extensive report on more than 4 million policies and 100,000 deaths published in *Build Study* (29). The data demonstrate that the mortality ratio follows a J- or U-shaped distribution (Fig. 8.2), with high mortality at both the very low and the very high BMIs and the lowest mortality at an intermediate zone. A quadratic equation defines each curve, the nadir of which can be computed for each age group. The nadir represents the BMI associated with the lowest mortality. The relationship between the nadir and age represents a progressive increase in the "best" BMI with age in both sexes (Fig. 8.3). There is no statistically significant difference between men and women across the age span of five decades.

Since a useful table of recommended weights must provide a range of weights rather than a single point, Andres and co-workers made an empirical decision based on the fact that the quadratic curve intersects the 100% mortality line at two points (Fig. 8.2). The BMI values at those two points represent the upper and lower BMI limits for mortality ratios, which are lower than the average. Since these BMI limits are very similar in men and women, the weight goals do not need to be sex-specific. Women, who are, on average, fatter than men across the age spectrum, evidently benefit from this adiposity.

A recommended height–weight table has been constructed (Table 8.5), which presents the computed weight ranges for each age decade from 20–29 through 60–69 yr. For comparison, the corresponding total weight ranges from the 1983 Metropolitan Tables are

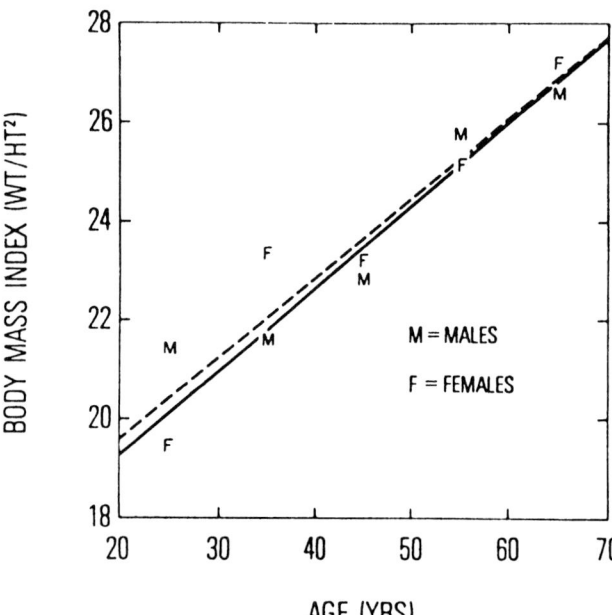

FIG. 8.3. The effect of age on the BMI associated with lowest mortality. Minimal mortality points were computed for each age-sex group as indicated in Table 8.5. The regression lines were computed separately for men (——) and for women (– – –). Note that there is a strong effect of age on the BMI associated with the lowest mortality and that the regression lines for men and women are nearly identical.

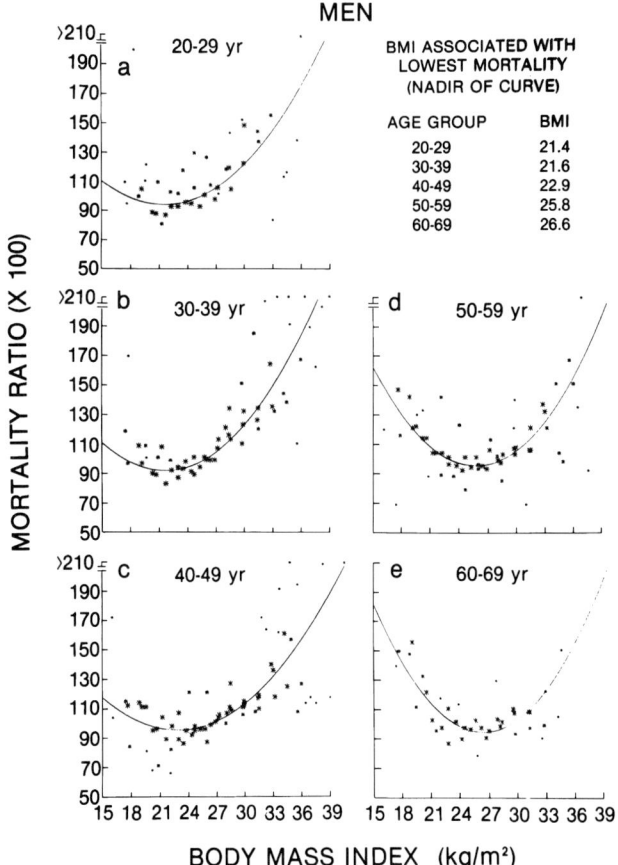

FIG. 8.2. The U-shaped relationships between BMI and mortality ratio. Data are derived from the Build Study (29). The curves were constructed from the quadratic relationship between the two variables. A mortality ratio of 100 represents the average or expected mortality for the specific age group. The nadirs of the curves represent BMI associated with minimal mortality. The two points at which the curves intersect the 100 mortality ratio line represent those BMIs associated with mortality ratios less than the average; those BMIs can, therefore, be used to define a recommended weight range.

TABLE 8.5. *Comparison of the Weight-for-Height Tables from Actuarial Data: Non-Age-Corrected Metropolitan Life Insurance Co. and Age-Specific Gerontology Research Center Recommendations*

Height (ft and in)	Metropolitan 1983 Weights* (25–59 yr)		Gerontology Research Center* (Age-Specific Weight Range for Men and Women)				
	Men	Women	20–29 yr	30–39 yr	40–49 yr	50–59 yr	60–69 yr
4'10"		100–131	84–111	92–119	99–127	107–135	115–142
4'11"		101–134	87–115	95–123	103–131	111–139	119–147
5'0"		103–137	90–119	98–127	106–135	114–143	123–152
5'1"	123–145	105–140	93–123	101–131	110–140	118–148	127–157
5'2"	125–148	108–144	96–127	105–136	113–144	122–153	131–163
5'3"	127–151	111–148	99–131	108–140	117–149	126–158	135–168
5'4"	129–155	114–152	102–135	112–145	121–154	130–163	140–173
5'5"	131–159	117–156	106–140	115–149	125–159	134–168	144–179
5'6"	133–163	120–160	109–144	119–154	129–164	138–174	148–184
5'7"	135–167	123–164	112–148	122–159	133–169	143–179	153–190
5'8"	137–171	126–167	116–153	126–163	137–174	147–184	158–196
5'9"	139–175	129–170	119–157	130–168	141–179	151–190	162–201
5'10"	141–179	132–173	122–162	134–173	145–184	156–195	167–207
5'11"	144–183	135–176	126–167	137–178	149–190	160–201	172–213
6'0"	147–187		129–171	141–183	153–195	165–207	177–219
6'1"	150–192		133–176	145–188	157–200	169–213	182–225
6'2"	153–197		137–181	149–194	162–206	174–219	187–232
6'3"	157–202		141–186	153–199	166–212	179–225	192–238
6'4"			144–191	157–205	171–218	184–231	197–244

*Values in this table are for height without shoes and weight without clothes.

also shown. Since no anthropometric data were available on the insured subjects other than height and weight, the individual weight ranges for each of the three body frames represent only a conjecture of the weight adjustment that should be permitted for frame size. It seems preferable to provide an age-adjusted table (for which data are available) and to avoid a frame-adjusted table (for which no data are available). Computation of BMI from the 1983 Metropolitan Tables of relative weight (Table 8.5) reveals that BMI decreases as height increases in both sexes (the 1959 Metropolitan Tables held BMI constant). The BMIs for an average height of 5'9" for men and 5'4" for women are 23.2 and 22.9 kg/m², respectively. BMI computed from the age-adjusted weight tables remains constant for all heights in each age category. The average BMIs for the third and fourth decades are 20.4 and 22.1 kg/m², respectively, and increase by 1.6 kg/m² each decade thereafter (Table 8.6).

Over the major portion of the height spectrum, the 1983 Metropolitan Life Insurance Co. weight range for men and women (12) falls near the weights in the age-adjusted table for individuals in their thirties or forties. Thus the 1983 Metropolitan Tables provide weights that are higher than the primary insurance data would justify for young adults and lower than the insurance data would dictate for older adults. The increased weight allowance in the age-specific table is close to 10 lb per decade of life or 1 lb per yr, somewhat in excess of the actual mean weight increase that occurs in American men and women across the age span of 20–70 yr.

It must be stressed that tables of recommended weight are applicable to healthy individuals only, void of medical conditions which may affect or be affected by body weight. Furthermore, it is difficult to recommend weights for individuals over the age of 70 yr. For men and women in their seventies and eighties, data from the American Cancer Society Study (86) suggest that the weight gain permitted with increasing age should be maintained into very old age. A number of other studies of elderly populations also suggest that the weights associated with lowest mortality remain on the relatively high side. The results of the effects of changes in

TABLE 8.6. *Computation of BMI from the 1983 Metropolitan Tables of Relative Weight*

Age Range	Lower Limit	Average	Upper Limit
20–29	17.6	20.4	23.3
30–39	19.2	22.1	25.0
40–49	20.8	23.7	26.6
50–59	22.4	25.3	28.2
60–69	24.0	26.9	29.8

body weight from thirteen studies conducted in eleven diverse populations have recently been summarized by Andres et al. (8).

Body surface area is also frequently calculated from height and weight. This parameter is commonly used as a reference base to normalize data and drug dosage, especially in clinical settings such as metabolic research. Body surface area (SA) is commonly estimated from an equation developed by DuBois and DuBois (39) based on direct measurements in nine subjects:

$$SA = 0.007184 \times W^{0.425} \times H^{0.725}$$

where W equals weight in kilograms, H equals height in centimeters, and SA equals surface area in meters squared. The accuracy of this equation, along with eight other equations, has recently been tested from the dissected skins of ten female and seven male cadavers in the Brussels Cadaver Analysis Study (92). The investigators concluded that, although seven of the equations used predicted SA with equal accuracy, the use of the time-honored equation of DuBois and DuBois should be continued.

Physiological functions are generally related to a parameter of physical size. Although estimation of obesity can be made from measurements of height and weight, the accuracy is questionable. In fact, it is well known that more accurate estimations of fat can be made by other techniques. Furthermore, many reports have provided clear evidence that patterns of regional fat distribution have differential consequences on health status. Techniques are available to make measurements (simple to complex) that will provide estimates of fat which are more predictive of risk conditions than weight and height alone.

Total Body Density. Total body density is the indirect gold standard technique of measuring body fat. The method is based on Archimedes' principle that any object in water displaces a mass of water equal to its own volume.

In humans, body volume is obtained by measuring weight in air and under water. Weight under water is computed after correction for residual volume of air in the lungs. The helium or nitrogen dilution method is used to estimate residual lung volume prior to or during underwater weighing (109). Intestinal gas can theoretically affect the estimate, although its magnitude is relatively small, especially in the fasted state. From measurement of body density, percent body fat and FFM are then calculated. A two-compartment model is used in estimating body fat. The density of fat is constant and equal to 0.9007 g/ml, and the density of FFM is assumed to be 1.10 g/ml (3, 28). The percent of body weight estimated to be fat mass may be calculated using the following equations of Brozek et al. and Siri, respectively (28, 120):

$$\% \text{ fat} = \frac{4.570}{D_b} - 4.142$$

or

$$\% \text{ fat} = \frac{4.95}{D_b} - 4.5$$

where D_b is body density. Fat mass is then calculated as percent fat $\times$ body weight. The density of FFM, however, is not constant and changes as a function of age, exercise, and gender. For example, density differences can be clearly demonstrated in bone, which is increased in athletes and decreased in postmenopausal women. Age- and sex-specific FFM density constants are available only for children and young adults (7–25 yr) (87).

Skin-fold Measurements. Determination of body density in the elderly may be difficult. A more convenient method, subcutaneous skin-fold thickness, has been most commonly used to estimate body fat content. Total body density and the sum of skin-fold thicknesses from four sites—biceps, triceps, subscapular, and suprailiac—were measured by Durnin and Womersley in 209 males and 272 females aged 16–72 yr (41). Percent fat was calculated from density using Siri's equation (120), and thus age- and sex-specific values for density of FFM were not used. From correlation analysis, a table was derived by gender for four separate age groups (Table 8.7). The fat content as a percentage of body weight can be estimated from the sum of the above four skin folds by referring to this table, which is the most frequently used table in adults. It should be noted that this table was derived from measurement of Glaswegian adults and therefore may not be applicable to other populations, especially non-Caucasians. In addition, although three age groups are provided for each sex (16–49 yr), all individuals above age 50 are grouped together. Thus the table may not be valid for the old-old age group.

Isotope Dilution. Skin-fold measurements use equations that estimate total body fat. Thus it is difficult to separate percentage of subcutaneous vs. internally deposited deep fat using this technique. In addition to the concerns raised regarding assumptions inherent in estimating percent fat from skin-fold thicknesses, the measurement itself requires an experienced anthropometrist to ensure that the correct sites and amounts of tissue are selected. This problem is further complicated in the elderly because skin-fold compressibility becomes greater in older people (41). Thus the measurement of body water

TABLE 8.7. *Equivalent Fat Content, as a Percentage of Body Weight, for a Range of Values for the Sum of Four Skin Folds (Biceps, Triceps, Subscapular, and Suprailiac) of Males and Females of Different Ages*

Skin fold (mm)	Males				Females			
	17–29 yr	30–39 yr	40–49 yr	50+	16–29 yr	30–39 yr	40–49 yr	50+
15	4.8	—	—	—	10.5	—	—	—
20	8.1	12.2	12.2	12.6	14.1	17.0	19.8	21.4
25	10.5	14.2	15.0	15.6	16.8	19.4	22.2	24.0
30	12.9	16.2	17.7	18.6	19.5	21.8	24.5	26.6
35	14.7	17.7	19.6	20.8	21.5	23.7	26.4	28.5
40	16.4	19.2	21.4	22.9	23.4	25.5	28.2	30.3
45	17.7	20.4	23.0	24.7	25.0	26.9	29.6	31.9
50	19.0	21.5	24.6	26.5	26.5	28.2	31.0	33.4
55	20.1	22.5	25.9	27.9	27.8	29.4	32.1	34.6
60	21.2	23.5	27.1	29.2	29.1	30.6	33.2	35.7
65	22.2	24.3	28.2	30.4	30.2	31.6	34.1	36.7
70	23.1	25.1	29.3	31.6	31.2	32.5	35.0	37.7
75	24.0	25.9	30.3	32.7	32.2	33.4	35.9	38.7
80	24.8	26.6	31.2	33.8	33.1	34.3	36.7	39.6
85	25.5	27.2	32.1	34.8	34.0	35.1	37.5	40.4
90	26.2	27.8	33.0	35.8	34.8	35.8	38.3	41.2
95	26.9	28.4	33.7	36.6	35.6	36.5	39.0	41.9
100	27.6	29.0	34.4	37.4	36.4	37.2	39.7	42.6
105	28.2	29.6	35.1	38.2	37.1	37.9	40.4	43.3
110	28.8	30.1	35.8	39.0	37.8	38.6	41.0	43.9
115	29.4	30.6	36.4	39.7	38.4	39.1	41.5	44.5
120	30.0	31.1	37.0	40.4	39.0	39.6	42.0	45.1
125	30.5	31.5	37.6	41.1	39.6	40.1	42.5	45.7
130	31.0	31.9	38.2	41.8	40.2	40.6	43.0	46.2
135	31.5	32.3	38.7	42.4	40.8	41.1	43.5	46.7
140	32.0	32.7	39.2	43.0	41.3	41.6	44.0	47.2
145	32.5	33.1	39.7	43.6	41.8	42.1	44.5	47.7
150	32.9	33.5	40.2	44.1	42.3	42.6	45.0	48.2
155	33.3	33.9	40.7	44.6	42.8	43.1	45.4	48.7
160	33.7	34.3	41.2	45.1	43.3	43.6	45.8	49.2
165	34.1	34.6	41.6	45.6	43.7	44.0	46.2	49.6
170	34.5	34.8	42.0	46.1	44.1	44.4	46.6	50.0
175	34.9	—	—	—	—	44.8	47.0	50.4
180	35.3	—	—	—	—	45.2	47.4	50.8
185	35.6	—	—	—	—	45.6	47.8	51.2
190	35.9	—	—	—	—	45.9	48.2	51.6
195	—	—	—	—	—	46.2	48.5	52.0
200	—	—	—	—	—	46.5	48.8	52.4
205	—	—	—	—	—	—	49.1	52.7
210	—	—	—	—	—	—	49.4	53.0

In two-thirds of the instances the error was within ±3.5% of the body weight as fat for the women and ±5% for the men. Reprinted from Durnin and Womersley (41) with permission.

has been increasingly used with the isotope dilution method. Radioactive or stable isotopes of water are usually administered orally. After equilibration, total body water can be estimated since the dilution of the isotope is proportional to the volume of body water:

$$C_1 \times V_1 = C_2 \times V_2$$

where C_1 equals the concentration of the ingested isotope, V_1 equals the volume of the ingested isotope, C_2 equals the concentration of the isotope in the body after equilibration (typically plasma, saliva, or urine), and V_2 equals the volume to be determined (that is, total body water).

The assumptions of this in vivo technique are (1) C_2 is completely at equilibrium in each body compartment at the time of measurement, (2) the isotope has not been incorporated with any body constituent other than the tracer (water), and (3) between administration of the tracer and its measurement, there has been a stable state with respect to influx and efflux of the tracee into the water compartments of the body. Fat mass or FFM may then be estimated using one of the body composition models. In all models, body weight is compartmentalized into two or more components. For estimation of body fat from body water, a two-compartmental model is commonly used, where $BW = F + FFM$ and it is assumed that the ratio of water weight to FFM is equal to 0.732 (0.732 = $WATER/FFM$). The derivation of 0.732 is discussed in detail in the review by Sheng and Huggins (116).

The isotopes most commonly used in the estimation of total body water are tritiated water (^3H_2O) or heavy isotopes of water (D_2O, $H_2^{18}O$, $D_2^{18}O$). Labeled hydrogen of water rapidly exchanges with hydrogen of several moieties (amide, carboxyl, hydroxyl) and is incorporated into carbohydrate, fat, and protein. This will result in overestimation of total body water by 3%–5%. Therefore, it has been suggested that the estimated total body water using ^3H or D be corrected by 5% to account for this exchange (47). The weight of water is further corrected by the density of water at 37°C (0.994 g/ml). Stable oxygen of water exchanges with oxygen of bicarbonate in blood. This results in overestimation of total body water by only 1%, and thus ^{18}O is the isotope of choice (138). However, the supply of ^{18}O-labeled water is very limited.

The errors associated with this technique increase with pathologic (nonsteady) states such as edema and dehydration. Schoeller has recently reviewed the principles and limitations of isotope dilution methods (110).

Total Body Potassium. All cells contain potassium, and from estimation of total body potassium, lean body mass can be calculated since the ratio of potassium to lean body mass is relatively constant for each species (48). Of the three naturally occurring isotopes of potassium (^{39}K, ^{40}K, and ^{41}K) ^{40}K is radioactive. It has a very long half-life (1.3 × 10^9 yr) and emits a high-energy gamma ray (1.46 MeV); 99% of the total body potassium is contained within cells. The abundance of naturally occurring ^{40}K is 0.0118%. Total body potassium can be measured in a shielded room with a sensitive gamma-ray detector. ^{40}K counts obtained from a whole-body counter are converted with a calibration factor to grams of potassium (48). Lean body mass can then be calculated using the equations of Forbes or Womersley et al., respectively (47, 137):

Men: LBM (kg) = $total\ body\ K$ (mEq)/68.1
LBM (kg) = $total\ body\ K$ (mmol) × 6.64

Women: LBM (kg) = $total\ body\ K$ (mEq)/64.2
LBM (kg) = $total\ body\ K$ (mmol) × 5.97

Isotope dilution methods can also be used to estimate total body potassium with the short-half-life (12.4 h) isotope ^{42}K. However, this isotope requires more than 24 h to equilibrate with total body potassium (67) and thus has no advantage over measurement of ^{40}K.

Moore and colleagues (98) have suggested that body cell mass (BCM) should be calculated instead of lean body mass. BCM includes those tissues that have a high turnover rate (brain, muscle, viscera, and blood), excluding bone and connective tissue. BCM represents the energy-metabolizing mass of the human body and is calculated as:

BCM (kg) = $total\ K$ (mEq) × 0.00833

It should be noted that, although ^{40}K can be accurately measured with sensitive whole-body counters, estimation of LBM or BCM may be erroneous in potassium-depleted states. Thus this technique should not be used in conditions of malnutrition or diarrhea or in patients medicated with diuretics without potassium supplementation.

In Vivo Neutron-Activation Analysis. In a nuclear reactor accident in Los Alamos, New Mexico (1945–1946), nine people were exposed to large doses of neutrons (59). The blood of these individuals contained radioactive sodium and phosphorus. The absorbed dose of radiation was calculated from measuring ^{24}Na in the blood. The interaction of neutrons with tissue produces radioactive elements which have gamma-ray decay products that can be used to measure neutron exposure. This principle was used by Anderson et al. (5) to estimate total body mass by bombardment of the body with neutrons and measurement of the induced activities of sodium, chloride, and calcium. Investigators at Brookhaven National Laboratory (BNL) and St. Luke's Roosevelt Hospital Center (Columbia University, New York, NY) have actively been refining this technique since establishment of their first whole-body counter in 1969 (32). Approximately a dozen elements can be measured. This technique has allowed direct estimation of total protein and bone mineral. The body is divided into four compartments: adipose tissue mass (ATM), BCM, extracellular water (ECW), and skeletal tissue (Fig. 8.4) (106). Each compartment represents a functional activity and can be measured: ATM = energy storage,

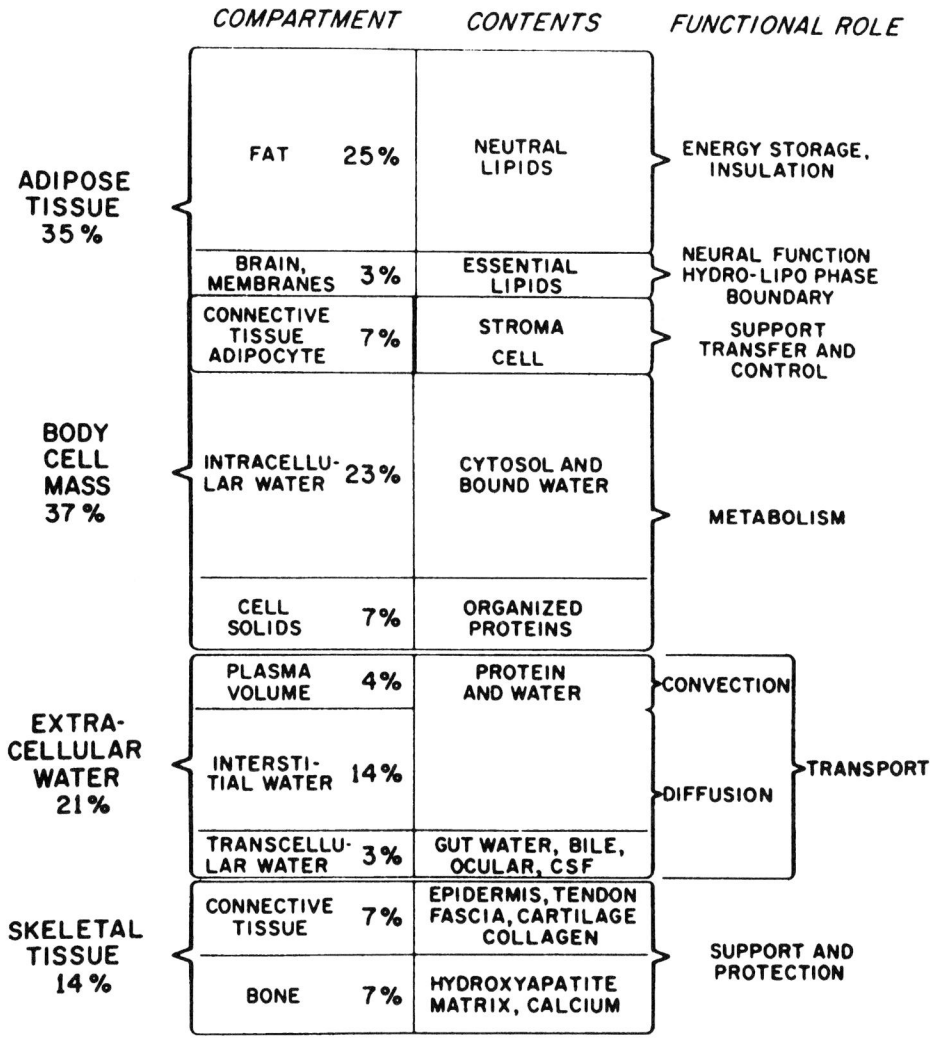

FIG. 8.4. A four-compartment functional model for body composition. From Pierson, R. N., Jr., Wang, J., *Body Composition,* 167, in Section A: *Nuclear Medicine,* Vol. I, Spencer, R. P., Sect. Ed., in Clinical Laboratory Science Series, Seligson, D., Editor-in-Chief. Boca Raton, Florida, 1977. With permission.

BCM = metabolism, ECM = transport, skeletal tissue = structure.

Protein contains 16% nitrogen, which accounts for 99% of all total body nitrogen. Thus *total body protein (kg) = 6.25 × total body nitrogen (kg)* (60). With ^{238}PuBe as the neutron source (37), nitrogen can be measured by the total body neutron–activation system at BNL. ^{14}N is excited, resulting in ^{15}N and gamma-rays. The latter product has a very short half-life (approximately 10^{-15} s) and therefore must be counted simultaneously with neutron activation. This is the PGNA technique mentioned earlier under FAT MASS. The BNL uses two sodium iodide (NaI) detectors positioned above the patient to measure gamma-rays generated. The radiation exposure is 0.26 mSv (26 mrem), and the procedure requires approximately 35 min. The technique is described in detail by Vartsky et al. (130, 131).

Neutron activation can also be used to measure total body minerals. The system uses 14 ^{238}PuBe sources to excite ^{48}Ca to ^{49}Ca and gamma-rays. The half-life of ^{49}Ca is 8.7 min, allowing the subject to be transported to a whole-body counter. This is the DGNA technique mentioned earlier under FAT MASS. The BNL counter has 32 NaI detectors, 16 placed above and 16 below the subject (37). The radiation exposure is 2.5 mSv, and the procedure requires approximately 20 min. The DGNA and whole-body counter system can also be used to estimate total body sodium and chloride. Estimation of total body water (TBW) with the isotope dilution method combined with estimations of total body protein (TBPr) by PGNA and bone mineral ash (BMA) allows calculation of total body fat (TBF):

$$TBF = body\ weight - (TBW + TBPr + BMA)$$

A semidirect method for estimation of body fat, was developed by Kehayias and colleagues from BNL and the Sandia National Laboratory (69). This system is based on the concept of determining total body carbon by measuring inelastic neutron scatter (INS) gamma-rays as reported by Kyere et al. (82). A miniature deuterium–tritium accelerator generates fast neutrons, which results in gamma rays produced from ^{12}C. The model assumes that total body carbon is distributed in fat, protein, glycogen, and bone ash. Carbon in protein and glycogen is estimated from the measurement of total body nitrogen (PGNA), with the assumption that protein contains 53% carbon by weight (74) and glycogen 44.4%. Bone ash contains 5% (18), and fat contains 77.4% carbon by weight (42). From measurement of total body carbon and with the above assumptions, total fat (TBF) can be estimated as follows:

$$Fat\ (kg) = [TBC - (3.43 \times TBN + 0.05 \times TBCa)]/0.774$$

where TBC, TBN, and TBCa are measured amounts of body carbon, nitrogen, and calcium in kilograms. The derivation of this equation can be obtained from the report by Kehayias et al. (70). The radiation exposure is 0.16 mSv, and the procedure requires approximately 45 min.

The estimation of nitrogen and chlorine by neutron-activation analysis has been validated in two human cadavers. The elements were then chemically measured after homogenization (75). The two cadavers weighed 58.6 and 25.9 kg. There were no significant differences between cadaver and homogenate estimates. In one cadaver, total body nitrogen averaged 1.51 ± 0.03 kg by chemical analysis and 1.47 ± 0.02 kg by neutron-activation analysis (mean ± SEM). Total body chlorine averaged 0.147 ± 0.002 and 0.144 ± 0.004 by the two methods, respectively. Similarities between the two methods were also observed in the other cadaver. This study demonstrates the accuracy of in vivo neutron-activation analysis over a wide range of body weights.

Dual Photon Absorptiometry. While in vivo neutron-activation analysis has precision of 3% or better for all measured elements (106), it is limited to only a few centers. A more frequently utilized method for estimation of body fat is based on dual photon absorptiometry (DPA). The early systems used the isotope ^{153}Gd, with peak energies of 44 and 100 keV, while the most recent systems, dual X-ray absorptiometry (DXA), use an X-ray source with peak energies of 40 and 80 keV. The latter is a more stable source of radiation and, unlike the ^{153}Gd source, does not have to be changed because of the decay of the radionuclide. Up to 32 NaI crystals coupled to a bialkali photomultiplier tube are used for detection of bone mass. With this procedure, both soft and skeletal tissues can be measured simultaneously. Soft tissue is separated into fat and fat-free components. The ratio of soft tissue attenuation, R_{st}, of the lower energy to the higher energy is a function of fat mass and lean body mass. Skeletal tissues attenuate photons in relation to their chemical composition. Thus total body weight, represented as a three-compartmental model, is composed of skeletal, fat, and fat-free components. The method is described in detail by Gotfredsen et al. (54, 55). The radiation exposure is 0.5 μSv, and the procedure requires approximately 10 min in normal subjects and 20 min in obese subjects. The relatively low-dose whole-body radiation and the fast speed of this method allow for examination of changes in fat and bone mineral density after metabolic interventions. Both DXA and DPA have been validated against several other methods of measuring body composition (56, 61, 94, 95). Studies are in progress at both the National Institute on Aging and the USDA Human Nutrition Research Center on Aging at Tufts University in Boston to validate this technique for assessment of body composition as a function of age.

Bioelectrical Impedance Analysis. Although DXA systems are more readily available than in vivo neutron-activation analysis, they are expensive and not available for routine analysis of body composition. An increasingly utilized, noninvasive, safe method for assessment of obesity is tetrapolar bioelectrical impedance analysis (BIA), introduced by Hoffer et al. (63). The principle involves the passage of a low-frequency electrical current through the extracellular fluid while a high-frequency electrical current penetrates the intra- and extracellular fluids (102). Fat is void of water and electrolytes and only fat-free tissues are good conductors of electricity. Body fluids and cell membranes are responsible for conductance and capacitance (low impedance), respectively, whereas bone, fat, and triglyceride are nonconductive and have high impedance. The conduction of an applied current in a system is a function of the volume of the conductor and the distribution of the fluid and its concentration. The impedance of the flow can be described as $Z = \sigma L^2/V$, where Z is impedance in ohms, σ is volume resistivity in ohm·cm, L is conductor length in cm, and V is volume in liters (63). When alternating current is administered to healthy volunteers, the ratio of height squared to impedance (Ht^2/Z) is highly correlated to total body water as determined by isotopically labeled water (81). Impedance can be partitioned into its components, resistance (R) and reactance (Xc): $Z^2 = R^2 + Xc^2$. Lukaski et al. (90) showed that resistance and impedance predicted total body water equally well and that reactance was not a good predictor. The ratio of Ht^2/R correlates with total body water ($r = 0.98$, $P<0.0001$) and is used for the prediction of total body water and FFM. Other investigators have confirmed this relationship (113, 129).

To validate estimation of FFM derived from bioelectrical impedance measurement, Lukaski et al. (91) examined body composition in 114 volunteers aged 18–50 yr, with body fat ranging from 4% to 41%. The regression equation for FFM developed for men was used to estimate FFM in women. This was similar to estimates made with the equation developed in women (low SEE) and not statistically different from FFM estimated by densitometry. In a different validation study with 312 adults, aged 18–73 yr, with body fat from 7% to 55%, FFM estimated by impedance or densitometry was similar and distributed very close to the line of identity ($r = 0.985$) with SEE 2.29 kg (89).

Kusher and Schoeller (79) developed a model for estimation of total body water in 40 healthy adults and validated it in 18 obese patients. The BIA-estimated total body water differed from the dilution technique with deuteriated water estimate by 0.6–1 liter. They further demonstrated that BIA is a good technique for assessment of changes in body composition. In 12 obese females undergoing weight loss, BIA was a better predictor of FFM than skin-fold anthropometry (80). More recently, they have combined their previously published data set comprised of 116 individuals and a cross-validation group of 59 (81). There were 62 adults (aged 23–67 yr) among the premature neonates, preschool, and prepubertal children. The ratio of height squared to resistance was the best single predictor of total body water and explained 99% of the variation (SEE = 1.67 kg). Segal et al. (114) also combined bioelectric impedance estimates of lean body mass from four laboratory studies comprised of 1,599 adults (1,089 men and 510 women). Comparisons were made to densitometrically determined lean body mass. These adults were 17–62 yr of age with 3%–56% body fat. This study also supports the use of BIA for prediction of FFM and suggests that estimation of FFM can be improved with sex- and obesity-specific equations. However, the average age of this population was less than 35 yr. BIA may overestimate percent fat in lean individuals and underestimate it in obese individuals (62, 113, 114). Estimation of percent fat with BIA has not been adequately validated in a large aging population with a wide range of obesity. Deurenberg et al. (36) estimated FFM by impedance measurements in a nonobese Dutch population. They compared the results to FFM determined by densitometry and skinfold thickness measurements. They studied 35 healthy men and 37 healthy women, aged 60–83 yr. BMI averaged 25 ± 2.2 kg/m² in men and 25.9 ± 3.2 kg/m² in women, mean ± SD. FFM was accurately predicted as:

$$FFM \text{ (kg)} = [6{,}710 \times (Ht^2(m^2)/R(\Omega)] + 3.1S + 3.9$$

with S representing gender with a value of 0 for females and 1 for males, (r = 0.94, SEE = 3.1 kg). This estimate can be improved with the addition of body weight (BW, kg) and thigh circumference (T):

$$FFM \text{ (kg)} = [3{,}600 \times (Ht^2(m^2)/R(\Omega)] \\ + 0.359BW + 4.5S - 20T + 7$$

(r = 0.96, SEE = 2.5 kg).

A study is currently in progress at the USDA Human Nutrition Research Center on Aging at Tufts University (V. Hughes and W. Evans, personal communication). FFM has been determined by BIA and hydrodensitometry. In a preliminary abstract, Hughes and Evans (65) reported their early analyses in 36 females and 30 males aged 49–74 yr. BMI ranged from 18 to 35 kg/m². FFM can be estimated as:

$$FFM \text{ (kg)} = -15.26 + 0.775 \, [Ht^2(cm^2)/R(\Omega)] \\ + 0.146wt(kg) + 0.185Xc$$

($r = 0.972$, SEE 2.65 kg).

It should be noted that bioelectrical impedance measurements have not been validated in patients with fluid and electrolyte imbalances. Furthermore, dehydration, skin temperature (cool or warm), and exercise affect estimates of resistance and reactance. However, bioelectrical impedance provides a simple and adequate estimate of FFM and is particularly useful in epidemiological studies.

Measurement of Body Fat Distribution

There are several studies which call for a total reconsideration of the recommendations for body weight (20, 21, 118). These concern not only weight itself but also epidemiological implications of the distribution of body fat—"where fat?" in addition to "how fat?", as it were. The suggestions have been made that when fat is distributed primarily in the lower part of the body (hips, buttocks, and thighs), the obesity is relatively benign; that is, associated abnormalities of blood pressure, glucose tolerance, and serum lipid levels may not occur. In contrast, when the fat is distributed intraabdominally or in the neck, shoulder, and arm areas, the obesity takes on a more "malignant" prognosis.

Anthropometric Measurements. A simple measure of fat distribution may be the ratio of waist circumference to hip circumference (WHR). In addition to measurements of waist and hip circumference, circumferences from other parts of the body as well as depth, breadth, and skinfold measurements may be useful in the determination of regional obesity. The World Health Organization has released recommendations for simple measurements, which should have better predictive power for the morbidity related to obesity than height and weight indices alone. They recommend twelve indices, of which the first five are thought to be the most important. The twelve measurements are presented in descending order of importance: height, weight, waist circumference, hip circumference, subscapular skin fold, upper thigh circumference, tricep skinfold, upper midarm circumference, bicep skinfold, suprailiac skinfold, waist and knee breadth, and abdominal and thigh skinfold (139).

A comprehensive manual written by members of the Airlie Conference Committee, experts on measurement techniques and the health consequences of obesity, and edited by Lohman et al. has been published (88). This reference manual provides details of measurement procedures and standardized techniques for more than 40 anthropometric measurements, and its recommendations should be followed. A second useful manual that should be consulted is Frisancho's *Anthropometric Standards* (52). The anthropometric data from the National Health and Nutritional Examination Surveys of 1971–1974 and 1976–1980 (NHANES I and II) have been compiled in this monograph. Anthropometric standards by age (1–74 yr), sex, height, and frame size are provided both in tabular and graphic forms. Separate tables for white and black populations are also provided.

The importance of fat distribution as an independent predictor of fat was first described by Vague in 1947 (127, 128) and reintroduced by Kissebah et al. in 1982 (73). Abdominal obesity is an independent risk factor for a variety of morbid conditions, including noninsulin-dependent diabetes mellitus, myocardial infarction, angina pectoris, and stroke (19). The effects of aging on the pattern of fat distribution have been reported by Shimokata et al. (118). A redistribution of fat toward the waist (abdominal area) occurs in men predominantly from early adulthood to the middle-aged years, while in women the same shift tends to occur mainly in the immediate postmenopausal years. Shimokata et al. (117) have also shown that the WHR pattern can be improved significantly in men by weight loss, but women tend to lose waist and hip circumferential dimensions at the same rate, thus making improvements in WHR relatively small. The reader is referred to several excellent reviews for the complex biological factors (endocrine, neurogenic), which on the one hand contribute to the fat pattern and on the other hand are responsible for the multiple deleterious effects (19, 25, 72).

Computerized Tomography and Magnetic Resonance. Although circumference measurements provide estimates of body fat distribution, they lack specificity with regard to depth, especially in the abdominal region, that is, subcutaneous vs. deep deposition. Fat deposition can be quantified with respect to localization through the application of electromagnetic waves, X-rays in computerized tomography (CT), and radio frequency in magnetic resonance imagining (MRI). Fat is usually quantified in selected portions of the body, for example, abdomen or midthigh.

In the CT procedure, X-rays are attenuated as they pass through tissues. Differential attenuation, due to density of adipose tissue, lean tissue, bone, and mineral organs, allows separation of image components. Computer software is used to quantify the relative abundance of each tissue from the graphic display. The radiation dose is 15–30 mGy, and each slice requires approximately 10 s (136). Borkan et al. showed that a single abdominal scan can give an accurate estimate of the overall abdominal adiposity (22). Using this technique, it has been shown that despite similar total body fat and total abdominal adipose tissue, older men (59–85 yr), have more intraabdominal fat than younger men (18–52 yr). In the same studies, analysis of thigh scans showed that older men have less muscle (24). This observation has been confirmed (111). The more central distribution of adipose tissue in older men is preferentially lost during endurance training (111, 112).

MRI can also be used to construct an image for evaluation of body composition. The general principle is that when a magnetic field is placed across the body, dipolar nuclei (for example, ^{23}Na, ^{13}C, ^{31}P, and ^{1}H) align their angular momentums with the external magnetic field. A radio frequency wave is used simultaneously to rotate the nuclei 90° to the magnetic field. The absorbed energy from the activated nuclei is released when the radio frequency is shut off. This radio signal is used to develop an image and to evaluate body composition. Most imaging uses the hydrogen proton ^{1}H since it is abundantly distributed in body water. MRI also allows sharp imaging and clear determination of adipose and muscle tissue. Figure 8.5 shows magnetic resonance images from the midthigh of a young and an older subject. Fat infiltration of muscle in the elderly can be readily observed.

In addition, nuclear magnetic resonance (NMR) can be used to monitor biochemical changes since identification of chemical compounds is possible (2). Although a distinct advantage of this technique is that it is not associated with radiation exposure, approximately 45 min is required for a regional scan. Since magnetic resonance and CT are both extensively used for diagnostic evaluation, limited time in the use of these instruments may be available for body composition analysis. We are not aware of any report on body composition with NMR in aging.

Recommendations on Fat Mass Measurements

We have provided a description of the available methods that can be used to measure body composition. No

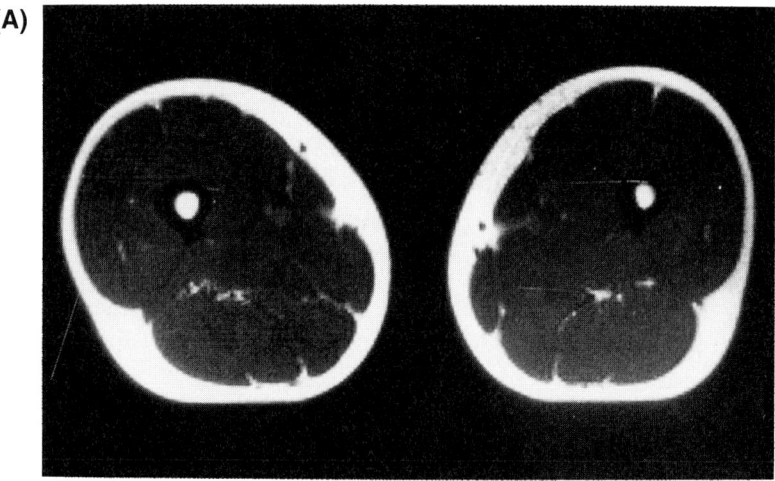

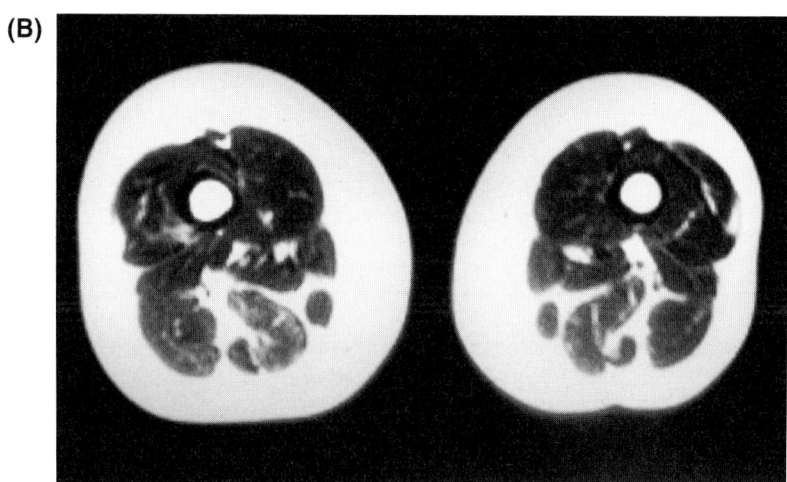

FIG. 8.5. Magnetic resonance images of the thigh showing differences in total muscle, intramuscular fat, subcutaneous fat, and bone between a young woman athlete (**A**) and an old sedentary woman (**B**). From Evans, W. J., Meredith, C. N., Exercise and Nutrition in the Elderly. In *Nutrition, Aging and the Elderly,* Munro H. N. and Danford, D. E., Eds. Plenum Publishing, New York, 1989. With permission.

single method can be recommended as superior in all respects to others for determination of body composition in the elderly. Some of the methods are very time-consuming, prohibitively expensive, and require extensive proficiency in their operation, for example, neutron-activation analysis. Currently, however, this analysis can only be used for limited numbers of elderly individuals and is not recommended for providing reference values for population studies. A very simple, quick, inexpensive, and easily learned method of estimating body composition is the bioelectrical impedance technique. However, the user must be very careful with this method. An important implicit assumption is that the subject's hydration status is in balance. Either dehydration or fluid overload can reduce the accuracy of the estimate of lean body mass. The correct placement of the electrodes is important. Even in a state of fluid balance, the measurement can be very inaccurate in some older residents of nursing homes who have contractures. Furthermore, there are measurement differences between the different bioelectrical impedance devices currently available. The inconsistencies associated with the measurement of body water with the use of these devices can be avoided by direct estimation of body water with tracers. This method is also relatively easily performed but requires a longer amount of time (at least 4 h), the use of isotopes, and special equipment for estimating radioactive or stable isotopes.

The generally acknowledged gold standard is the measurement of body density through underwater weighing. It is, however, very difficult to perform this technique in a large number of elderly individuals. An accurate estimate of body density can be achieved with dual energy absorptiometry devices. Limiting factors of this technique include the cost, technical expertise, and the subject's ability to lie in the supine position. The subject must fit comfortably in the scanning area, thus excluding the very obese. This technique and the estimation of body water with isotopes are sufficiently sensitive to discern small changes within an individual.

Skinfold measurements may be obtained easily in large numbers of elderly individuals to estimate body composition, but reproducibility among technicians has been notoriously poor. Nevertheless, measurement of skinfold thicknesses with the use of the appropriate age-specific equations to compute body fat is available as an alternative method to the more difficult ones noted above.

Assessment of the pattern of distribution of body fat is under active investigation. While the WHR has been most widely used, the possibility that the abdominal sagittal (anterior–posterior) diameter will be a better index of intraabdominal fat remains to be explored. The ratio of subscapular to triceps skinfolds does not appear to correlate with risk factors as highly as WHR.

ADIPOSITY AND AGE-ASSOCIATED DISEASES

Body composition alterations are associated with important structural and metabolic changes which increase the risk for significant illness in the elderly. Being overweight affects a larger percentage of females than males over 55 yr. Data from NHANES and the Framingham Heart Study (1, 15, 99) show that in men, Metropolitan relative weights (MRW), computed as the subject's weight divided by desirable weight based on Metropolitan Life Insurance Co. Tables (12) and the Build Study (29), increased with advancing age from 30 to 65 yr and then declined. In women, MRW increased with advancing age to about age 70 yr and then declined. Thus body weight generally increases with aging, reaches a peak in late middle age, and then tends to decline in old age. Old individuals with similar total body weight to young individuals will have approximately 40% more fat (85). Since body weight generally increases with age, the amount of body fat in the elderly is greater than that cited above. The prevalence of glucose intolerance, obesity, and atherosclerosis in the elderly is severalfold that of the general population, and each will be discussed briefly.

Glucose Intolerance

Harris and colleagues have examined the prevalence of glucose intolerance in the U.S. black and white populations for 20–74- yr-olds (57, 58, 97). The prevalence of diabetes, as assessed by the National Diabetes Data Group criteria (100) for this age group, was estimated to be 6.6%, and the prevalence of undiagnosed diabetics (approximately half the total) was nearly identical to the prevalence of previously diagnosed diabetics. Obesity was associated with significantly higher rates of glucose intolerance. Prevalence of previously diagnosed diabetics for the 65–74 yr age group in white and black populations for both sexes increased to 9.3% compared to 4.3% in the 45–54 yr age group. Furthermore, the prevalence of undiagnosed diabetes increased similarly for these two age groups (8.4% vs. 4.2%). The total prevalence of diabetes in the 65–74 yr age group for both races was 17.7% for men and 19.2% for women. Obesity and parental history of diabetes each doubled the prevalence of diagnosed and undiagnosed diabetes and impaired glucose tolerance. When both factors are present the rate increases fourfold. Age-related changes in glucose metabolism are reflected in hyperglycemia (7, 34) and a decreased ability of the peripheral tissue, especially muscle, to dispose of a glucose load (44). It has been suggested that this decline in glucose metabolism with age is not a primary biological aging effect but that it is secondary to such age-associated factors as increased presence of disease, medications, physical activity, obesity, or change in the pattern of fat distribution. A population study by Shimokata et al. (119), however, showed that when the above factors are accounted for, age per se still remains an independent risk factor in the decline of glucose tolerance.

Obesity

Obese humans have an increased risk of developing non-insulin-dependent diabetes due to a reduction in insulin sensitivity (132). Increased body fat has been associated with reduced rates of insulin-mediated glucose disposal (77, 108). For this reason, the increased obesity of advancing age is thought to be causally related to age-related decreases in glucose tolerance, especially if fat is accumulated in the upper body (that is, android obesity). In a recent report it was shown that for women with upper body obesity, aged 18–45 yr, the risk of developing diabetes or cardiovascular disease is stronger in Caucasians than in African Americans (38). Sparrow and colleagues have shown that intraabdominal fat content in 41 men (41–76 yr of age), as measured by CT, was significantly correlated with the 2-h serum glucose level following an oral glucose challenge (122). More recently, in healthy older men (47–73 yr of age), utilizing the euglycemic clamp, Coon et al. showed that insulin sensitivity and glucose tolerance are affected primarily by regional fat distribution, not age, physical fitness assessed as VO$_2$ max, or obesity (33). The same finding has been reported by Kohrt (76). However, Shimokata et al. (119) showed that, although fatness, fitness, and fat distribution can account for the decline in glucose tolerance from young (17–39 yr) to middle-aged (40–59 yr) subjects, age remains a significant determinant of further decline in glucose tolerance of healthy old (60–92 yr) subjects. Upper body fat accumulation is associated with insulin resistance, hyperinsulinemia, diminished glucose tolerance, lower sensitivity to insulin in skeletal muscle, and reduced rate of hepatic insulin extraction (43, 73, 105). The distribution of adipose tissue is a risk factor in the development of hypertension, gall bladder disease, NIDDM, cardiovascular disease, as well as some types of cancer (46, 68, 84, 103, 115, 122). The influence of body composition in aging humans has not been accurately studied since anthropometric measurements routinely used as a surrogate to estimate body fat do not reflect the intraabdominal accumulation of fat that occurs with aging (23).

Serum Lipoproteins and Atherosclerosis

Chronically elevated insulin levels may play a role in the development of atherosclerosis, as exogenous insulin enhances the synthesis of cholesterol, triglyceride, and fatty acids in the aorta (124, 125). It has been speculated that even the mild hyperinsulinemia seen in the elderly may play a role in the atherogenic process (45). High insulin levels have been shown to be an independent risk factor for the development and subsequent complications of coronary artery disease (40, 66). Impaired glucose tolerance is also associated with an increased risk of atherosclerotic disease and cataracts and a greatly increased risk of NIDDM (64); NIDDM increases the risk of intermittent claudication, microvascular disease leading to retinopathy and nephropathy, neuropathy, cataracts, and increased risk of infections.

The relationship of lipids and lipoproteins to age and as contributing factors for coronary heart disease (CHD) has been reported from several prevention trials and reviewed by Glueck and Margolin (53). As an example, changes in lipids and lipoproteins with respect to obesity and age can be illustrated from the results of The Prospective Cardiovascular Munster Study (Figure 8.6) (14). Over 12,000 men and 5,000 women, aged 20–59 yr, free of myocardial infarction and stroke, participated in this study. Total cholesterol increased with age, but the BMI in men had only a small effect and no effect in women. Nevertheless, triglycerides (TGs) showed a direct correlation with BMI in contrast to high-density lipoprotein (HDL) cholesterol, which showed a strong inverse relationship with BMI in all age subgroups in each sex. Low-density lipoprotein (LDL) cholesterol also increased with an increase in BMI and age; however, the effect of BMI decreased with increasing age.

Age, gender, and dietary habits appear to be the three most relevant factors responsible for variations in plasma lipoprotein levels. Women have higher HDL cholesterol levels until menopause, when concentrations decrease to those found in men (71). In men, TG concentrations increase until approximately 50 yr of age and then begin to decline. The TG concentrations in women tend to increase progressively with age, with levels slightly higher in women taking estrogens (78).

Strong associations have been made between elevated TG levels and CHD. An NIH Consensus Conference (101) reported that a strong positive relationship between TG and CHD was demonstrated in prospective cohort studies. When other risk factors (such as blood pressure, physical activity, and obesity) are controlled by multivariate analyses, the effect of TG is diminished.

Many studies have found that increased body weight associated with aging as well as fat distribution are accountable for abnormal lipid concentrations (dyslipidemia), thus increasing the risk for cardiovascular disease. Upper body obesity has been shown to be more strongly associated with diabetes, hypertension, altered lipid profiles, and gallbladder disease than lower body obesity (123). Upper body fat is associated with insulin resistance and hyperinsulinemia, which promotes the production of TGs and cholesterol-rich lipoproteins from the liver (17).

Alterations in lipid profiles have been observed with body fat concentrated in the abdominal area (android pattern) (4). In healthy men and women, adipose tissue distribution, assessed by the WHR, and obesity, assessed by the Quetelet Index, were found to be positively correlated to plasma levels of total and HDL cholesterol, TGs, and apolipoprotein B (apoB). The lowest HDL cholesterol was observed in the subjects in the highest tertile of the Quetelet Index (4).

Landin et al. (83) compared WHR and metabolism in lean and obese postmenopausal women. They found significant associations between WHR and metabolic alterations in obese women but no relationship of fat distribution to metabolic complications in lean women. Their data suggest that obesity is essential in order to associate metabolic abnormalities with fat distribution.

Despres et al. (35) have reviewed the relationship of intraabdominal accumulation of fat and obesity for risk factors of CHD. They studied three groups of premenopausal women: 25 nonobese, 10 obese with low levels of intraabdominal fat, and 10 obese with high levels of intraabdominal fat. Obese women with low levels of intraabdominal fat were found to have increased TG and insulin levels compared to the nonobese controls. The obese women with high levels of intraabdominal fat, however, exhibited several other metabolic complications compared to nonobese women, including increased plasma TG, cholesterol, LDL cholesterol, LDL apoB, and reduced HDL cholesterol. They concluded that in obese premenopausal women, the level of intraabdominal fat correlates more closely with an atherogenic profile than obesity per se (35).

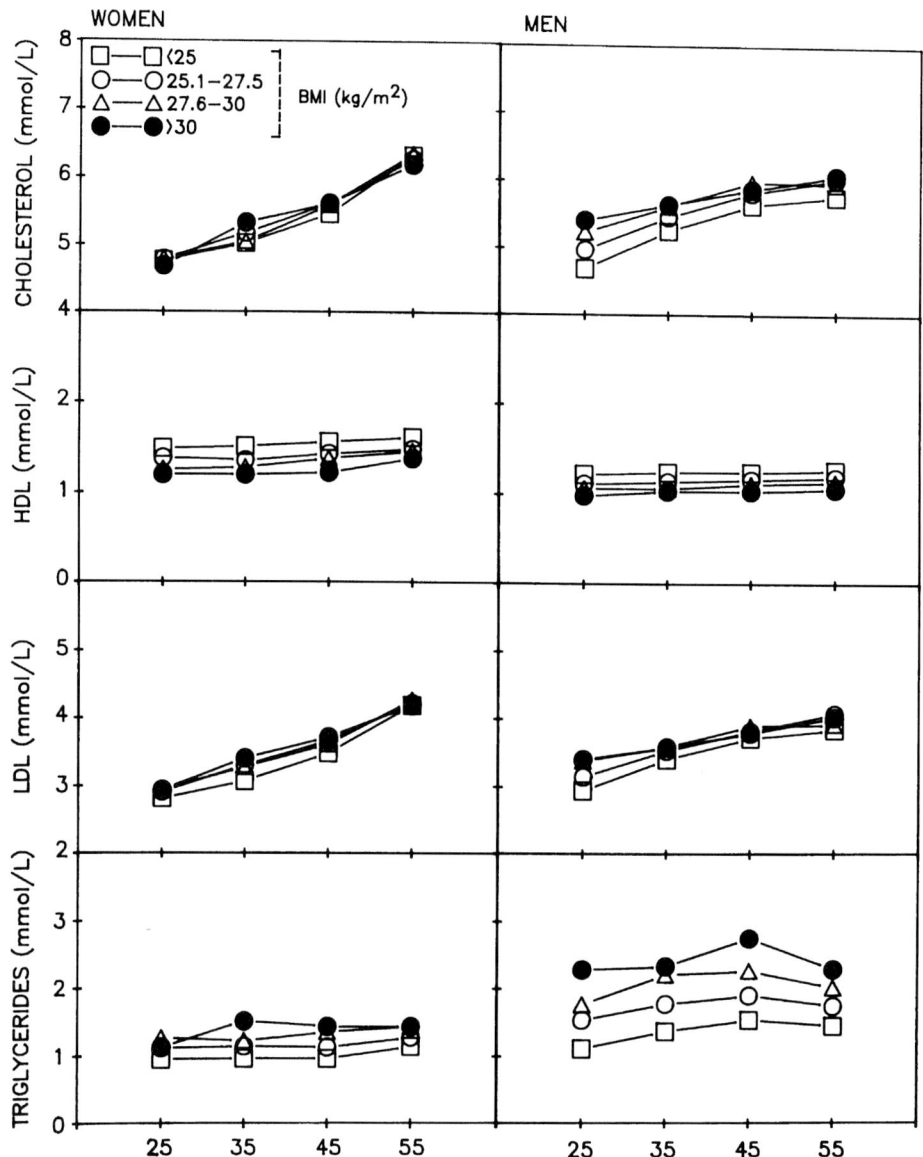

FIG. 8.6. Changes in lipids and lipoproteins in men and women with respect to age and obesity. Adapted from Assman, G., Schulte, H., Obesity and Hyperlipidemia: Results from the Prospective Cardiovascular Munster (PROCAM) Study. In *Obesity*, Bjorntorp, P. and Brodoff, B. N., Eds. J. P. Lippincott Philadelphia, 1992.

In a group of middle-aged, healthy men, Terry et al. (126) reported that WHR correlated positively with plasma TG, cholesterol, LDL cholesterol, and very low-density lipoprotein cholesterol (VLDLC). In addition, HDL cholesterol was inversely correlated with WHR. A subfraction of HDL cholesterol (HDL_2) and its association with metabolic complications was investigated by Ostlund et al. (104). Seventy-seven healthy men and 69 healthy women in the seventh decade of life were studied. In men, women, or the total population, they found no association between HDL_2 levels and obesity as measured by BMI or percent fat. However, this was after adjustment for the WHR. Independent of gender, the WHR predicted HDL_2 concentrations. Ostlund et al. (104) also found plasma insulin concentrations to be inversely correlated with the level of HDL_2 cholesterol. The WHR is widely used as a simple, convenient measure of intraabdominal fat, even though it does not differentiate subcutaneous from intraabdominal fat accumulation.

It remains controversial whether changes in lipoprotein levels that occur with age are, in fact, true biological aging changes or result from life-style factors (such as physical activity and diet). In the Bronx Aging Study (BAS), Zimetbaum et al. (140) studied 488 elderly subjects (75–85 yr) during a 10 yr period to determine risk factors for coronary and cerebrovascular diseases. The study found that in men low levels of HDL cholesterol are a coronary heart disease risk factor. In women elevated levels of LDL cholesterol are associated with myocardial infarction. In this study, however, factors such as medication use, nutrition, and exercise were not controlled for, which may have a significant impact on lipid metabolism.

The BAS is one of a few studies to evaluate a group of elderly subjects prospectively with respect to their lipid and lipoprotein profiles. Therefore, "premature" deaths from CHD are excluded since subjects below age 75 yr were not studied. The BAS suggests that treatment for CHD at advanced ages may improve the quality of life.

In the Framingham Heart Study (30), serum cholesterol was shown to be a risk factor for CHD in patients older than 65 yr. Sorkin et al. (121) demonstrated that cholesterol is a significant risk factor for CHD even in the age group of 75–97 yr. Unlike other studies, the Framingham Study controlled for other risk factors, such as obesity. A linear association of weight with coronary disease was found in men. The sample of women was smaller and showed a less than linear association. Nonetheless, the fact that an association exists between obesity and CHD needs further analysis since several risk factors occur as an individual gains weight. Obesity is associated with lower HDL cholesterol levels. With a weight increase of as little as 5 lb, a 5% decrease in HDL cholesterol level with increases in LDL cholesterol and VLDLC levels can occur (6). Recommendations from the Framingham Study include educating patients on how to increase their HDL cholesterol levels, such as through exercise and weight control (135).

The health consequences of regional adiposity is the subject of intense investigation at this time. Several recent studies suggest that this may have a higher predictive value than obesity per se. The National Institutes of Health convened a workshop to examine this issue. The summary of the proceedings has been published (25), and further publications are expected in the near future.

REFERENCES

1. ABRAHAM, S. Obese and overweight adults in the United States. In: *Vital and Health Statistics,* Washington, D.C.: U.S. Government Printing Service, 1983, series 11, no. 230, p. 1–93.
2. ALLEN, P. S. In vivo NMR spectroscopy. In: *In Vivo Body Composition Studies. Recent Advances,* edited by S. Yasumura, J. E. Harrison, K. G. McNeill, A. D. Woodhead, and F. A. Dilmanian. New York: Plenum Press, 1990, p. 419–426.
3. ALLEN, T. H., H. J. KRZYWICKI, and J. E. ROBERTS. Density, fat, water and solids in freshly isolated tissues. *J. Appl. Physiol.* 14: 1005, 1959.
4. ANDERSON, A. J., K. A. SOBOCINSKI, D. S. FREEDMAN, J. J. BARBORIAK, A. A. RIMM, and H. W. GRUCHOW. Body fat distribution, plasma lipids, and lipoproteins. *Arteriosclerosis* 8: 88–94, 1988.
5. ANDERSON, J., S. B. OSBORN, R. W. S. TOMLINSON, D. NEWTON, J. RUNDO, L. SALMON, and J. W. SMITH. Neutron-activation analysis in man in vivo: a new technique in medical investigation. *Lancet* 2: 1201–1205, 1964.
6. ANDERSON, K. M., P. W. F. WILSON, R. J. GARRISON, and W. P. CASTELLI. Longitudinal and secular trends in lipoprotein cholesterol measurements in a general population sample: the Framingham Offspring Study. *Atherosclerosis* 68: 59–66, 1987.
7. ANDRES, R. Aging and diabetes. *Med. Clin. North Am.* 55: 835–846, 1971.
8. ANDRES, R., D. C. MULLER, and J. D. SORKIN. Long-term effects of change in body weight on all-cause mortality. *Ann. Intern. Med.* 119: 737–743, 1993.
9. ANONYMOUS. Ideal weights for women. *Stat. Bull.* 23: 6–8, 1942.
10. ANONYMOUS. Ideal weights for men. *Stat. Bull.* 24: 6–8, 1943.
11. ANONYMOUS. New weight standards for men and women. *Stat. Bull.* 40: 1–3, 1959.
12. ANONYMOUS. Metropolitan height and weight tables. *Stat. Bull.* 64: 2–9, 1983.
13. ANONYMOUS. Methods for voluntary weight loss and control. *Ann. Intern. Med.* 119: 764–770, 1993.
14. ASSMANN, G., and H. SCHULTE. Obesity and hyperlipidemia: results from the Prospective Cardiovascular Munster (PROCAM) Study. In: *Obesity,* edited by P. Bjorntorp and B. N. Brodoff. Philadelphia: J. B. Lippincott Company, 1992, p. 502–511.
15. BELANGER, B. A., L. A. CUPPLES, and R. B. D'AGOSTINO. *The Framingham Study: an epidemiological investigation of cardiovascular disease,* NIH Publication No. 88-2970, (36th ed) 1988.
16. BENNETT, P. H. Recommendations on the standardization of methods and reporting of tests for diabetes and its microvascular complications in epidemiologic studies. *Diabetes Care* 2: 98–104, 1979.
17. BIERMAN, E. L. Aging and atherosclerosis. In: *Principles of Geriatric Medicine and Gerontology,* edited by W. R. Hazzard, R. Andres, E. L. Bierman, and J. P. Blass, New York: McGraw-Hill, 1990, p. 458–465.
18. BILTZ, R. M., and E. D. PELLIGRINO. The chemical anatomy of bone. *J. Bone Joint Surg.* 51A: 456–466, 1969.
19. BJORNTORP, P. Abdominal obesity and the development of non-insulin dependent diabetes mellitus. *Diabetes Metab. Rev.* 4: 615–622, 1988.
20. BJORNTORP, P. Regional obesity. In: *Obesity,* edited by P. Bjorntorp and B. N. Brodoff. New York: J. P. Lippincott, 1992, p. 579–586.
21. BJORNTORP, P., U. SMITH, and P. LONNROTH (Eds.) Health implications of obesity. *Acta Med. Scand.* 223(suppl. 723): 1, 1988.
22. BORKAN, G. A., S. G. GERZOF, A. H. ROBBINS, D. E. HULTS, C. K. SILBERT, and J. E. SILBERT. Assessment of abdominal fat content by computed tomography. *Am. J. Clin. Nutr.* 36: 172–177, 1982.
23. BORKAN, G., D. E. HULTS, S. G. GERZOF, A. H. ROBINS, and C. K. SILBERT. Age changes in body composition revealed by computed tomography. *J. Gerontol.* 38: 673–677, 1983.
24. BORKAN, G. A., D. E. HULTS, S. G. GERZOF, and A. H. ROBBINS. Comparison of body composition in middle-aged and elderly males using computed tomography. *Am. J. Anthropol.* 66: 289–295, 1985.
25. BOUCHARD, C., G. A. BRAY, and V. S. HUBBARD. Basic and clinical aspects of regional fat distribution. *Am. J. Clin. Nutr.* 52: 946, 1990.

26. BRAY, G. A., (Ed). *Obesity in Perspective,* Washington, D.C.: DHEW Publication No 75-708, 1975.
27. BRAY, G. A. (Ed). *Obesity in America,* Washington, D.C.: NIH Publication No. 79-359, 1979.
28. BROZEK, J., F. GRANDE, J. T. ANDERSON, and A. KEYS. Densitometric analysis of body composition: revision of some quantitative assumptions. *Ann. N.Y. Acad. Sci.* 110: 113–140, 1963.
29. *Build Study 1979.* Chicago: Society of Actuaries and Association of Life Insurance Medical Directors of America, 1980.
30. CASTELLI, W. P., P. W. WILSON, D. LEVY, and K. ANDERSON. Cardiovascular risk factors in the elderly. *Amer. J. Cardiol.* 63: 12h–19h, 1989.
31. CLARYS, J. P., A. D. MARTIN, and D. T. DRINKWATER. Gross tissue weights in the human body cadaver. *Hum. Biol.* 56: 459–473, 1984.
32. COHN, S. H., C. S. BOMBROWSKI, H. R. PATE, and J. S. ROBERTSON. A whole-body counter with an invariant response to radionuclide distribution and body size. *Phys. Med. Biol.* 14: 645–658, 1969.
33. COON, P. J., E. M. ROGUS, D. DRINKWATER, D. C. MULLER, and A. P. GOLDBERG. Role of body fat distribution in the decline in insulin sensitivity and glucose tolerance with age. *J. Clin. Endocrinol. Metab.* 75: 1125–1132, 1992.
34. DAVIDSON, M. B. The effect of aging on carbohydrate metabolism: a review of the English literature and a practical approach to the diagnosis of diabetes mellitus in the elderly. *Metabolism* 28: 688–705, 1979.
35. DESPRES, J., S. MOORJANI, P. J. LUPIEN, A. TREMBLAY, A. NADEAU, and C. BOUCHARD. Regional distribution of body fat, plasma lipoproteins, and cardiovascular disease. *Arteriosclerosis* 10: 497–511, 1990.
36. DEURENBERG, P., K. VAN DER KOOY, P. EVERS, and T. HULSHOF. Assessment of body composition by bioelectrical impedance in a population aged >60 y. *Am. J. Clin. Nutr.* 51: 3–6, 1990.
37. DILMANIAN, F. A., D. A. WEBER, S. YASUMURA, Y. KAMEN, L. LIDOFSKY, S. B. HEMYSFIELD, and R. N. PIERSON JR. Performance of the delayed- and prompt-gamma neutron activation systems at Brookhaven National Laboratory. In: *In Vivo Body Composition Studies,* edited by S. Yasumura, J. E. Harrison, K. G. McNeill, A. D. Woodhead, and F. A. Dilmanian. New York: Plenum Press, 1990, p. 309–316.
38. DOWLING, H. J., and X. PI-SUNYER. Race-dependent health risks of upper body obesity. *Diabetes* 42: 537–543, 1993.
39. DUBOIS, D., and E. F. DUBOIS. Clinical calorimeter. A formula to estimate the approximate surface if height and weight be known. *Arch. Intern. Med.* 17: 863–871, 1916.
40. DUCIMETIERE, P., L. ESCHWEGE, J. PAPOZ, J. L. RICHARD, J. R. CLAUDE, and G. ROSSELIN. Relationship of plasma insulin levels to the incidence of myocardial infarction and coronary heart disease mortality in a middle-aged population. *Diabetologia* 19: 205–210, 1980.
41. DURNIN, J. V. G. A., and J. WOMERSLEY. Body fat assessed from total body density and its estimation from skinfold thickness: measurements from 481 men and women aged from 16 to 72 years. *Br. J. Nutr.* 32: 77–97, 1974.
42. ELIA, M., and G. LIVESEY. Theory and validity of indirect calorimetry during net lipid synthesis. *Am. J. Clin. Nutr.* 47: 591–607, 1988.
43. EVANS, D. J., R. G. HOFFMANN, R. K. KALKHOFF, and A. H. KISSEBAH. Relationship of body fat topography to insulin sensitivity and metabolic profiles in premenopausal women. *Metabolism* 33: 68–75, 1984.
44. FINK, R. I., O. G. KOLTERMAN, J. GRIFFIN, and J. M. OLEFSKY. Mechanisms of insulin resistance in aging. *J. Clin. Invest.* 71: 1523–1535, 1983.
45. FINK, R. I., O. G. KOLTERMAN, and J. M. OLEFSKY. The physiological significance of the glucose intolerance of aging. *J. Gerontol.* 39: 273–278, 1984.
46. FOLSOM, A. R., S. A. KEYS, R. J. PRINEAS, S. D. POTTER, S. M. GAPSTUR, and R. B. WALLACE. Increased incidence of carcinoma of the breast associated with abdominal adiposity in postmenopausal women. *Am. J. Epidemiol.* 131: 794–803, 1990.
47. FORBES, G. B. *Human Body Composition,* New York: Springer-Verlag, 1987, p. 5–100.
48. FORBES, G. B., and A. M. LEWIS. Total sodium, potassium and chloride in adult man. *J. Clin. Invest.* 35: 596–600, 1956.
49. FORBES, R. M., A. R. COOPER, and H. H. MITCHEL. The composition of the adult human body as determined by chemical analysis. *J. Biol. Chem.* 203: 359–366, 1953.
50. FORBES, R. M., H. H. MITCHELL, and A. R. COOPER. Further studies on the gross composition and mineral elements of the adult human body. *J. Biol. Chem.* 223: 969–975, 1956.
51. FOSTER, W. R., and B. T. BURTON (eds.). Health implications of obesity. *Ann. Intern. Med.* 103: 977–1077, 1985.
52. FRISANCHO, A. R. *Anthropometric Standards for the Assessment of Growth and Nutritional Status,* Ann Arbor: The University of Michigan Press, 1990, p. 1–185.
53. GLUECK, C. J., and E. G. MARGOLIN. Lipoprotein metabolism. In: *The Merck Manual of Geriatrics,* edited by W. B. Abrams and R. Berkow. Rahway: Merck Sharp and Dohme Research Laboratories, 1990, p. 844–873.
54. GOTFREDSEN, A., C. CHRISTIANSEN, and R. B. MAZESS. Total body bone mineral in vivo by dual photon absorptiometry. I. Measurement procedures. *Clin. Physiol.* 4: 343–355, 1984.
55. GOTFREDSEN, A., J. JENSEN, J. BORG, and C. CHRISTIANSEN. Measurement of lean body mass and total body fat using dual photon absorptiometry. *Metabolism* 35: 88–93, 1986.
56. HAARBO, J., A. GOTFREDSEN, C. HASSAGER, and C. CHRISTIANSEN. Validation of body composition by dual energy X-ray absorptiometry (DEXA). *Clin. Physiol.* 11: 331–341, 1991.
57. HARRIS, M. I. Noninsulin-dependent diabetes mellitus in black and white Americans. *Diabetes Metab. Rev.* 6: 71–90, 1990.
58. HARRIS, M. I., W. C. HADDEN, W. C. KNOWLER, and P. H. BENNETT. Prevalence of diabetes and impaired glucose tolerance and plasma glucose levels in U.S. population aged 20–74 yr. *Diabetes* 36: 523–534, 1987.
59. HEMPELMANN, L. H., H. LISCO, and J. G. HOFFMANN. The acute radiation syndrome: a study of nine cases and a review of the problem. *Ann. Intern. Med.* 36: 279–510, 1952.
60. HEYMSFIELD, S. B., J. WANG, S. LICHTMAN, Y. KAMEN, J. KEHAYIAS, and R. N. PIERSON. Body composition in elderly subjects: a critical appraisal of clinical methodology. *Am. J. Clin. Nutr.* 50: 1167–1175, 1989.
61. HEYMSFIELD, S. B., J. WANG, M. AULET, J. J. KEHAYIAS, S. LICHTMAN, Y. KAMEN, and F. A. DILMANIAN. Dual photon absorptiometry: validation of mineral and fat measurements. In: *In Vivo Body Composition Studies,* edited by S. Yasumura, J. E. Harrison, K. G. McNeill, A. D. Woodhead, and F. A. Dilmanian, New York: Plenum Press, 1990, p. 327–337.
62. HODGDON, J. A., and P. I. FITZGERALD. Validity of impedance predictions at various levels of fatness. *Hum. Biol.* 59: 281, 1987.
63. HOFFER, E. C., C. K. MEADOW, and D. C. SIMPSON. Correlation of whole body impedance with total body water. *J. Appl. Physiol.* 27: 531–534, 1969.
64. OLLOSZY, J. D., J. SCHULTZ, J. KUSHIERKIEWICZ, J. M. HAGBERY, and A. A. EHSANI. Effects of exercise on glucose tolerance and insulin resistance. *Acta Med. Scand.* 711(suppl): 55–65, 1986.
HUGHES, V. A., and W. J. EVANS. Assessment of fat-free mass in an older population using bioelectrical impedance [Abstract]. *Fed. Proc.* 46: 1187A, 1987.
66. JARRETT, R. J., P. MCCARTNEY, and J. KEEN. The Bedford Sur-

vey: ten year mortality rates in newly diagnosed diabetics, borderline diabetics and normoglycemic controls and risk of indices for coronary heart disease in borderline diabetics. *Diabetologia* 22: 79–84, 1982.
67. JASANI, B. M., and C. J. EDMONDS. Kinetics of potassium distribution in man using isotope dilution and whole body counting. *Metabolism* 20: 1099–1106, 1971.
68. KAPLAN, N. M. The deadly quartet: upper body obesity, glucose intolerance, hypertriglyceridemia and hypertension. *Arch. Intern. Med.* 149: 14–20, 1989.
69. KEHAYIAS, J. J., K. J. ELLIS, S. H. COHN, S. YASUMURA, and J. WEINLEIN. Use of a pulsed neutron generator for in vivo measurement of body carbon. In: *In Vivo Body Composition Studies*, edited by K. J. Ellis, S. Yasumura, and W. D. Morgan. London: Institute of Physical Sciences in Medicine, 1987, p. 427–435.
70. KEHAYIAS, J. J., S. B. HEYMSFIELD, A. F. LoMONTE, J. WANG, and R. N. PIERSON, JR. In vivo determination of body fat by measuring total body carbon. *Am. J. Clin. Nutr.* 53: 1339–1344, 1991.
71. KIRBY, B. Lipoproteins in the elderly. *J. Int. Med. Res.* 19: 425–432, 1991.
72. KISSEBAH, A. H., and A. N. PEIRIS. Biology of regional fat distribution: relationship to non-insulin-dependent diabetes mellitus. *Diabetes Metab. Rev.* 5: 83–109, 1989.
73. KISSEBAH, A. H., N. VYDELINGUM, R. MURRAY, D. J. EVANS, A. J. HARTZ, R. K. KALKHOFF, and P. W. ADAMS. Relation of body fat distribution to metabolic complications of obesity. *J. Clin. Endocrinol. Metab.* 54: 254–260, 1982.
74. KLEIBER, M. *The Fire of Life: An Introduction to Animal Energetics*, Huntington, NY: Robert E. Krieger Publishing, 1975.
75. KNIGHT, G. S., A. H. BEDDOE, S. J. STREAT, and G. L. HILL. Body composition of two human cadavers by neutron activation and chemical analysis. *Am. J. Physiol.* 250 (*Endocrinol. Metab.* 8): E179–E185, 1986.
76. KOHRT, W. M., J. P. KIRWAN, M. A. STATEN, R. E. BOUREY, D. S. KING, and J. O. HOLLOSZY. Insulin resistance in aging is related to abdominal obesity. *Diabetes* 42: 273–281, 1993.
77. KOLTERMAN, O. G., J. INSEL, M. SAEKOW, and J. M. OLEFSKY. Mechanisms of insulin resistance in human obesity. Evidence for receptor and postreceptor defects. *J. Clin. Invest.* 65: 1272–1284, 1980.
78. KREISBERG, R. A., and S. KASIM. Cholesterol metabolism and aging. *Am. J. Med.* 82(suppl. 1B): 54–60, 1987.
79. KUSHNER, R. F., and D. A. SCHOELLER. Estimation of total body water by bioelectrical impedance analysis. *Am. J. Clin. Nutr.* 44: 417–424, 1986.
80. KUSHNER, R. F., A. KUNIGK, M. ALSPAUGH, P. T. ANDRONIS, C. A. LEITCH, and D. SCHOELLER. Validation of bioelectrical-impedance analysis as a measurement of change in body composition in obesity. *Am. J. Clin. Nutr.* 52: 219–223, 1990.
81. KUSHNER, R. F., D. SCHOELLER, C. R. FJELD, and L. DANFORD. Is the impedance index (ht^2/R) significant in predicting total body water? *Am. J. Clin. Nutr.* 56: 835–839, 1992.
82. KYERE, K., B. OLDROYD, C. B. OXBY, L. BURKINSHAW, R. E. ELLIS, and G. L. HILL. The feasibility of measuring total body carbon by counting neutron inelastic scatter gamma rays. *Phys. Med. Biol.* 27: 805–817, 1982.
83. LANDIN, K., M. KROTKIEWSKI, and U. SMITH. Importance of obesity for the metabolic abnormalities associated with abdominal fat distribution. *Metabolism* 38: 572–576, 1989.
84. LARSSON, B., K. SVARDSUDD, L. WELIN, L. WILHELMSEN, P. BJORNTORP, and G. TIBBLIN. Abdominal adipose tissue distribution, obesity and risk of cardiovascular disease and death: 13 year follow up of participants in the study of men born in 1913. *Br. Med. J.* 288: 1401–1404, 1984.

85. LESSER, G. T., S. DEUTSCH, and J. MARKOFSKY. Use of independent measurements of body fat to evaluate overweight and underweight. *Metabolism* 20: 792–804, 1971.
86. LEW, E. A., and L. GARFINKEL. Variations in mortality by weight among 750,000 men and women. *J. Chron. Dis.* 32: 563–576, 1979.
87. LOHMAN, T. G. Applicability of body composition techniques and constants for children and youths. *Exerc. Sport. Sci. Rev.* 14: 325–357, 1986.
88. LOHMAN, T. G., A. F. ROCHE, and R. MARTORELL. *Anthropometric standardization reference manual.* Champaign, IL: Human Kinetics Books, 1988, p. 1–164.
89. LUKASKI, H. C., and W. W. BOLONCHUK. Theory and validation of the tetrapolar bioelectrical impedance method to assess human body composition. In: *In Vivo Body Composition Studies*, edited by K. J. Ellis, S. Yasumura, and W. D. Morgan. London: Institute of Physical Sciences in Medicine, 1987, p. 410–414.
90. LUKASKI, H. C., P. E. JOHNSON, W. W. BOLONCHUK, and G. L. LYKKEN. Assessment of fat free mass using bioelectrical impedance measurements of the human body. *Am. J. Clin. Nutr.* 41: 810–817, 1985.
91. LUKASKI, H. C., W. W. BOLONCHUK, C. B. HALL, and W. A. SIDERS. Validation of tetrapolar bioelectrical impedance method to assess human body composition. *J. Appl. Physiol.* 60: 1327–1332, 1986.
92. MARTIN, A. D., D. T. DRINKWATER, and J. P. CLARYS. Human body surface area: validation of formulae based on a cadaver study. *Hum. Biol.* 56: 475–488, 1984.
93. MARTIN, A. D., L. F. SPENST, D. T. DRINKWATER, and J. P. CLARYS. Anthropometric estimation of muscle mass in men. *Med. Sci. Sports Exerc.* 22: 729–733, 1990.
94. MAZESS, R. B., W. W. PEPPLER, and M. GIBBONS. Total body composition by dual photon (^{153}Gd) absorptiometry. *Am. J. Clin. Nutr.* 40: 834–839, 1984.
95. MAZESS, R., B. COLLICK, J. TREMPE, H. BARDEN, and J. HANSON. Performance evaluation of a dual-energy X-ray bone densitometer. *Calcif. Tissue Int.* 44: 228–232, 1989.
96. MITCHELL, H. H., T. S. HAMILTON, F. R. STEGGERDA, and H. W. BEAN. The chemical composition of the adult human body and its bearing on the biochemistry of growth. *J. Biol. Chem.* 158: 625–637, 1945.
97. MODAN, M., M. I. HARRIS, and H. HALKIN. Evaluation of WHO and NDDG criteria for impaired glucose tolerance: results from two national samples. *Diabetes* 38: 1630–1635, 1989.
98. MOORE, F. D., K. H. OLESEN, J. D. McMURRAY, H. V. PARKER, M. R. BALL, and C. M. BOYDEN. *The Body Cell Mass and Its Supporting Environment.* Philadelphia: W. B. Saunders, 1963.
99. NAJJAR, M. F., and M. ROWLAND. Anthropometric reference data and prevalence of overweight, 1976–80. In: *Vital and Health Statistics*, Washington, D.C.: U.S. Government Printing Office, 1987, series 11, no. 238.
100. National Diabetes Data Group. Classification and diagnosis of diabetes mellitus and other categories of glucose intolerance. *Diabetes* 28: 1037–1057, 1979.
101. NIH Consensus Conference. Triglyceride, high-density lipoprotein, and coronary heart disease. *JAMA* 269: 505–510, 1993.
102. NYBOER, J. Workable volume and flow concepts of biosegments by electrical impedance plethysmography. *J. Life Sci.* 2: 1–13, 1972.
103. OHLSON, L. O., B. LARSSON, K. SVARDSUDD, L. WELIN, H. ERIKSSON, L. WILHELMSEN, P. BJORNTORP, and G. TIBBIN. The influence of body fat distribution on the incidence of diabetes mellitus: 13.5 years of follow-up of the participants in the study of men born in 1913. *Diabetes* 34: 1055–1058, 1985.

104. OSTLUND, R. E., JR., M. STATEN, W. M. KOHRT, J. SCHULTZ, and M. MALLEY. The ratio of waist-to-hip circumference, plasma insulin level, and glucose intolerance as independent predictors of the HDL2 cholesterol level in older adults. *N. Engl. J. Med.* 322: 229–234, 1990.
105. PEIRIS, B. N., R. A. MUELLER, G. A. SMITH, M. F. STRUVE, and A. H. KISSEBAH. Splanchnic insulin metabolism in obesity: influence of body fat distribution. *J. Clin. Invest.* 78: 1648–1657, 1986.
106. PIERSON, R. N. JR., J. WANG, S. B. HEYMSFIELD, F. A. DILMANIAN, and D. A. WEBER. High precision in-vivo neutron activation analysis: a new era for compartmental analysis in body composition. In: *In Vivo Body Composition Studies,* edited by S. Yasumura, J. E. Harrison, K. G. McNeill, A. D. Woodhead, and F. A. Dilmanian. New York: Plenum Press, 1990, p. 317–325.
107. QUETELET, M. A. *A Treatise on Man and the Development of his Faculties,* Edinburgh: William and Robert Chambers, 1842.
108. RABINOWITZ, D., and K. L. ZIERLER. Forearm metabolism in obesity and its response to intraarterial insulin: Characterization of insulin resistance and evidence for adaptive hyperinsulinism. *J. Clin. Invest.* 41: 2173–2182, 1962.
109. RAHN, H., W. O. FENN, and A. B. OTIS. Daily variation of vital capacity, residual air, and expiratory reserve including a study of the residual air methods. *J. Appl. Physiol.* 1: 725–743, 1949.
110. SCHOELLER, D. A. Isotope dilution methods. In: *Obesity,* edited by P. Bjorntorp, and B. N. Brodoff. Philadelphia: Lippincott Co., 1992, p. 80–88.
111. SCHWARTZ, R. S., W. P. SHUMAN, V. L. BRADBURY, K. C. CAIN, G. W. FELLINGHAM, J. C. BEARD, and S. KAHN. Body fat distribution in healthy young and older men. *J. Gerontol.* 45: M181–M185, 1990.
112. SCHWARTZ, R. S., W. P. SHUMAN, V. LARSON, K. C. CAIN, G. W. FELLINGHAM, J. C. BEARD, and S. E. KAHN. The effect of intensive endurance training on body fat distribution in young and older men. *Metabolism* 40: 545–551, 1991.
113. SEGAL, K. R., B. GUTIN, E. PRESTA, J. WANG, and T. B. VAN ITALLIE. Estimation of human body composition by electrical impedance methods: a comparitive study. *J. Appl. Physiol.* 58: 1565–1571, 1985.
114. SEGAL, K. R., M. VAN LOAN, P. I. FITZGERALD, J. A. HODGDON, and T. B. VAN ITALLIE. Lean body mass estimation by bioelectrical impedance analysis: a four-site cross-validation study. *Am. J. Clin. Nutr.* 47: 7–14, 1988.
115. SELBY, J. V., G. D. FREIDMAN, and C. P. QUESENBERRY. Precursors of essential hypertension. *Am. J. Epidemiol.* 129: 43–53, 1989.
116. SHENG, H. P., and R. A. HUGGINS. A review of body composition studies with emphasis on total body water and fat. *Am. J. Clin. Nutr.* 32: 630–647, 1979.
117. SHIMOKATA, H., R. ANDRES, P. J. COON, D. ELAHI, D. C. MULLER, and J. D. TOBIN. Studies in the distribution of body fat: II. Longitudinal effects of change in weight. *Int. J. Obes.* 13: 455–464, 1989.
118. SHIMOKATA, H., J. D. TOBIN, D. C. MULLER, D. ELAHI, P. J. COON, and R. ANDRES. Studies in the distribution of body fat: effect of age, sex and obesity. *J. Gerontol.* 44: M66–M73, 1989.
119. SHIMOKATA, H., D. C. MULLER, J. L. FLEG, J. SORKIN, A. W. ZIEMBA, and R. ANDRES. Age as independent determinant of glucose tolerance. *Diabetes* 40: 44–51, 1991.
120. SIRI, W. E. The gross composition of the body. In: *Advances in Biological and Medical Physics IV,* edited by C. A. Tobias and J. H. Lawrence. New York: Academic Press, 1956, p. 239–279.
121. SORKIN, J. D., R. ANDRES, D. C. MULLER, H. L. BALDWIN, and J. L. FLEG. Cholesterol as a risk factor for coronary heart disease in elderly men. The Baltimore Longitudinal Study of Aging. *Ann. Epidemiol.* 2: 59–67, 1992.
122. SPARROW, D., G. A. BORKAN, S. G. GERZOF, C. WISNIEWSKI, and C. W. SILBERT. Relationship of fat distribution to glucose tolerance. Results of computed tomography in male participants of the Normative Aging Study. *Diabetes* 35: 411–415, 1986.
123. STERN, M. P., and S. M. HAFFNER. Body fat distribution and hyperinsulinemia as risk factors for diabetes and cardiovascular disease. *Arteriosclerosis* 6: 123–130, 1986.
124. STOUT, R. W. The role of insulin in atherosclerosis in diabetics and nondiabetics: a review. *Diabetes* 30(suppl. 2): 54–57, 1981.
125. STOUT, R. W. Insulin and atheroma. *Diabetes Care* 13: 631–654, 1990.
126. TERRY, R. B., P. D. WOOD, W. L. HASKELL, M. L. STEFANICK, and R. M. KRAUSS. Regional adiposity patterns in relation to lipids, lipoprotein cholesterol, and lipoprotein subfraction mass in men. *J. Clin. Endocrinol. Metab.* 68: 191–199, 1989.
127. VAGUE, J. La differenciation sexuelle, factuer determinant des formes de l'obesitie. *Presse Med.* 30: 339, 1947.
128. VAGUE, J. The degree of masculine differentiation of obesities: a factor determining predisposition to diabetes, atherosclerosis, gout, and uric calculous disease. *Am. J. Clin. Nutr.* 4: 20–34, 1956.
129. VAN LOAN, M., and P. MAYCLIN. Bioelectrical impedance analysis: is it a reliable estimator of lean body mass and total body water? *Hum. Biol.* 59: 299–309, 1993.
130. VARTSKY, D., K. J. ELLIS, and S. H. COHN. In vivo quantification of body nitrogen by neutron capture prompt gamma-ray analysis. *J. Nucl. Med.* 20: 1158–1165, 1979.
131. VARTSKY, D., K. J. ELLIS, A. N. VASWANI, S. YASUMURA, and S. H. COHN. An improved calibration for the in vivo determination of body nitrogen, hydrogen and fat. *Phys. Med. Biol.* 29: 209–218, 1984.
132. WEST, K. M. *Epidemiology of Diabetes and Its Vascular Lesions.* New York: Elsevier, 1978, p. 231–248.
133. WIDDOWSON, E. M. Chemical analysis of the body. In: *Human Body Composition: Approaches and Applications, symposia for the Society for the Study of Human Biology,* edited by J. Brozek. Oxford: Pergamon Press, 1965, p. 31–55.
134. WIDDOWSON, E. M., R. A. MCCANCE, and C. M. SPRAY. The chemical composition of the human body. *Clin. Sci.* 10: 113–125, 1951.
135. WILSON, P. W. F. High-density lipoprotein, low-density lipoprotein and coronary artery disease. *Am. J. Cardiol.* 66: 7a–10a, 1990.
136. WINTER, J., and W. KING. Basic principles of computed tomography. In: *Essentials of body Computed Tomography,* edited by M. Greenberg and B. M. Greenberg. Philadelphia: W. B. Saunders, 1983, p. 1–23.
137. WOMERSLEY, J., K. BODDY, P. C. KING, and J. V. G. A. DURNIN. A comparison of the fat-free mass of young adults estimated by anthropometry, body density and total body potassium content. *Clin. Sci.* 43: 469–475, 1972.
138. WONG, W. W., W. J. COCHRAN, L. S. LEE, W. J. KLISH, and P. D. KLEIN. Deuterium and oxygen-18 isotope dilution spaces in normal adults. In: *In Vivo Body Composition Studies,* edited by K. J. Ellis, S. Yasumura, and W. D. Morgan. London: Institute of Physical Sciences in Medicine, 1987, p. 144–148.
139. World Health Organization. Measuring obesity: classification and description of anthropometric data. (Unpublished report on a WHO consultation on the epidemiology of obesity, October 1987). Copenhagen: Nutrition Unit, WHO Regional Office for Europe, 1989, p. 1–21.
140. ZIMETBAUM, P., W. H. FRISHMAN, W. L. OOI, M. P. DERMAN, M. ARONSON, L. I. GIDEZ, and H. A. EDER. Plasma lipids and lipoproteins and the incidence of cardiovascular disease in the very elderly: the Bronx Aging Study. *Arterio. Thromb.* 12: 416–423, 1992.

9. Gene expression and protein degradation

HOLLY VAN REMMEN
WALTER F. WARD
ROBERT V. SABIA
ARLAN RICHARDSON

Departments of Medicine and Physiology, University of Texas Health Science Center, and the Geriatric Research, Education and Clinical Center, Audie L. Murphy Memorial Veterans Hospital, San Antonio, Texas

CHAPTER CONTENTS

Transcription
    RNA synthesis
    mRNA levels
    Transcriptional and posttranscriptional processing of mRNA
    Factors that regulate transcription
        Chromatin structure
        DNA methylation
        Transcription factors
    Effect of dietary restriction on transcription
Translation
    Protein synthesis
    Effect of dietary restriction on protein synthesis
    Fidelity of protein synthesis
    Various steps of protein synthesis
Protein Degradation
    Degradation of mixed protein populations
    Degradation of individual proteins
    Degradation of abnormal proteins
    Effect of dietary restriction on protein degradation
Summary and Conclusions

GENETIC INFORMATION FLOWS IN ALL CELLS from DNA to RNA to protein. Regulation of the flow of information from DNA, that is, gene expression, is critical to a cell because it determines what biochemical processes a cell can or cannot perform by determining what proteins/polypeptides a cell can or cannot synthesize. The first step in the flow of genetic information is the production of RNA molecules from specific genes in the DNA, a process known as *transcription*. The regulation of transcription, that is, the process of determining which genes are or are not transcribed by a cell, represents a major method for regulating gene expression in all living organisms. The second step in the flow of information is the production of protein from the mRNA template, a process known as *translation* or *protein synthesis*. Translation is a complex process involving a large number of protein factors and a variety of RNA species (for example, rRNA and tRNA) in addition to mRNA molecules, which code for the specific polypeptides. Gene expression can be regulated at the level of translation; however, regulation at the level of transcription generally represents the primary method. Because a change in the level of the gene product, that is, the polypeptide, is the critical endpoint in gene expression, the degradation of proteins also is very important to a cell or organism.

A list of review articles that have been published on aging and various aspects of gene expression and protein degradation is given in Table 9.1. In this chapter, we present a comprehensive review of the research that has been conducted on aging in relation to transcription, translation, and protein degradation/turnover. We discuss the current view of alterations in transcription, translation, and protein degradation with increasing age in animal systems ranging from invertebrates to human subjects, excluding studies that measured gene expression or protein degradation during development or maturation. Studies of gene expression/protein degradation in the fibroblast model of cellular senescence are only mentioned where they are relevant to whole animal studies because this model is discussed in detail in Chapter 4.

TRANSCRIPTION

RNA Synthesis

Table 9.2 lists all the studies in which transcription has been measured in young and old organisms. In these studies, transcription (or RNA synthesis) was measured by incorporating a radioactively labeled precursor into RNA. Because the immediate precursors to RNA (the nucleotide triphosphates) cannot penetrate the cell membrane, it is difficult to accurately measure RNA synthesis by cells or tissues. Simply measuring the incorporation of a radiolabeled nucleoside or pyrimidine base into RNA is not an accurate measure of RNA synthesis because changes in uptake or metabolism of the processor or the pool size of the endogenous precursor

172 HANDBOOK OF PHYSIOLOGY—AGING

TABLE 9.1. *Recent Reviews on Aging and Gene Expression or Protein Degradation/Metabolism*

Chromatin proteins and cellular aging	Medvedev (237)
The relationship between aging and protein synthesis	Richardson (313)
RNA synthesis	Rothstein and Seifert (333)
Protein synthesis and degradation during aging and senescence	Makrides (215)
Aging and transcription	Richardson et al. (319)
Age-related changes in protein synthesis	Richardson and Birchenall-Sparks (315)
Enzymes, enzyme alteration, and protein turnover	Rothstein 332
Age-related changes in the structure and function of chromatin	Thakur (391)
Macromolecular methylation during aging	Mays-Hoopes (231)
The effect of age and nutrition on protein synthesis by cells and tissues from mammals	Richardson (314)
Levels of specific messenger RNA species as a function of age	Richardson (324)
Aging and gene expression	Richardson et al. (323)
Age-related changes of transcription and RNA processing	Medvedev (239)
Age-related changes in the synthesis of individual liver-specific proteins	Horbach et al. (148)
Effect of aging on translation and transcription	Richardson and Semsei (318)
Implication of protein oxidation in protein turnover, aging, and oxygen toxicity	Stadtman et al. (374)
Biochemical markers of aging	Stadtman (372)
Protein oxidation and aging	Stadtman (373)
DNA methylation in aging and cancer	Mays-Hoopes (232)
RNA and protein metabolism in the aging brain	Finch and Morgan (94)
Alterations in gene expression with aging	Danner and Holbrook (72)
Protein synthesis and the components of protein synthetic machinery during cellular ageing	Rattan (304)
Effect of age on liver protein synthesis and degradation	Ward and Richardson (414)
The next frontier: studies of the effects of age and diet on mammalian gene expression	Kristal and Yu (183)
Protein synthesis, posttranslational modifications, and aging	Rattan et al. (306)
Gene expression and aging	Thakur et al (394)

could have a significant impact on the amount of radioactivity incorporated. This might be a significant problem in aging research because changes in the nucleotide content of tissues have been reported with age (31). The problem of precursor uptake, pool size, and metabolism can be eliminated using isolated nuclei to measure RNA synthesis. In this system, the amount of a radioactively labeled nucleotide triphosphate, for example, uridine triphosphate (UTP), incorporated into RNA can be used to directly assess the level of RNA synthesis. While this system allows accurate measurement of RNA synthesis under defined conditions, the question remains as to whether isolated nuclei accurately reflect the transcriptional activity of a whole cell or tissue.

Most of the studies in this area have measured RNA synthesis as a function of age in the liver of rodents (Table 9.2). The studies in which RNA synthesis has been measured in vivo should be viewed with caution because neither the uptake of the precursor nor the specific activity of the precursor pool was measured. However, it is striking that eight of the nine studies that used isolated nuclei to measure transcription reported a significant decrease (33–88%) in RNA synthesis with age. Figure 9.1 shows an example of one of these studies in which liver nuclei isolated from rats of various ages were used to measure transcription. RNA synthesis decreased over 70% between 6 and 31 months of age. It appears that the age-related decrease in RNA synthesis observed in isolated nuclei accurately reflects the transcriptional status of the liver because Richardson et al. (320) reported that the rate of RNA synthesis, measured by suspension of rat hepatocytes, declined with age, as shown in Figure 9.1. In this study, Richardson et al. (320) measured the rates of RNA synthesis by hepatocytes isolated from rats of various ages by dividing the amount of radioactivity incorporated into RNA by the specific activity of the UTP precursor pool. Thus these measurements should be an accurate reflection of the ability of hepatocytes isolated from young and old rats to synthesize RNA. Park and Buetow (291) confirmed this observation and showed that RNA synthesis (the incorporation of uridine into RNA) declined significantly with age in isolated hepatocytes. Thus it appears fairly certain that the total transcriptional activity of rodent liver declines significantly with age.

Table 9.2 also lists the studies in which RNA synthesis was measured as a function of age in various rodent tissues and invertebrates. Over 75% of these studies showed an age-related decrease in RNA synthesis.

TABLE 9.2. *Effect of Age on RNA Synthesis*

Sex/Strain	Ages Studied (in months, unless specified)	System	Percent Change	Reference
Liver				
Rats				
Male strain unspecified	3–27	In vivo	+42	Samis et al. (336)
Male Wistar	12–31	Liver slices	No change	Beauchene et al. (14)
Female Wistar	12–31	Liver slices	No change	Beauchene et al. (14)
Male Sprague-Dawley	12–31	Liver slices	No change	Beauchene et al. (14)
Unspecified	1–22	Nuclei	No change	Gibas and Harmon (45)
Male Wistar	10–22	In vivo	−75	Kanungo et al. (166)
Female Sprague-Dawley	2–18	Nuclei	−85	Denckla (76)
Sex/species unspecified	3–20	In vivo	+48	Martin and Martin (222)
Male Fischer 344	13–31	Nuclei	−36	Castle et al. (46)
Male Sprague-Dawley	0.75–24	Hepatocytes	Decrease	Collins (62)
Female Sprague-Dawley	6–24	Nuclei	−75	Bolla and Denckla (30)
Male Fischer 344	12–30	Hepatocytes	−37	Kreamer et al. (182)
Sex/strain unspecified	4–27	Nuclei	−46	Lindell et al (205)
Male Fischer 344	12–32	Hepatocytes	−40 – 60	Richardson et al (320)
Female CYF	13–25	In vivo	No change	Semsei et al. (343)
Female CYF	13–26	In vivo	No change	Zs.-Nagy and Semsei (443)
Female Wistar	12–26	Nuclei	Decrease	Park and Buetow (290)
Female Wistar	12–25	Hepatocytes	Decrease	Park and Buetow (291)
Mice				
Unspecified	1–25	Nuclei	−43	Devi et al. (77)
Female C57B1/6J	3–28	Liver slices	No change	Beauchene et al. (14)
Male C57B1/6J	6–30	Nuclei	−33	Mainwaring (213)
Male C57B1/6J	3–25	Nuclei	−50	Britton et al (34)
Male NMRI	3–24	In vivo	−37	Fog and Pakkenberg (100)
Male C57B1/6J	4–15	In vivo	−20	Soriero (369)
Other Tissues				
Rats				
Bone Marrow				
Male Wistar	12 and 24	In vitro	No change	Menzies et al, (242)
Brain				
Female CYF	13–26	In vivo	−29	Semsei et al (343)
Female CYF	13–26	In vivo	−40	Zs.-Nagy and Semsei (443)
Heart				
Male strain unspecified	3–4 and 23–24	In vivo	−50	Meerson et al. (240)
Kidney				
Male Wistar	6 and 24	Nuclei	−37	Liang et al. (201)
Uterus				
Female Wistar	6–8 and 24	Nuclei	−25 to −50	Haji et al. (131)
Various tissues				
Male Wistar	3–22	In vivo	Increase in most tissues	Kanungo et al. (166)
Mice				
Cartilage				
Swiss albino sex unspecified	1–20	In vivo	−70	Tonna and Singh (396)
Human skin	0–82	Fibroblasts	−50	Chen et al. (55)

Again, one must be concerned with the accuracy in measuring RNA synthesis in the in vivo studies because the specific activities of the precursor pools were not measured. Figure 9.2 shows the effect of age on the synthesis of RNA by cultured fibroblasts isolated from the skin of human subjects over a wide spectrum of ages. RNA synthesis decreased approximately 50% after 20 y of age. More recently, Fernandez-Silva et al (92) reported that the in vitro synthesis of RNA by isolated mitochondria from rat brain decreased over 50% between 4 and 28 months of age. Thus the data suggest that an age-related decline in transcription occurs with increasing age in most tissues and organisms.

It should be noted that the studies listed in Table 9.2

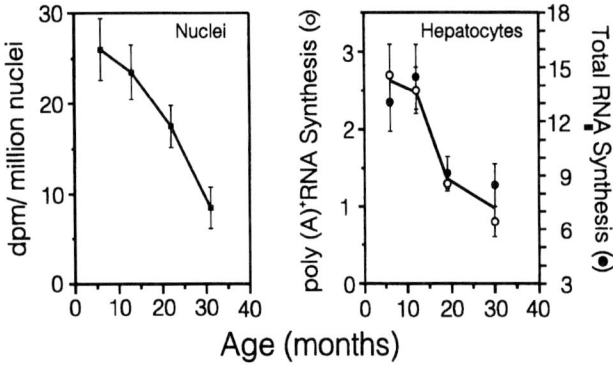

FIG. 9.1. Effect of age on RNA synthesis by rat liver. The graph on the *left* shows the rate of RNA synthesis by nuclei isolated from the livers of rats of various ages [data taken from Castle et al. (46)], and the graph on the *right* shows the rate of total RNA synthesis (●) and poly(A)⁺RNA synthesis (○) by hepatocytes isolated from rats of various ages [data taken from Richardson et al. (320)].

measured total RNA synthesis, that is, the synthesis of all RNA species (rRNA, tRNA, and mRNA). Because these three RNA species are synthesized in various amounts and because rRNA makes up the bulk of the RNA synthesized under the conditions used to measure transcription, it is impossible to conclude from these studies anything about how aging specifically affects the synthesis of a particular species of RNA, such as mRNA, which makes up only a small fraction of the newly synthesized RNA. The effect of aging on mRNA synthesis is of particular interest because mRNA plays a central role in gene expression, and gene expression is regulated primarily through changes in the synthesis of specific mRNA transcripts. Only five studies have expressly measured mRNA synthesis as a function of age. In these studies, synthesis was measured by incorporating a radiolabeled precursor into poly(A)⁺RNA; approximately 80% of the mRNA molecules in mammalian cells contain a 3′-poly(A) terminus (250). In the first study in this area, Richardson et al. (320) measured the rate of poly(A)⁺RNA synthesis by hepatocytes isolated from 6–30-month-old rats. A 65% decrease in the rate of poly(A)⁺RNA was observed, as shown in Figure 9.1. They also found that the rates of rRNA synthesis and tRNA synthesis declined with age. Park and Buetow (291) reported that the synthesis of poly(A)⁺RNA by rat hepatocytes decreased almost 50% between 12 and 25 months of age. Thus mRNA synthesis appears to decrease with increasing age in rat liver. Semsei et al. (343) and Zs.-Nagy and Semsei (443) reported that the in vivo incorporation of radioactive uridine into poly(A)⁺RNA in brain of rats decreased between 1.5 and 26 months of age. However, the specific activity of the UTP precursor pool was not measured. Liang et al. (201) found that the synthesis of poly(A)⁺RNA by nuclei from rat kidney decreased 39% between 6 and 24 months of age. In addition, Fernandez-Silva et al. (92) observed that the in vitro transcription of 12S and 16S rRNA and various poly(A)⁺RNA transcripts by mitochondria isolated from rat brain decreased over 50–80% between 4 and 28 months of age. The age-related decrease in RNA synthesis by mitochondria was correlated to a decrease in the levels of rRNA and various RNA transcripts in brain mitochondria (108).

Although there are only a few studies in which poly(A)⁺RNA synthesis has been measured as a function of age, there are several studies in which the poly(A)⁺RNA content of RNA has been measured in tissues of young and old rodents, for example, liver (22, 145, 262) and brain (61). These studies reported no age-related change in the poly(A)⁺RNA content of the RNA; only the study by Semsei et al. (343) found a significant decrease in poly(A)⁺RNA content with age. Thus the age-related decrease in poly(A)⁺RNA synthesis observed in hepatocytes by Richardson et al. (320) and Park and Buetow (291) does not appear to result in a significant reduction in the level of poly(A)⁺RNA in the liver. Based on these preliminary observations, one would predict that the degradation of the poly(A)⁺RNA would also decrease with age to compensate for the age-related decrease in its synthesis. The decrease in the synthesis and degradation of poly(A)⁺RNA would lead to an age-related increase in its turnover, or half-life. In 1980, Moore et al. (254) reported that the half-life of poly(A)⁺RNA in the liver of rats increased from 3.6 to 15.2 h between 3 and 30 months of age. Thus these very limited data suggest that the turnover of poly(A)⁺RNA

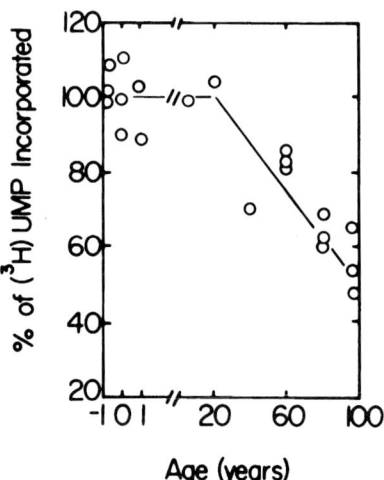

FIG. 9.2. Effect of donor age on RNA synthesis in human fibroblasts. Fibroblasts were obtained from the foreskin of normal white males of various ages and RNA synthesis measured as the incorporation of radioactive UTP into RNA [data taken from Chen et al. (55) and figure taken from Richardson et al. (319), with permission].

decreases with age because of an age-related decrease in its synthesis and degradation. These data are important to keep in mind because it has often been assumed that the degradation of RNA increases, not decreases, with age. Heydari et al. (138) compared the rate of degradation of a specific mRNA transcript, heat shock protein (hsp) 70, by hepatocytes isolated from young and old rats. As the data in Figure 9.3 show, the rate of hsp70 mRNA degradation was reduced in hepatocytes isolated from old rats. This is the first study to show that the degradation rate of a specific mRNA species is altered by aging. It would be interesting to know if the degradation/turnover of other mRNA species is altered with increasing age. Based on the data of Richardson et al. (320) and Moore et al. (254), one would predict that the turnover of most mRNA species would decrease with age in liver. This is interesting because a similar phenomenon appears to occur with proteins; that is, an age-related decrease in protein turnover arises from a decrease in protein synthesis and degradation. In the following sections on TRANSLATION and PROTEIN DEGRADATION, these experiments will be discussed in more detail.

Since the early 1970s several laboratories have studied the mechanism responsible for the age-related decline in RNA synthesis in rodent liver. Using [^{32}P]-labeled purine nucleoside triphosphates, Miller and co-workers (248) showed that the initiation of RNA synthesis decreased with age in nuclei isolated from livers of rats ranging from 3 to 30 months of age. A similar conclusion was reached by Park and Buetow (290) using a nuclear "runoff" transcription assay, which measured the number of active transcription complexes initiated in a cell. Thus it appears that the age-related decrease in RNA synthesis in rodent liver is due primarily to an inability of the hepatocytes from the old animals to initiate transcription. However, it appears that the age-related decrease in the initiation of transcription is not due to a deficiency in the enzymes involved in RNA synthesis, that is, the RNA polymerases. For example, Britton et al. (34) reported that the RNA polymerase activity of isolated liver nuclei from mice with exogenous DNA did not change significantly with increasing age. Subsequently, Benson and Harker (16) measured the activities of purified RNA polymerases isolated from the nuclei of liver and brain of 18- and 31-month-old mice and found no significant age-related change in the activities of RNA polymerases I and II, which catalyze the synthesis of rRNA and hnRNA (that is, mRNA), respectively. However, an age-related decrease in the activity of RNA polymerase III was observed. Bolla and Denckla (30) and Park and Buetow (290) also found that the total RNA polymerase activity of liver nuclei isolated from rats did not change with age. However, these two groups did observe a significant change in the amount of the RNA polymerase activity bound to chromatin; the percentage of this activity decreased significantly with age while the percentage of free RNA polymerase activity, that is, not bound to chromatin, increased with age. Therefore, the age-related decrease in RNA synthesis does not appear to be due to a decrease in the amount of RNA polymerase available to the cell to catalyze RNA synthesis but to the amount of RNA polymerase bound to DNA and actively synthesizing RNA.

mRNA Levels

With the advent of DNA recombinant technology, there has been a rapid explosion in the amount of data on specific mRNA transcript changes with age. Using cDNA probes to specific mRNAs, it is relatively simple to measure the level of an mRNA transcript in RNA preparations by RNA/DNA hybridization. Before cDNA probes were available to specific genes, a few investigators studied the effect of age on the level of a specific mRNA using cell-free translation assays [see review by Richardson et al. (318)]; however, these assays are difficult to perform and only indirectly measure the level of an mRNA transcript. In Tables 9.3–9.6, we list all of the published studies that have compared the level of mRNA transcripts in tissues of young and old animals. The data from these studies show that the effect of age on mRNA levels varies from mRNA to mRNA: the levels of many mRNA transcripts decline with age; however, some levels do not change significantly with age, and in a few cases, levels have been reported to increase with age. Figure 9.4 shows an

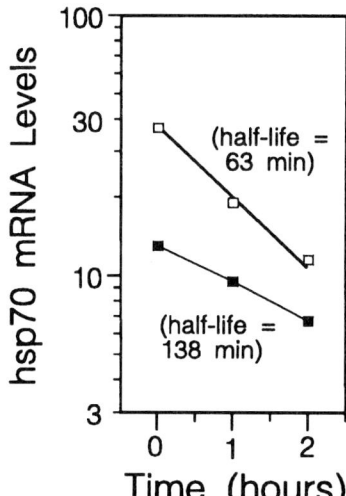

FIG. 9.3. Effect of age on the degradation of hsp70 mRNA. Levels of hsp70 transcript were measured in hepatocytes isolated from 6- (□) and 26- (■) month-old rats after a brief heat shock [data taken from Heydari et al. (138)].

TABLE 9.3. *Effect of Age on the mRNA Levels in Liver*

Sex/Strain	mRNA	Change with Age	Ages Studied (months, unless specified)	Reference
Rat				
Male Wistar	Acetyl CoA carboxylase $^{\Delta,+}$	Decrease	1.5–18	Fukuda and Iritani (105)
Male Sprague-Dawley	α_1-acid glycoprotein	Decrease	10 and 23	Sierra et al. (351)
Female WAG/Rij	α-actin	No change	6–36	Slagboom et al. (359)
Female WAG/Rij	Albumin$^+$	Increase	3–36	Horbach et al. (145)
Male Fisher 344	Albumin	Increase	6–29	Richardson et al. (324)
Male Sprague-Dawley	Albumin	Increase	10 and 25	Wellinger and Guigoz (428)
Female Wistar	Albumin	No change	6 and 24	Sato et al. (337)
Male Fischer 344	Aldolase$^\Delta$	Decrease	6–29	Richardson et al. (324)
Male Fischer 344	Androgen sulfotransferase	Increase	1–28	Chatterjee et al. (52)
Male Fischer 344	Androgen receptor	Decrease	12–27	Song et al. (364)
Male Fischer 344	Apolipoprotein A1	Increase	6–37	Waggoner et al. (408)
Male Fischer 344	Apolipoprotien B	Decrease	6–37	Waggoner et al. (408)
Male Fischer 344	Catalase$^\Delta$	Decrease	6–26	Rao et al. (301)
Male Fischer 344	Catalase$^\Delta$	Decrease	4–28	Rao et al. (300)
Male Fischer 344	Catalase$^\Delta$	Decrease	6–29	Semsei et al. (341)
Fischer 344 (sex unspecified)	Cytochrome oxidase I	No change	8 an 28	Gadaleta et al. (108)
Male Fischer 344	Cytochrome P450	Decrease	6–29	Richardson et al. (323)
Female Wistar	Cytochrome P450e$^+$	Increase	5 and 30	Rath and Kanungo (302)
Female Wistar	Cytochrome P450b$^+$	Increase	5 and 30	Rath and Kanungo (302)
Male BN/BiRij	Cytochromme P450IIB1	Decrease	3–36	Horbach et al. (146)
Male BN/BiRij	Cytochromme P450IIB2	Decrease	3–36	Horbach et al. (146)
Male BN/BiRij	Cytochromme P450IA1 (basal)	No change	3–36	Horbach et al. (147)
Male BN/BiRij	Cytochromme P450IA1 (induced)	No change	3–36	Horbach et al. (147)
Male BN/BiRij	Cytochromme P450IA2 (basal)	No change	3–36	Horbach et al. (147)
Male BN/BiRij	Cytochromme P450IA2 (induced)	No change	3–36	Horbach et al. (147)
Male Fischer 344	Dehydroepiandrosterone sulfotransferase	Increase	3 and 27	Demyan et al. (74)
Male Fischer 344	Elongation factor-1α	No change	3 and 26	Lee et al. (196)
Male Fischer 344	Estrogen sulfotransferase	Decrease	3 and 27	Demyan et al. (75)
Male Wistar	Fatty acid synthetase$^{\Delta,+}$	Decrease	1.5–18	Fukuda and Iritani (105)
Male Fischer 344	α-fetoprotein	No change	6–29	Richardson et al. (324)
Sex and strain unspecified	Fibronectin	Decrease	2–12	Singh and Kanungo (354)
Male/Female Wistar/Slc	c-fos	Increase	6–25	Fujita and Maruyama (104)
Male Fischer 344	α_{2u}-globulin	Decrease	1–28	Chatterjee et al. (52)
Male Fischer 344	α_{2u}-globulin	Decrease	2–28	Waggoner et al. (408)
Male Fischer 344	α_{2u}-globulin*	Decrease	2–30	Roy et al. (336)
Male Fischer 344	α_{2u}-globulin	Decrease	6–29	Richardson et al. (321)
Male Fischer 344	α_{2u}-globulin*,+	Decrease	6–30	Richardson et al. (321)
Male Fischer 344	α_{2u}-globulin$^+$	Decrease	1–26	Murty et al. (263)
Male Wistar	glut-2	Decrease	2–20	Lin et al. (204)
Male/Female Wistar/Slc	Glutathione S transferase	Increase	6–25	Fujita and Maruyama (104)
Male Fischer 344	Glutathione peroxidase$^\Delta$	Decrease	6–26	Rao et al. (301)
Male Fischer 344	Glutathione peroxidase$^\Delta$	No change	4–28	Rao et al. (300)
Female WAG/Rij	Glyceraldehyde phosphate dehydrogenase	No change	6–36	Slagboom et al. (359)
Male Fischer 344	Heat shock protein (hsp70)*,+	Decrease	4–28	Heydari et al. (138)
Female Wistar	Insulin growth factor-I	Decrease	6–25	Park and Buetow (292)
Male/Female Wistar/Slc	c-jun	Increase	6–25	Fujita and Maruyama (104)
Male Sprague-Dawley	Kininogen	Decrease	10 and 23	Sierra et al. (351)
Male/Female Wistar/Slc	LF-B	No change	6–25	Fujita and Maruyama (104)
Male Fischer 344	c-myc	Increase	3–23	Matocha et al. (227)
Male Fischer 344	c-myc	Increase	6–29	Waggoner et al. (408)
Female Fischer 344	c-myc (basal)	Decrease	2–3 and 22–24	Sawada (339)
Female Fischer 344	c-myc (induced)	No change	2–3 and 22–24	Sawada (339)
Male/Female Wistar/Slc	Poly A binding protein	No change	6–25	Fujita and Maruyama (104)
Male Fischer 344	Superoxide dismutase, Cu/Zn$^\Delta$	Decrease	6–26	Rao et al. (301)
Male Fischer 344	Superoxide dismutase, Cu/Zn$^\Delta$	Decrease	4–28	Rao et al. (300)
Male Fischer 344	Superoxide dismutase, Cu/Zn$^\Delta$	Decrease	6–29	Semsei et al. (341)
Male Fischer 344	Senescence marker protein-1	Decrease	1–28	Chatterjee et al. (52)
Male Sprague-Dawley	Tyrosine aminotransferase (basal)	Decrease	10–25	Wellinger and Guigoz (428)
Male Sprague-Dawley	Tyrosine and aminotransferase (induced)	Decrease	10 and 25	Wellinger and Guigoz (428)
Female WAG/Rij	Tyrosine aminotransferase (basal)	Decrease	6–35	Slagboom et al. (358)
Male Sprague-Dawley	Trytophan oxygenase (basal)	No change	10 and 25	Wellinger and Guigoz (428)
Male Sprague-Dawley	Tryptophan oxygenase (induced)	No change	10 and 25	Wellinger and Guigoz (428)
Male Wistar	Thyroid-binding globulin	Increase	2–30	Savu et al. (338)

Sex/Strain	mRNA	Change with Age	Ages Studied (months, unless specified)	Reference
Mouse				
BALB/c (sex unspecified)	α_1-acid glycoprotein 1 (basal)	Increase	2–24	Carter et al. (45)
BALB/c (sex unspecified)	α_1-acid glycoprotein 1 (induced)	No change	2–24	Carter et al. (45)
BALB/c (sex unspecified)	α_1-acid glycoprotein 2 (basal)	No change	2–24	Carter et al. (45)
BALB/c (sex unspecified)	α_1-acid glycoprotein 1 (induced)	Decrease	2–24	Carter et al. (45)
Male BALB/c	α_1-acid glycoprotein	Increase	2–24	Post et al. (297)
Female C57B1/6J	Actin	No change	2–26	Ono et al. (279)
Male C57B1/6J	Albumin	No change	4–48	Yang et al. (439)
Male BALB/c	Albumin	Decrease	2–24	Post et al. (297)
Male BALB/c	α-antitrypsin	Decrease	2–24	Post et al. (297)
Male SAM-R/1	Apolipoprotein B	No change	2–22	Higuchi et al. (140)
Male SAM-P/1	Apolipoprotein B	No change	2–22	Higuchi et al. (140)
Male C57B1/70	Catalase	Decrease	4–24	Mote et al. (259)
Male B10.RIII	Catalase	Decrease	4–28	Mote et al. (259)
Female C3B10RF$_1$	Catalase	Decrease	4–30	Mote et al. (261)
Female 3B10RF	C/EBP[a]	No change	4–30	Spindler et al. (371)
Male C57B1/10; B10.BR	C/EBP[a]	No change	4–28	Mote et al. (261)
Male B10.BR	C/ECP[a]	No change	4–28	Mote et al. (261)
Male B10.RIII	C/EBP[a]	No change	4–28	Mote et al. (261)
Male B10.RIII	Cytochrome P$_1$450 (basal)	Decrease	4–28	Mote et al. (259)
Male B10.RIII	Cytochrome P$_1$450 (induced)	Decrease	4–28	Mote et al. (259)
Male B10.RIII	Cytochrome P$_3$450 (basal)	Decrease	4–28	Mote et al. (259)
Male B10.RIII	Cytochrome P$_3$450 (induced)	Decrease	4–28	Mote et al. (259)
Male C57B1/10	Cytochrome P$_1$450 (basal)	No change	4–28	Mote et al. (259)
Male C57B1/10	Cytochrome P$_1$450 (induced)	No charge	4–28	Mote et al. (259)
Male C57B1/10	Cytochrome P$_3$450 (basal)	No change	4–28	Mote et al. (259)
Male C57B1/10	Cytochrome P$_3$450 (induced)	No change	4–28	Mote et al. (259)
Female C3B10RF$_1$	Cytochrome P$_3$450	Decrease	4–30	Mote et al. (260)
Female C3B10RF$_1$	Cytochrome P$_1$450	Decrease	4–30	Mote et al. (260)
Female C3b10RF$_1$	Epoxide hydrolase	No change	4–30	Mote et al. (260)
Male C57B1/10	Glucocorticoid receptor	No change	4–28	Mote et al. (261)
Male B10.BR	Glucocorticoid receptor	No change	4–28	Mote et al. (261)
Male B10.RII	Glucocorticoid receptor	No change	4–28	Mote et al. (261)
Female C3B10RF$_1$	Glucorticoid receptor	Increase	4–30	Spindler et al. (371)
Female C3B10RF$_1$	Gluathione peroxidase	No change	4–30	Mote et al. (260)
Female C3B10RF$_1$	Heat shock protein (grp-78)	No change	4–31	Spindler et al. (370)
Female C3B10RF$_1$	Heat shock protein (grp-94)	No change	4–31	Spindler et al. (370)
Male C57B1/10	Insulin growth factor I	No change	4–28	Mote et al. (261)
Male B10.BR	Insulin growth factor I	No change	4–28	Mote et al. (261)
Male B10.RIII	Insulin growth factor I	No change	4–28	Mote et al. (261)
Female C3B10RF$_1$	Insulin growth factor I	No change	4–30	Spindler et al. (371)
Male C57B1/10	Insulin receptor	Increase	4–28	Mote et al. (261)
Male B10.BR	Insulin receptor	Increase	4–28	Mote et al. (261)
Male B10.RIII	Insulin receptor	Increase	4–28	Mote et al. (261)
Female C3B10RF$_1$	Insulin receptor	Increase	4–30	Spindler et al. (371)
Male C57B1/6J	Intracisternal A- particle	Decrease	6–32	Gaubatz et al. (113)
Female C3B10RF$_1$	c-jun	No change	4–30	Spindler et al. (371)
Female C57B1/10; B10.BR and B10.RIII	c-jun	No change	4–28	Mote et al. (261)
Male C57B1/6J	c-myc	Decrease	2–26	Ono et al. (279)
Male C57B1/6J	c-my	Increase	2–32	Semsei et al. (340)
Male C57B1/6J	Parathymosin*	Decrease	2 and 18	Clinton et al. (60)
Male C57B1/6J	Prothymosin*	Decrease	2 and 18	Clinton et al. (60)
Male C57B1/10	S-11 protein	No change	4–28	Mote et al. (261)
Male B10.BR	S-11 protein	No change	4–28	Mote et al. (261)
Male B10.RIII	S-11 protein	No change	4–28	Mote et al. (261)
Female 3B10RF$_1$	S-11 protein	No change	4–30	Spindler et al. (371)
Female C3B10RF$_1$	Sp1	No change	4–30	Spindler et al. (371)
Male C57B1/10	Sp1	No change	4–28	Mote et al. (261)
Male B10.BR	Sp1	No change	4–28	Mote et al. (261)
Male B10.RIII	Sp1	No change	4–28	Mote et al. (261)
Male C57B1/10	Superoxide dismutase, Cu/Zn	Decrease	4–24	Mote et al. (259)
Male B10.RIII	Superoxide dismutase, Cu/Zn	Decrease	4–28	Mote et al. (259)
Female C3B10RF$_1$	Superoxide, Cu/Zn	No change	4–30	Mote et al. (260)
Female C3B10RF$_1$	Superoxide dismutase, Mn	Decrease	4–30	Mote et al. (260)
Male C57B1/6J	Transferrin	Increase	4–28	Yang et al. (439)

*Protein level was also measured in this study. [Δ]Activity was also measured in this study. [+]Nuclear transcription was also measured in this study. [a]CAAT enhancer binding protein.

TABLE 9.4. *Effect of Age on mRNA Levels in Brain*

Sex/Strain	mRNA	Change with Age	Ages Studied (months)	References
Whole Brain				
Rat				
Female WAB/Rij	α-actin	No change	6–36	Slagboom et al. (359)
Male Fischer 344	Catalase^Δ	Decrease	5–37	Semsei et al. (342)
Male Fischer 344	catalase^Δ	Decrease	6–26	Rao et al. (301)
Male Fischer 344	Elongation facto 1α	No change	3–26	Lee et al. (196)
Male Wistar	Ferritin	Decrease	4 and 30	Ammendola et al (1)
Male Wistar	Glut-1^Δ	No change	2–20	Oka et al. (275)
Male Fischer 344	Glutathione peroxidase	No change	6–26	Rao et al. (301)
Female WAG/Rij	Glyceraldehyde phosphate dehydrogenase	No change	6–36	Slagboom et al. (275)
Male Wistar	Heat shock protein (hsp70)	Decrease	5 and 25	Blake et al. (24)
Female Wistar	Insulin growth factor I	Decrease	6–25	Park and Buetow (292)
Female Wistar	Insulin growth factor II	Decrease	6–25	Park and Buetow (292)
Male Fischer 344	Muscarinic receptor, rm1	No change	5–8 and 24–28	Wang et al. (412)
Male Fischer 344	Muscarinic receptor, m2	Decrease	5–8 and 24–28	Wang et al. (412)
Female Wistar	Myelin basic protein	No change	6 and 24	Sato et al. (337)
Wistar (sex unspecified)	Neural cell adhesion molecule	No change	40 days–27 months	Linnemann et al. (206)
Male Fischer 344	S1 protein	No change	3–26	Lee et al. (196)
Male Fischer 344	Superoxide dismutase, Cu/Zn^Δ	Decrease	6–26	Rao et al. (301)
Male Fischer 344	Superoxide dismutase, Cu/Zn^Δ	Decrease	5–37	Semsei et al. (342)
Mouse				
Male C57B1/6J	Intracisternal A- particle	Decrease	2–32	Gaubatz et al. (113)
Male C57B1/6J	c-myc	No change	2–32	Semsei et al. (340)
Male C57B1/6J	Parathymosin*	Decrease	2 and 18	Clinton et al. (60)
Male C57B1/6J	Prothymosin a*	Decrease	2 and 18	Clinton et al. (60)
Cerebellum				
Rat				
Fischer 344 (sex unspecified)	Cytochrome oxidase I	Decrease	8 and 28	Gadaleta et al. (108)
Male Wistar	c-Fos	Decrease	3–5 to 18–20	Kitraki et al. (179)
Male Wistar	IGF-II	Decrease	3–5 to 18–20	Kitraki et al. (179)
Cerebral Cortex or Hemispheres				
Rat				
Fischer 344 (sex unspecified)	Cytochrome oxidase I	Decrease	8 and 28	Gadaleta et al. (108)
Male Wistar	c-fos	Decrease	3–5 to 18–20	Kitraki et al. (179)
Male Wistar	IGF-II	Decrease	3–5 to 18–20	Kitraki et al. (179)
Forebrain				
Rat				
Female Sprague-Dawley	Amyloid precursor product	Increase	7 and 25	Higgins et al. (139)
Fischer 344 (sex unspecified)	Nerve growth factor	Decrease	6 and 24	Larkfors et al. (190)
Frontal Lobe				
Rat				
Female Wistar	Somatostatin	Decrease	3–25	Florio et al. (99)
Hippocampus				
Rat				
Sprague-Dawley (sex unspecified)	B-50	Decrease	5 and 24	Bacci et al. (7)
Male Sprague-Dawley	Brain-derived neurotropic factor	No change	3–24	Lapchak et al. (189)
Male Fischer 344	Brain-derived neurotropic factor	No change	7–24	Lapchak et al. (189)

Sex/Strain	mRNA	Change with Age	Ages Studied (months)	References
Male Sprague-Dawley	D2 receptor	Decrease	2–29	Vedova et al. (405)
Male Wistar	D2 receptor	Decrease	2–29	Vedova et al. (405)
Male Long-Evans	Glucocorticoid receptor II	Decrease	6–24	Peiffer et al. (294)
Male Fischer 344	Heat shock protein (hsp70)	Decrease	4 and 30	Pardue et al. (289)
Male Wistar	IGF-II	Decrease	3–5 to 18–20	Kitraki et al. (179)
Male Fischer 344	N-cadherin	No change	6–24	Wagner et al. (409)
Male Fischer 344	Neural cell adhesion molecule	No change	6–24	Wagner et al. (409)
Sprague-Dawley (sex unspecified)	Synapsin I	Decrease	5 and 24	Bacci et al. (7)
Male Sprague-Dawley	Synaptosomal-associated protein 25	No change	3–24	Lapchak et al. (189)
Male Fischer 344	Synaptosomal-associated protein 25	No change	7–24	Lapchak et al. (189)
Male Sprague-Dawley	Tyrosine receptor kinase	No change	3–24	Lapchak et al. (189)
Male Fischer 344	Tyrosine receptor kinase	No change	7–24	Lapchak et al. (189)

Hypothalmus

Rat

Sex/Strain	mRNA	Change with Age	Ages Studied (months)	References
Male Sprague-Dawley	Antiotensinogen	Increase	3 and 18	Bunnemann et al. (37)
Male Fischer 344	α1 GABA receptor subunit	Decrease	6–25	Mhatre et al. (247)
Male Wistar	IGF-II	Decrease	3–5 to 18–20	Kitraki et al. (179)
Female Sprague–Dawley	Proopiomelanocortin	Decrease	3–20	Weiland et al. (425)
Female Wistar	Somatostatin	No change	3–25	Florio et al. (99)
Male Sprague- Dawley	Somatostatin	Decrease	3–22	Martinoli et al. (223)
Female Sprague- Dawley	Somatostatin	Decrease	3–22	Martinoli et al. (223)
Male Fischer 344	Vasopressin (basal)	Decrease	3 and 24	Dobie et al. (80)
Male Fischer 344	Vasopressin (induced)	No change	3 and 24	Dobie et al. (80)

Mouse

Sex/Strain	mRNA	Change with Age	Ages Studied (months)	References
Female C57B1/6J	Proopiomelanocortin	Decrease	7–31	Nelson et al (267)
Female C57B1/6J	Proopiomelanocortin (basal)	Decrease	4–25	Karelus and Nelson (167)
Female C57B1/6J	Proopiomelanocartin (induced)	No change	4–25	Karelus and Nelson (167)

Neocortex

Rat

Sex/Strain	mRNA	Change with Age	Ages Studied (months)	References
Sprague-Dawley (sex unspecified)	B-50	No change	5 and 24	Bacci et al. (7)
Sprague-Dawley (sex unspecified)	Synapsin I	No change	5 and 24	Bacci et al. (7)

Medulla Oblongata

Rat

Sex/Strain	mRNA	Change with Age	Ages Studied (months)	References
Male Sprague-Dawley	Angiotensinogen	No change	3 and 18	Bunnemann et al. (37)

Midbrain

Rat

Sex/Strain	mRNA	Change with Age	Ages Studied (months)	References
Male Sprague-Dawley	Angiotensinogen	No change	3 and 18	Bunnemann et al. (37)

Parietal Lobe

Rat

Sex/Strain	mRNA	Change with Age	Ages Studied (months)	References
Female Wistar	Somatostatin	Decrease	3–25	Florio et al. (99)

Pituitary

Rat

Sex/Strain	mRNA	Change with Age	Ages Studied (months)	References
Male Sprague-Dawley	Growth hormone	Decrease	3–22	Martinoli et al. (223)
Female Sprague-Dawley	Growth hormone	Decrease	3–22	Martinoli et al. (223)
Male Wistar/Tw	Growth hormone	Decrease	6–18	Takahashi et al. (387)
Female Wistar/Tw	Growth hormone	Decrease	6–18	Takahashi et al. (387)
Male Long-Evans	Glucorticoid receptor II	No change	6–24	Peiffer et al. (294)
Female Wistar	Leuteinizing hormone*	No change	6–7 and 23–25	Stewart et al. (378)

(*continued*)

TABLE 9.4. *Effect of Age on mRNA Levels in Brain—Continued*

Sex/Strain	mRNA	Change with Age	Ages Studied (months)	References
Male Wistar/Tw	Prolactin	Decrease	6–18	Takahashi et al. (387)
Female Wistar/Tw	Prolactin	Increase	6–18	Takahashi et al. (387)
Female Wistar	Prolactin*	No change	6–7 and 23–25	Stewart et al. (378)
Mouse				
Male C57B1/6J	Growth hormone	Decrease	3–27	Crew et al. (69)
Male C57B1/6J	Prolactin	Decrease	3–27	Crew et al. (69)
Female C5B1/6J	Proopiomelanocortin	Increase	7–31	Nelson et al. (267)
Male C57B1/6J	α-tubulin	No change	3–27	Crew et al. (69)
Striatum				
Rat				
Male Sprague-Dawley	β-actin	No change	2–29	Vedova et al. (405)
Male Wistar	β-actin	No change	2–29	Vedova et al. (405)
Male Wistar	Cannabinoid receptor	Decrease	3 and 24	Mailleux and Vanderhaeghen (212)
Male Wistar	D2 receptor	Decrease	6–25	Mesco et al. (246)
Male Sprague-Dawley	D2 receptor	Decrease	2–29	Vedova et al. (405)
Male Wistar	D2 receptor	Decrease	2–29	Vedova et al. (405)
Male Wistar	IGF-II	Decrease	3–5 to 18–20	Kitraki et al. (179)
Female Wistar	Somatostatin	Decrease	3–25	Florio et al. (99)
Trigeminal Ganglion				
Rat				
Male Fischer 344	Calcitonin gene regulated peptide*	No change	6–24	Salih et al. (336)

*Protein level was also measured in this study. ᐃActivity was also measured in this study. ⁺Nuclear transcription was also measured in this study.

example of an mRNA transcript, albumin, that increases with age in rat liver, and Figure 9.5 shows an example of an mRNA transcript, α_{2u}-globulin, that decreases with age in rat liver.

Unfortunately, the majority (approximately 80%) of the studies listed in Tables 9.3–9.6 did not measure the level (or enzyme activity) of the protein coded for by the mRNA transcript studied. It appears that investigators generally have assumed that the changes they observed with age in an mRNA transcript would be paralleled by similar changes in the protein coded for by the mRNA. In most of the studies that have measured both mRNA and protein (enzyme activity) levels, there appears to be a good correlation between changes in the two. For example, Figure 9.4 shows that both the mRNA level and the synthesis of albumin in rat liver increase with age. Figure 9.5 shows an excellent correlation between the age-related decline in the level of α_{2u}-globulin mRNA and the synthesis of α_{2u}-globulin by rat hepatocytes; the synthesis and mRNA levels of α_{2u}-globulin decreased approximately 85% between 5 and 24 months of age. A good correlation between the age-related changes in the mRNA levels of catalase and superoxide dismutase and the activities of these two enzymes in rat liver also has been observed (300, 341).

As Figure 9.6 shows, the age-related decrease in the induction of the mRNAs coding interleukins 2 and 3 and granulocyte/macrophage colony-stimulating factor by spleen lymphocytes isolated from mice has been correlated to a similar decrease in the levels of these proteins.

Although most of the studies show a good correlation between age-related changes in the mRNA transcript and its protein product, there are a few reports where these changes differ. For example, Figure 9.4 shows that both the synthesis and the mRNA level of albumin increase with age; however, the age-related increase in albumin synthesis is much less than that of the mRNA level, the increases in albumin mRNA being three-fold and in albumin synthesis only 1.5-fold between 3 and 36 months of age. Perhaps the best example of an inconsistency in mRNA and protein changes with age was reported by Strong et al. (380). They measured the activity and mRNA level of tyrosine hydroxylase in the adrenal gland of rats. As shown in Figure 9.7, tyrosine hydroxylase mRNA levels increased over sixfold between 2 and 27 months of age; however, tyrosine hydroxylase activity increased only 1.5-fold over this age range, with the major discrepancy occurring in the very old (27 months) rats. The inconsistency between

TABLE 9.5. *Effect of Age on mRNA Levels in Spleen, Thymus and Lymphocytes*

Sex/Strain	mRNA	Change with Age	Ages Studied	References
Spleen				
Mouse				
Female C57B1/6J	Actin	No change	2–26 months	Ono et al. (279)
Female C57B1/6J	c-myc	No change	2–26 months	Ono et al. (279)
Male C57B1/6J	c-myc	Increase	3–32 months	Semsei et al. (340)
Male C57B1/6J	Parathymosin*	Decrease	2 and 18 months	Clinton et al. (60)
Male C57B1/6J	Prothymosin*	Decrease	2 and 18 months	Clinton et al. (60)
Rat				
Female WAG/Rij	α-actin	Increase	6–36 months	Slagboom et al. (359)
Female WAG/Rij	Glyceraldehyde phosphate dehydrogenase	Increase	6–36 months	Slagboom et al. (359)
Thymus				
Mouse				
Male C57B1/6J	Parathymosin*	Decrease	2 and 18 months	Clinton et al. (60)
Male C57B1/6J	Prothymosin*	Decrease	2 and 18 months	Clinton et al. (60)
Lymphocytes				
Rat				
Female Wistar	K-immunoglobulin	No change	6 and 24 months	Sato et al. (337)
Male Fischer 344	Interleukin 2$^\Delta$	Decrease	5 and 29 months	Wu et al. (437)
Male Fischer 344	Interleukin 2$^\Delta$	No change	4–5 and 22–24 months	Holbrook et al. (143)
Mouse				
Male albino Swiss	c-fos	Decrease	3 and 18–20 months	Sikora et al. (352)
Male C57B1/6J	Interleukin 2$^\Delta$	Decrease	5–37 months	Li et al. (200)
Male C57B1/6J	Interleukin 2	Decrease	6–29 months	Cai et al. (42)
Male C57B1/6J	Interleukin 3$^\Delta$	Decrease	5–37 months	Li et al. (200)
Male C57B1/6J	Interleukin 3	Decrease	6–29 months	Cai et al. (42)
Male albino Swiss	c-jun	Increase	3 and 18–20 months	Sikora et al. (352)
Male C57B1/6J	MGCSF$^\Delta$	Decrease	6–29 months	Cai et al. (42)
Male C57B2/6J	cmyc+	Decrease	2–5 and 20–26 months	Buckler et al. (35)
Female BALB/cANN	Perforin	Decrease	2–3 and 24–33 months	Bloom et al. (28)
Female BALB/cANN	Serine esterase	Decrease	2–3 and 24–33 months	Bloom et al. (28)
Human				
	c-fos	No change	<40 and >60 yr	Song et al. (365)
	Histone H3	Decrease	20–35 to 70–85 yr	Travali et al. (397)
	Interleukin 2$^\Delta$	Decrease	<40 and >60 yr	Nagel et al. (264)
	Interleukin 2 receptor	Decrease	<40 and >60 yr	Nagel et al. (264)
	Interleukin 2 receptor	Decrease	20–35 to 70–85 yr	Travali et al. (397)
	c-jun	Decrease	<40 and >60 yr	Song et al. (365)
	junB	No change	<40 and >60 yr	Song et al. (365)
	c-myc+	Decrease	<35 and >65 yr	Gamble et al. (109)
	Nerve growth factor receptor (low-affinity p75^{NGFR})	No change	<40 and >60 yr	Kittur et al. (180)
	Thymidine kinase	Decrease	20–35 to 70–85 yr	Travali et al. (397)

*Protein level was also measured in this study. $^\Delta$Activity was also measured in this study. +Nuclear transcription was also measured in this study.

the age-related changes in tyrosine hydroxylase mRNA levels and activity was most obvious when rats were treated with reserpine, a drug that induces tyrosine hydroxylase expression. Reserpine administration induced both tyrosine hydroxylase activity and mRNA 1.5-fold in young rats. However, reserpine treatment did not induce significantly the activity of tyrosine hydroxylase in old rats even though it increased mRNA levels two- to threefold. Using a polyclonal antibody to tyrosine hydroxylase, Wessels-Reiker et al. (429) showed that the age-related changes in tyrosine hydroxylase activity in reserpine-treated and untreated rats were due to changes in the levels of the tyrosine hydroxylase protein. Thus it is clear that the induction of tyrosine hydroxylase transcription is uncoupled from tyrosine hydroxylase translation in the adrenal gland of old rats. This study points to the importance of measuring both the level of an mRNA transcript and the level or

TABLE 9.6. *Effect of Age on mRNA Levels in Various Tissues*

Sex/Species	mRNA	Change	Ages Studied (months unless specified)	References
Adipose Tissue				
Rat				
Male Wistar	Glut 4*	Decrease	2–20	Lin et al. (204)
Male Wistar	Glut 4*	Decrease	2 and 20	Oka et al. (275)
Adrenal				
Rat				
Male Wistar	Heat shock protein (hsp70)	Decrease	2–24	Blake et al. (25)
Male Fischer 344	Tyrosine hydroxylase$^\Delta$	Increase	2–23	Strong et al. (379, 380)
Female Fischer 344	Tyrosine hydroxylase$^\Delta$	Increase	5 and 25	Tumer et al. (398)
Bovine				
	Cytochrome P450 c11 (basal)	No change	1 to 10–12 yr	Ogo et al. (273)
	Cytochrome P450 c11 (induced)	No change	1 to 10–12 yr	Ogo et al. (273)
	Cytochrome P450 c17 (basal)	Decrease	1 to 10–12 yr	Ogo et al. (273)
	Cytochrome P450 c17 (basal)	Decrease	1 to 10–12 yr	Ogo et al. (273)
Aorta				
Human				
Endothelial cells	Fibronectin	Increase	5, 50, and 76 yr	Kumazaki et al. (185)
Hardarian Gland				
Rat				
Male Fischer 344	5-aminolevulinate synthase	Decrease	3 and 24	Rodriguez et al. (329)
Heart				
Rat				
Male Fischer 344	α-actin, cardiac (basal)	No change	9 and 18	Takahashi et al. (386)
Male Fischer 344	α-actin, cardiac (induced)	Decrease	9 and 18	Takahashi et al. (386)
Wistar (sex unspecified)	α-actin	No change	3–24	Carrier et al. (44)
Female Wistar	α-actin+	Increase	6–33	Jaiswal and Kanungo (162)
Wistar (sex unspecified)	α-actin	No change	3–24	Carrier et al. (44)
Male Fischer 344	α-actin, skeletal, (basal)	No change	9 and 18	Takahashi et al. (386)
Male Fischer 344	α-actin, skeletal (induced)	Decrease	9 and 18	Takahashi et al. (386)
Male Fischer 344	β-actin	No change	4–25	Kimball et al. (177)
Male Fischer 344	α- adrenoreceptor	Decrease	4–25	Kimball et al. (177)
Male Long-Evans	ATPase	No change	4 and 24	Buttrick et al. (40)
Male Fischer 344	ATPase (basal)	No change	9 and 18	Takahashi et al. (386)
Male Fischer 344	ATPase (induced)	Decrease	9 and 18	Takahashi et al. (386)
Wistar (sex unspecified)	ATPase	Decrease	1–24	Lompre et al. (209)
Male Wistar	ATPase (basal)	Decrease	6 and 22	Besse et al. (19)
Male Wistar	ATPase (induced)	Decrease	6 and 22	Besse et al. (19)
Female Wistar	Atrial natriuretic factor	No change	6 and 24	Sato et al. (337)
Male Fischer 344	Atrial natriuretic factor (basal)	Increase	9 and 18	Takahashi et al. (386)
Male Fischer 344	Atrial natriuretic factor (induced)	No change	9 and 18	Takahashi et al. (386)
Wistar (sex unspecified)	Calsequestrin	No change	1–24	Lompre et al. (209)
Male Fischer 344	Calsequestrin (basal)	No change	9 and 18	Takahashi et al. (386)
Male Fisher 344	Calsequestrin (induced)	Decrease	9 and 18	Takahashi et al. (386)
Male Fischer 344	Cytochrome c	Decrease	11 and 23	Biggs et al. (21)
Fischer 344 (sex unspecified)	Cytochrome oxidase I	Decrease	8 and 28	Gadaleta et al. (108)
Male Fischer 344	Elongation factor 1α	No change	3–26	Lee et al. (197)
Male Fischer 344	c-fos (basal)	No change	9 and 19	Takahashi et al. (386)
Male Fischer 344	c-fos (induced)	Decrease	9 and 18	Takahashi et al. (386)
Female Wistar	Insulin growth factor I	Decrease	6–25	Park and Buetow (292)
Female Wistar	Insulin growth factor II	Decrease	6–25	Park and Buetow (292)
Male Fischer 344	c-jun (basal)	No change	9 and 19	Takahashi et al. (386)
Male Fischer 344	c-jun (induced)	Decrease	9 and 18	Takahashi et al. (386)
Female Wistar	Myosin heavy chain+	No change	6–33	Jaiswal and Kanungo (162)
Wistar (sex unspecified)	Myosin heavy chain	No change	1–24	Lompre et al. (209)
Male Long-Evans	α-myosin heavy chain (basal)	Decrease	4 and 24	Buttruck et al. (40)

Sex/Species	mRNA	Change	Ages Studied (months unless specified)	References
Male Long-Evans	α-myosin heavy chain (induced)	Decrease	4 and 24	Buttrick et al. (40)
Male Fischer 344	α-myosin heavy chain (basal)	No change	9 and 18	Takahashi et al. (386)
Male Fischer Fischer 344	α-myosin heavy chain (induced)	No change	9 and 18	Takahashi et al, (386)
Male Long-Evans	β-myosin heavy chain (basal)	Increase	4 and 24	Buttrick et al. (40)
Male Long-Evans	β-myosin heavy chain (basal)	Increase	4 and 24	Buttrick et al. (40)
Male Fischer 344	β-myosin heavy chain (basal)	No change	9 and 18	Takahashi et al. (386)
Male Fischer 344	β-myosin heavy chain (induced)	No change	9 and 18	Takahashi et al. (386)
Male Long-Evans	β-myosin heavy chain	Increase	4 and 24	Buttrick et al. (40)
Male Fischer 344	β-myosin heavy chain	No change	9 and 18	Takahashi et al. (386)
Male Wistar	α-myosin heavy chain (basal)	Decrease	6 and 22	Besse et al. (19)
Male Wistar	α-myosin heavy chain (induced)	Decrease	6 and 22	Besse et al. (19)
Male Wistar	β-myosin heavy chain (basal)	Increase	6 and 22	Bessee et al. (19)
Male Wistar	β-myosin heavy chain (induced)	Increase	6 and 22	Besse et al. (19)
Wistar (sex unspecified)	Neural cell adhesion molecule*	Decrease	1–730 days	Gaardsvoll et al. (106)
Male Fischer 344	S1 protein	No change	3–26	Lee et al. (197)

Mouse

Sex/Species	mRNA	Change	Ages Studied	References
Male C57Bl/6J	Intracisternal A- particle	Decrease	2–32	Gaubatz et al. (113)
Male C57Bl/6J	c-myc	Increase	2–32	Semsei et al (340)

Intestine

Rat

Sex/Species	mRNA	Change	Ages Studied	References
Male Fischer 344	Calbindin-D- 9k*	Increase	13–24	Armbrecht et al. (4)

Mouse

Sex/Species	mRNA	Change	Ages Studied	References
Male SAM-R/1	Apolipoprotein B	Decrease	8–22	Higuchi et al. (140)
Male SAM-P/1	Apolipoprotein B	Decrease	8–22	Higuchi et al. (140)
Male C57Bl/6J	c-myc	Increase	2–32	Semsei et al. (340)

Kidney

Rat

Sex/Species	mRNA	Change	Ages Studied	References
Male Wistar	β-actin	No change	6 and 24	Liang et al. (201)
Male Fischer 344	Calbindin-D-28k*	No change	13–24	Armbrecht et al. (4)
Male Fischer 344	Catalase^Δ	Decrease	6 and 24	Rao et al. (301)
Male Sprague-Dawley	Collagen type I	Increase	5 and 22	Peleg et al. (295)
Male Wistar	$G_i\alpha 2$ protein	Increase	6 and 24	Liang et al. (201)
Male Wistar	$G_s\alpha$ protein*,+	Decrease	6 and 24	Liang et al. (201)
Male Fischer 344	Glutathione peroxidase^Δ	Decrease	6 and 24	Rao et al. (301)
Male Fischer 344	Superoxide dismutase Cu/Zn^Δ	Decrease	6 and 24	Rao et al. (301)

Mouse

Sex/Species	mRNA	Change	Ages Studied	References
Male C57Bl/6J	Intracisternal A-particle	Decrease	2 and 32	Gaubatz et al. (113)
Male C57Bl/6J	c-myc	Increase	2–32	Semsei et al. (340)
Male C57Bl/6J	Parathymosin*	Decrease	2 and 18	Clinton et al. (60)
Male C57Bl/6J	Prothymosin*	Decrease	2 and 18	Clinton et al. (60)
Male C57Bl/6J	Renin*	Decrease	5–37	Hung and Richardson (155)

Lung

Rat

Sex/Species	mRNA	Change	Ages Studied	References
Male Wistar	Heat shock protein (hsp70)	Decrease	5 and 24	Blake et al. (24)
Male Wistar	Heat shock protein (hsp70)*	Decrease	5 and 24	Fargnoli et al. (90)

Mouse

Sex/Species	mRNA	Change	Ages Studied	References
Male C57Bl/6J	Parathymosin*	Decrease	2 and 18	Clinton et al. (60)
Male C57Bl/6J	Prothymosin*	Decrease	2 and 18	Clinton et al. (60)

Muscle, Skeletal

Rat

Sex/Species	mRNA	Change	Ages Studied	References
Female Wistar	α-actin+	Decrease	6 and 33	Jaiswal and Kanungo (162)
Male Wistar	Glut 4	Increase	2 and 20	Oka et al. (275)
Male Wistar	Glut 4*	Increase	2–20	Lin et al. (204)
Female Wistar	Myosin heavy chain+	No change	6 and 33	Jaiswal and Kanungo (162)

(continued)

TABLE 9.6. *Effect of Age on mRNA Levels in Various Tissues—Continued*

Sex/Species	mRNA	Change	Ages Studied (months unless specified)	References
Mouse				
Male C57B1/6J	Parathymosin*	No change	2 and 18	Clinton et al. (60)
Male C57B1/6J	Prothymosin*	No change	2 and 18	Clinton et al. (60)
Pancreas				
Rat				
Male Sprague-Dawley	Actin	Decrease	2–24	Kim et al. (173)
Male Sprague-Dawley	α-amylase (basal)$^\Delta$	Increase	2–24	Kim et al. (173)
Male Sprague-Dawley	α-amylase (induced)$^\Delta$	Increase	2–24	Kim et al. (173)
Male Fischer 344	Pre-proinsulin	No change	3–4 and 18	Wang and Rowe (413)
Parotid Gland				
Rat				
Male Sprague-Dawley	Amylase (induced)	Decrease	2 and 24	Kim et al. (174)
Skin				
Rat				
Male Wistar	Heat shock protein (hsp70)	Decrease	5 and 25	Blake et al. (24)
Female Wistar	Keratin	No change	6 and 24	Sato et al. (337)
Male Wistar	Heat shock protein (hsp70)*	Decrease	5 and 24	Fargnoli et al. (90)
Mouse				
Male C57B1/6J	c-myc	No change	2–32	Semsei et al. (340)
Human				
Fibroblasts	Fibronectin	Increase	29–88yr	Kumazaki et al. (185)
Submandibular Gland				
Mouse				
Male C57B1/6	Epidermal growth factor*	Decrease	12 and 26–28	Gresik et al. (127)
Testes				
Rat				
Male Wistar	Heat shock protein (hsp70)	Decrease	4–27	Krawczyk and Szymik (181)
Thyroid				
Rat				
Male Fischer 344	Calcitonin*,+	Increase	6–24	Salih et al. (335)
Male Fischer 344	Calcitonin gene-regulated peptide*,+	Increase	6–24	Salih et al. (335)
Male Fischer 344	Somatostatin*,+	Increase	6–24	Salih et al. (335)
Uterus				
Rat				
Female Wistar	α-actin+	Decrease	6 and 33	Jaiswal and Kanungo (162)
Female Wistar	Myosin heavy chain+	No change	6 and 33	Jaiswal and Kanungo (162)

*Protein level was also measured in this study. $^\Delta$Activity was also measured in this study. +Nuclear transcription was also measured in this study.

enzyme activity of the protein coded for by the mRNA transcript in aging studies.

Transcriptional and Posttranscriptional Processing of mRNA

In eukaryotes, mRNA transcripts are synthesized from the DNA template as much larger molecules, hnRNA, by RNA polymerase II. After the hnRNA transcripts are synthesized in the nucleus, they are processed through a series of posttranscriptional steps before mature mRNA appears in the cytoplasm as templates to direct the synthesis of proteins. Age-related changes in mRNA levels could arise from changes at either the transcriptional or posttranscriptional level as well as from changes in the degradation of the mRNA. Although it

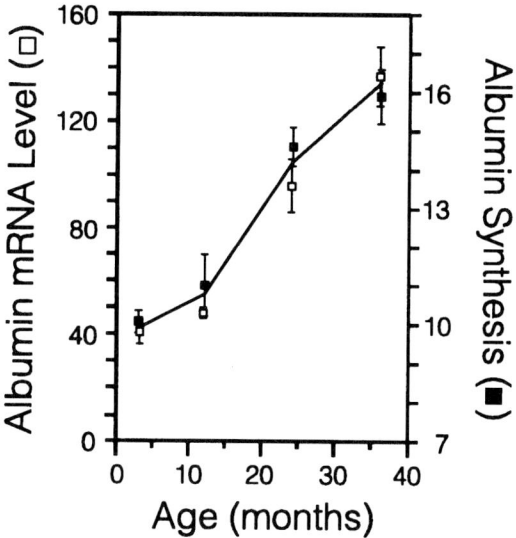

FIG. 9.4. Effect of age on the expression of albumin. Synthesis (■) and mRNA levels (□) of albumin were measured in the livers of rats of various ages [data taken from Horbach et al. (145)].

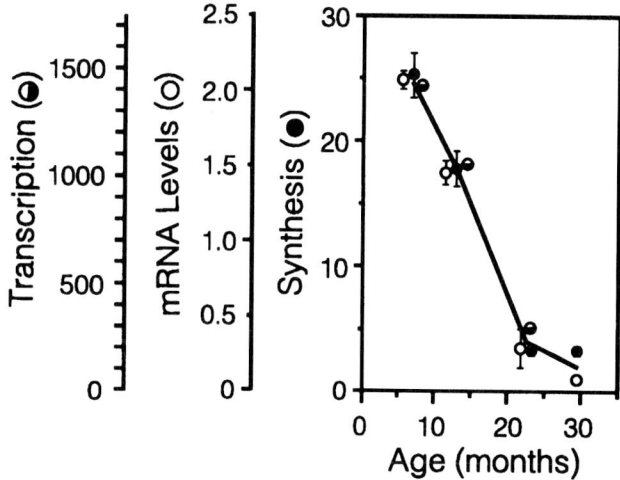

FIG. 9.5. Effect of age on the expression of α_{2u}-globulin. Synthesis (●), mRNA levels (○), and nuclear transcription (◐) of α_{2u}-globulin were measured in hepatocytes isolated from rats of various ages [data taken from Richardson et al. (321)].

has been quite popular to hypothesize that aging might alter the posttranscriptional processing of hnRNA, there is very little information on the effect of aging on this process. For example, there are only three studies that have measured the posttranscriptional splicing of hnRNA as a function of age. Each of the three exons in the fibronectin gene is known to undergo alternative splicing, and the effect of aging on the alternative splicing of the fibronectin transcript has been studied. Pagani et al. (285, 287) measured alternative splicing by the ribonuclease protection assay in various tissues from rats. They did not observe any generalized change in the relative amounts of the alternatively spliced transcripts of fibronectin. Using a reverse transcription-polymerase chain reaction assay, Magnuson et al. (211) measured alternative splicing in fibronectin hnRNA in various tissues of rats. They found statistically significant shifts (4–11%) in alternative splicing of the fibronectin transcript; all three alternatively spliced exons were spliced out at a higher frequency in tissues from 30-month-old rats compared to tissues from 15-month-old rats. Interestingly, similar changes in splicing of the fibronectin transcript were observed in human fibroblasts with increasing passage number. The changes in the splicing of the fibronectin transcript in senescent fibroblasts appeared to occur because of changes in the response of the senescent fibroblasts to growth factor stimulation.

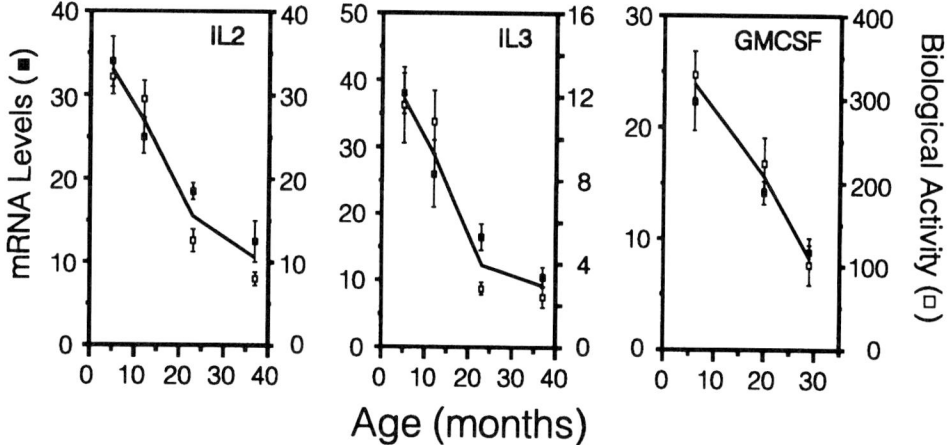

FIG. 9.6. Effect of age on the expression of genes by spleen lymphocytes. The biological activity (□) and mRNA levels (■) of interleukin 2 (IL2), IL3, and granulocyte/macrophage colony-stimulating factor (GMCSF) in mitogen-stimulated lymphocytes isolated from the spleen of mice of various ages is shown [data taken from Li et al. (201) and Cai et al. (42)].

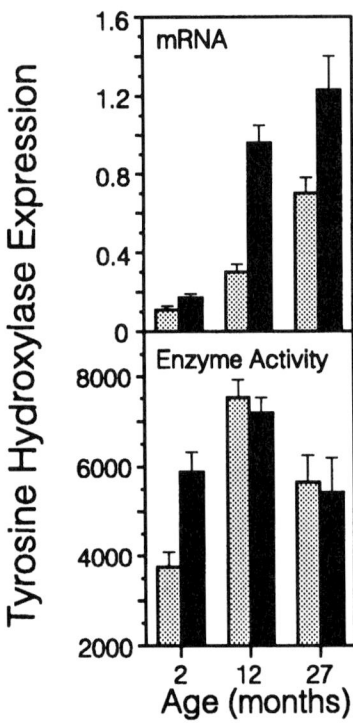

FIG. 9.7. Effect of age on the induction of tyrosine hydroxylase expression in the adrenal gland. The enzyme activity and the level of the mRNA transcript for tyrosine hydroxylase were determined in the adrenal gland of rats of various ages before (*shaded bars*) and after (*solid bars*) treatment with reserpine [data taken from Strong et al. (380)].

Because they did not observe any major alteration leading to the absolute predominance of one spliced form over another and because changes in alternative splicing in fibroblasts appeared to arise from changes in response to growth factors, Magnuson et al. (211) concluded that the integrity of the machinery involved in alternative splicing was preserved during aging both in vivo and in vitro. Data from a study by Singh and Kanungo (354) also suggest that the splicing of the fibronectin transcript does not change with age. They reported that the size of the fibronectin transcript was approximately 8 kb and that this did not change with age in rat liver.

Several investigators also have studied the effect of age on the size of the poly(A)-tail on the 3′-end of mRNA transcripts. Bernd et al. (18) and Horbach et al. (149) reported an age-related decrease in the poly(A)-tail size of poly(A)$^+$RNA isolated from tissues of quail and rat liver, respectively. However, Birchenall-Sparks et al. (22) did not observe any age-related change in either the size or the heterogeneity of the poly(A)-tails in poly(A)$^+$RNA isolated from rat hepatocytes. Using a more sensitive analytical technique for measuring poly(A)-tail size, Kristal et al. (184) recently reported no significant age-related change in the size of the poly(A)-tails of poly(A)$^+$RNA isolated from liver, kidney, and brain of rats. Thus there is no strong evidence that either the alternative splicing of hnRNA or the size of the poly(A)-tail on mRNA transcripts changes markedly with age.

Because there is no strong evidence that major changes occur with age in the posttranscriptional processing of hnRNA, it would appear that the age-related changes in mRNA levels arise primarily through changes in transcription. Although there are a large number of studies that have measured the mRNA levels with age, only a handful (less than 5%) have measured the effect of age on the transcription of the genes coding for the mRNA transcripts studied (see Tables 9.3–9.6). The few studies that have measured both the mRNA transcript and transcription suggest that the age-related change in the level of an mRNA transcript is due to an alteration in the transcription of the gene coding for the mRNA. For example, Figure 9.5 shows an excellent correlation between the age-related decrease in α_{2u}-globulin mRNA levels and the transcription of the α_{2u}-globulin genes in rat hepatocytes. The level of α_{2u}-globulin mRNA decreased 85% between 5 and 24 months of age, while the transcription of α_{2u}-globulin in a nuclear runoff assay decreased 80%. Semsei et al. (341) also found that the age-related decreases in the levels of superoxide dismutase and catalase mRNA in liver were paralleled by similar decreases in the nuclear transcription of these genes. More recently, Heydari et al. (138) reported that the age-related induction of the mRNA for the heat shock gene hsp70 in rat hepatocytes was due to a decrease in the nuclear transcription of hsp70. In addition, Liang et al. (201) showed that the age-related decline in the level of $G_s\alpha$ (stimulating guanine nucleotide-binding protein) arose from a decrease in the nuclear transcription of the $G_s\alpha$ gene (see Fig. 9.8). This study is very important because it is the first to show that age-related changes in signal transduction can arise from a change in the transcription of a gene coding for a component of the signal transduction machinery.

However, there are a few reports that have been unable to show any correlation between the age-related change in the level of an mRNA species and transcription of the gene coding for the mRNA. For example, Horbach et al. (149) reported that transcription of the albumin gene by liver nuclei isolated from rats did not change between 3 and 36 months of age, even though the level of albumin mRNA increased over twofold. They proposed that the increase in albumin mRNA was due to an age-related decrease in the turnover of albumin mRNA; however, they did not measure the turnover. Buckler et al. (35) also were unable to correlate the age-related decrease in the induction of c-*myc*

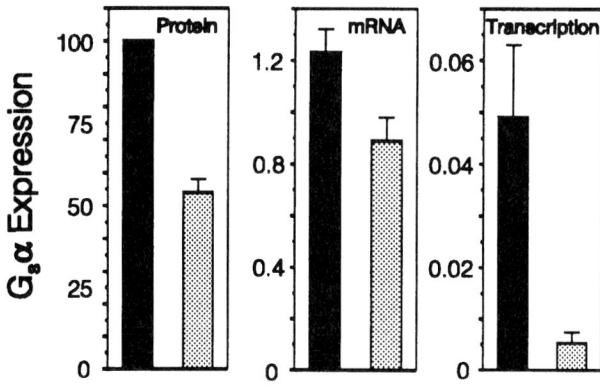
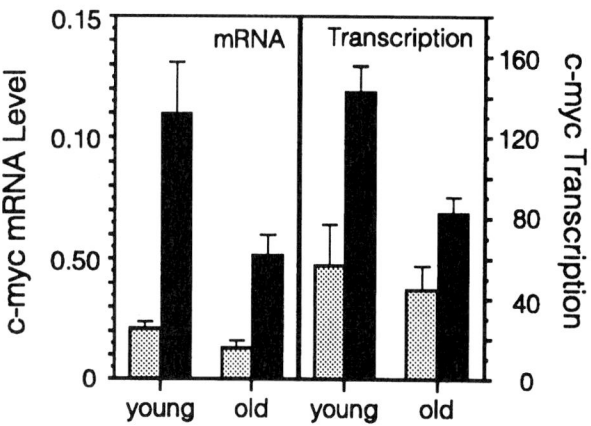

FIG. 9.8. Effect of age on the expression of $G_s\alpha$ and c-*myc*. The *left* graph shows the levels of $G_s\alpha$ protein, mRNA, and nuclear transcription by the renal cortex of 6- (*shaded bars*) and 24- (*solid bars*) month-old rats [data taken from Hanai et al. (132) and Liang et al. (201)]. The graph on the *right* shows the levels of the mRNA transcript and the nuclear transcription of c-*myc* in lymphocytes isolated from young and old human subjects before (*shaded bars*) and after (*solid bars*) mitogen stimulation [data taken from Gamble et al. (109)].

mRNA by a mitogen to a decrease in c-*myc* transcription. Induction of c-*myc* mRNA by lymphocytes from old mice was 50% of that observed for lymphocytes isolated from young mice. However, they found that the transcription of c-*myc* in a nuclear runoff assay was similar for mitogen-stimulated lymphocytes from young and old mice. Buckler et al. (35) also measured the degradation of c-*myc* mRNA in mitogen-stimulated lymphocytes and found no difference in the kinetics of degradation. They proposed that the age-related decrease in the induction of c-*myc* mRNA was due, therefore, to an alteration(s) in posttranscriptional processing. However, Gamble et al. (109) showed that the age-related decrease in the induction of c-*myc* mRNA in lymphocytes from human subjects was correlated to a decrease in the transcription of the c-*myc* gene, as shown in Figure 9.8. Induction of both mRNA and nuclear transcription of c-*myc* in peripheral T lymphocytes isolated from old (greater than 65 yr) human subjects was approximately 50% less than that observed for peripheral T lymphocytes from young (less than 35 yr) human subjects. Thus it appears that in most cases the age-related changes in an mRNA species probably arise from changes in transcription. Because of the difficulty in measuring the transcription of a specific gene using the nuclear runoff assay, investigators should be cautious in assuming that age-related changes arise from an alteration in either posttranscriptional processing or mRNA degradation when the age-related changes in the level of an mRNA transcript are not correlated to a change in the nuclear transcription of the gene, unless they clearly demonstrate that either the posttranscriptional processing of hnRNA or the mRNA degradation is altered by aging.

Factors That Regulate Transcription

Tables 9.3–9.6 illustrate that the expression of specific mRNA transcripts varies from mRNA to mRNA; therefore, it appears that the age-related changes in the transcription of specific genes are not due to a general up- or down-regulation of transcription. This view is supported by the studies described above in which the activities of the RNA polymerases were measured as a function of age; no major age-related decline in RNA polymerase II was found. Therefore, the age-related changes in the transcription of specific genes appears to be relatively unique and regulated at the level of the gene. It is currently known that transcription requires the recognition of numerous DNA sequences by a diverse group of proteins, *transcription factors*. Transcription factors form a complex with RNA polymerase that initiates the synthesis of RNA. Assembly of the transcription complex requires that the DNA in the chromatin be accessible to the transcription factors, RNA polymerase, and the progression of the RNA polymerase along the DNA. Therefore, age-related changes in chromatin structure or transcription factors could play a primary role in the changes in transcription with age. In addition, changes in chromatin structure or transcription factors could result in changes in gene expression that would affect only one gene or group of genes.

Chromatin Structure. In the 1960s and 1970s there was a great deal of research on the effect of age on the histone content of DNA, described in detail in early reviews (238, 319, 333). The general consensus from these studies was that the content of the nucleosome core histones (H2A, H2B, H3, and H4) in chromatin did not change with age, though several reports indicated that a change in the percentage of H1 in chromatin occurred with age. (H1 is associated with the linker region of the nucleosome structure.) In addition, several studies conducted in the 1970s indicated that the acetylation of histones decreased with age [see Richardson et al. (319)]. However, no one has shown that the age-related changes in H1 content or histone acetylation affect chromatin structure or function (that is, gene expression) in senescent animals.

Subsequent studies investigated the sensitivity of chromatin to nuclease digestion as a function of age because it appeared that active genes, that is, genes that can be expressed, were packaged in an altered nucleosome structure in which chromatin is less condensed, or more open, than inactive regions of chromatin. Therefore, active/expressed genes are more sensitive to nuclease digestion than inactive regions of chromatin. The initial studies in this area by Hill and Whelan (141) and Gaubatz et al. (110, 111) reported no age-related change in the sensitivity of liver chromatin from mice to digestion with either DNase I, DNase II, or micrococcal nuclease. However, Walford's laboratory (388, 389) reported that chromatin from the livers of old mice was less susceptible to digestion with either micrococcal nuclease or DNase I than chromatin from the liver of young mice. Berkowitz et al. (17) also observed an age-related decrease in the sensitivity of chromatin from cerebral and cerebellar neuronal cells of rats to micrococcal nuclease digestion. However, chromatin from cerebral neuroglial cells showed no age-related change in sensitivity to nuclease digestion. Chaturvedi and Kanungo (53) found that the rate of DNase I digestion of chromatin from the cerebral hemispheres of rats decreased with age, and Singh et al. (353) reported that the DNase I hypersensitive site in the albumin gene in liver becomes less sensitive to DNase I digestion with age. An age-related decrease in the sensitivity of chromatin to nuclease digestion would suggest that chromatin becomes more condensed with age, and this could result in decreased transcriptional activity, which appears to occur with increasing age. However, it is not clear if the sensitivity of chromatin to nuclease digestion decreases with age and becomes less accessible to the transcriptional apparatus.

DNA Methylation. It has been proposed that 5-Methylcytosine (5mC) in DNA plays a role in the regulation of gene expression at the level of transcription (49). In certain genes, decreased methylation (or *hypomethylation*) has been correlated to increased gene expression, and increased methylation (or *hypermethylation*), has been correlated to decreased gene expression. Alterations in DNA methylation also have been associated with cell differentiation and cancer (232). In early studies, in which the 5mC content of DNA hydrolysates was measured by thin-layer chromatography, no consistent pattern in DNA methylation was observed with age [see review by Mays-Hoopes (232)]. A list of studies which have employed a variety of highly sensitive techniques to measure DNA methylation is given in Table 9.7 These studies have measured 5mC content in DNA from a variety of tissues and animals, including humans. Almost all of these studies indicate that the genome becomes hypomethylated with age; that is, a loss of 5mC residues is observed in the DNA. In addition, Wilson et al. (434) showed a correlation between the loss of 5mC residues from the genome and life span. As Figure 9.9 shows, the rate of 5mC loss from DNA of the mucosa of the small intestine of mice (*Mus musculus*) was approximately twice as high as the rate of 5mC loss for DNA from the same cells of *Peromyscus leucopus*; *Peromyscus leucopus* generally lives twice as long as *Mus musculus*. Evidence that changes in DNA methylation play a role in aging also comes from studies on aging in vitro or cellular aging. A loss of 5mC residues from the genome of human fibroblasts is also observed with increasing passage number (433). More importantly, several investigators (88, 144, 427) have shown that incubating human fibroblasts with 5-azacytidine, a compound that inhibits the methylation of cytosine in DNA and results in the hypomethylation of DNA, shortens the in vitro life span of human fibroblasts; that is, the number of population doublings was reduced after 5-azacytidine treatment.

Although there is a great deal of evidence showing that the content of 5mC residues in the genome decreases with age, the functional significance of the age-related decrease in DNA methylation is not clear. For example, hypomethylation of DNA is generally believed to be associated with an increase in gene expression (49); however, most studies indicate that RNA synthesis decreases with age (see Table 9.2). Wilson et al. (434) suggested that the random loss of 5mC residues from promoter sequences of repressed genes would result in the inappropriate expression of these genes, which might alter the genetically programmed functions of old cells. This suggestion fits with the dysdifferentiation theory of aging originally advanced by Cutler in 1982 (71). He proposed that aging was a problem of improper gene regulation caused by mutation or epigenetic factors. Previous studies by Cutler's laboratory supported the dysdifferentiation theory; for example, the amount of RNA sequences complementary to the globin genes and the murine leukemic virus gene increased with age in brain and liver of mice, genes that normally are not expressed in brain and liver (98, 277). Gaubatz and Cutler (112) detected transcripts of the major satellite sequence in the heart of 12-month-old mice, and the level of these transcripts increased twofold

TABLE 9.7. *Effect of Age on DNA Methylation*

Methylation of the Whole Genome		Ages Studied (months, unless specified)	Assay	Change with Age	Reference
Sex/Species	Tissue				
Human					
	Bronchial epithelium	18–58 yr	^{32}P-postlabeling	Decrease	Wilson (434)
	Uncultured peripheral blood lymphocytes	25–75 yr	Restriction enzymes	Decrease	Drinkwater (81)
	Spleen	1–26	HPLC	Decrease	Tawa et al. (390)
Rat					
Female Wistar	Brain	4 and 22	Restriction enzymes	Increase	Rath and Kanungo (303)
Female Wistar	Uterus	5 and 24	HPLC and restriction enzymes	Decrease	Thakur and Kaur (393)
Mouse					
Male C57B1/6J	Liver	6–28	HPLC	Decrease	Singhal (357)
C57B1/6J (sex unspecified)	Liver, brain, small intestine	2–32	^{32}P-postlabeling	Decrease	Wilson (434)
White-footed (sex unspecified)	Liver, brain, small intestine	4–60	^{32}P-postlabeling	Decrease	Wilson (434)
C57B1/6NJcl	Liver	1–26	HPLC	No change	Tawa et al. (390)
Female C3H/SHNF1	Liver	2 to 21–27	HPLC	No change	Miyamura et al. (251)

Methylation of Specific Genes					
Gene	Sex/Species	Tissue	Ages Studied	Change with Age	Reference
Actin	Female C57B1/6NJcl mice	Liver, brain and spleen	2–26	No change	Ono et al (280)
β-actin	Female WAG/Rij rats	Spleen	6–36	Decrease	Slagboom et al. (360)
β-actin	Female WAG/Rij rats	Liver	6–36	No change	Slagboom et al. (360)
β-actin	Female WAG/Rij rats	Brain	6–36	No change	Slagboom et al. (360)
Albumin	Male Wistar rats	Liver	5 and 21	Increase	Singh et al. (353)
Dihydrofolate reductase	Female C57B1/6NJcl mice	Liver, brain and spleen	2–26	No change	Ono et al. (280)
c-*fos*	C57B1/6NJcl mice (sex unspecified)	Liver, brain and spleen	0.5–26	No change	Uehara et al. (400)
c-*fos*	Male Wistar rats	Brain	3–5 to 18–20	Increase	Kitraki et al. (179)
IGR-II	Male Wistar rats	Brain	3–5 to 18–20	Increase	Kitraki et al. (79)
Intracisternal particle A	Male C57B1/6J mice	Liver	3–26	Decrease	Mays-Hoopes (233)
LlMd	Male C57B1/6J mice	Liver	3–27	Decrease	Mays-Hoopes (230)
Major histocompatability complex I	Female WAG/Rij rats	Pituitary	3 and 25	No change	Slagboom et al. (360)
c-*myc*	Female C57B1/6NJcl mice	Spleen	2–26	Decrease	Ono et al. (280)
c-*myc*	Female C57B1/6NJcl mice	Liver	2–26	Increase	Ono et al. (280)
c-*myc*	Female C57B1/6NJcl mice	Brain	2–26	No change	Ono et al. (280)
c-*myc*	Human	Liver	0–93 yr	Increase	Ono et al. (281)
c-*myc*	Female C3H/SHNF1 mice	Liver	2 to 21–27	Decrease	Miyamura et al. (251)
v-Ki-*ras*	Female WAG/Rij rats	Pituitary	3 and 25	No change	Slagboom et al. (360)
rRNA (18S and 28S)	Male CBA/Ca mice	Liver, brain and spleen	6 and 18	Increase	Swisshelm (381)
S14	Male Sprague-Dawley rats	Liver	1–12	Increase	Wong et al. (436)
Tyrosine aminotransferase	Female WAG/Rij rats	Liver, brain and spleen	6–36	No change	Slagboom et al. (358)

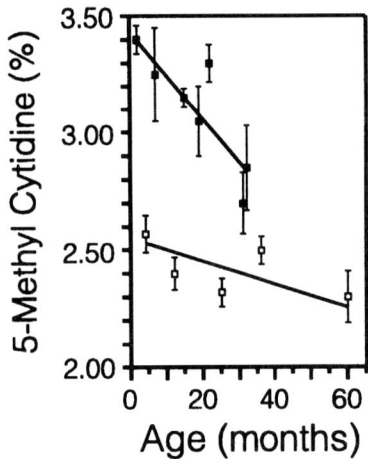

FIG. 9.9. Effect of age on DNA methylation. The percentage of 5mC in DNA isolated from the mucosa of the small intestine of *Mus musculus* (■) and *Peromyscus leucopus* (□) of various ages is shown [data taken from Wilson et al. (434)].

between 12 and 32 months of age. The satellite transcripts were not observed in heart tissue of young (2–6 months of age) mice. However, the expression of repressed genes in tissues from old animals is tissue-, species-, and gene-specific. For example, Ono et al. (278) found no evidence for the accumulation of RNA sequences complementary to the globin genes and the murine leukemic virus in tissues from a short-lived strain of mouse. In addition, Gaubatz and Cutler (112) did not detect satellite transcripts in brain, liver, and kidney tissue of mice at any age, and Richardson et al. (323) did not detect any age-related accumulation of α-fetoprotein transcripts in the liver of rats. Thus although the dysdifferentiation theory of aging is attractive and would explain how hypomethylation of the genome might be detrimental to an old organism, the evidence to support this theory is very limited. For example, it is not clear that the abnormal expression of repressed genes with age is due to hypomethylation because none of the studies measured the methylation of the genes in tissues from young and old animals.

To gain a greater insight into the importance of DNA methylation in aging, investigators have begun to study the methylation of specific regions of DNA using restriction enzymes specific for sequences containing 5mC (for example, Hpa II and Msp I). Table 9.7 lists the studies that have been conducted in this area. It is clear from the information in Table 9.7 that the effect of age on methylation of specific regions of the DNA or specific genes varies considerably from gene to gene and tissue to tissue. The initial studies by Mays-Hoopes et al. (230, 233) showed that the genes for the intracisternal A particle and the long interspersed repeated sequence L1Md were fully methylated in the liver of adult mice; however, these sequences were hypomethylated in liver DNA from senescent mice. In contrast, Rath and Kanungo (303) found that methylation of repetitive sequences in the DNA of brain increased with age in rats. Studies on c-*myc* showed that the effect of age on methylation of a gene varied considerably from tissue to tissue (280, 281). In mouse spleen, the c-*myc* gene became hypomethylated with age, while in the mouse and human liver it became hypermethylated. No appreciable age-related difference in methylation of the c-*myc* gene was observed in mouse brain.

Unfortunately, only a few of the studies listed in Table 9.7 measured both the methylation and the expression of the gene to determine if changes in methylation were functionally significant, that is, if changes in methylation could be correlated to changes in the expression of the gene. Singh et al. (353) reported that the age-related increase in methylation of the albumin gene in rat liver was correlated to a decrease in albumin mRNA transcripts and nuclear transcription of albumin. This observation is somewhat unexpected because most investigators have reported an age-related increase in albumin mRNA in rat liver (see Table 9.3). Swisshelm et al. (381) found that the age-related increase in methylation of rRNA genes was correlated to a decrease in the transcription of rRNA genes, and more importantly, 5-azacytidine treatment reactivated rRNA transcription and reduced rRNA gene methylation. Slagboom et al. (359) observed an age-related decrease in methylation of the β-actin gene and an increase in β-actin expression in the spleen of rats. These three studies support the view that during aging hypermethylation results in reduced expression and hypomethylation results in the increased expression of genes. However, several other studies suggest that the age-related changes in methylation are not linked to changes in gene expression. Slagboom et al. (359) observed no correlation between methylation and gene expression for either β-actin or glyceraldehyde-3-phosphate dehydrogenase in rat liver and brain. In addition, Wong et al. (436) found that the increase in methylation of the S14 gene in rat liver between 1 and 12 months of age was correlated to a fourfold increase in expression of the S14 mRNA and not a decrease in expression, as would have been predicted. Gaubatz et al. (113) found that expression of the intracisternal A particle gene does not change significantly with age in liver, brain, and kidney of mice. Thus the hypermethylation of the intracisternal A particle genes in mouse liver observed by Mays-Hoopes et al. (233) does not appear to alter expression of these genes. In addition, induction of c-*myc* expression in lymphocytes has been shown to decrease with age (35, 109), even though Ono et al. (280) observed that the c-*myc* gene in spleen became hypomethylated with age. Thus there is no direct evidence to show that age-related changes in methylation of a gene alter expression of the gene.

Transcription Factors. As our understanding of the mechanism of gene regulation has grown, it has become apparent that transcription factors play a critical role in cell development, differentiation, and growth. Transcription factors, which regulate the transcription of genes, represent one of the largest and most diverse classes of DNA-binding protein. These proteins bind specific DNA sequences, which are usually found distal to the 5′-end of the transcribed region of most genes. Therefore, age-related changes in the activities or levels of transcription factors could be the basis for age-related changes in gene expression. Because this is a new area of research, only a limited amount of information is available on how aging affects transcription factors; these studies are listed in Table 9.8. Two assays have been employed to study transcription factors with age. Using cDNA probes, the levels of the mRNA transcript coding for a transcription factor have been measured by cDNA/RNA hybridization. In addition, the activities of transcription factors in cell or nuclear extracts have been measured by binding the extracts to specific DNA sequences using the gel shift assay. However, one must be cautious in interpreting the data gathered from these assays. For example, one cannot be certain that the age-related changes in the level of an mRNA transcript coding for a transcription factor accurately reflect the changes in the transcription factor or its binding activity without actually measuring the level of the protein or the binding activity. In addition, the binding activity of a transcription factor in the gel shift assay does not necessarily reflect the activity of the factor in the transcription of a gene in the cell nucleus.

It is clear from the data presented in Table 9.8 that only a few transcription factors have been studied with respect to age. The majority of studies have focused on the fos-jun family, which encodes proteins that bind the AP-1 element (188). Three jun homologs have been identified: c-*jun*, *jun*-B, and *jun*-D. The jun proteins can form homo- or heterodimers that bind to the AP-1 element on DNA. In contrast, c-*fos* protein cannot form stable homodimers; however, it can interact with the jun family of proteins to form fos/jun heterodimers that show increased affinity for the AP-1 element. Interest in the effect of age on the fos-jun family of transcription factors was stimulated by the report from Seshadri and Campisi (344) on c-*fos* expression during aging in vitro. They showed that the induction of c-*fos* expression (mRNA levels and nuclear transcription) was blocked in late-passage fibroblasts and proposed that senescent fibroblasts were unable to proliferate because of, at least in part, the selective repression of c-*fos*. Subsequently, several investigators have measured the levels of the transcripts for the various members of the fos-jun family. Takahashi et al. (386) studied the effect of aging on the expression of c-*fos* and c-*jun* in rat heart. They measured the induction of c-*fos* and c-*jun* transcripts in the left ventricle of rats after ascending aortic constriction, which induces ventricular hypertrophy. As Figure 9.10 shows, the levels of c-*fos* and c-*jun* mRNA transcripts were induced dramatically immediately after ascending aortic constriction; however, induction of the c-*fos* and c-*jun* transcripts was approximately 80% lower in the hearts of old rats. Takahashi et al. (386) showed that the age-related decrease in c-*fos* and c-*jun* induction was not due to a difference in the hemodynamic stress applied to the heart and proposed that the age-related decline in the induction of c-*fos* and c-*jun* in the left ventricle might play a role in the diminished capacity of the heart of old animals to respond to hemodynamic stress and to develop left ventricular hypertrophy. D'Costa et al. (73) also observed an age-related decline in the induction of c-*fos* immunoreactivity by electroconvulsive shock in the brains of mice, and Sikora et al. (352) found a decrease in AP-1-binding activity with age in nuclear extracts from mitogen-stimulated lymphocytes isolated from mice that was correlated to the age-related decline in mitogen-induced lymphocyte proliferation. Thus the data from these studies suggest that a decrease in the expression of c-*fos* and c-*jun* occurs with aging, which might be related to a reduced ability of tissues from old animals to undergo cellular proliferation. However, it is clear from the studies listed in Table 9.8 that an age-related decline in the expression of c-*fos* and c-*jun* or the AP-1-binding activity is not always observed. For example, Fujita and Maruyama (104) reported that the transcripts for c-*fos* and c-*jun* increased dramatically with age in rat liver, and Ammendola et al. (1) found no age-related change in the AP-1-binding activity of nuclear extracts isolated from rat brain. Therefore, it is unclear how aging affects the transcription factors in the fos-jun family in animal tissues, even though human fibroblasts show a marked repression of c-*fos* expression during in vitro aging.

Several laboratories have studied the effect of age on the transcription factor Sp1, which is found in all mammalian cells and is required for the transcription of a large number of cellular genes (299). The data on Sp1 and age are also contradictory. Ammendola et al. (1) reported a marked decrease in Sp1-binding activity in nuclear extracts isolated from rat brain; however, they found that the Sp1 protein levels in brain did not change with age, as determined from immunoblots of nuclear extracts. In contrast, Heydari et al. (138) found no age-related change in the Sp1-binding activity of nuclear extracts from rat liver. In addition, Spindler's laboratory (261, 371) found no age-related change in the level of the mRNA transcript for Sp1 in mouse liver. Thus if

TABLE 9.8. *Effect of Age on Transcription Factors*

Sex/Species	Tissue	Ages Studied	Change with Age	Reference
AP-1				
Rat				
Male Wistar	Brain	4 and 30	No change in AP-1 binding	Ammendola et al. (1)
Wistar (sex unspecified)	Hippocampus (basal)	4 and 24	Increase in AP-1 binding	Kaminska and Kaczmarek (165)
	Hippocampus (induced)	4 and 24	Increase in AP-1 binding	Kaminska and Kaczmarek (165)
Mouse				
Swiss albino (sex unspecified)	Spleen lymphocytes (basal)	3 and 18–20	Decrease in AP-1 binding	Sikora et al. (352)
Swiss albino (sex unspecified)	Spleen lyphocytes (induced)	3 and 18–20	Decrease in AP-1 binding	Sikora et al. (352)
Fos-Jun Family				
c-*fos*, Human				
	Peripheral blood lymphocytes (PHA-activated)	32 and 75 yr	No change in c-*fos* mRNA	Song et al. (365)
c-*fos*, Rat				
Male/Female Wistar/Slc	Liver	6–25	Increase in c-*fos* mRNA	Fujita and Maruyama (102)
Male Fischer 344	Heart	2–18	No change in basal c-*fos* mRNA; decrease in induced c-*fos* mRNA	Takahashi et al. (386)
c-*fos*, Mouse				
Female C3B10RF$_1$	Liver	4–31	Increase in c-*fos* mRNA	Spindler et al. (371)
Female B6/C3	Amygdala (basal)	6–28	Decrease in c-*fos* protein	D'Costa et al. (73)
Female B6/C3	Amygdala (induced)	6–28	No change in c-*fos* protein	D'Costa et al. (73)
Female B6/C3	Cortex (basal)	6–28	Decrease in c-*fos* protein	D'Costa et al. (73)
Female B6/C3	Cortex (induced)	6–28	No change in c-*fos* protein	D'Costa et al. (73)
Female B6/C3	Hippocampus (basal)	6–28	Decrease in c-*fos* protein	D'Costa et al. (73)
Female B6/C3	Hippocampus (induced)	6–28	No change in c-*fos* protein	D'Costa et al. (73)
Swiss albino (sex unspecified)	Spleen lymphocytes (basal)	3 and 18–20	Decrease in c-*fos* mRNA	Sikora et al. (352)
Swiss albino (sex unspecified)	Spleen lymphocytes (induced)	3 and 18–20	Decrease in c-*fos* mRNA	Sikora et al. (352)
c-*jun*, Human				
	Peripheral blood lymphocytes (PHA-activated)	32 and 75 yr	Decrease in c-*jun* mRNA	Song et al. (365)
c-*jun*, Rat				
Male Wistar/Slc	Liver	6–25	Increase in c-*jun* mRNA	Fujita and Maruyama (102)
Female *Wistar/Slc	Liver	6–25	Increase in c-*jun* mRNA	Fujita and Maruyama (102)
Male Fischer 344	Heart	2–18	No change in basal c-*jun* mRNA, decrease in induced c-*jun* mRNA	Takahashi et al. (386)
c-*jun*, Mouse				
Male mice (three strains: B10RIII, C57Bl/10, and B10:BR	Liver	4–24	55% decrease in c-*jun* mRNA from 4 to 12 months, then return to 4-month levels by 24–25 months	Mote et al. (261)
Female C3B10RF$_1$	Liver	4–31	Increase in c-*jun* mRNA	Spindler et al. (371)
Swiss albino (sex unspecified)	Spleen lymphocytes (basal)	3 and 18–20	Increase in c-*jun* mRNA	Sikora et al. (352)
Swiss albino (sex unspecified)	Spleen lymphocytes (induced)	3 and 18–20	Decrease in c-*jun* mRNA	Sikora et al. (352)

CHAPTER 9: GENE EXPRESSION AND PROTEIN DEGRADATION 193

Sex/Species	Tissue	Ages Studied	Change with Age	Reference
jun-B, Human				
	Peripheral blood lymphocytes (PHA-activated)	32 and 75 yr	No change in *jun*-B mRNA	Song et al. (365)
C/EBP				
Mouse				
Male (three strains: B10RIII, C57B1/10, and B10:BR	Liver	4–24	No change in CEBP mRNA	Mote et al. (261)
Female C3B10RF₁	Liver	4–31	No change in CEBP mRNA	Spindler et al. (371)
CREB				
Rat				
Wistar (sex unspecified)	Hippocampus (basal)	4 and 24	No change in CRE binding	Kaminska and Kaczmarek (165)
	Hippocampus (induced)	4 and 24	No change in CRE binding	Kaminska and Kaczmarek (165)
(sex and strain unspecified)	Liver	2–110 wk	CRE binding decreases and CRE bands change	Singh and Kanungo (354)
Heat Shock Transcription Factor (HSF)				
Rat				
Male Fischer 344	Liver	4 and 25	Decrease in HSE binding	Heydari et al. (138)
LF-B1				
Rat				
Male/Female Wistar/Slc	Liver	6–25	Decrease in mRNA level	Fujita and Maruyama (104)
RNA Polymerase II Elongation Factor S-II				
Mouse				
Male mice (three strains: B10RIII, C57B1/10, and B10:BR		4–24	No change in S-II mRNA	Mote et al. (261)
Female C3B10RF₁	Liver	4–31	No change in S-II mRNA	Spindler et al. (371)
Sp1				
Rat				
Male Fischer 344	Liver	4 and 25	No change in the binding activity of Sp1	Heydari et al. (138)
Male Wistar	Brain	4 and 30	Decrease in the binding activity of Sp1	Ammendola et al. (1)
Mouse				
Male (three strains: B10RIII, C57B1/10, and B10:BR	Liver	4–24	No change in Sp1 mRNA	Mote et al. (261)
Female C3B10RF₁	Liver	4–31	No change in Sp1 mRNA	Spindler et al. (371)

Sp1 activity changes with age, it appears to be tissue-specific.

Although there have been several studies on the effect of age on the levels/activities of transcription factors, only one study has attempted to correlate changes in a transcription factor to changes in the expression of a gene. Studies on the heat shock transcription factor (HSF) suggest that an age-related decline in the ability of cells to express heat shock proteins may be due, at least partially, to alterations in the HSF. Induction of the transcription of heat shock genes is mediated by the binding of HSF to a highly conserved DNA sequence known as the heat shock element (HSE), which is found in the 5′-flanking sequence of all heat shock genes. An increase in temperature in mammalian cells results in the conversion of HSF from an inactive form that does not bind DNA to an active form that binds the HSE (368). Heydari et al. (138) showed that the age-related decrease in the transcription of the hsp70 gene in rat hepatocytes was correlated to a decrease in HSF-binding

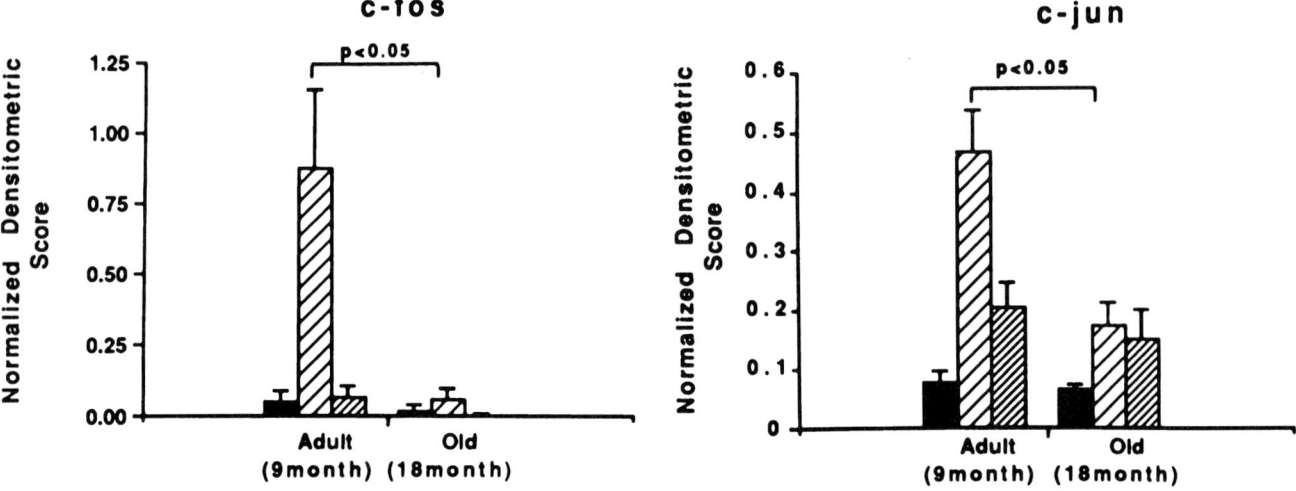

FIG. 9.10. Effect of age on the induction of c-*fos* and c-*jun* in rat heart. The levels of the mRNA transcripts for c-*fos* and c-*jun* were measured in the hearts of 9- and 18-month-old rats 90 (▨) and 180 (▨) minutes after acute pressure overload or in sham (■)-operated rats [data taken from Takahashi et al. (386)].

activity to HSE. Interestingly, Liu et al. (207) also observed a similar correlation during in vitro aging in human fibroblasts. Both the transcription of hsp70 and the HSF-binding activity to HSE were lower for fibroblasts with 48 population doublings compared to fibroblasts with 25 population doublings.

In summary, although it is quite attractive to propose that age-related changes in transcription factors are a major element underlying the age-related change in gene expression, the data are too limited to draw any conclusion. In addition, it is important in future studies that investigators correlate changes in transcription factors to changes in function, that is, to determine if the age-related changes in a transcription factor or transcription factors lead to changes in the expression of genes that require the transcription factor(s). In addition, one must keep in mind that modifications to the nucleosome might influence the binding of transcription factors to specific DNA sequences. Lee et al. (195) showed that the acetylation of the N-terminal tails of the core histones facilitated binding of the transcription factor TFIIIA to a model gene. Thus the age-related decline in histone acetylation, which was reported in studies in the 1970s [see Richardson et al. (20, 319)], might play a role in gene expression by reducing the binding of transcription factors to *cis*-acting sequences on genes.

Effect of Dietary Restriction on Transcription

Dietary restriction (restriction of total calories, not malnutrition) is the only experimental manipulation that has been shown consistently to increase the survival of mammals, and it is believed that dietary restriction increases survival by altering the aging process (224–226). Therefore, dietary restriction gives investigators a powerful tool to study how alterations in aging affect biological processes. The first report to show that dietary restriction altered the expression of a gene was published by Richardson et al. in 1987 (22, 321). They compared the expression (synthesis, mRNA levels, and nuclear transcription) of α_{2u}-globulin by hepatocytes isolated from 18-month-old rats fed ad libitum with those from rats on a calorie-restricted diet; the expression of α_{2u}-globulin decreased markedly with age (Fig. 9.5). Dietary restriction significantly retarded the age-related decline in α_{2u}-globulin expression. As shown in Figure 9.11, the expression (that is, the synthesis, mRNA levels, and transcription) of α_{2u}-globulin was increased two- to threefold by dietary restriction. Since this report a number of studies have compared the

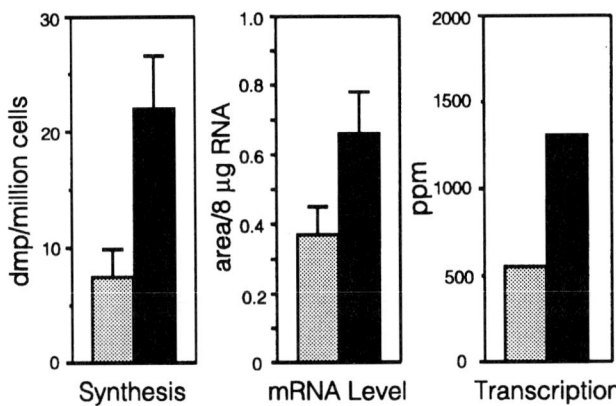

FIG. 9.11. Effect of dietary restriction on the expression of α_{2u}-globulin. The synthesis, mRNA levels, and nuclear transcription of α_{2u}-globulin by hepatocytes isolated from 18-month-old rats fed ad libitum (*shaded bars*) and a calorie-restricted diet (*solid bars*) are shown [data taken from Richardson et al. (321)].

expression of various mRNA transcripts in tissues from rodents fed ad libitum with those from rats on a calorie-restricted diet. A list of these studies is given in Table 9.9. It can be seen from this table that the effect of dietary restriction on the levels of mRNA transcripts varies significantly from transcript to transcript. The levels of many mRNA transcripts that decrease with age are increased by dietary restriction, for example, α_{2u}-globulin, catalase, superoxide dismutase, hsp70, androgen receptor, etc. However, dietary restriction has no effect on the levels of some mRNA transcripts (for example, albumin, c-*myc*, c-*jun*, Sp1, glutathione peroxidase, etc.) and reduces the levels of other mRNA transcripts (for example, grp78, calcitonin, somatostatin, apolipoprotein AI, etc.).

Although there are numerous studies on the effect of dietary restriction on the levels of mRNA transcripts, only a few have measured its effect on the transcription of specific genes. In general, it appears that the changes in the levels of the mRNA transcripts with dietary restriction are due to changes in transcription. As shown in Figure 9.11, both the level of the α_{2u}-globulin mRNA and the nuclear transcription of the α_{2u}-globulin gene in rat liver were increased by dietary restriction. In addition, Semsei et al. (341) showed that the increase in the mRNA transcripts for catalase and superoxide dismutase in the liver of calorie-restricted rats was paralleled by a similar increase in the transcription of the catalase and the superoxide dismutase genes. Heydari et al. (138) showed that dietary restriction increased induction of the expression of hsp70 in rat hepatocytes due to an increased transcription of the hsp70 gene.

The observation that dietary restriction alters the expression of genes at the level of transcription is quite exciting because it suggests that an alteration in the expression of one or more genes may be responsible for the decrease in pathology and the increased survival observed when rodents are maintained on a calorie-restricted diet (137). This suggestion is supported by the following: the expression of a variety of genes changes with age, and altering the expression of even one gene can have a profound effect on a cell or organism. It is interesting that dietary restriction enhances the expression of many genes (for example, catalase, superoxide dismutase, hsp70, interleukin 2, etc.) that play important roles in cellular protection. As more gene expressions are studied in tissues from calorie-restricted rats, we will gain a better appreciation for how dietary restriction alters gene expression in the whole organism.

Although research has demonstrated that dietary restriction alters gene expression at the level of transcription, the biological mechanism whereby dietary restriction alters the specific transcription of genes is not yet known. Heydari and Richardson (137) advanced the hypothesis that dietary restriction altered the transcription of genes through changes in the levels and/or activities of specific transcription factors. They proposed that dietary restriction induced the changes in the levels/activities of the transcription factors through changes in the hormonal status of the animal after it was placed on a calorie-restricted diet. Heydari et al. (138) supported this hypothesis by showing that the increase in hsp70 transcription in hepatocytes isolated from calorie-restricted rats was correlated to an increase in the binding activity of HSF in nuclear extracts from hepatocytes.

TRANSLATION

Protein Synthesis

Since 1967, many investigators have measured protein synthesis as a function of age in various tissues and organisms (see Tables 9.10–9.12). A variety of assays, ranging from cell-free assays to in vivo assays, have been used in these studies. The advantages and limitations of these assays have been discussed in detail in previous reviews (313, 315). In general, the data generated with in vivo assays are limited because most investigators have failed to measure the specific activity of the amino acid precursor pool. In contrast, one can carefully measure protein synthesis with cell-free assays; however, cell-free assays show only a fraction of the total protein synthesis with cell-free assays; however, cell-free assays show only a fraction of the total protein synthetic activity observed in vivo.

Most studies on the effect of age on protein synthesis were conducted in the 1970s and focused on protein synthesis in the liver of laboratory mice or rats (Table 9.11). In general, these studies (more than 80% of them) show an age-related decline in protein synthesis. For example, the data presented in Figures 9.12 and 9.13 show that an age-related decline in protein synthesis is observed in *Drosophila* and nematodes as well as in a variety of tissues from either F344 or Sprague-Dawley rats. The studies on liver protein synthesis in Table 9.11 generally demonstrate an age-related decrease in protein synthesis in both male and female rodents. Therefore, the age-related change in protein synthesis, at least in liver, does not appear to be sex-dependent.

An age-related decline in protein synthesis also appears to occur in humans (440). Welle et al. (426) carefully compared the rate of protein synthesis in the muscle of adult (21–31 yr) and healthy old (62–81 yr) men by measuring the in vivo incorporation of [^{13}C]-leucine into the *vastus lateralis* muscle. They observed that the rate of total myofibrillar protein synthesis was 44% lower in the muscle of old men and suggested that this decrease might be an important factor in muscle atrophy that is associated with aging and senescence.

In almost all of the studies listed in Tables 9.10–9.12, protein synthesis was determined using assays that mea-

TABLE 9.9. *Effect of Age and Dietary Restriction on mRNA Levels*

Sex/Species	mRNA	Ages Compared (months)	Change with Dietary Restriction	References
Adenal Gland				
Rat				
Male Fischer 344	Tyrosine hydroxylase	21	+60%[Δ]	Strong et al. (379)
Liver				
Rat				
Male Fischer 344	Androgen receptor	12–27	Increase	Song et al. (364)
Male Fischer 344	Apolipoprotein A1	18	−30%	Waggoner et al. (364)
Male Fischer 344	Apolipoprotein B	18	No change	Waggoner et al. (364)
Male Fischer 344	Catalase	18	+42%[Δ,+]	Semsei et al. (341)
Male Fischer 344	Catalase	4 and 12	No change [Δ]	Rao et al. (300)
		21 and 28	+12 to +49%[Δ]	
Male Fischer 344	Cytochrome P450 (P450IIB1/IIB2) induced by isosafrole	20	Increase*	Horbach et al. (150)
Male Fischer 344	α_{2u}-globulin	18	+78%[*,+]	Richardson et al. (320)
Male Fischer 344	α_{2u}-globulin	6 and 12	No change	Chatterjee et al. (51)
		18 and 27	50–1600%	
Male Fischer 344	α_{2u}-globulin	2	−80%	Waggoner et al. (364)
		4, 12, and 28	No change	
		21	800% increase	
Male Fischer 344	Glutathione peroxidase	4–28	No change [Δ]	Rao et al. (300)
Male Fischer 344	Heat shock protein (hsp70)	4–6 and 26–28	+27–+56%[*,+]	Heydari et al. (138)
Male Sprague-Dawley	T-kininogen	24	Decrease*	Sierra et al. (350)
Male Fischer 344	c-myc	18	No change	Waggoner et al. 364)
Male Fischer 344	Senesence marker protein (SMP-2)	6–24	No change*	Chatterjee et al. (51)
		27	−48%*	
Male Fischer 344	Superoxide dismutase (Cu/Zn)	18	+50%[Δ,+]	Semsei et al. (341)
Male Fischer 344	Superoxide dismutase (Cu/Zn)	4	No change[Δ]	Rao et al. (300)
		12–28	+20 to +64%[Δ]	
Mouse				
Female C3B10RF$_1$	CAAT enhancer binding protein (C/EBP)	4–31	No change	Spindler et al. (371)
Female C3B10RF$_1$	Glucorticoid receptor	4–31	No change	Spindler et al. (371)
Female C3B10RF$_1$	Heat shock protein (grp-78)	4–31	No change (20% restriction) −50% (40% restriction)	Spindler et al. (370)
	(grp-94	4–31	No change (20% restriction) −43% (40% restriction)	Spindler et al. (370)
Female C3B10RF$_1$	Insulin-like growth factor 1	4–31	+11% (20% restriction) +23% (52% restriction)	Spindler et al. (370)
Female C3B10RF$_1$	c-jun	4–31	No change	Spindler et al. (371)
B6CF$_1$	c-myc	30	−65%	Nakamura et al. (265)
Female C3B10RF$_1$	RNA polymerase II elongation factor SII	4–31	No change	Spindler et al. (371)
Female C3B10RF$_1$	Sp1	4–31	No change	Spindler et al. (371)
Spleen Lymphocytes				
Rat				
Male Fischer 344	Interleukin 2 (stimulated with conA)	5 and 12	No change[Δ]	Pahlavani et al. (283)
		21	+28%[Δ]	
		28	+50%[Δ]	
Thyroid				
Rat				
Male Fischer 344	Calcitonin	6	No change[*,pl]	Salih et al. (335)
		18 and 24	−30 to −36%[*,pl]	
Male Fischer 344	Calcitonin gene-related peptide	6	No change[*,+]	Salih et al. (335)
		18 and 24	−45 to −60%[*,+]	
Male Fischer 344	Somatostatin	6–24	−23 to −67%[*,+]	Salih et al. (335)
Trigeminal Ganglion				
Rat				
Male Fischer 344	Calcitonin gene-related peptide	6–24	No change*	Salih et al. (335)

*Protein level was also measured in this study. [Δ]Activity was also measured in this study. [+]Nuclear transcription was also measured in this study.

TABLE 9.10. *Effect of Age on Protein Synthesis in Invertebrates*

Animal/Tissue	Age Studied (days)	System	Percentage Change	Reference
Nematodes				
Turbatrix aceti	1 to 29–31	Cell-free	−75	Egilmez and Rothstein (85)
Turbatrix aceti	Not stated	In vivo	Decrease	Prasanna and Lane (298)
Insects				
Drosophila melanogaster				
Whole body	1–21	In vivo	−75	Webster et al. (423)
Whole body	1–21	In vivo	−68	Webster and Webster (422)
Whole body	3–50	In vivo	−60	Baumann et al. (13)
Abdomen	1–21	In vivo	−33	Webster et al. (423)
Head	1–21	In vivo	−15	Webster et al. (423)
Microsomes	1–21	Cell-free	−70	Webster and Webster (420)
Mitochondria	1–90	Cell-free	−40	Bailey and Webster (8)
Mitochondria	1–60	In vivo	−78	Bailey and Webster (8)
Mitochondria	6 and 38	In vivo	−29	Fleming et al. (96)
Ovaries	4–34	In vivo	−48	Wattiaux et al. (417)
Ovaries	12 and 72	In vivo	−74	Courtright et al. (68)
Thorax	4–34	In vivo	+16	Wattiaux et al. (417)
Thorax	1–21	In vivo	−96	Webster et al. (423)
Thorax	12 and 72	In vivo	+20	Courtright et al. (68)
Drosophila subobscura				
Whole body	20 and 60	In vivo	+95	Clarke and Smith (59)
Whole body	3 and 50	In vivo	−40	Chen et al. (56)
Musca domestica				
Isolated flight muscle	1–15	In vitro	−60 to −70	Rockstein and Baker (328)
Phormia regina				
Whole body	5–6 to 37–40	In vivo	−46 to −72	Levenbook and Krishna (197)
Schistocera gergaria				
Wings	1–14	In vivo	−44	Heslop (136)

sure cytoplasmic protein synthesis. However, a few groups have specifically studied protein synthesis in mitochondria as a function of age. An age-related decrease in mitochondrial protein synthesis has been observed in *Drosophila* (8), rat liver (156, 219, 220), mouse liver (8), rat heart (376), and mouse kidney (401). Thus it appears that both mitochondrial and cytoplasmic protein synthesis decrease with age in most tissues and organisms.

Several investigators have used two-dimensional gel electrophoresis to determine how aging alters the synthesis of individual proteins [for review see Richardson and Semsei (318)]. The most informative studies were conducted with nematodes (163), *Drosophila* (95, 96), and rat hepatocytes (39). In these studies, incorporation of radioactively labeled amino acids into hundreds of proteins was compared for young and old organisms. The major observation from these studies was that the qualitative pattern of protein synthesis did not change markedly with increasing age; for example, very few proteins either appeared or disappeared with age. In other words, it appears that the same proteins are synthesized by cells from young and old organisms. Thus aging is not a simple continuation of development in which a different spectrum of gene products is synthesized as an organism ages. Although the qualitative pattern of proteins synthesized by cells does not change with age, it appears that there are quantitative changes in the synthesis of proteins. Fleming et al. (96) observed a significant age-related increase in the heterogeneity of protein synthesis in *Drosophila*, that is, the age-related change in the synthesis varied significantly from protein to protein. When they compared the synthesis of 43 proteins by *Drosophila* of various ages, they found that the synthesis of 36 of them decreased with age, the synthesis of six did not change, and the synthesis of one increased over 200% (95). Butler et al. (39) carefully measured the rate of synthesis of 36 randomly chosen proteins by hepatocytes isolated from 5–30-month-old rats. The total decrease in the rate of synthesis of all 36 proteins was 40%, which was similar to the age-related decrease observed in the rate of total protein synthesis by the hepatocytes. The synthesis of 35 of the 36 proteins decreased with age, and this decrease was statistically

TABLE 9.11. *Effect of Age on Protein Synthesis in Liver*

Sex/Strain	Ages Studied (months)	System	Percentage Change	Reference
Rats				
Total Protein Synthesis				
Male/Female Wistar	12–31	Cell-free	No change	Beauchene et al. (14)
Male Sprague-Dawley	12–31	Cell-free	+33	Beauchene et al. (14)
Male/Female Wistar	12–31	Tissue slice	No change	Beauchene et al. (14)
Male Sprague-Dawley	12–31	Tissue slice	−16	Beauchene et al. (14)
Male albino	2–22	Cell-free	−74	Hrachovec (153)
Strain not given	11–28	In vivo	No change	Beauchene et al. (15)
Male Wistar	10–22	In vivo	+40–50	Kanungo et al. (166)
Male albino	2–25	Cell-free	−64	Hrachovec (154)
Male Wistar	1–26	In vivo	−18	Comolli et al. (64)
Female Fischer 344	1–20	In vivo	No change	Ove et al. (285)
Male Wistar	3–24	Cell-free	−10–20	Comolli (63)
Male Fischer 344	1.5–24	Cell-free	No change	Chen et al. (54)
Male Wistar	12–31	Cell-free	−20–40	Buetow and Gandhi (36)
Male Wistar	3–24	Cell-free	−40	Junghahn and Bielka (164)
Male Wistar	3–26	Cell-free	−30	Hellthaler et al. (132)
Female Sprague-Dawley	1–18	Cell-free	−56	Layman et al. (196)
Female Sprague-Dawley	2–12	Tissue slice	−45	Layman et al. (196)
Wistar (sex unspecified)	3–12	Cell-free	−30	Mariotti and Ruscitto (221)
Female WAG/Rij	3–24	Hepatocytes	−52	van Bezooijen et al. (402)
Male Sprague-Dawley	1–18	Hepatocytes	−64	Ricca et al. (312)
Male Sprague-Dawley	3–15	In vivo	−48	Ricca et al. (312)
Male Fischer 344	2.5–18	Hepatocytes	−44	Coniglio et al. (65)
Male Sprague-Dawley	2–28	Hepatocytes	−62	Viskup et al. (407)
Strain not given	2–30	Cell-free	−30	Moldave et al. (253)
Female Wistar	10–30	Cell-free	−48	Cook and Buetow et al. (66)
Male Sprague-Dawley	6–30	Cell-free	−75	Bolla and Greenblatt (32)
Holtzman (sex unspecified)	1–12	Cell-free	−63	Mallonee et al. (217)
DA/Han (sex unspecified)	1–28	Cell-free	−56	Gabius et al. (107)
Male CD	1–26	In vivo	No change	Goldspink and Kelly (118)
Male Fischer 344	2.5–19	Hepatocytes	−55	Birchnall-Sparks et al. (23)
Male CD	fetus–26	In vivo	−50	Goldspink et al. (121)
Male Sprague-Dawley	3.5–23	In vivo	−45	Neidermuller (269)
Male Fischer 344	9–29	Cell-free	−72	Sojar and Rothstein (363)
Male Fischer 344	5–30	Hepatocytes	−36	Butler et al. (39)
Male Sprague-Dawley	1–26	In vivo	−50	Merry et al. (244)
Fischer 344 (sex unspecified)	2–26.5	Cell-free	No change	Laughrea and Latulippe (191)
Male Fischer 344	3–24	Perfused liver	−59	Ward (415)
Female Sprague-Dawley	4 and 24	Hepatocytes	−50	Ferland et al. (91)
Male Sprague-Dawley	12 and 24	In vivo	No change	Mosoni et al. (258)
Mitochondrial Protein Synthesis				
Male Sprague-Dawley	3 and 26	Cell-free	−46	Ibrahim et al. (156)
Male Sprague-Dawley	2–3 and 26–30	Cell-free	−41	Marcus et al. (219)
Male Sprague-Dawley	1–2 to 28	Cell-free	−64	Marcus et al. (220)
Mice				
Total Protein Synthesis				
Female C57B1/6J	3–28	Tissue slice	No change	Beauchene et al. (14)
Male C57B1/6J	5–30	Cell-free	−53	Mainwaring (214)
Female C57B1/6J	2–31	Cell-free	−47	Kurtz *(186)
Male C57B1/6J	12–33	In vivo	0–+37	Du et al. (82)
Female C57B1/6J	11–28	Cell-free	−21	Kurtz et al. (187)
Male ddy	2–26	Cell-free	−20–−40	Mori et al. (256)
Male C57B1/6J	3–25	Cell-free	Slight increase	Reis (308)
Male C57B1/6J	2–21	Cell-free	−42	Vandenhaute et al. (403)
Male C57B1/6J	12–4	In vivo	−27	Barrows and Kokkonen (10)
Male 57B1/6J	5–24	In vivo	−33	Sonntag et al. (367)
Mitochondrial Protein Synthesis				
Female C57B1/6J	5–26	Cell-free	−65	Bailey and Webster (8)

TABLE 9.12. *Effect of Age on Protein Synthesis in Rodent Tissues Other Than Liver*

Tissue Sex/Strain	Ages Studied (months unless specified)	System	Percentage Change	Reference
Human				
Total Body	1 month–91 yr	In vivo	−88	Young et al. (440)
Lymphocytes	27–78 yr	Cell culture	−50	Tollesfsbol and Cohen (395)
Lens	8–95 yr	Organ culture	No change	De Vries et al. (74)
Rat				
Whole Body				
Male CD	1–26	In vivo	−65	Goldspink and Kelly (117)
Male Sprague-Dawley	1–26	In vivo	−66	Lewis et al. (198)
Various Tissues				
Male CD	2–26	In vivo	Decrease in most tissues	Goldspink et al. (121)
Brain				
Whole brain				
Male Wistar	10–22	In vivo	No change	Kanungo et al. (166)
Male Fischer 344	6–32	Cell-free	−56	Ekstrom et al. (86)
Male Fischer 344	1–16	Cell-free	−28 to 34	Fando et al. (89)
Male Fischer 344	1–16	Slices	−60	Fando et al. (89)
Male Fischer 344	1–24	In vivo	36 to 37	Fando et al. (89)
Male Sprague-Dawley	6–23	In vivo	−17	Ingvar et al. (157)
Male Fischer 344	3–23	Cell-free	No change	Cosgrove and Rapoport (67)
Male Sprague-Dawley (CFY)	2–25	In vivo	−58%	Goldspink et al. (117)
Brainstem				
Female Long-Evans	3–22.5	In vivo	−20	Dwyer et al. (84)
Cerebellum				
Male Wistar	4–24	In vivo	No change	Avola et al. (5)
Female Long-Evans	3–22.5	In vivo	−11	Dwyer et al. (84)
Cerebral cortex				
Male Wistar	4–24	In vivo	No change	Avola et al. (5)
Forebrain				
Female Long-Evans	3–22.5	In vivo	−20	Dwyer et al. (84)
Hippocampus				
Male Wistar	4–24	In vivo	No change	Avola et al. (5)
Hypothalamus				
Male Wistar	4–24	In vivo	No change	Avola et al. (5)
Microvessels				
Sex/strain unspecified	4–21	Organ culture	−60	Gozes et al. (126)
Striatum				
Male Wistar	4–24	In vivo	No change	Avola et al. (5)
Epididymal Fat Pad				
Male Fischer 344	9–26	Adipocytes	No change	Chang et al. (50)
Heart				
Male Wistar	10–22	In vivo	+150	Kanungo et al. (166)
Male (species unspecified)	3–24	Cell-free	−32	Meerson et al. (240)
Male (species unspecified)	3–24	In vivo	−46	Meerson et al. (240)
Male CFY hooded	1.5–24	In vivo	−67	Crie et al. (70)
Male CD	1–26	In vivo	−47	Lewis et al (199)
Male Sprague-Dawley	9 and 25	Perfused heart	−48	Starnes et al. (377)
Male Lewis	6–24	In vivo	No change	Mays et al (229)
Male Sprague-Dawley (CFY)	2–25	In vivo	−40	Goldspink et al. (122)
Male Fischer 344	12–25	In vivo	No change	Biggs and Booth (20)
Mitochrondria				
Male Sprague-Dawley	5–24	In vitro	Decrease	Starnes et al. (376)

(continued)

TABLE 9.12. *Effect of Age on Protein Synthesis in Rodent Tissues Other Than Liver—Continued*

Tissue Sex/Strain	Ages Studied (months unless specified)	System	Percentage Change	Reference
Intestine, large				
Male CD	1–26	In vivo	−44	Goldspink et al. (120)
Small				
Male CD	1–26	In vivo	−34	Goldspink et al. (120)
Male Sprague-Dawley	1–26	In vivo	−50	Goldspink (120)
Male Sprague-Dawley	1–26	In vivo	−50	Merry et al. (245)
Kidney				
Male Wistar	10–22	In vivo	+100	Kanungo et al. (166)
Male/Female Wistar	11–28	In vivo	−0 to 15	Beauchene et al. (5)
Male DA/Han	1–28	Cell-free	−67	Gabius et al. (107)
Male Fischer 344	4–31	Cell suspension	−60	Ricketts et al. (325)
Male CD	1–26	In vivo	−47	Goldspink and Kelly (118)
Male Fischer 344	4–31	Cell-free	−84	Hardwick et al. (133)
Lung				
Male CD	2–24	In vivo	−26	Goldspink (116)
Male Sprague-Dawley (CFY)*C*2–25	In vivo	−20	Goldspink and Merry (119)	
Male Lewis	6–24	In vivo	No change	Mays et al. (229)
Muscle				
Diaphragm				
Male CD	2–24	In vivo	−40	Kelley et al. (169)
Male Sprague-Dawley	3–21	Organ	−26	Sonntag et al. (366)
Male Sprague-Dawley (CFY)	2–24	In vivo	+13	Goldspink et al. (123)
Extensor digitorum longus				
Male CD	2–24	In vivo	−69	Kelley et al. (169)
Male Sprague-Dawley (CFY)	2–24	In vivo	−63%	Goldspink et al. (123)
Gastrocnemius				
Male CD	2–24	In vivo	−66%	Kelley et al. (169)
Male Sprague-Dawley	12 and 24	In vivo	No change	Mosoni et al. (258)
Oesophageal muscularis				
Male CD	1–26	In vivo	−67	Lewis et al. (199)
Skeletal				
Male Wistar	10–22	In vivo	−15	Kanungo et al. (166)
Male Sprague-Dawley	2–24	Cell-free	−40	Pluskal et al. (296)
Male Lewis	6–24	In vivo	No change	Mays et al. (229)
Soleus				
Male CD	1–26	In vivo	−70	Lewis et al. (199)
Male CD	2–24	In vivo	−58	Kelley et al. (169)
Male Sprague-Dawley (CFY)	2–25	In vivo	−62	el Haj et al. (87)
Tibialis anterior				
Male CD	1–26	In vivo	−67	Lewis et al. (199)
Male CD	2–25	In vivo	−56	el Haj et al. (87)
Pancreas				
Male Sprague-Dawley	2–30	Slices	−40	Kim et al. (175)
Parotid				
Male Sprague-Dawley	2–30	Tissue slices	−58	Kim et al. (176)
Male Sprague-Dawley	2–30	Tissue slices	−60	Kim et al. (175)
Male Sprague-Dawley	2 and 24	Tissue slices	−25	Kim et al. (172)
Male Sprague-Dawley	2 and 24	Tissue slices	−24	Kim and Caulkins (171)
Male Sprague-Dawley	2 and 24	Tissue slices	−30	Kim and Arisumi (170)
Skin				
Male Lewis	6–24	In vivo	Increase	Mays et al. (229)
Spleen				
Male Fisher 344	4–30	Lymphocytes	−74	Cheung et al. (57)

Tissue Sex/Strain	Ages Studied (months unless specified)	System	Percentage Change	Reference
Submandibular Gland				
Male Wistar	4–24	Cell-free	−25	Baum et al. (12)
Testes				
Male Wistar	10–22	In vivo	+800	Kanungo et al. (166)
Male Fischer 344	3–30	Cell-free	−47	Liu et al. (208)
Male Sprague-Dawley	6–30	Cell-free	−51	Richardson and Myers (317)
Mouse				
Brain				
Whole brain				
Male C57B1/6J	10–30	In vivo	No change	Finch (404)
Male C57B1/6J	9–28	In vivo	No change	Gordon and Finch (125)
Albino NYLAR	5–25	Tissue slices	No change	McMartin and Schedbauer (236)
Female C57B1/6J	5–26	Cell-free	−44	Blazejowski and Webster (26)
Kidney				
Mitochondria				
Female C57B1/6J	5–26	Cell-free	−47	Bailey and Webster (8)
Heart				
Male C5 B1/6J	8–25	Perfused heart	−50	Geary and Florini (114)
Male C57B1/6J	8–26	Perfused heart	−26	Florini et al. (99)
Male C57B1/6J	12–33	In vivo	No change	Du et al. (82)
Female C57B1/6J	5–16	Cell-free	−21	Blazejowski and Webster (26)
Female C57B1/6J	16–26	Cell-free	−50	Blazejowski and Webster (26)
Male 57B1/6J	5–24	In vivo	−40	Sonntag et al. (367)
Muscle				
Diaphragm				
Male 57B1/6J	5–24	In vivo	No change	Sonntag et al. (367)
Skeletal				
Male C57B1/6J	9–18	Cell-free	+80	Britton and Sherman (33)
Male C57B1/6J	18–29	Cell-free	−60	Britton and Sherman (33)
Female C57B1/6J	5–26	Cell-free	−83	Blazejowski and Webster (26)
Stratified squamous epithelium				
C57B1/6J (sex unspecified)	3–22	Tissue slices	No change	Hill and Karthigasan (142)
Testes				
Male C57B1/6J	6–30	Cell-free	−39	Richardson and Myers (317)
Thymus				
C57B1/6J (sex unspecified)	1–24	Cell-free	−90	Azelis et al. (6)
Uterus				
Female Wistar	5.5 and 25	In vitro	−40%	Thakur and Kaur (392)

significant for 19 of the proteins. As shown in Figure 9.14, the magnitude of the age-related decrease in the synthesis of the 35 proteins varied from 15 to 60%. Although the age-related change in the synthesis of individual proteins was not uniform, it is interesting that the synthesis of most proteins appears to decrease with age. This suggests that the age-related change in the synthesis of proteins might be controlled at two levels. One level would be pretranslational, which would depend on the level of the mRNA transcript coding for the protein. At this level, changes in the synthesis of individual proteins would be unique for each protein. The second level of control would be translational, that is, due to an age-related defect in the protein synthetic apparatus of the cell. At this level, similar changes in synthesis (that is, a decrease) would be observed for all proteins with increasing age. Thus changes at the translational level would be expected to give rise to a general decrease in the synthesis of all proteins. However, because of changes in the levels of the mRNA transcripts coding for the individual proteins, the age-related decrease in the synthesis of proteins would not be uniform, and the

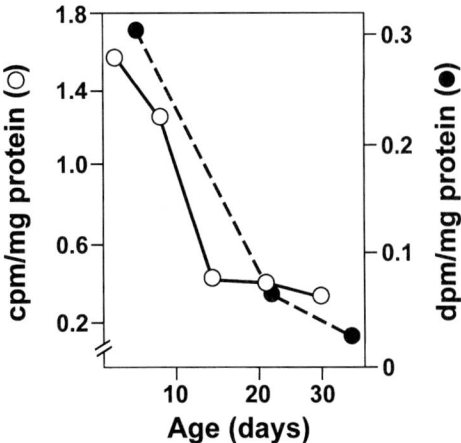

FIG. 9.12. Effect of age on protein synthesis by invertebrates. Cell-free incorporation of [³H]-leucine into protein by microsomes from *D. melanogaster* [○, data taken from Webster (420)] and the in vivo incorporation of [³H]-leucine into protein by nematodes [●, data taken from Sharma et al. (346)] are shown. [Figure taken from Richardson and Birchenall-Sparks (315) with permission.]

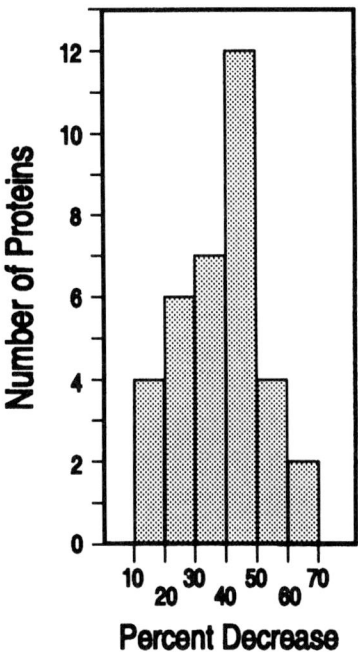

FIG. 9.14. Variation in the age-related decline in the synthesis of individual proteins by rat liver. A comparison of the decrease in the rate of synthesis of 35 proteins between 5 and 30 months of age is shown for rat hepatocytes [data taken from Butler et al. (39)].

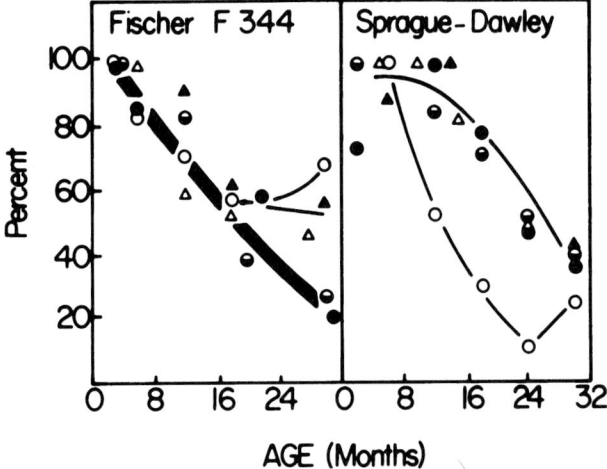

FIG. 9.13. Effect of age on protein synthesis by various tissues of rats. The *left graph* shows the relative protein synthetic activity of liver [○, data taken from Coniglio et al. (65)], brain [△, data taken from Ekstrom et al. (86)], kidney [●, data taken from Hardwick et al. (133)], testes [▲, data taken from Liu et al. (208)], and mitogen-stimulated spleen lymphocytes [◑, data taken from Cheung et al. (57)] of Fischer 344 rats. The *right graph* shows the relative protein synthetic activity of liver [◑, data taken from Bolla and Greenblatt (32)], pancreas [●, data taken from Kim et al. (175)], parotid gland [○, data taken from Kim et al. (176)], heart mitochondria [△, data taken from Starnes et al. (376)], and testes [▲, data taken from Richardson and Myers (317)] of Sprague-Dawley rats. [Figure taken from Richardson and Birchenall-Sparks (315) with permission.]

synthesis of some proteins could increase with age (for example, those proteins whose mRNA transcripts increase markedly with age).

Effect of Dietary Restriction on Protein Synthesis

One of the most exciting observations in the area of aging and protein synthesis is that dietary restriction alters the age-related decline in protein synthesis (Table 9.13). The first study in this area was conducted in 1985 by Birchenall-Sparks et al. (23). They showed that dietary restriction increased significantly the rate of protein synthesis by hepatocytes isolated from rats (Fig. 9.15). At 19 months of age, the rate of protein synthesis by hepatocytes isolated from rats fed the calorie-restricted diet was almost two times higher than that from rats fed ad libitum. Several investigators have subsequently confirmed the study by Birchenall-Sparks et al. (23); for example, dietary restriction has been reported to increase protein synthesis in hepatocytes (91), perfused liver (415), and liver in vivo (367) in rodents. Only in the study by Merry et al. (244) was it observed that dietary restriction did not affect protein synthesis in liver. It is unclear why this study is at variance with all of the other reports. Dietary restriction also appears to increase the rate of protein synthesis in tissues other than liver, as shown in Table 9.13. For example, whole-body protein synthesis (198) and pro-

TABLE 9.13. *Effect of Age and Dietary Restriction on Protein Synthesis*

Sex/Strain	Ages Compared (months)	Change with Dietary Restriction	Reference
Heart			
Rat			
Male Sprague-Dawley (CFY)	2	No change	Goldspink et al. (122)
Mouse			
C57B1/6J	2	98% increase	Sonntag et al. (367)
	12 and 25	No change	
Intestine (small)			
Rat			
Male Sprague-Dawley	2	No change	Merry et al. (245)
	12 and 25	60–90% increase	
Kidney			
Rat			
Male Fischer 344	19	45% increase	Ricketts et al. (325)
Liver			
Rat			
Male Fischer 344	4	No change	Birchenall-Sparks et al. (23)
	7–19	12–85% increase	
Male Sprague-Dawley	2	33% decrease	Merry et al. (244)
	12	No change	
		15% decrease	
Male Fischer 344	3	No change	Ward (415)
	6–24	35% increase	
Female Sprague-Dawley	4–6 and 20–24	20–30% increase	Ferland et al. (91)
Mouse			
Male C57B1/6J	5 and 24	No change	Sonntag et al. (367)
	15	66% increase	
Lung			
Rat			
Male Sprague-Dawley (CFY)	2 and 25	8–47% decrease	Goldspink and Merry (119)
	12	8% increase	
Muscle			
Extensor digitorum longus			
Rat			
Male Sprague-Dawley (CFY)	2 and 25	30–46% decrease	Goldspink et al. (123)
	12	20% increase	
Diaphragm			
Rat			
Male Sprague-Dawley (CFY)	2–25	15–58% decrease	Goldspink et al. (123)
Mouse			
C57B1/6J	5 and 24	66–100% increase	Sonntag et al. (367)
	12	No change	
Soleus			
Rat			
Male Sprague-Dawley (CFY)	2–25	6–36% decrease	el Haj et al. (87)
Tibialis anterior			
Rat			
Male Sprague-Dawley (CFY)	2 and 25	27–33% decrease	el Haj et al. (87)
	12	10% increase	

(continued)

TABLE 9.13. *Effect of Age and Dietary Restriction on Protein Synthesis—Continued*

Sex/Strain	Ages Compared (months)	Change with Dietary Restriction	Reference
Spleen Lymphocytes (mitogen-stimulated)			
Rat			
Male Fischer 344	5	32% decrease	Pahlavani et al. (288)
	12	No change	
	21 and 28	40–43% increase	
Testes			
Rat			
Male Fischer 344	19	50% increase	Richardson (314)
Whole Body			
Rat			
Male Sprague-Dawley	1.5	No change	Lewis et al. (198)
	12	45% increase	
	24	5% increase	

tein synthesis by kidney cells (325), mitogen-stimulated spleen lymphocytes (288), heart (367), diaphragm (367), small intestine (245), and testes (314) have been shown to be increased significantly by dietary restriction. Thus almost all studies indicate that dietary restriction significantly increases the rate of protein synthesis in most tissues of rodents. It is inviting to speculate that the increased rate of protein synthesis in most tissues of rodents. It is inviting to speculate that the increased rate of protein synthesis might in some way be responsible for the changes in survival and pathology observed in calorie-restricted rats.

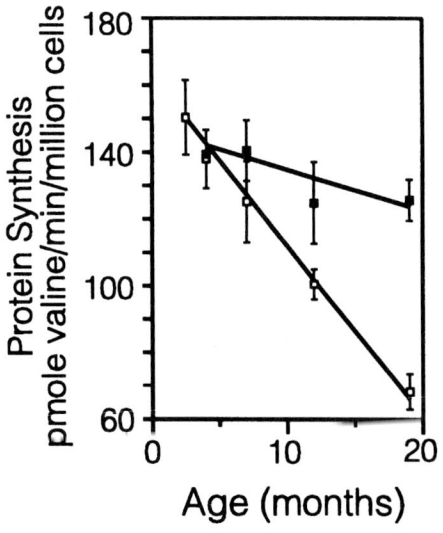

FIG. 9.15. Effect of dietary restriction on protein synthesis by rat liver. The rate of protein synthesis by hepatocytes isolated from rats fed ad libitum (□) or a calorie-restricted diet (■) is shown [data were taken from Birchenall-Sparks et al. (23)].

Fidelity of Protein Synthesis

In 1963, Orgel (282) advanced the error catastrophe hypothesis of aging and proposed that errors arising from the misincorporation of amino acids into proteins, which are involved in gene expression, give rise to increased errors in the products of these proteins. This would lead to an increasing number of errors with age, which cells eventually would not tolerate. Since the early 1970s, numerous investigators have compared the fidelity of protein synthesis in various cellular preparations from young and old organisms. Table 9.14 lists the studies that have been conducted on the effect of age on the fidelity of protein synthesis.

Using two-dimensional gel electrophoresis, investigators have studied the effect of aging on the fidelity of protein synthesis by looking for the appearance of new proteins and/or satellite spots, which would be indicative of random amino acid substitutions. Parker et al. (293) observed no heterogeneity in the migration of proteins from young and senescent *Drosophila*. Subsequently, similar observations were reported in nematodes and *Drosophila* by Johnson and McCaffrey (163) and Fleming et al. (96), respectively. However, this technique is limited by its sensitivity; therefore, a small increase in errors with age might escape detection. However, the fact that no major changes in the protein profiles have been observed in senescent organisms suggests that error catastrophe probably is not a major factor in senescence.

Fidelity has also been studied by measuring the errors produced at the various stages of protein synthesis. Several investigators have compared the fidelity of 80S monomeric ribosomes isolated from young and old

TABLE 9.14. *Effect of Age on the Fidelity of Protein Synthesis*

Sex/Strain	Tissue	Ages Studied (months, unless specified)	Observation	Reference
Nematodes				
Caenorhabditis elegans	Whole body	4–22 days	No change in the pattern of proteins synthesized as measured by two-dimensional gel electrophoresis	Johnson and McCaffrey (163)
Drosophila				
Drosophila melanogaster	Whole body	6–60 days	No change in the pattern of proteins synthesized as measured by two-dimensional gel electrophoresis	Parker et al. (293)
Rat				
Male Fischer 344	Liver	4 and 18	No change in errors in the aminoacylation of phe-tRNA	Coniglio et al. (65)
Male Fischer 344	Liver	6–10 to 23–24	No change in the capacity of ribosomes to accurately translate poly U	Butzow et al. (41)
Female Fischer 344	Kidney	4–31	Slight decrease in the accuracy of poly U translation	Hardwick et al. (133)
Male Sprague-Dawley	Liver	4 and 24	No alteration in tRNA function	Mays-Hoopes et al. (234)
Male Fischer 344	Hippocampus, liver	7–33	No change in the accuracy of poly U translation in post-mitochondrial supernatent	Filion and Laughrea (93)
Male Fischer 344/DuCrj	Liver	4–7 to 27–29	No change in the transitional fidelity of rat liver tyrosyl tRNA synthetase	Takahashi and Goto (383)
Mouse				
Female C57B1/6J	Liver	5–6 to 27–28	No change in the capacity of ribosomes to accurately translate poly U	Kurtz (186)
Female C57B1/6J	Liver	4–20	Decrease in the fidelty of cell-free translation	Ogrodnik (274)
Male C57B1/6J	Heart, kidney, liver, spleen	10 or 29	No change in the size or pattern of proteins synthesized as measured by two-dimensional gel electrophoresis or isoelectric focusing	Foote and Stulerg (102)
Male ddY	Liver	2–5 to 15–26	No change in the accuracy of poly U translation by liver ribosomes	Mori et al. (256)
Male ddy	Liver	2–29	No change in the accuracy of translation using a protamine mRNA template	Mori et al. (255)

organisms to translate the synthetic mRNA template polyuridylic acid. In these studies, errors were measured by the proportion of leucine (which is not coded in polyuridylic acid) and phenylalanine incorporated into acid-insoluble material. As shown in Table 9.14, most of these studies found no age-related change fidelity of polyuridylic acid translation. Only Butzow et al. (41) reported an age-related increase in errors in the translation of polyuridylic acid. However, this increase was observed in the presence of the aminoglycoside paromomycin, which decreases the fidelity of protein synthesis by ribosomes; no age-related change in the fidelity of polyuridylic acid translation was observed in the absence of paromomycin. Thus there does not appear to be any significant age-related decrease in the fidelity of ribosomes to translate polyuridylic acid. However, this assay is limited because polyuridylic acid might not be representative of natural mRNAs; that is, only one codon is being translated. Mori et al. (255) measured the fidelity of ribosomes from mouse liver to translate trout protamine mRNA by the incorporation of radioactive lysine, which is not present in protamine. No difference in the fidelity of ribosomes isolated from liver of 2- and 30-month-old mice was observed. Several laboratories have also measured the in vitro fidelity of aminoacylation of several tRNAs by extracts from liver of young and old rodents. In none of these studies, was there evidence that the fidelity of aminoacylation changed significantly with age.

Although the error catastrophe theory of aging is attractive, there is no evidence that errors in protein synthesis increase with age. In addition, the study by Libby (202) suggests that the misincorporation of amino acids into protein does not lead to an error catastrophe. Using bacteriophage T7–infected anucleate minicells of *Escherichia coli*, Libby (202) found that the misincorporation of amino acids into the early gene product T7 RNA polymerase did not suppress a nonsense mutation in a late gene product, the T7 gene. In other words, errors in the RNA polymerase did not alter the fidelity of transcription and result in increased mutations in the protein products ultimately derived from the action of the RNA polymerase. This observation does not support one of the basic tenets of the error catastrophe hypothesis of aging: errors that occur in proteins involved in gene expression will give rise to a decrease in the fidelity of gene expression and an increase in mutations in the protein product. Therefore, the experimental evidence indicates that an error catastrophe does not appear to be a viable hypothesis for the mechanism of aging.

Various Steps of Protein Synthesis

Because protein synthesis appears to decline significantly with age in most tissues and organisms, a great deal of research has gone into studying the mechanism responsible for the age-related decline in protein synthesis, that is, which step or steps of protein synthesis are altered with increasing age. Tables 9.15–9.17 list the studies that have been conducted in this area, covering various steps of protein synthesis. We will not discuss these studies individually but will summarize the generalizations that can be made on how aging affects specific steps in protein synthesis.

Although changes have been reported with age in various components of the system responsible for the aminoacylation of tRNA (see Table 9.15), the age-related decrease in protein synthesis does not appear to arise through a defect(s) in tRNA aminoacylation [see reviews by Richardson et al. (322) and Richardson and Semsei (318)]. It is unclear what effect aging has on the initiation of protein synthesis, but it is probably due to the difficulty in measuring accurately the initiation of protein synthesis (See Table 9.16). However, almost all studies have reported an age-related decrease in the aggregation of ribosomes to mRNA, that is, a decrease in polyribosomes and an increase in 80S monomeric ribosomes that are not associated with mRNA. Layman et al. (194) were the first investigators to show that a decline in ribosome aggregation to mRNA paralleled the age-related decrease in protein synthesis. Figure 9.16 shows the effect of age on ribosome profiles from the liver, brain, and skeletal muscle of rats. A decrease in ribosome aggregation to mRNA that has been observed with increasing age in a variety of rodent tissues. The decrease in the number of ribosomes associated with mRNA and actively synthesizing protein would be expected to be a major factor responsible for the age-related decrease in protein synthesis. One would predict that the age-related decline in ribosome aggregation to mRNA is due to a decrease in the initiation of protein synthesis, that is, the attachment of the ribosome subunits to the 5′-end of the mRNA. However, there is no strong evidence linking changes in initiation of protein synthesis to changes in either ribosome aggregation or protein synthesis. Kimball et al. (178) measured the activity and protein levels of eukaryotic initiation factor 2 (eIF-2) in various tissues of rats between 1 and 10 months of age. They showed that the eIF-2 content of a tissue was directly proportional to the rate of protein synthesis; that is, an excellent correlation was found between the age-related decrease in protein synthesis and the decrease in the level of eIF-2 between 1 and 10 months of age. Thus changes in initiation, for example, eIF-2, might play an important role in the age-related decrease in protein synthesis and ribosome aggregation to mRNA. Unfortunately, there is no information on the activity/level of eIF-2 in tissues of rodents older than 10 months of age.

The final general observation that can be made in this area is that the elongation step of protein synthesis appears to be reduced significantly with increasing age (see Table 9.17). As shown in Figure 9.17, Coniglio et al. (65) reported that the in vivo elongation of protein synthesis declined significantly with age. They measured the ribosome half-transit time (the elongation time required for the synthesis of an average half- length of a nascent polypeptide chain) in hepatocytes isolated from 4- and 18-month-old rats and found that it was 1.6 times higher for hepatocytes isolated from the old rats. More recently, Merry and Holehan (243) showed that the time to assemble the average peptide in vivo in rat liver increased significantly with age. Several laboratories have also measured the activity of the protein factors involved in the elongation step of protein synthesis as a function of age. In eukaryotes, two factors play a major role in the elongation of protein synthesis: elongation factor-1 (EF-1α), which catalyzes the GTP-dependent binding of aminoacyl-tRNA to the A site of the ribosome-mRNA complex, and elongation factor-2 (EF-2), which catalyzes the GTP-dependent translocation of the ribosome to the next codon on the mRNA template. There is no evidence to indicate that the activity of EF-2 changes significantly with age; however, a number of investigators have reported an age-related decrease in EF-1α activity in cell extracts obtained from a variety of organisms. The data presented in Figure 9.18 show how aging affects EF-1α activity in *Drosophila*, nematodes, and rat liver, demonstrating an age-related decrease in EF-1α activity in a wide variety of animals. Interestingly, Rattan et al. (307) found that dietary restriction, which results in increased protein synthesis in liver, had no effect on the age-related decrease in EF-1α activity.

Three other observations are relevant with respect to EF-1α and aging. First, Cavallius et al. (47) reported that the activity of EF-1α decreased significantly at the

TABLE 9.15. *Effect of Age on tRNA*

Sex/Species	Tissue	Ages Studied (months unless specified)	Change with Age	Reference
Drosophila				
Drosophila melanogaster	Whole body	1, 21, and 40 days	Decrease in tRNA content	Webster and Webster (421)
Rat				
Female albino	Liver	2, 10, 20	Highest concentration of tRNA in the adult (10 month) rats	Manjula and Sundari (218)
Mouse				
Female C57B1/6J skeletal muscle	Liver, kidney	1, 12, and 24	Decrease in tRNA content	Neumeister and Webster (268)
Female C57B1/6J 24 month	Brain, heart	1, 12, and 24	Increase in tRNA content	Neumeister and Webster (268)
Female C57B1/6J	Liver, kidney	1, 12, and 24	Decrease in tRNA synthesis	Neumeister and Webster (268)
Aminoacylation of tRNA				
Drosophila				
Drosophila melanogaster	Whole body	5 and 35 days	Decreased aminoacylation of tRNAs for ala arg, ile, pro, ser, thr, val, gly, and leu	Hosbach and Kubli (151)
Drosophila melanogaster	Whole body	5 and 35 days	Aminoacylation of ser tRNA decreased 25%	Hosbach and Kubli (152)
Drosophila melanogaster	Whole body	1, 21, and 40 days	Aminoacylation of tRNA by 20 amino acids decreased 40–50%	Webster and Webster (422)
Rat				
Male Charles River	Spleen	2–3 and 9–12	Over a 50% decrease in the aminoacylation of tRNA	Wust and Rosen (438)
Male Sprague-Dawley	Liver	3 and 24	a) The average decrease in the aminoacylation of phe, val, tyr, met, arg, ser, lys, leu, ala, asp, tyr, ile, glu, gly, pro, his, and thr tRNAs was 64% b) Very little decrease in the aminoacylation of tRNA in high-speed supernatant	Lawrence et al. (193)
Sex/strain unspecified	Liver	9, 18, and 27	Aminoacylation of lys tRNA increased with age	Singhal and Kopper (355)
Female Wistar	Liver	10–13 and 24–30	Decreased rate and extent of cell-free protein synthesis using tRNA from senescent cytosol	Cook and Buetow (66)
Female Wistar	Liver	10–13 and 24–30	a) Maximum aminoacylation of tRNAs for ala, arg, and asp increased and met decreased slightly b) Synthetase activity for met decreased	Cook and Buetow (66)
Female albino	Liver	2, 10, 20 month	a) Aminoacylation of ser and pro tRNAs increased from 2 to 10 months and decreased from 10 to 20 months b) Aminoacylation of ala, lys, arg, and glu tRNAs decreased continuously c) Little or no change in the aminoacylation of leu, gly, met, tyr, asp tRNAs	Manjula and Sundari (218)
Male DA/Han	Liver	1–28	Decreased binding of aminoacyl tRNA to ribosomes	Gabius et al. (107)
Male Sprague-Dawley	Liver	4 and 24	No change in the *in vivo* acylation of val and lys tRNAs	Mays-Hoopes et al. (234)

(*continued*)

TABLE 9.15. *Effect of Age on tRNA—Continued*

Sex/Species	Tissue	Ages Studied (months unless specified)	Change with Age	Reference
Male Fischer 344	Brain	7 and 33	No change in the endogenous amount of phe-tRNA or leu-tRNA	Filion and Laughrea (93)
Mouse				
BC3F (sex unspecified)	Brain, liver	5–9 and 28–36	Decreased aminoacylation of tRNAs for arg and tyr in liver and asp in brain	Frazer and Yang (103)
Male C57B16J	Liver, heart, kidney, spleen	10–12 and 29	No change in the aminoacylation capacities of tRNA preparations	Foote and Stulberg (102)
Aminoacylation of Isoaccepting tRNAs				
Nematodes				
Turbatrix aceti		8–15 to >20 days	Decrease in isoaccepting species of tyr- and art-tRNA	Reitz and Sanadi (309)
Rat				
Female albino	Skeletal muscle, liver	2–10 to 20	No change in the isoaccepting species of arg- or glut-tRNA	Vinayak et al. (406)
Male Sprague-Dawley	Liver	3 and 24	No change in lys$_5$- tRNA, increase in lys$_4$-tRNA, increase in ser$_2$-RNA and ser$_4$- tRNA	Mays et al. (228)
Male Sprague-Dawley	Liver	3 and 24	Increase in lys$_4$- tRNA	Lawrence et al. (193)
Sex/species unspecified)	Liver	1 wk and 10 month	Increase in asp$_2$-tRNA	Singhal and Kopper (355)
Female albino	Liver	2–20	a) Changes in the number and proportion of isoaccepting species of arg-tRNA b) Changes in the proportion of isoaccepting species of pro-tRNA c) No change in the isoaccepting species of glut-tRNA	Manjula and Sundari (218)
Mouse				
BC3F (sex unspecified)	Brain, liver	5–9 and 28–36	No change in the isoaccepting species of arg- or tyr-tRNA in the liver or asp-tRNA in the brain	Frazer and Yang (103)
Aminoacyl-tRNA Synthetases				
Drosophila				
Drosophila melanogaster	Whole body	5, 22, and 35 days	a) No change in the activities of synthetases for gly, thr, ile, and val b) Decrease in activities of synthetases for ala, arg, leu, pro, and ser, with the greatest decrease (50%) for leu synthetase	Hosbach and Kubli (151)
Drosophila melanogaster	Whole insect	5 and 35 days	Decrease in activities of synthetases for his, asn, leu, ala, met, and ser, with greatest decrease (60%) in ser synthetase activity	Hosbach and Kubli (152)
Rat				
Male Charles River	Spleen	2–3 and 9–12	Synthetase preparations from older animals are less active than preparations from young animals	Wust and Rosen (438)
Female Wistar	Liver	10–13 and 24–30	Decreased rate and extent of cell-free protein synthesis using tRNA synthetases from old animals	Cook and Buetow (66)

Sex/Species	Tissue	Ages Studied (months unless specified)	Change with Age	Reference
Female Han: NMRI	Various tissues	2 and 39	Age-related, organ-specific decrease of 20–70% in total and individual synthetase activities	Gabius et al. (107)
Male Wistar	Liver, brain, kidney	3–24	Increase in the proportion of heat-labile synthetases (0–20% in young, 15–40% in old)	Takahashi et al. (385)
Male Fischer 344	Liver, brain	4–30	Increase in the proportion of heat-labile synthetases	Takahashi and Goto (382)
Modification of tRNA Nucleosides				
Drosophila				
Drosophila melanogaster	Whole body	5 and 35 days	Increase in the contnet of queuine in asn, his, and tyr tRNAs	Hosbach and Kubli (152)
Drosophila melanogaster	Whole body	10, 20, and 30 days	Increase in the queuine content of tyr, his, and asp tRNAs	Owenby et al. (284)
Rat				
Male Fischer 344	Liver	0.25, 5, 9, 18, and 26	The queuine content of asn, his, tyr, and asp tRNAs increased from 0.25 to 9 months and then decreased	Singhal et al. (356)
Mouse				
Male C57Bl/6J	Brain activity	2–3, 12, 18, and 30	No change in tRNA methylase	Weber et al. (418)
Male BDFI/Crj	Liver, brain	4–30	Increase in the proportion of heat-labile synthetases	Takahashi and Goto (382)
Human				
	Skin fibroblasts	newborn, 20, 30, 40, 50, 60, 78, 80, and 100 yr	Decrease in tRNA methylase activity observed from newborn to 20 yr; no change after 20 yr	Lin and Chang (203)

end of the life span of serially passaged cultures of human fibroblasts. Second, Shepherd et al. (348) reported that *Drosophila* transformed with a P-element vector containing an EF-1α gene under the control of the hsp70 promoter had a longer life span than control flies. Both the mean and maximum survival of the flies were increased approximately 18% at 25°C and 40% at 29.5°C. This is one of only a few studies that have shown that the life span of *Drosophila,* or any animal, can be increased significantly by the overexpression of a gene, and it suggests that EF-1α might play a central role in aging. However, Shikana et al. (349) have found that the *Drosophila* transformed with the EF-1α gene did not show increased expression (either mRNA or protein) of EF-1α. Therefore, it does not appear that the increased life span of the *Drosophila* was due to EF-1α. Third, it has been shown that the human genome contains a family of at least twenty distinct EF-1α-like sequences, many of which are pseudogenes (210). Wang's laboratory (2) has found a high homology (>92%) in the amino acid sequence of the S1 gene in rat and the human EF-1 gene. This is relevant to aging because the S1 gene was identified by screening an expression library from rat brain with a monoclonal antibody specific to statin (3), a protein that is only present in the nuclei of nonproliferating human fibroblasts that accumulate with increasing passage number (411). In other words, statin appears to be associated with the in vitro phenomenon of cellular senescence, where human fibroblasts in culture lose their ability to divide and proliferate. The rat S1 protein, which is antigenically related to statin, appears to be a member of the EF-1α gene family; however, it is immunologically distinct from EF-1α because the sequence homology of the 5′- and 3′-untranslated regions and the introns of the S1 gene have less than 20% homology to the EF-1α gene. EF-1α and S1 also appear to be functionally different because S1 is only expressed in brain, heart, and muscle, while EF-1α is expressed in all tissues surveyed thus far (196). Lee et al. (196) suggested that S1 may be involved in specific control mechanisms of protein synthesis in tissues where cells are locked permanently in a state of nonproliferation, for example, neurons and myocytes.

TABLE 9.16. *Effect of Age on Ribosomes and the Initiation of Protein Synthesis*

Sex/Strain	Tissue	Ages Studied (months unless specified)	Observations	References
Ribosome Aggregation to mRNA				
Nematodes				
Turbatrix aceti	Whole body	5 and 53 days	Proportion of ribosomes in polyribosomes decreased from 63% at 5 days to 35% at 53 days	Wallach and Gershon (410)
Drosophila				
Drosophila melanogaster	Whole body	4–30 days	Decrease in the amount of 80S ribosomes	Baker and Scmidt (9)
Drosophila melanogaster	Whole body	1–48 days	Decrease in the amount of polyribosomes	Webster et al. (424)
Rat				
Female Sprague-Dawley	Liver	1–18	Increase in monomer- dimer sedimenting ribosomal material from 1 to 9 months and then no change to 18 months; decrease in polyribosomes	Layman et al. (195)
Female Wag/Rij	Liver	3–36	Monoribosomes increased 25% between 3 and 12 months, then decreased 27% by 36 months	Claes- Reckinger et al. (58)
Male Sprague-Dawley	Skeletal muscle	2–24	Decrease in the content of large polyribosomes	Pluskal et al. (296)
Male Fischer 344	Brain	3–30	No change in the percentage of polyribosomes or monoribosomes	Cosgrove and Rapoport (67)
Mouse				
Male C57B1/6J	Liver	1–3 and 18–24	50% increase in monoribosomes	Vandenhaute and Delcour (403)
Male C57B1/6J	Liver	10–35	Increase in the number of small polyribosomes and decrease in large polyribosomes	Makrides and Goldthwaite (216)
Biological Activity of Ribosomes				
Rat				
Male Fischer 344	Brain	6–28	Decrease in poly U-directed polypeptide synthesis by monoribosomes	Ekstrom et al. (86)
Mouse				
Male ddY	Muscle	18–19 to 25–30	Decrease in the ability of ribosomes to incorporate labeled amino acids into protein	Britton and Sherman (33)
Male ddY	Liver	2–5 to 15–26	30–40% decrease in the poly U-directed incorporation of radiolabeled phe and leu	Mori et al. (256)
Male C57B1/6J	Liver	3–25	No decrease in poly U-directed polypeptide synthesis by ribosomes	Reis (308)
Male ddY	Liver	2–27	60–70% decrease in ribosomal activity meausured in a cell-free translation system using a globin mRNA template	Nakazawa et al. (206)
Initiation of Protein Synthesis				
Drosophila melanogaster	Whole body	1–48 days	12% decrease in the binding of fmet-tRNA to the 40S subunit and 20% decrease in binding to the 80S subunit	Webster et al. (424)
Rat				
Male DA/Han	Liver, kidney	1–28	Slight decrease in binding of fmet-tRNA to 40S and 80S ribosomes	Gabius et al. (107)
Male ddY	Liver	4–27	14–19% decrease in the activity of 40S ribosomal subunits to form initiation complex	Nakazawa et al. (266)
Mouse				
C57B1/6J (sex unspecified)	Liver	11 and 28	Decreased poly U-stimulated polypeptide synthesis in parallel with a decrease in the number of functionally active ribosomes	Kurtz (187)
Male C57B1/6J	Liver	1–3 to 18–24	The effect of inhibitors of initiation suggests a reduced capacity of ribosomes from older animals to sustain reinitiation	Vandenhaute et al. (403)
Female C57B1/6J	Liver, kidney	3–27	Slight decrease in the formation of 80S initiation complex	Blazejowski and Webster (27)

TABLE 9.17. *Effect of Age of the Elongation Step of Protein Synthesis*

Sex/Species	Tissue	Ages Studied (months unless specified)	Observation	Reference
Nematodes				
Turbotrix aceti	Whole body	5–40 days	Increase in active or partialy active EF-1α molecules detected immunologically; shift from high- to low-molecular-weight species	Bolla and Brot (139)
Drosophila				
Drosophila melanogaster	Whole body	0–21 days	93% decrease in EF-1α synthesis; 61% decrease in the level of EF-1α protein	Webster and Webster (422)
Drosophila melanogaster	Whole body	0–21 days	95% decrease in EF-1α mRNA; no change in EF-2 activity	Webster (419)
Rat				
Male Fischer 344	Liver	4 and 18	60% increase in the ribosomal half-transit in hepatocytes	Coniglio et al. (65)
Sex/strain unspecified	Liver, brain	3 and 30	60–70% decrease in EF-1α activity and no change in EF-2 activity	Moldave et al. (253)
Male DA/Han	Liver	1–28	Decrease in EF-1α-dependent binding of aminoacyl tRNA to ribosomes; no change in EF-2-dependent translocation	Gabius et al. (107)
Male Wistar	Liver	5–22	Increase in percentage of heat-labile EF-2	Takahashi et al. (384)
Female WAG/Rij	Liver	2–33	40% decrease in EF-1α catalytic activity and 50% decrease in the amount of active EF-1α measured by binding of radiolabeled phe-tRNA to ribosomes	Cavallius et al. (48)
Female WAG/Rij	Liver	12–36	10% decrease in the amount of active EF-2	Riis et al. (326)
Male Sprague-Dawley	Liver	4–5 to 28	Polypeptide chain assembly time increased 27%	Merry and Holehan (243)
Male Fischer 344	Liver	3–24	Decrease in the activity and amount of EF-1α; no change in EF-2	Rattan et al. (307)
Mouse				
Female C57B1/6J	Brain, liver, kidney and skeletal muscle	3–27	67–85% decrease in the rate of elongation determined by incorporation of labeled phe into phe-tRNA	Blazekowski and Webster (27)
Male ddY	Liver	5–22	Increase in the percentage of heat-labile EF-2	Takahashi et al. (384)
Male C3H	Liver	2–33	20% decrease in EF-1α catalytic activity and a 25% decrease in the amount of active EF-1α measured by binding of radiolabeled phe-tRNA to ribosomes	Rattan et al. (305)

PROTEIN DEGRADATION

The level of a gene product, that is, a protein/enzyme, is determined by both the rate of synthesis and the rate of degradation of the protein. However, the area of aging and protein degradation has received much less attention than the areas of aging and transcription or translation. Indirect evidence (for example, the observation that protein synthesis decreases with age while the protein content of a cell/tissue remains relatively constant) has been used to support the view that protein degradation decreases with increasing age (316). However, the studies that have measured the rate of protein degradation or protein turnover as a function of age are somewhat contradictory. This is at least in part due to the complexity of protein degradation and the difficulty of accurately measuring protein degradation or turnover. As shown in Figure 9.19, proteins can be degraded by three pathways. Intracellular proteins are degraded by either the cytosolic or the autophagic pathway, and extracellular proteins are degraded by the heterophagic pathway, which appears to involve the lysosomal sys-

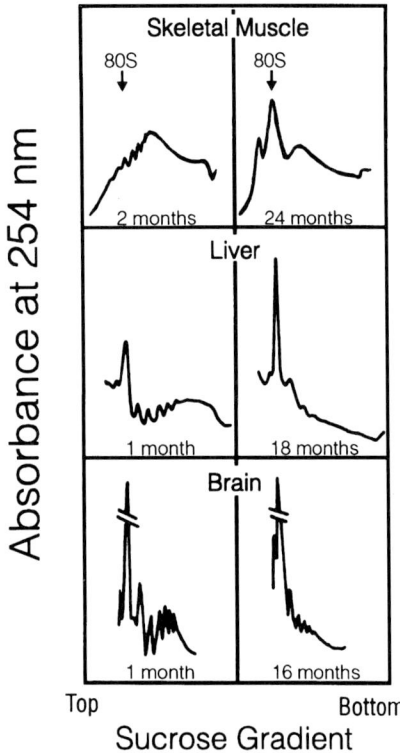

FIG. 9.16. Effect of age on ribosome aggregation to mRNA. The sedimentation of polyribosomes in sucrose gradients is shown for skeletal muscle [data taken from Pluskal et al. (296)], liver [data taken from Layman et al. (194)], and brain [data taken from Fando et al. (89)] of rats.

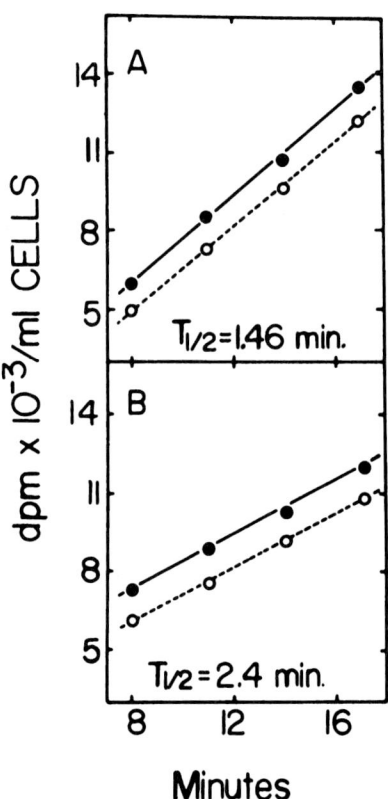

FIG. 9.17. Effect of age on the elongation of protein synthesis in rat liver. The ribosomal half-transit times for hepatocytes isolated from 4-month-old (A) and 18-month-old (B) rats are shown. [Figure taken rom Coniglio et al. (65) with permission.]

tem (135). The process of protein degradation is further complicated by the fact that the rate of degradation is relatively specific for a particular protein and varies considerably from protein to protein (257). The factors responsible for the specificity of protein degradation are still poorly understood.

Intracellular proteins are generally classified as either short-lived ($t_{1/2}$ < 1 h) or long-lived ($t_{1/2}$ > 1 h). The degradation of short-lived proteins is not responsive to physiological regulators (for example, insulin, glucagon, or amino acids) or lysosomal inhibitors (for example, chloroquine or leupeptin). Therefore, it is believed that short-lived proteins are degraded by the extralysosomal, cytoplasmic pathway. In the cytoplasmic pathway, it appears that proteins are degraded primarily by a complex that has been termed the "proteasome" or "multicatalytic proteinase complex." The proteasome consists of 10–20 polypeptide subunits and is involved in both ubiquitin-dependent and ubiquitin-independent protein degradation. The cytosolic pathway is also believed to play a primary role in the degradation of abnormal proteins, which can arise through either mutations/biosynthetic errors or postsynthetic modifications, such as oxidation. Long-lived proteins, which also are referred to as "resident proteins," are degraded primarily by the lysosomal system (the autophagic pathway). Their degradation is responsive to physiological

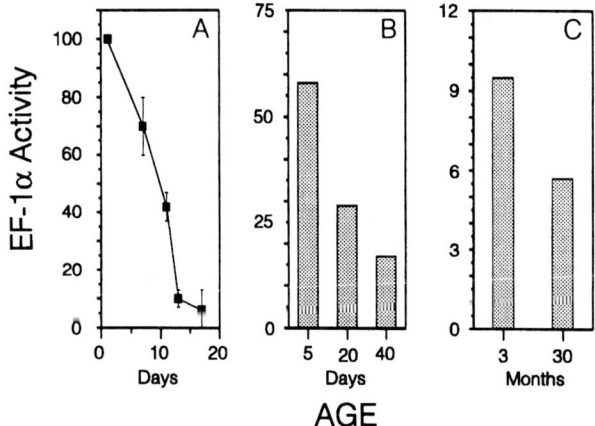

FIG. 9.18. Effect of age on the activity of EF-1α. The activity of EF-1α is shown for *D. melanogaster* [A, data taken from Webster and Webster (422)], nematodes [B, data taken from Bolla and Brot (29)], and rat liver [C, data taken from Moldave et al. (254)].

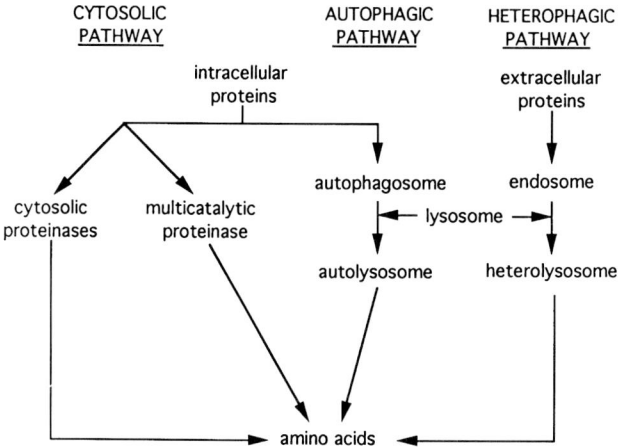

FIG. 9.19. Pathway of protein degradation in mammalian cells.

regulation and is inhibited by lysosomal inhibitors. Although the degradation of intracellular proteins is believed to occur by either the cytosolic or the autophagic pathway (that is, by either the extralysosomal or the lysosomal system) as presented in Figure 9.19, recent studies suggest that both pathways may be involved in the degradation of certain intracellular proteins (79).

Degradation of Mixed Protein Populations

The majority of studies on aging and protein degradation have measured the degradation of mixed protein populations in a tissue or whole organism (see Tables 9.18–9.23). The assay most commonly used to measure protein degradation or turnover in the studies with experimental animals involved following the rate of loss of radioactivity from a mixed population of proteins that were labeled previously with a radioactivity from a mixed population of proteins that were labeled previously with radioactive precursor, for example, an amino acid. However, Goldspink's laboratory (118) calculated protein degradation in rodents from the difference between the growth rate of the rodent or tissue and the fractional synthetic rate, which was measured by the in vivo incorporation of radioactive phenylalanine into protein (118). As Table 9.18 shows, the studies with nematodes and *Drosophila* consistently showed a decline in protein degradation with increasing age, resulting in a longer half-life of the mixed protein population in the old invertebrates. Evidence for a decrease in protein degradation with age also comes from studies on aging in vitro or cellular aging. A decline in protein degradation has been observed in human fibroblasts with increasing passage number (78, 124, 276). However, the data obtained with tissues from rodents vary from tissue to tissue and in some tissues from study to study. As Table 9.19 shows, all of the studies in which turnover or degradation of whole-body protein in rats was measured reported a decrease in protein degradation or an increase in the half-life of protein with age. In contrast, the data on whole-body protein degradation in human subjects are quite contradictory, as shown in Table 9.20. Almost equal numbers of studies have observed a decrease or an increase in protein degradation with age in human subjects. The contradictory data for humans are probably due to the techniques used to measure protein degradation. In the human studies listed in Table 9.19, the degradation of protein was estimated from the urinary excretion of [^{15}N]-urea after [^{15}N]-glycine was given to subjects in their meals to label protein. Therefore, the accuracy of this assay is limited because it is an indirect measure of protein degradation and because it is very difficult to prevent or minimize the reutilization of the [^{15}N]-glycine in human subjects.

Tables 9.21–9.23 list the studies that have measured protein degradation as a function of age in various tissues of rodents. The data from these studies suggest that aging may affect protein degradation differently in different tissues. For example, almost all studies that have measured protein degradation in the skeletal muscle or heart of rodents have observed a significant decrease with age (Table 9.22). However, all of the studies in the lung showed no age-related change in protein degradation (Table 9.23), and the studies in the liver are contradictory (Table 9.21). It is possible that technical differences in the assays used to measure protein degradation in the liver are partially responsible for the contradictory data. For example, different populations of mixed proteins were measured; that is, the degradation of either long- or short-lived proteins can be followed depending on the timing of the measurement of the release of radioactivity from protein. In addition, the inability to minimize the reutilization of the labeled amino acid(s) for protein synthesis would seriously limit the accuracy of comparing protein degradation by tissues from young and old animals if reutilization of amino acids changes with age. One of the most carefully controlled studies to measure the effect of age on protein degradation in liver was conducted by Ward (416). The rates of protein degradation (primarily short-lived proteins) were measured in perfused livers from rats of various ages under conditions where the reutilization of the radioactively labeled amino acid incorporated into the protein was minimal. As shown in Figure 9.20, Ward (416) found that the rate of protein degradation decreased continuously between 6 and 24 months of age. In addition, Ward (415) showed that the age-related decline in protein degradation was strongly correlated to the age-related decrease in protein synthesis observed in perfused liver. Thus the studies by Ward (415, 416) support the view that protein degradation and synthesis decrease in parallel with increasing age,

TABLE 9.18. *Age-Related Changes in Protein Degradation in Invertebrates*

Organism	Ages Studied (days)	Tissue	Observations	References
Nematodes				
Turbatrix aceti	7–35	Whole body	$t_{1/2}$ of total soluble proteins increased 400%	Resnick and Gershon (310)
Turbatrix aceti	2–20	Whole body	$t_{1/2}$ increased from 25 to 269 h	Prasanna and Lane (298)
Turbatrix aceti	5 and 22–30	Whole body	$t_{1/2}$ increased from 73 to 163 h	Sharma et al. (346)
Turbatrix aceti	7–9 and 24–26	Whole body	$t_{1/2}$ increased from 67.5 t 170 h	Karey and Rothstein (168)
Insects				
Drosophila melanogaster	4 and 32	Thorax	[^{3}H]-leucine-specific activity slightly lower in old, suggesting increased turnover	Wattiaux et al. (418)
Drosophila melanogaster	6–45	Thorax	Decreased relative turnover rate with age	Dubitsky et al. (83)
Drosophila melanogaster	7–10 and 49	Thorax	55% decrease in protein radioactivity after 30 h in young, no change in old	Niedzwiecki and Fleming (270)

TABLE 9.19. *Effect of Age on Whole Body Protein Degradation in Rodents*

Sex/Strain	Ages Studied (months)	Observations	References
Rat			
Male Holtzman	1–20	Protein turnover rate was decreased	Yousef and Johnson (441)
Hooded (sex unspecified)	0.8–23.3	Protein degradation decreased from 22.5%/day to 2.9%/day	Millward (249)
Sprague-Dawley (CFY) (sex unspecified)	0.8–10.7	Protein degradation decreased from 9.8%/day to 4.5%/day	Millward (249)
Male Sprague-Dawley (CFY)	0.7–24	Protein degradation decreased from 25.5%/day to 10.9%/day	Lewis et al. (198)
Male CD	1–26	Protein degradation decreased from 23.3%/day to 10.9%/day	Goldspink and Kelly (118)
Male Sprague-Dawley	1–10	Protein degradation decreased from 19.7%/day to 7.8%/day	Obled and Arnal (272)
Mouse			
Male Swiss	10 and 25	$t_{1/2}$ increased from 144.5 to 193.9 f	Sobel and Bowman (362)

TABLE 9.20. *Changes in Whole Body Protein Degradation in Aging Humans*

Sex	Ages Studied (yr)	Observations	References
Unspecified	24 and 59–70	50% decrease in the rate of release of [^{15}N] from protein	Sharp et al. (347)
Male/Female	20–23 and 69–91	37% decrease with age*	Young et al. (440)
Male	20–25 and 65–72	No change*	Winterer et al. (435)
Female	18–23 and 67–91	17% decrease with age*	Winterer et al. (435)
Male	20–25 and 65–72	41% increase with age†	Winterer et al. (435)
Female	18–23 and 67–91	61% increase with age†	Winterer et al. (435)
Male	20–25 and 68–72	10% decrease with age*	Uuay et al. (399)
Female	18–23 and 67–91	18% decrease with age*	Uuay et al. (399)
Male	20–25 and 68–72	42% increase with age†	Uuay et al. (399)
Female	18–23 and 67–91	61% increase with age†	Uuay et al. (399)

*Rate expressed per kg body weight.
†Rate expressed per g urinary creatinine excretion.

TABLE 9.21. *Effect of Age on Mixed Protein Degradation in the Liver of Rodents*

Sex/Strain	Ages Studied (months)	Observations	References
Rat			
Male Sprague-Dawley	12 and 24	No change	Barrows and Roeder (11)
Female Fischer 344	1–1.4 and 17	No change in $t^{1/2}$ of total protein	Ove et al. (271)
Male Wistar	4–6 to 18–27	20% decrease in the ability of lysosomal enzyme mixture to degrade liver cytosolic proteins	Wiederanders et al. (432)
Female Wistar	12 and 29	$t^{1/2}$ of total liver homogenate protein increased from 2.15 to 2.45	Weideranders and Oelke (431)
Female Wistar	4–5 to 27	$t^{1/2}$ of cytosolic proteins increased 50%	Weideranders and Oelke (430)
Male CD	1–26	No change	Goldspink and Kelly (118)
Male Fischer 344	3–24	50% decrease between 6 and 24 months of age	Ward (416)
Mouse			
Female C57B1/6J	4–28	500% increase in $t^{1/2}$ of puromycinyl peptides	Lavie et al. (192)
Male C57B1/6J	12 to 32–34	No change	Barrows and Kokkonen (10)

TABLE 9.22. *Effect of Age on Mixed Protein Degradation in Heart and Skeletal Muscle of Rats*

Sex/Strain	Ages Studied (months)	Observations	References
Heart			
Female Sprague-Dawley	12 and 24	No change	Barrows and Roeder (11)
Wistar (sex unspecified)	5–25	Increase in *in vitro* autocatalytic degradation	Mohan and Radha (252)
Male albino	3–24	$t_{1/2}$ of total protein increased from 12 to 16 days	Meerson et al. (240)
Sex/strain (unspecified)	1–2 and 10–14	Degradation rate decreased 27%	Wildethal and Crie (432)
Male albino (outbred)	1.25 to 10–14	Phenylalanine release decreased 27%	Crie et al. (70)
Male Sprague-Dawley (CFY)	1.5 and 12	Decreased from 14.6%/day to 10.8%/day	Crie et al. (70)
Male hooded	12 and 24	Decreased from 12.4%/day to 6.7%/day	Crie et al. (70)
Male albino	0.8–26.3	Decreased from 15%/day to 5.8%/day	Lewis et al. (199)
Male Sprague-Dawley (CFY)	0.8–25.8	Decreased from 17%/day to 6%/day	Goldspink et al. (122)
Male Lewis	1.2–24	No change	Mays et al. (229)
Skeletal Muscle			
Female Sprague-Dawley	12 and 24	No change	Barrows and Roeder (11)
Hooded (sex unspecified)	0.8–23.3	Decreased from 22.5%/day to 2.9%/day	Millward (249)
Wistar (sex unspecified)	5–25	Increase of 68.8% in red muscle and 53.7% in white muscle	Mohan and Radha (252)
Male CD	0.7–24.5	Decreased from 7.4%/day to 3.2%/day in diaphragm	Kelly et al. (169)
Male Sprague-Dawley (CFY)	0.8–25.7	Decreased from 17.6%/day to 4.5%/day in diaphragm	Goldspink et al. (123)
Male CD	0.7–24.5	Decreased from 9.3%/day to 4.4%/day extensor digitorum longus	Kelly et al. (169)
Male Sprague-Dawley (CFY)	0.8–25.7	Decreased from 7.9%/day to 2.8%/day extensor digitorum longus	Goldspink et al. (107)
Male CD	0.7–24.5	Decreased from 11.0%/day to 5.6%/day gastrocnemius	Kelly et al. (169)
Male CD	0–26.3	Decreased from 11.6%/day to 5.1%/day soleus	Lewis et al. (199)
Male/CD	0.7–24.5	Decreased from 11.4%/day to 5.0%/day soleus	Kelly et al. (169)
Male Sprague-Dawley (CFY)	0.8–25.8	Decreased from 22.2%/day to 5.1%/day soleus	el Haj et al. (87)
Male CD	0.8–26.3	Decreased from 7.3%/day to 1.8%/day tibialis anterior	Lewis et al. (199)
Male Sprague-Dawley (CFY)	0.8–25.8	Decreased from 6.7%/day to 2.7%/day tibialis anterior	el Haj et al. (87)

TABLE 9.23. *Effect of Age on Mixed Protein Degradation in Brain, Kidney, and Lung of Rats*

Sex/Strain	Ages Studied (months)	Observations	References
Brain			
Male Wistar	12 and 24	Protein degradation decreased from 36.4%/day to 4.1%/day	Goldspink (117)
Male Wistar	12 and 24	$t_{1/2}$ of mitochondrial bulk protein decreased from 26.8 to 23.5 days	Menzies and Gold (241)
Kidney			
Female Sprague-Dawley	12 and 24	No change	Barrows and Roeder (11)
Fischer 344 (sex unspecified)	3 and 24	Increased rate of degradation of labile proteins with age, no change with stable protein	Roberts and Griminger (327)
Male CD	0.8–24	Protein degradation decreased from 41.8%/day to 23.3%/day	Goldspink and Kelly (118)
Lung			
Male CD	0.8–26.3	No change	Goldspink (116)
Male Sprague-Dawley (CFY)	0.8–25.8	No change	Goldspink and Merry (119)
Male Lewis	1–24	No change	Mays et al. (229)

which would result in a reduced rate of protein turnover in the liver of senescent animals.

Degradation of Individual Proteins

The information gained from measuring the degradation or turnover of mixed protein populations is limited because one gets only an average value for the rate of thousands of proteins, which have quite different half-lives. Significant changes could occur with age in the degradation of specific proteins, and these changes could be masked when protein degradation is measured in a mixed protein population. Table 9.24 gives a list of the studies that have measured the effect of age on the degradation of specific proteins using a variety of techniques as described by Ward and Richardson (414). The

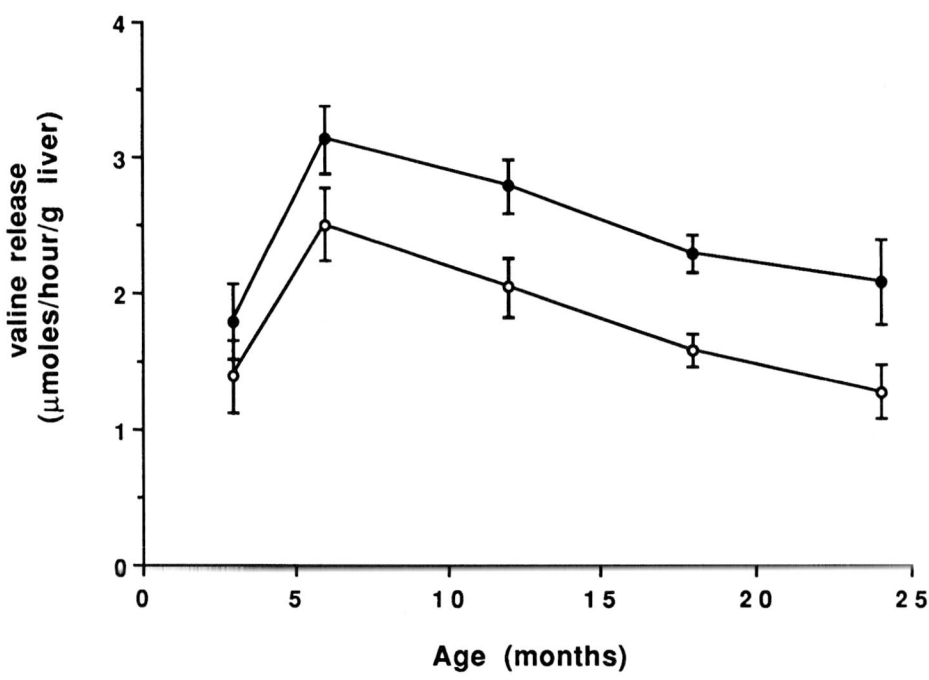

FIG. 9.20. Effect of age on protein degradation in rat liver. The rate of protein degradation by perfused liver from rats fed ad libitum (○) or a calorie-restricted diet (●) is shown as a function of age [data taken from Ward (416) with permission].

TABLE 9.24. *Effect of Age on the Degradation of Individual Proteins*

Sex/Strain	Ages Studied (months unless specified)	Protein/Organ	Observations	References
Nematode				
Turbatrix aceti	7–60 days	Aldolase	$t_{1/2}$ increased from 40 to 120 h	Zeelon et al. (442)
Turbatrix aceti	7 and 22–30 days	Enolase	$t_{1/2}$ increased from 58 to 161 h	Sharma et al. (346)
Rat				
Liver				
Male AXC	3–4 and 24–26	S-adenosylmethionine decarboxylase	No change	Shain and Moss (345)
Female Fischer 344	1.5–30	Catalase	k_d increased from 0.009 h^{-1} to 0.029 h^{-1} at 24 months decreasing to 0.019 h^{-1} at 30 months	Haining and Legan (130)
Sex/strain unspecified	3 and 18	Citrate cleavage	No change	Richter (324)
Female Sprague-Dawley	12 and 22–24	Cytochrome c	No change	Fletcher and Sanadi (97)
Female Fischer 344	1–1.4 to 17	Ferritin	$t_{1/2}$ increased from 1.9 to 4.0 days	Ove et al. (283)
Female Fischer 344	1–1.5 to 17–20	Ferritin	No change	Obenrader et al. (271)
Sex/strain unspecified	3 and 18	Glucose-6-phosphate dehydrogenase	No change	Richter et al. (324)
Sex/strain unspecified	3 and 18	α-glycerol phosphate dehydrogenase	No change	Richter et al. (324)
Male Wistar	1–26	Lysosomes	$^3H/^{14}C$ ratio decreased 21%	Comolli et al. (64)
Sex/strain unspecified	3 and 18	Malic enzyme	$t_{1/2}$ decreased from 43 to 25 h	Richter et al. (324)
Male Wistar	1–26	Microsomes	$^3H/^{14}C$ ratio decreased 24%	Comolli et al. (64)
Male Wistar	1–26	Mitochondria	No change	Comolli et al. (64)
Male Wistar	12 and 24	Mitochondria	No change for liver, brain, testes, small intestine, lung, and kidney	Menzies and Gold (241)
Female Sprague-Dawley	12 and 22–24	Mitochondria	No change in either soluble or insoluble protein	Fletcher and Sanadi (97)
Male AXC	3–4 and 24–26	Ornithine decarboxylase	No change	Shain and Moss (345)
Male Fischer 344	1–24	Tryptophane pyrolase	k^d decreased from 0.714 h^{-1} to 0.322 h^{-1}	Haining and Correll (129)
Male Fischer 344	1.5–24	Xanthine oxidase	$t^{1/2}$ decreased from 44 to 39 h	Haining and Legan (130)
Kidney				
Male Fischer 344	1.5–30	Catalase	No change	Haining and Legan (130)
Mouse				
Liver				
Female C57B1/6J	3–4 and 24	Aldolase	$t^{1/2}$ increased from 25.6 to 37 h	Reznick et al. (312)
Male C57B1/6J	3–4 and 24	Asialofetuin	No change	Burrows and Davison (38)
Male BDF1	3–8 and 28–30	Horseradish peroxidase	$t^{1/2}$ increased from 50 to 75 h	Ishigami and Goto (158)
Female C57B1/6J	3–4 and 24	Ornithine decarboxylase	$t^{1/2}$ increased from 15 to 30 min	Jacobus and Gershon (161)
Male BDF1	3.5–6.5 and 24.5–30.5	Ovalbumin	$t^{1/2}$ increased from 106 to 164 h	Ishigami and Goto (159)

half-lives of aldolase (310, 442) and enolase (346) are increased two- to sixfold with age in nematodes, and Sharma et al. (346) showed that the increase in the half-life of enolase paralleled the age-related decrease in the degradation of the mixed protein population. Table 9.24 also shows that the effect of age on the degradation of individual proteins varies greatly from protein to protein. However, it is clear that the degradation/turnover of some proteins decreases with increasing age. For example, in rodent liver, the half-lives of ferritin (283), ornithine decarboxylase (161), and aldolase (311) were 40–100% longer in the liver of old rodents than in the liver of young rodents. The study by Burrows and Davison (38) is of interest because they measured the degradation of a protein, asialofetuin, that is degraded by the heterophagic pathway. No age-related change in the degradation of asialofetuin by cultured hepatocytes isolated from young and old mice was observed, which suggests that aging has very little effect on the heterophagic pathway of protein degradation in hepatocytes. Gurley and Dice (128) also found that the rate of degradation of endocytosed proteins was similar in early- and late-passage human fibroblasts.

More recently, investigators have taken a unique approach by measuring the degradation of proteins microinjected into cells to study the effect of aging on protein degradation. In 1982, Dice (78) showed that the degradation of a variety of proteins (for example, RNase A, aldolase, and lysozyme) microinjected into human fibroblasts decreased with in vitro aging; the half-lives of these proteins were 40–200% lower in late-passage compared to early-passage fibroblasts. Ishigami and Goto (158, 159) measured the degradation of horseradish peroxidase and ovalbumin that were microinjected into cultured hepatocytes isolated from young and old mice. The degradation of both proteins was approximately 50% lower in hepatocytes isolated from old compared to young mice. Because both proteins were localized in the cytoplasmic fraction of the hepatocytes, it appears that the changes in protein degradation observed in these studies occurred in the cytoplasmic pathway of protein degradation. Thus the data from the studies that have measured the degradation of individual proteins support the view that protein degradation decreases with age, leading to a slower rate of protein turnover. However, the current data, which are limited, also suggest that the effect of age on protein degradation varies considerably from protein to protein and that aging might affect the three pathways of protein degradation differently.

Degradation of Abnormal Proteins

One of the characteristics of aging at the biochemical level is the accumulation of "abnormal" or "altered" proteins. The presence of abnormal proteins was demonstrated by immunotitration studies, which showed that the catalytic activity of several enzymes per unit of protein antigen decreased with age (333). Initially, it was believed that the appearance of abnormal proteins in tissues from senescent animals was due to an age-related decrease in the fidelity of translation and/or transcription as predicted by the error catastrophe hypothesis proposed by Orgel (282). However, it is now well established that the appearance of abnormal proteins in senescent animals is not due to errors in gene expression but arises posttranslationally by a variety of mechanisms, for example, oxidation of amino acid side chains, spontaneous deamidation of asparagine and glutamine residues, glycation of lysine residues, oxidation of sulfhydryl groups, racemization of aspartic acid residues, and spontaneous changes in protein conformation (372–374). Figure 9.21 shows examples of the age-related accumulation of one type of covalent modification to proteins, the accumulation of oxidized protein as determined by the presence of carbonyl groups in soluble protein.

The accumulation of abnormal proteins could arise from an age-related increase in the rate of formation of the abnormal proteins or to a decrease in the rate of degradation of the abnormal proteins, or both. In 1979, Rothstein (332) proposed that abnormal proteins appeared in tissues of senescent animals because of an age-related decrease in protein turnover, which increased the "dwell time" of the protein in a cell as well as the probability that the protein would become posttranslationally altered. Subsequently, Reznick et al. (311) estimated that the age-related decline in the turnover of aldolase in liver accounted for 40% of the inactive aldolase molecules found in the livers of senescent mice. The only study to compare the abilities of tissues from young and old animals to degrade abnormal proteins was conducted by Lavie et al. (192). They injected mice with puromycin, which becomes incorporated into the growing peptide chain and terminates the elongation of protein synthesis. The puromycinyl peptides are recognized by the cell as abnormal or aberrant proteins and are rapidly degraded (135). As shown in Figure 9.22, Lavie et al. (192) found that the half-life of the puromycinyl peptides in liver increased from 30 min in 6-month-old mice to 150 min in 24-month-old mice. Two other studies indicate that the degradation of altered proteins is slower in senescent cells. Using either puromycin or a lysine analog (aminoethyl-L-cysteine), McKay et al. (235) measured the degradation of altered proteins by rabbit reticulocytes separated into ten cell-age groups. They showed that the degradation of the puromycinyl peptides or the analog-containing proteins decreased with the age of the reticulocytes. Dice (78) measured the degradation of altered proteins microinjected into early- and late-passage human fibroblasts. He found that the rate of degradation of proteolytically cleaved RNase A (for example, RNase S and RNase B) by late-passage human fibroblasts was less than 50% of the rate of degradation by early-passage fibroblasts.

The study by Lavie et al. (194) suggests that the cytosolic pathway of protein degradation is significantly reduced in the liver with increasing age because this pathway is responsible for the degradation of aberrant or abnormal proteins (135). The studies by Ward (416) and Ishigami and Goto (158, 159) also support the view that aging alters the cytosolic pathway of protein deg-

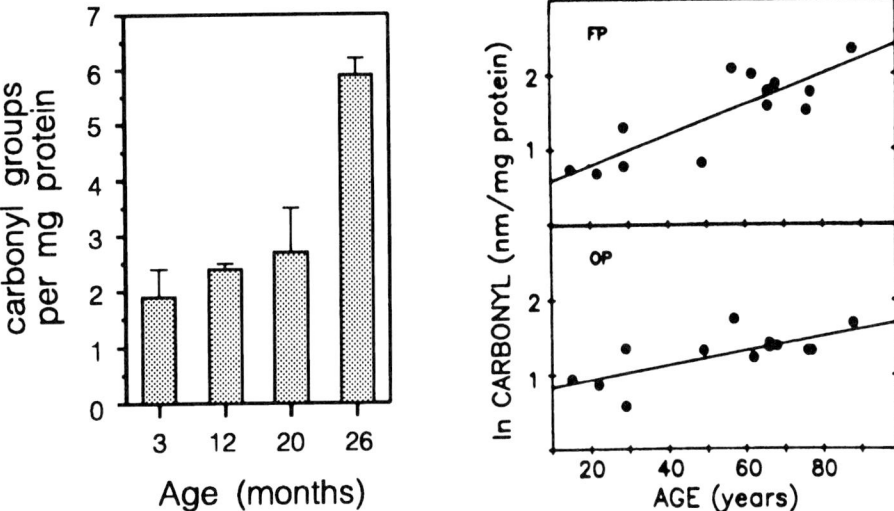

FIG. 9.21. Effect of age on the accumulation of oxidized proteins in rat liver. *Left*: levels of carbonyl groups in soluble proteins in the livers of rats of various ages is shown [data taken from Starke-Reed and Oliver (375)]. *Right*: levels of carbonyl groups in the frontal pole (*FP*) and occipital pole (*OP*) of brain obtained from 16 patients at autopsy [data taken from Smith et al. (361) with permission].

radation in the liver; for example, the degradation of short-lived proteins was reduced with increasing age in perfused liver, and cultured hepatocytes isolated from old mice showed a reduced rate of degradation of microinjected proteins that localized in the cytosol. Thus the data are consistent with the view that abnormal proteins accumulate with age because of a reduction in the cytosolic pathway of protein degradation. Two studies have correlated the age-related accumulation of abnormal proteins to a decline in protein degradation. As shown in Figure 9.23, Starke-Reed and Oliver (375) found that the age-related increase in the level of oxidized protein in hepatocytes was correlated to a decrease in the activity of alkaline protease, which is presumed to be a measure of the activity of the proteasome (or multicatalytic proteinase complex). Carney et al. (43) showed that the age-related increase in oxidized proteins in the brain of gerbils, as measured by an

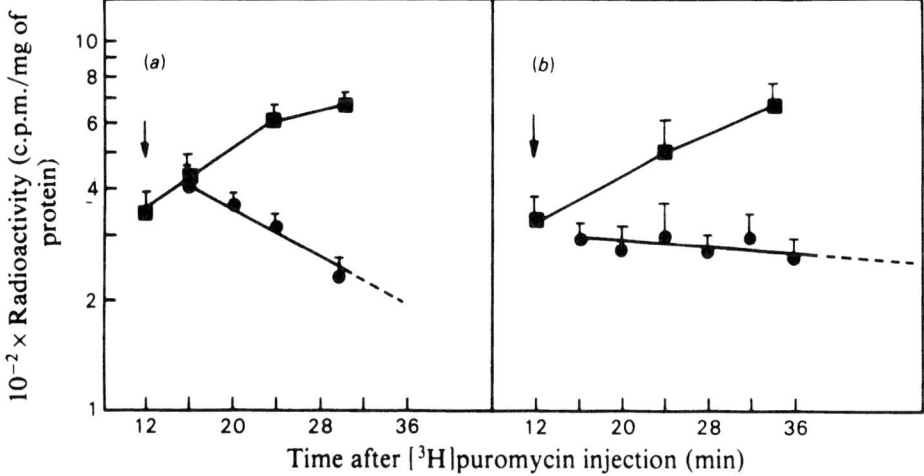

FIG. 9.22. Effect of age on the degradation of abnormal peptides by rat liver. After rats received an injection of [^{3}H]-puromycin, they were given unlabeled puromycin (●) or saline (■). The radioactivity in puromycinyl peptides in the liver of 6-month-old (*a*) and 24–25-month-old (*b*) rats is shown. [Figure taken from Lavie et al. (192) with permission.]

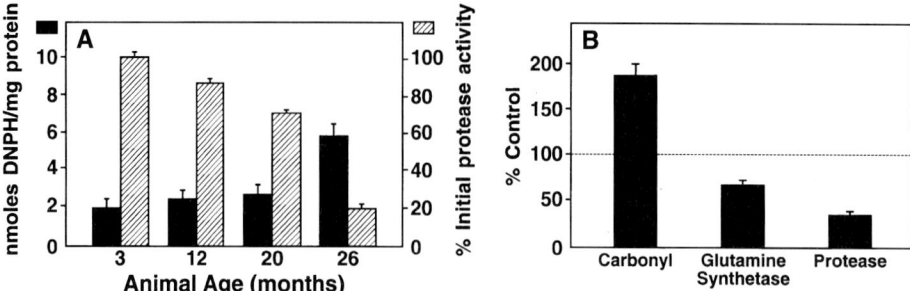

FIG. 9.23. Effect of age on the degradation of oxidized proteins. *A*: comparison of levels of carbonyl groups in soluble protein in livers of rats of various ages to activity of alkaline protease activity [taken from Starke-Reed and Oliver (375) with permission]. *B*: carbonyl content of protein, glutamine synthetase activity, and alkaline protease activity of brains from old (15–18 months) gerbils compared to brains of young (3 months) gerbils as 100% [data taken from Carney et al. (43) with permission].

increase in protein carbonyl groups or a decrease in glutamine synthetase activity, was correlated to a decrease in the activity of alkaline protease (Fig. 9.23).

Effect of Dietary Restriction on Protein Degradation

In 1985, Birchenall-Sparks et al. (23) proposed that dietary restriction enhanced protein degradation, based on their studies on protein synthesis in rat hepatocytes. Since 1985, several studies have compared protein degradation in various tissues of rodents fed either ad libitum or a calorie-restricted diet (Table 9.25). These data show that dietary restriction significantly increases the rate of protein degradation or protein turnover in the whole body of rodents as well as in liver, heart, diaphragm, and muscle. An example of the effect of dietary restriction on protein degradation is shown in Figure 9.20. Dietary restriction increased protein degradation 20–30% in perfused rat liver at 6, 12, 18, and 24 months of age. A study by Goto's laboratory suggests that dietary restriction alters protein degradation within a relatively short time after its implementation. Measuring the degradation of proteins (horseradish peroxidase and ovalbumin) microinjected into cultured hepatocytes, Ishigami and Goto (160) showed that the degradation of these proteins was increased significantly after only 70 days of caloric restriction. This observation is consistent with the report by Ward (416) shown in Figure 9.20, who found that protein degradation by perfused liver was significantly altered between 42 and 126 days after the initiation of caloric restriction. Thus the data indicate that dietary restriction enhances both the synthesis and the degradation of proteins, leading to an increase in the protein turnover. It is unclear what physiological impact increased protein turnover would have on the calorie-restricted rodents; however, one could predict that increased protein turnover would reduce the levels of abnormal proteins in tissues of rodents fed a calorie-restricted diet. Unfortunately, there is no information on how dietary restriction affects the age-related appearance of abnormal proteins.

SUMMARY AND CONCLUSIONS

As this review shows, there is a great deal of information on how gene expression and protein degradation are altered with increasing age in a variety of animal models. The majority of the research indicates that both total RNA synthesis and total protein synthesis decline with age in most tissues. The decrease in transcription and translation, however, does not appear to lead to a significant decrease in the RNA or protein content of a cell; therefore, it has been assumed that the degradation of RNA and protein also decline with age, resulting in a slower turnover (317, 414), and, in general, the studies on protein degradation support this view. The few studies on the degradation of mRNA also support the view that the degradation of RNA is reduced significantly with age; however, more research is needed in this area before this conclusion can be stated with any confidence. Thus the data suggest that a general decline in the synthesis and degradation of RNA and protein occurs with age and that this leads to a slower turnover of these macromolecules in the cells of senescent animals.

What are the physiological consequences of the age-related decrease in the turnover of protein and RNA? Richardson and Cheung (316) suggested that the slower rate of protein turnover might be physiologically important to an organism in two ways. First, the slower turnover of proteins might be a major factor in the age-related accumulation of abnormal proteins. The increased "dwell time" of proteins in a cell would lead to an increase in the probability that the protein would

TABLE 9.25. *Effect of Dietary Restriction on Protein Degradation*

Sex/Strain	Ages Compared (months)	Changes with Dietary Restriction	References
Rat			
Heart			
Male Sprague-Dawley (CFY)	2–25	22%–63% increase	Goldspink et al. (122)
Liver			
Male Fischer 344	3 and 6–24	No change 25% increase	Ward (416)
Lung			
Male Sprague-Dawley (CFY)	2 and 25 12	12%–42% decrease No change	Goldspink and Merry (119)
Skeletal Muscle			
Anterior tibialis			
Male Sprague-Dawley (CFY)	12 2 and 25	No change 41%–65% decrease	el Haj et al. (87)
Extensor digitorum longus			
Male Sprague-Dawley (CFY)	2 and 25 12	40%–50% decrease 37% increase	Goldspink et al. (119)
Diaphragm			
Male Sprague-Dawley (CFY)	2 and 12 25	13%–72% decrease 44%	Goldspink et al. (119)
Soleus			
Male Sprague-Dawley (CFY)	2–25	25%–46% decrease	el Haj et al (87)
Whole Body			
Male Sprague-Dawley (CFY)	24 1.5 and 12	No change 10%–59% increase	Lewis et al. (198)
Mouse			
Cultured hepatocytes			
Male BDI	23–25.3	$t_{1/2}$ for horseradish peroxidase and ovalbumin microinjected into cells decreased 40% after 70 days of dietary restriction	Ishigami and Goto (160)

become posttranslationally altered. This possibility is supported by several studies. For example, it has been estimated that a significant fraction of the altered aldolase molecules found in the livers of senescent mice arise from the decline in the turnover of aldolase (311). In addition, studies have shown a good correlation between the age-related decline in the proteolytic system involved in the accumulation and the degradation of abnormal (for example, oxidized) proteins (43, 375). Richardson and Cheung (316) also proposed that the decrease in protein turnover might reduce the ability of a cell/tissue to respond to intracellular or extracellular signals because it has been shown that the induction of proteins with short half-lives is much more rapid than the induction of proteins with long half-lives. Thus the age-related decrease in protein turnover could be predicted to lead to a decline in the ability of a cell/tissue to respond to signals that require the induction of gene expression. Although this hypothesis is quite appealing, there is currently no evidence that the decreased ability of senescent organisms to respond to stimuli or stresses arises from a decrease in the turnover of either protein or mRNA.

Our knowledge of aging has grown most rapidly in the area of changes in the expression of specific mRNA transcripts in tissues of animals. There have been several publications in which the level of one or more mRNA transcripts has been measured in a tissue as a function of age. Even though studies on total RNA synthesis indicate that the transcriptional activity of tissues declines with age, the effect of age on mRNA levels varies from mRNA transcript to mRNA transcript. While the levels of many mRNA transcripts decline with age, some do not change significantly, and in some cases, the level has been reported to increase with age. It appears that the age-related changes in the levels of most mRNA transcripts arise from changes in the transcription of the gene. However, the mechanism responsible for the age-related changes in the transcription of the genes is unknown. It appears clear that the changes in the transcription of mRNA transcripts are not due to a change in RNA polymerase II activity. Attention has been focused on studying regulatory mechanisms that would alter the expression of genes differentially. Because methylation of DNA has been proposed to play a role in the regulation of gene expression at the level of transcription, a number of investigators have studied the effect of aging on DNA methylation. Although most of the research indicates that the genomes of cells/tissues become more methylated with age, there is no evidence that age-related changes in the methylation of a specific gene are responsible for the age-related change in its transcription. Attention has also been focused on transcription factors that bind to specific DNA sequences and alter the transcription of genes. It seems highly probable that age-related changes in the levels/activities of transcription factors will be critical factors in altering the transcription of specific genes with age. Age-related changes in the nucleosome structure of chromatin also might influence the association of transcription factors to specific DNA sequences on genes. The only evidence for a transcription factor playing a role in the age-related change in the transcription of a gene has come from studies on the heat shock gene hsp70 (138).

One very interesting observation in this area is the effect of dietary restriction on gene expression and protein degradation. Dietary restriction is the only experimental manipulation known to retard aging and increase the life span of mammals. A variety of studies have shown that dietary restriction significantly increases the rate of protein synthesis in different rodent tissues. In addition, dietary restriction has been shown to enhance protein degradation. Thus the turnover of proteins in tissues of animals fed a calorie-restricted diet is significantly higher than in animals fed ad libitum. Dietary restriction has also been shown to alter the age-related changes in the expression of a variety of mRNA transcripts, and these alterations appear to occur at the level of transcription. It has been proposed that dietary restriction triggers the changes in gene transcription by altering the levels/activities of transcription factors through a change in the hormonal status of the animal (137).

In summary, the data clearly demonstrate that aging alters gene expression and protein degradation in animals. However, it is not known if the changes in gene expression and/or protein degradation play a causal role in aging and senescence or if the changes are simply secondary to the aging process. The data obtained with dietary restriction suggest that changes in gene expression might play a fundamental role in the aging process. For example, dietary restriction reverses the age-related decrease in protein turnover and the age-related decline in the expression of several genes that play important protective roles, for example, genes coding for antioxidant enzymes and heat shock proteins. These changes would be expected to be beneficial to an organism and lead to increased longevity. Thus it seems reasonable to hypothesize that some of the changes in gene expression and protein degradation that occur with age are important components in the biological mechanism underlying the aging process.

This work was supported in part by grants AG01548 and AG01188 from the National Institute on Aging and by the Office of Research and Development, Department of Veterans Affairs.

REFERENCES

1. AMMENDOLA, R., M. MESURACA, T. RUSSO, and F. CIMINO. Sp1 DNA binding efficiency is highly reduced in nuclear extracts from aged rat tissues. *J. Biol. Chem.* 267: 17944–17948, 1992.
2. ANN, D. K., H. H. LIN, S. LEE, Z. TU, and E. WANG. Characterization of the statin-like S1 and rat elongation factor 1 α as two distinctly expressed messages in rat. *J. Biol. Chem.* 267: 699–702, 1992.
3. ANN, D. K., I. K. MOUTSATSOS, T. NAKAMURA, H. H. LIN, P. MAO, M. LEE, S. CHIN, R. K. LIEM, and E. WANG. Isolation and characterization of the rat chromosomal gene for a polypeptide (pS1) antigenically related to statin. *J. Biol. Chem.* 266: 10429–10437, 1991.
4. ARMBRECHT, H. J., M. BOLTZ, R. STRONG, A. RICHARDSON, M. E. H. BURNS, and S. CHRISTAKOS. Expression of calbindin-D decreases with age in intestine and kidney. *Endocrinology* 125: 2950–2956, 1989.
5. AVOLA, R., D. F. CONDORELLI, N. RAGUSA, M. RENIS, M. ALBERGHINA, A. M. GIUFFRIDA STELLA, and A. LAJTHA. Protein synthesis rates in rat brain regions and subcellular fractions during aging. *Neurochem. Res.* 13: 337–342, 1988.
6. AZELIS, A. E., K. M. MCMULLEN, and G. C. WEBSTER. Progressive reduction in protein synthesis during involution and aging of the mouse thymus. *Mech. Ageing Dev.* 20: 361–368, 1982.
7. BACCI, B., L. PETRELLI, R. DAL TOSO, and M. G. NUNZI. Age-associated alteration in the expression of synapsin I mRNA in the rat central nervous system. *Ann. N.Y. Acad. Sci.* 663: 463–465, 1992.
8. BAILEY, P. J., and G. C. WEBSTER. Lowered rates of protein synthesis by mitochondria isolated from organisms of increasing age. *Mech. Ageing Dev.* 24: 233–241, 1984.
9. BAKER, G. T., and T. SCHMIDT. Changes in 80S ribosomes from *Drosophila melanogaster* with age. *Experientia* 32: 1505–1506, 1976.
10. BARROWS, C. H., and G. C. KOKKONEN. The effect of age and diet on the cellular protein synthesis of liver of male mice. *Age* 10: 54–57, 1987.
11. BARROWS, C. H., and L. M. ROEDER. Effect of age on protein synthesis in rats. *J. Gerontol.* 16: 321–325, 1961.
12. BAUM, B. J., B. L. KUYATT, and S. HUMPHREYS. Protein production and processing in young adult and aged rat submandibular gland cells in vitro. *Mech. Ageing Dev.* 23: 123–136, 1983.
13. BAUMANN, P., and P. S. CHEN. Alterung and proteinsynthese bei *Drosophila melanogaster*. *Rev. Suisse Zool.* 69: 1051–1055, 1969.
14. BEAUCHENE, R. E., L. M. ROEDER, and C. H. BARROWS. The effect of age and ethionine feeding on RNA and protein synthesis of rats. *J. Gerontol.* 22: 318–324, 1967.
15. BEAUCHENE, R. E., L. M. ROEDER, and C. H. BARROWS, JR. The

interrlelationships of age, tissue protein synthesis, and proteinuria. *J. Gerontol.* 25: 359–363, 1970.

16. BENSON, R. W., and C. W. HARKER. RNA polymerase activities in liver and brain tissue of aging mice. *J. Gerontol.* 33: 323–328, 1978.

17. BERKOWITZ, E. M., A. C. SANBORN, and D. W. VAUGHAN. Chromatin structure in neuronal and neuroglial cell nuclei as a function of age. *J. Neurochem.* 41: 516–523, 1983.

18. BERND, A., E. BATKE, P. K. ZAHN, and W. E. MULLER. Age-dependent gene induction in quail oviduct. XV. Alterations of the poly (A)-associated protein pattern and of the poly(A) chain length of mRNA. *Mech. Ageing Dev.* 19: 361–377, 1982.

19. BESSE, S., P. ASSAYAG, C. DELCAYRE, F. CARRE., S.-L. CHEAV, Y. LECARPENTIER, and B. SWYNGHEDAUW. Normal and hypertrophied senescent rat heart: mechanical and molecular characteristics. *Am. J. Physiol.* 265 (*Heart Circ. Physiol.* 36): H183–H190, 1993.

20. BIGGS, R. B., and F. W. BOOTH. Protein synthesis rate is not suppressed in rat heart during senescence. *Am. J. Physiol.* 258 (*Heart Circ. Physiol.* 29): H207–H211, 1990.

21. BIGGS, R. B., R. M. HANLEY, P. R. MORRISON, and F. W. BOOTH. Cytochrome *c* mRNA levels decrease in senescent rat heart. *Mech. Ageing Dev.* 60: 285–293, 1991.

22. BIRCHENALL-SPARKS, M. C., M. S. ROBERTS, M. S. RUTHERFORD, and A. RICHARDSON. The effect of aging on the structure and function of liver messenger RNA. *Mech. Ageing Dev.* 32: 99–111, 1985.

23. BIRCHENALL-SPARKS, M. C., M. S. ROBERTS, J. STAECKER, J. P. HARDWICK, and A. RICHARDSON. Effect of dietary restriction on liver protein synthesis in rats. *J. Nutr.* 115: 944–950, 1985.

24. BLAKE, M. J., J. FARGNOLI, D. GERSHON, and N. J. HOLBROOK. Concomitant decline in heat-induced hyperthermia and HSP70 and mRNA expression in aged rats. *Am. J. Physiol.* 260: 663–667, 1991.

25. BLAKE, M. J., R. UDELSMAN, G. J. FEULNER, D. D. NORTON, and N. J. HOLBROOK. Stress-induced heat shock protein 70 expression in adrenal cortex: an adrenocorticotropic hormone-sensitive, age-dependent response. *Proc. Natl. Acad. Sci. U.S.A.* 88: 9873–9877, 1991.

26. BLAZEJOWSKI, C. A., and G. C. WEBSTER. Decreased rates of protein synthesis by cell-free preparations from different organs of aging mice. *Mech. Ageing Dev.* 21: 345–356, 1983.

27. BLAZEJOWSKI, C. A., and G. C. WEBSTER. Effect of age on peptide chain initiation and elongation in preparations from brain, liver, kidney and skeletal muscle of the C57B/6J mouse. *Mech. Ageing Dev.* 25: 323–333, 1984.

28. BLOOM, E. T., H. UMEHARA, R. C. BLEACKLEY, K. OKUMURA, H. MOSTOWSKI, and J. T. BABBITT. Age-related decrement in cytotoxic T lymphocyte (CTL) activity is associated with decreased levels of mRNA encoded by two CTL-associated serine esterase genes and the perforin gene in mice. *Eur. J. Immunol.* 20: 2309–2316, 1990.

29. BOLLA, R., and N. BROT. Age dependent changes in enzymes involved in macromolecular synthesis in turbatrix aceti. *Arch. Biochem. Biophys.* 169: 227–236, 1975.

30. BOLLA, R., and W. D. DENCKLA. Effect of hypophysectomy on liver ribonucleic acid synthesis in aging rats. *Biochem. J.* 184: 669–674, 1979.

31. BOLLA, R., and J. MILLER. Endogenous nucleotide pools and protein incorporation into liver nuclei from young and old rats. *Mech. Ageing Dev.* 12: 107–118, 1980.

32. BOLLA, R. I., and C. GREENBLATT. Age-related changes in rat liver total protein and tranferrin synthesis. *Age* 5: 72–79, 1982.

33. BRITTON, G. W., and F. G. SHERMAN. Altered regulation of protein synthesis during aging as determined by in vitro ribosomal assays. *Exp. Gerontol.* 10: 67–77, 1975.

34. BRITTON, V. J., F. G. SHERMAN, and J. R. FLORINI. Effect of age on RNA synthesis by nuclei and soluble RNA polymerases from liver and muscle of C57BL/6J mice. *J. Gerontol.* 27: 188–192, 1972.

35. BUCKLER, A. J., H. VIE, G. E. SONENSHEIN, and R. A. MILLER. Defective T lymphocytes in old mice: diminished production of mature c-myc RNA after mitogen exposure not attributable to alterations in transcription or RNA stability. *J. Immunol.* 140: 2442–2446, 1988.

36. BUETOW, D. E., and P. S. GANDHI. Decreased protein synthesis by microsomes isolated from senescent rat liver. *Exp. Gerontol.* 8: 243–249, 1973.

37. BUNNEMANN, B., R. METZGER, K. FUXE, and D. GANTEN. Regional expression of angiotensinogen mRNA in the brain of one-week-old, adult and old male rats. *Dev. Brain Res.* 73: 41–45, 1993.

38. BURROWS, R. B., and P. F. DAVISON. Protein catabolism in cultures of hepatocytes derived from mice of various ages. *Mech. Ageing Dev.* 19: 85–94, 1982.

39. BUTLER, J. A., A. R. HEYDARI, and A. RICHARDSON. Analysis of effect of age on synthesis of specific proteins by hepatocytes. *J. Cell. Physiol.* 141: 400–409, 1989.

40. BUTTRICK, P., A. MALHOTRA, S. FACTOR, D. GEENEN, L. LEINWAND, and J. SCHEUER. Effect of aging and hypertension on myosin biochemistry and gene expression in the rat heart. *Circ. Res.* 68: 645–652, 1991.

41. BUTZOW, J. J., M. G. MCCOOL, and G. L. EICHHORN. Does the capacity of ribosomes to control translation fidelity change with age. *Mech. Ageing Dev.* 15: 203–216, 1981.

42. CAI, N. S., D. D. LI, H. T. CHEUNG, and A. RICHARDSON. The expression of granulocyte/macrophage colony-stimulating factor in activated mouse lymphocytes declines with age. *Cell. Immunol.* 130: 311–319, 1990.

43. CARNEY, J. M., P. E. STARKE-REED, C. N. OLIVER, R. W. LANDUM, M. S. CHENG, J. F. WU, and R. A. FLOYD. Reversal of age-related increase in brain protein oxidation, decrease in enzyme activity, and loss in temporal and spatial memory by chronic administration of the spin-trapping compound N-tert-butyl-α-phenylnitrone. *Proc. Natl. Acad. Sci. U.S.A.* 88: 3633–3636, 1991.

44. CARRIER, L., K. R. BOHELER, C. CHASSAGNE, D. DE LA BASTIE, C. WISNEWSKY, E. G. LAKATTA, and K. SCHWARTZ. Expression of the sarcomeric actin isogenes in the rat heart with development and senescence. *Circ. Res.* 70: 999–1005, 1992.

45. CARTER, K. C., D. J. POST, and J. PAPACONSTANTINOU. Differential expression of the mouse α_1-acid glycoprotein genes (AGP-1 and AGP-2) during inflammation and aging. *Biochim. Biophys. Acta.* 1089: 197–205, 1991.

46. CASTLE, T., A. KATZ, and A. RICHARDSON. Comparison of RNA synthesis by liver nuclei from rats of various ages. *Mech. Ageing Dev.* 8: 383–395, 1978.

47. CAVALLIUS, J., S. I. RATTAN, and B. F. CLARK. Changes in activity and amount of active elongation factor 1α in aging and immortal human fibroblast cultures. *Exp. Gerontol.* 21: 149–157, 1986.

48. CAVALLIUS, J., S. I. RATTAN, B. RIIS, and B. F. CLARK. A decrease in levels of mRNA for elongation factor-1α accompanies the decline in its activity and the amounts of active enzyme in rat livers during ageing. In: *The Liver, Metabolism and Ageing,* edited by K. W. Woodhouse, C. Yelland, and O. F. W. James. Rijswijk, Netherlands: INSERM-EURAGE/Libbey 1989, p. 125–132.

49. CEDAR, H. DNA methylation and gene activity. *Cell* 53: 3–4, 1988.

50. CHANG, W. C., M. T. HOOPES, and G. S. ROTH. Biosynthetic rates of protein having the characteristics of glucocorticoid

receptors in adipocytes of mature and senescent rats. *J. Gerontol.* 36: 386–390, 1981.
51. CHATTERJEE, B., G. FERNANDES, B. P. YU, C. SONG, J. M. KIM, W. DEMYAN, and A. K. ROY. Calorie restriction delays age-dependent loss in androgen responsiveness of the rat liver. *FASEB J.* 3: 169–173, 1989.
52. CHATTERJEE, B., S. T. NATH, and A. K. ROY. Differential regulation of the messenger RNA for three major senescence maker proteins in male rat liver. *J. Biol. Chem.* 256: 5939–5941, 1981.
53. CHATURVEDI, M. M., and M. S. KANUNGO. Analysis of conformation and function of the chromatin of the brain of young and old rats. *Mol. Biol. Rep.* 10: 215–219, 1985.
54. CHEN, J. C., P. OVE, and A. I. LANSING. In vitro synthesis of microsomal protein and albumin in young and old rats. *Biochim. Biophys. Acta* 312: 598–607, 1973.
55. CHEN, J. J., N. BROT, and H. WEISSBACH. RNA and protein synthesis in cultured human fibroblasts derived from donors of various ages. *Mech. Ageing Dev.* 13: 285–295, 1980.
56. CHEN, P. S. Amino acid pattern and rate of protein synthesis in aging drosophila. In: *Molecular Genetic Mechanisms in Development and Aging,* edited by M. Rockstein and G. T. Bakker. New York: Academic Press, 1972, p. 199–226.
57. CHEUNG, H. T., J. S. TWU, and A. RICHARDSON. Mechanism of the age-related decline in lymphocyte proliferation: role of IL-2 production and protein synthesis. *Exp. Gerontol.* 18: 451–460, 1983.
58. CLAES-RECKINGER, N., J. VANDENHAUTE, C. F. VAN BEZOOIJEN, and J. DELCOUR. Functional properties of rat liver protein synthesizing machinery in relation to aging. *Exp. Gerontol.* 17: 281–286, 1982.
59. CLARKE, J. M., and J. M. SMITH. Increase in the rate of protein synthesis with age in *Drosophila* subobscura. *Nature* 209: 627–629, 1966.
60. CLINTON, M., M. FRANGOU-LAZARIDIS, C. PANNEERSELVAM, and B. L. HORECKER. Prothymosin α and parathymosin: mRNA and polypeptide levels in rodent tissues. *Arch. Biochem. Biophys.* 269: 256–263, 1989.
61. COLEMAN, P. K., B. B. KAPLAN, H. H. OOSTERBURG, and C. E. FINCH. Brain poly (A) RNA during aging: stability of yield and sequence complexity in two rat strains. *J. Neurochem.* 34: 335–345, 1980.
62. COLLINS, J. M. RNA synthesis in rat liver cells with different DNA contents. *J. Biol. Chem.* 253: 5769–5773, 1978.
63. COMOLLI, R. Polyamine effects of carbon-14 leucine transfer to microsomal protein in a rat liver cell free system during aging. *Exp. Gerontol.* 8: 307–313, 1973.
64. COMOLLI, R., M. E. FERIOLI, and S. AZZOLA. Protein turnover of the lysosomal and mitochondrial fractions of rat liver during aging. *Exp. Gerontol.* 7: 369–376, 1972.
65. CONIGLIO, J. J., D. S. LIU, and A. RICHARDSON. A comparison of protein synthesis by liver parenchymal cells isolated from Fischer F344 rats of various ages. *Mech. Ageing Dev.* 11: 77–90, 1979.
66. COOK, J. R., and D. E. BUETOW. The complement of cytoplasmic tRNAs, including queuosine-containing tRNAs, in adult and senescent Wistar rat liver and their levels of aminoacylation. *Mech. Ageing Dev.* 20: 289–304, 1982.
67. COSGROVE, J. W., and S. I. RAPOPORT. Absence of age differences in protein synthesis by rat brain, measured with an initiating cell-free system. *Neurobiol. Aging* 8: 27–34, 1987.
68. COURTRIGHT, J. B., J. SONSTEIN, and A. K. KUMARAN. Age specific regulation of gene expression in *Drosophila*. In: *Molecular Biology of Aging: Gene Stability and Gene Expression,* edited by R. S. SOHAL, L. S. BIRNBAUM, and R. G. CUTLER. New York: Raven Press, 1985, p. 209–222.
69. CREW, M. D., S. R. SPINDLER, R. L. WALFORD, and A. KOIZUMI. Age-related decrease of growth hormone and prolactin gene expression in the mouse pituitary. *Endocrinology* 121: 1251–1255, 1987.
70. CRIE, J. S., D. J. MILLWARD, P. C. BATES, E. E. GRIFFIN, and K. WILDENTHAL. Age-related alterations in cardiac protein turnover. *J. Mol. Cell. Cardiol.* 13: 589–598, 1981.
71. CUTLER, R. G. The dysdifferentiative hypothesis of mammalian aging and longevity. In: *The Aging Brain,* edited by E. GIACOBINI, G. GIACOBINI, G. FILOGAMO, and A. VERNADAKIS. New York: Raven Press, 1982, p. 25–114.
72. DANNER, D. B., and N. J. HOLBROOK. Alterations in gene expression with aging. In: *Handbook of the Biology of Aging,* edited by E. L. SCHNEIDER and J. W. ROWE. San Diego: Academic Press, 1990, p. 97–115.
73. D'COSTA, A., C. R. BREESE, R. L. BOYD, R. M. BOOZE, and W. E. SONNTAG. Attenuation of fos-like immunoreactivity induced by a single electroconvulsive shock in brains of aging mice. *Brain Res.* 567: 204–211, 1991.
74. DEMYAN, W. F., C. S. SONG, D. S. KIM, S. HER, W. GALLWITZ, T. R. RAO, M. SLOMCZYNSKA, B. CHATTERJEE, and A. K. ROY. Estrogen sulfotransferase of the rat liver: complementary DNA cloning and age- and sex-specific regulation of messenger RNA. *Mol. Endocrinol.* 6: 589–597, 1992.
75. DENCKLA, W. D. System analysis of possible mechanisms of mammalian aging. *Mech. Ageing Dev.* 6: 143–152, 1977.
76. DEVI, A., P. LINDSAY, P. L. RAINA, and N. K. SARKAR. Effect of age on some aspects of the synthesis of ribonucleic acid. *Nature* 212: 474–475, 1966.
77. DE VRIES, A. C., M. A. VERMEER, A. L. HENDRIKS, H. BLOEMENDAL, and L. H. COHEN. Biosynthetic capacity of the human lens upon aging. *Exp. Eye Res.* 53: 519–524, 1991.
78. DICE, J. F. Altered degradation of proteins microinjected into senescent human fibroblasts. *J. Biol. Chem.* 257: 14624–14627, 1982.
79. DICE, J. F., and H. CHIANG. Peptide signals for protein degradation within lysosomes. *Biochem. Soc. Symp.* 55: 45–55, 1989.
80. DOBIE, D. J., M. A. MILLER, M. A. RASKIND, and D. M. DORSA. Testosterone reverses a senescent decline in extrahypothalamic vasopressin mRNA. *Brain Res.* 583: 247–252, 1992.
81. DRINKWATER, R. D., T. J. BLAKE, A. A. MORLEY, and D. R. TURNER. Human lymphocytes aged in vivo have reduced levels of methylation in transcriptionally active and inactive DNA. *Mutat. Res.* 219: 29–37, 1989.
82. DU, J. T., T. A. BEYER, and C. A. LANG. Protein biosynthesis in aging mouse tissues. *Exp. Gerontol.* 12: 181–191, 1977.
83. DUBITSKY, R., K. G. BENSCH, and J. E. FLEMING. Age-related changes on turnover and concentration of a subset of thorax polypeptides from *Drosophila melanogaster*. *Mech. Ageing Dev.* 32: 311–317, 1985.
84. DWYER, B. E., J. L. FANDO, and C. G. WASTERLAIN. Rat brain protein synthesis declines during postdevelopmental aging. *J. Neurochem.* 35: 746–749, 1980.
85. EGILMEZ, N. K., and M. ROTHSTEIN. The effect of aging on cell-free protein synthesis in the free-living nematode Turbatrix aceti. *Biochim. Biophys. Acta* 840: 355–363, 1985.
86. EKSTROM, R., D. S. LIU, and A. RICHARDSON. Changes in brain protein synthesis during the life span of male Fischer rats. *Gerontology* 26: 121–128, 1980.
87. EL HAJ, A. J., S. E. LEWIS, D. F. GOLDSPINK, B. J. MERRY, and A. M. HOLEHAN. The effect of chronic and acute dietary restriction on the growth and protein turnover of fast and slow types of rat skeletal muscle. *Comp. Biochem. Physiol. A* 85: 281–287, 1986.
88. FAIRWEATHER, D. S., M. FOX, and G. P. MARGISON. The in vitro lifespan of MRC-5 cells in shortened by 5-azacytidine-induced demethylation. *Exp. Cell Res.* 168: 153–159, 1987.

89. FANDO, J. L., M. SALINAS, and C. G. WASTERLAIN. Age-dependent changes in brain protein synthesis in the rat. *Neurochem. Res.* 5: 373–383, 1980.
90. FARGNOLI, J., T. KUNISADA, A. J. FORNACE, E. L. SCHNEIDER, and N. J. HOLBROOK. Decreased expression of heat shock protein 70 mRNA and protein after heat treatment in cells of aged rats. *Proc. Natl. Acad. Sci. U.S.A.* 87: 846–850, 1990.
91. FERLAND, G., M. AUDET, and B. TUCHWEBER. Effect of dietary restriction on lysosomal bodies and total protein synthesis in hepatocytes of aging rats. *Mech. Ageing Dev.* 64: 49–59, 1992.
92. FERNANDEZ-SILVA, P., V. PETRUZZELLA, F. FRACASSO, M. N. GADALETA, and P. CANTORE. Reduced synthesis of mtRNA in isolated mitochondria of senescent rat brain. *Biochem. Biophys. Res. Commun.* 176: 645–653, 1991.
93. FILION, A. M., and M. LAUGHREA. Translation fidelity in the aging mammal: studies with an accurate in vitro system on aged rats. *Mech. Ageing Dev.* 29: 125–142, 1985.
94. FINCH, C. E., and D. G. MORGAN. RNA and protein metabolism in the aging brain. *Annu. Rev. Neurosci.* 13: 75–87, 1990.
95. FLEMING, J. E., P. S. MELNIKOFF, G. I. LATTER, D. CHANDRA, and K. G. BENSCH. Age dependent changes in the expression of *drosophila* mitochondrial proteins. *Mech. Ageing Dev.* 34: 63–72, 1986.
96. FLEMING, J. E., E. QUATTROCKI, G. LATTER, J. MIQUEL, R. MARCUSON, E. ZUCKERKANDL, and K. G. BENSCH. Age-dependent changes in proteins of *Drosophila melanogaster*. *Science* 231: 1157–1159, 1986.
97. FLETCHER, M. J., and D. R. SANADI. Turnover of liver mitochondrial components in adult and senescent rats. *J. Gerontol.* 16: 255–257, 1961.
98. FLORINE, D. L., T. ONO, R. G. CUTLER, and M. J. GETZ. Regulation of endogenous murine leukemia virus-related nuclear and cytoplasmic RNA complexity in C57BL/6J mice of increasing age. *Cancer Res.* 40: 519–523, 1980.
99. FLORINI, J. R., S. GEARY, Y. SAITO, E. J. MANOWITZ, and R. S. SORRENTINO. Changes in protein synthesis in heart. *Adv. Exp. Med. Biol.* 61: 149–162, 1975.
100. FLORIO, T., C. VENTRA, A. POSTIGLIONE, and G. SCHETTINI. Age-related alterations of somatostatin gene expression in different rat brain areas. *Brain Res.* 557: 64–68, 1991.
101. FOG, R., and H. PAKKENBERG. Age-related changes in ^{3}H-uridine uptake in the mouse. *J. Gerontol.* 36: 680–681, 1981.
102. FOOTE, R. S., and M. P. STULBERG. Efficiency and fidelity of cell-free protein synthesis by transfer RNA from aged mice. *Mech. Ageing Dev.* 13: 93–104, 1980.
103. FRAZER, J. M., and W. K. YANG. Isoaccepting transfer ribonucleic acid in liver and brain of young and old BC3F1 mice. *Arch. Biochem. Biophys.* 153: 610–618, 1972.
104. FUJITA, T., and N. MARUYAMA. Elevated levels of c-jun and c-fos transcripts in the aged rat liver. *Biochem. Biophys. Res. Commun.* 178: 1485–1491, 1991.
105. FUKUDA, H., and N. IRITANI. Effects of aging on gene expression of acetyl-CoA carboxylase and fatty acid synthase in rat liver. *J. Biochem.* 122: 277–280, 1992.
106. GAARDSVOLL, H., L. KROG, D. ZHERNOSEKOV, A.-M. ANDERSSON, K. EDVARDSEN, M. OLSEN, E. BOCK, and D. LINNEMANN. Age-related changes in expression of neural cell adhesion molecule (NCAM) in heart: a comparative study of newborn, adult and aged rats. *Eur. J. Cell Biol.* 61: 100–107, 1993.
107. GABIUS, H. J., R. ENGELHARDT, F. DEERBERG, and F. CRAMER. Age-related changes in different steps of protein synthesis of liver and kidney of rats. *FEBS Lett.* 160: 115–118, 1983.
108. GADALETA, M. N., V. PETRUZZELLA, M. RENIS, F. FRACASSO, and P. CANTATORE. Reduced transcription of mitochondrial DNA in the senescent rat; tissue dependence and effect of L-carnitine. *Eur. J. Biochem.* 187: 501–506, 1990.
109. GAMBLE, D. A., R. SCHWAB, M. E. WEKSLER, and P. SZABO. Decreased steady state c-myc mRNA in activated T cell cultures from old humans is caused by a smaller proportion of T cells that transcribe the c-myc gene. *J. Immunol.* 144: 3569–3573, 1990.
110. GAUBATZ, J., M. ELLIS, and R. CHALKLEY. The structural organization of mouse chromatin as a function of age. *FASEB J.* 38: 1973–1978, 1979a.
111. GAUBATZ, J., M. ELLIS, and R. CHALKLEY. Nuclease digestion studies of mouse chromatin as a function of age. *J. Gerontol.* 34: 672–679, 1979b.
112. GAUBATZ, J. W., and R. G. CUTLER. Mouse satellite DNA is transcribed in senescent cardiac muscle. *J. Biol. Chem.* 265: 17753–17758, 1990.
113. GAUBATZ, J. W., B. ARCEMENT, and R. G. CUTLER. Gene expression of an endogenous retrovirus-like element during murine development and aging. *Mech. Ageing Dev.* 57: 71–85, 1991.
114. GEARY, S., and J. R. FLORINI. Effect of age on rate of protein synthesis in isolated perfused mouse hearts. *J. Gerontol.* 27: 325–332, 1972.
115. GIBAS, M. A., and D. HARMAN. Ribonucleic acid synthesis by nuclei isolated from rats of different ages. *J. Gerontol.* 25: 105–107, 1970.
116. GOLDSPINK, D. F. Pre- and post-natal growth and protein turnover in the lung of the rat. *Biochem. J.* 242: 275–279, 1987.
117. GOLDSPINK, D. F. Protein turnover and growth of the rat brain from the foetus to old age. *J. Neurochem.* 50: 1364–1368, 1988.
118. GOLDSPINK, D. F., and F. J. KELLY. Protein turnover and growth in the whole body, liver and kidney of the rat from the fetus to senility. *Biochem. J.* 217: 507–516, 1984.
119. GOLDSPINK, D. F., and B. J. MERRY. Changes in protein turnover and growth of the rat lung in response to ageing and long-term dietary restriction. *Mech. Ageing Dev.* 42: 253–262, 1988.
120. GOLDSPINK, D. F., S. E. LEWIS, and F. J. KELLY. Protein synthesis during the developmental growth of the small and large intestine of the rat. *Biochem, J.* 217: 527–534, 1984.
121. GOLDSPINK, D. F., S. E. LEWIS, and F. J. KELLY. Protein turnover and cathepsin B activity in several tissues of foetal and senescent rats. *Comp. Biochem. Physiol.* 82B: 849–853, 1985.
122. GOLDSPINK, D. F., S. E. LEWIS, and B. J. MERRY. Effects of aging and long term dietary intervention on protein turnover and growth of ventricular muscle in the rat heart. *Cardiovasc. Res.* 20: 672–678, 1986.
123. GOLDSPINK, D. F., A. J. EL HAJ, S. E. LEWIS, B. J. MERRY, and A. M. HOLEHAN. The influence of chronic dietary intervention on protein turnover and growth of the diaphragm and extensor digitorum longus muscles of the rat. *Exp. Gerontol.* 22: 67–78, 1987.
124. GOLDSTEIN, S., D. STOTLAND, and R. A. J. CORDEIRO. Decreased proteolysis and increased amino acid efflux in aging human fibroblasts. *Mech. Ageing Dev.* 5: 221–223, 1976.
125. GORDON, S. M., and C. E. FINCH. An electrophoretic study of protein synthesis in brain regions of senescent male mice. *Exp. Gerontol.* 9: 267–273, 1974.
126. GOZES, I., B. L. CRONIN, and M. A. MOSKOWITZ. Protein synthesis in rat brain microvessels decreases with aging. *J. Neurochem.* 36: 1311–1315, 1981.
127. GRESIK, E. W., K. WENK-SALAMONE, A. ONETTI-MUDA, R. M. GUBITS, and P. A. SHAW. Effect of advanced age on the induction by androgen or thyroid hormone of epidermal growth factor and epidermal growth factor mRNA in the submandibular glands of C57BL/6 male mice. *Mech. Ageing Dev.* 34: 175–189, 1986.
128. GURLEY, R., and J. F. DICE. Degradation of endocytosed proteins is unaltered in senescent human fibroblasts. *Cell Biol. Int. Rep.* 12: 885–894, 1988.
129. HAINING, J. L., and W. W. CORRELL. Turnover of tryptophan-

induced tryptophan pyrrolase in rat liver as a function of age. *J. Gerontol.* 24: 143–148, 1969.
130. HAINING, J. L., and J. S. LEGAN. Catalase turnover in rat liver and kidney as a function of age. *Exp. Gerontol.* 8: 85–91, 1973.
131. HAJI, M., R. S. CHUKNYISKA, and G. S. ROTH. Isolated uterine nuclei and cytosol receptors of aged rats exhibit impaired estrogenic stimulation of RNA polymerase II. *Proc. Natl. Acad. Sci. U.S.A.* 81: 7481–7484, 1984.
132. HANAI, H., C. T. LIANG, L. CHENG, and B. SACKTOR. Densensitization to parathyroid hormone in renal cells from aged rats is associated with alterations in G-protein activity. *J. Clin. Invest.* 83: 268–277, 1989.
133. HARDWICK, J., W. H. HSIEH, D. S. LIU, and A. RICHARDSON. Cell-free protein synthesis by kidney from the aging female Fischer F344 rat. *Biochim. Biophys. Acta.* 652: 204–217, 1981.
134. HELLTHALER, V. G., D. REIGEGERSTE, R. KOHLER, and W. ROTZSCH. Zur molekularbiologie des alterns 7 mitteilung: Einflub der cytosolfraktion auf die aminosaureinkorporation durch rattenlebermikrosomen in abhangigkeit vom lebensalter. *Z. Alfernsforseh* 31: 457–460, 1976.
135. HERSHKO, A., and A. CIECHANOVER. Mechanisms of intracellular protein breakdown. *Annu. Rev. Biochem.* 51: 335–364, 1982.
136. HESLOP, J. P. Effect of age on [^{14}C]valine turnover into locust wing proteins [Abstract]. *Biochem. J.* 104: 5P–6P, 1967.
137. HEYDARI, A. R., and A. RICHARDSON. Does gene expression play any role in the mechanism of the antiaging effect of dietary restriction. *Ann. N.Y. Acad. Sci.* 663: 384–395, 1992.
138. HEYDARI, A. R., B. WU, R. TAKAHASHI, R. STRONG, and A. RICHARDSON. Expression of heat shock protein 70 is altered by age and diet at the level of transcription. *Mol. Cell. Biol.* 13: 2909–2918, 1993.
139. HIGGINS, G. A., G. A. OYLER, R. L. NEVE, K. S. CHEN, and F. H. GAGE. Altered levels of amyloid protein precursor transcripts in the basal forebrain of behaviorally impaired aged rats. *Proc. Natl. Acad. Sci. U.S.A.* 87: 3032–3036, 1990.
140. HIGUCHI, K., K. KITAGAWA, K. KOGISHI, and T. TAKEDA. Developmental and age-related changes in apolipoprotein B mRNA editing in mice. *J. Lipid Res.* 33: 1753–1764, 1992.
141. HILL, B. T., and R. D. H. WHELAN. Studies of the degradation of ageing chromatin DNA by nuclear and cytoplasmic factors and deoxyribonucleases. *Gerontology* 24: 326–336, 1978.
142. HILL, M. W., and J. KARTHIGASAN. Glucose metabolism and protein synthesis in stratified squamous epithelia from young and old mice. *Exp. Gerontol.* 24: 331–340, 1989.
143. HOLBROOK, N. J., R. K. CHOPRA, M. T. MCCOY, J. E. NAGEL, D. C. POWERS, W. H. ADLER, and E. L. SCHNEIDER. Expression of interleukin 2 and the interleukin 2 receptor in aging rats. *Cell. Immunol.* 120: 1–9, 1989.
144. HOLLIDAY, R. Strong effects of 5-azacytidine on the in vitro lifespan of human diploid fibroblasts. *Exp. Cell Res.* 166: 543–552, 1986.
145. HORBACH, G. J., H. M. G. PRINCEN, M. VAN DER KROEF, C. F. VAN BEZOOIJEN, and S. H. YAP. Changes in the sequence content of albumin mRNA and in its translational activity in the rat liver with age. *Biochim. Biophys. Acta* 783: 60–66, 1984.
146. HORBACH, G. J., J. G. VAN ASTEN, and C. F. VAN BEZOOIJEN. The influence of ageing on the induction of the mRNAs of rat liver cytochromes P450IIB1 and P450IIB2. *Biochem. Pharmacol.* 40: 529–533, 1990a.
147. HORBACH, G. J., J. G. VAN ASTEN, and C. F. VAN BEZOOIJEN. The influence of age on the inducibility of rat liver cytochrome P450IA (CYPIA1) and P450IA2 (CYPIA2) mRNAs. *Mutat. Res.* 237: 117–121, 1990b.
148. HORBACH, G. J., C. F. VAN BEZOOIJEN, and D. L. KNOOK. Age-related changes in the synthesis of individual liver-specific proteins. In: *Review of Biological Research in Aging*, edited by M. Rothstein. New York: Alan R. Liss, 1987, vol. 3, p. 485–494.
149. HORBACH, G. J., H. VAN DER BOOM, C. F. VAN BEZOOIJEN, S. H. YAP. Molecular aspects of age-related changes in albumin synthesis in female WAG/Rij rats. *Life Sci.* 43: 1707–1714, 1988.
150. HORBACH, G. J., J. T. VENKATRAMAN, and G. FERNANDES. Food restriction prevents the loss of isosafrole inducible cytochrome P-450 mRNA and enzyme levels in aging rats. *Biochem. Int.* 20: 725–730, 1990.
151. HOSBACH, H. A., and E. KUBLI. Transfer RNA in aging *Drosophila*: I. Extent of aminoacylation. *Mech. Ageing Dev.* 10: 131–140, 1979a.
152. HOSBACH, H. A., and E. KUBLI. Transfer RNA in aging *Drosophila*: II. Isoacceptor patterns. *Mech. Ageing Dev.* 10: 141–149, 1979b.
153. HRACHOVEC, J. P. Age changes in amino acid incorporations by rat liver microsomes. *Gerontologia* 15: 52–63, 1969.
154. HRACHOVEC, J. P. The effect of age on tissue protein synthesis. I. Age changes in amino acid incorporation by rat liver purified microsomes. *Gerontologia* 17: 75–86, 1971.
155. HUNG, L., and A. RICHARDSON. The effect of aging on the genetic expression of renin by mouse kidney. *Aging Clin. Exp. Res.* 5: 193–198, 1993.
156. IBRAHIM, N. G., K. L. MARCUS, and M. L. FREEDMAN. Maintenance of cytochrome P_{450} content in old rat livers in spite of decreased mitochondrial protein synthesis. *J. Clin. Exp. Gerontol.* 3: 327–337, 1981.
157. INGVAR, M. C., P. MAEDER, L. SOKOLOFF, and C. B. SMITH. Effects of ageing on local rates of cerebral protein synthesis in Sprague-Dawley rats. *Brain* 108: 155–170, 1985.
158. ISHIGAMI, A., and S. GOTO. Inactivation kinetics of horseradish peroxidase microinjected into hepatocytes of mice of various ages. *Mech. Ageing Dev.* 46: 125–133, 1988.
159. ISHIGAMI, A., and S. GOTO. Age-related change in the degradation rate of ovalbumin microinjected into mouse liver parenchymal cells. *Arch. Biochem. Biophys.* 277: 189–195, 1990a.
160. ISHIGAMI, A., and S. GOTO. Effect of dietary restriction on the degradation of proteins in senescent mouse liver parenchymal cells in culture. *Arch. Biochem. Biophys.* 238: 362–366, 1990b.
161. JACOBUS, S., and D. GERSHON. Age-related changes in inducible mouse liver enzymes: ornithine decarboxylase and tyrosine amino-transferase. *Mech. Ageing Dev.* 12: 311–322, 1980.
162. JAISWAL, Y. K., and M. S. KANUNGO. Expression of actin and myosin heavy chain genes in skeletal, cardiac and uterine muscles of young and old rats. *Biochem. Biophys. Res. Commun.* 168: 71–77, 1990.
163. JOHNSON, T. E., and G. MCCAFFREY. Programmed aging or error catastrophe? An ecanination by two dimensional polyacrylamide gel electrophoresis. *Mech. Ageing Dev.* 30: 285–297, 1985.
164. JUNGHAHN, I., and H. BIELKA. Regulation der translation in eukaryotischen zellen. II. Uber die altersabhangige wirkung des zytosols der leber auf die in vitro proteinsynthese in einem polysomensystem. *Acta Biol. Med. Germ.* 32: 267–269, 1974.
165. KAMINSKA, B., and L. KACZMAREK. Robust induction of AP-1 transcription factor DNA binding activity in the hippocampus of aged rats. *Neurosci. Lett.* 153: 189–191, 1993.
166. KANUNGO, M. S., O. KOUL, and K. R. REDDY. Concomitant studies on RNA and protein syntheses in tissues of rats of various ages. *Exp. Gerontol.* 5: 261–269, 1970.
167. KARELUS, K., and J. F. NELSON. Aging impairs estrogenic suppression of hypothalamic proopiomelanocortin messenger ribonucleic acid in the mouse. *Neuroendocrinology* 55: 627–633, 1992.
168. KAREY, K. P., and M. ROTHSTEIN. Evidence for the lack of lyso-

somal involvement in the age-related slowing of protein breakdown in *Turbatrix aceti*. *Mech. Ageing Dev.* 35: 169–178, 1986.
169. KELLY, F. J., S. E. LEWIS, R. G. ANDERSON, and D. F. GOLDSPINK. Pre- and postnatal growth and protein turnover in four muscles of the rat. *Muscle Nerve* 7: 235–242, 1984.
170. KIM, S. K., and P. P. ARISUMI. The synthesis of amylase in parotid glands of young and old rats. *Mech. Ageing Dev.* 31: 257–266, 1985.
171. KIM, S. K., and D. W. CALKINS. Secretory protein synthesis in parotid glands of young and old rats. *Arch. Oral Biol.* 28: 1–4, 1983.
172. KIM, S. K., D. W. CALKINS, P. A. WEINHOLD, and S. S. HAN. Changes in the synthesis of exportable and nonexportable proteins in parotid glands during aging. *Mech. Ageing Dev.* 18: 239–250, 1982.
173. KIM, S. K., L. M. CUZZORT, and E. D. ALLEN. Effects of age on diabetes- and insulin-induced changes in pancreatic levels of α-amylase and its mRNA. *Mech. Ageing Dev.* 58: 151–161, 1991.
174. KIM, S. K., L. M. CUZZORT, and R. K. MCKEAN. Amylase mRNA synthesis and ageing in rat parotid glands following isoproterenol-stimulated secretion. *Arch. Oral Biol.* 37: 349–354, 1992.
175. KIM, S. K., P. A. WEINHOLD, D. W. CALKINS, and V. W. HARTOG. Comparative studies of the age-related changes in protein synthesis in the rat pancreas and parotid gland. *Exp. Gerontol.* 16: 91–99, 1981.
176. KIM, S. K., P. A. WEINHOLD, S. S. HAN, and D. J. WAGNER. Age-related decline in protein synthesis in the rat parotid gland. *Exp. Gerontol.* 15: 77–85, 1980.
177. KIMBALL, K. A., L. E. CORNETT, E. SEIFEN, and R. H. KENNEDY. Aging: changes in cardiac α_1- adrenoceptor responsiveness and expression. *Eur. J. Pharmacol. Mol. Pharmacol.* 208: 231–238, 1991.
178. KIMBALL, S. R., T. C. VARY, and L. S. JEFFERSON. Age-dependent decrease in the amount of eukaryotic initiation factor 2 in various rat tissues. *Biochem. J.* 286: 263–268, 1992.
179. KITRAKI, E., E. BOZAS, H. PHILIPPIDIS, and F. STYLIANOPOULOU. Aging-related changes in IGF-II and c-fos gene expression in the rat brain. *Int. J. Dev. Neurosci.* 11: 1–9, 1993.
180. KITTUR, S. D., L. SONG, H. ENDO, and W. H. ADLER. Nerve growth factor receptor gene expression in human peripheral blood lymphocytes in aging. *J. Neurosci. Res.* 32: 444–448, 1992.
181. KRAWCZYK, Z., and N. SZYMIK. Effect of age and busulphan treatment on the hsp70 gene-related transcript level in rat testes. *Int. J. Androl.* 12: 72–79, 1989.
182. KREAMER, W., N. ZORICH, D. S. LIU, and A. RICHARDSON. Effect of age on RNA synthesis by rat hepatocytes. *Exp. Gerontol.* 14: 27–36, 1979.
183. KRISTAL, B. S., and B. P. YU. The next frontier: studies of the effects of age and diet on mammalian gene expression. *Age Nutr.* 3: 217–224, 1992.
184. KRISTAL, B. S., C. C. CONRAD, A. RICHARDSON, and B. P. YU. Is poly(A) tail length altered by aging or dietary restriction? *Gerontology* 39: 152–162, 1993.
185. KUMAZAKI, T., M. KOBAYASHI, and Y. MITSUI. Enhanced expression of fibronectin during in vivo cellular aging of human vascular endothelial cells and skin fibroblasts. *Exp. Cell Res.* 205: 396–402, 1993.
186. KURTZ, D. I. The effect of ageing on in vitro fidelity of translation in mouse liver. *Biochim. Biophys. Acta* 407: 479–484, 1975.
187. KURTZ, D. I. A decrease in the number of active mouse liver ribosomes during aging. *Exp. Gerontol.* 13: 397–402, 1978.
188. LAMB, P., and S. MCKNIGHT. Diversity and specificity in transcriptional regulation: the benefits of heterotypic dimerization. *TIBS* 16: 417–422, 1991.
189. LAPCHAK, P. A., D. M. ARAUJO, K. D. BECK, C. E. FINCH, S. A. JOHNSON, and F. HEFTI. BDNF and trkB mRNA expression in the hippocampal formation of aging rats. *Neurobiol. Aging* 14: 121–126, 1993.
190. LARKFORS, L., T. EBENDAL, S. R. WHITTEMORE, H. PERSSON, B. HOFFER, and L. OLSON. Decreased level of nerve growth factor (NGF) and its messenger RNA in the aged rat brain. *Mol. Brain Res.* 3: 55–60, 1987.
191. LAUGHREA, M., and J. LATULIPPE. The poly(U) translational capacity of Fischer 344 rat liver does not deteriorate with age and is not affected by dietary regime. *Mech. Ageing Dev.* 45: 137–143, 1988.
192. LAVIE, L., A. Z. REZNICK, and D. GERSHON. Decreased protein and puromycinil-peptide degradation in livers of senescent mice. *Biochem. J.* 202: 47–51, 1982.
193. LAWRENCE, A. E., J. Z. READINGER, R. W. HO, S. ACKLEY, M. HOLLANDER, and L. L. MAYS. Age-related changes in lysine isoacceptor proportions and acylation capacity of rat liver transfer RNAs with little change in physical properties. *Age* 2: 56–62, 1979.
194. LAYMAN, D. K., G. A. RICCA, and A. RICHARDSON. The effect of age on protein synthesis and ribosome aggregation to messenger RNA in rat liver. *Arch. Biochem. Biophys.* 173: 246–254, 1976.
195. LEE, D. Y., J. J. HAYES, D. PRUSS, and A. P. WOLFFE. A positive role for histone acetylation in transcription factor access to nucleosomal DNA. *Cell* 72: 73–84, 1993.
196. LEE, S., A. FRANCOEUR, S. LIU, and E. WANG. Tissue-specific expression in mammalian brain, heart, and muscle of S1, a member of the elongation factor-1α gene family. *J. Biol. Chem.* 267: 24064–24068, 1992.
197. LEVENBOOK, L., and I. KRISHNA. Effect of ageing on amino acid turnover and rate of protein synthesis in the blowfly Phormia regina. *J. Insect Physiol.* 17: 9–12, 1971.
198. LEWIS, S. E., D. F. GOLDSPINK, J. G. PHILLIPS, B. J. MERRY, and A. M. HOLEHAN. The effects of aging and chronic dietary restriction on whole body growth and protein turnover in the rat. *Exp. Gerontol.* 20: 253–263, 1985.
199. LEWIS, S. E., F. J. KELLY, and D. F. GOLDSPINK. Pre- and postnatal growth and protein turnover in smooth muscle, heart and slow- and fast-twitch skeletal muscles of the rat. *Biochem. J.* 217: 517–526, 1984.
200. LI, D. D., Y. K. CHIEN, M. Z. GU, A. RICHARDSON, and H. T. CHEUNG. The age-related decline in interleukin-3 expression in mice. *Life Sci.* 43: 1215–1222, 1988.
201. LIANG, C. T., J. BARNES, H. HANAI, and M. A. LEVINE. Decrease in G_s protein expression may impair adenylate cyclase activation in old kidneys. *Am. J. Physiol.* 264 (*Renal Fluid Electrolyte Physiol.* 33): F770–F773, 1993.
202. LIBBY, R. T. Mistranslation in bacteriophage-infected anucleate minicells of *Escherichia coli*: a test for error propagation. *Mech. Ageing Dev.* 26: 23–35, 1984.
203. LIN, F. K., and S. H. CHANG. Differences between transfer RNA methylase activity in human diploid fibroblasts during in vitro and in vivo aging. *Mech. Ageing Dev.* 11: 383–392, 1979.
204. LIN, J. L., T. ASANO, Y. SHIBASAKI, K. TSUKUDA, H. KATAGIRI, H. ISHIHARA, F. TAKAKU, and Y. OKA. Altered expression of glucose transporter isoforms with aging in rats—selective decrease in GluT4 in the fat tissue and skeletal muscle. *Diabetologia* 34: 477–482, 1991.
205. LINDELL, T. J., J. J. DUFFY, and B. BYRNES. Transcription in aging: the response of rat liver nuclear RNA polymerases to cyclohexamide in vivo. *Mech. Ageing Dev.* 19: 63–71, 1982.
206. LINNEMANN, D., H. GAARDSVOLL, M. OLSEN, and E. BOCK.

Expression of NCAM mRNA and polypeptides in aging rat brain. *Int. J. Dev. Neurosci.* 11: 71–81, 1993.
207. LIU, A. Y., H. CHOI, Y. LEE, and K. Y. CHEN. Molecular events involved in transcriptional activation of heat shock genes become progressively refractory to heat stimulation during aging of human diploid fibroblasts. *J. Cell. Physiol.* 149: 560–566, 1991.
208. LIU, D. S., R. EKSTROM, J. W. SPICER, and A. RICHARDSON. Age-related changes in protein, RNA and DNA content and protein synthesis in rat testes. *Exp. Gerontol.* 13: 197–205, 1978.
209. LOMPRE, A. M., F. LAMBERT, E. G. LAKATTA, and K. SCHWARTZ. Expression of sarcoplasmic reticulum Ca^{2+}-ATPase and calsequestrin genes in rat heart during ontogenic development and aging. *Circ. Res.* 69: 1380–1388, 1991.
210. MADSEN, H. O., K. POULSEN, O. DAHL, B. F. CLARK, and J. P. HJORTH. Retropseudogenes constitute the major part of the human elongation factor 1α gene family. *Nucleic Acids Res.* 18: 1513–1516, 1990.
211. MAGNUSON, V. L., M. YOUNG, D. G. SCHATTENBERG, M. A. MANCINI, D. CHEN, B. STEFFENSEN, and R. J. KLEBE. The alternative splicing of fibronectin pre-mRNA is altered during aging and in response to growth factors. *J. Biol. Chem.* 266: 14654–14662, 1991.
212. MAILLEUX, P., and J. J. VANDERHAEGHEN. Age-related loss of cannabinoid receptor binding sites and mRNA in the rat striatum. *Neurosci. Lett.* 147: 179–181, 1992.
213. MAINWARING, W. I. Changes in the ribonucleic acid metabolism of aging mouse tissues with particular reference to prostate gland. *Biochem. J.* 110: 79–86, 1968.
214. MAINWARING, W. I. The effect of age on protein synthesis in mouse liver. *Biochem. J.* 113: 869–878, 1969.
215. MAKRIDES, S. C. Protein synthesis and degradation during aging and senescence. *Biol. Rev. Camb. Philos. Soc.* 58: 343–422, 1983.
216. MAKRIDES, S. C., and J. GOLDTHWAITE. The content and size distribution of membrane-bound and free polyribosomes in mouse liver during aging. *Mech. Ageing Dev.* 27: 111–134, 1984.
217. MALLONEE, R. J., N. E. GARRISON, and C. M. SELLERS. Quantity and translational efficiency of liver microsomes in young and old rats following partial hepatectomy. *Comp. Biochem. Physiol.* 72B: 275–281, 1982.
218. MANJULA, and R. M. SUNDARI. Variation in transfer ribonucleic acid population in liver of young, adult, and old female albino rats. *Indian J. Biochem. Biophys.* 18: 192–197, 1981.
219. MARCUS, D. L., N. G. IBRAHIM, and M. L. FREEDMAN. Age-related decline in the biosynthesis of mitochondrial inner membrane proteins. *Exp. Gerontol.* 17: 333–341, 1982.
220. MARCUS, D. L., G. LEW, N. GRUENSPECHT-FAHAM, and M. L. FREEDMAN. Effect of inhibitors and stimulators on isolated liver cell mitochondrial protein synthesis from young and old rats. *Exp. Gerontol.* 17: 429–435, 1982.
221. MARIOTTI, D., and R. RUSCITTO. Age-related changes of accuracy and efficiency of protein synthesis machinery in rat. *Biochim. Biophys. Acta* 475: 96–102, 1977.
222. MARTIN, H., and R. MARTIN. RNA metabolism and ageing. *Akt. Gerontol.* 7: 247–252, 1977.
223. MARTINOLI, M. G., J. OUELLET, E. RHÁEAUME, and G. PELLETIER. Growth hormone and somatostatin gene expression in adult and aging rats as measured by quantitative in situ hybridization. *Neuroendocrinology* 54: 607–615, 1991.
224. MASORO, E. J. Nutrition and aging: a current assessment. *J. Nutr.* 115: 842–848, 1985.
225. MASORO, E. J. Food restriction in rodents: an evaluation of its role in the study of aging. *J. Gerontol.* 43: B59–B64, 1988.
226. MASORO, E. J. Retardation of aging processes by food restriction: an experimental tool. *Am. J. Clin. Nutr.* 55: 1250S–1252S, 1992.
227. MATOCHA, M. F., J. W. COSGROVE, J. R. ATACK, and S. I. RAPOPORT. Selective elevation of c-myc transcript levels in the liver of the aging fischer-344 rat. *Biochem. Biophys. Res. Commun.* 147: 1–7, 1987.
228. MAYS, L. L., A. E. LAWRENCE, R. W. HO, and S. ACKLEY. Age-related changes in function of transfer ribonucleic acid of rat livers. *FASEB J.* 38: 1984–1988, 1979.
229. MAYS, P. K., R. J. MCANULTY, and G. J. LAURENT. Age-related changes in rates of protein synthesis and degradation in rat tissues. *Mech. Ageing Dev.* 59: 229–241, 1991.
230. MAYS-HOOPES, L., W. CHAO, H. C. BUTCHER, and R. C. HUANG. Decreased methylation of the major mouse long interspersed repeated DNA during aging and in myeloma cells. *Dev. Genet.* 7: 65–73, 1986.
231. MAYS-HOOPES, L. L. Macromolecular methylation during aging. In: *Review of Biological Research in Aging,* edited by M. Rothstein. New York: Alan R. Liss, 1985, p. 361–393.
232. MAYS-HOOPES, L. L. DNA methylation in aging and cancer. *J. Gerontol.* 44: 35–36, 1989.
233. MAYS-HOOPES, L. L., A. BROWN, and R. C. HUANG. Methylation and rearrangement of mouse intracisternal A particle genes in development, aging, myeloma. *Mol. Cell. Biol.* 3: 1371–1380, 1983.
234. MAYS-HOOPES, L. L., G. CLELAND, J. BOCHANTIN, D. KALUNIAN, J. MILLER, W. WILSON, M. K. WOND, and D. JOHNSON. Function and fidelity of aging tRNA: in vivo acylation, analog discrimination, synthetase binding, and in vitro translation. *Mech. Ageing Dev.* 22: 135–149, 1983.
235. MCKAY, J. J., R. S. DANIELS, and A. R. HIPKISS. Breakdown of aberrant protein in rabbit reticulocytes decreases with cell age. *Biochem. J.* 188: 279–283, 1980.
236. MCMARTIN, D. N., and L. M. SCHEDBAUER. Incorporation of [$_{14}$C]leucine into protein and tubulin by brain slices from young and old mice. *J. Gerontol.* 30: 132–136, 1975.
237. MEDVEDEV, Z. A. Chromatin proteins and cellular ageing. In: *Biomedical and Morphological Aspects of Ageing,* edited by J. W. Rohen, 1981, p. 125–148.
238. MEDVEDEV, Z. A. Age changes of chromatin. A review. *Mech. Ageing Dev.* 28: 139–154, 1984.
239. MEDVEDEV, Z. A. Age-related changes of transcription and RNA processing. In: *Drugs and Aging,* edited by D. Platt. New York: Springer-Verlag 1986, p. 1–19.
240. MEERSON, F. Z., M. P. JAVICH, and M. I. LERMAN. Decrease in the rate of RNA and protein synthesis and degradation in the myocardium under long-term compensatory hyperfunction and on aging. *J. Mol. Cell. Cardiol.* 10: 145–159, 1978.
241. MENZIES, R. A., and P. H. GOLD. The apparent turnover of mitochondria, ribosomes and sRNA of the brain in young adult and aged rats. *J. Neurochem.* 19: 1671–1683, 1972.
242. MENZIES, R. A., G. D. PRESS, and B. L. STREHLER. Nucleic acid synthesis by old and young adult rat marrow cells in vitro. *Biochim. Biophys. Acta* 145: 178–180, 1967.
243. MERRY, B. J., and A. M. HOLEHAN. Effect of age and restricted feeding on polypeptide chain assembly kinetics in liver protein synthesis in vivo. *Mech. Ageing Dev.* 58: 139–150, 1991.
244. MERRY, B. J., A. M. HOLEHAN, S. E. LEWIS, and D. F. GOLDSPINK. the effects of ageing and chronic dietary restriction on in vivo hepatic protein synthesis in the rat. *Mech. Ageing Dev.* 39: 189–199, 1987.
245. MERRY, B. J., S. E. LEWIS, and D. F. GOLDSPINK. The influence of age and chronic restricted feeding on protein synthesis in the small intestine of the rat. *Exp. Gerontol.* 27: 191–200, 1992.

246. MESCO, E. R., J. A. JOSEPH, M. J. BLAKE, and G. S. ROTH. Loss of D_2 receptors during aging is partially due to decreased levels of mRNA. *Brain Res.* 545: 355–357, 1991.
247. MHATRE, M. C., G. FERNANDES, and M. K. TICKU. Aging reduces the mRNA of α_1 $GABA_A$ receptor subunit in rat cerebral cortex. *Eur. J. Pharmacol. Mol. Pharmacol.* 208: 171–174, 1991.
248. MILLER, J. K., R. BOLLA, and W. D. DENCKLA. Age-associated changes in initiation of ribonucleic acid synthesis in isolated rat liver nuclei. *Biochem. J.* 188: 55–60, 1980.
249. MILLWARD, D. J. The regulation of muscle-protein turnover in growth and development. *Biochem. Soc. Trans.* 6: 494–499, 1978.
250. MINTY, A. J., and F. GROSS. Coding potential of non-polyadenylated messenger RNA in mouse friend cells. *J. Mol. Biol.* 139: 61–83, 1980.
251. MIYAMURA, Y., R. TAWA, A. KOIZUMI, Y. UEHARA, A. KURISHITA, H. SAKURAI, S. KAMIYAMA, and T. ONO. Effects of energy restriction on age-associated changes of DNA methylation in mouse liver. *Mutat. Res.* 295: 63–69, 1993.
252. MOHAN, S., and E. RADHA. Age related changes in muscle protein degradation. *Mech. Ageing Dev.* 7: 81–87, 1978.
253. MOLDAVE, K., J. HARRIS, W. SABO, and I. SADNIK. Protein synthesis and aging: studies with cell-free mammalian systems. *FASEB J.* 38: 1979–1983, 1979.
254. MOORE, R. E., T. L. GOLDSWORTHY, and H. C. PITOL. Turnover of 3'-polyadenylate-containing RNA in livers from aged, partially hepatectomized, neonatal, and Morris 5123C hepatoma-bearing rats. *Cancer Res.* 40: 1449–1457, 1980.
255. MORI, N., K. HIRUTA, Y. FUNATSU, and S. GOTO. Codon recognition fidelity of ribosomes at the first and second positions does not decrease during aging. *Mech. Ageing Dev.* 22: 1–10, 1983.
256. MORI, N., D. MIZUNO, and S. GOTO. Conservation of ribosomal fidelity during ageing. *Mech. Ageing Dev.* 10: 379–398, 1979.
257. MORTIMORE, G. E., and A. R. POSO. Intracellular protein catabolism and its control during nutrient deprivation and supply. *Annu. Rev. Nutr.* 7: 539–564, 1987.
258. MOSONI, L., M.-L. HOULIER, P. P. MIRAND, G. BAYLE, and J. GRIZARD. Effect of amino acids alone or with insulin on muscle and liver protein synthesis in adult and old rats. *Am. J. Physiol.* 264 (*Endocrinol. Metab.* 27): E614–E620, 1993.
259. MOTE, P. L., J. M. GRIZZLE, R. L. WALFORD, and S. R. SPINDLER. Age-related down regulation of hepatic cytochrome P_1-450, P_3-450, catalase and CuZn-superoxide dismutase RNA. *Mech. Ageing Dev.* 53: 101–110, 1990.
260. MOTE, P. L., J. M. GRIZZLE, R. L. WALFORD, and S. R. SPINDLER. Influence of age and caloric restriction on expression of hepatic genes for xenobiotic and oxygen metabolizing enzymes in the mouse. *J. Gerontol.* 46: B95–B100, 1991a.
261. MOTE, P. L., J. M. GRIZZLE, R. L. WALFORD, and S. R. SPINDLER. Aging alters hepatic expression of insulin receptor and c-*jun* mRNA in the mouse. *Mutat. Res.* 256: 7–12, 1991b.
262. MOUDGIL, P. G., J. R. COOK, and D. E. BUETOW. The proportion of ribosomes active in protein synthesis and the content of polyribosomal poly(A)-containing RNA in adult and senescent rat livers. *Gerontology* 25: 322–326, 1979.
263. MURTY, C. V., M. A. MANCINI, B. CHATTERJEE, and A. K. ROY. Changes in transcriptional activity and matrix association of α_{2u}-globulin gene family in the rat liver during maturation and aging. *Biochim. Biophys. Acta* 949: 27–34, 1988.
264. NAGEL, J. E., R. K. CHOPRA, F. J. CHREST, M. T. MCCOY, E. L. SCHNEIDER, N. J. HOLBROOK, and W. H. ADLER. Decreased proliferation, interleukin 2 synthesis, and interleukin 2 receptor expression are accompanied by decreased mRNA expression in phytohemagglutinin-stimulated cells from elderly donors. *J. Clin. Invest.* 81: 1096–1102, 1988.
265. NAKAMURA, K., P. H. DUFFY, M.-H. LU, A. TURTURRO, and R. W. HART. The effect of dietary restriction on MYC protooncogene expression in mice: a preliminary study. *Mech. Ageing Dev.* 48: 199–205, 1989.
266. NAKAZAWA, T., N. MORI, and S. GOTO. Functional deterioration of mouse liver ribosomes during aging: translational activity and activity for formation of the 47S initiation complex. *Mech. Ageing Dev.* 26: 241–251, 1984.
267. NELSON, J. F., M. BENDER, and B. S. SCHACHTER. Age-related changes in proopiomelanocortin messenger ribonucleic acid levels in hypothalamus and pituitary of female C57BL/6J mice. *Endocrinology* 123: 340–344, 1988.
268. NEUMEISTER, J. A., and G. C. WEBSTER. Changes in the levels and the rate of synthesis of transfer RNA in tissues of mice of different ages. *Mech. Ageing Dev.* 16: 319–326, 1981.
269. NIEDERMULLER, H. Effects of aging on the recycling via the pentose cycle on the kinetics of glycogen and protein metabolism in various organs of the rat. *Arch. Gerontol. Geriatr.* 5: 305–316, 1986.
270. NIEDZWIECKI, A., and J. E. FLEMING. Changes in protein turnover after heat shock are related to accumulation of abnormal proteins in aging *Drosophila melanogaster*. *Mech. Ageing Dev.* 52: 295–304, 1990.
271. OBENRADER, M., J. CHEN, P. OVE, and A. I. LANSING. Functional regeneration in liver of old rats after partial hepatectomy. *Exp. Gerontol.* 9: 181–190, 1974.
272. OBLED, C., and M. ARNAL. Age-related changes in whole-body amino acid kinetics and protein turnover in rats. *J. Nutr.* 121: 1990–1998, 1991.
273. OGO, A., M. HAJI, M. OHASHI, and H. NAWATA. Decreased expression of cytochrome P450 17α-hydroxylase mRNA in senescent bovine adrenal gland. *Gerontology* 37: 262–271, 1991.
274. OGRODNIK, J. P., J. H. WULF, and R. G. CUTLER. Altered protein hypothesis of mammalian ageing processes-II. Discrimination ratio of methionine vs. ethionine in the synthesis of ribosomal protein and RNA of C57BL/6J mouse liver. *Exp. Gerontol.* 10: 119–136, 1975.
275. OKA, Y., T. ASANO, K. TSUKUDA, H. KATAGIRI, H. ISHIHARA, K. INUKAI, and Y. YAZAKI. Expression of glucose transporter isoforms with aging. *Gerontology* 38: 3–9, 1992.
276. OKADA, A. A., and J. F. DICE. Altered degradation of intracellular proteins in aging human fibroblasts. *Mech. Ageing Dev.* 26: 341–356, 1984.
277. ONO, T., and R. G. CUTLER. Age-dependent relaxation of gene repression. Increase of endogenous murine leukemia virus-related RNA in brain and liver of mice. *Proc. Natl. Acad. Sci. U.S.A.* 75: 4431–4435, 1978.
278. ONO, T., R. DEAN, S. K. CHATTOPADHYAY, and R. G. CUTLER. Dysdifferentiative nature of aging: age-dependent expression of MULV and globin genes in thymus, liver and brain in the AKR mouse strain. *Gerontology* 31: 362–372, 1985.
279. ONO, T., N. TAKAHASHI, and S. OKADA. Age-associated changes in DNA methylation and mRNA level of the c-myc gene in spleen and liver of mice. *Mutat. Res.* 219: 39–50, 1989.
280. ONO, T., R. TAWA, K. SHINYA, S. HIROSE, and S. OKADA. Methylation of the c-myc gene changes during aging process of mice. *Biochem. Biophys. Res. Commun.* 139: 1299–1304, 1986.
281. ONO, T., S. YAMAMOTO, A. KURISHITA, K. YAMAMOTO, Y. YAMAMOTO, Y. UJENO, K. SAGISAKA, Y. FUKUI, M. MIYAMOTO, R. TAWA, S. HIROSE, and S. OKADA. Comparison of age-asso-

ciated changes of c-*myc* gene methylation in liver between man and mouse. *Mutat. Res.* 237: 239–246, 1990.
282. ORGEL, L. E. The maintenance of the accuracy of protein synthesis and its relevance to ageing. *Proc. Natl. Acad. Sci. U.S.A.* 49: 517–521, 1963.
283. OVE, P., M. OBENRADER, and A. I. LANSING. Synthesis and degradation of liver proteins in young and old rats. *Biochim. Biophys. Acta* 277: 211–221, 1972.
284. OWENBY, R. K., M. P. SULBERG, and B. JACOBSON. Alteration of the Q family of transfer RNAs in adult *Drosophila malanogaster* as a function of age, nutrition, and genotype. *Mech. Ageing Dev.* 11: 91–103, 1979.
285. PAGANI, F., L. ZAGATO, D. COVIELLO, and C. VERGANI. Alternative splicing of fibronectin pre-mRNA during aging. *Ann. N.Y. Acad. Sci.* 663: 477–478, 1992.
286. PAGANI, F., L. ZAGATO, J. A. M. MAIER, G. RAGNOTTI, D. A. COVIELLO, and C. VERGANI. Expression and Alternative splicing of fibronectin mRNA in human diploid endothelial cells during aging in vitro. *Biochim. Biophys. Acta* 1173: 172–178, 1993.
287. PAGANI, F., L. ZAGATO, C. VERGANI, G. CASARI, A. SIDOLI, and F. E. BARALLE. Tissue-specific splicing pattern of fibronectin messenger RNA precursor during development and aging in rat. *J. Cell Biol.* 113: 1223–1230, 1991.
288. PAHLAVANI, M. A., H. T. CHEUNG, N. S. CAI, and A. RICHARDSON. Influence of dietary restriction and aging and gene expression in the immune system of rats. In: *Biomedical Advances in Aging*, edited by A. L. Goldstein. New York: Plenum, 1990, p. 259–270.
289. PARDUE, S., K. GROSHAN, J. D. RAESE, and M. MORRISON-BOGORAD. Hsp70 mRNA induction is reduced in neurons of aged rat hippocampus after thermal stress. *Neurobiol. Aging* 13: 661–672, 1992.
290. PARK, G. H., and D. E. BUETOW. RNA synthesis by nuclei and chromatin isolated from adult and senescent Wistar rat liver. *Gerontology* 36: 61–75, 1990a.
291. PARK, G. H., and D. E. BUETOW. RNA synthesis by hepatocytes isolated from adult and senescent Wistar rat liver. *Gerontology* 36: 76–83, 1990b.
292. PARK, G. H., and D. E. BUETOW. Genes for insulin-like growth factors I and II are expressed in senescent rat tissues. *Gerontology* 37: 310–316, 1991.
293. PARKER, J., J. FLANAGAN, J. MURPHY, and J. GALLANT. On the accuracy of protein synthesis in *Drosophila melanogaster*. *Mech. Ageing Dev.* 16: 127–139, 1981.
294. PEIFFER, A., N. BARDEN, and M. J. MEANEY. Age-related changes in glucocorticoid receptor binding and mRNA levels in the rat brain and pituitary. *Neurobiol. Aging* 12: 475–479, 1991.
295. PELEG, I., Z. GREENFELD, H. COOPERMAN, and S. SHOSHAN. Type I and type III collagen mRNA levels in kidney regions of old and young rats. *Matrix* 13: 281–287, 1993.
296. PLUSKAL, M. G., M. MOREYRA, R. C. BURINI, and V. R. YOUNG. Protein synthesis studies in skeletal muscle of aging rats. I. alterations in nitrogen composition and protein synthesis using a crude polyribosome and pH 5 enzyme system. *J. Gerontol.* 39: 385–391, 1984.
297. POST, D. J., K. C. CARTER, and J. PAPACONSTANTINOU. The effect of aging on constitutive mRNA levels and lipopolysaccharide inducibility of acute phase genes. *Ann. N.Y. Acad. Sci.* 621: 66–77, 1991.
298. PRASANNA, H. R., and R. S. LANE. Protein degradation in aged nematodes (*Turbatrix aceti*). *Biochem. Biophys. Res. Commun.* 86: 552–559, 1979.
299. PUGH, B. F., and R. TIJAN. Mechanism of transcriptional activation by Sp1: evidence for coactivators. *Cell* 61: 1187–1197, 1990.
300. RAO, G., E. XIA, M. J. NADAKAVUKAREN, and A. RICHARDSON. Effect of dietary restriction on the age-dependent changes in the expression of antioxidant enzymes in rat liver. *J. Nutr.* 120: 602–609, 1990.
301. RAO, G., E. XIA, and A. RICHARDSON. Effect of age on the expression of antioxidant enzymes in male Fischer F344 rats. *Mech. Ageing Dev.* 53: 49–60, 1990.
302. RATH, P. C., and M. S. KANUNGO. Age-related changes in the expression of cytochrome P-450 (b+e) gene in the rat after phenobarbitone administration. *Biochem. Biophys. Res. Commun.* 157: 1403–1409, 1988.
303. RATH, P. C., and M. S. KANUNGO. Methylation of repetitive DNA sequences in the brain during aging of the rat. *FEBS Lett.* 244: 193–198, 1989.
304. RATTAN, S. I. Protein synthesis and the components of protein synthetic machinery during cellular ageing. *Mutat. Res.* 256: 115–125, 1991.
305. RATTAN, S. I., J. CAVALLIUS, G. K. HARTVIGSEN, and B. F. CLARK. Amounts of active elongation factor 1 and its activity in livers of mice during aging. In: *Modern Trends in Aging Research*, edited by Y. Courtois et al. Rijswijk, Netherlands: INSERM-EURAGE/Libbey, 1986, p. 135–147.
306. RATTAN, S. I., A. DERVENTZI, and B. F. CLARK. Protein synthesis, posttranslational modifications, and aging. *Ann. N.Y. Acad. Sci.* 663: 48–62, 1992.
307. RATTAN, S. I., W. F. WARD, M. GLENTING, L. SVENDSEN, B. RIIS, and B. F. CLARK. Dietary calorie restriction does not affect the levels of protein elongation factors in rat livers during aging. *Mech. Ageing Dev.* 58: 85–91, 1991.
308. REIS, R. J. Ribosomes from aging mice are not generally deficient in cell-free protein synthesis. *Mech. Ageing Dev.* 17: 311–320, 1981.
309. REITZ, M. S., JR., and D. R. SANADI. An aspect of translational control of protein synthesis in aging: changes in the isoaccepting forms of tRNA in Turbatrix aceti. *Exp. Gerontol.* 7: 119–129, 1972.
310. REZNICK, A. Z., and D. GERSHON. The effect of age on the protein degradation system in the nematode *Turbatrix aceti*. *Mech. Ageing Dev.* 11: 403–415, 1979.
311. REZNICK, A. Z., L. LAVIE, H. E. GERSHON, and D. GERSHON. Age-associated accumulation of altered FDP aldolase B in mice. *FEBS Lett.* 128: 221–224, 1981.
312. RICCA, G. A., D. S. LIU, J. J. CONIGLIO, and A. RICHARDSON. Rates of protein synthesis by hepatocytes isolated from rats of various ages. *J. Cell Physiol.* 97: 137–146, 1978.
313. RICHARDSON, A. The relationship between aging and protein synthesis, In: *CRC Handbook of Biochemistry in Aging*, edited by J. R. Florini. Boca Raton, FL: CRC Press, 1981, p. 79–101.
314. RICHARDSON, A. The effect of age and nutrition on protein synthesis by cells and tissues from mammals. In: *CRC Handbook of Nutrition and Aging*, edited by R. R. Watson. Boca Raton, FL: CRC Press, 1985, p. 31–48.
315. RICHARDSON, A., and M. C. BIRCHENALL-SPARKS. Age-related changes in protein synthesis. In: *Biological Research in Aging*, edited by M. Rothstein. New York: Alan R. Liss, 1983, p. 255–273.
316. RICHARDSON, A., and H. T. CHEUNG. The relationship between age-related changes in gene expression, protein turnover, and the responsiveness of an organism to stimuli. *Life Sci.* 31: 605–613, 1982.
317. RICHARDSON, A., and J. MYERS. A comparison of the cell-free protein synthetic activities of testicular tissue obtained from rats and mice of various ages. *Comp. Biochem. Physiol.* 71B: 709–712, 1982.
318. RICHARDSON, A., and I. SEMSEI. Effect of aging on translation and transcription. In: *Review of Biological Research in Aging*,

vol. 3, edited by M. Rothstein. New York: Alan R. Liss, 1987, p. 467–483.
319. RICHARDSON, A., M. C. BIRCHENALLNM-SPARKS, and J. L. STAECKER. Aging and transcription. In: *Biological Research in Aging,* edited by M. Rothstein. New York: Alan R. Liss, 1983, p. 275–294.
320. RICHARDSON, A., M. C. BIRCHENALL-SPARKS, J. L. STAECKER, J. HARDWICK, and D. S. LIU. The transcription of various types of ribonucleic acid by hepatocytes isolated from rats of various ages. *J. Gerontol.* 37: 666–672, 1982.
321. RICHARDSON, A., J. A. BUTLER, M. S. RUTHERFORD, I. SEMSEI, M. Z. GU, G. FERNANDES, and W. H. CHIANG. Effect of age and dietary restriction on the expression of α_{2u}-globulin. *J. Biol. Chem.* 262: 12821–12825, 1987.
322. RICHARDSON, A., M. S. ROBERTS, and M. S. RUTHERFORD. Aging and gene expression. In: *Review Biological Research in Aging,* vol. 2, edited by M. Rothstein. New York: Alan R. Liss, 1985, p. 395–419.
323. RICHARDSON, A., M. S. RUTHERFORD, M. C. BIRCHENALL-SPARKS, M. S. ROBERTS, W. T. WU, and H. T. CHEUNG. Levels of specific messenger RNA species as a function of age. In: *Molecular Biology of Aging: Gene Stability and Gene Expression,* edited by R. S. Sohal, L. Birnbaum, and R. G. Cutler. New York: Raven Press, 1985, p. 229–241.
324. RICHTER, V. Turnover of lipogenic enzymes of rat liver in dependence on age. *Acta. Biol. Med. Germ.* 36: 1833–1836, 1977.
325. RICKETTS, W. G., M. C. BIRCHENALL-SPARKS, J. P. HARDWICK, and A. RICHARDSON. Effect of age and dietary restriction on protein synthesis by isolated kidney cells. *J. Cell. Physiol.* 125: 492–498, 1985.
326. RIIS, B., S. I. RATTAN, J. CAVALLIUS, and B. F. CLARK. Levels of active elongation factor-2 in rat livers during ageing. In: *The Liver, Metabolism and Ageing,* edited by K. W. Woodhouse, C. Yelland, and O. F. W. James. Rijswijk, Netherlands: INSERM-EURAGE/Libbey, 1989, p. 117–124.
327. ROBERTS, D. M., and P. GRIMINGER. Studies concerning the protein metabolism of primary kidney cells isolated from rats of various ages. *Fed. Proc.* 37: 884, 1978.
328. ROCKSTEIN, M., and G. T. BAKER. Effects of X-irradiation of pupae on aging of the thoracic flight muscle of the adult house fly *Musca domestica* 1. *Mech. Ageing Dev.* 3: 271–278, 1974.
329. RODRIGUEZ, C., A. MENENDEZ-PELAEZ, K. A. HOWES, and R. J. REITER. Age and food restriction alter the porphyrin concentration and mRNA levels for 5-aminolevulinate synthase in rat harderian gland. *Life Sci.* 51: 1891–1897, 1992.
330. ROTHSTEIN, M. The formation of altered enzymes in ageing animals. *Mech. Ageing Dev.* 9: 197–202, 1979.
331. ROTHSTEIN, M. Enzymes and altered proteins. In: *Biochemical Approaches to Aging,* edited by M. Rothstein. New York: Academic Press, 1982, p. 213–255.
332. ROTHSTEIN, M. Enzymes, enzyme alteration, and protein turnover. In: *Review of Biological Research in Aging,* edited by M. Rothstein. New York: Alan R. Liss, 1983, p. 305–314.
333. ROTHSTEIN, M., and S. C. SEIFERT. RNA synthesis. In: *Handbook of Biochemistry in Aging,* edited by J. R. Florini. Boca Raton, FL: CRC Press, 1981, p. 51–63.
334. ROY, A. K., S. T. NATH, N. M. MOTWANI, and B. CHATTERJEE. Age-dependent regulation of the polymorphic forms of α_{2u}-globulin. *J. Biol. Chem.* 258: 10123–10127, 1983.
335. SALIH, M. A., D. C. HERBERT, and D. N. KALU. Evaluation of the molecular and cellular basis for modulation of thyroid c-cell hormones by aging and food restriction. *Mech. Ageing Dev.* 70: 1–21, 1993.
336. SAMIS, H. V., V. J. WULFF, and J. A. FALZONE. The incorporation of [H-3]-cytidine into ribonucleic acid of liver nuclei of young and old rats. *Biochim. Biophys. Acta* 91: 223–232, 1964.

337. SATO, A. I., E. L. SCHNEIDER, and D. B. DANNER. Aberrant gene expression and aging: examination of tissue-specific mRNAs in young and old rats. *Mech. Ageing Dev.* 54: 1–12, 1990.
338. SAVU, L., R. VRANCKX, M. ROUAZE-ROMET, M. MAYA, E. A. NUNEZ, J. TRÉTON, and I. L. FLINK. A senescence up-regulated protein: the rat thyroxine-binding globulin (TBG). *Biochim. Biophys. Acta* 1097: 19–22, 1991.
339. SAWADA, N. Hepatocytes from old rats retain responsiveness of c-myc expression to EGF in primary culture but do not enter s phase. *Exp. Cell Res.* 181: 584–588, 1989.
340. SEMSEI, I., S. MA, and R. G. CUTLER. Tissue and age specific expression of the myc proto-oncogene family throughout the life span of the C57BL/6J mouse strain. *Oncogene* 4: 465–471, 1989.
341. SENSEI, I., G. RAO, and A. RICHARDSON. Changes in the expression of superoxide dismutase and catalase as a function of age and dietary restriction. *Biochem. Biophys. Res. Commun.* 164: 620–625, 1989.
342. SEMSEI, I., G. RAO, and A. RICHARDSON. Expression of superoxide dismutase and catalase in rat brain as a function of age. *Mech. Ageing Dev.* 58: 13–19, 1991.
343. SEMSEI, I., F. SZESZAK, and I. ZS.-NAGY. In vivo studies on the age-dependent decrease of the rates of total and mRNA synthesis in the brain cortex of rats. *Arch. Gerontol. Geriatr.* 1: 29–42, 1982.
344. SESHADRI, T., and J. CAMPISI. Repression of c-fos transcription and an altered genetic program in senescent human fibroblasts. *Science* 247: 205–209, 1990.
345. SHAIN, S. A., and A. L. MOSS. Aging in the AXC rat: equivalence of the rates of inactivation of L-ornithine decarboxylase and S-adenosyl-L-methionine decarboxylase in prostate of young and aged rats. *Endocrinology* 109: 1192–1195, 1981.
346. SHARMA, H. K., H. R. PRASSANA, R. S. LANE, and M. ROTHSTEIN. The effect of age on enolase turnover in the free-living nematode, *Turbatrix aceti*. *Arch. Biochem. Biophys.* 194: 275–282, 1979.
347. SHARP, G. S., S. LASSEN, S. SHANKMAN, J. W. HAZLET, and M. S. KENDIS. Studies of protein retention and turnover using nitrogen-15 as a tag. *J. Nutr.* 63: 155–162, 1957.
348. SHEPHERD, J. C. W., U. WALLDORF, P. HUG, and W. J. GEHRING. Fruit flies with additional expression of elongation factor EF-1α live longer. *Proc. Natl. Acad. Sci. U.S.A.* 86: 7520–7521, 1989.
349. SHIKAMA, N., R. ACKERMANN, and C. BRACK. Protein synthesis elongation factor EF-1α expression and longevity in *Drosophila melanogaster*. *Proc. Natl. Acad. Sci. U.S.A.* In press, 1994.
350. SIERRA, F., S. COEYTAUX, M. JUILLERAT, C. RUFFIEUX, J. GAULDIE, and Y. GUIGOZ. Serum T-kininogen levels increase two to four months before death. *J. Biol. Chem.* 267: 10665–10669, 1992.
351. SIERRA, F., G. H. FEY, and Y. GUIGOZ. T-kininogen gene expression is induced during aging. *Mol. Cell. Biol.* 9: 5610–5616, 1989.
352. SIKORA, E., B. KAMINSKA, E. RADZISZEWSKA, and L. KACZMAREK. Loss of transcription factor AP-1 DNA binding activity during lymphocyte aging in vivo. *FEBS Lett.* 312: 179–182, 1992.
353. SINGH, A., S. SINGH, and M. S. KANUNGO. Conformation and expression of the albumin gene of young and old rats. *Mol. Biol. Rep.* 14: 251–254, 1990.
354. SINGH, S., and M. S. KANUNGO. Changes in expression and CRE binding proteins of the fibronectin gene during aging of the rat. *Biochem. Biophys. Res. Commun.* 193: 440–445, 1993.
355. SINGHAL, R. P., and R. A. KOPPER. Changes in transfer RNAs in development and aging. *FASEB J.* 39: 20–23, 1980.
356. SINGHAL, R. P., R. A. KOPPER, S. NISHIMURA, and N. SHINDO-

OKADA. Modification of guanine to queuine in transfer RNAs during development and aging. *Biochem. Biophys. Res. Commun.* 99: 120–126, 1981.
357. SINGHAL, R. P., L. L. MAYS-HOOPES, and G. L. EICHHORN. DNA methylation in aging of mice. *Mech. Ageing Dev.* 41: 199–210, 1987.
358. SLAGBOOM, P. E., W. J. DE LEEUW, and J. VIJG. mRNA levels and methylation patterns of the tyrosine aminotransferase gene in aging inbred rats. *FEBS Lett.* 269: 128–130, 1990a.
359. SLAGBOOM, P. E., W. J. DE LEEUW, and J. VIJG. Messenger RNA levels and methylation patterns of GAPDH and β-actin genes in rat liver, spleen and brain in relation to aging. *Mech. Ageing Dev.* 53: 243–257, 1990b.
360. SLAGBOOM, P. E., A. G. UITTERLINDEN, and J. VIJG. Methylation status of cKi-ras and MHC genes in rat pituitary glands during aging and tumorigenesis. *Aging* 3: 141–146, 1991.
361. SMITH, C. D., J. M. CARNEY, P. E. STARKE-REED, C. N. OLIVER, E. R. STADTMAN, R. A. FLOYD, and W. R. MARKESBERY. Excess brain protein oxidation and enzyme dysfunction in normal aging and in Alzheimer disease. *Proc. Natl. Acad. Sci. U.S.A.* 88: 10540–10543, 1991.
362. SOBEL, H., and R. BOWMAN. Protein metabolism in aging mice. *J. Gerontol.* 26: 558–560, 1971.
363. SOJAR, H. T., and M. ROTHSTEIN. Protein synthesis by liver ribosomes from aged rats. *Mech. Ageing Dev.* 35: 47–57, 1986.
364. SONG, C. S., T. R. RAO, W. F. DEMYAN, M. A. MANCINI, B. CHATTERJEE, and A. K. ROY. Androgen receptor messenger ribonucleic acid (mRNA) in the rat liver: changes in mRNA levels during maturation, aging, and calorie restriction. *Endocrinology* 128: 349–356, 1991.
365. SONG, L., J. M. STEPHENS, S. KITTUR, G. D. COLLINS, J. E. NAGEL, P. H. PEKALA, and W. H. ADLER. Expression of c-fos, c-jun, and jun B in peripheral blood lymphocytes from young and elderly adults. *Mech. Ageing Dev.* 65: 149–156, 1992.
366. SONNTAG, W. E., V. W. HYLKA, and J. MEITES. Growth hormone restores protein synthesis in skeletal muscle of old rats. *J. Gerontol.* 40: 689–694, 1985.
367. SONNTAG, W. E., J. E. LENHAM, and R. L. INGRAM. Effects of aging and dietary restriction on tissue protein synthesis: relationship to plasma insulin-like growth factor-1. *J. Gerontol.* 47: B159–B163, 1992.
368. SORGER, P. K. Heat shock factor and the heat shock response. *Cell* 65: 363–366, 1991.
369. SORIERO, A. A. Autoradiographic study of the effect of estrogen on in vivo incorporation of [H-3]-uridine into uterine smooth muscle and stromal RNA in the aging ovariectomized mouse. *J. Gerontol.* 35: 167–176, 1980.
370. SPINDLER, S. R., M. D. CREW, P. L. MOTE, J. M. GRIZZLE, and R. L. WALFORD. Dietary energy restriction in mice reduces hepatic expression of glucose-regulated protein 78 (BiP) and 94 mRNA. *J. Nutr.* 120: 1412–1417, 1990.
371. SPINDLER, S. R., J. M. GRIZZLE, R. L. WALFORD, and P. L. MOTE. Aging and restriction of dietary calories increases insulin receptor mRNA, and aging increases glucocorticoid receptor mRNA in the liver of female C3B10RF$_1$ mice. *J. Gerontol.* 46: B233–B237, 1991.
372. STADTMAN, E. R. Biochemical markers of aging. *Exp. Gerontol.* 23: 327–347, 1988.
373. STADTMAN, E. R. Protein oxidation and aging. *Science* 257: 1220–1224, 1992.
374. STADTMAN, E. R., C. N. OLIVER, R. L. LEVINE, L. FUCCI, and A. J. RIVETT. Implication of protein oxidation in protein turnover, aging, and oxygen toxicity. *Basic Life Sci.* 49: 331–339, 1988.
375. STARKE-REED, P. E., and C. N. OLIVER. Protein oxidation and proteolysis during aging and oxidative stress. *Arch. Biochem. Biophys.* 275: 559–567, 1989.
376. STARNES, J. W., R. E. BEYER, and D. W. EDINGTON. Effects of age and cardiac work in vitro on mitochondrial oxidative phosphorilation and [^{3}H]-leucine incorporation. *J. Gerontol.* 36: 130–135, 1981.
377. STARNES, J. W., D. W. EDINGTON, and R. E. BEYER. Myocardial protein synthesis during aging and endurance exercise in rats. *J. Gerontol.* 38: 660–665, 1983.
378. STEWART, D. A., M. R. BLACKMAN, M. A. KOWATCH, D. B. DANNER, and G. S. ROTH. Discordant effects of aging on prolactin and luteinizing hormone-β messenger ribonucleic acid levels in the female rat. *Endocrinology* 126: 773–778, 1992.
379. STRONG, R., M. A. MOORE, C. HALE, W. J. BURKE, H. J. ARMBECHT, and A. RICHARDSON. Age-related changes in adrenal catecholamine content and tyrosine hydroxylase gene expression: effects of dietary restriction. In: *Endocrine Function and Aging*, edited by J. A. Armbrecht, R. Coe, and N. Wongsurawat. Berlin: Springer-Verlag, 1990, p. 218–227.
380. STRONG, R., M. A. MOORE, C. HALE, M. WESSELS-REIKER, H. J. ARMBRECHT, and A. RICHARDSON. Modulation of tyrosine hydroxylase gene expression in the rat adrenal gland by age and reserpine. *Brain Res.* 525: 126–132, 1990.
381. SWISSHELM, K., C. M. DISTECHE, J. THORVALDSEN, A. NELSON, and D. SALK. Age-related increase in methylation of ribosomal genes and inactivation of chromosome-specific rRNA gene clusters in mouse. *Mutat. Res.* 237: 131–146, 1990.
382. TAKAHASHI, R., and S. GOTO. Age-associated accumulation of heat-labile aminoacyl-tRNA synthetases in mice and rats. *Arch. Gerontol. Geriatr.* 6: 73–82, 1987.
383. TAKAHASHI, R., and S. GOTO. Fidelity of aminoacylation by rat-liver tryosyl-tRNA synthetase. *Eur. J. Biochem.* 178: 381–386, 1988.
384. TAKAHASHI, R., N. MORI, and S. GOTO. Accumulation of heat-labile elongation factor 2 in the liver of mice and rats. *Exp. Gerontol.* 20: 325–331, 1985a.
385. TAKAHASHI, R., N. MORI, and S. GOTO. Alteration of aminoacyl tRNA synthetases with age: accumulation of heat-labile enzyme molecules in rat liver, kidney and brain. *Mech. Ageing Dev.* 33: 67–75, 1985b.
386. TAKAHASHI, R., H. SCHUNKERT, S. ISOYAMA, J. Y. WEI, B. NADAL-GINARD, W. GROSSMAN, and S. IZUMO. Age-related differences in the expression of proto-oconogene and contractile protein genes in response to pressure overload in the rat myocardium. *J. Clin. Invest.* 89: 939–946, 1992.
387. TAKAHASHI, S., S. KAWASHIMA, H. SEO, and N. MATSUI. Age-related changes in growth hormone and prolactin messenger RNA levels in the rat. *Endocrinol. Jpn.* 37: 827–840, 1990.
388. TAS, S., and R. L. WALFORD. Influence of disulfide-reducing agents on fractionation of the chromatin complex by endogenous nucleases and deoxyribonuclease I in aging mice. *J. Gerontol.* 37: 673–679, 1982.
389. TAS, S., C. F. TAM, and R. L. WALFORD. Disulfide bonds and the structure of the chromatin complex in relation to aging. *Mech. Ageing Dev.* 12: 65–80, 1980.
390. TAWA, R., S. UENO, K. YAMAMOTO, Y. YAMAMOTO, K. SAGISAKA, R. KATAKURA, T. KAYAMA, T. YOSHIMOTO, H. SAKURAI, and T. ONO. Methylated cytosine level in human liver DNA does not decline in aging process. *Mech. Ageing Dev.* 62: 255–261, 1992.
391. THAKUR, M. K. Age-related changes in the structure and function of chromatin: a review. *Mech. Ageing Dev.* 27: 263–286, 1984.
392. THAKUR, M. K., and J. KAUR. Estrogen-induced synthesis of uterine proteins declines during aging. *Mol. Biol. Rep.* 17: 29–34, 1992a.
393. THAKUR, M. K., and J. KAUR. Methylation of DNA and its modulation by estrogen in the uterus of aging rats. *Cell. Mol. Biol.* 38: 525–532, 1992b.

394. THAKUR, M. K., T. OKA, and Y. NATORI. Gene expression and aging. *Mech. Ageing Dev.* 66: 283–298, 1993.
395. TOLLEFSBOL, T. O., and H. J. COHEN. Decreased protein synthesis of transforming lymphocytes from aged humans. *Mech. Ageing Dev.* 30: 53–62, 1985.
396. TONNA, E. A., and I. J. SINGH. Autoradiographic investigation by aging mouse cartilage cells. *Exp. Gerontol.* 11: 231–241, 1976.
397. TRAVALI, S., G. CARNAZZO, A. M. DISTEFANO, P. MANCIAGLI, C. COSENZA, E. FIDONE, S. PETRALIA, A. BERNARDINI, L. MOTTA, and F. STIVALA. Expression of cell cycle-dependent genes and proliferative state of lymphocytes in aging. *Arch. Gerontol. Geriatr.* 11: 133–139, 1990.
398. TUMER, N., C. HALE, J. LAWLER, and R. STRONG. Modulation of tyrosine hydroxylase gene expression in the rat adrenal gland by exercise: effects of age. *Mol. Brain Res.* 14: 51–56, 1992.
399. UAUY, R., J. C. WINTERER, C. BILMAZES, L. N. HAVERBERG, N. S. SCRIMSHAW, H. N. MUNRO, and V. R. YOUNG. The changing pattern of whole body protein metabolism in aging humans. *J. Gerontol.* 33: 663–671, 1978.
400. UEHARA, Y., O. TETSUYA, A. KURISHITA, H. KOKURYU, and S. OKADA. Age-dependent and tissue-specific changes of DNA methylation within and around the c-fos gene in mice. *Oncogene* 4: 1023–1028, 1989.
401. VAN BEZOOIJEN, C. F., T. GRELL, and D. KNOOK. Albumin synthesis by liver parenchymal cells isolated from young, adult, and old rats. *Biochem. Biophys. Res. Commun.* 31: 513–519, 1976.
402. VAN BEZOOIJEN, C. F., T. GRELL, and D. L. KNOOK. The effect of age on protein synthesis by isolated liver parenchymal cells. *Mech. Ageing Dev.* 6: 293–304, 1977.
403. VANDENHAUTE, J., N. CLAES-RECKINGER, and J. DELCOUR. Age-related functional alteration of mouse liver ribosomes. *Exp. Gerontol.* 18: 355–363, 1983.
404. VAN DER VLIET, P. C., and C. P. VERRIJZER. Bending of DNA by transcription factors. *BioEssays* 15: 25–32, 1993.
405. VEDOVA, F. D., F. FUMAGALLI, G. SACCHETTI, G. RACAGNI, and N. BRUNELLO. Age-related variations in relative abundance of alternative spliced D_2 receptor mRNAs in brain areas of two rat strains. *Mol. Brain Res.* 12: 357–359, 1992.
406. VINAYAK, M. A comparison of tRNA populations of rat liver and skeletal muscle during aging. *Biochem. Int.* 15: 279–285, 1987.
407. VISKUP, R. W., M. BAKER, J. P. HOLBROOK, and R. PENNIALL. Age-associated changes in activities of rat hepatocytes. I. Protein synthesis. *Exp. Aging Res.* 5: 487–496, 1979.
408. WAGGONER, S. M., M. Z. GU, W. H. CHIANG, and A. RICHARDSON. The effect of dietary restriction on the expression of a variety of genes. In: *Genetic Effects on Aging II*, edited by D. E. Harrison. Cadwell, NJ: Telford Press, 1990, p. 255–272.
409. WAGNER, A. P., K. D. BECK, and G. RECK. Neural cell adhesion molecule (NCAM) and N-cadherin mRNA during development and aging: selective reduction in the 7.4-kb and 6.7-kb NCAM mRNA levels in the hippocampus of adult and old rats. *Mech. Ageing Dev.* 62: 201–208, 1992.
410. WALLACH, Z., and D. GERSHON. Altered ribosomal particles in senescent nematodes. *Mech. Ageing Dev.* 3: 225–234, 1974.
411. WANG, E. Characterization of the absence of an unique DNA-binding protein in senescent but not in their young growing and nongrowing counterparts provides the means to mark the final stage of the cellular aging process. *Exp. Gerontol.* 27: 503–517, 1992.
412. WANG, S., S. ZHU, J. A. JOSEPH, and E. E. EL-FAKAHANY. Comparison of the level of mRNA encoding m1 and m2 muscarinic receptors in brains of young and aged rats. *Neurosci. Lett.* 145: 149–152, 1992.
413. WANG, S. Y., and J. W. ROWE. Age-related impairment in the short term regulation of insulin biosynthesis by glucose in rat pancreatic islets. *Endocrinology* 123: 1008–1013, 1988.
414. WARD, W., and A. RICHARDSON. Effect of age on liver protein synthesis and degradation. *Hepatology* 14: 935–948, 1991.
415. WARD, W. F. Enhancement by food restriction of liver protein synthesis in the aging Fischer 344 rat. *J. Gerontol.* 43: B50–B53, 1988a.
416. WARD, W. F. Food restriction enhancement of the proteolytic capacity of aging rat liver. *J. Gerontol.* 43: B121–B124, 1988b.
417. WATTIAUX, J. M., M. LIBION-MANNAERT, and J. DELCOUR. Protein turnover and protein synthesis following actinomycin-D injection as a function of age in *Drosophila melanogaster*. *Gerontologia* 17: 289–299, 1971.
418. WEBER, G., J. MARGETAN, C. E. FINCH, and L. L. MAYS. Brain transfer ribonucleic acid methyltransferases in young adult and old mice. *Exp. Gerontol.* 14: 157–160, 1979.
419. WEBSTER, G. C. Protein synthesis in aging organisms. In: *Molecular Biology of Aging: Gene Stability and Gene Expression*, edited by R. S. Sohal, L. S. Birnbaum, and R. G. Cutler. New York: Raven Press, 1985, p. 263–290.
420. WEBSTER, G. C., and S. L. WEBSTER. Decreased protein synthesis by microsomes from aging *Drosophila melanogaster*. *Exp. Gerontol.* 14: 343–348, 1979.
421. WEBSTER, G. C., and S. L. WEBSTER. Aminocylation of tRNA by cell-free preparations from aging *Drosophila melanogaster*. *Exp. Gerontol.* 16: 487–494, 1981.
422. WEBSTER, G. C., and S. L. WEBSTER. Decline in synthesis of elongation factor one (EF-1) precedes the decreased synthesis of total protein in aging *Drosophila melanogaster*. *Mech. Ageing Dev.* 22: 121–128, 1983.
423. WEBSTER, G. C., V. T. BEACHELL, and S. L. WEBSTER. Differential decrease in protein synthesis by microsomes from aging *Drosophila melanogaster*. *Exp. Gerontol.* 15: 495–497, 1980.
424. WEBSTER, G. C., S. L. WEBSTER, and W. A. LANDIS. The effect of age on the initiation of protein synthesis in *Drosophila melanogaster*. *Mech. Ageing Dev.* 16: 71–79, 1981.
425. WEILAND, N. G., K. SCARBROUGH, and P. M. WISE. Aging abolishes the estradiol-induced suppression and diurnal rhythm of proopiomelanocortin gene expression in the arcuate nucleus. *Endocrinology* 131: 2959–2964, 1992.
426. WELLE, S., C. THORNTON, R. JOZEFOWICZ, and M. STATT. Myofibrillar protein synthesis in young and old men. *Am. J. Physiol.* 264 (*Endocrinol. Metab.* 27): E693–E698, 1993.
427. WELLER, E. M., M. POOT, and H. HOEHN. Induction of replicative senescence by 5-azacytidine: fundamental cell kinetic differences between human diploid fibroblasts and NIH-3T3 cells. *Cell Prolif.* 26: 45–54, 1993.
428. WELLINGER, R., and Y. GUIGOZ. The effect of age on the induction of tyrosine aminotransferase and tryptophan oxygenase genes by physiological stress. *Mech. Ageing Dev.* 34: 203–217, 1986.
429. WESSELS-REIKER, M., C. HALE, and R. STRONG. Molecular biology of information storage in the nervous system during aging. In: *Memory Function and Aging-Related Disorders*, edited by J. E. Morley, R. M. Coe, R. Strong, and G. T. Grossberg. New York: Springer, 1992, p. 22–37.
430. WIEDERANDERS, B., and B. OELKE. The turnover of liver cytosol proteins in very old rats. *Acta Biol. Med. Germ.* 40: 1243–1247, 1981.
431. WIEDERANDERS, B., S. ANSORGE, P. BOHLEY, H. KIRSCHKE, J. LANGNER, and H. HANSON. The age dependence of intracellular proteolysis: changes of the substrate proteins. *Mech. Ageing Dev.* 8: 355–362, 1978.
432. WILDENTHAL, K., and J. S. CRIE. The role of lysosomes and lysosomal enzymes in cardiac protein turnover. *FASEB J.* 39: 37–41, 1980.

433. WILSON, V. L., and P. A. JONES. DNA methylation decreased in aging but not in immortal cells. *Science* 220: 1055–1057, 1983.
434. WILSON, V. L., R. A. SMITH, S. MA, and R. G. CUTLER. Genomic 5-methyldeoxycytidine decreases with age. *J. Biol. Chem.* 262: 9948–9951, 1987.
435. WINTERER, J. C., W. P. STEFFEE, W. DAVY, A. PERERA, R. UAUY, N. S. SCRIMSHAW, and V. R. YOUNG. Whole body protein turnover in aging man. *Exp. Gerontol.* 11: 79–87, 1976.
436. WONG, N. C., H. L. SCHWARTZ, K. STRAIT, and J. H. OPPENHEIMER. Thyroid hormone-, carbohydrate-, and age-dependent regulation of a methylation site in the hepatic S14 gene. *Mol. Endocrinol.* 3: 645–650, 1989.
437. WU, W. T., M. A. PAHLAVANI, H. T. CHEUNG, and A. RICHARDSON. The effect of aging on the expression of interleukin 2 messenger ribonucleic acid. *Cell. Immunol.* 100: 224–231, 1986.
438. WUST, C. J., and L. ROSEN. Aminoacylation and methylation of tRNA as a function of age in the rat. *Exp. Gerontol.* 7: 331–343, 1972.
439. YANG, F., W. E. FRIEDRICHS, J. M. BUCHANAN, D. C. HERBERT, F. J. WEAKER, J. H. BROCK, and B. H. BOWMAN. Tissue specific expression of mouse transferrin during development and aging. *Mech. Ageing Dev.* 56: 187–197, 1990.
440. YOUNG, V. R., W. P. STEFFEE, P. B. PENCHARZ, J. C. WINTERER, and N. S. SCRIMSHAW. Total human body protein synthesis in relation to protein requirements at various ages. *Nature* 253: 192–194, 1975.
441. YOUSEF, M. K., and H. D. JOHNSON. ^{75}-Selenomethionine turnover rate during growth and aging in rats. *Proc. Soc. Exp. Biol. Med.* 133: 1351–1353, 1970.
442. ZEELON, P., H. GERSHON, and D. GERSHON. Inactive enzyme molecules in aging organisms. Nematode fructose-1,6-diphosphate aldolase. *Biochemistry* 12: 1743–1750, 1973.
443. ZS.-NAGY, I., and I. SEMSEI. Centrophenoxine increases the rates of total and mRNA synthesis in the brain cortex of old rats: an explanation of its action in terms of the membrane hypothesis of aging. *Exp. Gerontol.* 19: 171–178, 1984.

10. Aging of long-lived proteins: extracellular matrix (collagens, elastins, proteoglycans) and lens crystallins

DAVID R. SELL
VINCENT M. MONNIER

Institute of Pathology, Case Western Reserve University, Cleveland, Ohio

CHAPTER CONTENTS

Collagens
  Overview
  Methodological difficulties in the assessment of collagen changes during aging
  Hypertension and collagen deposition in relation to the aging process
  Turnover of collagen
    Methodological difficulties in the study of collagen turnover
    Collagen turnover as a function of tissue
    Collagen turnover as a function of age
    Cellular aging in culture in relation to population doublings
  Physical properties of aging collagen
    Solubility
    Thermostability
    Mechanical/tensile strength
    Stiffness
  Measurement of the physical properties of collagen as potential biomarkers of aging
    Biological markers
  Chemical properties of aging collagen
    Cross-links mediated by lysyl oxidase
    Cross-links originating from lipid peroxidation
    Cross-links derived from Maillard/glycation reactions
  Conclusions
Elastin
  Molecular contrasts between elastin and collagen
  Morphological changes in elastin with aging
  Quantitative changes in elastin with aging
    Elastin content and appearance
    Changes in physical properties
    Changes in chemical properties
    Changes in gene expression, synthesis, and turnover
  Conclusions
Proteoglycans
  Biochemical composition
  Aggregating and nonaggregating populations of proteoglycans
  Age-related changes in proteoglycans
  Conclusions
Lens Crystallins
  Overview
  Age-related changes in lens and lens crystallins
    Solubility
    Conformational changes
    Racemization and fragmentation
    Yellowing and fluorescence
    Oxidation
    Nondisulfide covalent cross-links
    Deamidation and deamination
    Glycation
  Changes in enzyme activity
  Mechanisms of crystallin aging
    Weakening of antioxidant defense
    Photooxidative mechanisms of damage to lens crystallins
    Maillard reaction by reducing sugars and ascorbate
  Conclusions
Summation

TISSUES RICH IN LONG-LIVED PROTEINS, such as those of the extracellular matrix (ECM) and the lens, show some of the most pronounced age-related physiological changes. For example, there is with increasing age an increase in arterial rigidity, a loss of lung and skin elasticity, a decrease in joint mobility, a decrease in basement membrane permeability to certain solutes, and loss of accommodation (311, 419). Although, for the most part, precise measurements of the turnover rates of ECM proteins are lacking, it is generally assumed that proteins composing the ECM, such as the collagens, the proteoglycans, and elastin, are very long-lived and undergo, therefore, qualitative changes which underlie the altered function of the aging tissue.

Whereas it has been relatively easy to determine experimentally turnover rates for many cellular proteins, it has been very difficult to demonstrate clear-cut impairments of cellular homeostatic functions in aging (312), except in cells that are postmitotically fixed, such as neurons, red blood cells, and the differentiated, fiber-like cells of the lens. This statement does not apply to cellular responses to specific stimuli such as the T-cell response to mitogens, which is clearly impaired in senescence.

The red blood cell and the fiber-like cells of the lens are unique in that they have to obtain their entire energy through glycolysis since they lack mitochondria. Both lack the machinery for protein synthesis, and their proteins are, therefore, extremely long-lived. In the case of the lens, for example, the nuclear proteins are as old as the individual and are thus prone to postsynthetic chemical and physical modifications. However, the milieu surrounding the ECM and the lens crystallins is very different in that a complex redox system together with a very low oxygen tension prevent oxidative modifications of lens crystallins. In contrast, ECM proteins are exposed to high oxygen tension, but the proteins are very resistant to nonphysiological oxidant changes, being poor in cysteine residues and highly rigid in their conformation. Thus marked differences in the nature of age-related damage are expected between ECM proteins and lens crystallins. Nevertheless, some modifications will be common to both, especially those related to glycation, racemization, fragmentation, and cross-linking.

One of the major focal points for the study of biochemical changes in the aging ECM is that the ECM is thought to provide a window into the fundamental mechanisms of aging. In the 1940s, Bjorksten formulated a cross-linking hypothesis of aging after noting that a protein gel in contact with free aldehyde–containing "tanning agents" caused increased tensile strength, thus reducing rhythmical stretching and relaxation of the gel, which he analogized to the aging process of human arteries (48). Similarly, Verzár (665, 666) demonstrated that the resistance to thermal denaturation of rat tail tendons, composed primarily of collagen, increased with advancing age.

In the 1970s, Kohn and his colleagues (227–229) made two important observations. First, they noted that insoluble collagen became progressively less digestible by collagenase with advancing age and that the loss of digestibility was accelerated by a factor of two in diabetes. Second, they found that the loss of digestibility was higher in short-lived species, dog, than in longer-lived species, such as monkey and human. These observations were of landmark significance in that they suggested *(1)* that study of the nature of collagen cross-linking in aging would reveal an important aspect of a biological aging clock and *(2)* that the ticking rate of such a clock was modulated along the glucose–insulin axis. These concepts have gained in importance in recent years with the demonstration that dietary restriction, which prolongs maximum life span, leads to a decrease in glycemia and insulin levels (384, 385) and that collagen cross-links originate in part from the glucose-mediated advanced Maillard reaction (see Cross-links Derived from Maillard/Glycation Reactions). Furthermore, many of the age-related processes are accelerated by diabetes, thereby implying a key role for glucose as a mediator of tissue aging (83).

In this chapter, we review systematically the changes affecting the ECM and the lens, focusing on the proteins of these tissues and their immediate function. Although this chapter discusses general changes affecting the ECM and the lens, other chapters review the physiological changes affecting the tissue as a whole.

A word of caution is necessary for the reader who will quite often face contradictory observations and great difficulties interpreting the voluminous data presented herein. Several factors are behind the contradictory studies. First, authors have at times compared very young, premature animals with very old ones, subsequently revealing only minor changes past sexual maturity. Obviously, growth is associated with a high protein turnover rate and rejuvenation of aged proteins. One typical example is the formation of newly synthesized collagen, which is accompanied by a large increase in lysyl oxidase–mediated cross-links that subsequently "mature" into more stable physiological cross-links. Second, the proportion of insoluble proteins in the ECM and the lens increases with age, and the insoluble fraction becomes very difficult to study accurately because of resistance to solubilization by chaotropic agents. Thus data will depend on the extraction procedure used, whereby an insoluble pellet generally remains, which may account for up to 90% of insoluble dura mater collagen. By and large, investigators have shunned the tedious and often unrewarding work of characterizing insoluble material, leaving behind an important gap in knowledge of tissue aging. Finally, profound species differences do exist. For example, clear-cut age-related changes in matrix solubility and digestibility are found in skin from most primates, cow, and dog, but such changes are absent in rodent skin. Throughout the chapter, we have attempted to provide explanatory comments for such discrepancies, whenever an obvious explanation was readily apparent. However, in several cases, the reader is advised to consult the primary literature and form his or her own opinion.

COLLAGENS

Overview

The collagens are a family of structural proteins. The number of genetically distinct collagens that have been structurally characterized has been increasing. By 1993, 16 collagen types had been defined (651) and approximately 30 genes with specific subunit structures had been identified (504, 652). Collagens are classified as either *fibrillar* or *nonfibrillar* (Table 10.1). Fibrillar collagens are characterized by an uninterrupted helical region with alternating polar and nonpolar domains, permitting lateral alignment of molecules in staggered arrays, a prerequisite for stabilization by lysine-derived

TABLE 10.1. *Collegen Molecules Involved in Fibril Formation*

Type	Chains	Molecules	Representative Tissues
Fibrillar collagens		Associated with type I	
I	α1(I), α2(I)	[α1(I)]$_2$, α2(I),	Skin, bone, tendon, dentin, etc.
		[α1(I)]$_3$	Dentin, skin (minor form)
III	α1(III)	[α1(III)]$_3$	Skin, vessels
V	α1(V),* α2(V), α3(V)	[α1(V)]$_3$	Hampster lung cell cultures
		[α1(V)]$_2$, α2(V)	Fetal membranes, skin, bone
		α1(V), α2(V), α3(V)	Placenta, synovial membranes
		Associated with type II	
II	α1(II)	[α1(II)]$_3$	Hyaline cartilage, vitreous body
XI†	α1(XI), α2(XI), α3(XI)‡	α1(XI), α2(XI), α3(XI)	Hyaline cartilage
Nonfibrillar collagens			
IV	α1(IV), α2(IV)	[α1(IV)]$_2$, α2(IV)	Basement membranes
	α3(IV), α4(IV), α5(IV)	(?)	Glomerular basement membranes
VI	α1(VI), α2(VI), α3(VI)	α1(VI), α2(VI), α3(VI)	Vessels, skin, intervertebral disc
VII	α1(VII)	[α1(VII)]$_3$	Dermoepidermal junction
VIII	α1(VIII), α2(VIII)	(?)	Descemet's membrane, endothelial cells
IX	α1(IX), α2(IX), α3(IX)	α1(IX), α2(IX), α3(IX)	Hyaline cartilage, vitreous humor
X	α1(X)	[α1(X)]$_3$	Growth plate
XII	α(XII)	[α1(XII)]$_3$	Embryonic tendon and skin periodontal ligament
XIII	α1(XIII)	(?)	Endothelial cells
XIV	α1(XIV)	[α1(XIV)]$_3$	Fetal skin and tendon

Reproduced with permission from van der Rest and Garrone (652).
*A chain similar in its triple helix, but different in its propeptides has been described and called α1(V)′ or α4(V).   † Often called 1α2α3α.   ‡α3(XI) is probably identical to α1(II), except for posttranslational modifications.

cross-links. Nonfibrillar collagens, in contrast, possess helical domains interrupted by nonhelical regions; regions of molecular overlap stabilized by covalent cross-links have been demonstrated in most of these collagens.

The nonfibrillar collagens are involved in complex interactions with other molecules of the ECM and often participate in stabilizing multidimensional networks composed of other collagens, proteoglycans, and laminin. For example, types XIII, XIV, and XI collagen are fibril-associated collagens which interact with each other (types XII and XIV) or with type II collagen and glycosaminoglycans (type IX). Types IV, VIII, and perhaps X collagen are sheet-forming collagens present in basement membranes of capillaries, glomeruli, and cornea. Type VI collagen forms bent filaments through interaction with itself. It has been found in several pathological conditions involving fibrotic diseases, osteoarthritis, and Down's syndrome. Finally, type VII collagen forms anchoring fibrils which play a role in stabilizing the dermoepithelial junction.

Splendid reviews of the types and structures of collagen molecules are contained in recent articles by van der Rest and colleagues (651, 652). In the next section, we will, as far as possible, refer to age-related changes affecting specific types of collagen. In all those cases where the collagen type is not mentioned, one can assume that the changes observed in aging refer to the fibrillary collagen type.

Methodological Difficulties in the Assessment of Collagen Changes during Aging

Table 10.2 summarizes the age-related changes in collagen content of tissues as reported by various independent investigators. Although a fairly large amount of data has accumulated over the years, the age-related patterns for most tissues are inconsistent even within the same species. The conflicts originate in part from different ways of expressing results, and also from technological difficulties and uncontrolled variables in the experimental design. Frequently, studies limit their samples to a very small number, thus making comparisons within and between laboratories difficult.

One of the main problems is the determination of the appropriate denominator term to express collagen levels. Expression of collagen on a whole-organ basis appears to be the most accurate method (324). However, frequently the whole organ is not available, thus an alternative denominator term, such as "dry weight,"

TABLE 10.2. Age-Associated Changes in Collagen Content of Tissues

Tissue	Species	Age Range	Assay*	Effect of Age	Expression of Results and Comments	Reference
Myocardium	Rat	5–29 months	Colorimetric (hyp)	Increases in males until 10 months, in females throughout life span	mg collagen/g dry tissue	141
Myocardium	Rat	1 day–26 months	Colorimetric (hyp)	Increases up to 18 months	mg Hyp/g protein tissue	78
Myocardium	Rat	0.5–24 months	Colorimetric (hyp)	Increases	mg collagen/g tissue (heart weight also increased)	390
Myocardium	Rat	1–26 months	Amino acid analysis (hyp)	Increases (plateaus at 22 months)	Total collagen of ventricles	144
Myocardium	Rat	4–29 months	Morphometric	Increases	Left and right ventricles expressed as volume of collagen (mm^3)	15
Myocardium	Rat	7–>32 months	Morphometric	Increases	Staining collagen deposition by visual grading 1–4	106
Papillary muscle	Rat	5, 23 months	Colorimetric (hyp)	Increases	Expressed as percent of Hyp of total amino acids of left ventricular papillary muscle	627
Myocardium	Human	0–90 yr	Colorimetric (hyp)	No change	Percent collagen of dry tissue	315
Myocardium	Human	20–>60 yr	Colorimetric (hyp)	No change	Percent collagen of dry tissue	427
Myocardium	Human	1–90 yr	Colorimetric (hyp)	No change	mg Hyp/g dry tissue	22
Myocardium Epicarcium Endocardium	Human	0–>60 yr	Colorimetric (hyp)	No change	mg Hyp/g dry tissue (in NaCl-soluble TCA-soluble and residual fractions)	556
Endocardium Papillary muscle	Human	0–90 yr	Colorimetric (hyp)	Increases	mg Hyp/g dry tissue	278
Aorta	Rat	5–36 months	Histomorphologic	Increases	Increased wall thickness with increased collagen content by staining	100
Aorta	Rat	1–24 months	Colorimetric (hyp)	Decreases	Total collagen decreases, elastin increases	671
Aorta	Human	8 days–78 yr	Colorimetric (hyp)	No change	Percent collagen of dry tissue (thoracic and abdominal aorta)	161
Blood vessels	Pig	2 days–10 yr	Histomorphologic	Increases	Thickening of wall of cerebral arteries. Replacement of smooth muscle cells by collagen and proteoglycan	441
Lung	Rat	1–39 months	Colorimetric (hyp)	Increases	mg Hyp/100 g dry tissue	559
Lung	Rat	12–24 months	Colorimetric (hyp)	Increase in Sprague-Dawley, no change in Fischer 344	mg Hyp/lung	300
Lung	Human	15–83 yr	Colorimetric (hyp)	Decreases	Expressed as µg total collagen/cc (per unit volume)	11, 12
Lung	Human	28–57 yr	Immunohistochemical (type III collagen)	Increases	Increase of type III collagen in alveolar walls	117
Liver	Rat	1 day–39 months	Colorimetric (hyp)	Increases	mg Hyp/100 g dry tissue	559
Liver	Rat	3–24 months	Colorimetric (hyp)	No change	mg collagen/g tissue (wet)	493

Tissue	Species	Age	Method	Change with age	Description	Ref.
Stomach	Rat	3–26 months	Amino acid analysis (hyp) / Colorimetric (hyp)	Increases	μg Hyp/mm² surface	213
Stomach	Rat	3–24 months	Histomorphologic	Increases	Increased total thickness of the gastric wall with age	255
Duodenum	Rat	3–26 months	Amino acid analysis (hyp)	No change	μg Hyp/mm² surface	213
Skin	Rat	2 wk–26 months	Colorimetric (hyp)	Maximum levels reached at 4 months and plateaus/declines slightly thereafter	Expressed as total skin collagen (g) and percent collagen of skin	699
Skin	Rat	5–39 months	Colorimetric (hyp)	Maximum reached at 10 months and declines	mg collagen/g dry tissue	134
Skin	Rat	3–25 months	Colorimetric (hyp)	Maximum reached at 3 months and plateaus	Percent collagen of dry tissue	164
Skin	Rat	0.5–24 months	Hyp/ gel electrophoresis for type III collagen	Maximum at 12 months and declines thereafter, no change in percent type III collagen with age	mg collagen/g tissue	390
Skin	Mouse	2–28 months	Colorimetric (hyp)	Maximum levels reached at 10 months and declines thereafter	Percent collagen in skin	49
Skin	Mouse.	2–23 months	Colorimetric (hyp)	Decreases	mg Hyp/mg wet weight	60
Skin	Human	3 months–82 yr	Amino acid analysis (hyp)	No change	Collagen expressed two ways: per cm² surface area and, as a percent of dry tissue, percentage of type III collagen in skin increases after age 65 yr	368
Skin	Human	16–75 yr / 15–93 yr	Colorimetric (hyp)	Decreases	μg collagen per sq. mm surface area	578, 579
Skin	Human	17–81 yr	Colorimetric (hyp)	Decreases	Percent collagen of skin (also elastin decreases)	481
Skin	Human	20–75 yr (female)	Colorimetric (hyp)	Decreases (after age 40 yr)	μg collagen/mg protein (decrease prevented by estrogen hormone replacement therapy)	81
Skeletal muscle	Rat	5–25 months	Colorimetric (hyp)	Increases (slight)	Total collagen mg/g wet tissue	411
Skeletal muscle	Rat	1–24 months	Radioimmunoassay colorimetric (hyp)	Increases (slight)	7-S domain of basement membrane type IV collagen, μg Hyp/mg dry tissue	318–320
Tendon	Rabbit	2 months–4 yr	Colorimetric (hyp)	Increases	Achilles tendon, collagen expressed as a percent of dry tissue	275
Tendon	Rabbit	0–4 yr	Colorimetric (hyp)	Increases until 2 months reaching steady-state levels	Achilles tendon, collagen expressed as a percent of dry tissue	85
Tendon	Rat	9–28 months	Colorimetric (hyp)	Increases	Patellar tendon expressed μg Hyp/ mg dry tissue	647
Tendon	Rat	3–24 months	Immunohistochemical	Increases	Type II collagen of suprapatella	36
Tendon	Rat	1–24 months	Colorimetric (hyp)	Decreases	Tail tendon expressed as mg Hyp/g wet tissue	671, 673
Tendon	Rat	13–52 wk	Amino acid analysis (hyp)	No change	Tail tendon expressed as mg collagen/cm unit length	115

(continued)

TABLE 10.2. Age-Associated Changes in Collagen Content of Tissues—continued

Tissue	Species	Age Range	Assay*	Effect of Age	Expression of Results and Comments	Reference
Cartilage	Rabbit	Newborn, 4wk, 4yr	Colorimetric (hyp)	Increases (very slight)	Costal cartilage expressed as mg/g dry tissue	499
Cartilage	Sheep	0–7 yr	Colorimetric (hyp)	Rapid increase until 12 months, slow increase thereafter	mg collagen/g wet weight of nasal cartilage	626
Cartilage	Human	3–86 yr	Colorimetric (hyp)	Decreases (slight)	Femoral head expressed as percent collagen of wet tissue	379
Cartilage	Human	17–60 yr	Colorimetric (hyp)	Decreases	mg collagen/mg dry weight of tracheal cartilage	502
Cartilage	Human	5–86 yr	Immunohistochemical	No change for type II collagen (80% of the collagen for cartilage), decrease for type IX collagen	Articular cartilage	132
Bone	Rat	6–30 months	Colorimetric (hyp)	No change	Tibial bone μg Hyp/mg	448
Bone	Human	1–80 yr	Colorimetric (hyp)	No change	mg collagen/g undecalcified cortical bone	121
Bone	Rat	9–2 months	Colorimetric (hyp)	No change	Cortical femur mg collagen/mm surface	113
Bone	Mouse	1–32 months	Ninhydrin	Decreases (slight)	μg Hyp/g femur dry weight	386
Bone	Rat	1–24 months	Colorimetric (hyp)	Decreases	mg Hyp/g wet weight	671
Bone	Mouse	6–27 months	Amino acid analysis (hyp)	Increases	Percent Hyp of total protein	581
Intervertebral disc	Human	14–91 yr	Colorimetric (hyp)	No change	g collagen/g dry tissue	646a
Intervertebral disc	Human	0–90 yr	Colorimetric (hyp)	Increases until 40 yr, plateaus and slightly decreases thereafter	mmol Hyp/g dry tissue	465
Kidney	Rat	1–39 months	Colorimetric (hyp)	Increases	mg Hyp/100 g dry tissue	559
Kidney	Human	23–90 yr	Radioimmunoassay Colorimetric (hyp)	Increases	Type IV collagen expressed as μg/mg wet weight	295
Intraocular fluid (vitreous and aqueous)	Rat	1–16 months	Colorimetric (hyp)	Total amount decreases after 15 months	Total Hyp (μg) per eyeball	576
Vitreous	Human	0–90 yr	Colorimetric (hyp)	Concentration increases after 50 yr, but total collagen content does not change from 30 to 90 yr	mg/ml vitreous (change may be due to a decrease in gel volume)	565
Vas deferens	Human	2–84 yr	TCA extract/Lowry's method	Increases	mg collagen/g tissue	438

*hyp:hydroxyproline.

"wet weight," or "protein level" must be used. Expressing results on a dry or wet weight basis makes it difficult to compare data between laboratories, because of differences in the experimental approaches, such as sampling and handling methods. Tissues within an organ are heterogeneous in structure, and since collagen is distributed unevenly, even in the same tissue, the results may depend upon sample location (144). If wet tissue weights are to be compared, the results may depend upon the water content of the specimen, which in turn may depend upon handling methods.

Andreotti et al. (11) advocated that collagen content for certain extensible tissues like lung, skin, or blood vessels be expressed in reference to a spatial unit of measurement. Thus this group reported no difference in total collagen content of human lung when results were expressed per unit tissue mass but decreased levels of collagen when expressed per unit surface area (11, 12). However, their results are in conflict with results of other groups who have reported an age-related increase in lung collagen when expressed per unit mass (Table 10.2) (324). In other studies with other tissues, the results are just as conflicting. For example, Shuster et al. (578, 579) reported that the collagen content of human skin decreases with age when results are expressed per unit surface area (Table 10.2). However, Lovell et al. (368) found no age-related change in the collagen content of human skin when results were expressed either per unit surface area or as a percentage of dry weight (Table 10.2). This latter group claimed that the results of Shuster et al. were confounded due to tissue sampling from a sun-exposed site (the extensor forearm). Uitto (645) concluded that the conflicting results in human skin collagen with age appear to be due to different ways of expressing results, but even in studies which have shown differences with age, the changes have been relatively small.

A frequently used marker for collagen is hydroxyproline (Table 10.2). The assumption is that the total hydroxyproline content of a tissue reflects collagen and comprises an average level of 10–14% of the total amino acid residues of this structure. Indeed, proteins other than collagen contain hydroxyproline, although under most circumstances this assumption is true (see 392). However, in certain tissues (for example, aorta and arteries), elastin is a major component and hydroxyproline content contributed by elastin is significant (161). Thus results in these tissues may depend upon the methods used to separate and assay collagen and elastin.

Quantitation of collagen is difficult due to its insolubility. Extraction methods used to solubilize collagen, such as 10% hot trichloracetic acid for protein assay, also extract noncollagenous proteins (324). Methods to isolate collagen by extracting all noncollagenous proteins and leaving behind the insoluble protein may also leave behind other insoluble proteins, such as elastin. However, by far the major portion of collagen found in most tissues is the insoluble form (324). Unless the collagen is solubilized, expressing it on a per protein basis may be impossible. Equally unfeasible is the expression of collagen on a per DNA basis, since cell loss may increase with age in collagen-enriched tissues (15).

The influence of whole-organ/tissue dynamics is equally important to assess when reporting age-related changes. For example, expressing collagen on a whole-organ basis may be misleading unless the age-related changes in the weight of the organ are also reported. Also, these changes may simply be due to an age-related atrophy of any particular tissue, such as muscle, with reciprocated replacement by connective tissue components, such as collagen. Hormonal influence can also not be neglected. For example, skin biopsies taken from the lower abdomen of pre- and postmenopausal women showed a significant decrease in collagen after the age of 40 yr, which was preventable by the use of estrogen hormone replacement therapy (81).

Collagen assessment obtained by quantitative biochemical assays must be distinguished from semiquantitative approaches, such as immunohistochemical or histological staining (Table 10.2), that purport to be specific for certain collagen types. Limiting factors for immunohistochemical approaches include purity of collagen antigens and inadequate knowledge of the epitopes (456).

By far the most frequent method in the quantitation of collagen is the colorimetric assay for hydroxyproline (Table 10.2), based upon the oxidation of imino acid by chloramine-T prior to chromogen formation with Ehrlich's reagent (p-dimethylamino-benzaldehyde). This assay does not work well for urine samples or tissues very low in hydroxyproline due to reactive contaminants, such as the putative intermediate Maillard-reactive products (see Cross-links Derived from Maillard/Glycation Reactions). Assays based on Lowry's method (369) are inadequate unless the collagen can be solubilized.

Hypertension and Collagen Deposition in Relation to the Aging Process

Many studies have dealt with collagen deposition in relation to hypertension and arteriosclerosis. Many of the arterial changes induced by hypertension are mimicked by those occurring as a result of aging, including intimal thickening, shape and appearance of arterial endothelial cells, adherence of circulating blood cells originating from smooth muscle and blood-borne sources, and an increase in medial mass, including elastin and collagen (80, 96). Studies with spontaneously

TABLE 10.3. *Comparison of Tissue Turnover*

Tissues Compared	Species	Age	Technique	Turnover Effect of Tissue	Reference
Skin, muscle, tendon, bone, kidney, intestine, liver	Rat	Not specified but reference to young weighing 128 ± 4 g	I.P. injection of ^{14}C-Pro; killed at interval 1–15 days later; assay for radioactivity in Pro and Hyp of isolated collagen fractions	Turnover rate fastest for intestine > liver > bone > muscle > skin > tendon > kidney	202
Lung, skin, bone	Rat	1–17 months	I.P. injection of ^{14}C-Pro for 21 consecutive days starting at suckling; tissues collected at intervals 5–17 months of age	One-third decrease in specific activity of lung and bone over time interval; two-thirds decrease in skin	485
Renal glomerular basement membrane, tendon	Rat	Young (age not specified)	I.P. injection of tritiated labeled Pro, Lys, Gly, Phe, and Leu; rats killed at interval 4–504 h later	Half-life turnover time of Pro and Hyp for glomerular basement membrane (GBM) determined to be > 100 days in contrast with turnover of Pro in other glomerular proteins (9 days) turnover of Pro, Hyp, and Gly in GBM slower than other amino acids (23–65 days); turnover of Pro and Hyp in tail tendon also slow (> 100 days)	496
Mesenteric artery, aorta, skin, tail, tendon	Rat	12 wk	I.P. injection of ^{3}H-Pro followed 24 h later by chase injection of unlabeled Pro given twice daily for 12 consecutive days	Turnover times for all tissues studied determined to be approximately the same (60–70 days); increase in turnover of collagen in aorta and artery during hypertension	449
Dorsal skin, tail skin, bone, skeletal muscle, gut	Rat	Weanling (age not specified)	Exposure to $^{18}O_2$ in chamber; measured ^{18}O in Hyp of tissues by isotope ratio mass spectrometry	Half-lives of dorsal skin, tail skin, cortical bone muscle, and gut determined to be 55, 74, 47, 45, and 244 days, respectively	547

hypertensive rats have shown increases in aortic diameter, thickness, weight, and collagen content compared with normotensive control rats (217). However, Ehrhart and Ferrario (145) concluded that although the rates of aortic collagen synthesis declined with age in hypertrophied intima media of thoracic aortas from 10-, 15-, and 20-wk-old spontaneously hypertensive rats, the dry weight and total collagen content increased proportionally; thus the total collagen concentration remained unchanged. This would suggest that aortic collagen has a significant turnover.

Essential hypertension develops with age, and its complication, arteriosclerosis, seems to be an accelerated form of the aging process in blood vessels (472). Work with spontaneously hypertensive rats demonstrated that deposition of collagen fibers in the vessel wall may represent an aspect of the aging phenomenon occurring in normal vasculature (472). Although the mechanism is uncertain, increased arterial mechanical stress induced by hypertension may be a direct stimulus for smooth muscle cells to synthesize more collagen (486).

Turnover of Collagen

Reviews of collagen turnover have been made by Kivirikko (305), Prockop et al. (497), and Laurent (339). It has been known for many years that the turnover rates of collagen in all age groups are low compared with those of other proteins, and this is especially true in the studies with old rats where the turnover seemed to be almost negligible. However, although the bulk of body collagen is remarkably stable, it is believed that a fraction of the collagen in all tissues is continuously being degraded and replaced even into old age (497).

The traditional view that collagen is a totally inert protein is questionable in light of the important discoveries on the rapid turnover of newly synthesized collagens (45, 46, 339, 392, 396). However, the view that the total collagen pool is metabolically active with frequent turnover is erroneous and probably is limited to the short-lived, newly synthesized procollagen intermediates that occur intracellularly (547).

Changes in the view of collagen turnover are due primarily to the important discoveries concerning different genetically distinct types of collagens (Table 10.1), as well as important discoveries in the posttranslation processing and modification of collagen occurring both intracellularly and extracellularly (339). In the review below, two important things to note are that turnover of collagen varies from one tissue to another (Table 10.3), although the extent of this turnover is controversial, and that, despite the different methodologies, in almost all species and tissues studied so far, it has been consistently found that collagen synthesis and degradation decrease with age (Table 10.4).

Methodological Difficulties in the Study of Collagen Turnover. The study of collagen turnover is a particularly difficult one. Experiments utilizing radiolabeling to track turnover must take into account both the extensive intracellular degradation of newly synthesized procollagen molecules and the very long half-life of collagen molecules that are stabilized by covalent cross-linking in the ECM. Indeed, because of this long half-life, there are serious problems with label recycling. Thus an understanding of radiolabeling techniques as a realistic estimate of collagen half-life is necessary in the interpretation of the literature on turnover in aging studies, as presented in Table 10.4.

Early studies on measurements of collagen turnover were questioned by Jackson and Heininger (279–281). Their initial study (279) with rat granuloma tissue suggested that introducing a radiolabel into collagen-bound proline to measure turnover was not valid since proline was capable of being recycled during collagen catabolism. To circumvent this problem of reutilization, they introduced the label on the 4-hydroxy position of hydroxyproline with the stable isotope $^{18}O_2$ (280). Since hydroxyproline itself cannot be incorporated into collagen and since the ^{18}O-labeled hydroxyproline cannot be produced by de novo synthesis of the collagen from systemic amino acids, a more realistic measurement of collagen turnover was obtained. A further advantage of this technique is that the free oxygen pool turns over very quickly, within minutes, such that there is no possibility of relabeling with $^{18}O_2$. Hence, this label is not reutilizable. In application, Jackson and Heininger (281) compared the half-life of rat skin collagen using this ^{18}O-labeling technique to the more traditional method of radiolabeling hydroxyproline through proline (see discussion below on pulse-chase experiments). Their results showed that half-life measurements of this tissue using ^3H radiolabeling was twice that of the stable isotope technique (53 vs. 27 days, respectively). Thus significant and efficient recycling of proline occurred during collagen turnover, and therefore, measurements using recyclable labels were inaccurate by underestimating collagen turnover.

Since the study of Jackson and Heininger (281) dealt with a single rat, additional studies using the stable isotope technique to evaluate collagen turnover were made by Molnar et al. (415, 417). In these studies (415), three weanling, 25-day-old rats were subjected to $^{18}O_2$ by chamber exposure for 36 h. Immediately following this exposure, the rats were additionally labeled by multiple subcutaneous injections of the stable isotope [^2H]proline. Skin biopsies were taken at various intervals for up to 392 days (13 months) following the pulse. In turn, the labels bound to hydroxyproline were monitored in extracted soluble and insoluble collagen samples.

The results of Molnar et al. (415) essentially agreed with those of Jackson and Heininger (281) in that significant reutilization of labeled proline was determined. During the monitoring period, a significant removal of the soluble collagen occurred, regardless of the label used. Most importantly, however, the insoluble collagen pool did not show any measurable loss of the label (that is, no measurable turnover); in fact, the amount of labeling tended to increase with time, most probably due to the conversion of soluble collagen to the insoluble pool. Similar observations were made by Molnar et al. (417) with malnourished rats fed a protein-deficient diet.

These studies (281, 415) involved derivatization of isolated, collagen-derived hydroxyproline and the estimation of ^{18}O enrichment of these samples by gas chromatography–mass spectrometry (GC–MS) using peak-ratio detection. In a further refinement, Rucklidge et al. (547) described an isotope ratio mass spectrometry method (IRMS) for the analysis of even smaller amounts of collagen-derived ^{18}O-hydroxyproline, thus achieving higher sensitivity (1,000-fold) than that of the previous GC–MS method. The disadvantage of IRMS is that the hydroxyproline must be purified prior to mass spectrometry. However, in both methods, correction must be made for the dilution effect incurred by the growth of the animal subsequent to pulse labeling.

The results of Rucklidge et al. (547) using IRMS suggested a large variation in turnover rates between different sites of the same tissue. However, in this study, turnover rate of rat dorsal skin collagen was determined to be 55 days compared with 27 days by Jackson and Heininger (281). Half-life determinations for other tissues by Rucklidge et al. (547) are given in Table 10.3. Although the exact cause is uncertain, the discrepancy over the measurable turnover rate for skin may be due to variations in the sample site and/or the sequential removal of biopsies, as used by the previous investigators, which potentially introduces further complications due to the effects of wound healing (547). Obviously, this point needs further investigation.

Since the use of $^{18}O_2$ is not feasible for all laboratories, other techniques have been developed in an attempt to circumvent the problem of label recycling. Of these, the most commonly described utilize variations of pulse-chase protocols, the so-called pool expansion approach (339, 392). Undoubtedly, proline is the source of the radiolabel because of its incorporation into collagen as radiolabeled hydroxyproline. Reutilization is minimized or eliminated by "flooding" with large amounts of unlabeled proline. For example, Nissen et al. (449) described the injection of radiolabeled proline to rats followed

TABLE 10.4. *Age-Associated Changes in Turnover of Collagen*

Tissue(s) Studied	Species	Age Range	Technique	Effect of Age	Reference
Liver, bone, skin, tendon	Rat	Not specified, categorized as young, adult, and old rats (> 14 months)	I.P. injection of ^{14}C-Gly; killed at interval 1–9 wk after injection; measured derivatized ^{14}C-Gly in tissues	Greater synthetic rates for young compared with old for all tissues; turnover rates greatest for bone collagen	443
Aorta, uterus, tendon	Rat	5 wk, 8 months, 2 yr	I.P injection of ^{14}C-Lys, killed at interval 1–40 days after injection; measured incorporation and removal of ^{14}C-Lys in tissues	Synthesis most rapid in young (5 wk) rats; no detectable synthesis in tendon at 2 yr; appreciable synthesis and turnover of collagen in older rats; no turnover in unsoluble collagen of tendon and skin at 8 months and 2 yr, respectively	294
Skin	Mice	6–60 wk	I.P. injection of ^{3}H-Pro at 4 wk of age; animals killed at interval 6–60 wk of age; measured ^{3}H-Hyp 60 wk in collagen	Half-life of collagen increased with age; 80 days at 18–30 wk, 200 days at 45–60 wk	463
Lung	Rabbit	0–24 month	Tissue explant incubated with ^{14}C-Pro; incorporation of ^{14}C-Pro and ^{14}C-Hyp into collagen	Rate and percent collagen synthesis decreased with age	61
Skin, tendon	Rat	3–24 month	^{3}H-Pro injection, ^{3}H-Hyp present in tissue at interval 1–864 h post-injection	Synthesis and degradation greater in young vs. old rats; turnover greater for skin than tendon	444
Liver	Rat	4–22 month	I.P. injection of ^{14}C-Pro, killed 24 h later; analysis of ^{14}C-Hyp in liver	Specific activity of Hyp decreased with age	216
Skin	Human	19–94 yr	Tissue explant incubated with ^{3}H-Pro for 4 h at 37°C; measured uptake of radioactivity	Decreased incorporation of ^{3}H-Pro into elastase and collagenase digested extracts in bedridden elderly subjects compared with young normal control subjects	388
Skin	Rat	3–25 months	I.P. injection of ^{3}H-Pro with 72-h postsampling; ^{3}H-Pro and ^{3}H-Hyp incorporation into collagen	Decreased synthesis and turnover with age; sevenfold decrease in ^{14}C-Hyp incorporation into collagen	164
Bone	Mice	6–27 months	Tissue explant of femur incubated with ^{3}H-Pro and ^{14}C-Pro; results expressed as incorporation of radio-labeled Pro per mg protein or per mg wet tissue weight	Decreased synthesis in old vs. young mice; decrease in old mice corrected by physical training	581
Intestine	Rat	3 and 7 wk, 13 months	Tissue explant of colon or ileum incubated with ^{3}H-Pro for ^{3}H with and without unlabeled Pro; ^{3}H-Pro incorporation into collagen	Percent collagen synthesis relative to all other non-collagenous proteins decreased with age; decrease was more pronounced in colon than in ileum	380
Lung	Rat	1–24 months	I.P. or I.V. injection of ^{14}C-Pro with a flood dose of unlabeled Pro; rats killed approximately 30 min later	Net collagen fractional synthesis and degradation expressed as %/day decreased with age	393
Bone	Rat	6, 12, 52 wk	I.P. injection of ^{14}C-Pro; rats killed 24 h later; incorporation of label into Hyp of collagen	Decreased synthesis with age expressed as a ratio of ^{14}C-Hyp:total Hyp	273
Skin	Mice	2–23 months	Tissue explant incubated with ^{3}H-Pro for 24 h incorporation of radiolabel into collagen-bound Hyp	Total collagen synthesis expressed as a percentage of total protein synthesis did not vary with age but, expressed on a per skin weight basis, decreased by about 30% between 2 and 22 months	60
Liver	Rat	1–24 months	I.P. or I.V. injection of ^{14}C-Pro with a flood dose of unlabeled Pro; rats killed approximately 30 min later	No difference in synthesis rate at 1 and 15 months; increased at 24 months	394
Heart, lung, skeletal muscle, skin	Rat	1–24 months	I.P. or I.V. injection of ^{14}C-Pro with a flood dose of unlabeled Pro; rats killed approximately 30 min later	Progressive decrease in synthesis with age in lung and skin; decrease occurred at 24 months only in heart and muscle	392

24 h later by a series of flood doses of unlabeled proline given 3 g/day, half of which was injected twice daily for 12 consecutive days. Rats in turn were killed at various intervals between 0 and 100 days after the initial injection to measure the specific activity of collagen-bound hydroxyproline of various tissues. Besides being tedious and requiring long periods of time, this method is only partially effective in preventing reutilization (341). Another approach used by Laurent's group (392) involved simultaneous administration of the radioisotope with a flood dose of unlabeled proline (approximately 0.2 g/100 g body weight). In this case, collagen-bound hydroxyproline was measured in tissues collected over an extremely short time (30–60 min) after the injection (392).

In the assessment of this latter technique, early studies by Laurent's group (338, 340, 342) suggested that collagen turnover rates were extremely high, far higher than had been determined using $^{18}O_2$ labeling, primarily because no distinction was made between intracellular and extracellular breakdown. Later studies (392, 396) acknowledged that some of the turnover was accounted for by intracellular degradation (see discussion below on intracellular degradation), yet reported rates of matrix collagen turnover were still inconsistent with other studies. This is most likely due to measurements made over a very short time period, which essentially reflect turnover of the newly synthesized procollagen molecules occurring intracellularly. The turnover contribution to this measurement made by the insoluble collagens present extracellularly is not clear but would be expected to be negligible.

Limitations, including the validity of the basic assumptions of the pool expansion techniques, have been made by Laurent's group (338, 339, 392). It suffices to say that the effects of such high doses of proline on collagen metabolism have not been adequately addressed, although some evidence suggests that collagen synthesis is not affected (392).

Collagen Turnover as a Function of Tissue. Early studies showed that different organs and tissues turn over at different rates. This turnover was highly affected by the collagen content, which was found uniquely inert and apparently, at least for the rat, not replaced at all during the lifetime of the animal (628). Long since, many other studies have shown that turnover varies according to the tissue (Table 10.3), with the collagen of some tissues (uterus, intestine, liver) showing rapid turnover and others (tendon, kidney) showing slower turnover. However, as we know, the rates of turnover reported by different studies are inconsistent due to technological difficulties.

Collagen Turnover as a Function of Age. Turnover consists of net synthesis and net degradation. Table 10.4 summarizes investigations, listed in chronological order, made on collagen turnover in aging research.

Synthesis. Studies measuring radiolabeled amino acid incorporation (glycine, lysine, proline) into collagen have consistently showed a greater rate of synthesis for young compared with old rat skin, bone, lung, and intestine (Table 10.4). Collagen synthesis in rat heart and muscle is reported to be decreased only at the late age of 24 months (392). Synthesis and turnover of collagen are very rapid in the liver, and fractional rates of collagen synthesis were found to be equivalent between 1- and 24-month-old rats (394).

The effects of age and endurance training on collagen synthesis and accumulation in the femur bone of mice were reported by Silbermann and co-workers (581). Radiolabeled proline incorporation into long bone was significantly decreased in old (27 months) compared with young (6 months) mice, expressed per tissue weight, while physical training significantly increased incorporation in both young and old mice. Both collagen and total protein content of femurs were significantly increased in old, untrained mice, compared with controls, while training significantly decreased total bone collagen even below untrained control (young) mice. Thus physical training appeared to alleviate the age-related effects on collagen turnover in the long bone of mice (581).

It was noted that ^{3}H-proline incorporation into collagenous extracts of human skin biopsies decreased with increasing age, and the results agreed in part with changes observed by light and electron microscopy, which revealed an increase in ground substance and fragmentation of collagen bundles in the dermis of older subjects (388).

Although many studies emphasized here and presented in Table 10.4 have shown decreased collagen synthesis with age by pulse-labeling and pulse-chasing experiments, many other studies have shown that rates of procollagen expression and levels of posttranslational enzymes involved in the biosynthesis of collagen are also decreased with age (reviewed in 497). The relationship of proline hydroxylation with aging is important because some of the previously mentioned techniques assume no variation with age (392). However, this has not been conclusive. For example, Barnes et al. (29) reported no change in hydroxylation of proline from 4 to 18 months of age in chickens. Conversely, Grasedyck et al. (216) reported a progressive decrease with age in the activity of propyl hydroxylase and the specific activity of hydroxyproline after pulse-labeling rat liver with C-14 proline for 24 h. Hydroxylation of collagen was also noted to be decreased with age in mouse skin; however, total collagen synthesis expressed as a percentage of total protein synthesis did not vary with age but decreased by about 30% between 2 and 22 months of age when expressed on a per skin weight basis (Boyer, 60). Likewise, Prockop et al. (497) conclude that the activity of this enzyme decreases with age, though this conclusion is based on the results of enzyme immunoassay and activity studies by Tuderman and Kivirikko (642). A closer look at their data, however, showed only a slight decrease, at most, in the amount of immunoreactive protein and essentially no change in the level of enzyme activity in human skin after the age of 10 yr.

Degradation. The degradation of collagen is also adversely affected by the aging process. Urinary excretions of hydroxylysine (321) and especially hydroxyproline (412) have been widely used as an index of collagen catabolism, especially in many collagen-associated disease processes (305). Although it is assumed that the bulk of measurable hydroxyproline is derived from collagen in these studies, other proteins contain hydroxyproline as well, including elastin among others. However, these compounds probably contribute negligibly to the total pool of hydroxyproline in tissues, and unless they turn over very rapidly, measurements based on the turnover of tissue hydroxyproline probably represent collagen metabolism (392).

The rate of hydroxyproline excretion (Fig. 10.1) decreases with age (reviewed in 305, 412). However, it is not known whether the urinary hydroxyproline originates from the degradation of newly synthesized soluble collagens or from the degradation of mature insoluble collagen fibers (305).

The degradation of collagen is more rapid in young than in old animals (Table 10.4). At the molecular level, collagen is catabolized both intracellularly and extracellularly.

Intracellular Degradation. Early in vivo work showed the rapid appearance of radiolabeled hydroxyproline in urine within 1 h after injection of ^{14}C-proline to rats (302, 334). These findings were in addition to in vivo studies with soluble collagens which suggested unusually high turnover rates (446). Thus such studies led to the speculation that recently synthesized collagen was more susceptible to specific degradation processes and also helped to explain why large amounts of peptide-bound hydroxyproline appeared in the urine during periods of rapid collagen synthesis (446).

The degradation of newly synthesized collagen was studied in vitro by Bienkowski et al. (45, 46). Using radiolabel incorporation into peptide-bound hydroxyproline and measuring the retainment of these peptides by dialysis membranes, they estimated that between 20% and 40% of the newly synthesized collagen was destroyed within minutes of its synthesis, as studied in rabbit lung explants (45). Further work with cultures of human fetal lung fibroblasts revealed that within 30 min after introducing the tracer to these cells, even though the newly synthesized collagen had not yet been secreted, approximately 30% of the labeled collagen in the cell layer was already degraded into peptides small enough to pass through a dialysis membrane (46). Such a fast time course supported a mechanism for intracellular degradation.

A further look into this prospect in vivo was made by McAnulty and Laurent (396), who found extensive degradation of newly synthesized collagen taking place in the tissues of adult rats. Employing the flooding technique to negate the effects of isotope reutilization, their results (392, 396) established that, at least for soluble collagens, turnover in adult tissues was more rapid than traditionally believed and apparently occurred intracellularly for cells in various tissues (396). Intracellular degradation has been reported to account for the fate of approximately one-third of newly synthesized collagen in the lung (45, 46, 340). However, the extent of the process is believed to vary in different tissues (396).

An investigation of this process (392) described an age-related increase in the degradation of newly synthesized collagen, maximal values ranging from 57% in skin to 96% in heart. These authors concluded that there were marked age-related changes in rates of collagen metabolism in rats, with synthesis active even in old animals where the bulk of the collagen produced was destined for degradation (392).

Such large degradation rates of newly synthesized collagen in old animals has not been verified by Laurent's group. The limitations of their work, including the technique employed to study turnover, have been previously

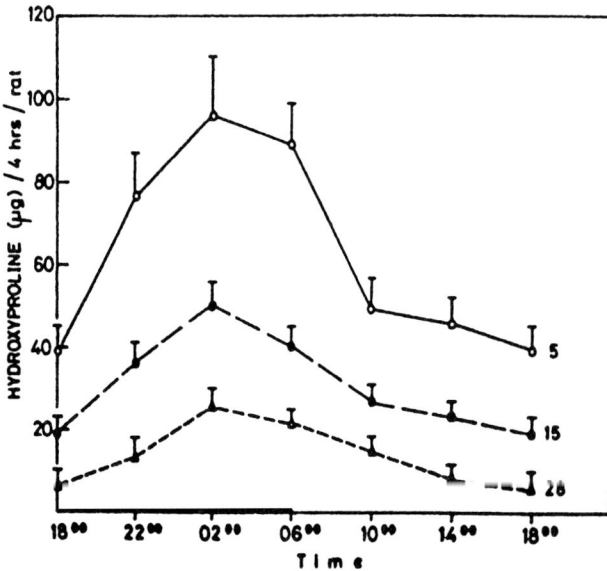

FIG. 10.1. Age-related change in the excretion of hydroxyproline in 5-, 15-, and 28-month-old Wistar rats. [From Mohan and Radha (412), by copyright permission from Academic Press.]

discussed (see under Methodological Difficulties in the Study of Collagen Turnover). From the results of urinary excretion of hydroxyproline (Fig. 10.1) and synthesis of collagen by this group among others (Table 10.4), it appears that the scenario in the older animal is one of depressed collagen synthesis. Of the limited amount of collagen that is actually produced during this time, most of it is highly subject to degradation.

Extracellular Degradation. Collagen is in a triple-helical configuration when it is secreted from the cell (497). In the ECM, cleavage of the molecule in its triple-helical state is primarily accomplished by collagenase, although serine proteinases, such as trypsin and elastase, have been shown to cleave certain native collagens (608). Collagen-bound collagenase is present on the periphery of collagen bundles, suggesting that collagen molecules arranged in deeper or more centrally located fibrils within the bundle are not accessible to the enzyme unless the outer fibrils are first removed (428). It was hypothesized that continuous displacement of the enzyme to the more recently synthesized and superficial collagen molecules on the fiber surface would allow deeper molecules the time needed to establish the degree and type of cross-links needed for the high stability of the fibril structure and for its proper function (428). In support of this proposition is the age-related resistance of native collagen to collagenolytic attack, attributed to the degree of cross-linking which increases with age (228).

The age distribution of collagenase has not been studied in great detail, but it is safe to assume that the level of activity decreases with age since remodeling of tissues takes place more frequently in the young than in the old (225). Furthermore, products of collagenolysis appear more abundantly in the urine of the young. Hall (225) hypothesized that the production of collagenase may continue into old age but that once cross-links are introduced into collagen, fusion of main chain peptide linkages no longer results in the production of low-molecular-weight material which can be excreted from the body but instead results in the accumulation of an amorphous material called "pseudoelastin," which is no longer susceptible to attack by collagenase. However, there has been no evidence for the presence of this material in tissues. Also, proteolytic degradation of collagen is further complicated by the fact that many age-related disease processes induce and/or activate collagenase (236).

The relationship of collagenase activity with age in vivo has not been established, though it has been concluded that fibroblasts maintained in culture for long periods of time (for example, 35–40 population doublings) show a decline in their ability to express this enzyme (608). However, other in vitro studies with early- and late-passage human skin fibroblasts have shown overexpression of collagenase associated with increased collagenolytic activity during the senescent phase (407, 678).

Cellular Aging in Culture in Relation to Population Doublings. The modification in the amount of collagen observed in cell culture during passaging and donor-related aging appears to be primarily the result of regulation at the levels of genomic expression and intracellular biosynthesis and degradation.

Expression of RNA for various collagens has been measured in relation to passage number and donor age. The levels of both collagen types, I, α1 and α2 mRNA, were significantly decreased in senescent WI-38 fibroblasts, suggesting that one factor contributing to decreased collagen content of aging skin in vivo may be a decreased expression of these collagen mRNAs by senescent fibroblasts (187). Similarly, mRNA concentrations for the same collagens declined during continuous passaging of fetal fibroblasts from humans and were also found lower in fibroblasts from older donors (615). The expression of mRNA for collagen type I in the culture of pig skin fibroblasts exhibited a slight decrease with aging, but conversely, the level of type III collagen mRNA rose markedly during the senescence phase (382). Levels of collagen mRNA in culture of skin cells from hamster were increased for type III collagen as the cells reached the end of their in vitro proliferative life span, followed by an increase in mRNA for type I collagen when the cells entered the postmitotic senescent phase (97).

The relative changes of total collagen and its synthesis during in vitro aging are controversial (382). Primary explant cultures initiated from rat lung (414) and human skin (4) showed a proportional increase in the level of collagen synthesis with increasing donor age. In a similar fashion, fibroblasts from rat, cultured from early to late passage, revealed that the rate of collagen synthesis increased proportionally with cumulative population doubling level (PDL) (317).

Conversely, many other researchers have claimed a decrease in collagen production with aging in vitro. Fibroblasts cultured from the skin of rats (391), pigs (382), and humans (615) showed a progressive decrease in collagen synthesis from early to late passage. Similar results were reported for skin fibroblasts obtained from donors of increasing age in rats (243) and humans (615).

Total collagen content of pig aortic endothelial cells and its culture medium reportedly reached maximal levels at passage 6 and thereafter progressively decreased with further passaging (47).

Mays et al. (391) studied the rates of synthesis and degradation of newly synthesized collagen in rat skin in vivo compared with rat skin fibroblasts in vitro and reported that collagen synthesis decreased with age in vivo and passage level in vitro. However, they noted that much of this newly synthesized collagen was immediately degraded, especially at late age and passage. Thus these authors concluded that a large portion of newly synthesized collagen appears to be destined for intracellular degradation, especially in old cells. Similar results and conclusions were reached by Martin et al. (382) working with pig skin fibroblasts.

The reasons for the apparent conflicts concerning the relative proportion of collagen synthesized are not apparent but most certainly concern the many pitfalls that exist in interpreting cell culture work due to the large number of variables that affect both gene expression and posttranslational steps in collagen biosynthesis in vitro.

Physical Properties of Aging Collagen

A detailed list of reviews concerning the physical changes of collagen with aging is provided in publications by Kohn (311) and Asghar and Henrickson (17). Hence, in this chapter only a brief synopsis will be given.

Solubility. The amount of collagen solubilized by extraction with neutral salt, acetic acid, and digestion with pepsin at 4°C decreases with age in rat skin, bone, tendon, and muscle (411, 416, 671) and human skin (408). The amount of collagen solubilized by guanidine hydrochloride and pepsin was very little (5%–10%) and decreased after the age of 25 yr in the annulus fibrosus of human intervertebral disc (465). In this same study, a larger proportion of tissue collagen was solubilized by pepsin in the nucleus pulposus and the amount solubilized after the age of 40 yr decreased only slightly. In contrast, almost the total collagen content of the nucleus pulposus during prolapse of the disc was solubilized by these treatments (465).

With age, human skin collagen becomes progressively more resistant to digestion by pepsin at either 4°C or 18°C (408). Likewise, bone matrix of rats is described to be more resistant to digestion by collagenase with age (395). Hamlin et al. (229) compared the rates of collagen digestion by collagenase for pooled fascia and tendon from jaw and neck muscles of rat and dura mater of dog, macaque, and human (Fig. 10.2). Dura mater samples from all species showed a progressive age-related resistance to digestion which was inversely related to the maximum life span. However, the rat tissue was uniformly and readily digested at all ages and only a slight resistance was noted. Human dura mater (313) and Bruch's membrane from the eye (296) showed a progressive, age-related resistance to digestion by cyanogen bromide.

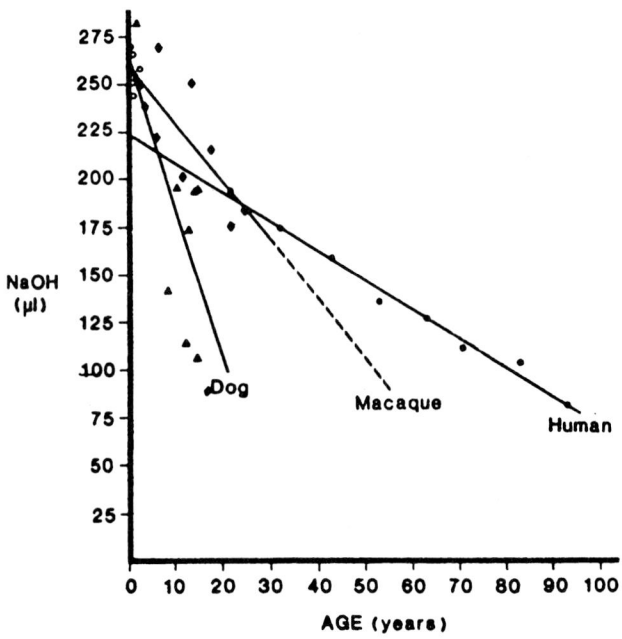

FIG. 10.2. Rates of collagen digestion vs. age for rat (○), dog (▲), macaque (♦), and human (●). NaOH required (μl as shown of a 0.01M solution) to maintain pH 7.8 at 37°C during the initial 35 min of collagenase digestion. [From Hamlin et al. (229) Copyright 1980, with kind permission from Pergamon Press Ltd., Headington Hill Hall, Oxford OX3 OBW, UK.]

Thermostability. The ability of collagen to resist deformation, denaturation, and rupturing after application of heat, known as *thermostability,* generally increases with age. Increased thermostability with age has been described for rat (109, 163, 344a), pig, and human skin (344a) and tail tendon of rat (689) and mouse (49). Snowden et al. (587) compared the relative thermal stabilities of bovine vitreous, articular cartilage, and Achilles tendon collagens to the effects of increasing heat (50°–97°C) and a combination of heat and trypsin digestion. The amount of tendon collagen solubilized by heat alone decreased with age, whereas very small quantities of vitreous and cartilage were rendered soluble by heat at all ages. By application of a combination of heat and trypsin digestion, a substantial quantity of tendon and vitreous collagens were solubilized at all ages and levels of heat, whereas partial solubilization of cartilage collagen was achieved at a significantly higher temperature.

Mechanical/Tensile Strength. Mechanical properties of rat skin have been reviewed by Vogel (672). This is a measure of the ability of a mechanical load to rupture a collagen fiber. Davison (115) showed that tensile strength of rat tail tendon increases with age but varies with the weight of the animal, the vertebra to which the tendon is attached, the pH of the tendon, and finally the chemical treatment. For the latter, treatment of tail tendon by reduction with sodium borohydride significantly increased tensile strength at all ages but did not diminish the age-related effect.

Stiffness. This property is related to tensile strength and is a measure of deformation, tension, or strain (sometimes as elastic modulus) on the fiber or tissue after a given amount of mechanical stress. Stiffness of rat tail tendon (42) and skeletal muscle (5) are reported to increase with age. Human intracranial cerebral arteries were found to be much stiffer than the extracranial arteries of all ages studied (245). Age-related increases were noted for both types of artery with greater magnitude of increase for intra- compared with extracranial arteries. However, Borg et al. (56) reported no difference among young, adult, and old rats or hamsters on the stiffness of myocardial collagen, although the left ventricles of rats at all ages were considerably more stiff than those of hamsters.

Utilizing crimp as a measure of the periodic waviness of collagen fibers in tissues subjected to tensile stress, Betsch and Baer (42) described increased crimp wavelength and decreased crimp angle for tail tendons of rats of increasing age. Crimp measurements involve a combination of polarizing optical microscopy and low-angle X-ray diffraction methodology.

Extensive studies on the physical properties of collagen have been made by Danielsen (109–112). The studies by Danielsen showed three things: *(1)* the physical properties of soft tissue collagen (skin, tendon) responded differently to the aging process than those of bone, *(2)* dissociation of age-related mechanisms causing increased mechanical strength with enzymatic resistance, particularly in bone, and *(3)* incubation of collagen with buffer or exposure to air catalyzed the age-related stability of collagen. For the latter point, if it is assumed that the age-related increase in thermostability and stiffness of collagen is due to increased cross-linking, then possibly the precursors of these cross-links preexist in the collagen, and exposure to an aqueous medium or air simply catalyzes cross-link formation by oxidation. Although we do not have full knowledge of these precursors, aside from the possible origins and mechanisms of cross-link formation, the section below on nonenzymatic glycation (Cross-links Derived from Maillard/Glycation Reactions) provides a very detailed look at several well-characterized compounds arising from glycoxidative events.

Measurement of the Physical Properties of Collagen as Potential Biomarkers of Aging

Biological Markers. There has been recent interest in the development of biological markers, or biomarkers, of aging in the hope of establishing reproducible scientific criteria for assessing the effectiveness of intervention on the processes of aging. Although many interventions have been proposed, the only one which is currently scientifically valid in altering aging is food restriction (24). The question of what constitutes a biomarker of aging is controversial (429). However, there is general agreement that different individuals age at different rates, thus chronological age does not accurately reflect biological age (24, 383, 397, 429). Indeed, even within the same individual, different tissues may age at different rates (383). Since biological age bears the most importance in explaining the aging phenomenon, interest has been kindled in the development of biomarkers of aging. Undoubtedly, the usefulness of biomarkers of aging in research is clear-cut: to estimate chronological and biological age and to predict future occurrence of age-associated diseases, impending mortality, and maximum longevity of species (383). However, criteria for identification of these biomarkers is not clear-cut. Here, the reasoning and logic involved in explaining these criteria are philosophical in nature and come from an incomplete understanding of the aging process. Some of the criteria for identifying biomarkers of aging have been summarized by Mooradian (429).

In this light, physiological parameters involving the measurement of physical changes in collagen have been among the most promising biomarkers of the aging process, especially in rodent models. Age-related changes in the solubility of rat skin (141, 416) and the thermomechanical properties of tail tendon (253, 274) have shown high correlations with chronological age and thus may be useful as predictors of biological age (141, 253) and life span (274). However, these parameters used independently do not explain the total variation in life spans of species and thus are used in combination with other physiological measurements.

Various investigators have dealt with the relationship between tail tendon breaking time as a measure of collagen aging and the subsequent life span of rodent species. The assumption in these studies is that the resistance of the tendon to break in 7-M urea as measured by breaking time reflects collagen aging. The cause of the resistance to break is not fully understood but is directly related to the amount of insoluble collagen and the cross-links of the collagen (149). When breaking time is measured a rate is obtained and, hence, aging rate is expressed. Indeed, it has been known for many years that tail tendon breaking time correlates well with chronological age (468, 665). In this regard, another expression often used is "accelerated aging," a generic expression coined by Hamlin et al. (227). It originally referred to the normal age-related increases in the processes that characterize the aging phenomena (for example, thickening of basement membrane, arterial-wall stiffness, etc.) but occur at a faster rate in diabetes mellitus.

Comparison of tail fiber breaking strength with age in males of the shorter-lived Sprague-Dawley strain with that for the longer-lived Fischer 344 strain showed that aging rate of tendon collagen occurred faster for the shorter-lived strain and strongly correlated with maximum life span but not with average life span (54). Likewise, similar studies by Harrison and colleagues with inbred strains of mice have shown that tail tendon denaturation rates correlate very well with chronological age (Fig. 10.3) but again not with average life span (238, 241). The lack of a correlation in these studies between the rate of collagen aging and average life span tends to refute the hypothesis that changes in tail tendon characteristics with age are an accurate measure of biological age. However, in the study of two species of wild mice by Harrison et al. (241), the shorter-lived species *(Mus Musculus)* showed a faster aging rate of collagen than the longer-lived species *(Peromyscus leucopus)*, suggesting that tail collagen age in this case reflects biological age.

Cross-sectional studies by Higgins et al. (251) and longitudinal studies by Heller and McClearn (248) showed two things. First, tail tendon breaking times for two strains of inbred mice correlated well with chronological age. Second, the aging rate of tail collagen was faster for the shorter-lived strain (DBA/2) than the longer-lived strain (C57BL/6). Substantial genetic influence on the phenotype was determined, accounting for between 25% and 43% of the variance from 300 to 450 days of age (248). However, since the average and maximum life spans were not reported in these studies, no conclusions could be drawn on the correlation between these parameters and tail tendon breaking times.

Other findings in the above studies revealed that tail tendon collagen in females tended to age faster than that in males (241, 248), as well as notable differences in the aging rates of tendons taken from the dorsal and ventral sides of the tail (253), with the ventral being greater than the dorsal side (251). Some of the work by Bochantin and Mays (54) with rats suggested that the presence of certain tumors may be correlated with abnormally high tendon fiber breaking time. This has not been substantiated.

The effects of high-fat diets on the aging rate of collagen fibers as measured by tail tendon breaking times have been described in the literature with conflicting results. Rats consuming a low-fat (5%) diet showed an age-related acceleration of collagen compared with rats fed diets high in fat (28%), with the difference being most marked in the older animals (261a). Conversely, Everitt et al. (150) found accelerated collagen aging in mice consuming high-fat (21%) vs. low-fat (7%) diets.

Food restriction of rats (151) and mice (239) begun

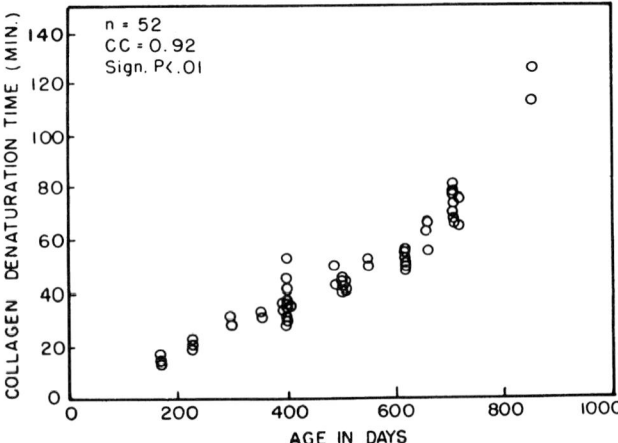

FIG. 10.3. Relationship between tail tendon denaturation (measured by tendon breaking time) and age of B6 male mice. [From Harrison et al. (238), copyright permission from Taylor and Francis.]

early in life consistently increases average and maximum life spans and at the same time decreases the aging rate of tail tendon collagen (Fig. 10.4). In a study of the effects of lifelong food restriction in genetically obese and normal mice of the same inbred strain, Harrison et al. (240) showed that a decrease in food consumption, not a decrease in adiposity, was the most important factor in increasing longevity of the obese mice. Hypophysectomy begun at early age was found to have a negative effect on collagen aging compared to intact rats (Fig. 10.4) at equivalent food-intake levels (152).

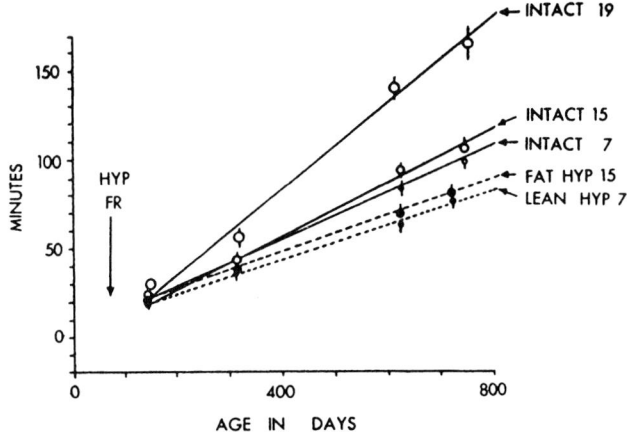

FIG. 10.4. Effect of hypophysectomy (LEAN HYP 7) and hypophysectomy with hypothalamic lesions (FAT HYP 15) at age 70 days on the aging of tail tendon collagen measured by tendon breaking time in minutes. INTACT 19 refers to ad libitum fed rats eating 19 g of food per day. INTACT 15 and 7 refer to rats fed 15 and 7 g of food per day. The collagen aging rate (slope of the regression line) in hypophysectomized rats is slower than that in intact rats eating the same amount of food. [From Everitt et al. (152), copyright permission from Elsevier Scientific Publishers Ireland Ltd.]

Chemical Properties of Aging Collagen

Early on, Verzár (665, 666) reported that the number of striations in the rat tail tendon and the thermal contraction force exerted by it increased with age; however, the solubility of the tendon decreased at the same time. Thus these physical changes indicated to Verzár that the polypeptide chains of collagen became increasingly cross-linked in old age and led him to propose a collagen-based theory of aging (see review in 293). Ever since, the exact chemical structures for these putative cross-links of senescence have long been sought after (74) and have been the subject of much speculation, investigation, and, at times, controversy. In the following discussion, we review some of these age-associated cross-links according to their proposed molecular origins.

Cross-Links Mediated by Lysyl Oxidase. Difunctional lysine-derived intermolecular cross-links of collagen were originally described in the late 1960s and early 1970s. They were demonstrated to be present in type I collagen from various tissues and derived from the interaction of hydroxylysine with either lysine aldehyde (allysine) to form aldimine bonds (23) or hydroxylysine aldehyde (hydroxyallysine) to form oxoamine bonds (403, 525). Further work showed that these divalent cross-links were also precursors of more complex multifunctional intermolecular cross-links, which form spontaneously in the tissue and may be responsible for the noted increase in collagen stability with maturation and aging (28, 364, 525, 527).

Biosynthetic pathways. The in vivo effects of lysyl oxidase and subsequent reactions in the formation of physiological cross-links have been described and reviewed in detail (see reviews in 17, 156, 337, 514, 515, 523, 683); hence, only some of these reactions are discussed here. In these reaction schemes (see reviews), lysyl oxidase oxidatively deaminates the epsilon amino group of lysine or hydroxylysine to form allysine and hydroxyallysine. These in turn can further react with the corresponding aldehydes present on adjacent polypeptide chains to form aldol condensation product (ACP) or, alternatively, with another lysine or hydroxylysine residue to form difunctional cross-links dehydrolysinonorleucine (ΔLNL), dehydrohydroxylysinonorleucine (ΔHLNL), or dehydrodihydroxylysinonorleucine (ΔHLNL). ACP can further react with histidine, which in turn can react with another lysine residue to form the tetrafunctional cross-link histidinohydroxymerodesmosine (ΔHHMD). These reactions result in the formation of Schiff base double bonds and hence are reducible with sodium borohydride or borotritide (NaB^3H_4) for the purpose of radiolabeling for tracing.

Both ΔHLNL and ΔDHLNL have been found to undergo further reactions to form nonreducible trifunctional compounds. For example, ΔDHLNL can react with hydroxylysine to form hydroxypyridinoline (HP), originally discovered by Fujimoto et al. (185), followed by the reaction mechanism given by Fujimoto and Moriguchi (183) and Eyre and Oguchi (153). Two minor analogs of HP have been described: *(1)* lysylpyridinoline (LP), which lacks the aliphatic hydroxyl group, was referred to by Eyre et al. (155) and elucidated by Ogawa et al. (460); and *(2)* 3-deoxypyridinoline (3DP), which lacks the hydroxyl group in the phenolic ring, was isolated and characterized by Barber et al. (26). Tilson (631) further described this analog to be the most abundant cross-link in human skin, where the two other pyridinium compounds are virtually absent (155).

Yamauchi et al. (684) described condensation reaction between ΔHLNL and histidine to form the trifunctional nonreducible cross-link histidinohydroxylysinonorleucine (HHL).

Changes in lysyl oxidase activity and lysyl oxidase-derived cross-links. Sanada et al. (554) reported that after an initial increase in the activity of lysyl oxidase from 2–4 wk in bone of mice, activity levels progressively decreased through 99 wk of age. Similarly, in the study by Poole et al. (492), lysyl oxidase activity was shown to decrease by over 72% in rat lungs between 10 and 34 wk of age. However, of this decrease, over 70% occurred during the first 12 wk of the study. These results were similar to those reported by Brody et al. (66) in rabbit lung. In a more recent study, lysyl oxidase activity of rat aorta reached maximal levels during the first 2 months of life, decreased rapidly until 8 months, and thereafter decreased only slightly, reaching minimum levels at 2 yr. Thus lysyl oxidase remained very active even in old age (170).

The age-related changes of total aldehyde content, supposedly attributed to the activity of lysyl oxidase, were described by Olczyk (465) in solubilized fractions of human invertebral disc collagen. In the normal disc, higher levels were found in the annulus fibrosus compared with the nucleus pulposus. However, in both anatomical parts, levels increased rapidly until 30 yr of age and thereafter declined steadily throughout the remainder of life. Elevated levels were found in the nucleus pulposus of prolapsed discs compared with normal controls (465).

The effects of aging on the precursor isoforms of lysyl oxidase are not known (531, 619), nor is it known to what extent the distribution of the 40 kd vs. 32 kd forms is influenced by aging. In addition, lysyl oxidase undergoes considerable posttranslational modification, including proteolytic processing, glycation, quinolation or quinone addition, and copper addition (108, 531, 619). The effects of aging on these posttranslational steps are also unknown.

Reducible Cross-Links. The age-related changes of the reducible and nonreducible cross-links have been rigorously described (see reviews cited above). Despite conclusions to the contrary (293), it has consistently been shown that the reducible cross-links decrease with age (Fig. 10.5).

In the skin collagen of rat (164, 513), cow (527), and monkey (513), ΔDHLNL levels were shown to be highest in the fetus and to decrease immediately after birth to trace levels. In other tissues, including rat and monkey lungs (513), rabbit joint ligaments (7), and human bone (154) and dentin (Fig. 10.5) (445, 675), the highest levels were at birth and declined throughout the life span.

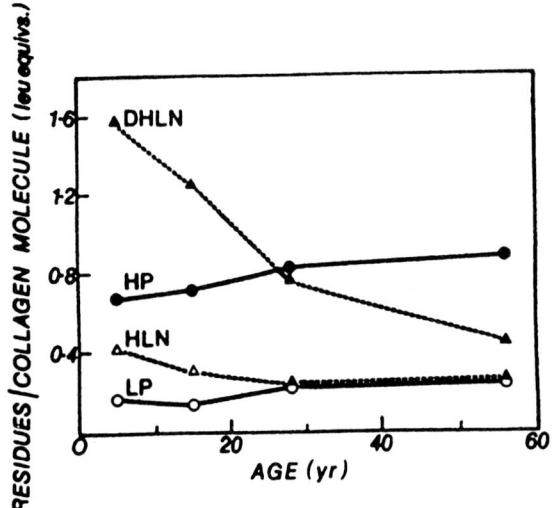

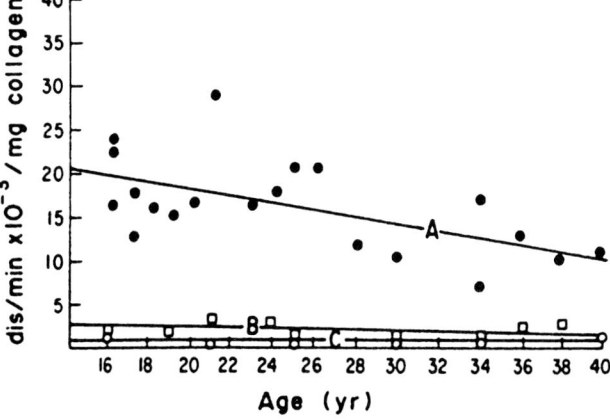

FIG. 10.5. Age-related changes in content of collagen cross-links in human tooth tissue. **Upper:** dentin; DHLN, dehydrodihydroxylysinonorleucine; HLN, dehydrohydroxylysinonorleucine; HP, hydroxypyridinoline; LP, lysylpyridinoline. **Lower:** pulp. *Line A* (●) represents DHLNL; *line B* (□) represents HLNL; *line C* (○) represents LNL. [**Upper** from Walters and Eyre (675) by copyright permission from Springer-Verlag, New York; **Lower** from Nielsen et al. (445) Copyright 1983, with kind permission from Pergamon Press Ltd., Headington Hill Hall, Oxford OX3 OBW, UK.]

Trace levels of ΔHLNL were found in dentin of cow (675) and human (Fig. 10.5) (445), and remain approximately the same throughout the life span. In rat skin (164, 513), levels were highest at birth and decreased slightly thereafter. A much larger decline throughout the life span is seen in monkey skin, monkey and rat lung (513), rabbit ligament (7), and human bone (154). ΔHLNL is a major cross-link in bovine skin, with levels reaching a maximum at 1 yr of age and declining thereafter (523, 527).

ΔHHMD is a major reducible cross-link in bovine skin, increasing sharply after birth to maximal levels at 1–2 yr and thereafter declining slowly with age (523, 527). In rat skin, levels increased until 10 months of age and thereafter declined slightly with age (164). However, Reiser et al. (513) reported a large decline of this cross-link in rat and monkey skin, reaching levels of approximately 20% of fetal values in both species at late age. Levels in lung for these two species were very minor but appeared to increase slightly with age (513).

Nonreducible Cross-Links. By far the major form of pyridinoline found in tissues is HP. Since this compound is autofluorescent, very low levels can be detected in tissues, which makes quantitation relatively easy (155). There appears to be no overall general pattern of change with aging, but instead, levels tend to be related to species and tissue type. There is virtually no HP (or LP) in human and bovine skin and rat tail tendon (155). HP has been noted to increase from birth throughout the life span in various tissues of rats, including mandibular bone (Fig. 10.6) (574), lung (513), costal cartilage, and Achilles tendon (Fig. 10.6) (430). A similar trend is reported for joint ligaments of rabbits (Fig. 10.6) (7) and aorta of humans (Fig. 10.7) (181). However, by far the most consistent trend is for levels to increase from birth until maturity and to remain constant or to decrease thereafter. This latter trend has been reported for skeletal and cardiac muscles of rabbits (288), lungs of monkeys (513), and most tissues of humans, including cartilage (Fig. 10.8) (154, 430, 644), bone (154), lung (513), dentin (675), Bruch's membrane of the eye (296), and Achilles tendon (Fig. 10.8) (430).

HP was significantly elevated (5×) in the left ventricular cardiac muscle in old (23 months) rats compared with younger (5 months) controls. However, after 10 wk of treadmill running, a significant decline of HP in the heart muscle of old rats was noted, resulting in levels comparable to that for the younger rats, where levels remained unaffected by training (627).

A significant portion of pyridinoline (HP + LP) found in human urine was in the free form and when expressed as a ratio to creatinine was found to be highly elevated in young children, significantly decreased with growth, low and constant in adults, and slightly increased with old age (186).

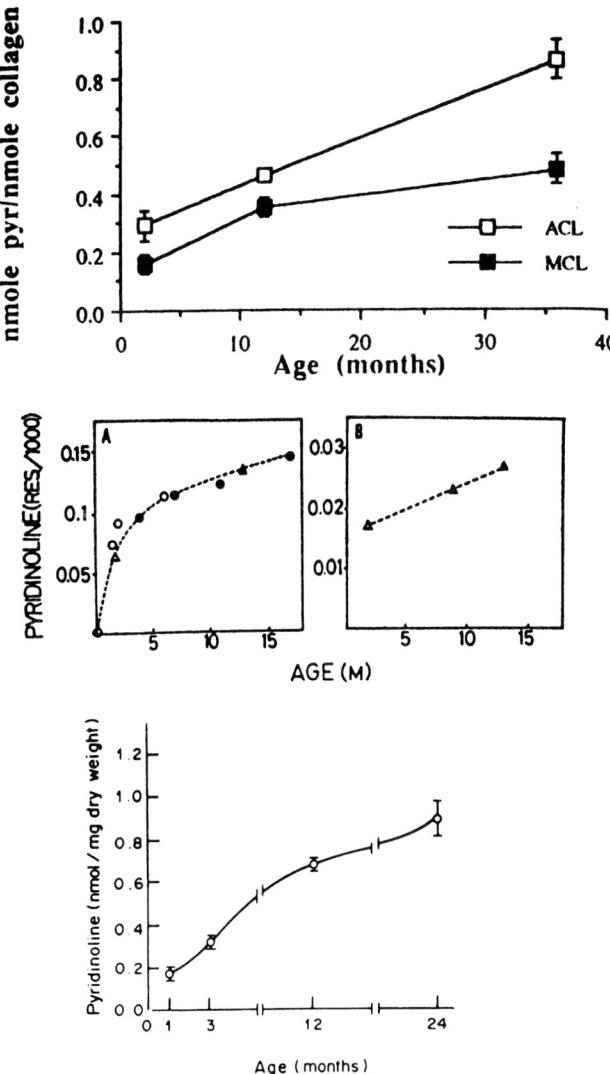

FIG. 10.6. Age-related changes in the nonreducible cross-link pyridinoline of collagen. **Upper:** Medial (**MCL**) and anterior (**ACL**) cruciate ligament of rabbits. **Middle:** Contents in rat (**A**) costal cartilage and (**B**) Achilles tendon. **Lower:** Rat mandibular bone. [**Upper** from Amiel et al. (7) by copyright permission from The Gerontological Society of America; **middle** from Moriguchi and Fujimoto (430) by permission; **Lower** from Shikata et al. (574) Copyright 1985, with kind permission from Pergamon Press Ltd., Headington Hill Hall, Oxford OX3 OBW, UK.]

When collagen from chick bone was aerobically or anaerobically aged by in vitro incubation for 4 wk in buffer at 37°C, the subsequent solubility of the collagen significantly decreased and, at the same time, the pyridinoline (HP + LP) content of the collagen increased for both the $-O_2$ (fourfold elevation)- and $+O_2$ (12-fold elevation)-incubated collagens in comparison with unincubated controls (643). The authors concluded that both nonoxidative and oxidative processes participated in the maturation of these cross-links, which in turn caused the noted increase in collagen fiber stability.

However, a more likely explanation is that the total oxygen content of the tubes failed to be removed by their evacuation technique (water-aspirator for 15 min), thus oxidative processes still occurred in these sealed tubes but at a much slower rate. In support, oxidation has previously been proposed for involvement in the formation mechanism of pyridinoline (526).

LP has been found in minor concentrations in tissues in comparison to HP, with the ratio of these two cross-links remaining the same (155). Reiser et al. (513) studied concentrations in lung tissue of rat and monkey and found that the HP:LP ratio remained constant at about 10:1 throughout the life span in both species. Similarly, an approximate 4:1 ratio was reported for human dentin by Walters and Eyre (675), which did not change after the age of 5 yr.

Tilson (631) reported 3-DP to be the most abundant amine in the cross-link region of the HPLC chromatogram for human skin. Despite this finding, Reiser et al. (513) found 3-DP concentrations in skin of rats and monkeys to be 10–50 times less than that noted for HP. Levels remained approximately the same throughout the life span in ages from fetal to old (513).

HHL, originally described by Yamauchi et al. (684), is reported to be one of the major cross-links of skin, together with ΔHLNL and ΔHHMD (470, 685). However, unlike the latter two cross-links, levels increase with age, although the rate of increase is biphasic (Fig. 10.9), occurring relatively fast up to the ages of 4 and 55 yr in cows and humans, respectively, and thereafter at much slower rates (470).

Other Potential Lysyl Oxidase-Derived Cross-Links. Barnard et al. (28) partially characterized a putative cross-link of mature collagen. Evidence was presented of a new amino acid of high molecular weight derived from lysine and present in acid hydrolysates of the poly-α_1CB6 oligomeric peptide complex (363) from cyanogen bromide digests of mature bovine tendon collagen. Levels were described to increase with aging in rabbit skin in vitro and sheep tendon in vivo in proportion to the respective decrease in some of the previously mentioned reducible cross-links. However, the exact chemical structure of this cross-link has not been determined (28).

A trisubstituted pyrrole-type cross-link has been described by Kuypers et al. (329). Isolated from the highly cross-linked peptides of insoluble collagen from bovine tendon, this cross-link may be the Ehrlich chromogen of elastin and collagen described by Scott and colleagues (299, 564). The proposed mechanism of formation involves condensation of a ketoamine, hydroxylysine-5- oxonorleucine, with allysine, cyclization, and ring closure to produce a 1,3,4-trisubstituted pyrrole cross-link (329). The proposed mechanistic origin of this pyrrole to lysyl oxidase activity is in conflict with

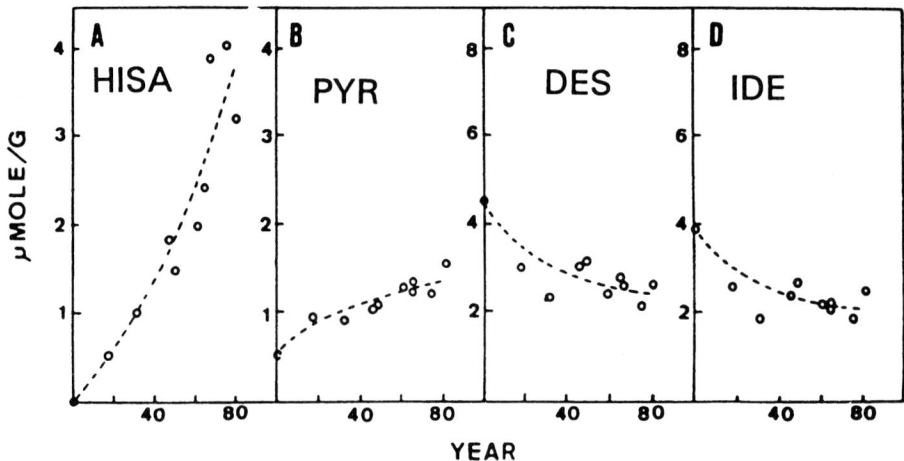

FIG. 10.7. Changes in the contents of cross-linking amino acids of human aorta with age. A: Histidinoalanine (HISA), B: pyridinoline (PYR), C: desmosine (DES), and D: isodesmosine (IDE). [From Fujimoto (181), by copyright permission from Academic Press.]

that of the formation mechanism of the pyrrole described by Monnier and colleagues (244, 409); however, these may be different substances present in the same tissue. In the latter studies, a pyrrole adduct derived from glucose was described (244), rather than a cross-link, which was immunohistochemically detected in the ECM of various tissues in diabetes and aging (409). It remains to be determined whether the pyrrole described by Kuypers et al. (329) is a true cross-link of aging or, rather, a cross-link of maturation similar to that described for pyridinoline.

Histidinoalanine was structurally elucidated by Fujimoto et al. (184) from hydrolysates of human dentin and bone. Although collagen contains this amino acid, a substantial portion has been found in noncollagenous proteins, particularly and putatively in proteoglycans from costal cartilage (182). The mechanism of formation has not been determined, but it has been suggested that the reaction may proceed nonenzymatically under physiological conditions by the condensation reaction of the histidine residue of one peptide chain with the dehydroxylated serine or desulfated cysteine residue of another peptide chain (182).

Levels were reported to increase with age (Fig. 10.10) in various human tissues, including skin, aorta, Achilles tendon, and costal cartilage (181, 182) as well as in the mandibular bone of rat (574). Thus histidinoalanine is a true cross-link of aging. However, quantitation of this amino acid in aging tissues by independent investigators has been lacking.

Cross-Links Originating from Lipid Peroxidation. Originally hypothesized by Chio and Tappel (91), oxidation of polyunsaturated lipids results in the release of malondialdehyde (MDA) and other reactive carbonyl compounds, which in turn are capable of reacting with proteins, such as collagen, with resultant formation of intra- and intermolecular cross-links. These polymerized proteins are further described as yellow and fluorescent (92).

Evidence that such reactions occur with collagen mainly comes from in vitro studies. Amino acid sequence determinations for three peptide fragments isolated from calf skin collagen modified in vitro by MDA showed that lysine residues participated in cross-linking (114). When gelatin films containing unsaturated lipids were exposed to ultraviolet and visible irradiation, cross-linking of collagen occurred, as measured by increasing melting points. The increase was inhibited by the presence of free radical scavengers (610). Tail tendon thermal rupture times of rats were increased, indicative of accelerated collagen aging when tendons were incubated in the presence of peroxidized lipid or MDA (250). However, the increase was much greater for the former (38-fold) than the latter (2.7-fold), indi-

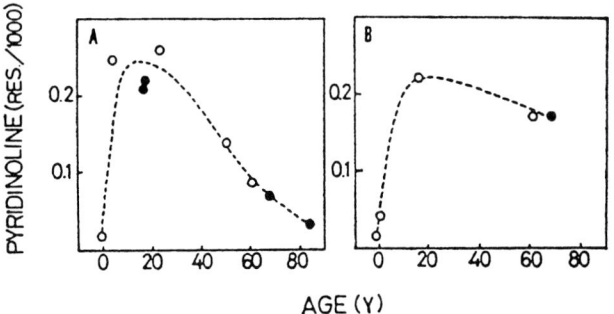

FIG. 10.8. Age-related changes in pyridinoline content of cartilage from human (A) costal cartilage and (B) Achilles tendon: ○, male; ●, female. [From Moriguchi and Fujimoto (430), by permission.]

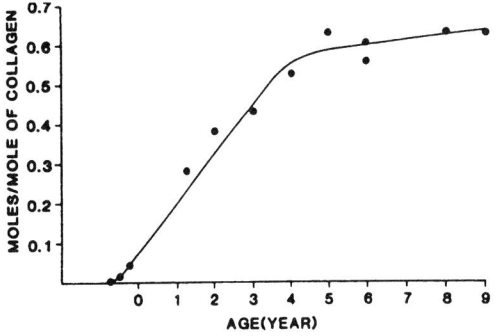

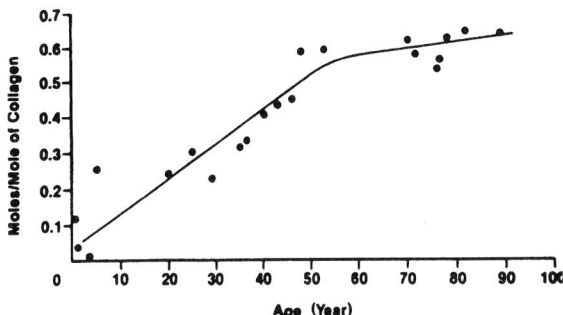

FIG. 10.9. Changes in the content of histidinohydroxylysinonorleucine with age in bovine (**upper**) and human (**lower**). [From Yamauchi et al. (685), by copyright permission from Academic Press.]

cating that a range of monofunctional aldehydes arising from lipid hydroperoxide decomposition, as described by Kikigawa and Beppu (303), were more important in cross-link formation than MDA. Even these increases, however, were relatively minor in comparison to those which occurred when the tendons were nonenzymatically glycosylated prior to these experiments (250). Thus evidence suggests that lipid peroxidation may contribute to cross-linking in two general ways: *(1)* by reactions with early glycation products on collagen through non-Maillard reactions and *(2)* by reactions that do not involve glycated residues.

To date, none of the cross-links derived from lipid peroxidation have been isolated and structurally elucidated, thus evidence that such a mechanism actually occurs in vivo with aging is circumstantial. The level of MDA significantly increases in human plasma with age (529). Also, measurement of the levels of hydroperoxides and of oxidized collagen in epidermal skin of mice, rabbits, and humans showed a direct correlation, both increasing dramatically during the senescent phase of aging (365). However, in both of these studies, the measurements were nonspecific with thiobarbituric acid used for MDA and near-infrared spectroscopy used for both hydroperoxides and oxidized collagen.

A somewhat different mechanism of fluorophore formation resulting from the oxidation of aromatic amino acid residues has been proposed by Lunec et al. (370). They have noted that human immunoglobulin (IgG) undergoes fluorescent and sulfhydryl-related damage when exposed to free radical reactions originating from various sources, including peroxidizing lipids, ultraviolet irradiation, and activated human neutrophils. Several of the fluorescent oxidation products of tryptophan generated by these reactions have been tentatively identified by this group, with structures presented which include 5-hydroxy tryptophan, formed by a hydroxylation reaction on the aromatic ring, and *N*-formyl-*L*-kynurenine, formed by bond breaking of the pyrrole ring (370).

The relationship of ECM aging to that of cellular

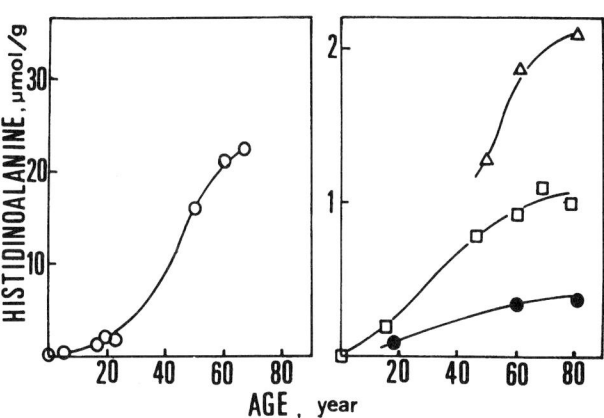

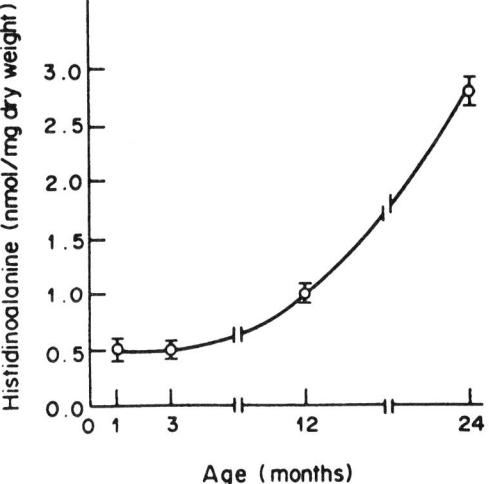

FIG. 10.10. Histidinoalanine content as a function of age. **Upper:** Human costal cartilage (○), Achilles tendon (□), aorta (△), and skin (●). **Lower:** Rat mandibular bone. [**Upper** from Fujimoto (182); by copyright permission from Academic Press. **Lower** from Shikata et al. (574) Copyright 1985, with kind permission from Pergamon Press Ltd., Headington Hill Hall, Oxford OX3 OBW, UK.]

aging in regard to lipid peroxidation has been the subject of much speculation. Cellular aging is associated with the accumulation of lipofuscin granules, lysosomal in origin, and containing various unsaturated fatty acids, reactive aldehydes, phospholipids, and amino acids (93). These granules are known to be derived from the reaction of substances having an amino base, such as proteins and MDA (91, 93). Lipofuscin-overloaded lysosomes might be unable to handle further peroxidized material formed during oxidative stress, resulting in increased intracellular concentration of products of lipid peroxidation, such as MDA, impairing critical cellular functions (69). Also, it has been speculated that lipofuscin-containing lysosomes contain high levels of free radicals, which in turn could result in increased fragility of these organelles and possible excessive leakage of lysosomal contents, including lytic enzymes, into the cytosol (69). Perhaps lipofuscin is released outside the cell or flows into the matrix during cellular degeneration and necrosis (277). One of the consequences of the extracellular release of lipofuscin would be the cross-linking of collagen. In a study of histochemical and ultrastructural features of brown degeneration of human intervertebral disc by Ishii et al. (277), it was noted that numerous amorphous electron-dense materials showing the different shapes of lipofuscin granules lying between collagen fibrils were markedly increased in the degenerative brown tissue. However, these granules, which contributed to discoloration of the disc, did not emit the characteristic fluorescence at excitation 365 nm and emission 470 nm of lipofuscin as reported by Chio et al. (93). Hence, these investigators concluded that these pigments were not truly lipofuscin. Instead, this material was still morphologically considered to be cell debris. They suggested possible chemical alteration in the cell debris by nonenzymatic browning processes involving reducing sugars. Ordinarily these materials would be metabolized by wandering leukocytes or histiocytes, but since this disc was avascular, the granules remained in the matrix and became diffused (277).

Cross-Links Derived from Maillard/Glycation Reactions. Vast amounts of new information have accumulated on the posttranslational modifications of collagen by sugars. Progress in this rapidly changing field is attributable to, and in part expedited by, the fact that certain complications of diabetes mellitus resemble those of aging (72, 207, 210, 421, 423). Because of the excessive level of sugars present in the diabetic state, it was hypothesized that these sugars could react under physiological conditions with long-lived proteins, like collagen, to form fluorescent, yellow-colored protein adducts and cross-links such as those occurring in normal aging and accelerated by diabetes (83, 420, 421, 424). These modifications were found to resemble those that occur in stored and heated foods and were attributed to the nonenzymatic browning, or Maillard reaction (420, 421, 424).

This area has received considerable attention, as reflected by extensive review articles in recent years (84, 511, 514). Amino-carbonyl reactions of the Maillard type occur essentially in three stages—early, intermediate, and late (Fig. 10.11)—associated with the formation of thermodynamically stable products (420, 424, 514).

Initial products of the Maillard reaction. The complex series of reactions collectively known as nonenzymatic browning begins as nonenzymatic glycosylation and involves the initial condensation of a sugar aldehyde or ketone with a free amino group of proteins by nucleophilic addition, resulting in the rapid formation of a

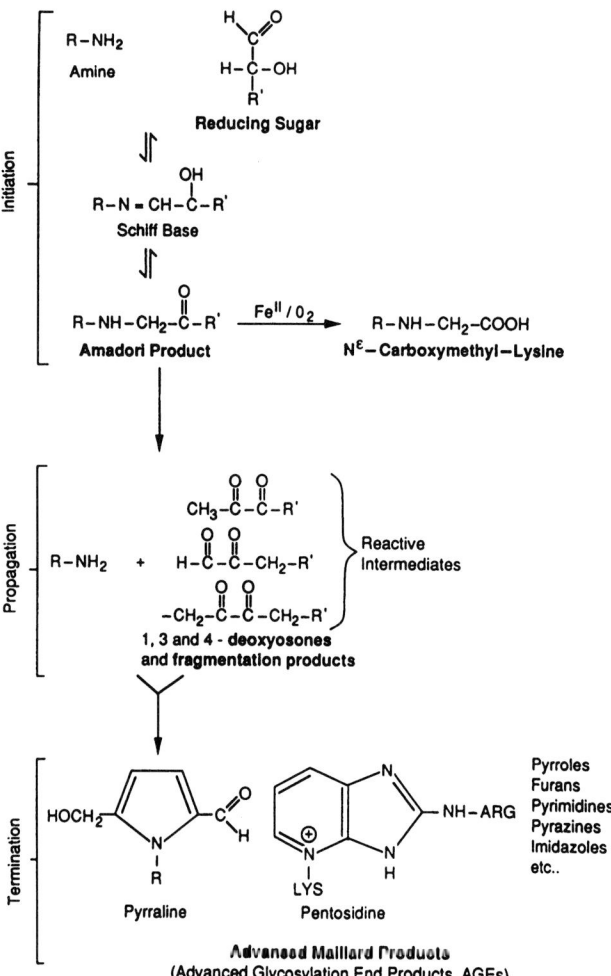

FIG. 10.11. Scheme representing potential stages of the Maillard reaction (nonenzymatic browning) corresponding to initiation, propagation, and termination events, respectively. [From Monnier et al. (424), by permission.]

Schiff base (Fig. 10.11) (420, 424). In essence, only the open chain form of the sugar is reactive. The total percentage of the sugar existing in the open chain form in solution is indeed very minor (<0.05%), which is characteristic of any particular and contributable sugar, mainly by carbon chain length (13). Thus different sugars show different rates of reactivity in the formation of a Schiff base, with glucose reacting very slowly in comparison to most other sugars (73, 420).

Structure and Specificity of Collagen Glycation. The Schiff base can undergo rearrangement to form the more stable Amadori product. Both Schiff base formation and Amadori rearrangement reactions are reversible, but the latter is less so based on increased stability (34). In collagen, trapping the Schiff base by reduction with cyanoborohydride prevents reversibility and increases the extent of glycation in comparison to unreduced collagen. However, in the study by Rogozinski et al. (530) 8% vs. 15% of the potential glycation sites in each α chain were modified in the nonreduced and reduced calf skin collagen, respectively. Thus these investigations showed two important things. First, even though modified lysyl + hydroxylysyl residues by glycation were found to occur along the entire length of the collagen chains, most of the potential residues were not available for reaction with glucose. Second, in the absence of cyanoborohydride, most of the residues that were glycated had undergone Amadori rearrangement. This was in marked contrast to poly-L-lysine in which between 3% and 50% of potential sites were glycated in the absence and presence of cyanoborohydride, respectively.

Ubiquity combined with site-specificity of glucose adducts on collagen was also reported by Reiser et al. (512). In this study, specific lysyl residues present in two isolated cyanogen bromide peptides of type I collagen of rat tail tendon were found to be preferential sites for glycation. Unexpectedly, however, these same sites were found to be highly conserved with aging, even in extremely old (36 months) rats, despite significant structural changes taking place in old collagen fibrils. The mechanism responsible for the specificity is uncertain, but local acid-base catalysis of Amadori rearrangement by proximity to other electrostatic or charged residues is likely involved for other noncollagenous proteins (34, 575). Also in this study, experiments conducted in vitro suggested that the primary structure of collagen was the major determinant of selectivity, while the influence of a higher order structure remained questionable.

Glycation of Collagen and the Effects of Aging. Whether or not glycosylation of collagen increases with aging in vivo is controversial, the results being highly dependent upon methodology (reviewed in 34, 511).

As early as 1972, Robins and Bailey (524) isolated a reducible fraction from bovine skin, shown to increase with age and later identified by a combination of radiolabeling and peroxidase degradation techniques as a condensation product between lysine and hexoses.

Studies using the thiobarbituric acid method (TBA) to measure glycation of collagen as 5-hydroxymethyl furfural (HMF) have consistently shown increased levels with age, although this method has been widely criticized for being nonspecific (34, 138, 511). These studies include investigations with human skin and tendon by Kohn and Schnider (316), glomerular and lens basement membranes by Cohen and Yu-Wu (103), cornea and sclera by Malik et al. (378), and rodent skin and aorta by Deyl et al. (118). In the study by Malik et al. (378), glycation of corneal collagen increased until 30 yr, while that of scleral collagen increased modestly throughout the human life span.

Techniques based on boronate affinity chromatography and/or amino acid analysis have shown inconsistent results. Glycation of skin collagen, as measured by total counts eluting from a boronate affinity column following tritiated borohydride reduction of collagen and its subsequent acid hydrolysis, showed no increase between the ages of 20 and 40 yr in the study of Vishwanath et al. (667). Conversely, using this same method, Deyl et al. (118) reported increased glycation with age expressed as total hexosyllysine content in aortic and skin collagens of mice and rats when measured at 2 and 24 months. These results were consistent when measuring HMF with TBA in this same study (118), but twice the values obtained by boronate affinity chromatography. Application of the same method, plus high performance liquid chromatography (HPLC) of the eluate from the affinity column to identify specific glycated residues, showed that glycation in human glomerular basement membranes did not correlate with age between 20 and 91 yr (192). However, in this same study, analysis of calf and adult bovine glomerular basement membranes and lens capsules indicated that glycation was several times greater in older animals. Studies using the amino acid analyzer to separate glycated amino acids have shown no age-related increases for collagen from human skin (276) or glomerular basement membrane (583).

Human studies measuring glycation by assaying for furosine by HPLC or GC–MS in collagens from tendon (560), aorta (447, 560), and skin (Fig. 10.12) (138) have all shown modest increases with age. The magnitude of the differences in glycation of aorta during the human life span was much greater in the study of Nishimoto et al. (447) than in that of Schleicher and Wieland (560), where the increase was very modest.

Studies investigating the age-related changes in glycation of rodent tissues have also been conflicting.

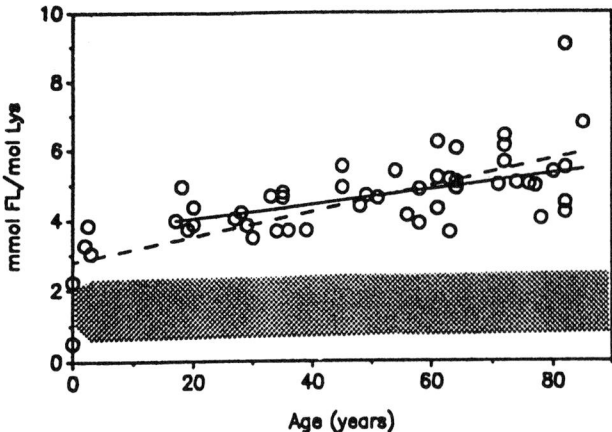

FIG. 10.12. Age-dependent changes in glycation of human skin collagen measured by fructose-lysine (**FL**) content (acid-hydrolyzed product is furosine). Shaded area at the bottom includes 95% confidence limits for similar analyses of normal lens proteins. [Reprinted with permission from Dunn et al. (138). Copyright 1991, American Chemical Society.]

Hofecker et al. (253) reported total hexosamine content of rat skin collagen to be highly, but surprisingly, negatively correlated with age. However, it is uncertain to what degree and specificity this parameter was a measure of glycated collagen. Reiser (511) found no significant age-associated increase in glycation of rat skin collagen. This is in marked contrast with the results of Deyl et al. (118), where glycation of collagen from aorta and skin, expressed as HMF or hexosyllysine were reported to be greater at 24 months than at 2 months. In a further report from Deyl's group (406), levels expressed either way progressively increased from 4 to 24 months of age in both aortic and skin collagens of Wistar rats. Continuous food restriction throughout this time period or food restriction for the first year followed by ad libitum feeding for the second year, but not vice versa, significantly inhibited collagen glycation in both tissues (406). In a study reported by Oimomi et al. (464), peak levels of glycation, measured by furosine, occurred at approximately 13 months in aortic collagen from rats, thereafter declining progressively throughout the remainder of the life span.

In regard to the conflicting studies concerning the relationship between aging and nonenzymatic glycation of collagen, Baynes and colleagues appear to have reached the best conclusions so far. They believe that the more rigorous chemical analyses tend to indicate that there is, at best, only a slight age-dependent increase in glycation (Fig. 10.12). Their results (138), among others (560), support the notion that the extent of glycation of long-lived proteins is in an equilibrium, or steady-state, relationship with ambient glucose concentrations. However, the possibility remains that some of the differences in accumulation of glycated collagen are species- or tissue-specific.

Intermediate products of the Maillard reaction. Propagative Maillard reactions following glycation have been extensively reviewed by Monnier (420), Monnier et al. (424), Reiser (511), and Reiser et al. (514). Although glycated residues as Amadori products may undergo further reactions to form advanced Maillard products, like pyrroles and the cross-link pentosidine, current evidence suggests that the bulk of these glycated residues degrade and fragment (424). The ketoamine bond of the Amadori product can split, leading to the regeneration of the free amine but at the same time releasing highly reactive α-dicarbonyl compounds called "deoxyglucosones" (DG), upon the reaction conditions of which the predominance of the chemical subspecies depends (424). In turn, DG can react further with other free amines of proteins to form chromophores, fluorescent adducts, and cross-links.

Evidence in support of DG existence in vivo has come from various metabolic studies from Kato's and Baynes's groups. When 3-DG was administered orally or injected intravenously into rats, 3-deoxyfructose (3-DF) was found to be a major metabolite (298). A potential enzyme involved in the metabolism of 3-DG was recently purified and characterized from porcine liver (362). Other evidence has come from the work of Knecht et al. (307), where a sensitive assay based on GC–MS was developed to detect 3-DG and its metabolites in human plasma and urine. Their results suggest that several milligrams of 3-DG are generated in the body each day and detoxified by reduction to 3-DF. This supports the role of 3-DG as an intermediate in the browning of protein in vivo via the Maillard reaction.

Since the α-dicarbonyl compounds like 3-DG produced during cleavage of the Amadori product are more reactive than the original sugar from which they derive, they act and are referred to as propagators of the Maillard reaction. However, the Amadori product can also undergo various oxidative reactions to produce fragmented products and free radicals, which in turn can act as propagators.

Interface between glycation and oxidation. Amadori products can undergo oxidative fragmentation in the presence of transition metals and oxygen to form carboxyalkylated lysine residues. Fragmentation of the Amadori product of glucose between carbons 2 and 3 gave rise to N^ϵ-carboxymethyl lysine (CML) and erythronic acid (3), whereas fragmentation between carbons 3 and 4 resulted in the formation of 3-(N^ϵ-lysino)-lactic acid and glyceric acid (2). These reactions were found to involve a free radical mechanism, since inhibition occurred in the presence of metal chelators and free radical scavengers and failed to occur in the absence of oxygen (2, 3).

Investigations of CML in human skin collagen showed that levels increase linearly over the life span (Fig. 10.13) but only at approximately one-tenth of the levels found in human lens (138). The reason for the differences in CML accumulation between the two tissues is unclear (Fig. 10.13) but may relate either to less oxidative stress in skin, possibly due to lower exposure to ionizing radiation, lower concentrations of oxygen, or metal catalysts in the collagenous matrix of skin (138), or to the fact that the CML precursor in the lens is ascorbate and not glucose. It was speculated that the increased levels with age were due to the decreasing rate of turnover of insoluble collagen of skin with age but not to the increased oxidative stress, since urinary excretion of CML did not vary with age (138, 306).

Levels of N^ϵ-(carboxymethyl) hydroxylysine also increased with age in human skin but at rates three times faster than for CML. The reason for the differences is not known but has been attributed to either preferential glycation of hydroxylysine or preferential oxidation of this glycated residue (138).

A mechanism of glucose autoxidation that is not dependent upon glycation but results in the production of protein-reactive dicarbonyl compounds and free radicals has been proposed by Wolff and Dean (681). Proteins exposed to autoxidizing glucose undergo fragmentative damage and conformational changes attributed to hydroxyl radical formation (269, 682). Although Wolff et al. (682) negate the effects of the superoxide radical produced during the reaction on structural damage to noncollagenous proteins, the investigations by Monboisse and Borel (418) emphasized the importance of both radical types in the fragmentation of collagens, which was thought to be especially important during inflammation. The fragmentation and conformational changes of proteins occurring during autoxidation of glucose were in addition to covalent modifications of proteins producing fluorophores and cross-links (682). Covalent modifications, which were found to be substantial, can be dissociated from described structural changes due to fragmented protein (682) and are probably most important in the aging process (418).

Such a mechanism of sugar autoxidation has been verified to occur in vitro and to cause cross-linking and aggregation of corneal type I collagen in short-term incubation with glucose for 72 h at 37°C in the presence of iron or copper (88). However, autoxidation of the Amadori product could not be excluded in this study (88). In both cases, cross-linking of collagen was attributable to hydroxyl radicals produced during oxidation.

Evidence suggests that glycated proteins are a potential source of free radicals, independent of transition metal catalysis. As previously mentioned, the study by Hicks et al. (250) showed a substantial increase in tendon stability as measured by thermal rupture of rat tail exposed to peroxidized lipid only when the tissue was glycosylated by preincubation with glucose. Previous work by Gillery et al. (208) showed that glycated ferricytochrome c prepared by incubation with various reducing sugars or glycated proteins isolated from diabetic blood serum showed the ability to generate the superoxide radical, observed in the reduction of the dye nitroblue tetrazolium (NBT).

Using the same dye, Mullarkey et al. (433) reported a substantial increase in the reduction rate of the dye

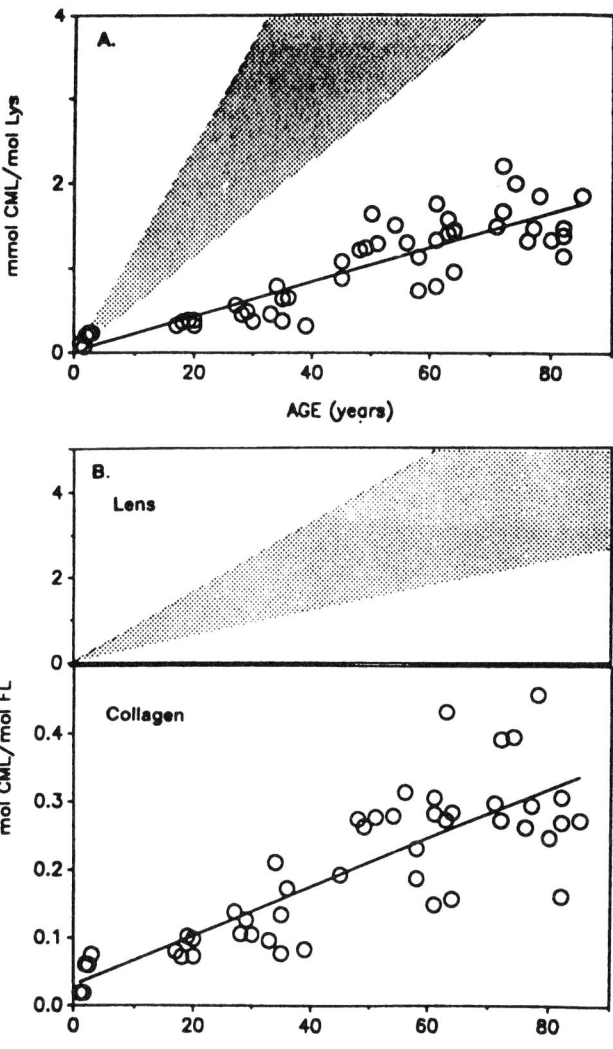

FIG. 10.13. Age-dependent changes in the concentration of N^ϵ-CML in human skin collagen. **A:** Concentration of CML, normalized to the lysine content of collagen. Shaded area represents 95% confidence limits for similar analyses of normal lens proteins. **B:** Concentration of CML normalized to the fructose-lysine (FL) content of collagen. Shaded area at top represents 95% confidence limits for similar analyses of normal lens proteins. Note that the slope for the lens data vs. age is approximately 20 times that observed for skin collagen. [Reprinted with permission from Dunn et al. (138). Copyright 1991, American Chemical Society.]

when RNAase or collagen was incubated for up to 4 wk at 37°C in the presence of the chelating agent EDTA. In similar experiments, progressive increases occurred for both proteins, with glucose concentrations increasing from 50 to 500 mM. Reduction of the Schiff base with sodium cyanoborohydride or the Amadori product with sodium borohydride decreased free radical production to undetectable levels in both cases. Their results demonstrated that both species of early glycosylation product were capable of generating free radicals. However, the relative reactivity of the Amadori product was 1.5-fold greater than that of the Schiff base.

Cyanogen bromide peptides prepared from rat tail tendon collagen upon exposure to singlet oxygen generated by a chemical system consisting of sodium hypochlorite and hydrogen peroxide immediately underwent oxidation, as assessed by polymerization and fluorescence (excitation/emission at 370/440 nm). Glycation of these peptides with subsequent exposure to the singlet oxygen was found to accelerate the oxidative process. In contrast, exposure of these peptides to hydroxyl radicals generated by a chemical system of cuprous chloride and ascorbate degraded predominantly polymeric peptides (180).

From the above results, sugar-derived modifications of collagen appeared to be mediated by a combination of mechanisms, including free radical, glycation, and Maillard reactions. Even though these mechanisms were formulated independently of each other (83, 235, 420), there is growing evidence that all three are synergistic in the aging process (323).

Advanced products of the glycation reaction. Products of nonenzymatic glycation consisting of the Schiff base and Amadori product have been clearly shown to be reversible reactions (34). However, attempts to measure the reversibility, especially the Amadori rearrangement, are in part hampered by further side-reactions, including fragmentation, dehydration, and late browning reactions (34). In fact, in studies of the model compound for fructosamine, N^ϵ-(1-deoxy-D-fructos-1-yl) hippuryl-lysine, reversal of the Amadori rearrangement was not found to be a major fate of glycation (585).

Late-stage Maillard reactions consist of further reactions of intermediate products to form fluorescent, pigmented adducts and cross-links, referred to as "advanced glycosylation end-products" (AGE) (83). Whether these reactions are reversible is questionable. Although there are no age-related studies on this topic, studies with streptozotocin-induced diabetes in mice suggest that AGE formation measured by fluorescence accumulation in glomerular basement membranes may be a reversible process (107). However, in short-term (4 months) periods of intensive therapy to improve glycemic control in the diabetic state, Lyons et al. (371) noted a significant decrease in glycation of skin collagen but failed to show changes in browning, oxidation, and fluorescence. Further work by Fu et al. (177) showed that oxidative cross-linking of collagen and AGE formation in vitro by glucose was essentially an irreversible process.

Fluorescence. Early studies by Deyl et al. (120) showed higher levels of fluorescence accumulation in old (26 months) rat skin collagen in comparison with that from young (3 months) animals. Although the origin of fluorescence was not investigated, it was speculated to be derived from oxidative reactions producing fluorescent dityrosine cross-links. Later studies by Monnier et al. (423) showed that fluorescence progressively increased with age in digests from human dura mater collagen (Fig. 10.14) and accelerated in patients with type I diabetes. Likewise, the origin of the fluorescence was uncertain but hypothesized to be sugar-derived. This was due in part to the higher levels of sugars present in the diabetic state but also to UV and fluorescent spectroscopic profiles produced by collagen samples that underwent nonenzymatic browning with glucose in vitro that were identical to those of de novo samples from aged and diabetic individuals. Other studies have confirmed that fluorescence increases with age in human tissues from various sources. These sources include skin (405, 426), subcutaneous tissue (458), intervertebral disc (261), aorta (405, 447), mesenteric artery (373), and scleral and corneal collagens (378).

Hormel and Eyre (261) described the isolation of a

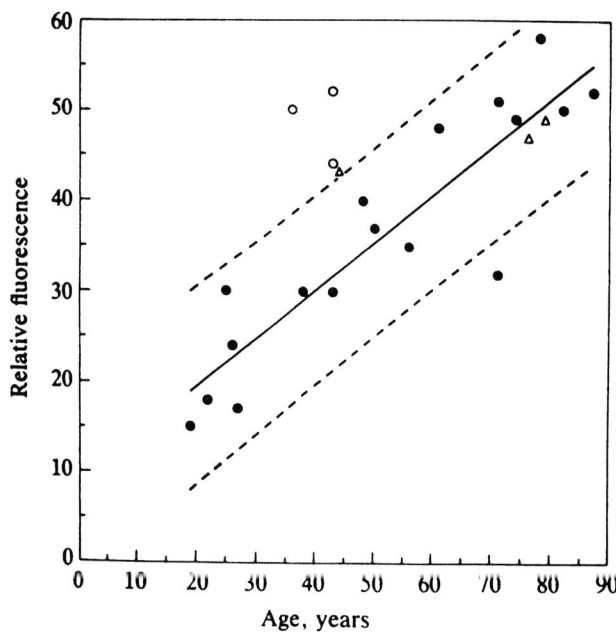

FIG. 10.14. Age-related increase in fluorescence (excitation/emission at 370/440 nm) in human dura mater. Nondiabetic (●), type I diabetic (○), type II diabetic (△); 95% confidence limits for nondiabetic control subjects. [From Monnier et al. (423), by permission.]

fluorescent peptide from human disc tissue and showed that peptide-associated fluorescence increased with age. Upon sequencing the peptide, fluorescence was identified to one particular cycle of Edman degradation and confirmed to contain a lysine residue. These researchers concluded that much of the yellow color and characteristic fluorescence that accumulated in aging discs represented covalent adducts linked to the collagen and probably to other long-lived matrix proteins. However, the cross-linking nature and origins of the covalent adducts were not discernible in this study.

Age-related increases in fluorescence have been described for various tissues from rats. These include tail tendon (516) and skin (118, 405, 406, 457). Similar age-related trends in fluorescence have been described for mouse skin and aorta by Miksik and Deyl (405).

Fluorescence in skin and aortic collagens of rats was found to increase progressively with age in the study by Miksik et al. (406). Food restriction from 3 months of age to the end of the study at 24 months most dramatically suppressed fluorescence accumulation in both tissues. In contrast, food restriction during the first year of the study with subsequent ad libitum feeding thereafter and, conversely, ad libitum feeding followed by dietary restriction also decreased tissue fluorescence, though in both cases significantly less compared to rats under continuous dietary restriction throughout the study. Dietary restriction in the second part of life had the least effect on suppressing tissue fluorescence.

Problems with Fluorescence as a Measure of Advanced Glycation In Vivo. Fluorescence has been commonly used as a measure of advanced glycation in vivo but has also been frequently criticized for this purpose. The most widely held criticism is its nonspecificity since its formation can occur through reactions other than with sugars, especially lipids (303). Another criticism is that proteins other than collagen are also modified by the Maillard reaction and show fluorescence (261). Thus fluorescence needs to be shown to be actually collagen-linked. The matter is further complicated due to age-related interactions between different ECM components, such as collagen with proteoglycans (563). Some of these may result from the entrapment and covalent cross-linking of plasma proteins to ECM, particularly to glycated ECM (68). Interestingly, covalent attachment of AGE-modified proteins present in plasma to ECM of rabbit and rat aortic tissues has been described in vivo (670). Another problem with fluorescence is the noted variability in measurements, particularly between different arteries (376). This may be due in part to contributions from non-AGE protein adducts, which fluoresce at similar wavelengths, and interference by nonprotein tissue components (376). Finally, Baynes (33) concluded that fluorescence accounts for only a small portion of the total cross-links which increase with age.

That is, the major AGE cross-links yet to be discovered are nonfluorescent. This claim tends to be substantiated by the results from radioreceptor and immunological assays for AGE formation in vitro and in vivo, where the differences between experimental groups and controls have been of a much larger magnitude than the differences based on fluorescence alone (376, 439, 500).

AGEs as Biomarkers of Aging. An enormous amount of effort has been made to structurally elucidate some of these late Maillard products so that they may serve as markers for the study of these reactions in vitro and in vivo. Fluorescence has sometimes been used to follow purification of these compounds partly because it has been shown to increase with age and partly because it is highly sensitive for the minute quantities of these products found in vivo.

Various fluorescent compounds that have been partially characterized but have yet to be structurally elucidated include late peak 1 (peak L_1) by Oimomi et al. (464), which increases in rat aorta; compound M (Maillard) by Sell and Monnier (566), shown to increase with age in human dura mater; and lens Maillard product 1 (LM-1) by Nagaraj and Monnier (436), which increases with age in human lens. Compound P (pyridinium) by Sell and Monnier (566) and Maillard reaction product 1 (MRP-1) by Dyer et al. (140) have been shown to be pentosidine.

The fluorescent compound FFI [1-(2-furoyl)-4(5)-(2-furanyl)-1H-imidazole] (491) and the nonfluorescent adduct pyrraline (5-hydroxymethyl-1-alkylpyrrole-2-carbaldehyde) (452) have not been isolated directly from tissues but instead have been detected immunologically by the methods of Chang et al. (86) and Hayase et al. (244), respectively. The actual presence of FFI in tissues could not be confirmed and has been found to be a breakdown product of acid-hydrolyzed Amadori product (260, 267, 335, 451). Other novel pyrroles hypothesized to be present in vivo have been described by Farmar et al. (157).

Pentosidine was structurally elucidated as a late-stage Maillard product and fluorescent cross-link consisting of arginine, lysine, and a pentose (567). The role of pentosidine formation in diabetes, aging, and uremia was recently reviewed by Sell et al. (571). Levels have been shown to increase progressively with age in human dura mater (Fig. 10.15) (567), skin (568–570), and cartilage (Fig. 10.16) (644). Levels in skin correlate with severity of complication in individuals with long-standing insulin-dependent diabetes (570) and are highly elevated during end-stage renal disease (568, 569). Although originally isolated from the highly insoluble fraction of collagen-enriched dura mater (566), pentosidine has also been identified in various other tissues and proteins (567). Elevated plasma protein levels have been found in diabetes (459, 570) and uremia (265, 459). Kidney

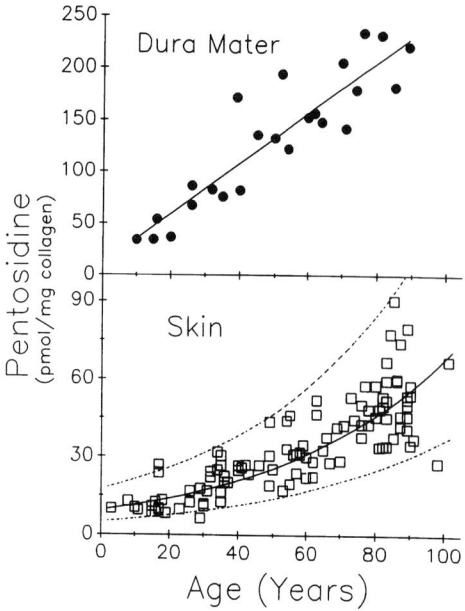

FIG. 10.15. Age-related changes of pentosidine in human dura mater and skin. [Upper from Sell and Monnier (567) by permission; Lower from Sell et al. (569), by permission.]

and kidney–pancreas transplantations were accompanied by a dramatic, but incomplete, reduction of plasma pentosidine concentrations within 3 months after transplantation (265).

Levels of pentosidine ranged from approximately 0.01 to 0.1 mol/mol triple-helical collagen, enough to impart a two- to threefold decrease in collagen digestibility at higher levels (567). In a comparative study in human articular cartilage by Uchiyama et al. (644), pentosidine increased linearly from 0.01 to 0.08 mol/mol collagen throughout the human life span, while pyridinoline did not change (Fig. 10.16). However, approximately 10 times more pyridinoline was present at very old age in comparison to pentosidine (85 yr, 0.8 mol/mol collagen). Baynes (33) observed that less than 1% of the level of natural enzymatic cross-links in skin collagen could be accounted for by pentosidine and concluded that, although it is not a major cross-link, it may be useful as a marker for the Maillard reaction in vivo (33, 140).

Original studies showed pentosidine formation by pentoses (567). However, subsequent work also showed formation through glucose by fragmentation reactions of carbohydrates (140, 215). In a set of in vitro experiments by Fu et al. (177), rat tail tendon collagen showed progressive polymerization of collagen (as assessed by gel electrophoresis) with simultaneous formation of fluorescence, CML, and pentosidine upon incubation with increasing concentrations of glucose (0–800 mM). However, under anaerobic conditions in the presence of chelating agents, cross-linking did not occur. Further work showed that the addition of chelators even under aerobic conditions effectively inhibited the cross-linking reaction. Baynes's group thus concluded that oxidative chemistry, that is, "glycoxidation," is absolutely essential in the irreversible chemical modification and cross-linking of collagens by the Maillard reaction. The same conclusion was reached by Chase et al. (88) in free radical studies of cross-linking of corneal collagen incubated with glucose.

Receptor-Mediated Uptake and Immunological Assay for AGEs. There is evidence for receptor-mediated uptake of AGE-modified proteins by various cell types, including macrophages, hepatic sinusoidal cells, and endothelial cells (148, 561, 614, 668, 669). Binding of protein to the macrophage receptor may induce uptake and removal of AGE proteins. However, the main event of this binding appears to be the release of cytokines, with the resultant cascading effects of stimulating pro-

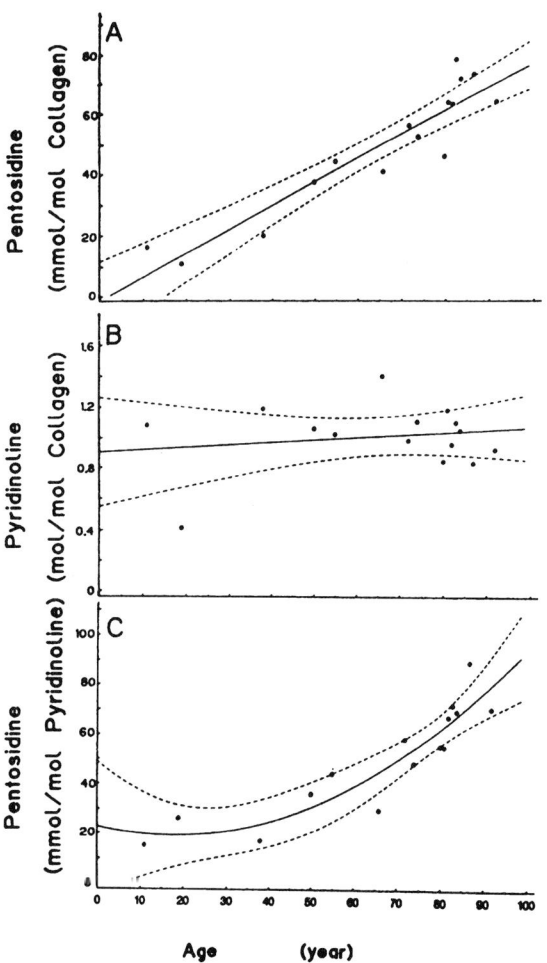

FIG. 10.16. Pentosidine and pyridinoline contents of human articular cartilage as a function of age. [From Uchiyama et al. (644), by permission.]

teolytic enzyme release by nearby mesenchymal cells (67). Binding of AGE protein to the endothelial receptor appears to have different effects. Here, binding may promote uptake, degradation, and/or transcytosis of the ligand, as well as modulation of cellular function (561).

Radoff et al. (500) described a competitive whole-cell radioreceptor assay for AGE-modified protein. The assay makes use of a specific surface-binding activity expressed by the immortal macrophage-like tumor cell line RAW 264.7 based on competition for binding between AGE protein and I-125-labeled bovine serum albumin (BSA). The assay has been used for the assessment of AGE formation in vitro as a function of collagen concentration (500) as well as in vivo to measure AGE accumulation on human arterial wall collagen, with significant elevation occurring in diabetes and end-stage renal disease (376). In these latter studies, the magnitude of the differences noted between nondiabetic and diabetic tissues was much greater using the radioreceptor assay than by measuring relative fluorescence.

Since the binding of AGE protein to the macrophage receptor has been found to be inhibited by many polyanionic compounds such as heparin and chondroitin sulfate, which are totally unrelated to AGE structures, the radioreceptor assay has been criticized as not being specific enough for AGE structures (16).

Recent attempts have been made to structurally elucidate compounds from model systems of the nonenzymatic browning reaction occurring under physiological conditions (450, 452). One of the major extractable products in the reaction mixture of glucose with the simple amine neopentylamine in phosphate buffer at 37°C was a nonfluorescent pyrrole–aldehyde (5-hydroxymethyl-1-alkylpyrrole-2-carbaldehyde) later named "pyrraline" (244). Attempts to directly isolate the chromophore from tissues proved impossible due to its lability to acid hydrolysis, with further attempts to stabilize the molecule by borohydride reduction or through reductive alkylation methods proving futile due to the presence of an amide in the ring (244). Thus an immunological assay was developed in which the molecule was quantitated by an enzyme-linked immunosorbent assay (ELISA) and a radioimmunoassay (RIA) for quantitation of pyrraline in intact proteins by a polyclonal antibody (244). Further work led to the development of a monoclonal antibody for the detection of pyrraline by an immunohistochemical staining technique (409).

Although pyrraline levels clearly increased in plasma of rats and humans during diabetes (244, 409), the age-related changes, and thus the importance of the chromophore, of the ECM, particularly with regard to collagen, are unclear. Studies on the immunoreactivity of pyrraline in human kidney tissue showed staining confined to the ECM, with the most intense staining in tissue from the oldest (87 yr) nondiabetic subject examined but no difference in staining patterns between young (22 yr) and middle-aged (36 yr) subjects. Immunostaining intensity appeared to be related to the presence of sclerosis and thickening of the ECM. Age-related changes in pyrraline staining in human coronary arteries, aortas, or nerves were not reported.

The mechanism of pyrrole formation in vivo is unclear. Pyrroles could form either through a lysyl oxidase pathway, resulting in an Ehrlich chromophore, as hypothesized by Kuypers et al. (329), or through a Maillard pathway to form pyrraline, as proposed by Miyata and Monnier (409). However, an attempt to detect pyrraline immunoreactivity in another laboratory using a polyclonal antibody has been unsuccessful, and thus the actual presence of this molecule in vitro and in vivo has been questioned (584). Differences in the methodologies may underlie the discrepancy. In the latter study, the authors had used an immunogen containing a pyrraline:protein incorporation ratio of 92:1, where only 59 lysyl residues are available for coupling. Thus the polyclonal antibody may contain antibodies toward other determinants, such as the coupling of the agent itself.

As we know, many problems have been encountered in elucidating structures of AGE products, including low abundance, chemical heterogeneity, hydrolytic lability, and artifactual species. As opposed to developing antibodies against specific haptens like FFI or pyrraline, other studies have approached these difficulties from a different perspective. This includes developing antibodies against modified proteins produced by the incubation of glucose over long periods of time (1–3.4 M glucose for approximately 90 days at 37°C) with various proteins, such as keyhole limpet hemocyanin (KLH) (440), BSA (259), and bovine ribonuclease (RNase) (377).

The procedures result in the production of antisera which recognize specifically cross-reactive AGE epitopes that form in vivo and have included studies with human and rat lens (16, 439), human serum (377), and rat collagens (377, 670). The results have indicated the presence of a dominant AGE epitope of a common structure which forms in vivo and, surprisingly, also in vitro from the reaction of glucose with various proteins, amino acids, and monoaminocarboxylic acids (259, 377).

Interestingly, kinetic studies by Makita et al. (377) showed that immunoreactive AGE-product formation in vitro occurred after fluorescent changes developed, suggesting that their antibody specifically recognized very late AGE products thought to represent terminal events. It was previously hypothesized that the development of fluorescence represented the terminal stages of the Maillard reaction (421).

In the studies of Makita et al. (377), it was noted that fluorescence of aortic collagen in normal rats increased very slightly between approximately 7 and 17 months of age (Fig. 10.17). However, AGE formation in this tissue, measured immunochemically by AGE antibody, increased significantly during this time period in a much larger magnitude than fluorescence. As expected, streptozocin-induced diabetes significantly increased both aortic collagen fluorescence and immunoreactive AGE-collagen formation during this time in far greater proportions than that noted for the nondiabetic control rats (Fig. 10.17).

In another study, daily injections of AGE-modified serum albumin into rats for 2–4 wk caused immediate attachment and deposition to heart muscle by putative covalent cross-linking to ECM proteins. This cross-linking was preventable by coinjections of aminoguanidine over this time period (670).

Conclusions

One of the most ubiquitous and reproducible phenomena in relation to collagen aging is its progressive loss of digestibility and resistance to denaturation with advancing age. The precise cause of these changes has yet to be elucidated. The finding of fluorescent molecules and the presence of pentosidine cross-links, which accumulate during aging of collagen-rich tissues, strongly suggests that amino-carbonyl reactions play a role in these modifications, especially since the collagen "aging rate" is modulated by metabolic diseases such as diabetes and uremia. Yet, the structure of the major collagen cross-link that forms during aging remains to be discovered. Although the Maillard reaction is thought to play an important role in aging of interstitial connective tissue, oxidized lipids are thought to play an important role in aging of the vascular bed matrix. In addition, the relationship of collagen aging to age-associated changes in other matrix macromolecules needs to be considered. The effects of age on two other key constituents of matrix, elastin and glycosaminoglycans, are discussed in the sections below.

ELASTIN

Elastin fibers consist of two components: elastin and elastic microfibrils. The elastic microfibrils are genetically distinct proteins, which include fibrillin and the so-called microfibrillar-associated proteins (99, 534). There is at present little information about how these microfibrillar components interact with elastin structure.

Molecular Contrasts between Elastin and Collagen

Elastin, like collagen, is a long-lived fibrous connective tissue protein that is strengthened by the development of cross-links. It is thought to undergo similar age-related events. Besides these similarities, many molecular differences exist between the two, which have been reviewed by Robert and Hornebeck (520).

Elastin is present in greatest amounts in tissues subjected to regular and periodic deformation, such as arteries, lung, and skin. As opposed to collagen, elastin is extensible and contributes little to the mechanical support and stability of tissues. Type I collagen exists as bundles of parallel fibers, each composed of linear aggregates of triple-helical polypeptide chains, which are in turn stabilized by covalent and noncovalent bonds. In contrast, elastin is composed of aggregates of randomly coiled, linear peptide chains laterally connected by covalent cross-links. These aggregates, for example, exist in many different arrangements, such as the sparse bundles of fibers in skin, the large, densely packed elastic fibers found in parallel bundles in ligaments, and the concentric sheets of elastic fibers in arterial walls. The ability of elastin to be stretched and then to recoil to its original configuration is dependent upon strategically placed cross-links and relatively weak

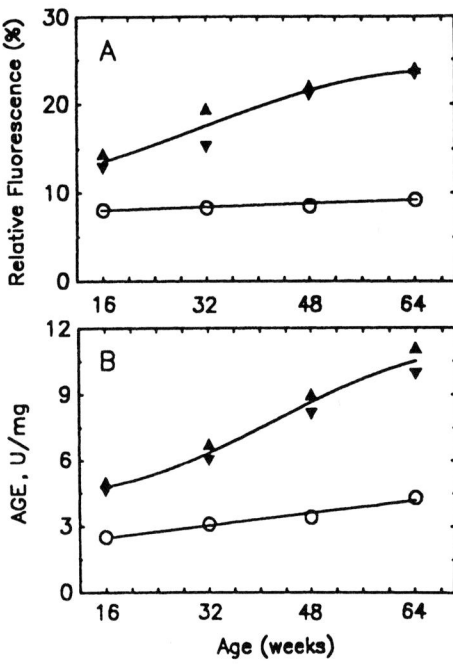

FIG. 10.17. Determination of AGE in aortic collagen of male Lewis rats with and without diabetes. Diabetes was induced in Lewis rats with either alloxan or streptozotocin at 8 wk of age. At 16 wk intervals, six animals were killed and the aortic collagen analyzed for hydroxyproline, fluorescence, and AGE content by ELISA. Values are expressed per mg of hydroxyproline. A: Relative fluorescence at excitation/emission 370/440 nm. B: Collagen-bound AGEs measured by ELISA. ○, Control rats; ▲, rats with alloxan-induced diabetes; ▼, rats with streptozotocin-induced diabetes. Each value shown is the mean of six experimental animals. [From Makita et al. (377), by permission.]

interchain hydrogen bonding. Stretching and recoiling is also most importantly dependent upon the ability of the molecule to be hydrated and subsequently dehydrated. It follows that dried elastin is brittle and cannot be stretched.

The amino acid composition of elastin and collagen has a similar content of glycine (the predominant amino acid), alanine, and proline (17, 480). However, hydroxyproline, which predominates in collagen, is present in elastin at only one-fifth to one-tenth the level found in collagen. Unlike collagen, elastin does not contain hydroxylysine (17, 156, 330, 480, 523).

The nonhelical arrangement of the polypeptide chains of elastin is essentially due to its noncollagenous sequences. This includes the absence of the basic repeating unit $(Gly-X-Y)_n$ and the minor quantities of hydroxyproline found in elastin, both of which stabilize the triple helix of collagen (17, 330). Elastin also contains a high content of hydrophobic sequences (156, 514).

A common mechanism of cross-link formation during growth and maturation involving lysyl oxidase has been described for both collagen and elastin (514). These connective tissues share a common intermediate in the pathway, the aldol condensation product, and contain the cross-link lysinonorleucine (17, 156, 514). Since hydroxylysine is not present in elastin, all cross-links are hence derived from lysine via allysine formation through lysyl oxidase. Thus pyridinoline is not found in elastin. However, elastin is unique in containing the cross-links desmosine and isodesmosine, the first cross-links discovered in connective tissues (156). The exact mechanism of formation of these cross-links is uncertain as to condensations involving dehydrolysinonorleucine or dehydromerodesmosine (156). However, one likely mechanism involving oxidation was proposed by Raju and Anwar (503) and recently reviewed by Reiser et al. (514).

Morphological Changes in Elastin with Aging

Human aging has been characterized by marked fragmentation and degeneration of elastic fibers in both aorta and skin (57–59, 64, 211, 343, 645). The progression of lysis is accelerated by conditions of diabetes and arteriosclerosis (521).

Changes in elastic fibers of the aorta begin as early as the second decade of human life (57, 518). In this tissue, the first sign of aging is a thickening of the intima (due to increased glycosaminoglycan content), which occurs simultaneously with lysis of the elastic layers. Separation between the intima and the media, which is initially most dramatic in the descending aorta below the diaphragm, becomes obscure with age (389). These changes progress throughout life, with the remaining elastic layers of the media becoming irregular and fragmented while glycosaminoglycans and collagen fibers accumulate continuously (57).

Morphological changes in aging skin are highly dependent upon exposure (57, 64, 173, 645). In sun-exposed skin, there is an excessive deposition of abnormal elastotic material. However, in nonexposed skin, there is fragmentation and loss of elastic fibers. These changes appear to be minor between the ages of 30 and 70 yr but thereafter become major (64, 645). Wrinkling and laxity of the skin are most prevalent in sun-exposed areas (676), but even in sun-protected areas, such as the buttocks, cutaneous laxity and subtle wrinkling occur and become most prevalent at late age (517). The causes of the latter sequela of aging are uncertain but may be due in part to a regression of the subepidermal elastic network of skin. Age-related increased avascularity, atrophy, and subcutaneous fat deposition of the dermis may also play a role in wrinkle formation (517). Two distinct structures within elastic fibers can be observed at the electron microscopic level: amorphous material containing elastin and microfibril (534). In the adult human dermis, over 90% of the total content of the fiber is represented by elastin (645). Degenerative changes in the elastic fibers begin as early as 30 yr of age with the loss of microfibrils and the appearance of cavities (343). An increase in electron-dense inclusions is noted, followed by the appearance of vesicular structures (641). Elastic fibers synthesized after the age of 50 yr appear to be loosely arranged. Moreover, the fibers that are deposited show increased complexity in shape, with granularity at the surface. The granularity partially obscures individual fibers and gives them a fuzzy or blurred appearance during scanning electron microscopy (64, 343, 641).

It is apparent then that there are serious difficulties in interpreting morphological data. This has to do with the fact that histological and ultrastructural properties of elastic fibers have not been proved to be equivalent to biochemically defined elastin. Thus assessment of elastin content by morphological methods remains at best qualitative.

Quantitative Changes in Elastin with Aging

Elastin Content and Appearance. The elastin content of human lung has been reported to either increase (82), decrease (237), or remain the same (490) with age. Conversely, levels in the aorta have consistently been reported to decrease with age (57, 490, 494, 521). Hypertension markedly increases the percentage of elastin in lung and arterial tissues (96, 490). However, much of this synthesized material is histologically abnormal (57, 521). Elastic fibers in the submucosa of the eustachian tube undergo hypertrophy and hyperplasia with age and also become more brittle (135). In rodents, histological comparison of aortas from 10-wk-old rats with those at 1 yr by Guyton et al. (224) showed a 28% increase in thickness in the innermost elastic lamina of the media in older rats. However, most of this increase was due to deposition of collagen since elastin concentration remained approximately the same during this time, although these trends were not studied beyond 1 yr. Similar findings were made by Hashimoto et al. (242) using a biochemical approach to measure elastin and collagen contents in aortic tissue from rats ranging in ages from 9 to 30 wk. However, in a more recent study by Fornieri et al. (170), morphometric analysis showed that elastin in rat aorta reached maximal levels at approximately 2 months of age and progressively declined through 24 months.

Age-related changes in arrangements of elastic fibers in relation to collagen fibers of skin were studied in rats of 2 wk and 24 months of age (270). A close association between these two sets of fibers was noted. However, at late age, individual elastic fibers became deformed, wrapping around collagen bundles and producing a disordered pattern. A further fine-branch system of elastic fibers then developed and irregularly interconnected the tortuous system of elastic fibers. In turn, this caused a mesh-like appearance consisting of interwoven elastic fibers interlocked around collagen bundles. The interlocking phenomenon between elastin and collagen fibers was hypothesized to cause a decrease in tissue compliance and to explain some of the age-related manifestations of human skin, such as laxity, sagging, and wrinkling.

Some of the abnormal histological features of aged elastic fibers, including the blurred appearance under scanning electron microscopy as well as the surface granularity, have been attributed to the effects of elastolytic enzymes on the fibers (64, 262, 343, 518, 519, 521). Early evidence came from histological studies noting that a progressive disappearance of the elastic framework occurred with aging in human aorta and skin (57). These events occurred simultaneously in both tissues and were attributed at that time to increased degradation of elastin. Further evidence came from the laboratory of Robert and colleagues, who noted that elastase activity progressively increased with age in human aortic tissue and correlated with the degree of atheromatous lesions (262, 518, 519, 521). These age-related histological changes in the elastic fibers could also be mimicked by the incubation of young elastin with various proteases, such as elastase, trypsin, and chymotrypsin (64, 290). It was found that old elastin is more susceptible to proteolysis than young elastin (209, 221) and that elastolysis was accelerated in diseases such as diabetes (65, 518), arteriosclerosis (521), aortic rupture (474), and emphysema (521).

Changes in Physical Properties. Generally, the extensibility and recoil properties of elastin decline with age. Harris et al. (237) noted that the extensibility of the human pulmonary trunk progressively decreased with age. This was attributed to the decreased elastin and the simultaneous increased collagen contents. Similarly, the relationship between age and folding of the elastin lamellae and collagen fibers per modular stretch (extension) was studied in human carotid artery by Samila and Carter (552). The residual folding of elastic fibers after recoiling upon stress release increased with age. This was essentially due to tissue specimens from subjects over 70 yr of age. However, the significance of this finding was thought to be of minor quantitative importance for the elastic properties of the vessels. In contrast, the residual folding of collagen fibers significantly decreased with age, indicative of increased stiffness.

Changes in Chemical Properties. Isolation of elastin from tissues has been difficult due to its insolubility. In arterial tissue, for example, over 99% of the elastin is insoluble (546). Thus harsh procedures have been frequently used to prepare elastins from tissues, including autoclaving, formic acid extraction, and hot alkali treatments (606). Unfortunately, the use of these procedures causes some degradation of the elastin and undoubtedly the destruction and possible alteration of the cross-links (156, 480, 523, 546). In morphological studies, for example, the method of boiling a tissue in 0.1 N sodium hydroxide to enable visualization of the internal structure of elastic fibers (amorphous component) for electron microscopy is quite controversial. This controversy stems from the possibility that the observed fibrillar structure could be an artifact (533).

In our own work, hot alkali treatment of tissues (0.1 NaOH at 95°C for 45 min) has been found to generate fluorescence, including pentosidine-like material. Undoubtedly, the generated fluorescence is artifactual due to a combination of events, including sugar fragmentation, known to be catalyzed under alkaline conditions, with the resultant generation of highly reactive carbonyl compounds and the accelerated Maillard reaction, all of which are greatly enhanced by elevated temperatures.

The above methodological problems may be avoided by the use of proteolytic enzymes to isolate elastin. However, the disadvantage of this route, besides expense, is that preparations may contain contaminating proteins other than elastin (546). Improved techniques have recently been described for the isolation of elastin from tissues without heat treatment (494, 573).

Another approach for avoiding the difficulties encountered in elastin extraction is to use desmosine and isodesmosine as markers for elastin content. For example, Starcher and Mecham (602) described the use of a desmosine RIA to study elastogenesis in cultures of fibroblasts and chondroblasts. However, in a study by Gunja-Smith et al. (222), it was concluded that desmosines could not be used as a direct measure of elastin, at least in the uterus, since during pregnancy and the subsequent post-partum period, levels continuously changed in relation to total elastin isolated by autoclaving.

Amino acid composition. Studies with elastin prepared from human aorta have shown age-related changes in the amino acid composition, shifting from hydrophobic to more polar residues, particularly in the shift from glycine to aspartate and glutamate (289, 332, 442, 494, 598). Similar findings have been made with lung tissues from humans (289). In all these studies, there was a tendency for an age-related shift toward the basic amino acids as well; however, these changes appeared to be much smaller than those noted for the acidic amino acids. As explained below (Changes in the Chemical Cross-Links), these shifts are likely due to age-related interactions between elastin and contaminating glycoproteins.

Racemization of L-aspartate. Studies indicate that aspartic acid in elastin undergoes progressive racemization with age, converting it from the L-form to the D-form. This conversion was conclusively shown to be age-related and not just an artifact created by thermal effects used during the isolation of elastin from tissues (494, 573). A linear increase occurs with age in elastin isolated from human aorta (Fig. 10.18) (494). However, the increase noted for aortic collagen was insignificant, indicative of a higher turnover rate. This reaction in human lung parenchyma correlated highly ($r = 0.98$) with the age of the patient at death (Fig. 10.18) (573). Racemization of aspartate occurs in essentially all mammalian proteins and has been used to date long-lived proteins such as dentin and lens crystallins (494).

Changes in the chemical cross-links. The age-related change of lysine is of particular interest since it is involved in the cross-linking process, particularly in the formation of desmosine and isodesmosine in elastins. Francis et al. (174) reported that lysine, together with its aldol condensation product, progressively decrease with age in elastin prepared from ligamentum nuchae of cattle. This decline is analogous to the decrease in the reducible cross-links dehydromerodesmosine and dehydrolysinonorleucine, except that these latter cross-links reached undetectable levels in cattle at a late age (12 yr). In comparison, the nonreducible cross-links lysinonorleucine, desmosine, and isodesmosine showed very slight increases with age (174).

The age-related trend in merodesmosine is not understood. Starcher et al. (603) reported substantial quantities of this cross-link in the hydrolysis products of borohydride-reduced elastin in young but not old cattle.

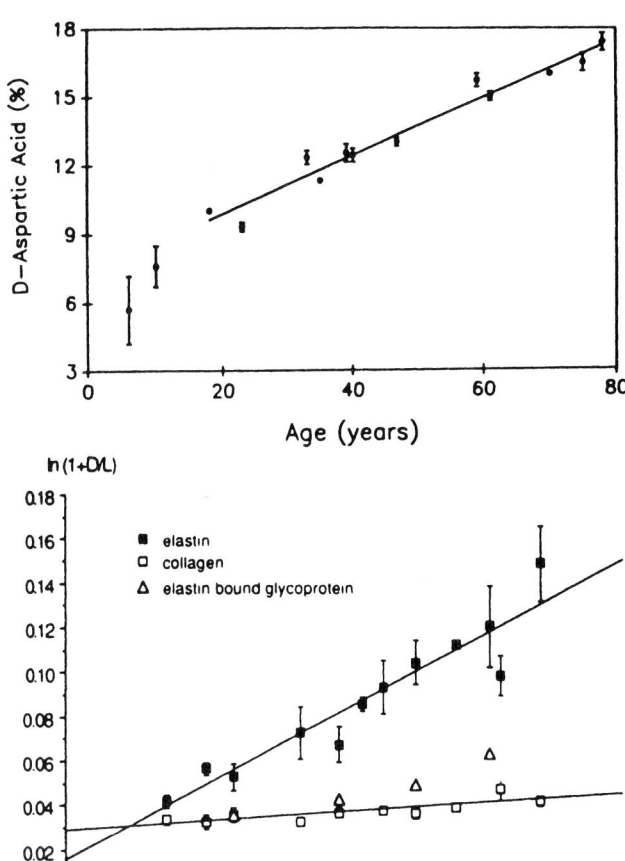

FIG. 10.18. D-Aspartate accumulation in human elastin as a function of age. **Upper:** Lung parenchymal elastin. **Lower:** Aorta. (■) Elastin, (□) collagen, (△) elastin-bound glycoprotein. [**Upper** from Shapiro et al. (573), by copyright permission of the American Society for Clinical Investigation. **Lower** from Powell et al. (494), by copyright permission from Portland Press Ltd., Colchester, UK.]

However, Francis et al. (174) showed that the level of this cross-link did not vary with cattle age.

Deyl et al. (119) found similar age-related decreases in lysine content in various elastin preparations from rats and cattle, including aorta and ligamentum nuchae. Also in agreement with the above results, lysinonorleucine increased slightly with age in the elastins from both species, but desmosine and isodesmosine essentially did not vary. Surprisingly, Deyl et al. (119) reported that pyridinoline increased most significantly in these preparations. However, since hydroxylysine is not found in elastin, this raises doubt concerning the purity of their elastin preparations and the possibility of contamination by collagen. Further analysis by Eyre et al. (156) showed that elastin did not contain pyridinoline.

In contrast to the above results with animals, elastins prepared from human tissues, such as aorta and lung, showed a tendency for lysine to increase with age (289, 442, 598). This is in agreement with the noted trend for the amino acid composition of elastin to shift toward increased polarity with aging, as previously discussed (see section on Amino Acid Composition of Elastin), and is most likely due to age-related interactions with other proteins. However, the lysine-derived cross-links desmosine and isodesmosine (Fig. 10.7) have been found to decrease with age in these tissues (181, 262, 289, 442, 494, 518). The one exception was the study of Spina et al. (598), where levels did not vary with age in thoracic aorta. Other cross-links described for human elastins include lysinonorleucine by John and Thomas (289) and histidinoalanine by Fujimoto (181, 182), where levels were reported to either slightly or significantly increase with age, respectively. However, in the study by Fujimoto (181), aortic elastin prepared by elastase digestion was substantially contaminated by collagen, as evidenced by the presence of pyridinoline.

Studies with human aorta suggest age-related changes in the amino acid profiles that reflect persistent contamination of the elastin preparations by more polar proteins, which are somehow related to the mineralization process (that is, calcium deposition) of this tissue (597). Analysis of the gene sequence of human tropoelastin showed that it encoded approximately four aspartate residues per 1,000 amino acid residues (158, 272), far lower than the 10–21 residues determined for old human elastins (289, 442, 598). Such findings suggested the presence of other proteins in elastin preparations (494, 573).

The avoidance of elevated temperatures in the preparation of elastin lengthened purification procedures, which included extensive extractions and digestions with pepsin and cyanogen bromide, but preparations still were impure, as indicated by amino acid analysis showing excessive levels of polar amino acids (494). Further cleavage of the insoluble residue by trypsin resulted in insoluble elastin and a solubilized elastin-bound glycoprotein fraction. Analysis of this insoluble elastin revealed that the polar amino acids did not vary significantly with age (494).

The nature and origin of the elastin-associated glycoprotein have not been investigated. Previously, John and Thomas (289) reported significant age-related increases in the carbohydrate content of human elastins from lung and aorta. However, it is not known whether the noted increase is due strictly to this association with glycoprotein. Powell et al. (494) suspected the origin of the glycoprotein to be the microfibrillar component of elastic fibers, since it is rich in hydrophilic amino acids and amino sugars (206).

It was hypothesized by Indik et al. (271) that the shift in the amino acid composition noted with age in human aorta and lung elastins was due to age-related changes in the splicing patterns of nucleotides encoded by elastin mRNA subjected to alternative splicing. The phenomenon resulted in sequences encoding disproportionately large numbers of polar amino acids. Evidence was presented by Indik et al. (271) that a particular exon from elastin mRNA, human exon 10a, isolated from human aorta of elderly subjects, encoded for such amino acid sequences. Interestingly, this exon could not be found in fetal tissue.

Fluorescence. Autofluorescence of elastin has been hypothesized to be caused by many factors, which include pyridinoline, dityrosine, products of lipid peroxidation and aldehyde lipid, aromatic-like compounds, quinones, and reactive carbonyl compounds such as carbohydrate (330, 546, 632). Analyses of elastins from various sources, including aorta, lung, and various arterial tissues, have shown age-related increases in fluorescence (52, 53, 289, 331, 588). Also, elastic fibers from lung viewed under a microscope showed age-related increases in autofluorescence (519). However, in all these studies, elastins were prepared by autoclaving, hot alkali extraction, and/or acid hydrolysis before measurements, methods which are known to cause fluorescent artifacts (633). Thus caution should be used in the interpretation.

Changes in Gene Expression, Synthesis, and Turnover.
Studies with cultures of human skin fibroblasts of increasing donor age showed that levels of mRNA for elastin remained fairly constant during early and middle ages (between 15 and 45 yr), but drastically declined after 60 yr (158). Similar studies by Quaglino et al. (498) revealed a rapid decline in the rate of elastin gene expression with age in both skin and blood vessels of rats as measured over a 2-year period. However, measurable amounts still occurred at late age. In another study, it was noted that much greater levels of DNA were present in lung than in aortic tissues of rats, but higher steady-state levels of tropoelastin mRNA were found in the aorta, probably reflecting greater elastin biosynthesis in this tissue (171, 172). Total DNA content of aorta progressively declined from 2 to 25 months of age but remained fairly constant in the lung. In contrast, tropoelastin mRNA dramatically declined, especially for lung, between 2 and 9 months but thereafter remained fairly constant with age in both tissues (172).

From the above results, a controversy has ensued over whether gene expression is actually rate-limiting for elastin biosynthesis. Uitto et al. (646) concluded that it is limiting, especially at late age, and that it may explain some of the loss of elastic fibers occurring in the dermis of the elderly. However, the results of Foster and Curtiss (171) showed detectable levels of tropoelastin mRNA throughout the life span of rats. Thus they concluded that elastin gene transcription is active even in old animals where the potential for elastin synthesis is still quite present. This conclusion is supported by the results of Quaglino et al. (498), who showed that although gene expression for elastin is drastically lower in older than in newborn rats, it is nevertheless still present in old age (170). To add further complexity to this issue are the findings that connective tissue-synthesizing cells, such as smooth muscle cells, have the ability to produce large amounts of elastin and other matrix proteins upon stimulation, especially during injury and pathological processes such as atherosclerosis or hypertension (170).

Studies of human skin fibroblasts showed that in vitro synthesis of tropoelastin remained high up to the age of 60 yr and thereafter declined (572). Morphological studies of human skin, which tend to confirm these results, showed that continuous synthesis of elastic fibers occurred even at late ages. However, abnormal features, consisting of loosely assembled fibers began to appear after the age of 50 yr (64).

Whole-organ cultures of rabbit aorta showed that, although incorporation of radiolabeled lysine into desmosine occurred in both young and adult animals (3 vs. 6 months), levels were greatly reduced in the adult (410). Similarly, in studies by Myers et al. (435) where synthesis was measured by labeled valine incorporation into soluble elastins from lung explants, the maximal rate of synthesis occurred in explants for 7–12-day-old rats but was comparatively reduced by five to eight times as much in the adult rat explants. These results agreed with earlier findings by this group which showed that elastin synthesis measured in vivo occurred predominantly during the first 2 weeks of life in mouse and rat lungs (133).

These results suggest that active synthesis of elastins still occurs in the adult. Although the rate of synthesis is maintained at high levels into late ages in skin, in other tissues, like aorta or lung, maximal rate occurred at a very young age and thereafter progressively declined. The rate of synthesis of elastin cross-links measured by absolute amounts of desmosine and isodesmosine in the aorta also progressively declined with age (410, 519). The data are in concert with the noted age-related decline in the activity of lysyl oxidase in the aorta of rat (170).

Animal studies suggest that the turnover of elastin is indeed very slow, with a half-life best measured in years. Evidence for this conclusion has come from experiments measuring turnover rates following an initial pulse of radiolabeled lysine incorporation into elastin and desmosine from rodent lung (133) and aorta of Japanese quail (344). In earlier experiments, Pierce et al. (485) used radiolabeled proline incorporation to study elastin turnover in several rat tissues and measured specific activity of elastin in animals between the ages of 4 and 17 months. Their results showed that some turnover of elastin did occur and that turnover rates varied among tissues. For example, the rate of turnover was greater for skin than for lung (62% vs. 39% decrease, respectively).

Human studies tend to support the hypothesis of slow elastin turnover. Estimation of the rate of elastin turnover in lung parenchyma by measurement of aspartate racemization (Fig. 10.18) and prevalence of carbon-14 originating from atmospheric testing of nuclear weapons indicates that elastin is a protein of remarkable longevity (573). In these experiments, it was concluded that total elastin synthesis essentially occurred during the periods of fetal and postnatal growth. Similarly, Powell et al. (494) showed that human aortic elastin turned over at a much slower rate than collagen based on aspartate racemization (Fig. 10.18). Whereas the degree of aspartate racemization occurring during the human life span was found to be minor for collagen, it was major for elastin (Fig. 10.18). Thus, based on the results of the rate of racemization and the specific accumulation of D-aspartate in elastin, Powell et al. (494) concluded that there is essentially no synthesis in the adult aorta. However, this conclusion did not apply to aortic collagen.

Conclusions

Biochemical evidence as presented above suggests that the turnover of elastin is very slow. Further support for this conclusion has come from the age-related accumulation of elastin-associated fluorescence. However, morphological as well as elastolytic studies indicate increased degradation of elastin during aging (519). Turnover of elastin does indeed occur since immunoreactive elastin peptides could be found in plasma and measurable amounts of desmosines have been found in human urine (573). However, the exact origin of these degradation products is not known. The findings of decreased desmosine content in tissues during aging could be due to one or more causes, including decreased synthesis of desmosine, decreased availability of tropoelastin, and/or increased rate of elastolysis (519). Fornieri et al. (170) concluded that the observed decrease in elastin content of tissues with age is difficult to interpret due to the incomplete knowledge of the mechanisms involved in the regulation of elastin synthesis.

PROTEOGLYCANS

Biochemical Composition

Proteoglycan consists of a core protein with at least one or more glycosaminoglycan (GAG) side chains covalently attached. The proteoglycan structure resembles that of a bottle-cleaning brush with a central stem, representing the core protein, and the attached bristles, each representing a single GAG chain. However, instead of being rigid, the entire proteoglycan molecule is highly flexible.

Core proteins elucidated so far have varied in size from 11,000 to 220,000 daltons (d), and the number of GAG chains attached has varied from one to approximately 100. In the large aggregating type of proteoglycan found in cartilage, the basic unit consisting of core protein and GAG is frequently referred to as a monomer, or sometimes as a subunit. Also, these structures may contain the core protein with attached oligosaccharide side chains. Thus the total weight of each monomer could be up to 10 million daltons or more. In turn, in some tissues, like cartilage, many of these large monomers may be noncovalently bound or "aggregated" to a central "string-like" filament consisting of a disaccharide repeating unit of hyaluronic acid. Thus the total weight of these large conglomerates may be in the tens of millions of Dalton units (77, 79, 246, 548, 630).

Progress in recent years has led to the complete elucidation of the coding sequence for the large aggregating proteoglycan of human and rat cartilage (129, 130). In the absence of a methodical nomenclature, it is common practice to indicate a member of the proteoglycan class by appending the suffix "an" to the name of the molecule once the primary structure of its protein core has been determined. Thus the large aggregating proteoglycan of cartilage has recently been referred to as "aggrecan" (130).

In the past, GAGs have frequently been referred to as acid mucopolysaccharides (304). The basic building block and repeating unit is composed of a varying number of identical or nearly identical disaccharide units consisting of hexuronic acid and a N-substituted hexosamine moiety. In many cases, these units may be modified by attached sulfated ester groups. Reviews of important structures, including those of hyaluronic acid, chondroitin, 4- and 6-sulfated derivatives of chondroitin, heparin, heparan sulfate, dermatan sulfate, and keratan sulfate, have been made by Kittlick (304) and Carney and Muir (79).

Some comments are noteworthy here. First, keratan sulfate is actually not a GAG but a sulfated glycoprotein. Its basic repeating disaccharide consists of a galactose-6-sulfate and N-acetyl-glucose-6-sulfate but not hexuronic acid. Second, the repeating units of GAG are built up into a polymer-like chain which may vary greatly in size anywhere from 20,000 to approximately 10 million daltons. The common properties of GAG usually dominate the physical behavior of proteoglycans and thus are frequently used to classify these molecules (548).

Less is known about the structure of core proteins, but investigations have suggested a large diversity in sizes and configurations (79). Molecular weights have ranged up to 20 kd, with structures consisting of one or more linear polypeptide chains arranged in lengths up to 400 nm (304). The amino acid composition of these polypeptides varies greatly according to the species and tissue but usually lacks cysteine and shows an abundance of glutamate, glycine, serine, and threonine (304). Furthermore, amino acid sequence analyses have indicated the existence of functional domains (548). For example, aggrecan contains a core protein organized into multidomains consisting of three globular regions (referred to as G1, G2, and G3) and two extended regions (E1, E2) (234, 246). The functions of these domains are unclear, but most appear to be involved in some sort of binding or adhesion. This is especially true for the NH_2- terminal globular (G1) domain of the core protein for aggrecan, which is capable of binding to hyaluronic acid to form large aggregates.

Long-branched chains of oligosaccharide residues have frequently been found attached to the core protein. This is especially true for aggrecan (77, 79). Sugars frequently found in these chains include fructose, N-acetylglucosamine, mannose, galactose, and sialic acid. These chains are N- or O-linked to the core protein by either asparagine or serine residues, respectively. The function of the N-linked oligosaccharides is not known; however, their high abundance suggests involvement in the biosynthesis and assembly of the proteoglycan. The function of the O-linked oligosaccharides is also not known, but they are believed to represent keratan sulfate chains in varying stages of completion (79).

Aggregating and Nonaggregating Populations of Proteoglycans

Proteoglycans have been classified according to their physical properties of buoyancy during centrifugation (630). The *low buoyant density* species are composed of nonaggregating molecules of low molecular weight predominantly consisting of a core protein with one or two GAG chains and possibly N-linked oligosaccharides covalently attached (630). These represent major species in cartilage (630) and are of the types of proteoglycan described as binding to extracellular components such as collagen and fibronectin (548).

The *high buoyant density* proteoglycans are of much larger molecular weights than the low buoyant types and have in turn been classified as nonaggregating and aggregating (630). In bovine articular cartilage, the nonaggregating type is relatively minor, accounting for less than 15% of the high buoyant density proteoglycans. They are structurally analogous to the aggregating type except that their hyaluronate binding domain is nonfunctional (630). However, by far the largest species, at least in cartilage, is the aggregating type, which consists of numerous proteoglycan subunits. These bind to hyaluronic acid and form extremely large supramolecular structures (79).

One mechanism of binding proteoglycans involves the link proteins. This is a group of heterogenous proteins of low molecular weight (40–50 kd) which function to stabilize the interaction of the proteoglycan subunit with hyaluronic acid in aggregate formation. The primary structure for link protein of aggrecan has been determined (135) and found to contain numerous disulfide-bonded loops (540).

Age-Related Changes in Proteoglycans

Care must be used in equating the changes occurring with growth and development with those occurring at late age. This is especially true in the case of proteoglycans where many investigators frequently refer to changes occurring in the early years of life as age-related. Although for a broad definition of aging this is true (630), this discussion presents aging henceforth by the criteria of Strehler (607), in that these changes must be universal, intrinsic, progressive, and deleterious (that is, senescence). Thus the events of aging to be discussed are those occurring after maturation, especially during the latter years of life.

Hydration. Because of their large size and high contents of sulfated and carboxylated carbohydrate groups, proteoglycans and their highly polyanionic GAG chains are capable of binding large volumes of water and thus have large swelling capacities. In cartilage, for example, the ability to withstand a compressive load is greatly dependent upon the ability of proteoglycans to expel and imbibe water (79). In other tissues, like skin, the maintenance of normal turgor and viscoelastic properties has been attributed to the water-binding properties of proteoglycans (211).

The percent hydration of cartilages from various tissues of human and animal species progressively declines with age (379, 502, 613, 626, 629). An age-related decline in hydration proportional to the decline in the fixed charge density (FCD) was also noted in human intervertebral disc (646a). However, in one study with human hip cartilage, the FCD was found to increase while loss of fluid under the effect of externally applied compression diminished with age (220).

Whether the age-related decrease in water content of cartilage is actually due to changes in proteoglycan structure remains questionable. A more likely explanation is the increase in cross-linking of collagen with age which restricts the ability of embedded proteoglycans to swell (630). In support, tensile stiffness, an attribute of collagen aging, is inversely correlated with percent water of tracheal cartilage (502).

Proteoglycan tissue content. Because of its low extractability, similar methodological problems in quantitation of glycosaminoglycan content in aging connective tissue are encountered for proteoglycans as for elastin and collagen.

A consistent finding in cartilage studies is that the extraction yield of proteoglycans by guanidine hydrochloride significantly decreases with age (31, 471, 680). This is especially true in studies where young and adult tissues were compared (613, 680). However, longevity studies have shown that essentially little change occurs after maturation (499, 539, 626, 636). Only in several studies with human and sheep cartilages was the extraction yield noted to decline after maturation into old age, but even in these studies, the major percentage of this decline essentially occurred during the very early years of life (142, 604). The yield was also found to vary according to the degree of cartilage disruption contributed to the amount of surface area exposed to the extractant (31). Changes in the collagen network with age rather than changes in proteoglycan structure (31) may have created a barrier to diffusion. Thus there is a need in this type of study to report total rather than extractable proteoglycan concentration of the cartilage.

Several methods of quantitative assessment of proteoglycan and GAG levels have been used. While most studies have used uronic acid concentrations as an index, others have measured hexosamine, galactosamine, chondroitin sulfate, or total GAG or have used histochemical evaluation (79).

Age-related trends in the total proteoglycan content of the intervertebral disc are similar to those noted for cartilage. In a comparison of disc tissue from young and old beagle dogs (2 vs. 10 yr), Cole et al. (104) noted that levels were decreased in the older tissues as determined by uronic acid concentrations in total tissue and guanidine hydrochloride extracts. Similar findings were made by Adams and Muir (1) with a guanidine hydrochloride extract of human disc tissue, except that the amount of proteoglycan remaining in the residue after extraction was higher in tissue from an older patient (44 yr) than in that from a younger patient (16 yr). Analyses of proteoglycan content of human disc evaluated over the life span (4.5–76 yr) showed that levels declined from 4.5 years to approximately 30 yr of age and thereafter varied very little with age (214).

Changes occurring in other tissues are inconsistent. For example, levels in the human meniscus increased until the second decade of life and thereafter remained approximately the same (401). Conversely, total GAG contents of skeletal and cardiac muscles of rats (413) and renal tissues of dogs (664) progressively decreased over the life spans. However, levels did not vary with age in human glomerular basement membranes (102).

The age-related changes occurring in GAG contents

of ligaments and tendon tissues are also not clear. Levels have been reported to either increase in bovine tendon (258) or decrease in rabbit Achilles tendon (85), but they do not vary in rabbit collateral ligament (175).

Just as unclear are changes in GAG concentrations of skin during aging. Biochemical studies have shown that levels as measured by uronic acid concentrations progressively declined over the human life span (169). Yet in another study, levels drastically declined during growth, remained approximately the same during middle ages, and slightly increased at old age (333). Conversely, morphological studies with elderly human subjects have suggested that levels increase with aging (388). In these studies, it is unclear whether the site of skin sampling had any influence on the results. Whereas one study used nonexposed abdominal skin (169), the other dealt with sun-exposed skin from the arm (388).

Studies of age-related changes in GAG concentrations in arterial and aortic tissues have given conflicting results (304, 486). Morphological studies suggest that GAG accumulates in these tissues especially in arteriosclerotic disease (57). This accumulation is believed to be due in part to the degenerative changes known to occur with aging in these tissues and in part to an age-related increase in permeability which allows blood-borne GAG penetration of the arterial wall (57). However, biochemical studies using different methods to assess GAG accumulation in these tissues have been conflicting. In these studies, levels have either increased (219, 256, 434), decreased (609), or remained unchanged during middle and late ages (223, 686). In a study with rabbit aorta, GAG content estimated by total hexosamine did vary from 5 to 15 months of age (247).

Interestingly, extensive deposition of periodic acid–Schiff (PAS)- positive material has been noted to occur with aging of the vasculature (38, 116, 255, 589). The positive staining of vessel tissues is indicative of vicinal hydroxyl groups, suggesting the presence of carbohydrate. However, it is not known whether this observation contributed to the age-related accumulation of GAG or some other carbohydrate, such as glycoprotein or Maillard-modified proteins, as hypothesized by Vlassara et al. (670).

Structural changes in the aggregating type of proteoglycan (aggrecan). Structural changes described for aggrecan which are attributed to aging include: *(1)* decrease in size and number of chondroitin sulfate residues, *(2)* increase in the 6-sulfation relative to the 4-sulfation of chondroitin sulfate, *(3)* increase in size and number of keratan sulfate and O-linked oligosaccharide chains attached to the core protein, and *(4)* increase in the protein to uronate ratios. These changes, which are essentially associated with the synthetic capacity of chondrocytes, are completed by the end of growth, and thus relatively minor changes have been noted to occur during the remainder of life (31, 79, 142, 537, 538, 626, 636). However, some human studies have indicated that some of these changes may continue well after growth into old age (32, 146, 379). Thus whether these changes actually occur progressively over the life span is far from conclusive.

In papain digests of human articular cartilage, it was noted that uronic acid when used as an index of aggrecan content decreased slightly from birth until the age of 25 yr and thereafter remained unchanged. Conversely, hyaluronic acid, as determined by a specific radiosorbent assay and expressed as a percentage of this total proteoglycan estimate, progressively increased over human life (Fig. 10.19) (32, 234, 257). Similar findings were made by Elliott and Gardner (146) when levels were expressed as a percentage of total GAG concentration. However, in a limited number of samples, Pearson and Mason (482) noted that levels did not vary over the human life span when expressed on the basis of dry tissue weight.

The most important changes in the structure of aggrecan during human aging result from the degradative processes due to proteolysis (537, 538). Electrophoretic studies of cartilage extracts showed a progressive increase in heterogeneity of aggrecan subunit size over

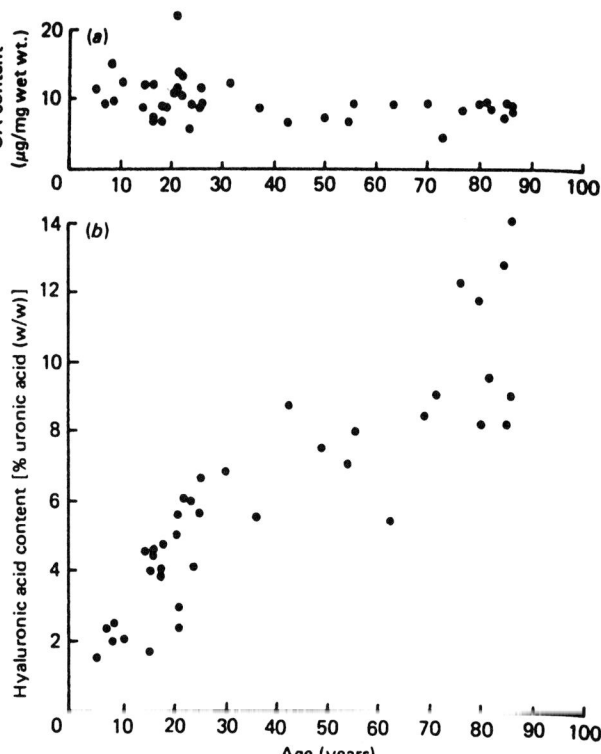

FIG. 10.19. Total uronic acid (as a measure of total proteoglycan estimate) and hyaluronic acid contents in papain digest of human articular cartilage. [From Holmes et al. (257), by copyright permission from Portland Press Ltd., Colchester, UK.]

the human life span (234). Although other mechanisms, such as age-related changes in gene expression and variation in activity of posttranslational modification enzymes, could explain this heterogeneity, the most likely cause based upon available evidence is due to an age-related increase in the proteolytic modification of aggrecan (234).

The N-terminal region of the core protein adjacent to the hyaluronic acid–binding region (HABR) appears to be especially susceptible to proteolytic cleavage (538). This results in the generation of aggrecan fragments bearing GAG chains, which are presumably able to diffuse from the cartilage, leaving behind hyaluronic acid and filaments bearing the HABR with the attached link proteins. Consistent with this hypothesis is the accumulation of poorly glycosylated species of N-terminal HABR in adult cartilage (234, 538), although in the studies by Bayliss and colleagues (32, 234) an asymptotic increase in this binding region occurred, with a plateau reached after the fifth decade of human life. Other evidence has come from the identification of a potential cleavage site within the interglobular region between the G1 and G2 domains of the core protein adjacent to the HABR. This cleavage by the enzyme stromelysin results in the separation of the G1 domain with the attached HABR from the remainder of the molecule (165).

Another potential site of cleavage is the C-terminal region of the G3 globular domain of the core protein (166). This results in cleavage of the G3 domain, allowing the C-terminal fragments to freely diffuse from the tissue (234). Evidence in support of this mechanism comes from electron microscopy studies which show a large proportion of aggrecan in the mature cartilage matrix from various animal species which lack an intact G3 domain, thus leading to the core proteins of shorter average length than those in which the G3 domain remained attached (479). Also, another investigation showed that the molar yield of a marker peptide for the G3 domain of aggrecan was markedly reduced in mature bovine cartilage (166).

The above studies revealed that changes in aggrecan subunits due to proteolysis result in shorter core proteins which lack the G1 and/or the G3 globular domains, thus leading to the accumulation of the N-terminal HABR. However, other studies suggest that structural changes, which may contribute to proteolysis, also occur within the hyaluronic acid filament. As previously explained, there is an age-related accumulation of hyaluronic acid which is unable to escape from the cartilage matrix. The work of Bayliss and colleagues suggests that this increase cannot be explained on the basis of increased synthesis. Further work showed that the average chain size of hyaluronic acid progressively decreased over the human life span (Fig. 10.20) (257).

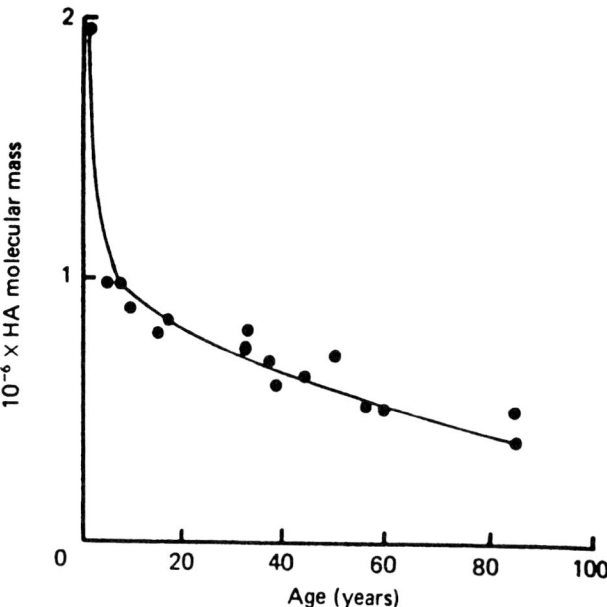

FIG. 10.20. Changes in molecular weight of hyaluronic acid over human life span. [From Holmes et al. (257), by copyright permission from Portland Press Ltd., Colchester, UK.]

Thus there is a slow accumulation of partially degraded hyaluronic acid that, together with the smaller aggrecan subunits, results in a lower-molecular-weight aggregate in the adult cartilage. The change in the overall size of aggrecan occurring during the human life span has been estimated to be over 14-fold (234).

Link proteins are also subjected to proteolysis. Evidence for such age-related fragmentation of link proteins has come from work using SDS-polyacrylamide gel electrophoresis/Western blot analysis of human cartilage extracts (32, 431). Using a polyclonal antibody to localize link proteins on the transfer blots, fragmentation was most noticeable in extracts from humans aged 44 yr and older (32). However, in this study, there appeared to be no difference in the fragmentation pattern in the extracts from a 44- and an 85-yr-old subject.

In similar studies, an age-related shift was noted in the proportion of two major molecular weight forms of link protein of rabbits up to approximately 2 yr of age (167). However, these changes appeared to be more related to development and maturation since the shift was not noticeably different at 1 and 2 yr and only slightly different from 20-wk-old animals (167). Further evidence that these changes were essentially events of maturation was that the total amount of link protein quantitated in guanidine extracts of cartilage did not differ at 22 and 80 wk of age. In these rabbit studies, some fragmentation of link proteins was also noticeable, though it represented a very minor fraction of total link proteins (< 5%) and did not differ at 20, 50 or 100 wk of age.

Proteolytic cleavage of link protein in the adult is limited to specific sites near the N-terminus region of the molecule and the adjacent disulfide-bonded loop (540). However, evidence suggests that further internal fragmentation of the molecule may be mediated by a free radical mechanism involving hydroxyl radicals formed from H_2O_2 by trace transition-metal catalysis (522). Intact disulfide bonds in the molecule tend to favor an interaction of the link protein with HABR in a pseudonative configuration even after proteolytic fragmentation occurs (536). Furthermore, its participation in proteoglycan aggregation appears to cause the link protein to be more resistant to proteolysis. These factors result in the accumulation of modified link proteins throughout life (540).

The significance of these fragmentative changes of the link proteins in the formation and stability of aggrecan in human aging is unclear. During normal aging, there appears to be no impairment in the ability of individual subunits to participate in aggregation (538). However, aggrecan preparations from mature human cartilage were shown to be considerably less stable to competitive disassociation than those from young cartilage (541). This instability may be explained on the basis of competition for the link protein between endogenous aggrecan and the excessive build-up of HABR in older human cartilage (79). The total amount of link protein in aggrecan preparations from human cartilage was found to be limiting at all ages, as evidenced by the molar amounts of the HABR being always in excess of the link protein. However, the molar ratio between the two did not vary after the second decade of human life (234).

Thus proteolytic changes occurring in proteoglycan structure of cartilage during normal aging are significant. However, these changes are probably even more significant during the processes of osteoarthritis, where the extent of the degradation may vary at different anatomical sites depending on mechanical stresses. In animal species other than human, these degradative changes are not believed to be as significant due to the shorter life spans. Therefore, there appears to be less propensity to accumulate such products of degradation (538, 540).

Structural changes in proteoglycans. Studies by Stanescu et al. (601) described a small, rapidly migrating proteoglycan species of low buoyant density with a protein core of Mr = 47 kd in extracts from young human cartilage. This proteoglycan was not present in extracts from humans over the age of 40 yr. Instead, the extracts from older subjects contained a low-buoyant-density proteoglycan with a core protein of heterogenous size, molecular weight ranging from 100 to 170 kd. Thus two distinct species of nonaggregating proteoglycans were found in human cartilage. The one found in the younger tissues was not expressed in the older tissues.

However, the higher-molecular-weight, heterogeneous species found in the older cartilage was believed to originate as a fragmented product of aggrecan. In support of this supposition, immunoreactivities for keratan sulfate and HABR were found for the higher-molecular-weight species from older subjects but not for the species prepared from younger subjects. Interestingly, the lower-molecular-weight proteoglycan was identified with osteoarthritis in the newly formed cartilage occurring in older patients.

In separate studies, Sampaio et al. (553) described the isolation of a low-molecular-weight (LMW) proteoglycan from human articular cartilage with a core protein of M_r = 40–44 kd. This proteoglycan was found to cross-react with antibodies raised against dermatan sulfate-proteoglycan II (DS-PG II) isolated from bovine cartilage by Rosenberg et al. (532) and was subsequently named human DS-PG II. This species appears to be similar to the LMW proteoglycan described by Stanescu et al. (601). However, the relationship between the two, or indeed whether they are the same proteoglycan, has not been verified. Age-related changes of DS-PG II were studied by Sampaio et al. (553) by competitive RIA. This study showed that levels expressed per weight cartilage increased until maturation and thereafter progressively declined throughout the remainder of the human life span. In contrast, total glycosaminoglycan content of this tissue expressed in a similar fashion did not vary with age (553). The function of DS-PG II is uncertain but is probably related to rates of deposition and maintenance of the collagen fibril network shown for other proteoglycans (234).

Age-Related Changes of Proteoglycans in Specific Tissues. The meniscus of the human adult was found to contain proteoglycan molecules of similar size and GAG content to those of cartilage, although the tissue concentrations were considerably lower (401). Another difference with cartilage is that there are fewer GAG chains covalently bound to the core protein (401). Although the large aggregating proteoglycans are the dominant species in the meniscus, this tissue is also believed to differ from cartilage by containing a substantially greater amount of nonaggregating proteoglycans enriched in dermatan sulfate (398).

In human meniscus, the molar ratio of galactosamine/glucosamine indicative of chondroitin sulfate/keratan sulfate contents decreases into the middle of the second decade of life and thereafter remains the same throughout old age (70 yr) (401). However, the ratio of 6-sulfation to 4-sulfation of chondroitin sulfate progressively increases between the ages of 4 and 70 yr.

In general, the age-related changes described for the intervertebral disc are similar to those for cartilage. Mild extraction of human disc tissue from a 44-yr-old subject with 0.15 M sodium acetate revealed that the majority of the proteoglycans were of a smaller size in comparison to those extracted from younger (8- and 16-yr-old) disc tissue. This was not noted in subsequent extractions with magnesium chloride and guanidine hydrochloride (1). Similarly, comparison of young vs. old (2 vs. 10 yr) canine intervertebral disc tissues showed a significant decrease in the percentage of proteoglycans, which could aggregate in older animals. This occurred simultaneously with an increase in the average size of nonaggregating proteoglycans, which was most prominent in the annuli fibrosis of older dogs (104). Thus, as previously mentioned for cartilage, it would appear that some, if not all, of this LMW material present in the older disc tissues may represent fragmentation products of the larger aggregating type of proteoglycans.

In the previously mentioned studies, it was found that the extracted proteoglycans from the older tissues contained greater amounts of GAG chains with a high content of keratan sulfate, which was most prominent in nonaggregating proteoglycans (104). However, in other studies with human and canine disc tissues, keratan sulfate content of GAG chains essentially did not vary after maturation (71, 203, 214).

Dermatan sulfate–containing proteoglycans were found to be a major component in both newborn and adult (5-yr-old) bovine tendons. Analyses showed that these proteoglycans were relatively small in size, with a core protein averaging 53 kd. The amount found in older animals was greater than that in newborn. Whereas chondroitin sulfate was not detected in the newborn, a large amount of this GAG was present in the older tendons. Conversely, more hyaluronic acid was detected in tendons from the newborn (258).

Age-related changes described for various GAGs present in aortic and arterial tissues are conflicting, with no consistent patterns discernable. This may be due in part to the source of the tissue and the degree of arteriosclerosis and/or atherosclerotic plaque formation (223, 304, 434, 486, 609, 686).

Studies by Willen et al. (679), using antibodies raised against specific proteoglycans of the human dermis, showed that changes in the type of proteoglycans occurred essentially after the age of 50 yr. These changes were progressive, highly dependent upon the dermal layer, and consisted of the following: increased keratan sulfate in the epidermis, increased dermatan sulfate but decreased chondroitin sulfate in the papillary dermis, and decreased chondroitin-6-sulfate in the basal lamina.

Synthesis. Human studies measuring [^{35}S]sulfate incorporation into proteoglycans as a measure of synthesis have generally shown that the rate of incorporation is maximum at birth, decreases rapidly until the second decade, and thereafter declines at greatly reduced rates throughout the remainder of the life span.

These studies have generally used both cell and explant cultures from tissues of donors of increasing age. These have included studies with cartilage explants (636), gingival fibroblasts (30), and bone cells (160). In the study of Bartold et al. (30), the rate of incorporation into the cell layers of cultures derived from gingival fibroblasts essentially did not vary from donors of ages 25 yr and older. However, when secreted proteoglycans were also considered, the rate of decline over the life span was much more noticeable and significant.

The rate of incorporation of [^{35}S]sulfate into cartilage explants from calves (4–6 wk) and mature (7–10 yr) cows was measured at various time intervals during 18 h of incubation (176). When results were expressed on the basis of dry tissue weight, the rates were significantly reduced in older animals. However, when corrected for cell densities, thus reflecting the decreased number of chondrocytes present in older cartilage, these rates did not vary with age.

The problem of using [^{35}S]sulfate incorporation into proteoglycans as a measure of its synthesis is obvious. What is actually measured is the rate of proteoglycan sulfation, which may or may not be synonymous with its synthesis. However, some investigators have argued that this measurement is actually a good indicator of synthesis, especially in culture studies (30).

Whether the total sulfation of proteoglycans varies with aging in vivo is not clear. In glomerular basement membranes, it was found that the proteoglycan content, measured by uronic acid concentration, did not vary with human age (102). When total sulfation of these proteoglycans was expressed as a ratio to total uronic acid, levels initially increased up to the age of 25 yr and thereafter declined sharply throughout the remainder of human life. This suggests that the reduction in net negative charge may alter the permeability/selective properties of these membranes (102). However, using staining methods with the cationic dye Alcian blue as an index of sulfation in human intervertebral disc, Taylor et al. (624) noted that essentially all increases in sulfation occurred during the early years of development. Whereas sulfation increased during the first decade of life, thereafter it did not change with age. Interestingly, the major part of the increase occurred only after the disappearance of blood vessels from the disc. Thus these researchers hypothesized that the replacement of chondroitin sulfate by keratan sulfate is initiated by the loss of vascularity in this disc, causing a condition of depleted oxygen supply. This would support the notion that the shift from chondroitin sulfate to keratan sulfate in proteoglycan structure is essentially a developmental event.

Turnover. Turnover of proteoglycans is believed to be considerably more rapid than that of collagen. Whereas the half-life of collagen may be measured in years, that for proteoglycans is measured in days (63). If urinary excretion of uronic acid is any indication of this turnover, human studies have shown that urinary levels are highest at birth, progressively decline with age until 20 yr, and thereafter remain at constant low values throughout middle and old ages (266, 301, 336). These results suggest that the major rate of turnover of proteoglycans occurs essentially during development. Although the exact metabolic events occurring after maturation are uncertain, these results further suggest that turnover is maintained at relatively constant levels throughout old age and/or that the degraded products are immediately, systemically, or locally reutilized.

Half-life studies of sulfated GAG in various tissues of rats show a progressive increase throughout the life span (304). GAG of cartilage have the longest half-life, followed respectively by skin and liver. However, even in the oldest (24 months) rats in this study, measurable half-lives were still very short in all tissues (< 16 days), suggesting that turnover remained continuous and very rapid even into old age.

The primary mode of proteoglycan turnover in vivo is believed to be through degradation mediated by proteolysis (234). In cartilage, for example, normal turnover involves the release of mainly large aggrecan fragments, such as those cleaved at the G1 and G2 domains of the core protein (506). These large fragments are believed to be able to diffuse slowly out of the tissue. However, other fragments, such as HABR, may be retained by the tissue, as previously discussed (234).

In vitro studies suggest that normal turnover of proteoglycans tends to involve the release of components into the surroundings. Explants of cartilage, when maintained in culture, released into the medium small amounts of proteoglycan components, particularly GAG chains, as the result of normal turnover (506). The amount released progressively increased over time in proportion to the amount of time maintained in culture and greatly accelerated in the presence of interleukin 1 (506). In explants of bovine cartilage, it was noted that the half-life of proteoglycan populations was considerably shorter in tissues from mature (1–5 yr) cattle than from immature (3 days–6 months) calves (62, 76). In the study by Brand et al. (62), the amount of proteoglycan released into the medium increased only slightly with age (6%). However, in cultured chondrocytes from rabbit donors of increasing age (1 wk–30 months), the amount of newly synthesized proteoglycan released into the medium did not vary in donors 4 wk or older (374). Thus the significance of this release as a measure of proteoglycan turnover in culture during cellular aging appears, at best, to be minor.

Conclusions

Several observations confirm the progressive decline in water content of aging cartilage. However, the biochemical basis of this phenomenon is highly controversial. Changes in glycosaminoglycan composition have indeed been observed, but most are based on studies of extractable proteoglycan, the content of which becomes increasingly cross-linked to collagen with age until it appears to vanish. One of the most reproducible and significant findings is the progressive fragmentation of aggrecan during aging. Where the process is generally attributed to proteolysis, metal-catalyzed oxidation reactions could be involved as well. However, since proteoglycan turnover is much higher than that of collagen, the possibility exists that chondrocytes from older mammals synthesize proteoglycan isoforms that are not as mechanically efficient as those synthesized during growth phase (77). Obviously, the role of proteoglycans in aging of cartilage and other tissues is yet poorly understood.

LENS CRYSTALLINS

Overview

The unusual morphological, biological, and metabolic aspects of the lens together with the fact that its proteins, once synthesized, do not turn over have made it a subject of intense study in aging research. The long life of lens proteins predisposes them to aggregation and light scattering, which, if extensive, will impair vision through clouding of the lens. The incidence of age-related cataract begins to rise after 50 yr. Over 45% of persons between the ages of 75 and 85 yr have cataract, and nearly 70% beyond the age of 85 yr suffer from this debilitating disease (687). Thus cataract is an important disease of old age, and because of overlap in biochemical abnormalities, some investigators have proposed that it may represent an exaggeration of changes found in normal aging (654).

We review biochemical age-related changes in crystallins and their mechanisms of formation, focusing primarily on the human lens. The reader with particular interest in the overall problem of cataract as a disease is referred to the comprehensive monograph by Young (687), which provides a full account of the pathogenesis, epidemiology, and clinical significance of age-related cataracts. Throughout the text we will use the term "cataract" to indicate changes in the senile type of cataract, which is characterized by changes occurring predominantly in the nuclear region of the lens. There are, however, other types of cataract, such as cortical and posterior subcapsular cataracts, which may differ from nuclear cataracts in natural history (687).

The lens consists of an onion-shaped system of cellular structures held together by a permeable capsule of type IV collagen (Fig. 10.21). The core of the lens, also called the nucleus, contains the oldest fibers. The epithelial cells at the anterior pole divide and migrate to the bow region, where they differentiate into elongated, "fiber-like" cells which lose nuclei, mitochondria, and other organelles (254, 308, 328, 375, 501). Consequently, the metabolic activity is highest in the lens epithelium and cortex and decreases toward the nucleus. Lens metabolism is in various respects similar to that of the red cell, as ATP synthesis needed for Na^P, K^P- pump and other reactions is largely dependent on anaerobic glycolysis and the hexose monophosphate shunt (89, 136, 654). Oxygen tension is negligible in the lens (469), and this has led some investigators to propose that the lens is "canned" (143).

The lens crystallins comprise approximately 90% of total soluble protein of the lens, which can be separated by gel filtration into three major classes, the α-, β-, and γ-crystallins (Fig. 10.22). The α-crystallins account for 50%–60% of the total soluble protein and are present as aggregates of 600–800 kd, consisting of 20,000 dalton subunits held together by noncovalent bonds. Beta-crystallins range from 10,000 to 60,000 d in weight, with a major polypeptide of 24 kd (βBp). The γ-crystallins are a group of seven or more cysteine-rich proteins with an average weight of 20,000 d. Interestingly, taxonomic studies have shown that several crystallins, although structural proteins, have sequence homology with enzymes, such as lactate dehydrogenase, α-enolase, or alcohol dehydrogenase, from which they arose through gene duplication or gene sharing (484). Only in a few instances in selected species, however, have these enzymatic activities been preserved in the lens.

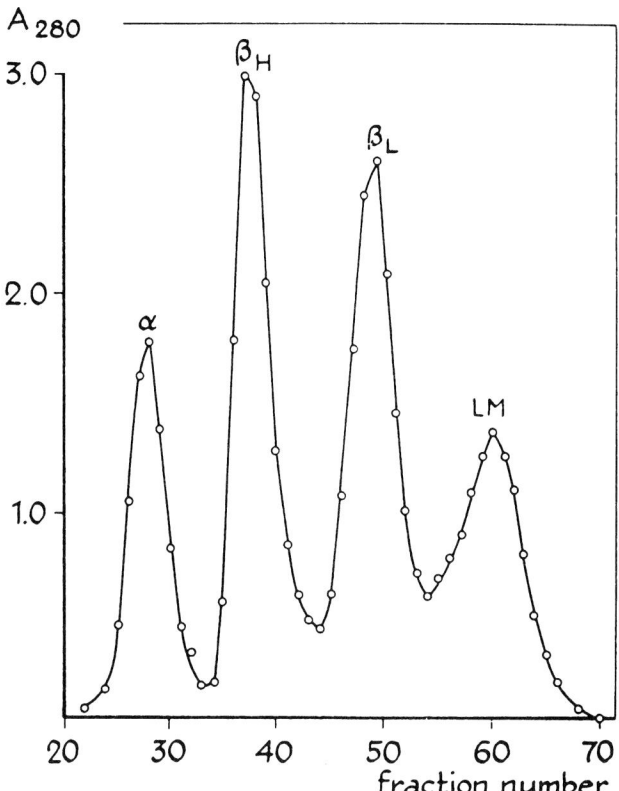

FIG. 10.22. Separation by gel filtration of the water-soluble lens proteins on an Ultrogel AcA 34 column. [From Bloemendal and Zweers (51), by permission.]

Protein conformation and supramolecular assembly of lens crystallins together with a tight control of the lens water content appear to play a crucial role in minimizing light scattering, since the latter increases invariably when the lens structure is disrupted through

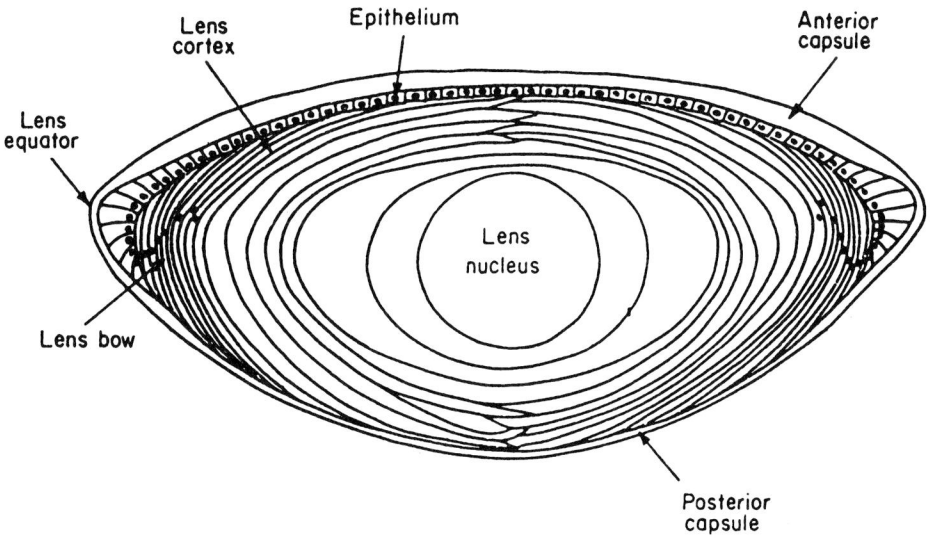

FIG. 10.21. Diagrammatic section of dog lens. [From van Heyningen, (654), by permission.]

mechanical means or acute metabolic stress, as in experimental diabetes, galactosemia, and other interventions (310, 535, 551, 520).

Age-Related Changes in Lens and Lens Crystallins

The lens grows throughout the life span. However, the growth rate decreases with age (453, 455, 557), and by the age of 70, the formation of new fibers is significantly reduced (528). However, the weight of the lens continues to increase (232, 557), as does the permeability of the lens capsule and the nuclear water content (162, 580). Aging lenses lose their ability to accommodate, and the loss is almost complete by the age of 50 yr. Aging lenses become progressively more yellow due to the formation of chromophores which absorb in the blue region (350–400 nm) (Fig. 10.23) (550). Lens fluorescence and opacity also increase as a function of age, regardless of the ethnic background of the population studied. In Japan, for example, opacities are found in nearly 90% of individuals above 80 yr of age (634). Since atherosclerosis linked to dietary factors is much less prevalent in Japan than in the United States (325), it is likely that dietary factors do not play a major role in the pathogenesis of cataracts. However, the intake of certain vitamins may have favorable effects on the prevalence and progression of cataracts (353).

Solubility. The hallmark of lens aging is a progressive discoloration and a loss of solubility of lens crystallins (Fig. 10.24). Lens crystallins can be fractionated into water-soluble and urea-soluble and -insoluble proteins. In the newborn lens, 95% of total proteins are soluble (9, 101, 128, 345). After the age of 50 yr, there is a rapid increase in the insoluble proteins (557, 697), and by the age of 80 yr, approximately half of the total protein is insoluble (9, 18). Nuclear proteins are generally less soluble than cortical proteins (8, 322), but the insolubilization process affects the entire lens (9) and all three crystallin fractions (98, 697). Similar changes have been noted in animal lenses, such as the bovine lens (39).

High-molecular-weight (HMW) aggregates form in the aging lens (286, 591). These are rich in α-crystallins and can be broken apart in urea, indicating that hydrogen bonds play a role in their formation. They increase beyond age 60 yr and account for approximately 15% of the total soluble protein in very old lenses (286, 596, 697). HMW aggregates are present in high concentrations in the nucleus, and covalent disulfide bonds are involved in their formation (557). In some lenses, HMW aggregates of 150 million daltons are detected, which are thought to represent native proteins in the process of becoming urea-insoluble (25, 543, 590, 697). Such aggregates may be sufficiently large to produce opaci-

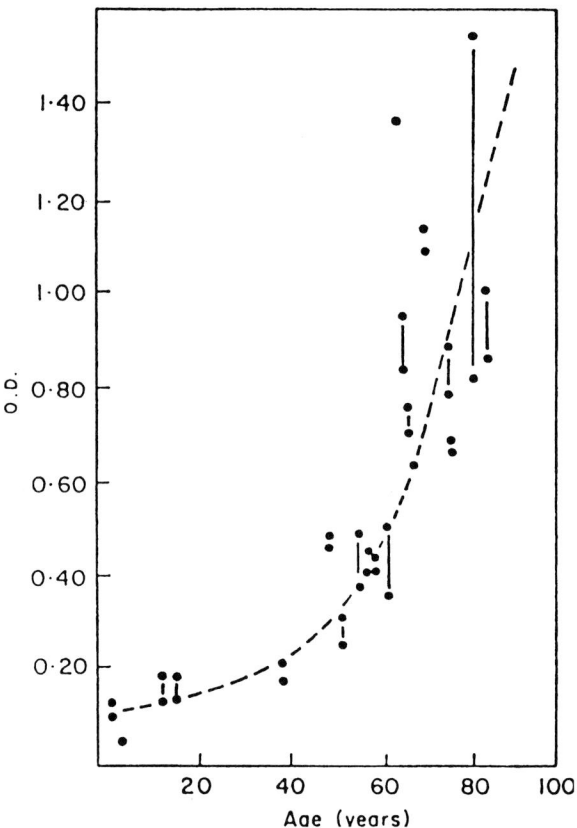

FIG. 10.23. Intensification of blue light absorption (at 440 nm) of noncataractous human lenses with increasing age. Points for the paired lenses of one individual are joined by a vertical line. [From Zigman (693), by permission.]

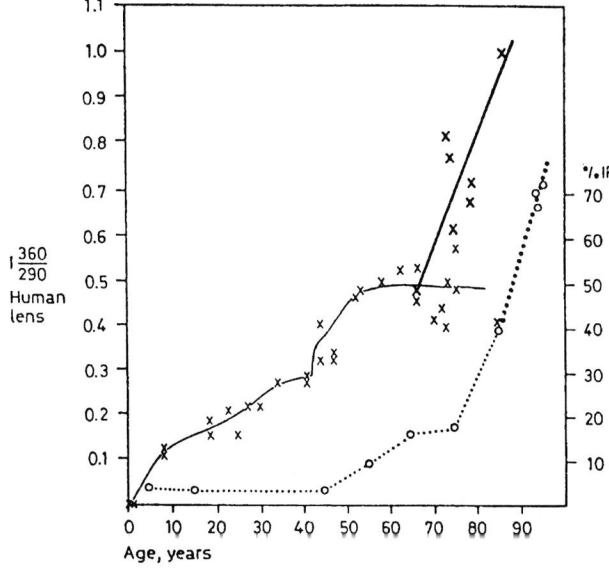

FIG. 10.24. Fluorescence intensity ratios of 360-nm fluorogen (I 360/290) in normal aging lens *(solid line)*, nuclear cataracts *(heavy solid line)*, and percent insoluble protein in normal aging lens *(dotted line)* and nuclear cataracts *(heavy dotted line)*. [From Lerman and Borkman (347), by permission.]

ties, since the critical threshold appears to be at 50 million daltons (35).

Conformational Changes.
Evidence for the unfolding of crystallins has been documented by several investigators. Liang and colleagues (357, 360) isolated HMW and LMW α-crystallins from normal young and old human lenses and obtained evidence for partial unfolding of LMW α- and γ-crystallins. However, in bovine lenses, whereas evidence was obtained for the unfolding of α-crystallins, no such changes were observed in β- and γ-crystallins. The suggestion that lens crystallins undergo unfolding during aging is based on observations that crystallins from old lenses have increased thiol reactivity and increased susceptibility to trypsin digestion (231). The increased exposure of sulfhydryl groups may favor protein aggregation by increasing hydrophobic protein interactions and the formation of intermolecular disulfide bonds. Indeed, as discussed below (see Oxidation of Crystallins), disulfide bonds are present in increased quantities in senile cataractous lenses.

Racemization and Fragmentation.
The absence of turnover of lens crystallins predisposes them to posttranslational, nonenzymatic modifications. An age-related increase in the enantiomeric D/L ratio of aspartic acid in the nuclear protein fraction from normal human lenses was first noted in 1977 (387) and confirmed soon after (194) (Fig. 10.25). Recent studies show that racemization occurs at specific sites in α-crystallins (179, 218), especially at residue 151, which, interestingly, is also an in vivo fragmentation site. A detailed study revealed that racemization increased linearly with age but that it did not correlate with the presence of cataract (649). This does not exclude the possibility that the racemized crystallins may have a higher tendency toward aggregation in aging.

Proteolysis of crystallins has been reported both in aging animal and human lenses. Degradation of αA and αB chains with elevated polypeptides gradually increasing with age has been documented in bovine lenses (658, 659). In aging human lenses, a 9,600 dalton cleavage product of a α-crystallin A chain increased to 36% of the insoluble proteins (544) and a similar 10 kd polypeptide showing cross-linking with α-crystallins increased with age and cataract formation (198, 199). Several investigators obtained evidence for proteolytic degradation of β-crystallins (249, 399) as well as for proteolysis of the membranous lens protein MIP26 (263, 542, 617).

Degradation of crystallins is increased during cataractogenesis and correlates with the severity of cataract (27). Gamma-crystallins are lost from the water-soluble fraction during cataract formation, a process that has been attributed to leakage from the lens, degradation, or insolubilization (232, 549, 555). LMW peptides (4–8 kd) have been reported in brunescent cataracts (195, 264).

In studies of normal lenses from 50-yr-old donors, Srivastava (599) obtained evidence for the presence of degraded peptides ranging between 3 and 18 kd in size. Interestingly, these peptides, which belonged to α- and γ-crystallins, showed a high tendency to self-aggregation.

Thus there is overwhelming evidence for lens crystallin degradation in aging, especially during cataractogenesis, and it would appear that the degraded crystallin polypeptides have a higher propensity to self-aggregation. Mechanisms underlying this phenomenon are discussed below.

Yellowing and Fluorescence.
Aging human lenses and lens crystallins undergo progressive yellowing (404) and acquire fluorescence in the blue region (400–450 nm) when excited at 350 nm. This blue fluorescence is often referred to as "nontryptophan" fluorescence in the lens literature. As for the insolubilization, the yellowing process appears to accelerate beyond the age of 50 yr (697, 698), especially for crystallin-linked fluorescence (Fig. 10.23). Fluorescence formation was found to be increased in diabetes (50), suggesting that hyperglycemia is involved in the accelerated browning process of the lens. The yellow color is primarily associated with the nucleus, and the absorbance at 360 nm increases three- to five-fold in the water-insoluble protein fraction from 20 to 80 yr (126, 347, 349, 558).

Although tryptophan fluorescence remains constant with age (558), several fluorescent pigments are believed to be products of tryptophan degradation. These include kynurenines, β-carbolines, and anthranilic acid (126, 640, 655–657). However, as discussed later under Glycation, there may be multiple mechanisms leading to production of crystallin-associated fluorescence.

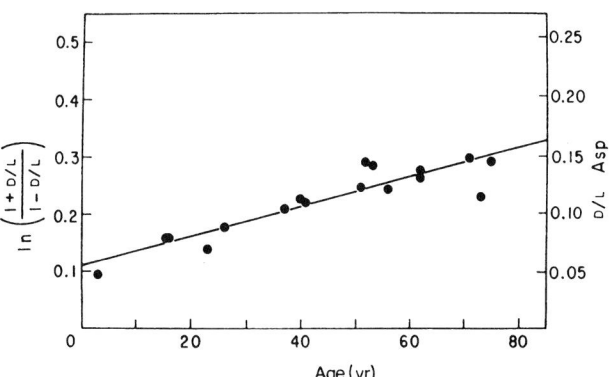

FIG. 10.25. Racemization of L-aspartic acid expressed as D/L aspartic acid in human lens crystallins as a function of age. [From Masters et al. (387), by permission.]

There appears to be a close relationship between the degree of fluorescence and the extent of insolubilization. Color and fluorescence are lowest in the soluble crystallin fraction, higher in the HMW and the urea-insoluble fractions, and highest in the totally insoluble protein fraction from the nucleus (19, 489, 697). This suggests that fluorophores may be involved in crystallin cross-linking and aggregation.

Interestingly, whereas blue fluorescence is the major fluorescent modification in the aging lens, molecules of unknown origin which emit green and red fluorescence (226, 558, 688) have been reported after the age of 70 yr. Such fluorophores could stem from vitamin C oxidation products (see topic below on Maillard Reaction by Reducing Sugars and Ascorbate).

Oxidation. The role of free sulfhydryl groups in the maintenance of lens transparency has been, and continues to be, an important research field. Decreased levels of LMW sulfhydryl compounds such as glutathione (GSH) are observed in human cataractous lens (230, 638), and a correlation between elevated protein disulfides and loss of free sulfhydryl content has been reported by several authors (21, 625).

Several in-depth studies on the relationship between oxidation, crystallin yellowing, and insolubilization have been carried out. In age-matched senile lenses, a progressive decrease in protein sulfhydryl of both cortical and nuclear lens crystallins was found to correlate inversely with the intensity of lens color (639). Free sulfhydryls were almost undetectable in the nucleus of cataractous lenses but were only moderately decreased in the cortex (638, 639). Anderson and Spector (8) found that more than 90% of the water-insoluble protein-SH groups are oxidized in advanced cataracts. In a subsequent study (9), the authors examined in detail the status of protein-sulfhydryl groups in normal lenses as a function of age. Disulfides were not detectable in 18-yr-old lens cortex but accumulated by 63 yr of age to 9% and 17% of total protein-sulfhydryl groups in cortex and nucleus, respectively. A strong correlation between degree of lens color, disulfide bond formation, and loss of free sulfhydryl groups was noted. Subsequent studies revealed the presence of protein-disulfides in HMW aggregates involving membrane-associated peptides (595). Using two-dimensional diagonal electrophoresis and immune blotting technique, Kodama and Takemoto (309) characterized disulfide-linked crystallins in lens membranes and obtained evidence for disulfide-bonded β- and especially γ-crystallins to purified fiber cell membranes from cataractous human lenses. Very few disulfide-bonded components were found in normal lenses. The role and consequences of disulfide bonding of cytosolic proteins to lens membrane proteins during cataract formation, as proposed by Spector (592), are depicted in Figure 10.26.

Additional evidence for the involvement of oxidative processes in cataracts is the detection of higher states of sulfhydryl oxidation, such as methionine sulfone and sulfoxide (637). In one group of elderly lenses, 19% of methionine was oxidized and 57% of cysteine was converted to disulfides (196). Obviously, protein unfolding in aging, as described by Harding (231), leads to exposure of sulfhydryl groups and methionine residues, which become more susceptible to oxidation. However, aging by itself, that is, in the absence of cataract, is associated with only mild and limited sulfhydryl oxidation, and the latter was noted only in membrane proteins (196). In contrast, extensive advanced oxidative

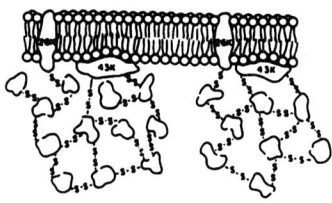

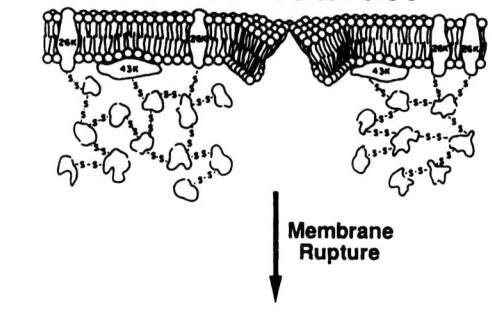

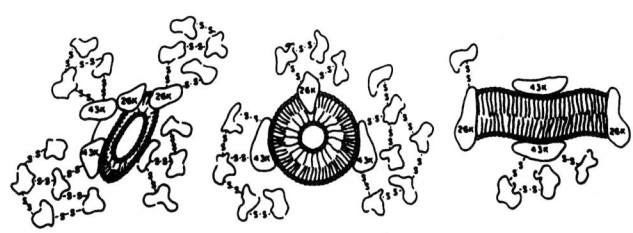

FIG. 10.26. Schematic representation of lens membrane-cytosol protein aggregates. **A:** Depiction of aggregates in the nuclear (inner) region of the lens. Intrinsic and extrinsic membrane proteins are disulfide-linked to cytosol protein units, which are in turn disulfide-linked to each other. Such giant aggregates scatter light and contribute to the loss of transparency. **B:** Aggregates in the outer cortical region of the lens. While nuclear fiber cell membranes appear to be rigid and do not break with aggregate formation, in the cortical region the formation of the aggregates causes membrane to rupture and the appearance of the membrane fragments linked to cytosol protein, as well as the nuclear region type of aggregate. [From Spector (592), by copyright permission from Academic Press.]

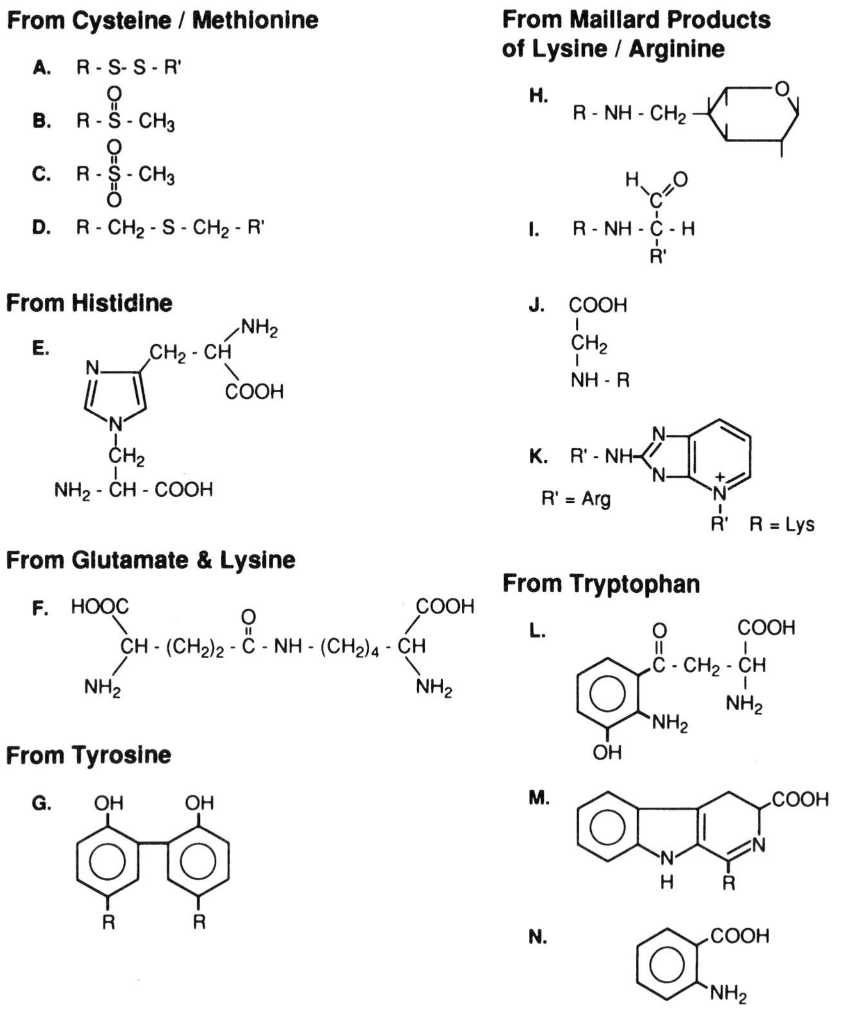

FIG. 10.27. Structures of postsynthetic modifications of amino acid residues in aging human lens. **A**: Cysteine disulfide, **B**: methionine sulfoxide, **C**: methionine sulfone, **D**: lanthionine, **E**: histidinoalanine, **F**: γ- glutamyl-lysine, **G**: dityrosine, **H**: ε-fructosyllysine, **I**: Heyns rearrangement of fructose lysine adduct, **J**: carboxymethyllysine, **K**: pentosidine, **L**: kynurenine, **M**: β-carboline, **N**: anthranilic acid.

changes are observed in cataractous lenses, suggesting that a breakdown of antioxidant defense mechanisms occurs in these lenses.

Nondisulfide Covalent Cross-links. Initial evidence for the involvement of nondisulfide covalent cross-links was based on the finding that lenses with a deep brown nucleus were only partially soluble in 6-M guanidinium chloride containing 50 mM dithiothreitol (489). Subsequent reports confirmed the presence of nonreducible HMW proteins in pigmented and cataractous lenses and revealed an association between cross-linking and yellowing of the crystallins in lenses classified according to Pirie (70, 637). Nontryptophan fluorescence was also associated with highly insoluble protein (19), suggesting that the fluorescent molecules may act as cross-links. Indeed, highly cross-linked yellow fluorescent material could be isolated from pigmented lenses following extensive proteolytic treatment (653). Borohydride reducibility of the material suggested the presence of an imino-propene structure. Evidence for the formation of nondisulfide cross-links has been found in several studies. Roy et al. (545) described a 43,000 dalton peptide containing components of β- and γ-crystallins. Previous studies by the same group showed that a similar 43 kd peptide was membrane-associated and served as an anchor for disulfide-linked proteins in senile cataractous lenses (618) (Fig. 10.26). Additional evidence for the involvement of γ-crystallins in covalent changes has been brought by Takemoto and colleagues (618), who found extensive covalent modification of γ-crystallins during aging of the normal human lens. Several structures (Fig. 10.27) have been proposed to explain the formation of nondisulfide covalent cross-links. Products with β-carboline structure (655), bityrosine, and anthranilic acid (188, 640) have been isolated from human lenses, but whether they serve as cross-linking structures is unknown. There is also concern that some of these products may have been artifactually created during isolation.

Currently, four types of nonfluorescent covalent cross-link have been detected in human lenses. Gamma-glutamyl-ε-lysine cross-links have been detected in significant amounts in cross-linked protein fraction of human cataracts (367). The formation of these cross-links is catalyzed by transglutaminase, a zinc- and Ca^{2+}-activated enzyme which has been detected in lenses of five different species. Histidinoalanine, a cross-link originally discovered in the ECM, was found to be particularly elevated in protein from human brown cataractous lens (292). Histidinoalanine is thought to result from a condensation of β-eliminated serine residue with histidine residue in an alkali-catalyzed reaction. Lanthionine, a thioether cross-link of cysteine naturally present in chick embryo and skin, was detected in acid hydrolysate of yellow protein fraction from human lens (40). Like histidinoalanine, lanthionine formation is catalyzed under alkaline conditions. Finally, pentosidine, an advanced Maillard reaction cross-link involving lysine and arginine residues, was detected in elevated amounts in highly pigmented lenses (437). Thus several apparently unrelated mechanisms, some of which are discussed in this chapter, may be responsible for the formation of nondisulfide covalent cross-links. Clearly, the most difficult task will be to assess the relative importance of individual cross-links and their mechanisms of formation.

Deamidation and Deamination. For several years it had been thought that lens crystallins were deamidated during aging based on observations of charge differences between the αA_1, αA_2, αB_2 subunits of α-crystallins (475, 562, 650, 658). Because no difference in the amino acid sequence was found between the more acidic subunits, A_1 and A_2 or B_1 and B_2, it was concluded that deamidation had occurred. More recently, however, it became clear that the more negative charge was, in fact, due to phosphorylation and not deamidation (594). Phosphorylation of α-crystallins appears to be developmentally regulated, and no evidence points toward its role in the aging of postmature lens. However, true deamidation of asparagyl and glutamyl residues has been documented in aging crystallins (387, 586, 674).

Deamination per se has not been reported in aging human lens crystallins. However, some investigators noted a decrease in lysyl residues in some lenses (489, 616) and others found an age-related decrease in titratable NH_2-groups (505). These observations do not allow the conclusion that lysyl residues are actually deaminated. It is likely that they are postsynthetically modified by advanced products of the Maillard reaction, by lipid peroxidation products, or by isopeptide bonds formed by transglutaminase (367).

Glycation. Like other proteins, lens crystallins are glycated, that is, they contain ketoamine-linked reducing sugars originating from the Maillard reaction with glucose (94, 476, 477, 605, 611), fructose (402), and oxidation products of ascorbate such as threose and xylosone (577). The structure of glycated proteins (Amadori product) is depicted in Figure 10.27. Because glycation is in part reversible, one would expect negligible accumulation of glycated proteins in the aging lens. Using tritium incorporation following sodium [^{3}H]borohydride reduction as a measure for 1-deoxyglucitolyl-lysine, Pande et al. (476) found no difference in glycation in young vs. senile cataractous lens and no correlation with extent of disulfide bond formation in normal, senile, or diabetic lens homogenates. In contrast, Garlick et al. (193), utilizing a specific assay for glucitolyl-lysine, found a modest age-related increase in glycation in lens homogenate which was three- to fivefold higher in diabetic lenses. The extent of glycation varied from 3% to 10% of total crystallins, assuming $M_r = 20,000$. Patrick et al. (477), however, quantitated borohydride-reduced, acid-hydrolyzed material retained by boronate affinity column, that is, representative of 1-deoxyglucitolyl-lysine, and found no change with age in human lens homogenate. With this method, the extent of crystallin glycation was only in the order of 1%–2%.

In most of the studies described above, measurements were performed in unfractionated lens homogenate. In studies of rat lenses, Swamy and Abraham (611) found a threefold increase in tritium incorporation in α-crystallins in old vs. young lenses. Extent of incorporation was higher in HMW aggregates and the αB chain. In contrast, it was higher in the αA chain from human lens crystallins (612). Overall, similar results were obtained by affinity chromatography and revealed that 5%–10% of crystallins were glycated. Chiou et al. (95) also found an increase in glucitolyl-lysine in aging bovine lens crystallins, particularly in HMW α-crystallins, and Kamei and Kato (291) reported a significant increase in NBT-reactive material in aging human lenses, which was associated with the degree of pigmentation of the lens. Although NBT is reactive with glycated protein, it is not specific for Amadori products.

Several reports not reviewed in this chapter have documented increased glycation in lenses from diabetic humans and experimental animals. Studies by Liang et al. (356, 361) confirm the preferential glycation of HMW α-crystallins and suggest that conformational changes such as unfolding may be linked to glycation, as originally proposed by Stevens et al. (604).

In summary, there is conflicting evidence for an increase in glycation of crystallins in aging. Borohydride reduction as well as NBT reduction have low specificity for glycation. Nevertheless, the more specific assays in which 1-deoxyglucitolyl-lysine was quantitated revealed only shallow increases in glycation, especially when lens homogenate was not fractionated. At least two studies, however, revealed preferential glycation of α-crystallins and especially HMW α-crystallins. Such modification may increase protein unfolding and favor aggregation of the protein. The overall role of the advanced glycation/Maillard reaction in lens aging will be discussed later (see Maillard Reaction by Reducing Sugars and Ascorbate).

Changes in Enzyme Activity

The activity of many lens enzymes studied so far decreases with age. Sodium-potassium ATPase (454), aldose reductase (285), and several other enzymes of carbohydrate metabolism (461) have decreased activities which contribute to decreasing glycolytic activity and rate of ATP production (582). Glutathione reductase and other enzymes become increasingly heat labile (462), suggesting conformational changes or changes in glycosylation. Such changes may explain the progressive heterogeneity of glycolytic enzymes in the aging lens (284). Enzyme activities, however, do not necessarily change in the same direction across animal species. Lactate dehydrogenase, for example, decreases with age in bovine lenses but increases in chicken and guinea pig lens (252).

Enzymes with antioxidant activities also decrease with age. GSH reductase, GSH peroxidase, and superoxide dismutase (SOD) activities decrease in the aging bovine lens (462), and both glucose-6-phosphate dehydrogenase and SOD were found to decrease in aging rat lens (131). During cataract formation the activities of SOD, catalase, and GSH peroxidase drop below normal and the electrical charge of the proteins is more heterogeneous (284, 462).

Most of the proteolytic enzymes that have been studied decrease in activity with age, including the ubiquitin conjugation system, the calpains, neutral endopeptidase, cathepsin B, and the aminopeptidases (168, 282, 621, 622). This may indicate that the age-related fragmentation of lens crystallins is primarily due to oxidative processes rather than to proteolytic activity. It may, however, also indicate that the removal of modified crystallins is impaired, thus leading to accumulation of crystallin, with high propensity to self-aggregation and light scattering.

Of considerable interest is the question of whether or not aldehyde metabolism is impaired in aging and cataractous lenses, since aldehydes are expected to play a role in the lens protein browning and cross-linking. Jedziniak and Rokita (283) found that enzymes capable of oxidizing glyceraldehyde, acetaldehyde, propionaldehyde, formaldehyde, and malonyldialdehyde are present in the human lens and that their activity is not impaired in deeply pigmented lenses compared to clear lenses. Such findings, however, do not exclude a significant role for these substrates in crystallin pigmentation and cross-linking. Since the O_2 content of the lens is very low, it is likely that these metabolic pathways which utilize oxygen are not fully functional. In contrast, pyridine dinucleotide–dependent reductases may be more important for the inactivation of reactive aldehydes. Altogether, little information on the level of these enzymes, their substrates, and reaction products is available in the aging lens, although these enzymes have been thoroughly studied in diabetic and galactosemic lenses. Obviously, research in this field should be pursued with priority if the molecular basis of the impaired defense mechanisms that underlie lens aging is to be understood.

Mechanisms of Crystallin Aging

The changes described above strongly suggest that chemical mechanisms play a major role in the aging of lens crystallins and cataractogenesis. Three mechanisms are currently under investigation: oxidative, photooxidative, and ketoaldehyde reactions, the latter resulting from amino-carbonyl reactions of the Maillard type. As demonstrated below, all three mechanisms can induce the changes described above, that is, protein unfolding and fragmentation, yellowing, fluorescence, disulfide and nondisulfide covalent bonding, and HMW aggregate formation.

Weakening of Antioxidant Defense. The aging lens becomes more susceptible to oxidative damage, although overall damage is mild in senile, noncataractous lenses. The increased susceptibility to oxidation is likely linked to decreased activity of antioxidant enzymes, especially GSH reductase, GSH peroxidase, and SOD (159, 462). As we have seen, other enzymes, such as Na^+,K^+-ATPase, aldose reductase, enzymes of glycolysis and carbohydrate metabolism, and enzymes involved in ATP production, also decrease. The lens enzyme involved in NADPH production, glucose 6-phosphate dehydrogenase, is remarkably well conserved during aging, and its activity is lost only in the most severe cases of human senile cataracts (87). However, its activity is detected only in the cortical and not the nuclear part of the lens (131), and levels of free radical scavengers such as ascorbic acid (20) and reduced glutathione (230) are reduced in senile lens, whereby small amounts of GSH are disulfide-linked (230, 510, 600). These changes in antioxidant levels including ascorbic acid are further accentuated in cataracts (127, 230, 508), but the decline of GSH in most cataracts represents an early change.

Role of GSH. GSH as an anticataractogenic agent has received considerable attention. Lens opacities develop within 2–3 days in mice in whom GSH biosynthesis was depleted with L-buthionine sulfoximine (75). It appears that lowering of lens GSH has an adverse effect on both active transport and permeability of lens membranes (147). As with several metabolites, its concentration is higher in the cortex than the nucleus and highest in the epithelium (509), reflecting the localization of oxidative stress in the normal lens.

Some information on the role of GSH in protecting against cataractogenesis comes from experiments with X-ray-induced cataracts in which protein thiols appear to become oxidized only when the level of GSH drops below some critical level (204). The NADPH:NADP ratio and the activity of hexose monophosphate shunt were significantly decreased just prior to maturation of X-ray-induced cataract, suggesting that the ability of the lens to regenerate reduced GSH is critical for the preservation of its transparency.

GSH can prevent protein aggregation by forming mixed disulfide bonds, which can be cleaved by GSH reductase and NADPH (600). Protein GSH appears to form from the oxidized form of GSH (GSSG) rather than from GSH itself (432). In the aging human lens, GSH levels are lower in the nucleus than in the cortex and protein disulfides appear to form in a concentration inversely related to GSH concentration (509). Furthermore, studies using intact cultured human lenses have shown an age-related decrease in L-cysteine uptake which could account for the decrease in GSH synthesis in the aging lens (507).

GSH may play an important role in protecting membrane sulfhydryl groups. Studies reviewed elsewhere (509) have shown that membrane sulfhydryl groups are involved in cation transport, Na^+,K^+-ATPase activity, and lens volume regulation. It would appear that one critical function of GSH is to protect the lens against oxidation by H_2O_2 since GSH-depleted rat lenses became cloudy upon incubation in H_2O_2 (14). In summary, GSH preserves the integrity of the aging human lens in several ways. Its presence in millimolar concentrations clearly suggests that it is a major antioxidant. Furthermore, the presence of GSH reductase in the lens is critical for regeneration of free GSH and sulfhydryl-groups at a minimum cost of energy.

Role of hydrogen peroxide. Hydrogen peroxide is thought to be an important mediator of oxidative damage in the lens. Traces of H_2O_2 are found in the normal aqueous humor, apparently when ascorbic acid is spontaneously oxidized (487, 488). Levels in the lens are influenced by levels in the aqueous humor (593). Several age- and cataract-related changes can be reproduced by treatment with H_2O_2. Oxidation of cysteine and methionine, formation of fluorescent blue and green chromophores, insolubilization, and disulfide bond formation were produced by exposing human lens proteins to H_2O_2 (400). Both Ca^{2+}-ATPase (55) and $Na^+;K^+$-ATPase (200) are susceptible to inactivation by H_2O_2. Following intravenous administration of 3-aminotriazol to rabbits, an inhibitor of catalase, Bhuyan and Bhuyan (43, 44) noticed a two- to threefold increase in the H_2O_2 concentration in the lens and the aqueous humor. However, GSH and protein sulfhydryl groups of the lens were unchanged and cataracts were not reported. In contrast, cataracts were observed in weanling littermate Dutch rabbits fed 3-aminotriazol for 2–4 wk. Both SOD and catalase were markedly inhibited (43).

When lens epithelial cells with fully active catalase but inhibited GSH reductase were exposed to H_2O_2, cellular damage was observed after 1.5 h (205). In contrast, damage was observed only after 3 h when catalase was completely inhibited but the GSH redox cycle left intact. Thus intactness of the GSH redox cycle appears to play a primary role in protecting lens crystallins and lens epithelial function from oxidative stress. This finding is further emphasized by recent experiments in which in vivo inhibition of GSH synthesis by buthionine sulfoximine led to cataract formation (381).

Role of metal-catalyzed oxidation reactions. Previously referred to as mixed function oxidation reactions (178, 355), metal-catalyzed oxidation reactions have been implicated in various diseases and in aging (466, 467).

In these reactions, metal components, such as Cu(II) or Fe (III), are bound to specific sites in protein, DNA, or lipid and carry out oxidation reactions following reduction by reductants such as GSH, ascorbate, and superoxide radicals. In proteins, the side chains of histidine, lysine, arginine, and proline are most susceptible to modification (6, 105).

In the lens, systems that are likely to act as catalysts of metal oxidation include xanthine oxidase, cytochrome C reductase, NAD(P)H oxidase, ascorbate/Fe(III)/O_2, Fe(II)/H_2O_2, and Fe(II)/O_2 (189). Hydrogen peroxide levels are 20–30 μM and may be increased in some cataracts (593). Both GSH and ascorbate are present in millimolar concentrations. Iron and copper concentrations are both in the nano- to low micromolar range, and small increases in cataractous vs. noncataractous lenses have been noted in some studies (189).

Widely cited as evidence in support of metal-catalyzed oxidation is the formation of carbonyl groups in proteins (354, 623). A small but significant increase in protein carbonyl groups was found in normal lenses as a function of age (190). In some cataractous lenses, these were elevated severalfold. Unfortunately, the assays used to establish the presence of carbonyl groups currently do not provide information on the source of these carbonyl groups. As discussed later, carbonyl groups could result from the Maillard reaction with reducing sugars or ascorbate.

Although the lens contains all the necessary components to catalyze metal oxidation and damage to crystallins, it is unclear factors are responsible for accelerated oxidative damage in some individuals. Are some individuals born with weaker antioxidant defense? Do nutritional factors play a role? Is sunlight exposure a factor in triggering damage to membranes?

Photooxidative Mechanisms of Damage to Lens Crystallins. The hypothesis that sunlight is involved in producing damage to lens crystallins is based, on the one hand, on epidemiological studies indicating that cataract is more common in tropical countries and in workers with greater sunlight exposure (204) and, on the other hand, on studies showing that age-related changes in the lens can be duplicated through photooxidation in vitro. A detailed analysis of epidemiological factors associating sunlight with cataract formation is contained in the monograph of Young (687). We discuss selected studies on the effects of light on lens crystallins.

In vitro exposure of human lenses to UV radiation increases the yellow color of the nucleus (350). In some experiments in which the lens was irradiated in vitro, both the cortex and the nucleus showed increased pigmentation (122, 232, 233).

The precise mechanism by which light mediates damage to the lens in vivo is unclear. Irradiation of lens crystallins leads to a loss of tryptophan residues. However, two reports have failed to confirm the loss of tryptophan residues (123, 692), thereby suggesting that tryptophan may not be involved in radiation effects in vivo. Tryptophan, however, may act as a photosensitizer (346, 677), and it has also been suggested that it is free lens tryptophan that is primarily oxidized (690). Interestingly, with increasing protein concentration, tryptophan acquires greater protection against destruction by UV radiation (125).

Photoirradiation of lens proteins leads to the formation of free radicals similar to those found in the lens (326, 327). Human lenses exposed to UV-A or UV-B photons at lens temperature acquired free radicals (347, 677, 697), and it appears that the deeper the pigmentation, the greater the free radical signal intensity (698).

In several experiments, investigators have been able to duplicate both the pigmentation and the fluorescence characteristic of the aging human lens (350–352, 696). Addition of ascorbic acid decreased the pigmentation (696), whereas addition of 3-aminotriazole, an inhibitor of catalase, enhanced fluorescence formation, suggesting that H_2O_2 is involved in the modification of crystallins (348).

Oxygen appears to play an important role in the destruction of tryptophan, since irradiation under anaerobic conditions or in the presence of free radical scavengers such as penicillamine markedly inhibited the damage (124, 351, 352).

In addition to its ability to duplicate fluorescence and pigmentation, irradiation of crystallins can induce conformational changes and protein cross-linking (10). Damage to Na^+,K^+-ATPase was noted when lenses were exposed to light in the presence of the photosensitizer riboflavin (287, 662). Again, prevention by vitamin C, as well as by SOD and catalase, was noted (662). Similarly, formation of lipid peroxides and malonyldialdehyde was also found in irradiated specimens (660, 661). Antioxidants such as ascorbic acid, tocopherol, catalase, and SOD diminished the damage (660, 661, 663).

Interestingly, the same enzymes that are involved in protecting the lens against photooxidative damage, such as catalase and GSH reductase, may become inactivated by irradiation, especially in the presence of tryptophan degradation products (694, 695).

Thus photosensitizers appear to play a key role in mediating damage to crystallins during irradiation. Goosey and colleagues (212) were able to duplicate all the major changes observed in the aging lens, that is, blue fluorescence, yellow pigmentation, covalent cross-linking, and high-molecular aggregate formation, by irradiating α and β bovine crystallins with light in the presence of photosensitizers such as riboflavin, methylene blue, or rose bengal. The data strongly implicate singlet oxygen as the culprit, since the process could be inhibited by singlet oxygen scavengers such as sodium azide but not by scavengers of H_2O_2, superoxide, or hydroxyl radical. Most interestingly, the brown insoluble protein fraction from human brunescent lenses was also able to generate singlet oxygen and to induce cross-linking of soluble crystallins (691).

In summary, it would appear that light mediates damage to the lens through an oxidative mechanism such that the older and the more pigmented the lens becomes, the more it is susceptible to photodamage. The role of tryptophan as a photosensitizer involved in cross-links in vivo remains speculative as no convincing evidence for a loss of tryptophan residues has emerged. Given the central role of oxygen-reactive species in the light-mediated damage to the lens, it might be very difficult in the absence of specific probes to delineate the precise role of sunlight exposure compared to other mechanisms of crystallin aging. It is likely that all merge into oxidative damage.

Maillard Reaction by Reducing Sugars and Ascorbate.
Evidence for occurrence in the lens of the initial stage of the Maillard reaction, that is, nonenzymatic glycosylation, was presented above. In vitro experiments have shown that incubation of the lens proteins with glucose or glucose-6-phosphate can duplicate most, if not all, age- and cataract-related changes. These include conformational changes (41, 356, 358, 359, 691); formation of HMW protein aggregates involving hydrophobic, disulfide-, and non-disulfide covalent bonds (421, 425, 483, 604, 648); and formation of yellow and blue fluorescent protein-linked molecules (291, 421, 422, 648). Proteolysis has not been reported in lens crystallins incubated with sugars but has been observed in other proteins when trace metals such as copper were added during glycation experiments (90, 269). Furthermore, Garner and colleagues (197, 201) have shown that Na^+,K^+-ATPase is inhibited by incubation with glucose, as well as in diabetes, and their data suggest that the glycated lens epithelial enzyme can be stimulated by inhibitors of aldose reductase. Thus the data above show that age-related damage to crystallins and lens can be duplicated by incubation with glucose or its analogs.

Whereas glucose and advanced glycation end-products derived from glucose are expected to be the major Maillard reactants in the ECM, a number of observations suggest that ascorbate could be the major culprit in the postsynthetic modification of crystallins, especially in those changes that involve deep pigmentation of the lens. When ascorbate was reacted with lens crystallins, rapid formation of the fluorescence characteristic of aging human lenses was observed (37, 191). Formation of nondisulfide covalent cross-links and protein fragments was also noted, especially in the presence of metal ions (191). In mechanistic studies, Ortwerth and colleagues (495) noted that ascorbate can bind to lens crystallins but that it first needs to be oxidized to dehydroascorbate (Fig. 10.28). Dehydroascorbate itself can delactonize to form the potent 2,3-diketogulonate from which xylosone and threose are formed spontaneously (366, 577). These oxidation compounds of ascorbate are likely to form covalent cross-links. This would explain why, in contrast to collagen cross-linking by glucose (177), no oxygen free radical is necessary for lens crystallin cross-linking by ascorbate once the latter has been oxidized to dehydroascorbate (495).

This initial oxidation step is thought to be a spontaneous process catalyzed by oxygen-reactive species. Evidence for the involvement of ascorbate in lens pigmentation stems from the demonstration that the protein cross-link pentosidine can be formed from ascorbate and its degradation products and that its levels increase in aging and correlate with the degree of pigmentation in senile cataractous human lenses (437) (Fig. 10.29). Further support comes from the demonstration of accu-

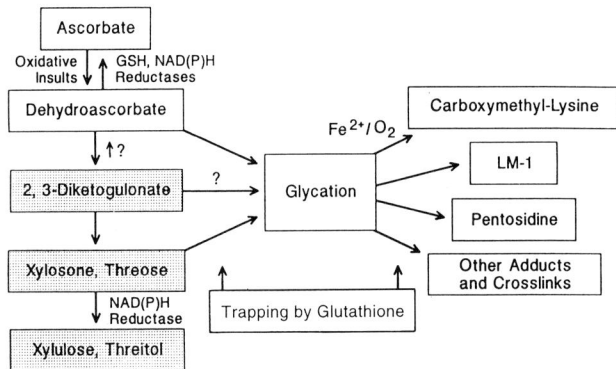

FIG. 10.28. Hypothetical mechanisms of protection against damage to lens crystallins by the ascorbate-mediated advanced Maillard reaction.

mulation in lens proteins of carboxymethyllysine, an oxidative degradation product of glycated proteins formed in proteins incubated with ascorbate (137, 139). It should be mentioned, however, that although ascorbate is likely to be the major precursor of pentosidine and carboxymethyllysine in the lens, these latter modi-

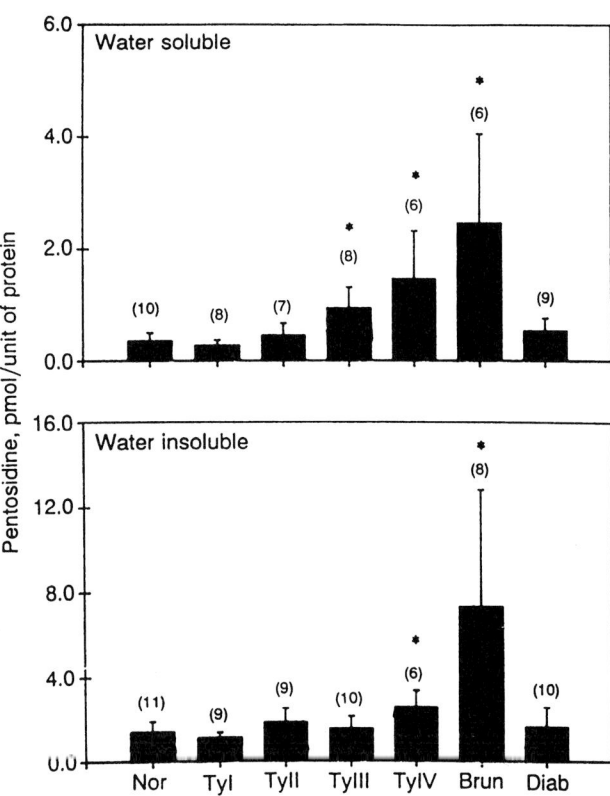

FIG. 10.29. Pentosidine levels in cataractous lenses classified on the basis of pigmentation. Results are expressed as the mean ± SD. Statistical significance was calculated using Student's nonpaired t test. *Significantly different compared to normal lenses ($P < 0.005$). *Nor*, normal; *Ty*, type; *Brun*, brunescent; *Diab*, diabetic. [From Nagaraj et al. (437), by permission.]

fications are not specific for ascorbate since they can be obtained by a variety of sugars (3, 140, 215). In the diabetic lens, it is likely that "glucated" or "fructated" protein would contribute to the increased formation of carboxymethyllysine and pentosidine (372), but there is currently no rationale to implicate glucose or fructose in the extensive pigmentation and protein-cross-linking seen in brunescent, nondiabetic cataracts.

If ascorbate-mediated Maillard reaction is to explain the greatly accelerated pigmentation of crystallins in the lens nucleus and in brunescent lenses, a breakdown in the redox state within the cell must be implicated. Under physiological conditions, dehydroascorbate is reduced back to ascorbate by NADH or GSH, possibly with the help of a reductase, although the existence of the latter is debatable. In cataractous lenses, however, the redox state is severely altered, as evidenced by a drop in free GSH level, the extent of which is inversely related to the severity of cataract (478). GSH itself has been found to have potent properties against Maillard reaction by ascorbate and reducing sugars (268, 473). Furthermore, GSH reductase activity is also decreased in the aging lens (462), thus further compromising the regeneration of free GSH.

As implied in Figure 10.27, GSH, which is present in millimolar concentration in the lens, is expected to also have the ability to scavenge advanced Maillard reaction products by reacting directly with them through their amino groups. Taurine could exert a similar function since it is present in very high concentrations in the lens. Interestingly, both amino acids are rapidly lost in experimental galactosemia (297), a condition associated with high pentosidine levels.

A second line of defense against ascorbate degradation products is anticipated distally from 2,3-diketogulonic acid, which would inactivate the highly reactive xylosone and threose (Fig. 10.27). Such reduction could be carried out by the NAPDH-dependent aldose reductase, an enzyme whose physiological function has not been clearly identified. Thus it may well be that detoxification of ascorbate oxidation products could be one of the physiological functions of aldose reductase.

Conclusions

The mechanisms of lens crystallin aging are heterogeneous. Oxidation, sunlight, and Maillard reaction–mediated modifications all can duplicate the age-related changes noted in senescent and cataractous lenses. This suggests that a common mechanistic pathway, most likely involving oxygen-reactive species, is responsible for some of the modifications. The greatest protection of the lens against this oxidative stress is its anaerobic metabolism coupled with the ascorbate–glutathione antioxidant system. As we know, when the latter is impaired, ascorbate's double-edged sword is likely to become activated and result in damage to lens crystallins through mechanisms expected to involve a combination of metal-catalyzed oxidation and amino-carbonyl reactions of the Maillard type. As the pigmentation of the lens increases, increased photosensitization occurs, leading to a vicious amplification of oxidative damage and further weakening of antioxidant defense mechanisms.

Although oxidative protein modifications are intense in cataracts, they are comparatively minimal in noncataractous lenses. Furthermore, several investigators have reported that some lenses display minimal or no sign of clouding even at an advanced age in spite of some degree of yellowing. This clearly suggests that conformational changes, protein fragmentation, yellowing, fluorescence, glycation, aggregation, and formation of mixed disulfide bonds involving GSH should be considered precataractous changes. The question arises as to why cataracts develop much faster in some individuals than in others. Although the mechanisms leading from precataractous to cataractous states are expected to be heterogeneous, as reviewed above, it is tempting to speculate that a greater defect in one or several components controlling the redox state of the lens may precipitate the demise of the lens. Such defects could have a genetic basis.

SUMMATION

In this chapter, we have reviewed several aspects of biochemical aging which affect long-lived proteins. Many of them have in common postsynthetic modifications which involve sulfhydryl groups, amino groups, and aromatic residues. Proteins become insoluble, acquire fluorescent chromophores and cross-links, and become racemized and fragmented. Strong evidence implicates oxidative, glycoxidative, and Maillard-type reactions. In the ECM, the amplitude of the oxidation stress, although never measured per se, is assumed to remain constant, being primarily dictated by the oxygen tension of interstitial fluid, which is in equilibrium with that of capillary blood. In contrast, the pO_2 of the lens is very low and so is the oxidative stress as long as the cell membrane and metabolic pathways are intact. Once these are disrupted, new biochemical pathways are activated which lead to intense oxidation and, most likely, the participation of ascorbate oxidation products in crystallin pigmentation and cross-linking.

One of the most difficult questions is the extent to which changes occurring in long-lived tissues account for age-related pathologies. Because of the multifactorial nature of these processes, evidence may remain circumstantial rather than direct. As a general rule, the authors have adopted the prudent opinion that age-related changes in long-lived proteins predispose rather than cause age-related diseases. In support of this statement are observations showing that the magnitude of degenerative changes varies considerably among old individuals, although cumulative damage to long-lived molecules overall appears similar. Nevertheless, except for those cases in which a clear-cut genetic predisposition exists, diseases such as nuclear cataract and osteoarthritis do not occur at a young age, most likely because the tissue is not vulnerable to trivial insults. In the elderly, these trivial insults are sufficient to precipitate catastrophic events (314) that may culminate in death.

We thank Dr. Karen Reiser for her critical review of the manuscript. Some of the work reviewed in this chapter was supported by grants EY07099 and AG05601 from the National Eye Institute and the National Institute on Aging, respectively. We thank Ms. Gina McVey for outstanding secretarial assistance.

REFERENCES

1. ADAMS, P., and H. MUIR. Qualitative changes with age of proteoglycans of human lumbar discs. *Ann. Rheum. Dis.* 35: 289–296, 1976.
2. AHMED, M. U., J. A. DUNN, M. D. WALLA, S. R. THORPE, and J. W. BAYNES. Oxidative degradation of glucose adducts to protein: formation of 3-(N^ϵ- lysino)-lactic acid from model compounds and glycated proteins. *J. Biol. Chem.* 263: 8816–8821, 1988.
3. AHMED, M. U., S. R. THORPE, and J. W. BAYNES. Identification of N^ϵ-carboxymethyllysine as a degradation product of fructoselysine in glycated protein. *J. Biol. Chem.* 261: 4889–4894, 1986.
4. ALBINI, A., B. PONTZ, M. PULZ, G. ALLAVENA, H. MENSING, and P. K. MÜLLER. Decline of fibroblast chemotaxis with age of donor and cell passage number. *Coll. Relat. Res.* 8: 23–37, 1988.
5. ALNAQEEB, M. A., N. S. AL ZAID, and G. GOLDSPINK. Connective tissue changes and physical properties of developing and ageing skeletal muscle. *J. Anat.* 139: 677–689, 1984.
6. AMICI, A., R. L. LEVINE, L. TSAI, and E. R. STADTMAN. Conversion of amino acid residues in proteins and amino acid homopolymers to carbonyl derivatives by metal catalyzed oxidation reactions. *J. Biol. Chem.* 264: 3341–3346, 1989.
7. AMIEL, D., S. D. KUIPER, C. D. WALLACE, F. L. HARWOOD, and J. S. VANDEBERG. Age-related properties of medial collateral ligament: a morphologic and collagen maturation study in the rabbit. *J. Gerontol.* 46: B159–B165, 1991.
8. ANDERSON, E., and A. SPECTOR. The state of sulfhydryl groups in normal and cataracous lens proteins. I. Nuclear region. *Exp. Eye Res.* 26: 407–417, 1978.
9. ANDERSON, E. I., D. D. WRIGHT, and A. SPECTOR. The state of sulfhydryl groups in normal and cataractous human lens proteins. II. Cortical and nuclear regions. *Exp. Eye Res.* 29: 233–243, 1978.
10. ANDLEY, U. Spectroscopic studies on the riboflavin-sensitized conformational changes of calf lens α-crystallin. *Exp. Eye Res.* 46: 531–544, 1988.
11. ANDREOTTI, L., A. BUSSOTTI, D. CAMMELLI, E. AIELLO, and S. SAMPOGNARO. Connective tissue in aging lung. *Gerontology* 29: 377–387, 1983.
12. ANDREOTTI, L., D. CAMELLI, A. BUSSOTTI, and P. ARCANGELI. Biochemical measurement of lung connective tissue. *Bull. Eur. Physiopathol. Respir.* 16: 83–90, 1980.
13. ANGYAL, S. J. The composition of reducing sugars in solution. *Adv. Carbohydr. Chem. Biochem.* 42: 15–68, 1984.
14. ANSARI, N. H., and S. K. SRIVASTAVA. Role of glutathione in the prevention of cataractogenesis in rat lenses. *Curr. Eye Res.* 2: 271–275, 1982–1983.
15. ANVERSA, P., T. PALACKAL, E. H. SONNENBLICK, G. OLIVETTI, L. G. MEGGS, and J. M. CAPASSO. Myocyte cell loss and myocyte cellular hyperplasia in the hypertrophied aging rat heart. *Circ. Res.* 67: 871–885, 1990.
16. ARAKI, N., N. UENO, B. CHAKRABARTI, Y. MORINO, and S. HORIUCHI. Immunochemical evidence for the presence of advanced glycation end products in human lens proteins and its positive correlation with aging. *J. Biol. Chem.* 267: 10211–10214, 1992.
17. ASGHAR, A., and R. L. HENRICKSON. Chemical, biochemical, functional and nutritional characteristics of collagen in food systems. *Adv. Food Res.* 28: 231–372, 1982.
18. AUGUSTEYN, R. C. Human lens albuminoid. *Jpn. J. Ophthalmol.* 18: 127–134, 1974.
19. AUGUSTEYN, R. C. Distribution of fluorescence in the human cataractous lens. *Ophthalmic Res.* 7: 217–224, 1975.
20. AUGUSTEYN, R. C. Protein modification in cataract: possible oxidative mechanism. In: *Mechanisms of Cataract Formation in Human Lens*, edited by G. Duncan. New York: Academic Press, 1981, p. 72–115.
21. AURICCHIO, G., and M. TESTA. Some biochemical differences between cortical (pale) and nuclear (brown) cataracts. *Ophthalmologica* 164: 228–235, 1972.
22. AYISI, K., J. LINDNER, J. KROHN, and I. MANGOLD. Investigations on connective tissue metabolism: ageing of the human heart. *Mech. Ageing Dev.* 14: 325–331, 1980.
23. BAILEY, A. J., and C. M. PEACH. Isolation and structural identification of a labile intermolecular crosslink in collagen. *Biochem. Biophys. Res. Commun.* 33: 812–189, 1968.
24. BAKER, G. T., III, and R. L. SPROTT. Biomarkers of aging. *Exp. Gerontol.* 23: 223–239, 1988.
25. BARBER, G. W. Biochemistry of cataracts. In: *Pathobiology of Ocular Disease*, edited by A. Garner and G. K. Klintworth. New York: Marcel Dekker, 1982, p. 1273–1302.
26. BARBER, M., R. S. BORDOLI, G. J. ELLIOTT, D. FUJIMOTO, and J. E. SCOTT. The structure(s) of pyridinoline(s). *Biochem. Biophys. Res. Commun.* 109: 1041–1046, 1982.
27. BARBER, W. C. Human cataractogenesis: a review. *Exp. Eye Res.* 16: 985–991, 1973.
28. BARNARD, K., N. D. LIGHT, T. J. SIMS, and A. J. BAILEY. Chemistry of the collagen crosslinks: origin and partial characterization of a putative mature crosslink of collagen. *Biochem. J.* 244: 303–309, 1987.
29. BARNES, M. J., B. J. CONSTABLE, L. F. MORTON, and P. M. ROYCE. Age-related variations in hydroxylation of lysine and proline in collagen. *Biochem. J.* 139: 461–468, 1974.
30. BARTOLD, P. M., R. R. BOYD, and R. C. PAGE. Proteoglycans synthesized by gingival fibroblasts derived from human donors of different ages. *J. Cell Physiol.* 126: 37–46, 1986.
31. BAYLISS, M. T. Proteoglycan structure in normal and osteoarthritic human cartilage. In: *Articular Cartilage Biochemistry*, edited by K. E. Kuettner, R. Schleyerbach, and V. C. Hascall. New York: Raven Press, 1986, p. 295–310.
32. BAYLISS, M. T. Proteoglycan structure and metabolism during maturation and ageing of human articular cartilage. *Biochem. Soc. Trans.* 18: 799–802, 1990.

33. BAYNES, J. W. Role of oxidative stress in development of complications in diabetes. *Diabetes* 40: 405–412, 1991.
34. BAYNES, J. W., N. G. WATKINS, C. I. FISHER, C. J. HULL, J. S. PATRICK, M. U. AHMED, J. A. DUNN, and S. R. THORPE. The Amadori product on protein: structure and reactions. In: *The Maillard Reaction in Aging, Diabetes, and Nutrition*, edited by J. W. Baynes and V. M. Monnier. New York: Alan R. Liss, 1989, p. 43–67.
35. BENEDEK, G. B. Theory of transparency of the eye. *Appl. Optics* 10: 459–473, 1971.
36. BENJAMIN, M., R. N. S. TYERS, and J. R. RALPHS. Age-related changes in tendon fibrocartilage. *J. Anat.* 179: 127–136, 1991.
37. BENSCH, K. G., J. E. FLEMING, and W. LOHMAN. The role of ascorbic acid in senile cataract. *Proc. Natl. Acad. Sci. USA* 82: 7193–7196, 1985.
38. BERNICK, S., and R. CAILLIET. Vertebral end-plate changes with aging of human vertebrae. *Spine* 7: 97–102, 1982.
39. BESSEMS, G. J. H., B. M. DEMAN, J. BOURS, and H. J. HOENDERS. Age-related variations in the distribution of crystallins within the bovine lens. *Exp. Eye Res.* 43: 1019–1030, 1986.
40. BESSEMS, G. J. H., H. J. J. M. RENNEN, and H. J. HOENDERS. Lanthionine, a protein crosslink in cataractous human lenses. *Exp. Eye Res.* 44: 691–695, 1987.
41. BESWICK, H. T., and J. J. HARDING. Conformational changes induced in the α- and γ-crystallins by modification with glucose 6-phosphate. *Biochem. J.* 246: 761–769, 1987.
42. BETSCH, D. F., and E. BAER. Structure and mechanical properties of rat tail tendon. *Biorheology* 17: 83–94, 1980.
43. BHUYAN, K. C., and D. K. BHUYAN. Regulation of hydrogen peroxide in eye humors. Effect of 3-amino-1H-1,2,4-triazole on catalase and GSH peroxidase in rabbit eye. *Biochim. Biophys. Acta* 497: 641–651, 1977.
44. BHUYAN, K. C., and D. K. BHUYAN. Mechanism of cataractogenesis induced by 3-aminotriazole. I. Morphology and histopathology of cataract and the role of catalase in the regulation of H_2O_2 in the eye. In: *Biochemical and Clinical Aspects of Oxygen*, edited by W. S. Caughey. New York: Academic Press, 1979, p. 789–796.
45. BIENKOWSKI, R. S., B. J. BAUM, and R. G. CRYSTAL. Fibroblasts degrade newly synthesized collagen within the cell before secretion. *Nature* 276: 413–416, 1978.
46. BIENKOWSKI, R. S., M. J. COWAN, J. A. MCDONALD, and R. G. CRYSTAL. Degradation of newly synthesized collagen. *J. Biol. Chem.* 253: 4356–4363, 1978.
47. BIHARI-VARGA, M., E. CSONKA, E. GRUBER, and H. JELLINEK. Age-related changes in the glycosaminoglycans and collagen of cultured pig endothelial cells. *Pathol. Biol. (Paris)* 29: 555–561, 1981.
48. BJÖRKSTEN, J., and W. J. CHAMPION. Mechanical influence upon tanning. *J. Am. Chem. Soc.* 64: 868–869, 1942.
49. BLACKETT, A. D., and D. A. HALL. Vitamin E—its significance in mouse ageing. *Age Ageing* 10: 191–195, 1981.
50. BLEEKER, J. C., J. A. VAN BEST, L. VRIJ, and E. A. VAN DER VELDE. Autofluorescence of the lens in diabetic and healthy subjects by fluorometry. *Invest. Ophthalmol. Vis. Sci.* 27: 791–794, 1986.
51. BLOEMENDAL, H., and A. ZWEERS. Improved separation of low molecular weight crystallins. In: *Progress of Lens Biochemistry Research*, edited by Doc. Ophthalmol. (The Hague) 15: 91–104, 1976.
52. BLOMFIELD, J., and J. F. FARRAR. Fluorescence spectra of arterial elastin. *Biochem. Biophys. Res. Commun.* 28: 346–351, 1967.
53. BLOMFIELD, J., and J. F. FARRAR. The fluorescent properties of maturing arterial elastin. *Cardiovasc. Res.* 3: 161–170, 1969.
54. BOCHANTIN, J., and L. L. MAYS. Age-dependence of collagen tail fiber breaking strength in Sprague-Dawley and Fischer 344 rats. *Exp. Gerontol.* 16: 101–106, 1981.
55. BORCHMAN, D., C. A. PATERSON, and N. A. DELAMERE. Oxidative inhibition of Ca^{2+}-ATPase in the rabbit lens. *Invest. Ophthalmol. Vis. Sci.* 30: 1633–1637, 1989.
56. BORG, T. K., and J. B. CAULFIELD. The collagen matrix of the heart. *Fed. Proc.* 40: 2037–2041, 1981.
57. BOUISSOU, H., and T. PIERAGGI. Changes in the morphology and chemistry of connective tissues during aging. In: *Collagen*, edited by M. E. Nimni. Boca Raton, FL: CRC Press, 1988, vol. II, p. 95–111.
58. BOUISSOU, H., T. PIERAGGI, M. JULIAN, and L. DOUSTE-BLAZY. Cutaneous aging. Its relation with arteriosclerosis and atheroma. In: *Frontiers of Matrix Biology*, edited by L. Robert. New York: Karger, 1973, vol. I, p. 190–211.
59. BOUISSOU, H., T. PIERAGGI, M. JULIAN, and L. DOUSTE-BLAZY. Simultaneous degradation of elastin in dermis and in aorta. In: *Frontiers of Matrix Biology*, edited by L. Robert. New York: Karger, 1976, vol. III, p. 242–255.
60. BOYER, B., P. KERN, A. FOURTANIER, and J. LABAT-ROBERT. Age-dependent variations of the biosynthesis of fibronectin and fibrous collagens in mouse skin. *Exp. Gerontol.* 26: 375–383, 1991.
61. BRADLEY, K. H., S. D. MCCONNELL, and R. G. CRYSTAL. Lung collagen composition and synthesis. *J. Biol. Chem.* 244: 2674–2683, 1974.
62. BRAND, H. S., M. H. M. T. DE KONING, G. P. J. VAN KAMPEN, and J. K. VAN DER KORST. Age-related changes in the turnover of proteoglycans from explants of bovine articular cartilage. *J. Rheumatol.* 18: 599–605, 1991.
63. BRANDT, K. D., and R. S. FIFE. Ageing in relation to the pathogenesis of osteoarthritis. *Clin. Rheum. Dis.* 12: 117–130, 1986.
64. BRAVERMAN, I. M., and E. FONFERKO. Studies in cutaneous aging: I. The elastic fiber network. *J. Invest. Dermatol.* 78: 434–443, 1982.
65. BRAVERMAN, I. M., and A. KEH-YEN. Ultrastructural abnormalities of the microvasculature and elastic fibers in the skin of juvenile diabetics. *J. Invest. Dermatol.* 82: 270–274, 1984.
66. BRODY, J. S., H. KAGAN, and A. MANALO. Lung lysyl oxidase activity: relation to lung growth. *Am. Rev. Respir. Dis.* 120: 1289–1295, 1979.
67. BROWNLEE, M., A. CERAMI, and H. VLASSARA. Advanced glycosylation end products in tissue and the biochemical basis of diabetic complications. *N. Engl. J. Med.* 318: 1315–1321, 1988.
68. BROWNLEE, M., S. PONGOR, and A. CERAMI. Covalent attachment of soluble proteins by nonenzymatically glycosylated collagen. *J. Exp. Med.* 158: 1739–1744, 1983.
69. BRUNK, U. T., C. B. JONES, and R. S. SOHAL. A novel hypothesis of lipofuscinogenesis and cellular aging based on interactions between oxidative stress and autophagocytosis. *Mutat. Res.* 275: 395–403, 1992.
70. BUCKINGHAM, R. H. The behavior of reduced proteins from normal and cataractous lenses in highly dissociating media: crosslinked protein in cataractous lenses. *Exp. Eye Res.* 14: 123–129, 1972.
71. BUDDECKE, E., and M. SZIEGOLEIT. Isolierung, chemische zusammensetzung und altersabhangige verteilung von mucopolysaccharinden menschlicher zwischenwirbelscheiben. *Hoppe Seyler Physiol. Chem.* 337: 66–78, 1964.
72. BUNN, H. F. Non-enzymatic glycosylation of protein: a form of molecular aging. *Schweiz. Med. Wochenschr.* 111: 1503–1507, 1981.
73. BUNN, H. F., and P. J. HIGGINS. Reaction of monosaccharides with proteins: possible evolutionary significance. *Science* 213: 222–224, 1981.

74. CALKINS, E. Aging of cells and people. *Clin. Obstet. Gynecol.* 24: 165–179, 1981.
75. CALVIN, H. I., C. MEDVEDOVSKI, J. C. DAVID, T. M. BROGLIO, J. L. HESS, S. C. J. FU, and B. V. WORGUL. Rapid deterioration of lens fibers in GHS-depleted mouse pups. *Invest. Ophthalmol. Vis. Sci.* 32: 1916–1924, 1991.
76. CAMPBELL, M. A., C. J. HANDLEY, V. C. HASCALL, R. A. CAMPBELL, and D. A. LOWTHER. Turnover of proteoglycans in cultures of bovine articular cartilage. *Arch. Biochem. Biophys.* 234: 275–289, 1984.
77. CAPLAN, A. Cartilage. *Sci. Am.* 251: 84–94, October 1984.
78. CAPPELLI, V., R. FORNI, C. POGGESI, C. REGGIANI, and L. RICCIARDI. Age-dependent variations of diastolic stiffness and collagen content in rat ventricular myocardium. *Arch. Int. Physiol. Biochem.* 92: 93–106, 1984.
79. CARNEY, S. L., and H. MUIR. The structure and function of cartilage proteoglycans. *Physiol. Rev.* 68: 858–910, 1988.
80. CASARETT, G. W. Acceleration of aging by ionizing radiations. In: *The Biology of Aging*, edited by B. Strehler. Washington D.C.: Institute of Biological Sciences, 1960, p. 147–152.
81. CASTELO-BRANCO, C., M. DURAN, and J. GONZÁLEZ-MERLO. Skin collagen changes related to age and hormone replacement therapy. *Maturitas* 15: 113–119, 1992.
82. CASTILLO, Y., H. KRUGER, J. ARAIS-STELLA, A. HURTADO, P. HARRIS, and D. HEATH. Histology, extensibility, and chemical composition of pulmonary trunk in persons living at sea level and at high altitude in Peru. *Br. Heart J.* 29: 120–128, 1967.
83. CERAMI, A. Hypothesis: glucose as a mediator of aging. *J. Am. Geriatr. Soc.* 33: 626–634, 1985.
84. CERAMI, A., H. VLASSARA, and M. BROWNLEE. Glucose and aging. *Sci. Am.* 257: 90–96, May 1987.
85. CETTA, G., R. TENNI, G. ZANABONI, G. DELUCA, E. IPPOLITO, C. DE MARTINO and A. A. CASTELLANI. Biochemical and morphological modifications in rabbit Achilles tendon during maturation and ageing. *Biochem. J.* 204: 61–67, 1982.
86. CHANG, J. C. F., P. C. ULRICH, R. BUCALA, and A. CERAMI. Detection of an advanced glycosylation product bound to protein in situ. *J. Biol. Chem.* 260: 7970–7974, 1985.
87. CHARLTON, J. M., and R. VAN HEYNINGEN. Glucose 6-phosphate dehydrogenase in the mammalian lens. *Exp. Eye Res.* 11: 351–355, 1971.
88. CHASE, K. V., R. CARUBELLI, and R. E. NORDQUIST. The role of nonenzymatic glycosylation, transition metals, and free radicals in the formation of collagen aggregates. *Arch. Biochem. Biophys.* 288: 473–480, 1991.
89. CHENG, H. M., and L. T. CHYLACK. Lens metabolism. In: *The Ocular Lens*, edited by H. Maisel. New York: Marcel Dekker, 1985, p. 223–264.
90. CHENG, R.-Z., J. TSUNEHIRO, K. UCHIDA, and S. KAWAKISHI. Oxidative damage of glycated protein in the presence of transition metabolism. *Agric. Biol. Chem.* 55: 1993–1988, 1991.
91. CHIO, K. S., and A. L. TAPPEL. Synthesis and characterization of the fluorescent products derived from malonaldehyde and amino acids. *Biochemistry* 8: 2821–2827, 1969.
92. CHIO, K. S., and A. L. TAPPEL. Inactivation of ribonuclease and other enzymes by peroxidizing lipids and by malonaldehyde. *Biochemistry* 8: 2827–2832, 1969.
93. CHIO, K. S., U. REISS, B. FLETCHER, and A. L. TAPPEL. Peroxidation of subcellular organelles: formation of lipofuscinlike fluorescent pigments. *Science* 166: 1535–1536, 1969.
94. CHIOU, S. H., L. T. CHYLACK, H. F. BUNN, and J. H. KINOSHITA. Role of nonenzymatic glycosylation in experimental cataract formation. *Biochem. Biophys. Res. Comm.* 95: 894–890, 1980.
95. CHIOU, S. H., L. T. CHYLACK, W. H. TUNG, and H. F. BUNN. Nonenzymatic glycosylation of bovine lens crystallins. *J. Biol. Chem.* 256: 5176–5180, 1981.
96. CHOBANIAN, A. V., M. F. PRESCOTT, and C. C. HAUDENSCHILD. Recent advances in molecular pathology: the effects of hypertension on the arterial wall. *Exp. Mol. Pathol.* 41: 153–169, 1984.
97. CHOI, A. M. K., D. R. OLSEN, K. G. COOK, S. F. DEAMOND, J. UITTO, and S. A. BRUCE. Differential extracellular matrix gene expression by fibroblasts during their proliferative life span in vitro and at senescence. *J. Cell. Physiol.* 151: 147–155, 1992.
98. CLARK, H. M., S. ZIGMAN, and S. LERMAN. Studies on the structural proteins of the human lens. *Exp. Eye Res.* 8: 172–182, 1969.
99. CLEARY, E. G. The microfibrillar component of the elastic fibers. Morphology and biochemistry. In: *Connective Tissue Disease: Molecular Pathology of the Extracellular Matrix*, edited by J. Uitto and A. J. Perejda. New York: Marcel Dekker, 1987, p. 55–81.
100. CLIFF, W. J. The aortic tunica media in aging rats. *Exp. Mol. Pathol.* 13: 172–189, 1970.
101. COGHLAN, S. D., and R. C. AUGUSTEYN. Changes in the distribution of proteins in the aging human lens. *Exp. Eye Res.* 25: 603–611, 1977.
102. COHEN, M. P., and L. KU. Age-related changes in sulfation of basement membrane glycosaminoglycans. *Exp. Gerontol.* 18: 447–450, 1983.
103. COHEN, M. P., and V. YU-WU. Age-related change in non-enzymatic glycosylation of human basement membranes. *Exp. Gerontol.* 18: 461–469, 1983.
104. COLE, T. C., P. GHOSH, and T. K. F. TAYLOR. Variations of the proteoglycans of the canine intervertebral disc with ageing. *Biochim. Biophys. Acta* 880: 209–219, 1986.
105. COOPER, B., J. M. CREETH, and A. S. R. DONALD. Studies of the limited degradation of mucus glycoproteins. *Biochem. J.* 228: 615–626, 1985.
106. CORNWELL, G. G., III, B. P. THOMAS, and D. L. SNYDER. Myocardial fibrosis in aging germ-free and conventional Lobund-Wistar rats: the protective effect of diet restriction. *J. Gerontol.* 46: B167–B170, 1991.
107. CRAIGHEAD, J. E. Editorial: Is advanced basement membrane glycosyaltion reversible? *Lab. Invest.* 60: 471–472, 1989.
108. CRONLUND, A. L., and H. M. KAGAN. Comparison of lysyl oxidase from bovine lung and aorta. *Connect. Tissue Res.* 15: 173–185, 1986.
109. DANIELSEN, C. C. Thermal stability of reconstituted collagen fibrils. Shrinkage characteristics upon in vitro maturation. *Mech. Ageing Dev.* 15: 269–278, 1981.
110. DANIELSEN, C. C. Mechanical properties of native and reconstituted rat tail tendon collagen upon maturation in vitro. *Mech. Ageing Dev.* 40: 9–16, 1987.
111. DANIELSEN, C. C. Age-related thermal stability and susceptibility to proteolysis of rat bone collagen. *Biochem. J.* 272: 697–701, 1990.
112. DANIELSEN, C. C., T. T. ANDREASSEN, and L. MOSEKILDE. Mechanical properties of collagen from decalcified rat femur in relation to age and in vitro maturation. *Calcif. Tissue Int.* 39: 69–73, 1986.
113. DANIELSEN, C. C., L. MOSEKILDE, and T. T. ANDREASSEN. Long-term effect of orchidectomy on cortical bone from rat femur: bone mass and mechanical properties. *Calcif. Tissue Int.* 50: 169–174, 1992.
114. DAVIDKOVA, E., and I. SVADLENKA. Interactions of malonaldehyde with collagen. IV. Localisation of malonaldehyde binding site in collagen molecule. *Lebensm. Unters. Forsch.* 158: 279–283, 1975.
115. DAVISON, P. F. The contribution of labile crosslinks to the tensile behavior of tendons. *Connect. Tissue Res.* 18: 293–305, 1989.
116. DE MIGNARD, V. A., and S. BERNICK. Microvascular changes in

aging human osseous tissue [Abstract]. *Microvasc. Res.* 17: S11, 1979.
117. D'ERRICO, A., P. SCARANI, E. COLOSIMO, M. SPINA, W. F. GRIGIONI, and A. M. MANCINI. Changes in the alveolar connective tissue of the ageing lung: an immunohistochemical study. *Virchows Archiv [A]*. 415: 137–144, 1989.
118. DEYL, Z., G. M. BUTENKO, J. HAUSMANN, M. HORAKOVA, and K. MACEK. Increased glycation and pigmentation of collagen in aged and young parabiotic rats and mice. *Mech. Ageing Dev.* 55: 39–47, 1990.
119. DEYL, Z., M. HORAKOVA, and O. VANCIKOVA. Changes in pyridinoline content of elastin during ontogeny. *Mech. Ageing Dev.* 17: 321–325, 1981.
120. DEYL, Z., H. SULCOVA, R. PRAUS, and J. N. GOLDMAN. A fluorescent compound in collagen and its relation to the age of the animal. *Exp. Gerontol.* 5: 57–62, 1970.
121. DICKSON, I. R., and M. K. BAGGA. Changes with age in the non-collagenous proteins of human bone. *Connect. Tissue Res.* 14: 77–85, 1985.
122. DILLEY, K. J. Ultraviolet light and human cataract [Letter]. *Nature* 257: 71, 1975.
123. DILLEY, K. J., and A. PIRIE. Changes to the proteins of human lens nucleus in cataract. *Exp. Eye Res.* 19: 59–72, 1974.
124. DILLON, J. Photolytic changes in lens proteins. *Curr. Eye Res.* 3: 145–150, 1984.
125. DILLON, J., M. GARNER, D. ROY, and A. SPECTOR. The photolysis of lens protein: molecular changes. *Exp. Eye Res.* 34: 651–658, 1982.
126. DILLON, J., A. SPECTOR, and K. NAKANISHI. Identification of β-carbolines isolated from fluorescent human lens proteins. *Nature* 259: 471–483, 1976.
127. DISCHE, Z. and H. ZIL. Studies on the oxidation of cysteine to cystine in lens proteins during cataract formation. *Am. J. Ophthalmol.* 34: 104–113, 1951.
128. DISCHE, Z., E. BORENFREUND, and G. ZELMENIS. Changes in lens proteins of rats during aging. *Arch. Ophthalmol.* 55: 471–483, 1956.
129. DOEGE, K. J., M. SASAKI, E. HORIGAN, J. R. HASSELL, and Y. YAMADA. Complete primary structure of the rat cartilage proteoglycan core protein deduced from cDNA clones. *J. Biol. Chem.* 262: 17757–17767, 1987.
130. DOEGE, K. J., M. SASAKI, T. KIMURA, and Y. YAMADA. Complete coding sequence and deduced primary structure of the human cartilage large aggregating proteoglycan, aggrecan. *J. Biol. Chem.* 266: 894–902, 1991.
131. DOVRAT, A., and D. GERSHON. Rat lens superoxide dismutase and glucose 6-phosphate dehydrogenase: studies on the catalytic activity and fate of antigen as a function of age. *Exp. Eye Res.* 33: 651–661, 1981.
132. DUANCE, V. C., and S. F. WOTTON. Changes in the distribution of mammalian cartilage collagens with age. *Biochem. Soc. Trans.* 19: 376S, 1991.
133. DUBICK, M. A., R. B. RUCKER, C. E. CROSS, and J. A. LAST. Elastin metabolism in rodent lung. *Biochim. Biophys. Acta* 672: 303–306, 1981.
134. DUBINA, T. L., V. A. DYUNDIKOVA, and E. V. ZHUK. Biological age and its estimation. II. Assessment of biological age of albino rats by multiple regression analysis. *Exp. Gerontol.* 18: 5–18, 1983.
135. DUDHIA, J., and T. E. HARDINGHAM. The primary structure of human cartilage link protein. *Nucleic Acids Res.* 18: 1292, 1990.
136. DUESSEN, A., and H. PAU. Nucleotide levels in human lens: regional distribution in different forms of senile cataract. *Exp. Eye Res.* 48: 37–47, 1989.
137. DUNN, J. A., M. U. AHMED, M. H. MURTIASHAW, J. M. RICHARDSON, M. D. WALLA, S. R. THORPE, and J. W. BAYNES. Reaction of ascorbate with lysine and protein under oxidizing conditions. Formation of N-(carboxymethyl)-lysine by reaction between lysine products of autooxidation of ascorbate. *Biochemistry* 29: 10964–10970, 1990.
138. DUNN, J. A., D. R. MCCANCE, S. R. THORPE, T. J. LYONS, and J. W. BAYNES. Age-dependent accumulation of N ε-(carboxymethyl)lysine and N ε-(carboxymethyl)-hydroxylysine in human skin collagen. *Biochemistry* 30: 1205–1210, 1991.
139. DUNN, J. A., J. S. PATRICK, S. R. THORPE, and J. W. BAYNES. Oxidation of glycated proteins. Age-dependent accumulation of N^{ϵ}-(carboxymethyl) lysine in lens proteins. *Biochemistry* 28: 9464–9468, 1990.
140. DYER, D. G., J. A. BLACKLEDGE, S. R. THORPE, and J. W. BAYNES. Formation of pentosidine during nonenzymatic browning of proteins by glucose. Identification of glucose and other carbohydrates as possible precursors of pentosidine in vivo. *J. Biol. Chem.* 266: 11654–11660, 1991.
141. DYUNDIKOVA, V. A., Z. K. SILVON, and T. L. DUBINA. Biological age and its estimation. I. Studies of some physiological parameters in albino rats and their validity as biological age tests. *Exp. Gerontol.* 16: 13–24, 1981.
142. DZIEWIATKOWSKI, D. D., J. LAVALLEY, and A. G. BEAUDOIN. Age-related changes in the composition of proteoglycans in sheep cartilages. *Connect. Tissue Res.* 19: 103–120, 1989.
143. EATON, J. W. Is the lens canned? *Free Radic. Biol. Med.* 11: 207–213, 1991.
144. EGHBALI, M., M. EGHBALI, T. F. ROBINSON, S. SEIFTER, and O. O. BLUMENFELD. Collagen accumulation in heart ventricles as a function of growth and aging. *Cardiovasc. Res.* 23: 723–729, 1989.
145. EHRHART, L. A., and C. M. FERRARIO. Collagen metabolism and reversal of aortic hypertrophy in spontaneously hypertensive rats treated with methyldopa. *Hypertension* 3: 479–484, 1981.
146. ELLIOTT, R. J., and D. L. GARDNER. Changes with age in the glycosaminoglycans of human articular cartilage. *Ann. Rheum. Dis.* 38: 371–377, 1979.
147. EPSTEIN, D. L., and J. H. KINOSHITA. The effect of diamide on lens glutathione and lens membrane function. *Invest. Ophthalmol.* 9: 629–638, 1970.
148. ESPOSITO, C., H. GERLACH, J. BRETT, D. STERN, and H. VLASSARA. Endothelial receptor-mediated binding of glucose-modified albumin is associated with increased monolayer permeability and modulation of cell surface coagulant properties. *J. Exp. Med.* 170: 1387–1407, 1989.
149. EVERITT, A. V., and L. DELBRIDGE. Two phases of collagen ageing in the tail tendon of hypophysectomized rats. *Exp. Gerontol.* 7: 45–51, 1972.
150. EVERITT, A. V., B. D. PORTER, and M. STEELE. Dietary, caging and temperature factors in the ageing of collagen fibres in rat tail tendon. *Gerontology* 27: 37–41, 1981.
151. EVERITT, A. V., N. J. SEEDSMAN, and F. JONES. The effects of hypophysectomy and continuous food restriction, begun at ages 70–400 days, on collagen aging, proteinuria, incidence of pathology and longevity in the male rat. *Mech. Ageing Dev.* 12: 161–172, 1980.
152. EVERITT, A. V., J. R. WYNDHAM, and D. L. BARNARD. The antiaging action of hypophysectomy in hypothalamic obese rats: effects on collagen aging, age-associated proteinuria development and renal histopathology. *Mech. Ageing Dev.* 22: 233–251, 1983.
153. EYRE, D. R., and H. OGUCHI. The hydroxypyridinium crosslinks of skeletal collagens: their measurement, properties and a proposed pathway of formation. *Biochem. Biophys. Res. Commun.* 92: 403–410, 1980.

154. EYRE, D. R., I. R. DICKSON, and K. VAN NESS. Collagen crosslinking in human bone and articular cartilage: age-related changes in the content of mature hydroxypyridinium residues. *Biochem. J.* 252: 495–500, 1988.

155. EYRE, D. R., T. J. KOOB, and K. P. VAN NESS. Quantitation of hydroxypyridinium crosslinks in collagen by high-performance liquid chromatography. *Anal. Biochem.* 137: 380–388, 1984.

156. EYRE, D. R., M. A. PAZ, and P. M. GALLOP. Cross-linking in collagen and elastin. *Annu. Rev. Biochem.* 53: 717–748, 1984.

157. FARMAR, J. G., P. C. ULRICH, and A. CERAMI. Novel pyrroles from sulfite-inhibited Maillard reactions: insight into the mechanism of inhibition. *J. Org. Chem.* 53: 2346–2349, 1988.

158. FAZIO, M. J., D. R. OLSEN, H. KUIVANIEMI, M.-L. CHU, J. M. DAVIDSON, J. ROSENBLOOM, and J. UITTO. Isolation and characterization of human elastin cDNAs, and age-associated variation in elastin gene expression in cultured skin fibroblasts. *Lab. Invest.* 58: 270–277, 1988.

159. FECONDO, J. V., and R. C. AUGUSTEYN. Superoxide dismutase, catalase and glutathione peroxidase in human cataractous lens. *Exp. Eye Res.* 36: 15–23, 1983.

160. FEDARKO, N. S., U. K. VETTER, S. WEINSTEIN, and P. G. ROBEY. Age-related changes in hyaluronan, proteoglycan, collagen and osteonectin by human bone cells. *J. Cell. Physiol.* 151: 215–227, 1992.

161. FELDMAN, S. A., and S. GLAGOV. Transmedial collagen and elastin gradients in human aortas: reversal with age. *Atherosclerosis* 13: 385–394, 1971.

162. FISHER, R. F. The changes with age in the biophysical properties of the capsule of the human crystalline lens in relation to cataract. *Interdiscipl. Top. Gerontol.* 13: 131–142, 1978.

163. FLANDIN, F., C. BUFFEVANT, and D. HERBAGE. A differential scanning calorimetry analysis of the age-related changes in the thermal stability of rat skin collagen. *Biochim. Biophys. Acta* 791: 205–211, 1984.

164. FLANDIN, F., C. BUFFEVANT, and D. HERBAGE. Age-related changes in the biochemical and physiocochemical properties of rat skin. Collagen synthesis and maturation and mechanical parameters (uniaxial tension). *Cell. Mol. Biol.* 32: 565–571, 1986.

165. FLANNERY, C. R., M. W. LARK, and J. D. SANDY. Identification of a stromelysin cleavage site within the interglobular domain of human aggrecan. *J. Biol. Chem.* 267: 1008–1014, 1992.

166. FLANNERY, C., V. STANESCU, M. MÖRGELIN, R. BOYNTON, J. GORDY, and J. SANDY. Variability in the G3 domain and content of bovine aggrecan from cartilage extracts and chondrocyte cultures. *Arch. Biochem. Biophys.* 297: 52–60, 1992.

167. FLANNERY, C. R., P. J. URBANEK, and J. D. SANDY. The effect of maturation and aging on the structure and content of link proteins in rabbit articular cartilage. *J. Orthop. Res.* 8: 78–85, 1990.

168. FLEISHMAN, K. R., S. C. MARGOLIS, J. FU, and B. J. WAGNER. Age changes in bovine lens endopeptidase activity. *Mech. Ageing Dev.* 31: 37–47, 1985.

169. FLEISCHMAJER, R., J. S. PERLISH, and R. I. BASHEY. Human dermal glycosaminoglycans and aging. *Biochim. Biophys. Acta* 279: 265–275, 1972.

170. FORNIERI, C., D. QUAGLINO, Jr., and G. MORI. Role of the extracellular matrix in age-related modifications of the rat aorta: ultrastructural, morphometric, and enzymatic evaluations. *Arterioscler. Thromb.* 12: 1008–1016, 1992.

171. FOSTER, J. A., and S. W. CURTISS. The regulation of lung elastin synthesis. *Am. J. Physiol.* 259: L13–L23, 1990.

172. FOSTER, J. A., C. B. RICH, M. MILLER, M. R. BENEDICT, R. A. RICHMAN, and J. R. FLORINI. Effect of age and IGF-1 administration on elastin gene expression in rat aorta. *J. Gerontol.* 45: B113–B118, 1990.

173. FOURTANIER, A., and C. BERREBI. Miniature pig as an animal model to study photoaging. *Photochem. Photobiol.* 50: 771–784, 1989.

174. FRANCIS, G., R. JOHN, and J. THOMAS. Biosynthetic pathway of desmosines in elastin. *Biochem. J.* 136: 45–55, 1973.

175. FRANK, C., D. MCDONALD, R. LIEBER, and P. SABISTON. Biochemical heterogeneity within the maturing rabbit medial collateral ligament. *Clin. Orthop.* 236: 279–285, 1988.

176. FRONT, P., F. APRILE, D. R. MITROVIC, and D. A. SWANN. Age-related changes in synthesis of matrix macromolecules by bovine articular cartilage. *Connect. Tissue Res.* 19: 121–133, 1989.

177. FU, M.-X., K. J. KNECHT, S. R. THORPE, and J. W. BAYNES. Role of oxygen in crosslinking and chemical modification of collagen by glucose. *Diabetes* 41(suppl. 2): 42–48, 1992.

178. FUCCI, L., C. N. OLIVER, M. J. COON, and E. R. STADTMAN. Inactivation of key metabolic enzymes by mixed-function oxidation reactions: possible implication in protein turnover and ageing. *Proc. Natl. Acad. Sci. USA* 80: 1521–1525, 1983.

179. FUJII, N., S. MURAOKA, K. SATHO, K. HORI, and K. HANADA. Racemization of aspartic acids at specific sites in αA-crystallins from aged human lens. *Biomed. Res.* 12: 315–321, 1991.

180. FUJIMORI, E. Crosslinking and fluorescence changes of collagen by glycation and oxidation. *Biochim. Biophys. Acta* 998: 105–110, 1989.

181. FUJIMOTO, D. Aging and crosslinking in human aorta. *Biochem. Biophys. Res. Commun.* 109: 1264–1269, 1982.

182. FUJIMOTO, D. Aging of human connective tissue: increase in the content of a crosslinking amino acid, histidinoalanine. *Biochem. Int.* 5: 743–746, 1982.

183. FUJIMOTO, D., and T. MORIGUCHI. Pyridinoline, a non-reducible crosslink of collagen. *J. Biochem.* 83: 863–867, 1978.

184. FUJIMOTO, D., M. HIRAMA, and T. IWASHITA. Histidinoalanine, a new crosslinking amino acid, in calcified tissue collagen. *Biochem. Biophys. Res. Commun.* 104: 1102–1106, 1982.

185. FUJIMOTO, D., T. MORIGUCHI, T. ISHIDA, and H. HAYASHI. The structure of pyridinoline, a collagen crosslink. *Biochem. Biophys. Res. Commun.* 84: 52–57, 1978.

186. FUJIMOTO, D., M. SUZUKI, A. UCHIYAMA, S. MIYAMOTO, and T. INOUE. Analysis of pyridinoline, a crosslinking compound of collagen fibers, in human urine. *J. Biochem.* 94: 1133–1136, 1983.

187. FURTH, J. J. The steady-state levels of type I collagen mRNA are reduced in senescent fibroblasts. *J. Gerontol.* 46: B122–B124, 1991.

188. GARCIA-CASTINEIRAS, S., J. DILLON, and A. SPECTOR. Non-tryptophan fluorescence associated with human lens protein; apparent complexity and isolation of bityrosine and anthranilic acid. *Exp. Eye Res.* 26: 461–476, 1978.

189. GARLAND, D. Role of site-specific, metal catalyzed oxidation in lens aging and cataract: a hypothesis. *Exp. Eye Res.* 50: 677–682, 1990.

190. GARLAND, D., P. RUSSELL, and J. S. ZIGLER, JR. The oxidative modification of lens proteins. In: *Oxygen Radicals in Biology and Medicine*, edited by Simic Fig et al. New York: Plenum Press, 1988, vol. 49. p. 347–352.

191. GARLAND, D., J. S. ZIGLER, JR., and J. KINOSHITA. Structural changes in bovine lens crystallins induced by ascorbate, metal and oxygen. *Arch. Biochem. Biophys.* 251: 771–776, 1986.

192. GARLICK, R. L., H. F. BUNN, and R. G. SPIRO. Nonenzymatic glycation of basement membranes from human glomeruli and bovine sources. *Diabetes* 37: 1144–1150, 1988.

193. GARLICK, R. L., J. S. MAZER, and H. F. BUNN. Characterization of glycosylated hemoglobins: relevance to monitoring of diabetic control and analysis of other proteins. *J. Clin. Invest.* 71: 1062–1072, 1982.

194. GARNER, W. H., and A. SPECTOR. Racemization in human lens.

Evidence of rapid insolubilization of specific polypeptides in cataract formation. *Proc. Natl. Acad. Sci. USA* 75: 3618–3620, 1978.
195. GARNER, W. H., and A. SPECTOR. A preliminary study of dynamic aspects of age-dependent changes in the abundance of human lens polypeptides. *Doc. Ophthalmol. (The Hague)* 18: 91–99, 1979.
196. GARNER, W. H., and A. SPECTOR. Selective oxidation of cysteine and methionine in normal and senile cataractous lenses. *Proc. Natl. Acad. Sci. USA* 77: 1274–1277, 1980.
197. GARNER, W. H., A. BAHADOR, and G. SACHS. Nonenzymatic glycation of Na,K-ATPase: effects on ATP hydrolysis and K^+ occlusion. *J. Biol. Chem.* 265: 15058–15063, 1990.
198. GARNER, W. H., M. H. GARNER, and A. SPECTOR. Comparison of the 10,000 and 43,000 dalton polypeptide populations isolated from the water soluble and insoluble fractions of human cataractous lenses. *Exp. Eye Res.* 29: 257–276, 1979.
199. GARNER, W. H., M. H. GARNER, and A. SPECTOR. Gamma-crystallin, a major cytoplasmic polypeptide disulfide linked to membrane proteins in human cataract. *Biochem. Biophys. Commun.* 98: 439–447, 1981.
200. GARNER, W. H., M. H. GARNER, and A. SPECTOR. H_2O_2-induced uncoupling of bovine lens Na^+, K^+-ATPase. *Proc. Natl. Acad. Sci. USA* 80: 2044–2048, 1983.
201. GARNER, W. H., G. M. WANG, and A. SPECTOR. Stimulation of glucosylated lens epithelial Na,K-ATPase by an aldose reductase inhibitor. *Exp. Eye Res.* 44: 339–345, 1987.
202. GERBER, G., G. GERBER, and K. I. ALTMAN. Studies on the metabolism of tissue proteins. I. Turnover of collagen labeled with proline-U-C^{14} in young rats. *J. Biol. Chem.* 235: 2653–2656, 1960.
203. GHOSH, P., T. K. F. TAYLOR, and K. G. BRAUND. The variation of the glycosaminoglycans of the canine intervertebral disc with ageing. I. chondrodystrophoid breed. *Gerontology* 23: 87–98, 1977.
204. GIBLIN, F. J., B. CHAKRAPANI, and V. N. REDDY. The effects of x-irradiation on lens reducing systems. *Invest. Ophthalmol. Vis. Sci.* 18: 468–475, 1979.
205. GIBLIN, F. J., J. R. REDDAN, L. SCHRIMPSHER, D. C. DZIEDZIC, and V. N. REDDY. The reactive roles of glutathione redox cycle and catalase in the detoxification of H_2O_2 by cultured rabbit epithelial cells. *Exp. Eye Res.* 50: 795–804, 1990.
206. GIBSON, M. A., J. S. KUMARATILAKE, and E. G. CLEARY. The protein components of the 12-nanometer microfibrils of elastic and nonelastic tissues. *J. Biol. Chem.* 264: 4590–4598, 1989.
207. GILCHREST, B. A. Premature aging syndromes affecting the skin. *Birth Defects* 17: 227–241, 1981.
208. GILLERY, P., J. C. MONBOISSE, F. X. MAQUART, and J. P. BOREL. Glycation of proteins as a source of superoxide. *Diabetes Metab.* 14: 25–30, 1988.
209. GODEAU, G., and W. HORNEBECK. Morphometric analysis of the degradation of human skin elastic fibres by human leukocyte elastase (EC 3-4-21-37) and human skin fibroblast elastase (EC 3- 4-24). *Pathol. Biol. (Paris)* 36: 1133–1138, 1988.
210. GOLDSTEIN, S. Human genetic disorders that feature premature onset and accelerated progression of biological aging. In: *The Genetics of Aging*, edited by E. L. Schneider. New York: Plenum Press, 1978, p. 171–224.
211. GOMEZ, E. C., and B. BERMAN. The aging skin. *Clin. Geriatr. Med.* 1: 285–305, 1985.
212. GOOSEY, J. D., J. S. ZIGLER, JR., I. B. C. MATHESON, and J. H. KINOSHITA. Effects of singlet oxygen on human lens crystallins in vitro. *Invest. Ophthalmol. Vis. Sci.* 20: 679–683, 1981.
213. GOTTRUP, F. Healing of incisional wounds in the stomach and duodenum. *Dan. Med. Bull.* 31: 32–48, 1984.
214. GOWER, W. E., and V. PEDRINI. Age-related variations in protein polysaccharides from human nucleus pulposus, annulus fibrosus, and costal cartilage. *J. Bone Joint Surg.* 51A: 1154–1162, 1969.
215. GRANDHEE, S. K., and V. M. MONNIER. Mechanism of formation of the Maillard protein crosslink pentosidine. Glucose, fructose, and ascorbate as pentosidine precursors. *J. Biol. Chem.* 266: 11649–11653, 1991.
216. GRASEDYCK, K., M. JAHNKE, O. FRIEDRICH, D. SCHULZ, and I. LINDNER. Aging of liver: morphological and biochemical changes. *Mech. Ageing Dev.* 14: 435–442, 1980.
217. GREENWALD, S. E., C. L. BERRY, and R. E. RAMSEY. The static elastic properties and chemical composition of the rat aorta in spontaneously occurring and experimentally induced hypertension: the effect of an anti-hypertensive drug. *Br. J. Exp. Path.* 66: 633–642, 1985.
218. GROENEN, P. J. T. A., P. R. L. A. VAN DEN IJSEEL, C. E. M. VOORTER, H. BLOEMENDAL, and W. W. DE JONG. Site-specific racemization in aging αA-crystallin. *FEBS Lett.* 269: 109–112, 1990.
219. GRUNDBOECK-JUSCO, J., A. BINETTE, A. KIMURA, L. TALARICO, R. KAELIN, and K. SCHMID. The glycosaminoglycan composition of the lung with acute and chronic pathology and in senescence. *Clin. Chim. Acta* 208: 77–84, 1992.
220. GRUSHKO, G., R. SCHNEIDERMAN, and A. MAROUDAS. Some biochemical and biophysical parameters for the study of the pathogenesis of osteoarthritis: a comparison between the processes of ageing and the degeneration in human hip cartilage. *Connect. Tissue Res.* 19: 149–176, 1989.
221. GUANTIERI, V., A. M. TAMBURRO, and D. D. GORDINI. Interactions of human and bovine elastins with lipids: their proteolysis by elastase. *Connect. Tissue Res.* 12: 79–83, 1983.
222. GUNJA-SMITH, Z., J. LIN, and J. F. WOESSNER. Changes in desmosine and pyridinoline crosslinks during rapid synthesis and degradation of elastin and collagen in the rat uterus. *Matrix* 9: 21–27, 1989.
223. GUTIERREZ, P. S., I. C. DE ALMEIDA, H. B. NADER, M. DE LOURDES HIGUCHI, N. STOLF, and C. P. DIETRICH. Decrease in sulphated glycosaminoglycans in aortic dissection—possible role in the pathogenesis. *Cardiovasc. Res.* 25: 742–748, 1991.
224. GUYTON, J. R., K. L. LINDSAY, and D. T. DAO. Comparison of aortic intima and inner media in young adult versus aging rats. Stereology in a polarized system. *Am. J. Pathol.* 111: 234–246, 1983.
225. HALL, D. A. The metabolism of connecttissue. In: *The Ageing of Connective Tissue*, edited by D. A. Hall. New York: Academic Press, 1976, p. 145–171.
226. HAM, W. T., JR., H. A. MUELLER, J. J. RUFFALO, JR., D. GUERRY, III, and R. K. GUERRY. Action spectrum for retinal injury from near-ultraviolet radiation in the aphakic monkey. *Am. J. Ophthalmol.* 93: 299–306, 1982.
227. HAMLIN, C. R., R. R. KOHN, and J. L. LUSCHIN. Apparent accelerated aging of collagen in diabetes mellitus. *Diabetes* 24: 902–904, 1975.
228. HAMLIN, C. R., J. H. LUSCHIN, and R. R. KOHN. Partial characterization of the age-related stabilizing factor of post-mature human collagen-I. By use of bacterial collagenase. *Exp. Gerontol.* 13: 403–414, 1978.
229. HAMLIN, C. R., J. H. LUSCHIN, and R. R. KOHN. Aging of collagen: comparative rates in four mammalian species. *Exp. Gerontol.* 15: 393–398, 1980.
230. HARDING, J. J. Free and protein-bound glutathione in normal and cataractous human lenses. *Biochem. J.* 117: 957–960, 1970.
231. HARDING, J. J. Conformational changes in human lens proteins in cataract. *Biochem. J.* 129: 97–103, 1972.
232. HARDING, J. J., and K. J. DILLEY. Structural proteins of the

mammalian lens: a review with emphasis on changes in development, aging and cataract. *Exp. Eye Res.* 22: 1–73, 1976.
233. HARDING, J. J., and R. VAN HEYNINGEN. Epidemiology and risk factors for cataract eye. *Eye* 1: 537–541, 1987.
234. HARDINGHAM, T., and M. BAYLISS. Proteoglycans of articular cartilage: changes in aging and in joint disease. *Semin. Arthritis Rheum.* 20(suppl. 1): 12–33, 1990.
235. HARMAN, D. Aging: a theory based on free radical and radiation chemistry. *J. Gerontol.* 11: 289–300, 1956.
236. HARRIS, E. D., and S. M. KRANE. Collagenases. *N. Engl. J. Med.* 291: (Parts 1–3), 557–564, 605–610, 652–661, 1974.
237. HARRIS, P., D. HEATH, and A. APOSTOLOPOULOS. Extensibility of human pulmonary trunk. *Br. Heart J.* 27: 651–659, 1965.
238. HARRISON, D. E., and J. R. ARCHER. Physiological assays for biological age in mice: relationship of collagen, renal function, and longevity. *Exp. Aging Res.* 9: 245–251, 1983.
239. HARRISON, D. E., and J. R. ARCHER. Genetic differences in effects of food restriction on aging in mice. *J. Nutr.* 117: 376–382, 1987.
240. HARRISON, D. E., J. R. ARCHER, and C. M. ASTLE. Effects of food restriction on aging: separation of food intake and adiposity. *Proc. Natl. Acad. Sci. USA* 81: 1835–1838, 1984.
241. HARRISON, D. E., J. R. ARCHER, G. A. SACHER, and F. M. BOYCE, III. Tail collagen aging in mice of thirteen different genotypes and two species: relationship to biological age. *Exp. Gerontol.* 13: 63–73, 1978.
242. HASHIMOTO, S., T. YOKOKURA, and M. MUTAI. Effect of age and dietary composition on aortic collagen to elastin ratio and on lipid metabolism in F-344 rat. *Exp. Gerontol.* 16: 35–39, 1981.
243. HATA, R. Age-dependent changes in collagen metabolism and response to hypertonic culture conditions of rat aortic smooth muscle cells in skin fibroblasts. *Cell Biol. Int. Rep.* 14: 25–33, 1990.
244. HAYASE, F., R. H. NAGARAJ, S. MIYATA, F. G. NJOROGE, and V. M. MONNIER. Aging of proteins: immunological detection of a glucose-derived pyrrole formed during Maillard reaction in vivo. *J. Biol. Chem.* 263: 3758–3764, 1989.
245. HAYASHI, K., S. NAGASAWA, Y. NARUO, A. OKUMURA, K. MORITAKE, and H. HANDA. Mechanical properties of human cerebral arteries. *Biorheology* 17: 211–218, 1980.
246. HEINEGARD, D., and A. OLDBERG. Structure and biology of cartilage and bone matrix noncollagenous macromolecules. *FASEB J.* 3: 2042–2051, 1989.
247. HELIN, P., C. GARBARSCH, G. HELIN, and I. LORENZEN. Vascular injury compared to ageing of normal rabbit aorta. Biochemical and histochemical studies on time-dependent alterations of vascular connective tissue. *Blood Vessels* 22: 94–105, 1985.
248. HELLER, D. A., and G. E. McCLEARN. A longitudinal genetic study of tail tendon fibre break time. *Age Ageing* 21: 129–134, 1992.
249. HERBRINK, P., and H. BLOEMENDAL. Studies on β-crystallin. I. Isolation and partial characterization of the principal polypeptide chain. *Biochim. Biophys. Acta* 336: 370–382, 1974.
250. HICKS, M., L. DELBRIDGE, D. K. YUE, and T. S. REEVE. Increase in crosslinking of nonenzymatically glycosylated collagen induced by products of lipid peroxidation. *Arch. Biochem. Biophys.* 268: 249–254, 1989.
251. HIGGINS, K. A., J. T. STOUT, D. A. HELLER, and R. F. PARKER. Individual variability in tail tendon fiber break time in three age cohorts of different strains of mice. *Exp. Gerontol.* 26: 467–477, 1991.
252. HOCKWIN, O. Enzyme activities in relationship to age and phosphorylated intermediates in energy metabolism. *Invest. Ophthalmol.* 4: 496–501, 1965.

253. HOFECKER, G., M. SKALICKY, A. KMENT, and H. NIEDERMÜLLER. Models of biological age of the rat. I. A factor model of age parameters. *Mech. Ageing Dev.* 14: 345–359, 1980.
254. HOGAN, M. J., J. A. ALVARADO, and J. E. WEDDELL (Eds). In: *Histology of the Human Eye,* Philadelphia: W. B. Saunders, 1971, p. 435.
255. HOLLANDER, D., A. TARNAWSKI, J. STACHURA, and H. GERGELY. Morphologic changes in gastric mucosa of aging rats. *Dig. Dis. Sci.* 34: 1692–1700, 1989.
256. HOLLMANN, J., A. SCHMIDT, D.-B. VON BASSEWITZ, and E. BUDDECKE. Relationship of sulfated glycosaminoglycans and cholesterol content in normal and arteriosclerotic human aorta. *Arteriosclerosis* 9: 154–158, 1989.
257. HOLMES, M. W. A., M. T. BAYLISS, and H. MUIR. Hyaluronic acid in human cartilage: age-related changes in content and size. *Biochem. J.* 250: 435–441, 1988.
258. HONDA, T., K. KATAGIRI, E. KURODA, E. MATSUNAGA, and H. SHINKAI. Age-related changes of the dermatan sulfate containing small proteoglycans in bovine tendon. *Collagen Rel. Res.* 7: 171–184, 1987.
259. HORIUCHI, S., N. ARAKI, and Y. MORINO. Immunochemical approach to characterize advanced glycation end products of the Maillard reaction. *J. Biol. Chem.* 266: 7329–7332, 1991.
260. HORIUCHI, S., M. SHIGA, N. ARAKI, K. TAKATA, M. SAITOH, and Y. MORINO. Evidence against in vivo presence of 2-(2-furoyl)-4(5)-(2-furanyl)-1H-imidazole, a major fluorescent advanced end product generated by nonenzymatic glycosylation. *J. Biol. Chem.* 263: 18821–18826, 1988.
261. HORMEL, S. E., and D. R. EYRE. Collagen in the ageing human intervertebral disc: an increase in covalently bound fluorophores and chromophores. *Biochim. Biophys. Acta* 1078: 243–250, 1991.
261a. HORN, P. L., J. J. LAVER, and J. T. WOOD. Changes of aging parameters among rats on diets differing in fat quantity and quality. *J. Gerontol.* 36: 285–293, 1981.
262. HORNEBECK, W., J. J. ADNET, and L. ROBERT. Age-dependent variation of elastin and elastase in aorta and human breast cancers. *Exp. Gerontol.* 13: 293–298, 1978.
263. HOROWITZ, J., and M. M. WONG. Peptide mapping by limited proteolysis in sodium dodecyl sulfate of the main intrinsive polypeptides isolated from human and bovine lens plasma membranes. *Biochim. Biophys. Acta* 622: 134–143, 1980.
264. HOROWITZ, J., J. S. HANSEN, C. C. CHENG, L. L. DING, B. R. STRAATSMA, D. O. LIGHTFOOT, and L. J. TAKEMOTO. Presence of low molecular weight polypeptides in human brunescent cataracts. *Biochem. Biophys. Res. Commun.* 113: 65–71, 1983.
265. HRICIK, D. E., J. A. SCHULAK, D. R. SELL, J. F. FOGARTY, and V. M. MONNIER. Effects of kidney or kidney–pancreas transplantation on plasma pentosidine. *Kidney Int.* 43: 398–403, 1993.
266. HUANG, K.-C., K. SUKEGAWA, and T. ORII. Glycosaminoglycan excretion in random samples of urine. *Clin. Chim. Acta* 151: 141–146, 1985.
267. HUBER, B., F. LEDL, T. SEVERIN, A. STANGL, and G. PFLEIDERER. Formation of 2-(2-furoyl)-4(5)-(2-furyl)-1H-imidazole in the Maillard reaction. *Carbohydr. Res.* 182: 301–306, 1988.
268. HUBY, R., and J. J. HARDING. Nonenzymatic glycosylation (glycation) of lens proteins by galactose and protection by aspirin and reduced glutathione. *Exp. Eye Res.* 47: 53–59, 1988.
269. HUNT, J. V., R. T. DEAN, and S. P. WOLFF. Hydroxyl radical production and autoxidative glycosylation: glucose autoxidation as the cause of protein damage in the experimental glycation model of diabetes mellitus and ageing. *Biochem. J.* 256: 205–212, 1988.
270. IMAYAMA, S., and I. M. BRAVERMAN. A hypothetical explanation for the aging of skin: chronologic alteration of the three-

dimensional arrangement of collagen and elastic fibers in connective tissue. *Am. J. Pathol.* 134: 1019–1025, 1989.
271. INDIK, Z., H. YEH, N. ORNSTEIN-GOLDSTEIN, U. KUCICH, W. ABRAMS, J. C. ROSENBLOOM, and J. ROSENBLOOM. Structure of the elastin gene and alternative splicing of elastin mRNA: implications for human disease. *Am. J. Med. Genet.* 34: 81–90, 1989.
272. INDIK, Z., H. YEH, N. ORNSTEIN-GOLDSTEIN, P. SHEPPARD, N. ANDERSON, J. C. ROSENBLOOM, L. PELTONEN, and J. ROSENBLOOM. Alternate splicing of human elastin mRNA indicated by sequence analysis of cloned genomic and complementary DNA. *Proc. Natl. Acad. Sci. USA* 84: 5680–5684, 1987.
273. INDREKVAM, K., I. VIKOYR, R. T. LIE, L. B. ENGESAETER, and N. LANGELAND. Age-related differences in chemical composition of rat femur as determinants for strain. *Acta Orthop. Scand.* 62: 455–458, 1991.
274. INGRAM, D. K., J. R. ARCHER, and D. E. HARRISON. Physiological and behavioral correlates of lifespan in aged C57BL/6J mice. *Exp. Gerontol.* 17: 295–303, 1982.
275. IPPOLITO, E., P. G. NATALI, F. POSTACCHINI, L. ACCINNI, and C. DE MARTINO. Morphological, immunochemical and biochemical study of rabbit Achilles tendon at various ages. *J. Bone Joint Surg.* 62: 583–598, 1980.
276. ISEMURA, M., K. TAKAHASHI, and T. IKENAKA. Comparative study of carbohydrate-protein complexes. II. Determination of hydroxylysine and its glycosides in human skin and scar collagens by an improved method. *J. Biochem.* 80: 653–658, 1976.
277. ISHII, T., H. TSUJI, A. SANO, Y. KATOH, H. MATSUI, and N. TERAHATA. Histochemical and ultrastructural observations on brown degeneration of human intervertebral disc. *J. Orthop. Res.* 9: 78–90, 1991.
278. ITO, A., H. YAMAGIWA, and R. SASAKI. Effects of aging on hydroxyproline in human heart muscle. *J. Am. Geriatr. Soc.* 28: 398–404, 1980.
279. JACKSON, S. H., and J. A. HEININGER. A reassessment of the collagen reutilization theory by an isotope ratio method. *Clin. Chim. Acta* 46: 153–160, 1973.
280. JACKSON, S. H., and J. A. HEININGER. A study of collagen reutilization using an $^{18}O_2$ labeling technique. *Clin. Chim. Acta* 51: 163–171, 1974.
281. JACKSON, S. H., and J. A. HEININGER. Proline recycling during collagen metabolism as determined by concurrent $^{18}O_2$-and ^{3}H-labeling. *Biochim. Biophys. Acta* 381: 359–367, 1975.
282. JAHNGEN, J. H., A. L. HAAS, A. CIECHANOVER, J. BLONDIN, D. EISENHAUER, and A. TAYLOR. The eye lens has an active ubiquitin-protein conjugation system. *J. Biol. Chem.* 261: 13760–13767, 1986.
283. JEDZINIAK, J., and J. ROKITA. Aldehyde metabolism in the human lens. *Exp. Eye Res.* 37: 119–127, 1983.
284. JEDZINIAK, J. A., L. M. ARREDONDO, and L. MEYS. Human lens enzyme alterations with age and cataract. Glyceraldehyde-6-P dehydrogenase and triose phosphate isomerase. *Curr. Eye Res.* 119–126, 1986.
285. JEDZINIAK, J. A., L. T. CHYLACK, JR., H.-M. CHENG, M. K. GILLIS, A. A. KALUSTIAN, and W. H. TUNG. The sorbitol pathway in the human lens: aldose reductase and polyol dehydrogenase. *Invest. Ophthalmol. Vis. Sci.* 20: 314–326, 1981.
286. JEDZINIAK, J. A., J. H. KINOSHITA, E. M. YATES, L. O. HOCHER, and G. B. BENEDEK. On the presence and mechanism of formation of heavy molecular weight aggregates in human normal and cataractous lenses. *Exp. Eye Res.* 15: 185–192, 1973.
287. JERNIGAN, H. M., JR., H. N. FUKUI, J. D. GOSSEY, and J. H. KINOSHITA. Photodynamic effects of rose bengal or riboflavin on carrier-mediated transport systems in rat lens. *Exp. Eye Res.* 32: 461–466, 1981.
288. JHA, M. Age-related changes in pyridinoline content of rabbit collagen. *Exp. Gerontol.* 17: 7–9, 1982.
289. JOHN, R., and J. THOMAS. Chemical compositions of elastins isolated from aortas and pulmonary tissues of humans of different ages. *Biochem. J.* 127: 261–269, 1972.
290. KADAR, A. Scanning electron microscopy of purified elastin with and without enzymatic digestion. *Adv. Exp. Med. Biol.* 79: 71–96, 1977.
291. KAMEI, A., and M. KATO. Contribution of glycation to human lens coloration. *Chem. Pharm. Bull.* 39: 1272–1276, 1991.
292. KANAYAMA, T., Y. MIYANAGA, K. HORIUCHI, and D. FUJIMOTO. Detection of the crosslinking amino acid, histidinoalanine, in human brown cataractous protein. *Exp. Eye Res.* 44: 165–169, 1987.
293. KANUNGO, M. S. Changes in collagen. In: *Biochemistry of Ageing*, edited by M. S. Kanungo. New York: Academic Press, 1980, p. 129–157.
294. KAO, K.-Y., D. M. HILKER, and T. H. MCGAVACK. Connective tissue V. Comparison of synthesis and turnover of collagen and elastin in tissues of rat at several ages. *Proc. Soc. Exp. Biol. Med.* 106: 335–338, 1961.
295. KARTTUNEN, T., J. RISTELI, H. AUTIO-HARMAINEN, and L. RISTELI. Effect of age and diabetes on type IV collagen and laminin in human kidney cortex. *Kidney Int.* 30: 586–591, 1986.
296. KARWATOWSKI, W. S., T. E. JEFFERIES, V. C. DUANCE, J. ALBON, A. J. BAILEY, and D. L. EASTY. Collagen and ageing in Bruch's membrane. *Biochem. Soc. Trans.* 19: 349S, 1991.
297. KASUYA, M., M. ITOI, S. KOBAYASHI, H. SUNAGA, and K. T. SUZUKI. Changes of glutathione and taurine concentrations in lenses of rat eye induced by galactose-cataract formation or aging. *Exp. Eye Res.* 54: 49–53, 1992.
298. KATO, H., N. VAN CHUYEN, T. SHINODA, F. SEKIYA, and F. HAYASE. Metabolism of 3-deoxyglucosone, an immediate compound in the Maillard reaction, administered orally or intravenously to rats. *Biochim. Biophys. Acta* 1035: 71–76, 1990.
299. KEMP, P. D., and J. E. SCOTT. Ehrlich chromogens, probable cross-links, in elastin and collagen. *Biochem. J.* 252: 387–393, 1988.
300. KERR, J. S., S. Y. YU, and D. J. RILEY. Strain specific respiratory air space enlargement in aged rats. *Exp. Gerontol.* 25: 563–574, 1990.
301. KETTELHUT, B. V., and D. D. METCALFE. Quantitation and characterization of urinary glycosaminoglycans in healthy subjects and patients with mastocytosis. *Clin. Chim. Acta* 171: 29–36, 1988.
302. KIBRICK, A. C., and K. D. SINGH. Hydroxyproline excreted in the urine: its source from collagen of tissues after ^{14}C-proline in rats with and without administration of prednisone. *J. Clin. Endocrinol. Metab.* 38: 594–601, 1974.
303. KIKUGAWA, K., and M. BEPPU. Involvement of lipid oxidation products in the formation of fluorescent and crosslinked proteins. *Chem. Phys. Lipids* 44: 277–296, 1987.
304. KITTLICK, P.-D. Glycosaminoglycans. Recent biochemical results in the fields of growth and inflammation. *Exp. Pathol.* 10 (suppl): 1–174, 1985.
305. KIVIRIKKO, K. I. Urinary excretion of hydroxyproline in health and disease. *Int. Rev. Connect. Tissue Res.* 5: 93–163, 1970.
306. KNECHT, K. J., J. A. DUNN, K. F. MCFARLAND, D. R. MCCANCE, T. J. LYONS, S. R. THORPE, and J. W. BAYNES. Effect of diabetes and aging on carboxymethyllysine levels in human urine. *Diabetes* 40: 190–196, 1991.
307. KNECHT, K. J., M. S. FEATHER, and J. W. BAYNES. Detection of 3-deoxyfructose and 3-deoxyglucosone in human urine and plasma: evidence for intermediate stages of the Maillard reaction in vivo. *Arch. Biochem. Biophys.* 294: 130–137, 1992.
308. KOBAYASHI, Y., and T. SUZUKI. The aging lens: ultrastructural changes in cataract. In: *Cataract and Abnormalities of the Lens*,

edited by J. G. Bellows. New York: Grune and Stratton, 1975, p. 313–343.

309. KODAMA, T., and L. TAKEMOTO. Characterization of disulfide-linked crystallins associated with human cataractous lens membranes. *Invest. Ophthalmol. Vis. Sci.* 29: 145–149, 1988.

310. KODAMA, T., V. N. REDDY, F. J. GIBLIN, J. H. KINOSHITA, and C. HARDING. Scanning electron microscopy of x-ray induced cataract in mice on normal and galactose diet. *Ophthalmol. Res.* 15: 324–333, 1983.

311. KOHN, R. R. *Principles of Mammalian Aging.* Englewood Cliffs, NJ: Prentice-Hall, 1978.

312. KOHN, R. R. Evidence against cellular aging theories. In: *Testing the Theories of Aging,* edited by R. C. Adelman and G. S. Roth. Boca Raton, FL: CRC Press, 1982, p. 221–232.

313. KOHN, R. R. Effects of age and diabetes mellitus on cyanogen bromide digestion of human dura mater collagen. *Connect. Tissue Res.* 11: 169–173, 1983.

314. KOHN, R. R., and V. M. MONNIER. Normal aging and its parameters. In: *Clinical Pharmacology in the Elderly,* edited by C. G. Swift. New York: Marcel Dekker, 1987.

315. KOHN, R. R., and E. ROLLERSON. Age changes in swelling properties of human myocardium. *Proc. Soc. Exp. Biol. Med.* 100: 253–256, 1959.

316. KOHN, R. R., and S. L. SCHNIDER. Glucosylation of human collagen. *Diabetes* 31 (suppl 3): 47–51, 1982.

317. KONTERMANN, K., and K. BAYREUTHER. The cellular aging of rat fibroblasts in vitro is a differentiation process. *Gerontology* 25: 261–274, 1979.

318. KOVANEN, V. Effects of ageing and physical training on rat skeletal muscle. An experimental study on the properties of collagen, lamini, and fibre types in muscles serving different functions. *Acta Physiol. Scand.* 577 (suppl): 1–56, 1989.

319. KOVANEN, V., H. SUOMINEN, and L. PELTONEN. Effects of aging and life-long physical training on collagen in slow and fast skeletal muscle in rats. *Cell Tissue Res.* 248: 247–255, 1987.

320. KOVANEN, V., H. SUOMINEN, J. RISTELI, and L. RISTELI. Type IV collagen and laminin in slow and fast skeletal muscle in rats—effects of age and life-time endurance training. *Coll. Relat. Res.* 8: 145–153, 1988.

321. KRANE, S. M., F. G. KANTROWITZ, M. BYRNE, S. R. PINNELL, and F. R. SINGER. Urinary excretion of hydroxylysine and its glycosides as an index of collagen degradation. *J. Clin. Invest.* 59: 819–827, 1977.

322. KRAUSE, A. C. Chemistry of the lens. V. Relation of the anatomic distribution of the lenticular proteins to their chemical composition. *Arch. Ophthalmol.* 10: 788–792, 1933.

323. KRISTAL, B. S., and B. P. YU. An emerging hypothesis: synergistic induction of aging by free radicals and Maillard reactions. *J. Gerontol.* 47: B107–B114, 1992.

324. KRUMPE, P. E., R. J. KNUDSON, G. PARSONS, and K. REISER. The aging respiratory system. *Clin. Geriatr. Med.* 1: 143–175, 1985.

325. KULLER, L. H. Epidemiology of cardiovascular disease: current perspectives. *Am. J. Epidemiol.* 104: 425, 1976.

326. KURZEL, R. B., M. L. WOLBARSHT, and B. S. YAMANASHI. Spectral studies on normal and cataractous intact human lenses. *Exp. Eye Res.* 17: 65–71, 1973.

327. KURZEL, R. B., M. L. WOLBARSHT, and B. S. YAMANASHI. Ultraviolet radiation effects on the human eye. *Photochem. Photobiol. Rev.* 2. 133–167, 1977.

328. KUWABARA, T. The maturation of the lens cell: a morphologic study. *Exp. Eye Res.* 20: 427–443, 1975.

329. KUYPERS, R., M. TYLER, L. B. KURTH, I. D. JENKINS, and D. J. HORGAN. Identification of the loci of the collagen-associated Ehrlich chromogen in type I collagen confirms its role as a trivalent crosslink. *Biochem. J.* 283: 129–136, 1992.

330. LABELLA, F. S. Cross-links in elastin and collagen. In: *Biophysical Properties of the Skin,* edited by H. R. Elden. New York: John Wiley and Sons, 1971, p. 243–301.

331. LABELLA, F. S. Enzymatic vs. nonenzymatic factors in the deterioration of connective tissue. *Adv. Exp. Med. Biol.* 43: 377–402, 1974.

332. LABELLA, F. S., S. VIVIAN, and D. P. THORNHILL. Amino acid composition of human aortic elastin as influenced by age. *J. Gerontol.* 21: 550–555, 1966.

333. LAGIER, P. R., and B. EXER. Etude de la composition chimique de tissus humains de nature conjonctive en rapport avec l'age: derme et aponevrose de la paroi abodominale, tendon d'Achille. *Gerontologia* 4: 39–59, 1960.

334. LAITINEN, O. The metabolism of collagen and its hormonal control in the rat: III. Collagen as a precursor of urinary hydroxyproline. *Acta Endocrinologia [Suppl.] (Copenha)* 120: 1–86, 1967.

335. LAPOLLA, A., C. GERHARDINGER, B. PELLI, A. STURARO, E. DEL FAVERO, P. TRALDI, G. CREPALDI, and D. FEDELE. Absence of brown product FFI in nondiabetic and diabetic rat collagen. *Diabetes* 39: 57–61, 1990.

336. LARKING, P. W., B. W. MCDONALD, M. L. TAYLOR, and A. D. KIRKLAND. Urine glycosaminoglycans in a reference population: effects of age, body surface area, and postmenopausal status. *Biochem. Med. Metab. Biol.* 37: 246–254, 1987.

337. LAST, J. A., L. G. ARMSTRONG, and K. M. REISER. Biosynthesis of collagen crosslinks. *Int. J. Biochem.* 22: 559–564, 1990.

338. LAURENT, G. J. Rates of collagen synthesis in lung, skin, and muscle obtained in vivo by a simplified method using [^{3}H]proline. *Biochem. J.* 206: 535–544, 1982.

339. LAURENT, G. J. Dynamic state of collagen: pathways of collagen degradation in vivo and their possible role in regulation of collagen mass. *Am. J. Physiol.* 252: C1–C9, 1987.

340. LAURENT, G. J., and R. J. MCANULTY. Protein metabolism during bleomycin-induced pulmonary fibrosis in rabbits: in vivo evidence for collagen accumulation because of increased synthesis and decreased degradation of the newly synthesized collagen. *Am. Rev. Respir. Dis.* 128: 82–88, 1983.

341. LAURENT, G. J., and M. P. SPARROW. Changes in RNA, DNA and protein content and the rates of protein synthesis and degradation during hypertrophy of the anterior latissimus dorsi muscle of the adult fowl *(Gallus domesticus)*. *Growth* 41: 249–262, 1977.

342. LAURENT, G. J., R. J. MCANULTY, and J. GIBSON. Changes in collagen synthesis and degradation during skeletal muscle growth. *Am. J. Physiol.* 249: C352–C355, 1985.

343. LAVKER, R. M., P. ZHENG, and G. DONG. Morphology of aged skin. *Clin. Geriatr. Med.* 5: 53–67, 1989.

344. LEFEVRE, M., and R. B. RUCKER. Aorta elastin turnover in normal and hypercholesterolemic Japanese quail. *Biochim. Biophys. Acta* 630: 519–529, 1980.

344a. LE LOUS, M., L. COHEN-SOLAL, J. C. ALLAIN, J. BONAVENTURE, and P. MAROTEAUX. Age-related evolution of stable collagen reticulation in human skin. *Connect. Tissue Res.* 13: 145–155, 1985.

345. LERMAN, S. Composition and formation of the insoluble protein fraction in the ocular lens. *Can. J. Ophthalmol.* 5: 152–159, 1970.

346. LERMAN, S. Biophysical aspects of corneal and lenticular transparency. *Curr. Eye Res.* 3: 3–14, 1984.

347. LERMAN, S., and R. BORKMAN. Spectroscopic evaluation and classification of the normal, aging and cataractous lens. *Ophthalmol. Res.* 8: 335–353, 1976.

348. LERMAN, S., and R. BORKMAN. Ultraviolet radiation in the aging and cataractous lens. *Acta Ophthalmol.* 58: 139–149, 1977.

349. LERMAN, S., and R. F. BORKMAN. Photochemistry and lens aging. *Interdiscipl. Top. Gerontol.* 13: 154–182, 1978.
350. LERMAN, S., K. GARDNER, J. MEGAW, and R. BORKMAN. Prevention of direct photosynthesized ultraviolet radiation to the ocular lens. *Ophthalmic Res.* 13: 284–292, 1981.
351. LERMAN, S., F. K. KUCK, R. BORKMAN, and E. SAKER. Acceleration of an aging parameter (fluorogen) in the ocular lens. *Ann. Ophthalmol.* 8: 558–562, 1976.
352. LERMAN, S., F. K. KUCK, R. BORKMAN, and E. SAKER. Induction, acceleration and prevention (in vitro) of an aging parameter in the ocular lens. *Ophthalmic Res.* 13: 154–182, 1976.
353. LESKE, M. C., L. T. CHYLACK, JR., and S. Y. WU. The lens opacities case-control study. Risk factors of cataract. *Arch. Ophthalmol.* 109: 244–251, 1991.
354. LEVINE, R. L. Oxidative modification of glutamine synthetase. I. Inactivation is due to the loss of one histidine residue. *J. Biol. Chem.* 258: 11823–11827, 1983.
355. LEVINE, R. L., C. N. OLIVER, M. J. COON, and E. R. STADTMAN. Turnover of bacterial glutamine synthatase: oxidative inactivation precedes proteolysis. *Proc. Natl. Acad. Sci. USA* 78: 2120–2124, 1981.
356. LIANG, J. N., and B. CHAKRABARTI. Sugar-induced change in near ultraviolet circular dichroism of α-crystallin. *Biochem. Biophys. Res. Commun.* 102: 180–189, 1981.
357. LIANG, J. N., and L. T. CHYLACK, JR. Age-related change in protein conformation of normal human α-crystallin. *Lens Res.* 2: 189–206, 1984.
358. LIANG, J. N., and L. T. CHYLACK. Spectroscopic study on the effects of nonenzymatic glycation in human α-crystallin. *Invest. Ophthalmol. Vis. Sci.* 28: 790–794, 1987.
359. LIANG, J. N., and M. T. ROSSI. In vitro nonenzymatic glycation and formation of browning products in the bovine lens α-crystallin. *Exp. Eye Res.* 50: 367–371, 1990.
360. LIANG, J. N., S. K. BOSE, and B. CHAKRABARTI. Age-related changes in protein conformation in bovine lens crystallins. *Exp. Eye Res.* 40: 461–469, 1983.
361. LIANG, J. N., L. L. HERSHORIN, and L. T. CHYLACK. Nonenzymatic glycosylation in human diabetic crystallins. *Diabetologia* 29: 225–228, 1986.
362. LIANG, Z.-Q., F. HAYASE, and H. KATO. Purification and characterization of NADPH-dependent 2-oxoaldehyde reductase from porcine liver: a self-defense enzyme preventing the advanced stage of the Maillard reaction. *Eur. J. Biochem.* 197: 373–379, 1991.
363. LIGHT, N. D., and A. J. BAILEY. The chemistry of the collagen cross-links. Purification and characterization of cross-linked polymeric peptide material from mature collagen containing unknown amino acids. *Biochem. J.* 185: 373–381, 1980.
364. LIGHT, N. D., and A. J. BAILEY. Molecular structure and stabilization of the collagen fibre. In: *Biology of Collagen*, edited by A. Viidik and J. Vuust. New York: Academic Press, 1980, p. 15–38.
365. LIPPMAN, R. D. Rapid in vivo quantification and comparison of hydroperoxides and oxidized collagen in aging mice, rabbits and man. *Exp. Gerontol.* 20: 1–5, 1985.
366. LOPEZ, M. G., and M. S. FEATHER. The production of threose as a degradation product from L-ascorbic acid. *J. Carbohydr. Chem.* 11: 799–806, 1992.
367. LORAND, L., L. K. H. HSU, G. E. SIEFRING, JR., and N. S. RAFFERTY. Lens transglutaminase and cataract formation. *Proc. Natl. Acad. Sci. USA* 78: 1356–1360, 1981.
368. LOVELL, C. R., K. A. SMOLENSKI, V. C. DUANCE, N. D. LIGHT, S. YOUNG, and M. DYSON. Type I and III collagen content and fibre distribution in normal human skin during ageing. *Br. J. Dermatol.* 117: 419–428, 1987.
369. LOWRY, O., N. J. ROSEBROUGH, A. L. FARR, and R. J. RANDALL. Protein measurement with the folin phenol reagent. *J. Biol. Chem.* 193: 265–275, 1951.
370. LUNEC, J., D. R. BLAKE, S. J. MCCLEARY, S. BRAILSFORD, and P. A. BACON. Self-perpetuating mechanisms of immunoglobulin G aggregation in rheumatoid inflammation. *J. Clin. Invest.* 76: 2084–2090, 1985.
371. LYONS, T. J., K. E. BAILIE, D. G. DYER, J. A. DUNN, and J. W. BAYNES. Decrease in skin collagen glycation with improved glycemic control in patients with insulin-dependent diabetes mellitus. *J. Clin. Invest.* 87: 1910–1915, 1991.
372. LYONS, T. J., G. SILVESTRI, J. A. DUNN, D. G. DYER, and J. W. BAYNES. Role of glycation in modification of lens crystallins in diabetic senile cataracts. *Diabetes* 40: 1010–1015, 1991.
373. MACDONALD, E., W. K. LEE, S. HEPBURN, J. BELL, P. J. W. SCOTT, and M. H. DOMINICZAK. Advanced glycosylation end products in the mesenteric artery. *Clin. Chem.* 38: 530–533, 1992.
374. MADSEN, K., S. MOSKALEWSKI, K. VON DER MARK, and U. FRIBERG. Synthesis of proteoglycans, collagen, and elastin by cultures of rabbit auricular chondrocytes—relation to age of the donor. *Dev. Biol.* 96: 63–73, 1983.
375. MAISEL, H., C. V. HARDING, J. R. ALCALA, J. KUSZAK, and R. BRADLEY. The morphology of the lens. In: *Molecular and Cellular Biology of the Eye Lens,* edited by H. Bloemendal. New York: John Wiley and Sons, pp. 49–84, 1981.
376. MAKITA, Z., S. RADOFF, E. J. RAYFIELD, Z. YANG, E. SKOLNIK, V. DELANEY, E. A. FRIEDMAN, A. CERAMI, and H. VLASSARA. Advanced glycosylation endproducts in patients with diabetic nephropathy. *N. Engl. J. Med.* 325: 836–842, 1991.
377. MAKITA, Z., H. VLASSARA, A. CERAMI, and R. BUCALA. Immunochemical detection of advanced of glycosylation end products in vivo. *J. Biol. Chem.* 267: 5133–5138, 1992.
378. MALIK, N. S., S. J. MOSS, N. AHMED, A. J. FURTH, R. S. WALL, and K. M. MEEK. Ageing of the human corneal stroma: structural and biochemical changes. *Biochim. Biophys. Acta* 1138: 222–228, 1992.
379. MAROUDAS, A., M. T. BAYLISS, and M. F. VENN. Further studies on the composition of human femoral head cartilage. *Ann. Rheum. Dis.* 39: 514–523, 1980.
380. MARTENS, M. F. W. C., and T. HENDRIKS. Collagen synthesis in explants from rat intestine. *Biochim. Biophys. Acta* 993: 252–258, 1989.
381. MARTENSON, J., A. JAIN, E. STOLE, W. FRAYER, P. A. M. AULD, and A. MEISTER. Inhibition of glutathione synthesis in the newborn rat. A model for endogenously produced oxidative stress. *Proc. Natl. Acad. Sci. USA* 88: 9360–9364, 1991.
382. MARTIN, M., R. E. NABOUT, C. LAFUMA, F. CRECHET, and J. REMY. Fibronectin and collagen gene expression during in vitro ageing of pig skin fibroblasts. *Exp. Cell Res.* 191: 8–13, 1990.
383. MASORO, E. J. Physiological system markers of aging. *Exp. Gerontol.* 23: 391–394, 1988.
384. MASORO, E. J., M. S. KATZ, and C. A. MCMAHAN. Evidence for the glycation hypothesis of aging from the food-restricted rodent model. *J. Gerontol.* 44: B20–B22, 1989.
385. MASORO, E. J., R. J. M. MCCARTER, M. S. KATZ, and C. A. MCMAHAN. Dietary restriction alters characteristics of glucose fuel use. *J. Gerontol.* 47: B202–B208, 1992.
386. MASSIE, H. R., V. R. AIELLO, M. E. SHUMWAY, and T. ARMSTRONG. Calcium, iron, copper, boron, collagen and density changes in bone with aging in C57BL/6J male mice. *Exp. Gerontol.* 25: 469–481, 1990.
387. MASTERS, P. M., J. L. BADA, and J. S. ZIGLER. Aspartic acid racemization in the human lens during aging and in cataract formation. *Nature* 268: 71–73, 1977.

388. MAUREL, E., H. BOUISSOU, M. T. PIERAGGI, M. JULIAN, M. MOCZAR, and L. ROBERT. Age-dependent biochemical changes in dermal connective tissue. Relationship to histological and ultrastructural observations. *Connect. Tissue Res.* 8: 33–39, 1980.

389. MAUREL, E., C. A. SHUTTLEWORTH, and H. BOUISSOU. Interstitial collagens and ageing in human aorta. *Virchows Arch [A].* 410: 383–390, 1987.

390. MAYS, P. K., J. E. BISHOP, and G. J. LAURENT. Age-related changes in the proportion of types I and III collagen. *Mech. Ageing Dev.* 45: 203–212, 1988.

391. MAYS, P. K., R. J. MCANULTY, J. S. CAMPA, A. D. CAMBREY, and G. J. LAURENT. Similar age-related alterations in collagen metabolism in rat tissues in vivo and fibroblasts in vitro. *Biochem. Soc. Trans.* 18: 957, 1990.

392. MAYS, P. K., R. J. MCANULTY, J. S. CAMPA, and G. J. LAURENT. Age-related changes in collagen synthesis and degradation in rat tissues. Importance of degradation of newly synthesized collagen in regulating collagen production. *Biochem. J.* 276: 307–313, 1991.

393. MAYS, P. K., R. J. MCANULTY, and G. J. LAURENT. Age-related changes in lung collagen metabolism: a role for degradation in regulating lung collagen production. *Am. Rev. Respir. Dis.* 140: 410–416, 1989.

394. MAYS, P. K., R. MCANULTY, and G. J. LAURENT. Age-related changes in total protein and collagen metabolism in rat liver. *Hepatology* 14: 1224–1229, 1991.

395. MBUYI-MUAMBA, J. M., and J. DEQUEKER. Age and sex variations on bone matrix proteins in Wistar rats. *Growth* 47: 301–315, 1983.

396. MCANULTY, R. J., and G. J. LAURENT. Collagen synthesis and degradation in vivo. Evidence for rapid rates of collagen turnover with extensive degradation of newly synthesized collagen in tissues of the adult rat. *Coll. Relat. Res.* 7: 93–104, 1987.

397. MCCLEARN, G. E. Strategies for biomarker research: experimental and methodological design. *Exp. Gerontol.* 23: 245–255, 1988.

398. MCDEVITT, C. A., and R. J. WEBBER. The ultrastructure and biochemistry of meniscal cartilage. *Clin. Orthop.* 252: 8–18, 1990.

399. MCFALL-NGAI, M., J. HOROWITZ, L. L. DING, and L. LACEY. Age-dependent changes in the heat-stable crystallin, βBp, of the human lens. *Curr. Eye Res.* 5: 387–394, 1986.

400. MCNAMARA, M., and R. C. AUGUSTEYN. The effects of hydrogen peroxide on lens proteins: a possible model for nuclear cataract. *Exp. Eye Res.* 38: 45–56, 1984.

401. MCNICOL, D., and P. J. ROUGHLEY. Extraction and characterization of proteoglycan from human meniscus. *Biochem. J.* 185: 705–713, 1980.

402. MCPHERSON, J. D., D. H. SHILTON, and D. J. WALTON. Role of fructose in glycation and crosslinking of proteins. *Biochemistry* 27: 1901–1907, 1988.

403. MECHANIC, G., P. M. GALLOP, and M. L. TANZER. The nature of crosslinking in collagens from mineralized tissues. *Biochem. Biophys. Res. Commun.* 45: 644–653, 1971.

404. MELLERIO, J. Yellowing of the human lens. Nuclear and cortical contributions. *Vision Res.* 27: 1581–1587, 1987.

405. MIKSIK, I., and Z. DEYL. Change in the amount of ε-hexosyllysine, UV absorbance, and fluorescence of collagen with age in different animal species. *J. Gerontol.* 46: B111–B116, 1991.

406. MIKSIK, I., R. STRUZINSKY, and Z. DEYL. Change with age of UV absorbance and fluorescence of collagen and accumulation of ε-hexosyllysine in collagen from Wistar rats living on different food restriction regimes. *Mech. Ageing Dev.* 57: 163–174, 1991.

407. MILLIS, A. J. T., J. SOTTILE, M. HOYLE, D. M. MANN, and V. DIEMER. Collagenase production by early and late passage of cultures of human fibroblasts. *Exp. Gerontol.* 24: 559–575, 1989.

408. MIYAHARA, T., A. MURAI, T. TANAKA, S. SHIOZAWA, and M. KAMEYAMA. Age-related differences in human skin collagen: solubility in solvent, susceptibility to pepsin digestion, and the spectrum of the solubilized polymeric collagen molecules. *J. Gerontol.* 37: 651–655, 1982.

409. MIYATA, S., and V. M. MONNIER. Immunohistochemical detection of advanced glycosylation end products in diabetic tissues using monoclonal antibody to pyrraline. *J. Clin. Invest.* 89: 1102–1112, 1992.

410. MOCZAR, M., J. OUZILOU, Y. COURTOIS, and L. ROBERT. Age dependence of the biosynthesis of intercellular matrix macromolecules of rabbit aorta in organ culture and cell culture. *Gerontology* 22: 461–472, 1976.

411. MOHAN, S., and E. RADHA. Age-related changes in rat muscle collagen. *Gerontology* 26: 61–67, 1980.

412. MOHAN, S., and E. RADHA. Hydroxyproline excretion and collagen catabolism in rats of different age groups. *Biochem. Med.* 24: 1–5, 1980.

413. MOHAN, S., and E. RADHA. Age-related changes in muscle connective tissue: acid mucopolysaccharides and structural glycoprotein. *Exp. Gerontol.* 16: 385–392, 1981.

414. MOLLENHAUER, J., and K. BAYREUTHER. Donor-age-related changes in morphology, growth potential, and collagen biosynthesis in rat fibroblasts subpopulations in vitro. *Differentiation* 32: 165–172, 1986.

415. MOLNAR, J. A., N. M. ALPERT, J. F. BURKE, and V. R. YOUNG. Synthesis and degradation rates of collagens in vivo in whole skin of rats, studies with $^{18}O_2$ labeling. *Biochem. J.* 240: 431–435, 1986.

416. MOLNAR, J. A., N. M. ALPERT, J. F. BURKE, and V. R. YOUNG. Relative and absolute changes in soluble and insoluble collagen pool size in skin during normal growth and with dietary protein restriction in rats. *Growth* 51: 132–145, 1987.

417. MOLNAR, J. A., N. M. ALPERT, D. A. WAGNER, S. MIYATANI, J. F. BURKE, and V. R. YOUNG. Synthesis and degradation of collagens of skin of healthy and protein-malnourished rats in vivo, studied by $^{18}O_2$ labeling. *Biochem. J.* 250: 71–76, 1988.

418. MONBOISSE, J. C., and J. P. BOREL. Oxidative damage to collagen. In: *Free Radicals and Aging,* edited by I. Emerit and B. Chance. Boston: Birkhäuser Verlag, 1992, p. 323–327.

419. MONNIER, V. M. Nonenzymatic glycosylation, the Maillard reaction and the aging process. *J. Gerontol.* 45: B105–B111, 1990.

420. MONNIER, V. M. Toward a Maillard reaction theory of aging. In: *The Maillard Reaction in Aging, Diabetes, and Nutrition,* edited by J. W. Baynes and V. M. Monnier. New York: Alan R. Liss, 1989, p. 1–22.

421. MONNIER, V. M., and A. CERAMI. Nonenzymatic browning in vivo: possible process for aging of long-lived proteins. *Science* 211: 491–493, 1981.

422. MONNIER, V. M., and A. CERAMI. Detection of nonenzymatic browning products in the human lens. *Biochim. Biophys. Acta* 760: 97–103, 1983.

423. MONNIER, V. M., R. R. KOHN, and A. CERAMI. Accelerated age-related browning of human collagen in diabetes mellitus. *Proc. Natl. Acad. Sci. USA* 81: 583–587, 1984.

424. MONNIER, V. M., D. R. SELL, R. H. NAGARAJ, and S. MIYATA. Mechanisms of protection against damage mediated by the Maillard reaction in aging. *Gerontology* 37: 152–165, 1991.

425. MONNIER, V. M., V. J. STEVENS, and A. CERAMI. Nonenzymatic glycosylation, sulfhydryl oxidation and aggregation of lens protein in experimental sugar cataracts. *J. Exp. Med.* 50: 1098–1107, 1970.

426. MONNIER, V. M., V. VISHWANATH, K. E. FRANK, C. A. ELMETS, P. DAUCHOT, P., and R. R. KOHN. Relation between complications of type I diabetes mellitus and collagen-linked fluorescence. *N. Engl. J. Med.* 314: 403–408, 1986.

427. MONTFORT, I., and R. PÉREZ-TAMAYO. The muscle–collagen ratio in normal and hypertrophic human hearts. *Lab. Invest.* 11: 463–470, 1962.

428. MONTFORT, I., and R. PÉREZ-TAMAYO. The distribution of collagenase in normal rat tissues. *J. Histochem. Cytochem.* 23: 910–920, 1975.

429. MOORADIAN, A. D. Biomarkers of aging: do we know what to look for? *J. Gerontol.* 45: B183–B186, 1990.

430. MORIGUCHI, T., and D. FUJIMOTO. Age-related changes in the content of the collagen crosslink, pyridinoline. *J. Biochem.* 84: 933–935, 1978.

431. MORT, J. S., B. CATERSON, A. R. POOLE, and P. J. ROUGHLEY. The origin of human cartilage proteoglycan link-protein heterogeneity and fragmentation during aging. *Biochem. J.* 232: 805–812, 1985.

432. MOSTAPAFOUR, M. K., and V. N. REDDY. Interactions of glutathione disulfide with lens crystallins. *Curr. Eye Res.* 2: 591–596, 1982–1983.

433. MULLARKEY, C. J., D. EDELSTEIN, and M. BROWNLEE. Free radical generation by early glycation products: a mechanism for accelerated atherogenesis in diabetes. *Biochem. Biophys. Res. Commun.* 173: 932–939, 1990.

434. MURATA, K., and Y. YOKOYAMA. Acidic glycosaminoglycans in human atherosclerotic cerebral arterial tissues. *Atherosclerosis* 78: 69–79, 1989.

435. MYERS, B., M. DUBICK, J. A. LAST, and R. B. RUCKER. Elastin synthesis during perinatal lung development in the rat. *Biochim. Biophys. Acta* 761: 17–22, 1983.

436. NAGARAJ, R. H., and V. M. MONNIER. Isolation and characterization of a blue fluorophore from human eye lens crystallins: in vitro formation from Maillard reaction with ascorbate and ribose. *Biochim. Biophys. Acta* 1116: 34–42, 1992.

437. NAGARAJ, R. H., D. R. SELL, M. PRABHAKARAM, B. J. ORTWERTH, and V. M. MONNIER. High correlation between pentosidine protein crosslinks and pigmentation implicates ascorbate oxidation in human lens senescence and cataractogenesis. *Proc. Natl. Acad. Sci. USA* 88: 10257–10261, 1991.

438. NAKADA, T., I. SASAGAWA, H. FURUTA, T. KATAYAMA, and J. SHIMAZAKI. Age-related differences in norephinephrine and non-collagenous protein in human vas deferens. *J. Urol.* 141: 998–1002, 1989.

439. NAKAYAMA, H., T. MITSUHASHI, S. KUWAJIMA, S. AOKI, Y. KURODA, T. ITOH, and S. NAKAGAWA. Immunochemical detection of advanced glycation end products in lens crystallins from streptozocin-induced diabetic rat. *Diabetes* 42: 345–350, 1993.

440. NAKAYAMA, H., S. TANEDA, S. KUWAJIMA, S. AOKI, Y. KURODA, K. MISAWA, and S. NAKAGAWA. Production and characterization of antibodies to advanced glycation products on proteins. *Biochem. Biophys. Res. Commun.* 162: 740–745, 1989.

441. NANDA, B. S., and R. GETTY. Age-related histomorphological changes in the cerebral arteries of domestic pig. *Exp. Gerontol.* 6: 453–460, 1971.

442. NEJJAR, I., M.-T. PIERAGGI, J. C. THIERS, and H. BOUISSOU. Age-related changes in the elastic tissue of the human thoracic aorta. *Atherosclerosis* 80: 199–208, 1990.

443. NEUBERGER, A., and H. G. B. SLACK. The metabolism of collagen from liver, bone, skin and tendon in the normal rat. *Biochem. J.* 53: 47–52, 1953.

444. NIEDERMÜLLER, H., M. SKALICKY, G. HOFECKER, and A. KMENT. Investigations on the kinetics of collagen-metabolism in young and old rats. *Exp. Gerontol.* 12: 159–168, 1977.

445. NIELSEN, C. J., J. P. BENTLEY, and F. J. MARSHALL. Age-related changes in reducible crosslinks of human dental pulp collagen. *Arch. Oral. Biol.* 28: 759–764, 1983.

446. NIMNI, M. E., E. DEGUIA, and L. A. BAVETTA. Synthesis and turnover of collagen precursors in rabbit skin. *Biochem. J.* 102: 143–147, 1967.

447. NISHIMOTO, S., M. OIMOMI, and S. BABA. Glycation of collagen in the aorta and the development of aging. *Clin. Chim. Acta* 182: 235–238, 1989.

448. NISHIMOTO, S. K., S. M. PADILLA, and D. L. SNYDER. The effect of food restriction and germ-free environment on age-related changes in bone matrix. *J. Gerontol.* 45: B164–B168, 1990.

449. NISSEN, R., G. J. CARDINALE, and S. UDENFRIEND. Increased turnover of arterial collagen in hypertensive rats. *Proc. Natl. Acad. Sci. USA* 75: 451–453, 1978.

450. NJOROGE, F. G., and V. M. MONNIER. The chemistry of the Maillard reaction under physiological conditions: a review. In: *The Maillard Reaction in Aging, Diabetes and Nutrition*, edited by J. W. Baynes and V. M. Monnier. New York: Alan R. Liss, 1989, p. 85–107.

451. NJOROGE, F. G., A. A. FERNANDES, and V. M. MONNIER. Mechanism of formation of the putative advanced glycosylation end product and protein crosslink 2-(2-furoyl)-4(5)-2(furanyl)1H-imidazole. *J. Biol. Chem.* 263: 10646–10652, 1988.

452. NJOROGE, F. G., L. M. SAYRE, V. M. MONNIER. Detection of D-glucose-derived pyrrole compounds during Maillard reaction under physiological conditions. *Carbohydr. Res.* 167: 211–220, 1987.

453. NORDMANN, J. Au sujet du vieillissement du cristallin humain et de la pathogenie de la cataracte senile. *Adv. Ophthalmol.* 34: 1–73, 1977.

454. NORDMANN, J., and J. KLETHI. L'activite Na-K-ATPasique dans le cristallin normal vieillissant et dans la cataracte senile. *Arch. Ophthalmol. (Paris)* 36: 523–552, 1976.

455. NORDMANN, J., H. FINK, and O. HOCKWIN. Die Wachstumskurve der menschlichen Linse. *Albrecht Von Graefes Arch. Klin. Exp. Ophthalmol.* 191: 165–175, 1974.

456. NOWACK, H., S. GAY, G. WICK, U. BECKER, and R. TIMPL. Preparation and use in immunohistology of antibodies specific for type I and type III collagen and procollagen. *J. Immunol. Methods* 12: 117–124, 1976.

457. ODETTI, P., A. BORGOGLIO, A. DE PASCALE, R. ROLANDI, and L. ADEZATI. Prevention of diabetes-increased aging effect on rat collagen-linked fluorescence by aminoguanidine and rutin. *Diabetes* 39: 796–801, 1990.

458. ODETTI, P., A. BORGOGLIO, and R. ROLANDI. Age-related increase of collagen fluorescence in human subcutaneous tissue. *Metabolism* 41: 655–658, 1992.

459. ODETTI, P., J. FOGARTY, D. R. SELL, and V. M. MONNIER. Chromatographic quantitation of plasma and erythrocyte pentosidine in diabetic and uremic subjects. *Diabetes* 41: 153–159, 1992.

460. OGAWA, T., T. ONO, M. TSUDA, and Y. KAWANISHI. A novel fluorophore in insoluble collagen: a crosslinking moiety in collagen molecule. *Biochem. Biophys. Res. Commun.* 107: 1252–1257, 1982.

461. OHRLOFF, C. Age changes of enzyme properties in crystalline lens. *Interdiscipl. Top. Gerontol.* 12: 158–179, 1978.

462. OHRLOFF, C., O. HOCKWIN, R. OLSON, and S. DICKMAN. Glutathione peroxidase, glutathione reductase and superoxide dismutase in the aging lens. *Curr. Eye Res.* 3: 109–111, 1984.

463. OHUCHI, K., and S. TSURUFUJI. Degradation and turnover of collagen in the mouse skin and the effect of whole body x-irradiation. *Biochim. Biophys. Acta* 208: 475–481, 1970.

464. OIMOMI, M., Y. MAEDA, F. HATA, Y. KITAMURA, S. MATSUMOTO, H. HATANAKA, and S. BABA. A study of the age-related

acceleration of glycation of tissue proteins in rats. *J. Gerontol.* 43: B98–B104, 1988.
465. OLCZYK, K. Age-related changes in collagen of human intervertebral discs. *Gerontology.* 38: 196–204, 1992.
466. OLIVER, C. N. Inactivation and oxidative modifications of proteins by stimulated neutrophils. *Arch. Biochem. Biophys.* 253: 62–67, 1987.
467. OLIVER, C. N., B. W. AHN, M. E. WITTENBERGER, R. L. LEVINE, and E. R. STADTMAN. Age-related alterations of enzymes may involve mixed function oxidation reactions. In: *Modern Aging Research: Modifications of Proteins During Aging,* edited by R. C. Adelman, and E. R. Dekker. New York: Alan R. Liss, 1985, vol 7, p. 39–52.
468. OLSEN, G. G., and A. V. EVERITT. Retardation of the aging process in collagen fibers from the tail tendon of the old hypophysectomized rat. *Nature* 206: 307–308, 1965.
469. OMEROD, C. D., M. A. C. EDELSTEIN, G. L. SCHMIDT, R. S. JAUREZ, S. M. FINEGOLD, and R. E. SMITH. The intraocular environment and experimental anaerobic bacterial endophthalmitis. *Arch. Ophthalmol.* 105: 1571–1575, 1987.
470. ONO, S., and M. YAMAUCHI. Collagen crosslinking of skin in patients with amyotrophic lateral sclerosis. *Ann. Neurol.* 31: 305–310, 1992.
471. OOHIRA, A., and H. NOGAMI. Age-related changes in physical and chemical properties of proteoglycans synthesized by costal and matrix-induced cartilages in the rat. *J. Biol. Chem.* 255: 1346–1350, 1980.
472. OOSHIMA, A., and Y. YAMORI. Hypertension, vasculature and aging. *Adv. Exp. Med. Biol.* 129: 99–110, 1980.
473. ORTWERTH, B. J., and P. R. OLESEN. Glutathione inhibits the glycation and crosslinking of lens proteins by ascorbic acid. *Exp. Eye Res.* 52: 439–444, 1988.
474. OSBORNE-PELLEGRIN, M. J., J. FARJANEL, and W. HORNEBECK. Role of elastase and lysyl oxidase activity in spontaneous rupture of internal elastic lamina in rats. *Arteriosclerosis* 10: 1136–1146, 1990.
475. PALMER, W. G., and J. PAPACONSTANTINOU. Aging of α-crystallins during development of the lens. *Proc. Natl. Acad. Sci. USA* 64: 404–408, 1969.
476. PANDE, A., W. H. GARNER, and A. SPECTOR. Glycosylation of human lens protein and cataractogenesis. *Biochem. Biophys. Res. Commun.* 89: 1260–1266, 1979.
477. PATRICK, J. S., S. R. THORPE, and J. W. BAYNES. Nonenzymatic glycosylation of protein does not increase with age in normal human lenses. *J. Gerontol.* 45: B18–B23, 1990.
478. PAU, H., P. GRAF, and H. SIES. Glutathione levels in human lens: regional distribution in different forms of cataract. *Exp. Eye Res.* 50: 17–20, 1990.
479. PAULSSON, M., M. MÖRGELIN, H. WIEDEMANN, M. BEARDMORE-GRAY, D. DUNHAM, T. HARDINGHAM, D. HEINEGARD, R. TIMPL, and J. ENGEL. Extended and globular protein domains in cartilage proteoglycans. *Biochem. J.* 245: 763–772, 1987.
480. PAZ, M. A., D. A. KEITH, and P. M. GALLOP. Elastin isolation and cross-linking. *Methods Enzymol.* 82: 571–587, 1982.
481. PEARCE, R. H., and B. J. GRIMMER. Age and the chemical constitution of normal human dermis. *J. Invest. Dermatol.* 58: 347–361, 1972.
482. PEARSON, J. P., and R. M. MASON. Proteoglycan aggregates in adult human costal cartilage. *Biochim. Biophys. Acta* 583: 512–526, 1979.
483. PERRY, R. E., M. S. SWAMY, and E. C. ABRAHAM. Progressive changes in lens crystallin glycation and high molecular weight aggregate formation leading to cataract development in streptozocin-diabetic rats. *Exp. Eye Res.* 44: 269–282, 1987.
484. PIATIGORSKY, J. Lens crystallins: innovation associated with changes in gene regulation. *J. Biol. Chem.* 267: 4277–4280, 1992.
485. PIERCE, J. A., H. RESNICK, and P. H. HENRY. Collagen and elastin metabolism in the lungs, skin, and bones of adult rats. *J. Lab. Clin. Med.* 69: 485–492, 1967.
486. PIETILÄ, K., and T. NIKKARI. Role of the arterial smooth muscle cell in the pathogenesis of atherosclerosis. *Med. Biol.* 61: 31–44, 1983.
487. PIRIE, A. Glutathione peroxidase in lens and a source of hydrogen peroxide in aqueous humour. *Biochem. J.* 96: 244–253, 1965.
488. PIRIE, A. A light-catalysed reaction in the aqueous humour of the eye. *Nature* 205: 500–501, 1965.
489. PIRIE, A. Color and solubility of the proteins of human cataracts. *Invest. Ophthalmol.* 7: 634–649, 1968.
490. PLANK, L., J. JAMES, and C. A. WAGENVOORT. Caliber and elastin content of the pulmonary trunk. *Arch. Pathol. Lab. Med.* 104: 238–241, 1980.
491. PONGOR, S., P. C. ULRICH, F. A. BENCSATH, and A. CERAMI. Aging of proteins: isolation and identification of a fluorescent chromophore from the reaction of polypeptides with glucose. *Proc. Natl. Acad. Sci. USA* 81: 2684–2688, 1984.
492. POOLE, A., R. MYLLYLA, J. C. WAGNER, and R. C. BROWN. Collagen biosynthesis enzymes in lung tissue and serum of rats with experimental silicosis. *Br. J. Exp. Pathol.* 66: 567–575, 1985.
493. PORTA, E. A., L. KEOPUHIWA, N. S. JOUN, and R. T. NITTA. Effects of the type of dietary fat at two levels of vitamin E in Wistar male rats during development and aging. III. Biochemical and morphometric parameters of the liver. *Mech. Ageing Dev.* 15: 297–335, 1981.
494. POWELL, J. T., N. VINE, and M. CROSSMAN. On the accumulation of D-aspartate in elastin and other proteins of the ageing aorta. *Atherosclerosis* 97: 201–208, 1992.
495. PRABHAKARAM, M., and B. J. ORTWERTH. The glycation-associated crosslinking of lens proteins by ascorbic acid is not mediated by oxygen free radicals. *Exp. Eye Res.* 53: 261–268, 1991.
496. PRICE, R. G., and R. G. SPIRO. Studies on the metabolism of the renal glomerular basement membrane. *J. Biol. Chem.* 252: 8597–8602, 1977.
497. PROCKOP, D. J., K. I. KIVIRIKKO, L. TUDERMAN, and N. A. GUZMAN. The biosynthesis of collagen and its disorders. *N. Engl. J. Med.* 301: (Parts 1 and 2) 13–23, 77–85, 1979.
498. QUAGLINO, D., JR., R. KENNEDY, C. FORNIERI, L. NANNEY, I. PASQUALI, D. RONCHETTI, and J. M. DAVIDSON. Matrix gene expression during aging process revealed by in situ hybridization. *J. Histochem. Cytochem.* 37: 933, 1989.
499. QUINTARELLI, G., E. IPPOLITO, and L. RODEN. Age-dependent changes on the state of aggregation of cartilage matrix. *Lab. Invest.* 32: 111–123, 1975.
500. RADOFF, S., Z. MAKITA, and H. VLASSARA. Radioreceptor assay for advanced glycosylation endproducts. *Diabetes* 40: 1731–1738, 1991.
501. RAFFERTY, N. S., and W. GOOSENS. Growth and aging of the lens capsule. *Growth* 42: 375–389, 1978.
502. RAINS, J. K., J. L. BERT, C. R. ROBERTS, and P. D. PARÉ. Mechanical properties of human tracheal cartilage. *J. Appl. Physiol.* 72: 219–225, 1992.
503. RAJU, K., and R. A. ANWAR. Primary structures of bovine elastin a,b,c deduced from the sequences of cDNA clones. *J. Biol. Chem.* 262: 5755–5762, 1987.
504. RAMIREZ, E., and M. DI LIBERTO. Complex and diversified regulatory programs control the expression of vertebrate collagen genes. *FASEB J.* 4: 1616–1623, 1990.
505. RAO, G., and E. COTLIER. Free ε-amino groups and 5-hydroxy-

methyl-furfuraldehyde content in clear and cataractous human lenses. *Invest. Ophthalmol.* 27: 98–102, 1986.

506. RATCLIFFE, A., J. A. TYLER, and T. E. HARDINGHAM. Articular cartilage cultured with interleukin 1: increased release of link protein, hyaluronate-binding region and other proteoglycan fragments. *Biochem. J.* 238: 571–580, 1986.

507. RATHBAN, W. B., and D. C. MURRAY. Age-related cysteine uptake as rate-limiting in glutathione synthesis and glutathione half-life in the cultured human lens. *Exp. Eye Res.* 53: 205–212, 1991.

508. REDDY, V. N. Metabolism of glutathione in the lens. *Exp. Eye Res.* 11: 310–328, 1971.

509. REDDY, V. N. Glutathione and its function in the lens—an overview. *Exp. Eye Res.* 50: 771–778, 1990.

510. REDDY, V., F. J. GIBLIN, and H. MATSUDA. Defense system of the lens against oxidative damage. In: *Red Blood Cell and Lens Metabolism*, edited by S. K. Srivastava. Amsterdam: Elsevier, 1980, p. 139–154.

511. REISER, K. M. Nonenzymatic glycation of collagen in aging and diabetes. *Proc. Soc. Exp. Biol. Med.* 196: 17–29, 1991.

512. REISER, K. M., M. A. AMIGABLE, and J. A. LAST. Nonenzymatic glycation of type I collagen: the effects of aging on preferential glycation sites. *J. Biol. Chem.* 267: 24207–24216, 1992.

513. REISER, K. M., S. M. HENNESSY, and J. A. LAST. Analysis of age-associated changes in collagen crosslinking in the skin and lung in monkeys and rats. *Biochim. Biophys. Acta* 926: 339–348, 1987.

514. REISER, K., R. J. MCCORMICK, and R. B. RUCKER. Enzymatic and nonenzymatic crosslinking of collagen and elastin. *FASEB J.* 6: 2439–2449, 1992.

515. RICARD-BLUM, S., and G. VILLE. Collagen crosslinking. *Cell. Mol. Biol.* 34: 581–590, 1988.

516. RICHARD, S., C. TAMAS, D. R. SELL, and V. M. MONNIER. Tissue-specific effects of aldose reductase inhibition on fluorescence and cross-linking of extracellular matrix in chronic galactosemia. *Diabetes* 40: 1049–1056, 1991.

517. RICHEY, M. L., H. K. RICHEY, and N. A. FENSKE. Aging-related skin changes: development and clinical meaning. *Geriatrics* 43: 49–64, 1988.

518. ROBERT, L. Aging of connective tissue. *Mech. Ageing Dev.* 14: 273–282, 1980.

519. ROBERT, L. Aging of connective tissues. *Experientia* 37: 1055–1058, 1981.

520. ROBERT, L. and W. HORNEBECK (Eds). *Elastin and Elastasis*. Boca Raton, FL: CRC Press, 1989.

521. ROBERT, L., M. P. JACOB, C. FRANCES, G. GODEAU, and W. HORNEBECK. Interaction between elastin and elastases and its role in the aging of the arterial wall, skin and other connective tissues. A review. *Mech. Ageing Dev.* 28: 155–166, 1984.

522. ROBERTS, C. R., J. S. MORT, and P. J. ROUGHLEY. Treatment of cartilage proteoglycan aggregate with hydrogen peroxide: relationship between observed degradation products and those that occur naturally during aging. *Biochem. J.* 247: 349–357, 1987.

523. ROBINS, S. P. Analysis of the crosslinking components in collagen and elastin. *Methods Biochem. Anal.* 28: 329–379, 1982.

524. ROBINS, S. P., and A. J. BAILEY. Age-related changes in collagen: the identification of reducible lysine-carbohydrate condensation products. *Biochem. Biophys. Res. Commun.* 48: 76–84, 1972.

525. ROBINS, S. P., and A. J. BAILEY. The chemistry of the collagen crosslinks: the mechanism of stabilization of the reducible intermediate cross-links. *Biochem. J.* 149: 381–385, 1975.

526. ROBINS, S. P., and A. DUNCAN. Cross-linking of collagen: location of pyridinoline in bovine articular cartilage at two sites of the molecule. *Biochem. J.* 215: 175–182, 1983.

527. ROBINS, S. P., M. SHIMOKOMAKI, and A. J. BAILEY. The chemistry of the collagen cross-links: age-related changes in the reducible components of intact bovine collagen fibers. *Biochem. J.* 131: 771–780, 1973.

528. RODRIGUEZ-CABALLERO, M. L., J. P. GERHARD, and J. NORDMANN. L'epaisseur cortical du cristallin humain. *Doc. Ophthalmol.* 35: 287–295, 1973.

529. RODRIGUEZ-MARTINEZ, M. A., and A. RUIZ-TORRES. Homeostasis between lipid peroxidation and antioxidant enzyme activities in healthy human aging. *Mech. Ageing Dev.* 66: 213–222, 1992.

530. ROGOZINSKI, S., G. O. BLUMENFELD, and S. SEIFTER. The nonenzymatic glycosylation of collagen. *Arch. Biochem. Biophys.* 221: 428–437, 1983.

531. ROMERO-CHAPMAN, N., J. LEE, D. TINKER, J. Y. URIU-HARE, C. L. KEEN, and R. R. RUCKER. Purification, properties and influence of dietary copper on accumulation and functional activity of lysyl oxidase in rat skin. *Biochem. J.* 275: 657–662, 1991.

532. ROSENBERG, L. C., H. U. CHOI, L.-H. TANG, T. L. JOHNSON, S. PAL, C. WEBBER, A. REINER, and A. R. POOLE. Isolation of dermatan sulfate proteoglycans from mature bovine articular cartilages. *J. Biol. Chem.* 260: 6304–6313, 1985.

533. ROSENBLOOM, J. Elastin: biosynthesis, structure, degradation and role in disease processes. *Connect. Tissue Res.* 10: 73–91, 1982.

534. ROSENBLOOM, J., W. R. ABRAMS, and R. MECHAM. Extracellular matrix 4: the elastic fiber. *FASEB J.* 7: 1208–1218, 1993.

535. ROSS, W. M., M. O. CREIGHTON, J. R. TREVITHICK, P. J. STERAT-DETLAAN, and M. SANWAL. Modelling cataractogenesis: VI. Induction by glucose in vitro or in diabetic rats: prevention and reversal by glutathione. *Exp. Eye Res.* 37: 559–573, 1983.

536. ROUGHLEY, P. J. Changes in cartilage proteoglycan structure during ageing: origin and effects—a review. *Agents Actions* [Suppl.] 18: 19–29, 1986.

537. ROUGHLEY, P. J. Structural changes in the proteoglycans of human articular cartilage during aging. *J. Rheumatol.* 14(suppl): 14–15, 1987.

538. ROUGHLEY, P. J., and J. S. MORT. Ageing and the aggregating proteoglycans of human articular cartilage. *Clin. Sci.* 71: 337–344, 1986.

539. ROUGHLEY, P. J., and R. J. WHITE. Age-related changes in the structure of the proteoglycan subunits from human articular cartilage. *J. Biol. Chem.* 255: 217–224, 1980.

540. ROUGHLEY, P. J., Q. NGUYEN, and J. S. MORT. Mechanisms of proteoglycan degradation in human articular cartilage. *J. Rheumatol.* [Suppl.] 27: 52–54, 1991.

541. ROUGHLEY, P. J., R. J. WHITE, A. R. POOLE, and J. S. MORT. The inability to prepare high-buoyant density proteoglycan aggregates from extracts of normal adult human articular cartilage. *Biochem. J.* 221: 637–644, 1984.

542. ROY, D. Age-dependent changes in the abundance of the major polypeptides of human lens membrane. *Biochem. Biophys. Res. Commun.* 88: 30–36, 1979.

543. ROY, D., and A. SPECTOR. Human insoluble lens protein. I. Separation and partial characterization of polypeptides. *Exp. Eye Res.* 26: 429–443, 1978.

544. ROY, D., and A. SPECTOR. Human insoluble lens protein II. Isolation and characterization of a 9600 dalton polypeptide. *Exp. Eye Res.* 26: 445–459, 1978.

545. ROY, D., J. DILLON, E. WADA, W. CHANEY, and A. SPECTOR. Nondisulfide polymerization of γ- and β-crystallins in the human lens. *Proc. Natl. Acad. Sci. USA* 81: 2878–2881, 1984.

546. RUCKER, R. B., and D. TINKER. Structure and metabolism of arterial elastin. *Int. Rev. Exp. Pathol.* 17: 1–47, 1977.

547. RUCKLIDGE, G. J., G. MILNE, B. A. MCGAW, E. MILNE, and S. P. ROBINS. Turnover rates of different collagen types measured by isotope ratio mass spectrometry. *Biochim. Biophys. Acta* 1156: 57–61, 1992.
548. RUOSLAHTI, E. Structure and biology of proteoglycans. *Annu. Rev. Cell Biol.* 4: 229–255, 1988.
549. RUSSEL, P., S. G. SMITH, D. A. CARPER, and J. H. KINOSHITA. Age- and cataract-related changes in the heavy molecular weight proteins and gamma crystallin composition of the mouse lens. *Exp. Eye Res.* 29: 245–255, 1979.
550. SAID, F. S., and R. A. WEALE. The variation with age of the spectral transmissivity of the living human crystalline lens. *Gerontologia* 3: 213–231, 1959.
551. SAITO, S., Y. TAKAHASHI, M. WYMAN, and P. F. KADOR. Progression of sugar cataract in the dog. *Invest. Ophthalmol. Vis. Sci.* 32: 1925–1931, 1991.
552. SAMILA, Z. J., and S. A. CARTER. The effect of aging on the unfolding of elastin lamellae and collagen fibers with stretch in human cartoid arteries. *Can. J. Physiol. Pharmacol.* 59: 1050–1057, 1981.
553. SAMPAIO, L. DE O., M. T. BAYLISS, T. E. HARDINGHAM, and H. MUIR. Dermatan sulphate proteoglycan from human articular cartilage. *Biochem. J.* 254: 757–764, 1988.
554. SANADA, H., J. SHIKATA, H. HAMAMOTO, Y. UEBA, T. YAMAMURA, and T. TAKEDA. Changes in collagen cross-linking and lysyl oxidase by estrogen. *Biochim. Biophys. Acta* 541: 408–413, 1978.
555. SANDBERG, H. O., and O. CLOSS. The alpha and gamma crystallin content in aqueous humor of eyes with clear lenses and with cataracts. *Exp. Eye Res.* 28: 601–610, 1979.
556. SASAKI, R., S. ICHIKAWA, H. YAMAGIWA, A. ITO, and S. YAMAGATA. Aging and hydroxyproline content in human heart muscle. *Tohoku J. Exp. Med.* 118: 11–16, 1976.
557. SATOH, K. Age-related changes in the structural proteins of human lens. *Exp. Eye Res.* 14: 53–57, 1972.
558. SATOH, K., M. BANDO, and A. NAKAJIMA. Fluorescence in human lens. *Exp. Eye Res.* 16: 167–172, 1973.
559. SCHAUB, M. C. Qualitative and quantitative changes of collagen in parenchymatous organs of the rat during ageing. *Gerontologia* 8: 114–122, 1963.
560. SCHLEICHER, E., and O. H. WIELAND. Kinetic analysis of glycation as a tool for assessing the half-life of proteins. *Biochim. Biophys. Acta* 884: 199–205, 1986.
561. SCHMIDT, A. M., M. VIANNA, M. GERLACH, J. BRETT, J. RYAN, J. KAO, C. ESPOSITO, H. HEGARTY, W. HURLEY, M. CLAUSS, F. WANG, Y.-C. E. PAN, T. C. TSANG, and D. STERN. Isolation and characterization of two binding proteins for advanced glycosylation end products from bovine lung which are present on the endothelial cell surface. *J. Biol. Chem.* 267: 14987–14997, 1992.
562. SCHOENMAKERS, J. J. G., J. J. T. GERDING, and H. BLOEMENDAL. The secondary structure of α-crystallin. *Eur. J. Biochem.* 11: 472–480, 1969.
563. SCOTT, J. E. Proteoglycan: collagen interactions and subfibrillar structure in collagen fibrils. Implications in the development and ageing of connective tissues. *J. Anat.* 169: 23–35, 1990.
564. SCOTT, J. E., R.-G. QIAN, W. HENKEL, and R. W. GLANVILLE. An Ehrlich chromogen in collagen cross-links. *Biochem. J.* 209: 263–264, 1983.
565. SEBAG, J. Ageing of the vitreous. *Eye* 1: 254–262, 1987.
566. SELL, D. R., and V. M. MONNIER. Isolation, purification and partial characterization of novel fluorophores from aging human insoluble collagen-rich tissue. *Connect. Tissue Res.* 19: 77–92, 1989.
567. SELL, D. R., and V. M. MONNIER. Structure elucidation of a senescence cross-link from human extracellular matrix: implication of pentoses in the aging process. *J. Biol. Chem.* 264: 21597–21602, 1989.
568. SELL, D. R., and V. M. MONNIER. End-stage renal disease and diabetes catalyze the formation of a pentose-derived crosslink from aging human collagen. *J. Clin. Invest.* 85: 380–384, 1990.
569. SELL, D. R., E. C. CARLSON, and V. M. MONNIER. Differential effects of type 2 (non-insulin-dependent) diabetes mellitus on pentosidine formation in skin and glomerular basement membrane. *Diabetologia* 36: 936–941, 1993.
570. SELL, D. R., A. LAPOLLA, P. ODETTI, J. FOGARTY, and V. M. MONNIER. Pentosidine formation in skin correlates with severity of complications in individuals with long-standing IDDM. *Diabetes* 41: 1286–1292, 1992.
571. SELL, D. R., R. H. NAGARAJ, S. K. GRANDHEE, P. ODETTI, A. LAPOLLA, J. FOGARTY, and V. M. MONNIER. Pentosidine: a molecular marker for the cumulative damage to proteins in diabetes, aging, and uremia. *Diabetes Metab. Rev.* 7: 239–251, 1991.
572. SEPHEL, G. C., and J. M. DAVIDSON. Elastin production in human skin fibroblast cultures and its decline with age. *J. Invest. Dermatol.* 86: 279–285, 1986.
573. SHAPIRO, S. D., S. K. ENDICOTT, M. A. PROVINCE, J. A. PIERCE, and E. J. CAMPBELL. Marked longevity of human lung parenchymal elastic fibers deduced from prevalence of D-aspartate and nuclear weapons-related radiocarbon. *J. Clin. Invest.* 87: 1828–1834, 1991.
574. SHIKATA, H., M. HIRAMATSU, T. MASUMIZU, D. FUJIMOTO, and N. UTSUMI. Age-related changes in the content of non-reducible crosslinks in rat mandibular bone. *Arch. Oral. Biol.* 30: 451–453, 1985.
575. SHILTON, B. H., and D. J. WALTON. Sites of glycation of human and horse liver alcohol dehydrogenase in vivo. *J. Biol. Chem.* 266: 5587–5592, 1991.
576. SHIMIZU, K., T. FURUYA, Y. TAKEO, K. SHIRAMA, and K. MAEKAWA. Decrease of collagen content in the intraocular fluid of senile rats. *Acta Anat.* 109: 44–46, 1981.
577. SHIN, D. B., and M. S. FEATHER. 3-deoxy-L-glycero- pentos-2-ulose (3-deoxy-L-xylosone) and L-threo- pentosulose (L-xylosone) as intermediates in the degradation of L-ascorbic acid. *Carbohydr. Res.* 208: 246–250, 1990.
578. SHUSTER, S., M. M. BLACK, and E. MCVITIE. The influence of age and sex on skin thickness, skin collagen and density. *Br. J. Dermatol.* 93: 639–643, 1975.
579. SHUSTER, S., E. J. RAFFLE, and E. BOTTOMS. Skin collagen in rheumatoid arthritis, and the effect of corticosteroids. *Lancet* 1: 525–527, 1967.
580. SIEBINGA, S., G. F. J. M. VRENSEN, F. F. M. DE MAL, and J. GREVE. Age-related change in local water and protein content of human eye lenses measured by Raman microspectroscopy. *Exp. Eye Res.* 53: 233–239, 1991.
581. SILBERMANN, M., K. VON DER MARK, M. VAN MENXEL, and old A. Z. REZNICK. Effect of short-term physical stress on DNA and collagen synthesis in the femur of young and old mice. *Gerontology* 33: 49–56, 1987.
582. SIPPEL, T. O. Energy metabolism in the lens during aging. *Invest. Ophthalmol. Vis. Sci.* 4: 502–513, 1965.
583. SMALLEY, J. W. Age-related changes in hydroxylysylglycosides of human glomerular basement membrane collagen. *Exp. Gerontol.* 15: 65–66, 1980.
584. SMITH, J. B., G. A. SHUN-SHIN, L. J. MIESBAUER, and D. L. SMITH. Posttranslational modifications of the water soluble α-crystallins from renal failure patients. *Invest. Ophthalmol.* 34: 1341, 1993.
585. SMITH, P. R., and P. J. THORNALLEY. Mechanism of the degradation of non-enzymatically glycated proteins under physiological conditions: studies with the model fructosamine, N^ϵ-(1-

deoxy-D-fructos-1-yl) hippuryl-lysine. *Eur. J. Biochem.* 210: 729–739, 1992.

586. SMITH, P. R., H. H. SOMANI, P. J. THORNALLEY, J. BENN, and P. H. SONKSEN. Evidence against the formation of 2-amino-6-(2-formyl-5-hydroxymethyl-pyrrol-l-yl)-hexanoic acid ("pyrraline") as an early-stage product or advanced glycation end product in non-enzymic protein glycation. *Clin. Sci.* 84: 87–93, 1993.

587. SNOWDEN, J. M., D. R. EYRE, and D. A. SWANN. Vitreous structure. VI. Age-related changes in the thermal stability and cross-links of vitreous, articular cartilage and tendon collagens. *Biochim. Biophys. Acta* 706: 153–157, 1982.

588. SOBEL, H. Ageing and age-associated disease. *Lancet* II: 1191–1192, 1970.

589. SOBIN, S. S. Landis Award lecture. Questions and signposts in microvascular research. *Microvasc. Res.* 21: 1–18, 1981.

590. SPECTOR, A. Aggregation of α-crystallin and its possible relationship to cataract formation. *Isr. J. Med. Sci.* 8: 1577–1582, 1972.

591. SPECTOR, A. Aging of the lens and cataract formation. In: *Aging and Human Visual Function*, edited by R. Sekuler, D. Kline and K. Dismukes. New York: Alan R. Liss, 1982, p. 27–43.

592. SPECTOR, A. The lens and oxidative stress. In: *Oxidative Stress. Oxidants and Antioxidants*, edited by H. Sies. London: Academic Press, 1991, p. 529–558.

593. SPECTOR, A., and W. H. GARNER. Hydrogen peroxide and human cataract. *Exp. Eye Res.* 33: 673–681, 1981.

594. SPECTOR, A., R. CHIESA, J. SREDY, and W. GARNER. cAMP-dependent phosphorylation of bovine lens α-crystallin. *Proc. Natl. Acad. Sci. USA* 82: 4712–4716, 1985.

595. SPECTOR, A., M. H. GARNER, W. H. GARNER, D. ROY, P. FARNSWORTH, and S. SHYNE. An extrinsic membrane polypeptide associated with high-molecular aggregates in human cataract. *Science* 204: 1323–1326, 1978.

596. SPECTOR, A., S. LI, and J. SIGELMAN. Age-dependent changes in the molecular size of human lens proteins and their relationship to light scatter. *Invest. Ophthalmol.* 13: 795–798, 1974.

597. SPINA, M., and G. GARBIN. Age-related chemical changes in human elastins from non-atherosclerotic areas of thoracic aorta. *Atherosclerosis* 24: 267–279, 1976.

598. SPINA, M., S. GARBISA, J. HINNIE, and J. C. HUNTER, A. SERAFINI-FRACASSINI. Age-related changes in composition and mechanical properties of the tunica media of the upper thoracic human aorta. *Arteriosclerosis* 3: 64–76, 1983.

599. SRIVASTAVA, O. P. Age-related increase in concentration and aggregation of degraded polypeptides in human lenses. *Exp. Eye Res.* 47: 525–543, 1988.

600. SRIVASTAVA, S. K. and E. BEUTLER. Cleavage of lens protein-GSH mixed disulfide by GSH reductase. *Exp. Eye Res.* 17: 33–42, 1973.

601. STANESCU, V., F. CHAMINADE, and M.-P. MURIEL. Age-related changes in small proteoglycans of low buoyant density of human articular cartilage. *Connect. Tissue Res.* 17: 239–252, 1988.

602. STARCHER, B. C., and R. P. MECHAM. Desmosine radioimmunoassay as a means of studying elastogenesis in cell culture. *Connect. Tissue Res.* 8: 255–258, 1981.

603. STARCHER, B. C., S. M. PARTRIDGE, and D. F. ELSDEN. Isolation and partial characterization of a new amino acid from reduced elastin. *Biochemistry* 6: 2425–2432, 1967.

604. STEVENS, V. J., C. A. ROUZER, V. M. MONNIER, and A. CERAMI. Diabetic cataract formation: potential role of glycosylation of lens crystallins. *Proc. Natl. Acad. Sci. USA* 75: 2918–2922, 1978.

605. STIDWORTHY, G., Y. F. MASTERS, and M. R. SHETLAR. The effect of aging on mucopolysaccharide composition of human costal cartilage as measured by hexosamine and uronic acid content. *J. Gerontol.* 13: 10–13, 1958.

606. STONE, P. J., C. FRANZBLAU, and H. M. KAGAN. Proteolysis of insoluble elastin. *Methods Enzymol.* 82: 588–605, 1982.

607. STREHLER, B. L. Definitions, criteria, categories, and origins of age changes. In: *Time, Cells, Aging*, (2nd Ed.) edited by B. L. Strehler. New York: Academic Press, 1977, p. 5–30.

608. STRICKLIN, G. P., and M. S. HIBBS. Biochemistry and physiology of mammalian collagenases. In: *Collagen*, edited by M. E. Nimni. Boca Raton, FL: CRC Press, 1988, vol. I, p. 187–205.

609. STUHLSATZ, H. W., H. LÖFFLER, V. MOHANARADHAKRISHNAN, S. COSMA, and H. GREILING. Topographic and age-dependent distribution of the glycosaminoglycans in human aorta. *J. Clin. Chem. Clin. Biochem.* 20: 713–721, 1982.

610. SUNDHOLM, F., A. VISAPÄÄ, and J. BJÖRKSTEN. Cross-linking of collagen in the presence of oxidizing lipid. *Lipids* 13: 755–757, 1978.

611. SWAMY, M. S., and E. C. ABRAHAM. Lens protein composition, glycation and high molecular weight aggregation in aging rats. *Invest. Ophthalmol. Vis. Sci.* 28: 1693–1701, 1987.

612. SWAMY, M. S., A. ABRAHAM, and E. C. BARAHAM. Glycation of human lens proteins. Preferential glycation of αA subunits. *Exp. Eye Res.* 54: 337–345, 1992.

613. SWEET, M. B. E., E. J.-M. A. THONAR, and J. MARSH. Age-related changes in proteoglycan structure. *Arch. Biochem. Biophys.* 198: 439–448, 1979.

614. TAKATA, K., S. HORIUCHI, N. ARAKI, M. SHIGA, M. SAITOH, and Y. MORINO. Endocytic uptake of nonenzymatically glycosylated proteins is mediated by a scavenger receptor for aldehyde-modified proteins. *J. Biol. Chem.* 263: 14819–14825, 1988.

615. TAKEDA, K., A. GOSIEWSKA, and B. PETERKOFSKY. Similar, but not identical, modulation of expression of extracellular matrix components during in vitro and in vivo aging of human skin fibroblasts. *J. Cell Physiol.* 153: 450–459, 1992.

616. TAKEMOTO, L., and P. AZARI. Amino acid composition of normal and cataractous human lens protein. *Exp. Eye Res.* 23: 1–7, 1976.

617. TAKEMOTO, L., and M. TAKEHANA. Major intrinsic polypeptide (MIP 26K) from human lens membrane: characterization of low-molecular weight forms in the aging human lens. *Exp. Eye Res.* 43: 661–667, 1986.

618. TAKEMOTO, L., T. KODAMA, and D. TAKEMOTO. Covalent changes at the N- and C-terminal regions of γ-crystallins during aging of the normal human lens. *Exp. Eye Res.* 45: 207–274, 1987.

619. TANG, S.-S., P. C. TRACKMAN, and H. M. KAGAN. Reaction of aortic lysyl oxidase with β-aminopropionitrile. *J. Biol. Chem.* 258: 4331–4338, 1983.

620. TAO, R. V., Y. TAKAHASHI, and P. F. KADOR. Effect of aldose reductase inhibitors on naphthalene cataract formation in the rat. *Invest. Ophthalmol. Vis. Sci.* 32: 1630–1637, 1991.

621. TAYLOR, A., and K. J. A. DAVIES. Protein oxidation and loss of protease activity may lead to cataract formation in the aged lens. *Free Radic. Biol. Med.* 3: 371–377, 1987.

622. TAYLOR, A., J. H. JAHNGEN, J. BLONDIN, and E. G. JAHNGEN, JR. Ascorbate delays ultraviolet-induced, age-related damage to lens protease and the effect of maturation and aging on the function of the ubiquitin-lens protein conjugating apparatus. *Proteases Biol. Control Biotech.* 57: 283–293, 1987.

623. TAYLOR, H. R., S. K. WEST, F. S. ROSENTHAL, B. MUNOZ, H. S. NEWLAND, H. ABBEY, and E. A. EMMETT. Effect of ultraviolet radiation on cataract formation. *N. Engl. J. Med.* 319: 1429–1433, 1988.

624. TAYLOR, J. R., J. E. SCOTT, A. M. CRIBB, and T. R. BOSWORTH. Human intervertebral disc acid glycosaminoglycans. *J. Anat.* 180: 137–141, 1992.

625. TESTA, M., C. FIORE, N. BOCCI, and S. CALABRO. Effect of the

oxidation of sulfhydryl groups on lens proteins. *Exp. Eye Res.* 7: 276–290, 1968.
626. THEOCHARIS, D. A. Comparisons between extracted and residual proteoglycans on the glycosaminoglycan level and changes with ageing. *Int. J. Biochem.* 17: 155–160, 1985.
627. THOMAS, D. P., R. J. MCCORMICK, S. D. ZIMMERMAN, R. K. VADLAMUDI, and L. E. GOSSELIN. Aging- and training-induced alterations in collagen characteristics of rat ventricle and papillary muscle. *Am. J. Physiol.* 263: H778–H783, 1992.
628. THOMPSON, R. C., and J. E. BALLOU. Studies of metabolic turnover with tritium as a tracer. V. The predominantly nondynamic state of body constituents in the rat. *J. Biol. Chem.* 223: 795–809, 1956.
629. THONAR, E. J.-M. A., and M. B. E. SWEET. Maturation-related changes in proteoglycans of fetal articular cartilage. *Arch. Biochem. Biophys.* 208: 535–547, 1981.
630. THONAR, E. J.-M. A., S. BJORNSSON, and K. E. KUETTNER. Age-related changes in cartilage proteoglycans. In: *Articular Cartilage Biochemistry*, edited by K. Kuettner, R. Schleyerbach and V. C. Hascall. New York: Raven Press, 1986, p. 273–288.
631. TILSON, M. D. Further studies of a putative cross-linking amino acid (3-deoxypyridinoline) in skin from patients with abdominal aortic aneurysms. *Surgery* 98: 888–891, 1985.
632. TINKER, D. H., and A. L. TAPPEL. A partial characterization of the major fluorophore of bovine ligamentum elastin. *Connect. Tissue Res.* 11: 309–319, 1983.
633. TINKER, D. H., R. B. RUCKER, and A. L. TAPPEL. Variation of elastin fluorescence with method of preparation: determination of the major fluorophore of fibrillar elastin. *Connect. Tissue Res.* 11: 299–308, 1983.
634. TOBARI, I. Aging and eye diseases II. *Nippon Ganka Gakkai Zasshi.* 47: 341–344, 1976.
635. TOMODA, K., S. MORII, T. YAMASHITA, and T. KUMAZAWA. Histologic architecture of submucosal connective tissues in human eustachian tube with supplemental reference to the effects of aging. *Arch. Otorhinolaryngol.* 232: 57–63, 1981.
636. TRIPHAUS, G. F., A. SCHMIDT, and E. BUDDECKE. Age-related changes in the incorporation of [^{35}S] sulfate into two proteoglycan populations from human cartilage. *Hoppe Seylers Z. Physiol. Chem.* 361: 1773–1779, 1980.
637. TRUSCOTT, R. J. W., and R. C. AUGUSTEYN. Oxidative changes in human lens proteins during senile nuclear cataract formation. *Biochim. Biophys. Acta* 492: 43–52, 1977.
638. TRUSCOTT, R. J. W., and R. C. AUGUSTEYN. The state of sulfhydryl groups in normal and cataractous human lenses. *Exp. Eye Res.* 25: 139–148, 1977.
639. TRUSCOTT, R. J. W., and R. C. AUGUSTEYN. Changes in human lens proteins during nuclear cataract formation. *Exp. Eye Res.* 24: 159–170, 1977.
640. TRUSCOTT, R. J. W., K. FUALL, and R. C. AUGUSTEYN. The identification of anthranilic acid in proteolytic digest of cataractous lens proteins. *Ophthalmic Res.* 9: 263–268, 1977.
641. TSUJI, T., and T. HAMADA. Age-related changes in human dermal elastic fibers. *Br. J. Dermatol.* 105: 57–63, 1981.
642. TUDERMAN, L., and K. I. KIVIRIKKO. Immunoreactive prolyl hydroxylase in human skin, serum and synovial fluid: changes in the content and components with age. *Eur. J. Clin. Invest.* 7: 295–299, 1977.
643. UCHIYAMA, A., T. INOUE, and D. FUJIMOTO. Synthesis of pyridinoline during in vitro aging of bone collagen. *J. Biochem. (Tokyo)* 90: 1795–1798, 1981.
644. UCHIYAMA, A., T. OHISHI, M. TAKAHASHI, K. KUSHIDA, T. INOUE, M. FUJIE, and K. HORIUCHI. Fluorophores from aging human articular cartilage. *J. Biochem.* 110: 714–718, 1991.
645. UITTO, J. Connective tissue biochemistry of the aging dermis. *Clin. Geriatr. Med.* 5: 127–147, 1989.

646. UITTO, J., M. J. FAZIO, and D. R. OLSEN. Molecular mechanisms of cutaneous aging. *J. Am. Acad. Dermatol.* 21: 614–622, 1989.
646a. URBAN, J. P. G., and J. F. MCMULLIN. Swelling pressure of the intervertebral disc: influence of proteoglycan and collagen contents. *Biorheology* 22: 145–157, 1985.
647. VAILAS, A. C., V. A. PEDRINI, A. PEDRINI- MILLE, and J. O. HOLLOSZY. Patellar tendon matrix changes associated with aging and voluntary exercise. *J. Appl. Physiol.* 58: 1572–1576, 1985.
648. VAN BOEKEL, M. A. M., and J. HOENDERS. Glycation-induced crosslinking of calf-lens crystallins. *Exp. Eye Res.* 52: 90–94, 1991.
649. VAN DEN OETELAAR, P. J. M., and H. J. HOENDERS. Racemizaton of aspartyl residues in proteins from normal and cataractous human lenses: an aging process without involvement in cataract formation. *Exp. Eye Res.* 48: 209–214, 1989.
650. VAN DER OUDERAA, F. J., W. W. DE JONG, A. HILDERINK, and H. BLOEMENDAL. The amino acid sequence of the αB$_2$ chain of bovine α-crystallin. *Eur. J. Biochem.* 49: 157–168, 1984.
651. VAN DER REST, M., and P. BRUCKNER. Collagens: diversity at the molecular and supramolecular levels. *Curr. Opinion Struct. Biol.* 3: 430–436, 1993.
652. VAN DER REST, M., and R. GARRONE. Collagen family of proteins. *FASEB J.* 5: 2814–2823, 1991.
653. VAN HAARD, P. M. M., J. A. KRAMPS, H. J. HOENDERS, and J. WOLLENSAK. Development of nondisulfide covalent crosslinks in nuclear cataractogenesis. *Interdiscipl. Top. Gerontol.* 13: 212–224, 1978.
654. VAN HEYNINGEN, R. The lens: metabolism and cataract. In: *The Eye* (2nd ed.), edited by H. Davson. New York: Academic Press, 1969, vol. 1, p. 381–488.
655. VAN HEYNINGEN, R. Fluorescent glucoside in the human lens. *Nature* 230: 393–394, 1971.
656. VAN HEYNINGEN, R. Assay of fluorescent glucosides in the human lens. *Exp. Eye Res.* 15: 121–126, 1973.
657. VAN HEYNINGEN, R. The glucoside of 3- hydroxykynurenine and other fluorescent compounds in the human lens. In: *The Human Lens—In Relation to Cataract*, edited by B. T. Philipson and P. P. Fagerholm. Amsterdam: Elsevier, 1973, p. 151–171.
658. VAN KLEEF, F. S. M., W. W. DE JONG, and H. J. HOENDERS. Stepwise degradations and deamination of the eye lens protein α-crystallin in aging. *Nature* 258: 264–266, 1975.
659. VAN KLEEF, S. M., W. WILLEMS-THIJSSEN, and H. J. HOENDERS. Intracellular degradation and deamidation of alpha-crystallin subunits. *Eur. J. Biochem.* 66: 477–483, 1976.
660. VARMA, S. D., N. A. BEACHY, and R. D. RICHARDS. Photoperoxidation of lens lipids: prevention by vitamin E. *Photochem. Photobiol.* 36: 623–626, 1982.
661. VARMA, S. D., D. CHAND, Y. R. SHARMA, J. F. KUCK, JR., and R. D. RICHARDS. Oxidative stress on lens cataract formation: role of light and oxygen. *Curr. Eye Res.* 3: 35–57, 1984.
662. VARMA, S. D., S. KUMAR, and R. D. RICHARDS. Light-induced damage to ocular lens cation pump: prevention by vitamin C. *Proc. Natl. Acad. Sci. USA* 76: 3504–3506, 1979.
663. VARMA, S. D., V. K. SRIVASTAVA, and R. D. RICHARDS. Photoperoxidation in lens and cataract formation: preventative role of superoxide dismutase, catalase and vitamin C. *Ophthalmic Res.* 14: 167–175, 1982.
664. VASAN, N. S., R. A. SAPORITO, JR., S. SAVASWATHI, J. V. TESORIERO, and S. MANLEY. Alterations of renal cortex and medullary glycosaminoglycans in aging dog kidney. *Biochim. Biophys. Acta* 760: 197–205, 1983.
665. VERZÁR, F. Veranderungen der thermoelastichen Knontrakfion der Sehnenfasern im Alter. *Helv. Physiol. Pharmacol. Acta.* 13: C64, 1955.

666. VERZÁR, F. The aging of collagen. *Sci. Am.* 208: 104–114, April 1963.
667. VISHWANATH, V., K. E. FRANK, C. A. ELMETS, P. J. DAUCHOT, and V. M. MONNIER. Glycation of skin collagen in type I diabetes mellitus: correlation with long-term complications. *Diabetes* 35: 916–921, 1986.
668. VLASSARA, H., M. BROWNLEE, and A. CERAMI. High-affinity receptor-mediated uptake and degradation of glucose-modified proteins: a potential mechanism for the removal of senescent macromolecules. *Proc. Natl. Acad. Sci. USA* 82: 5588–5592, 1985.
669. VLASSARA, H., M. BROWNLEE, and A. CERAMI. Macrophage receptor-mediated processing and regulation of advanced glycosylation endproduct (AGE)-modified proteins: role in aging and diabetes. In: *The Maillard Reaction in Aging, Diabetes and Nutrition*, edited by. J. W. Baynes and V. M. Monnier. New York: Alan R. Liss, 1989, p. 205–218.
670. VLASSARA, H., H. FUH, Z. MAKITA, S. KRUNGKRAI, A. CERAMI, and R. BUCALA. Exogenous advanced glycosylation end products induce complex vascular dysfunction in normal animals: a model for diabetic and aging complications. *Proc. Natl. Acad. Sci. USA* 89: 12043–12047, 1992.
671. VOGEL, H. G. Influence of maturation and aging on mechanical and biochemical properties of connective tissue in rats. *Mech. Ageing Dev.* 14: 283–292, 1980.
672. VOGEL, H. G. Mechanical properties of rat skin with aging. In: *Aging and the Skin*, edited by A. K. Balin and A. M. Kligman. New York: Raven Press, 1989, p. 227–275.
673. VOGEL, H. G. Species differences of elastic and collagenous tissue—influence of maturation and age. *Mech. Ageing Dev.* 57: 15–24, 1991.
674. VOORTER, C. E. M., W. A. DEHAARD-HOEHMAN, P. J. M. OETELAAR, H. BLOEMENDAL, and W. W. DE JONG. Spontaneous peptide bond cleavage in aging α-crystallin through a succinimide intermediate. *J. Biol. Chem.* 263: 19020–19023, 1988.
675. WALTERS, C., and D. R. EYRE. Collagen crosslinks in human dentin: increasing content of hydroxypyridinium residues with age. *Calcif. Tissue Int.* 35: 401–405, 1983.
676. WARREN, R., V. GARTSTEIN, A. M. KLIGMAN, W. MONTAGNA, R. A. ALLENDORF, and G. M. RIDDER. Age, sunlight, and facial skin: a histologic and quantitative study. *J. Am. Acad. Dermatol.* 25: 751–760, 1991.
677. WEITER, J. J. and E. D. FINCH. Paramagnetic species in cataractous human lenses. *Nature* 254: 536–537, 1975.
678. WEST, M. D., O. M. PEREIRA-SMITH, and J. R. SMITH. Replicative senescence of human skin fibroblasts correlates with a loss of regulation and overexpression of collagenase activity. *Exp. Cell Res.* 184: 138–147, 1989.
679. WILLEN, M. D., J. M. SORRELL, C. C. LEKAN, B. R. DAVIS, and A. I. CAPLAN. Patterns of glycosaminoglycan proteoglycan immunostaining in human skin during aging. *J. Invest. Dermatol.* 96: 968–974, 1991.
680. WOLF, B., A. M. GRESSNER, Z. NEVO, and H. GREILING. Age-related decrease in the activity of UDP-xylose: core protein xylosyltransferase in rat costal cartilage. *Mech. Ageing Dev.* 19: 181–190, 1982.
681. WOLFF, S. P., and R. T. DEAN. Glucose autoxidation and protein modification: the potential role of autoxidative glycosylation in diabetes. *Biochem. J.* 245: 243–250, 1987.
682. WOLFF, S. P., Z. A. BASCAL, and J. V. HUNT. Autoxidative glycosylation: free radicals and glycation theory. In: *Maillard Reaction in Aging, Diabetes, and Nutrition*, edited by J. W. Baynes and V. M. Monnier. New York: Alan R. Liss, 1989, p. 259–275.
683. YAMAUCHI, M., and G. L. MECHANIC. Cross-linking of collagen. In: *Collagen*, edited by M. E. Nimni. Boca Raton, FL: CRC Press, 1988, vol. I, p. 157–172.
684. YAMAUCHI, M., R. E. LONDON, C. GUENAT, F. HASHIMOTO, and G. L. MECHANIC. Structure and formation of a stable histidine-based trifunctional cross-link in skin collagen. *J. Biol. Chem.* 262: 11428–11434, 1987.
685. YAMAUCHI, M., D. T. WOODLEY, and G. L. MECHANIC. Aging and cross-linking of skin collagen. *Biochem. Biophys. Res. Commun.* 152: 898–903, 1988.
686. YLÄ-HERTTUALA, S., H. SUMUVUORI, K. KARKOLA, M. MÖTTÖNEN, and T. NIKKARI. Glycosaminoglycans in normal atherosclerotic human coronary arteries. *Lab. Invest.* 54: 402–407, 1986.
687. YOUNG, R. W. *Age-Related Cataract*. New York: Oxford University Press, 1991, p. 290.
688. YU, N. T., J. F. R. KUCK, and C. C. ASSKREN. Red fluorescence in older and brunescent human lenses. *Invest. Ophthalmol. Vis. Sci.* 18: 1278–1280, 1979.
689. YUE, D. K., S. MCLENNAN, L. DELBRIDGE, D. J. HANDELSMAN, T. REEVE, and J. R. TURTLE. The thermal stability of collagen in diabetic rats: correlation with severity of diabetes and nonenzymatic glycosylation. *Diabetologia* 24: 282–285, 1983.
690. ZIGLER, J. S., JR., and J. D. GOOSEY. Aging of protein molecules: lens crystallins as a model system. *Trends Biochem. Sci.* 6: 133–136, 1981.
691. ZIGLER, J. S., JR., and J. D. GOOSEY. Singlet oxygen as a possible factor in human senile nuclear cataract development. *Curr. Eye Res.* 3: 59–65, 1984.
692. ZIGLER, J. S., JR., J. B. SIDBURY, JR., B. S. YAMANASHI, and M. WOLBARSHT. Studies on brunescent cataracts. *Ophthalmic Res.* 8: 379–387, 1976.
693. ZIGMAN, S. Coloration of human lenses by near ultraviolet photo-oxidized tryptophan. *Exp. Eye Res.* 13: 70–76, 1972.
694. ZIGMAN, S. Tryptophan excited states in the lens. *Doc. Ophthalmol.* 8: 267–274, 1976.
695. ZIGMAN, S. Photochemical mechanisms in cataract formation. In: *Mechanisms of Cataract Formation in the Human Lens*, edited by G. Duncan. New York: Academic Press, 1981, p. 117–149.
696. ZIGMAN, S., G. GRIESS, T. YULO, and J. SCHULTZ. Ocular protein alterations by near UV light. *Exp. Eye Res.* 23: 555–567, 1973.
697. ZIGMAN, S., T. GROFF, T. YULO, and G. GRIESS. Light extinction and protein in lens. *Exp. Eye Res.* 23: 555–567, 1976.
698. ZIGMAN, S., T. YULO, and G. A. GRIESS. Inactivation of catalase by near ultraviolet light and tryptophan photoproducts. *Mol. Cell. Biochem.* 11: 149–154, 1976.
699. ZIKA, J. M., and L. KLEIN. Relative and absolute changes in skin collagen mass in the rat. *Biochim. Biophys. Acta* 229: 509–515, 1971.

IV ORGAN SYSTEM AND ORGANISMIC AGING

11. Skin

ANJALI CHUTTANI
BARBARA A. GILCHREST

Department of Dermatology, Boston University School of Medicine, Boston, Massachusetts

CHAPTER CONTENTS

In Vitro Studies
Intrinsic Aging
    Clinical Features
    Histopathology
        Epidermis
        Basement membrane zone
        Dermis
        Subcutaneous fat
Extrinsic Aging
    Photoaging
        Clinical features
        Histopathology
        Pathophysiology
        Relationship to skin cancer
    Cigarette smoking
Physiological Changes
    Barrier function
    Immune function
        Cell-mediated immunity
        Humoral responses
        Epidermal immune function
    Inflammatory response
    Wound healing
    Vitamin D production
Summary

ALL ORGAN SYSTEMS IN THE HUMAN BODY are subject to the ravages of time, but the effects of aging on the skin are most visible. Certainly, our earliest appraisal of age is often based on cutaneous clues. For physicians, the skin may also provide information regarding internal disease, nutritional status, and general well-being. The tremendous variation in the apparent aging processes of skin among individuals results from the interplay of genetic programming with a multitude of environmental factors, especially sun exposure. Intrinsic or chronological aging is based on the years since birth and produces clinical, histological, and functional changes that can be observed in sun-protected regions of the skin. Photoaging, by definition, is the superposition of cumulative sun damage on the intrinsic aging process and is responsible for most of the unwanted changes in skin appearance and for skin cancer, an extremely common and medically significant disorder of the elderly.

The dermatological significance of aging is evident in the fact that 7% of all physician visits in the United States are prompted by disorders of the skin, and the prevalence of such problems increases with age throughout adulthood (171). In a federally sponsored study of more than 20,000 noninstitutionalized Americans, 40% of the oldest (65–74 yr) cohort surveyed suffered from skin diseases sufficiently severe in the opinion of the consulting dermatologist to warrant at least one physician visit, and the average affected individual had 1.5 such disorders (87). Moreover, smaller studies (9) and anecdotal impressions strongly suggest a far higher prevalence of skin disease among those aged 75 yr and older. Such figures do not include the essentially universal "normal" changes in aging skin, which in themselves may reduce self-esteem, inhibit social interactions, and adversely affect subjective physical and mental health (63). In addition to disfigurement, skin conditions may cause itching or pain and may substantially interfere with daily activities. Finally, although hospitalization is infrequently the consequence of cutaneous disease, disorders such as decubitus ulcers and drug rashes may complicate and prolong hospitalization in the elderly.

IN VITRO STUDIES

The cellular basis of aging, initially studied in fetal lung fibroblasts (72, 73), has also been explored in cultured dermal fibroblasts, keratinocytes, and melanocytes (44, 56). A detailed discussion of this work is beyond the scope of this chapter, and the interested reader is referred to recent reviews (47, 51, 143, 170). The purpose of this section is to link the major findings at the cellular level with observations at the clinical and histological levels.

The literature to date focuses strongly on age-associated changes in cellular proliferative capacity, at least in part by default, as other major cellular functions are poorly understood or difficult to study in vitro for technical reasons. Initial studies demonstrated an inverse relationship between donor age and culture life span (115), by definition the number of cumulative cell divisions before proliferative senescence (72), and between donor age and short-term mitogenic responsiveness (139, 170). The former in vitro phenomenon may explain the progressive reduction in certain cutaneous cell populations with age, notably proliferatively competent basilar keratinocytes, epidermal and follicular melanocytes, and dermal fibroblasts. It is hypothesized that proliferative senescence of epidermal stem cells may compromise wound healing, while a similar loss of melanocytes may underlie the graying of hair. Poor mitogenic responsiveness of the remaining cells might also contribute directly to these problems.

The mechanism of proliferative senescence in human cells, including those in the skin, remains poorly understood (60). Indeed, it is even unclear how proliferative senescence (in vitro "aging") relates to the age-associated changes in cell function observed in vivo, including changes in proliferative behavior. One recent example involves the progressive loss of fibroblast ability to divide in response to stimulation by epidermal growth factor (EGF) (149). Refractoriness to EGF occurs both at late passage (in vitro aging) and with advanced donor age (in vivo aging). However, in the latter instance, there are changes in EGF receptor number, binding affinity, and internalization rate that appear to account for the loss of mitogenic responsiveness (93, 149); such changes cannot be implicated in late-passage vs. early-passage cells (136, 149).

The general molecular mechanisms underlying skin aging are, if anything, even less understood than the more proximate changes in receptor function and second-messenger pathways (14). However, patterns of change in gene expression recognized to date with increasing donor age in cultured keratinocyte suggest that aging may consist, at least in part, of a more advanced state of differentiation that may be modified by environmental influences (41).

With increasing age, the synthesis of autocrine and paracrine factors that stimulate the growth of cells in the skin may also be reduced. For instance, adult keratinocytes produce less epidermal thymocyte activating factor (interleukin-1) per cell than do newborn keratinocytes (158). Increased sensitivity to growth inhibitors may also be partly responsible for the age-associated loss in mitogenic potential. For example, an interferon-like molecule in the basal layer of the epidermis thought to act as a physiological inhibitor of cellular proliferation (191) has been shown to have greater effect on cultured adult donor keratinocytes than on newborn keratinocytes (135).

INTRINSIC AGING

Clinical Features

The clinical changes associated with normal skin aging are dryness, laxity, and fine wrinkling. In addition, a variety of benign proliferative lesions, including acrochordons (skin tags), seborrheic keratoses, cherry angiomas, and lentigines (age spots), become more numerous with age. Nearly every adult beyond the age of 65 yr has at least one such benign lesion, and most individuals have dozens.

Histopathology

The skin is comprised of three interrelated compartments, each demonstrating specific aging changes (Fig. 11.1; Table 11.1). These histological and functional changes appear to predispose old skin to injury and various disease processes.

Epidermis. The outermost compartment is the epidermis, of which the stratum corneum is the most superficial layer. The stratum corneum consists of 10–15 layers of tightly adherent, terminally differentiated, enucleated, flattened keratinocytes with cornified or cross-linked protein envelopes. This so-called barrier layer protects the body from excess water loss, prevents the entry of harmful chemicals or microbial pathogens, and scatters or reflects much of the incident UV light. Corneocytes are constantly shed from the skin surface and replaced by differentiating cells from viable epidermis below. A study of desquamation rates of corneocytes at selected body sites estimated a 30%–50% increase in the epidermal transit time between the third and eighth decades (66, 67), with the most pronounced changes occurring after the age of 50 yr (70). Also, tritiated thymidine studies have shown a 50% decline in epidermal labeling index (95), with a corresponding 100% prolongation in stratum corneum replacement (6). Thus the age-associated decrease in epidermal turnover rate increases the time spent by individual corneocytes at the skin surface. Perhaps because cells must reside on the surface where they are exposed to the environment for longer periods, they are more "weatherbeaten" in appearance and the stratum corneum appears less organized, manifest clinically by irregular fine surface lines (105). Barrier layer thickness is essentially unchanged, however (101).

Keratinocytes. Keratinocytes comprise more than 90% of the epidermis. They form a stratified transparent epithelium of perhaps 15 cell layers below the stratum corneum. In addition to creating the barrier layer

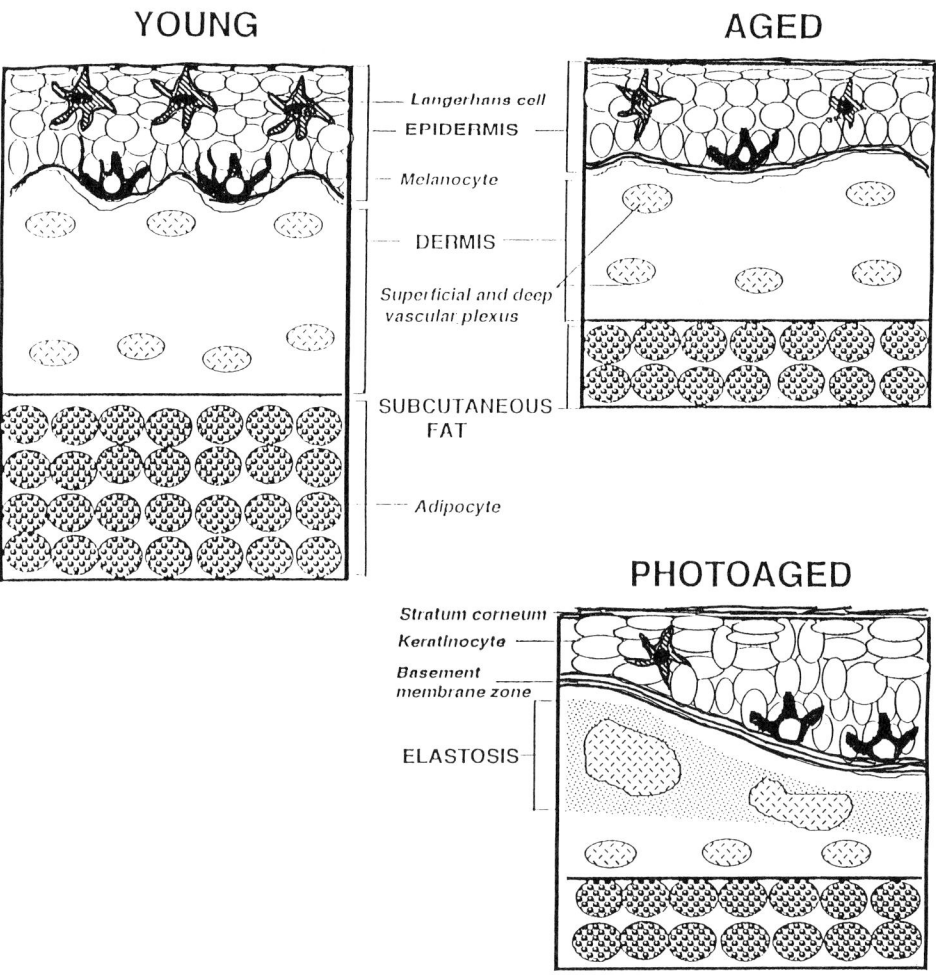

FIG. 11.1. Schematic drawings of young, aged, and photoaged skin. With aging alone, the interface between the dermis and the epidermis becomes flatter due to loss of the rete ridges. There is also a loss of Langerhans cells (suprabasilar dendritic cells) and melanocytes (dendritic pigment-producing cells) in basal layer and reductions in dermal thickness, vascularity, and subcutaneous fat. In photoaged skin there is variable epidermal atrophy and hyperplasia, a further reduction in Langerhans cells, and an increase in melanocytes compared to age-matched sun-protected skin. Vessels in the superficial dermis are dilated, and there is a striking change in the quality of the dermal elastic tissue that is termed "elastosis." Overall, aging alone results in skin that is less cellular and relatively atrophic, while photoaged skin may display either compensatory hypertrophy or further atrophy, depending on the severity of the cumulative UV injury. [Modified from Gilchrest (48) with permission.]

described above, the epidermis is known to be a major participant in immunological and inflammatory reactions through the production of numerous cytokines (156); there is possible in endocrine pathways as well (78, 91). As an individual ages, there is greater heterogeneity in keratinocyte size and shape. Above the basal layer, keratinocytes show decreased vertical height but increased volume (114, 137). Ultrastructural characteristics remain similar to young skin, although adhesion between corneocytes seems poorer and gaps separating cells seem wider (101).

Some investigators have reported overall atrophy of the epidermis in older skin (160), but other studies have emphasized preferential loss of the deep rete ridges extending into the dermis (101, 187), perhaps reflecting a reduction in the proportion of actively dividing keratinocytes (103).

Melanocytes. Melanocytes originate in the neural crest and migrate during embryogenesis to the epidermis, where they constitute 2%–4% of epidermal cells. They function primarily in the production and transfer of melanin pigment to keratinocytes, thus determining basal skin color and tanning response (133). The density of melanocytes in habitually exposed skin is twice that in nonexposed skin (52), presumably an adaptive response to UV injury; however, with each decade, the surviving population is reduced 10%–20%, regardless of the site (52, 145). Loss of enzymatically active me-

TABLE 11.1. *Age-Associated Skin Changes*

Component	Anatomic or Functional Change	Impacted Function
Epidermis		
Keratinocytes	Decreased proliferation	Wound healing; vitamin D_3
Melanocytes	Decreased 10% per decade	Photoprotection; color
Langerhans cells	Decreased up to 40%	Delayed hypersensitivity reactions; immune recognition
Basement membrane zone	Flattens, reducing dermo–epidermal interface	Epidermal–dermal adhesion
Dermis		
Fibroblasts	Decreased collagen/elastin synthesis	Tensile strength and elasticity
Microvasculature	Decreased vascular area	Thermoregulation and inflammatory response
Mast cells	Decreased	Immediate hypersensitivity reactions
Neural elements	Decreased by one-third	Sensation, pain threshold
Subcutis		
Fat	Decreased	Insulation and mechanical protection
Appendages		
Eccrine glands	Decreased number and output	Thermoregulation
Apocrine glands	Decreased number and output	Unknown
Sebaceous glands	Increased size; and decreased output	Unknown
Hair follicles	Decreased number and growth rate	Cosmetic

lanocytes results in less protection from UV light, since melanin absorbs carcinogenic UV radiation. Because of this, elderly patients often complain that they no longer tan as evenly or as deeply as they did when they were younger.

Aging affects not only the proliferative capacity of melanocytes (56) but also the degree of differentiation, as reflected in their morphology. Under culture conditions in which newborn melanocytes tend to be polygonal with a large cytoplasmic area, adult melanocytes are more dendritic, mimicking their differentiated in vivo appearance (50). In vivo, over several decades, melanocytes within melanocytic nevi change from small melanin-producing cells to neuroid forms in the deep dermis. Clinically, the number of detectable melanocytic nevi is reduced (112).

Langerhans cells. The remaining 1%–2% of the epidermis consists of Langerhans cells, immunocompetent cells that function primarily in antigen recognition and presentation. They originate in the bone marrow and, like melanocytes, migrate to the epidermis early in development. Also like melanocytes, they diminish in number with age. By late adulthood, there are 20%–50% fewer Langerhans cells in sun-protected skin (53), and more profound reductions are evident in sun-exposed skin. Because these cells are intimately involved in T cell–mediated immunological functions, their loss may contribute to the decreased ease of allergic sensitization in the elderly (125). The rather marked reduction of Langerhans cells in sun-exposed skin has also been postulated to contribute to photocarcinogenesis.

Basement Membrane Zone. In young skin, the epidermis is separated from the dermis by an intricate border that provides an extensive contact region for communication between the compartments. In addition, well-developed, villous-like cytoplasmic projections of the basal cells extend into the dermis, further augmenting the connection between the two. The most consistent finding in aged skin is a flattening of the dermal–epidermal junction, with effacement of the dermal papillae and the rete ridges (74, 119), as well as loss of the microfoot projections (101, 104). Some studies have estimated nearly a 50% reduction in the number of interdigitations per unit length of skin surface between the ages of 30 and 90 yr (2). Consequently, there is less surface area between the dermis and the epidermis, providing a smaller proliferative compartment, a diminished communicative exchange, as well as an increased propensity for separation with injury. Recent studies also suggest a reduction with age in the number of anchoring fibrils along the basement membrane. These changes may explain in part why the elderly are more susceptible to certain bullous diseases and abrasions following minimal injury (37). Interestingly, electron microscopy has demonstrated duplication of the lamina densa and the anchoring fibril complex periodically beneath basal keratinocytes and melanocytes, perhaps either as a compensation for the dermal–epidermal junction flattening or as a response to injury (101).

Dermis. Below the epidermis lies the dermis, consisting of supportive connective tissue, microvasculature, nerves, appendageal structures, and various cellular components, notably fibroblasts.

Collagen. Loss of dermal thickness approaches 20% in the elderly (15), perhaps accounting for the fragile, nearly translucent quality of older skin. One study using pulsed ultrasound reported an almost linear decline in skin thickness after the age of 20 yr (176). Although the majority of changes in collagen metabolism occur during fetal and neonatal growth (179), a loss of nearly 1% of dermal collagen content per year of adult life has been estimated (163). A reduction in collagen synthesis, as demonstrated by measuring the rate of incorporation of radioactive hydroxyproline (178) and prolyhydroxylase activity (180), probably accounts for this loss. Structurally, individual collagen fibers are thickened, less soluble, and more resistant to digestion by collagenase (147, 154). Higher amounts of ketosamine-linked, glycosylated, insoluble collagen are present, reflecting either slower collagen turnover or effects of elevated glucose levels in the tissue (168). Ultrastructurally, collagen fibers are coarser and arranged in "ropelike" bundles in relative disarray compared to those in young skin (95). Changes in cohesive bonding increase both the stability and the tensile strength of collagen. Consequently, older collagen is stiffer, less malleable, and hence, more vulnerable to injury (11).

Glycosaminoglycans. Less studied are the age-associated changes in ground substance of the dermal matrix. These substances, primarily glycosaminoglycans and proteoglycans, comprise only 0.1–0.3% of the dry weight of the normal dermis, although they may hold up to 1,000 times their weight in water (164). Thus even small losses of these substances may substantially reduce skin turgor. Some investigators reported a reduction with age in the amount of hyaluronic acid and dermatin sulfate in the dermis (38), but there is no recent work in this area and the existing literature does not clearly distinguish between aged and photoaged skin.

Elastic tissue. Major alterations also affect the elastin network during normal cutaneous aging. In young skin, fine, delicate fibers of elastic tissue extend to the top of the papillary dermis; these fibers progressively diminish with age (40, 119) and are replaced by fibers that are smaller, fragmented, and more loosely organized (101). These changes are probably responsible for the fine wrinkling of aged skin, which readily disappears when the skin is stretched. In the reticular or deeper dermis, elastic fibers are generally thicker, more abundant, more branched, and haphazardly arranged. These fibers also change with age, developing small cysts or lacunae after the fifth decade, with complete fragmentation observed in subjects over 70 yr of age (16). These changes have been reproduced experimentally by incubating dermal slices with elastase or chymotrypsin, implicating enzymatic digestion of elastin as a possible mechanism (16).

Cellular and vascular changes. Accompanying the changes in the connective tissue, specific changes in the cellular and vascular components of the dermis have also been described (31). Fibroblasts produce collagen, elastin, and ground substance. In old skin, electron microscopic studies reveal fibroblasts with extensive rough endoplasmic reticulum and dilated cisternae filled with flocculent material (101), presumably producing altered connective tissue.

One study comparing buttock skin from young and old subjects showed a 50% reduction in mast cells and a 30% reduction in venular cross-sections in the papillary dermis (54). Fewer mast cells may account for the infrequency of immediate hypersensitivity reactions (7) and acute urticaria seen in older patients. Also, the loss of mast cells may be related to the reduced vasculature, since heparin, a product of mast cells, promotes angiogenesis (4). There is a 30% decrease in adulthood of the vertical capillary loops extending into the dermal papillae (43); also reduced is the microvasculature surrounding hair bulbs and eccrine, sebaceous, and apocrine glands (95). In fact, this reduction in vasculature may contribute to the age-associated atrophy and fibrosis of these appendageal structures. Electron microscopic examination of these vessels shows normal appearing or slightly thickened walls in subjects below the age of 80 yr; however, the oldest subjects, aged 80–93 yr, had thinning of the vessel walls and fewer perivascular veil cells (17). These changes may explain why older skin is more easily bruised. Also, clinically, these patients are more susceptible to extremes in temperature (12), presumably because the loss of microvasculature interferes with thermoregulation.

Appendageal structures. The appendageal structures, including eccrine glands, apocrine glands, and pilosebaceous units, are also influenced by the aging process.

Hair. Perhaps the most clinically apparent are the changes related to hair, specifically its color, density, and distribution. The maximum density of hair follicles occurs at birth, and with somatic growth, these follicles are distributed over an increased surface area. Advancing age is also accompanied by a gradual reduction in the number of follicles, averaging a near 20% loss in density after age 60 yr (42). The residual follicles have a longer telogen (resting) phase, causing the hairs to grow more slowly and to be smaller in diameter. This diffuse loss and thinning of the hair is independent of hormonally mediated, male-pattern hair loss, which is typically seen in the bitemporal and the vertex regions (8). In this process, which also occurs in women, albeit to a lesser degree, androgen stimulation irreversibly converts follicles from producing dark terminal hairs to producing almost invisible vellous hairs.

Graying of hair is due to the progressive loss of melanocytes from the hair bulb as well as decreased melanogenic activity, perhaps due to lack of dopa oxidase activity in the remaining melanocytes (169). Ultrastructurally, the residual melanocytes show marked vacuolization, and the melanosomes are not fully melanized (52). There are fewer melanin granules in the matrix and shaft. The mechanism for these changes is not established, but heredity is a significant factor (127). Loss of melanocytes is thought to occur more rapidly in hair than in skin because the cells proliferate and manufacture melanin at maximal rates during the anagen (growth) phase of the hair cycle, whereas epidermal melanocytes are comparatively inactive throughout their life span. Scalp hair may gray more rapidly than other body hair because the ratio of anagen to telogen is much greater (48).

Eccrine Glands. There is a reduction in both the number and the functional capacity of eccrine glands in aging skin (165). Oberste-Lehn (123) estimated a 15% reduction with aging in eccrine glands at most body sites, excluding the scalp. Histologically, the remaining glands show a disorganization, with shrinkage of secretory cells and dilatation of the lumina (96). Also, lipofuscin, or "aging pigment," accumulates in the secretory cells (23).

Apocrine Glands. The secretory epithelium of aged apocrine glands is thinned with ballooning of the secretory tubules (118). Hurley and Shelley (83) reported an age-associated reduction in apocrine secretion experimentally following intradermal injection of epinephrine. Apocrine glands are known to be stimulated by androgens, and these changes are probably related to reduced production of endogenous androgen with age (97).

Sebaceous Glands. The number of sebaceous glands remains fairly constant with age, although glands may increase somewhat in size (138). Functionally, their output declines about 23% per decade in men and 32% per decade in women (85). Autoradiographic studies have demonstrated reduced cell turnover in sebaceous glands with age (140, 141). These changes, like those in the apocrine glands, may be due to decreased production of adrenal and gonadal androgens in advanced age (46).

Nerves and Nerve Endings. Pacinian and Meissner's corpuscles are the end organs responsible for cutaneous touch perception. Between the second and ninth decades, they are reduced by one-third their original number, as determined histochemically at two different body sites (189). Furthermore, they display greater variations in size and irregularities in structure, although free nerve endings are relatively unchanged (22). Clinically, patients are less sensitive to light touch, vibration, and radiant heat, and hence, they are less capable of reacting appropriately (162). The pain threshold also increases with age (20% in one study; 159). Clearly these changes leave elderly patients much more vulnerable to injury. There are very few histological changes with aging in Merkel's corpuscles or in free nerve endings (22).

Subcutaneous Fat. Subcutaneous fat undergoes aging changes also. Certain body regions are subject to increased fat deposition, including the waist in men and the thighs in women. In contrast, the face, the dorsal aspect of the hands, and the shins lose subcutaneous fat, predisposing these areas to injury following trauma. In addition, loss of subcutaneous fat on the plantar foot increases the risk of ulceration and other foot problems in the elderly. Atrophy of fat in general increases the risk of hypothermia because of the loss of insulative capacity (37).

EXTRINSIC AGING

The environment strongly influences the apparent aging process throughout the body, but this phenomenon is especially evident in the skin (48). The major contributor is sunlight. Another suspected gerontogen (agent capable of mimicking or accelerating aspects of normal aging) is cigarette smoke, interacting with chronic sun exposure in as yet undefined ways. Climactic extremes and various chemical substances are known to accelerate photocarcinogenesis, but their impact on extrinsic aging has not been studied.

Photoaging

Photoaging refers to those changes identified in the habitually sun-exposed skin of older individuals which are the combined result of intrinsic aging and chronic photodamage. The terms "dermatoheliosis" and "heliodermatitis" are also used, the latter implying an inflammatory component. Those with fair complexions, and hence, a minimal melanin barrier to sun damage, are the most vulnerable. In general, following UV injury, skin cells initially respond with hyperplasia, hypertrophy, or increased function, but eventually repeated damage leads to atrophy, reduced function, and/or cell loss (49). For instance, the coarse, pebbly elastosis seen in dark-skinned individuals with extensive sun exposure may represent increased fibroblastic activity. In contrast, light-skinned individuals, who are more vulnerable to severe photodamage, commonly manifest atrophy and pseudoscars due to decreased fibroblast number and protein synthetic capacity. Similarly, early alterations in cutaneous pigmentation include tanning, ephiledes, lentigines, and an increase in melanocyte number, while severely sun-damaged skin often has depigmented areas as well (48). These biphasic changes account for the literature's sometimes contradictory descriptions of histological changes due to photoaging (Table 11.2).

Clinical Features. Features of sun-damaged skin include coarseness, telangectasia, irregular pigmentation, and deep wrinkles or furrows. A variety of benign and malignant neoplasms may also be seen. A National Health and Nutrition Exam Survey involving 20,000 Americans aged 1–74 yr showed a positive association between sun exposure and xerosis, seborrheic keratoses, spider nevi, and superficial varicosities, among other lesions (32). Sun-induced skin damage is estimated to account for greater than 90% of age-associated cosmetic problems in the skin (46). The psychosocial implications of photoaging are apparent in the $20 billion per year cosmetic industry aimed at camouflaging, reversing, or preventing these changes (177).

Histopathology

Elastin and glycosaminoglycans. The most striking histological feature of chronically sun-exposed skin is altered elastic tissue, so-called "elastosis." As we know, in chronological aging, elastic fibers are smaller and more fragmented; in contrast, in photoaging, elastic tissue is increased in amount, initially appearing thickened and tangled and later more granular and amorphous at the ultrastructural level (94). Initially there is an increase in the microfibrillar component of elastin as well as enlargement of the fibers, which later evolves into severe disorganization with a fine granular matrix and homogenous inclusions. In mildly photodamaged skin, elastic fiber diameter increases up to 20-fold, with slight changes in fibrillar ultrastructure. In skin with severe actinic damage, elastic fibers are moth-eaten, with disruption of the normal architecture (16). Also increased with photodamage is the amount of glycosaminoglycans, in contrast to the reduction in sun-protected skin (155).

Collagen. In addition to the increase in elastic tissue and mucopolysaccharides seen in photoaged skin, changes in dermal collagen have also been described. A "grenz" or border zone lies between the dermal elastosis and the epidermis. Initially believed to represent a layer inexplicably spared from UV damage because of its relatively normal light microscopic appearance, it is now known to be comprised of densely packed collagen fibrils and to represent an area of scarring (101). Collagen elsewhere in the dermis decreases in amount (155). Animal studies suggest that collagen may be enzymatically hydrolyzed by the inflammatory cells that infiltrate UV-irradiated skin (100). The dermis demonstrates its earliest and most severe changes in the superficial layer with elastosis later involving the deeper layer consistent with the attenuation of solar energy as it passes through the skin (167).

Microvasculature. The microvasculature is also affected by photoaging. In sun-protected old skin the area of the horizontal vascular plexus is reduced, but vessel morphology is unaffected (54). In photoaged skin, however, the remaining vessels often become dilated and tortuous, perhaps due to the lack of support in the elastotic dermis. Direct injury to the endothelial cells and other components of the vessel wall are also possible. Electron microscopic studies of sun-damaged skin show thickening of the postcapillary venular walls due to concentric deposition of basement membrane–like material synthesized by perivenular veil cells (17), a recognized injury response.

Cellular components. The cellular infiltrate in the dermis differs between sun-protected and sun-exposed regions of the skin. In contrast to the hypocellularity seen in chronological aging (2), the dermis of actinically damaged skin is often characterized by inflammatory cells, numerous mast cells, and hyperplastic fibroblasts (102), particularly on the face (13). It is postulated that the inflammation accompanying UV injury may generate free radicals that further injure other cells, collagen, and the extracellular matrix.

Langerhans cells are reduced in number by approximately 50% in habitually sun-exposed compared to sun-protected skin (28, 55), possibly a perpetuation of the acute, initially reversible changes induced by a single UV exposure.

Keratinocytes in photoaged epidermis show marked irregularities in cell size and staining properties, and

TABLE 11.2. *Chronological Aging vs. Photoaging*

Component	Chronological Aging	Photoaging
Epidermis	Decreased thickness	Variable thickness; nuclear atypia
Dermis		
Fibroblasts	Inactive	Active
Collagen	Decreased	Decreased
Fibers	Thickened	Basophilic degeneration
Solubility	Decreased	Decreased
Synthesis	Decreased	Not known
Elastin	Decreased	Increased
Fibers	Disintegration and degeneration	Abnormal
Microfibrils	Decreased	Increased (early)
Glycosaminoglycans	Decreased	Increased
Inflammatory cells	Generally absent	Increased
Mast cells	Decreased	Increased
Microvasculature	Decreased	Dilated

both keratinocytes and melanocytes in the basal layer have variable levels of nuclear atypia (115).

Pathophysiology. The action spectrum for photoaging is difficult to determine experimentally, primarily because of the long delay between exposure and clinical effects. Epidemiological evidence, however, strongly implicates the short UV portion of sunlight in both photoaging and photocarcinogenesis (89). UVB (290–320 nm) photons, the shortest and most biologically active wavelengths to reach the earth's surface, are established inducers of erythema, DNA damage, and cutaneous neoplasms and presumably cause photoaging as well (98). In mice, large cumulative UVB doses produce elastic hyperplasia and an inflammatory response in the dermis, mimicking photodamage in human skin (98, 99, 155).

UVA (320–400 nm) is 500–1000 times more abundant in sunlight than UVB and penetrates the dermis more deeply because of its longer wavelength (132). In experimental animals, UVA produces less dense elastosis that extends deeper into the dermis than that produced by UVB (98), and both UVA and UVB similarly increase production of mucopolysaccharides. However, the glycosaminoglycans produced by UVB are localized to the upper dermis, whereas those produced by UVA are deposited throughout the dermis (98). Moreover, adults receiving psoralen-photosensitized UVA therapy for psoriasis demonstrate a dose-dependent increase in photoaging within 5 yr in treated skin (193). Thus both UVB and UVA produce photoaging-like changes in animal models, and although UVB is thought to be the primary offender, UVA may also promote photoaging.

Relationship to Skin Cancer. There is a strong epidemiological relationship between chronological aging and neoplasia that is well documented for all organ systems (79, 122). This is equally true in the skin, which shows an exponential increase in cancer incidence after 30 yr of age. However, 90% of these cancers arise in the approximately 10% of skin that is habitually sun-exposed, suggesting that age alone does not strikingly predispose to cancer in the absence of an exogenous carcinogen, in this case UV irradiation. Possible mechanisms include a disruption of proliferative homeostasis (18) or an altered state of differentiation leading to over-responsiveness to growth factors (41, 43, 109), compounded by cumulative environmental damage to the genome.

In the United States, basal cell carcinoma (BCC) and squamous cell carcinoma (SCC) are the leading forms of cancer (59, 185). Experimentally, SCC develop in a dose-dependent manner in animals exposed to UV irradiation (34, 35), and in humans, the incidence of both BCC and SCC increases with decreased latitude and increased sun exposure (3, 26, 43).

UV irradiation both initiates and promotes skin cancer. The multiple hit theory proposes that carcinogenesis is more likely when an individual cell has repeated exposures to a known carcinogen, each of which may produce a mutation; certainly, the number of sun exposures increases with age. With increasing age, however, dysregulation of growth from loss of feedback responsiveness to environmental signals may also contribute to tumor development (124, 134). Some have also postulated a decline in the DNA repair system in the elderly, increasing the risk of a mutagenic event during sun exposure (33, 161, 184). In addition, prolonged latency time with advanced age (182), gradual loss of the protective melanin barrier, and reduced immunosurveilence (36) may contribute to cancer development. The skin thus provides an important and probably underutilized model for examining the relationship between aging and carcinogenesis.

Physical influences may also enhance photocarcinogenesis. Specifically, animals kept in environments where heat is administered concurrently with UV irradiation (UVR) are more prone to develop neoplasms than are animals living in temperate climates (128). The mechanism is unclear, possibly related to biochemical reactions following the photochemical response or an additive injury. In addition, wind and increased humidity may cause acute UVR damage and accelerate tumor formation (129, 130). The cutaneous injury induced by these physical forces may stimulate epidermal hyperplasia, promoting the carcinogenic process. A number of other external chemical carcinogens have also been identified that accelerate carcinogenesis from UVR, including tar, nitrogen mustard, croton oil, and phorbol esters, among others (33).

Cigarette Smoking

Another environmental risk factor for extrinsic cutaneous aging is cigarette smoking. Ippen and Ippen (84) first suggested the connection between smoking and wrinkling by describing the skin of a 40-yr-old smoker and a 70-yr-old nonsmoker as comparable in appearance. More recently, Kadence (90) examined 132 adult smokers and control subjects and found the degree of facial wrinkling directly proportional to cigarette use, independent of age, sex, pigmentation, or previous sun exposure. In addition, the subset of patients with a greater than 50-pack/year history of smoking were almost five times as likely to be severely wrinkled as were nonsmokers. Also, smoking and sun exposure appear to act synergistically in accelerating wrinkles (90, 117). Other aspects of skin aging, such as functional changes, have not been examined with regard to smoking.

Although the exact mechanism by which cigarette smoking worsens wrinkles is still unknown, several theories have been proposed. Alterations in the microvasculature induced by the toxic by-products of cigarette smoke have been shown in several studies (150, 151). This may reduce cutaneous oxygenation and nutrient transfer, possibly impairing connective tissue metabolism and thus increasing wrinkles. Alternatively, cigarette smoke may directly damage connective tissue, as in the lungs where smoking leads to chronic obstructive lung disease. Interestingly, the development of lung cancer in patients has been reported to be inversely related to prior vitamin A consumption, as well as retinol levels (188). Joffe postulates that smoking, by reducing vitamin A levels that otherwise protect against oxygen radical damage, may exacerbate UV-induced skin injury (86). Finally, mechanical factors, such as squinting due to the irritant effects of the smoke, may also contribute to facial wrinkling.

PHYSIOLOGICAL CHANGES

In addition to the morphological and histopathological alterations in the skin associated with aging and photoaging, there is a gradual decline in many of the physiological functions of the skin (Table 11.3). The more extensively studied changes are discussed below.

Barrier Function

Human terrestrial life requires a covering that protects from desiccation, as well as from invasion of foreign substances. The stratum corneum thus plays a dual role, first in regulating water loss to the dry, outside environment and second in acting as a barrier through which exogenous agents must penetrate prior to entry into the human body. Whether or not the functions of transepidermal water loss (TEWL) and percutaneous absorption alter with age has been an area under investigation.

Because skin often appears drier with age, scientists

TABLE 11.3. *Cutaneous Functions that Decline with Age*

Barrier function	Sensory perception
Dermal clearance	Sweat production
Immune clearance	Thermoregulation
Injury response	Vascular response
Sebum production	Vitamin D_3 production

have questioned whether its water-holding capacity deteriorates in time. Initial studies by Kligman (94) demonstrated a reduced TEWL measured on the extensor arm and the lateral leg in a small number of patients. More recently, Potts (142) used transducers to measure the propagation and attenuation of shear waves in the skin and demonstrated that the stratum corneum from older skin has a lower water content than younger skin. Other investigators found a decrease in TEWL by measuring the change in absorbance of monochromatic light (570 nm) after applying cobalt chloride under occlusion for 10 min (175). Confounding variables that may influence TEWL studies include intrinsic factors, such as diminished eccrine activity with age, as well as extrinsic factors, such as humidity and temperature effects.

Early studies in percutaneous absorption of the stratum corneum showed variable results. Christopher (24) demonstrated by residual analysis studies that carbon-14-labeled testosterone applied to the stratum corneum suffered no functional loss in absorption with time. Tagami (175) found that older subjects required 50% longer to absorb fluoroscein-tagged tetrachlorosalycynanilide than younger individuals, suggesting a greater barrier function in the elderly. Guy (153) measured percutaneous absorption of a series of compounds labeled with carbon-14 and found that permeability of lipophilic substances, such as testosterone and estradiol, did not significantly differ with age, in contrast to more hydrophilic substances such as benzoic acid or salicylic acid. He thus concluded that permeability is largely dependent on the physicochemical properties of the substance contacting the skin surface, where those substances which are less lipid-soluble are more severely impacted. The diminished lipid content of older skin (141) offers less medium for dissolution of topically administered agents. In addition, reduced water content (142) of aged stratum corneum likely impairs absorption further for substances that are less lipophilic.

Immune Function

The immune system deteriorates with age (75) presumably leading to the increased incidence of cutaneous infections, certain autoimmune diseases, and neoplasms in the elderly (45, 144). Changes in systemic factors contributing to this loss in immune competence are covered in Chapter 19. The following section reviews only selected findings of direct relevance to the skin, particularly those pertaining to the epidermis itself as a component of the immune system.

Cell-Mediated Immunity. Of the major components of the immune system, T cells are perhaps the most vulnerable to the aging process (71). Partly responsible is the gradual, postpubertal involution of the thymus (107, 167). In addition, shifts within the subpopulations of T cells (10, 108), with greater numbers of T helper cells and fewer suppressor (121) and cytotoxic cells (62), impair function further. These changes are translated clinically into the less vigorous delayed hypersensitivity reactions in the elderly to common antigens, including candida, mumps, and purified protein derivative (152). Also, patients beyond 40 yr of age show a progressive decline in reactivity to the varicella zoster test (19). Patch tests may require 4 days or more rather than the 2–3 days required for standard patch test antigens to demonstrate positive reactivity, with less intense responses (88, 183). In addition, the degree of impairment of cellular immunity as manifested in the skin seems to correlate with survival in that subjects who do not react to any of five recall antigens have decreased survival over a 2-year follow-up period (70). Response to neoantigens is also reduced, perhaps due to the involution of the thymus, with fewer naive T cells produced. In one study, 95% of patients less than 70 yr of age developed contact sensitivity to dinitrochlorbenzene (DNCB), compared with 66% of patients over 70 yr of age (58).

The age-associated decrease in cytotoxic T cells presumably predisposes to reactivation of latent varicella virus infections; the incidence of zoster is ten times higher in the elderly as in the young (106). Older patients show impaired ability to elicit both skin graft rejection (64) and graft vs. host reactions (61).

Humoral Responses. Although the total number of B cells remains unchanged with age (192), their functional capacity lessens in time (131). Changes in regulatory T cells (113), as well as an intrinsic deterioration in B cell function with alterations in subsets of B cells, all contribute to this decline.

Antibody response to neoantigens is reduced with age, particularly for the IgG subset (1). In the skin, immediate hypersensitivity reactions decrease in incidence with age. Fifty-three percent of 20-yr-old subjects responded to at least one antigen in a standard battery of prick tests vs. 16% of patients 75 yr of age (7). In addition, in a subset of patients with a known history of urticarial reaction to penicillin, 69% of patients less than 30 yr old had reproducible positive results on intradermal testing, in contrast to 39% of patients greater than 30 yr old (174). Also decreased in the elderly are radioallergosorbent test (RAST) results for measurement of specific IgE antibody to a variety of allergens (172). Increased production of autoantibodies occurs in older patients (113, 146) and may explain the increased incidence of some autoimmune disorders, such as bullous pemphigoid, within this age group (191).

Epidermal Immune Function. Langerhans cells and keratinocytes produce numerous cytokines and other modulators of immune function (57, 110). Although the impact of age on this aspect of epidermal immune function is virtually unexplored, with increasing donor age, keratinocytes in culture have been shown to produce less interleukin-1 (20, 158).

Langerhans cells, involved in antigen presentation and stimulation of T cells, also produce a substance with IL-1-like activity (157). With advanced age, Langerhans cells decline in number and have shorter and fewer dendrites (54), presumably impairing their immune function.

The skin serves a role analogous to that of the thymus in immune function. As with the thymus, precursor lymphocytes have been shown to migrate between the blood and the skin and to become committed to a specific line of differentiation in the skin (173). Further support for the thymus/skin analogy is the fact that keratinocytes appear to synthesize serum thymic factor (92) and a thymic hormone, thymopoietin (25). Thymic involution, including decreased hormone production, is well documented to occur with aging, (186) but the impact of aging on this aspect of epidermal function has not yet been studied.

Inflammatory Response

Many studies have found that aging individuals are less reactive to noxious stimuli. As discussed previously, positive patch test reactions are generally less severe and slower to evolve in the elderly. Carlizza and Bologna (21) analyzed the blister fluid produced from the application of cantharidin topically and demonstrated fewer inflammatory cells in older subjects. Also, Grove demonstrated attenuated reactions in the elderly to harsh solvents such as croton oil, dimethyl sulfoxide (DMSO), and kerosene (69). UVR also produces less intense inflammation that evolves more slowly with advancing age. In a study that compared young and old subjects' responses to a standard erythemogenic dose, older subjects mounted less of a clinical sunburn reaction and fewer sunburn cells were seen histologically. Also, less histamine and slower prostaglandin E_2 release were found in suction blister aspirates from older skin (54). Because inflammation serves as a warning to avoid noxious stimuli, these results suggest that older subjects are more prone to tissue injury from harmful exposures

Wound Healing

Early in this century, DuNouy (29) reported a nearly linear increase in the time required for healing in World

War I soldiers aged 20–44 yr. Although numerous variables were uncontrolled, including concurrent infections, anatomical sites, and wound depths, more recent observations continue to suggest that healing is delayed with increased age. Grove studied the healing of blisters produced by ammonium hydroxide on the volar forearm and upper arm and found a significant lag in healing time for older subjects at both sites (65, 68). Reepithelialization postdermabrasion takes almost twice as long in elderly patients (126). Tensile strength of wounds also seems to diminish with age. Mendoza (116) reported that the rate of wound dehiscence was 0.9% in persons aged 30–39 yr, 2.5% in those aged 50–59 yr, and 5.5% in those over 70 yr of age.

Wound healing is a complex series of events that can be separated into three stages: inflammation, cellular proliferation, and matrix formation/maturation (27). Following injury to the skin, blood vessels are disrupted, leading to activation of platelets and coagulation pathways. Activated platelets also trigger a variety of other chemotactic factors that promote cell migration and growth. Neutrophils arrive first, followed by monocytes and lymphocytes. The arrival of macrophages marks the transition into the granulation stage. These cells, like neutrophils, scavenge bacteria, but they also digest other debris. Furthermore, they release a variety of biologically active substances, including vasoactive substances, chemotactic growth factors, enzymes, and proteases. Fibroblasts respond to these stimuli by proliferation, migration, and matrix deposition. The matrix produced by the fibroblasts functions as a substrate on which macrophages, new blood vessels, and fibroblasts migrate. Late in the granulation stage, collagen is laid down, increasing the tensile strength of wounds. The final stage, the maturation stage, primarily involves the remodeling of collagen along the lines of tension. Collagen is continually synthesized and broken down. Progressive cross-linking occurs, and covalent bonds form between the collagen fibrils, enhancing the tensile strength further. Gradually, the cellularity and vascularity of the wound diminishes (27).

Aging affects all stages of wound healing. As we have seen, the inflammatory response in the elderly is muted, and hence, the initial stage of the repair process is often compromised. Animal studies show that cell migration and proliferation decline with age. In rat palate burns, peak DNA content is earlier and greater in young animals (39). Holm-Pederson analyzed the specific activity of DNA in wounds using tritiated thymidine and found it to be higher in young animals for the first 7 days (82). Human studies demonstrate that monocytes and fibroblasts migrate to the site of injury 1–2 days earlier in younger subjects (181). The granulation phase is characterized by an age-associated decrease in metabolic activity, as measured by oxygen consumption and glucose metabolism. Viljanto and Raekallio (181) found that levels of isocitrate dehydrogenase and lactate dehydrogenase, key enzymes in glucose metabolism, were higher in younger individuals. Holm-Pederson and Zederfeldt (81) also found increased oxygen consumption in wounds of young animals by demonstrating lower pO_2 values in the dead space of lesions undergoing repair. The rate of capillary ingrowth, as demonstrated by transparent chambers in rat wounds, also decreases with age (190).

Studies focused on the maturation phase have shown similar amounts of collagen in the young and old; however, wound strength is generally reduced with increasing age (80). This is clinically evident in the higher rates of wound dehiscence seen in the elderly postoperatively (30). Animal studies demonstrate increased collagenase activity in wounds of young rats, suggesting that increased remodeling and collagen turnover may produce collagen of greater strength (126). In aged persons, synthesis and remodeling of collagen also decrease. Collagen cross-links are more stable (5), and the amount of glycosylated hydroxylysine decreases with age (120). The resultant collagen is more resistant to catabolism, and tissue remodeling is thus impaired (148).

Vitamin D Production

Vitamin D production is an endocrine function of the skin. In epidermal keratinocytes, provitamin D_3 (7-dehydrocholesterol) absorbs UVB radiation (290 and 315 nm) and is photoconverted to previtamin D_3. A slow process of thermal isomerization subsequently converts previtamin D_3 to vitamin D_3, which is then translocated to the dermal vasculature and transported to the liver and kidney for hydroxylation to $1,25\text{-}(OH)_2$, vitamin D_3, the biologically active form responsible for calcium homeostasis (77).

Aging is associated with a 75% linear decline in concentration of provitamin D_3 per unit skin area. The reduction in provitamin D_3 is due to a decreased rate of production rather than to a decrease in epidermal mass associated with aging (111). In addition, MacLaughlin and Holick (111) showed a marked decline in the capacity of aged skin to photoconvert provitamin D_3 to previtamin D_3 (76). The combination of less available precursor, a decline in synthetic capacity, and less exposure to sunlight predisposes the elderly to vitamin-D_3 deficiency and increased risk of boney fractures secondary to osteomalacia. The elderly also commonly have reduced intake of dairy products, the only dietary source of vitamin D_3. Darkly pigmented subjects are at greater risk, because melanin absorbs the UVB, making it less available for photoconversion of provitamin D_3 (78), although the greater initial bone density characteristic of blacks protects against boney fractures in the elderly.

SUMMARY

The aging process, a phenomenon shared by all living organisms, is the summation of intrinsic and extrinsic forces. Intrinsic skin aging encompasses certain genetically controlled changes, many of which are well described at the clinical and histological levels but generally poorly understood at the molecular level. Superimposed on these alterations are environmental effects, sun exposure and cigarette smoking having the greatest impact. Physiological decline accompanies cutaneous senescence, impacting on the injury response, immunosurveilence, wound healing, vitamin D_3 production, and many other functions. These changes in turn predispose the elderly to injury and various skin diseases. Its easy accessibility, the extensive background data now available both in vivo and in vitro, and the identification of major environmental gerontogens make the skin a valuable model for studies of aging throughout the body.

REFERENCES

1. AMMANN, A. J., G. SCHIFFMAN, and R. AUSTRIAN. The antibody responses to pneumococcal capsular polysaccharides in aged individuals. *Proc. Soc. Exp. Biol. Med.* 164: 312–317, 1980.
2. ANDREW, W., R. H. BEHNKE, and T. SATO. Changes with advancing age in the cell population of the human dermis. *Gerontologia* 10: 1–19, 1964.
3. AUERBACH, H. Geographic variation in incidence of skin cancer in the United States. *Public Health Rep.* 7: 143–171, 1982.
4. AZIZKHAM, R. B., J. C. AZIZKHAM, and B. R. ZETTER. Mast cell heparin stimulates migration of capillary endothelial cells in vitro. *J. Exp. Med.* 152: 931–944, 1980.
5. BAILEY, A. J., S. P. ROBINS, and G. BALIAN. Biological significance of the intermolecular crosslinks of collagen. *Nature* 251: 105–109, 1974.
6. BAKER, H., and C. P. BLAIR. Cell replacement in the human stratum corneum. *Br. J. Dermatol.* 80: 367–372, 1968.
7. BARBEE, R. A. Immediate skin test reactivity in a general population sample. *Ann. Intern. Med.* 84: 129–133, 1976.
8. BARMAN, J. M., V. PERCORARO, and I. ASTORE. Biological bases of the inception and evolution of baldness. *J. Gerontol.* 24: 163–170, 1969.
9. BEAUREGARD, S., and B. A. GILCHREST. A survey of skin problems and skin care regimens in the elderly. *Arch. Dermatol.* 123: 1638–1643, 1987.
10. BECKER, M. J., R. FARKO, and M. SCHNEIDER. Cell mediated cytotoxicity in humans: age related decline as measured by xenographic assay. *Clin. Immunol. Immunopathol.* 14: 204–210, 1979.
11. BENTLEY, J. P. Aging of collagen. *J. Invest. Dermatol.* 73: 80–83, 1979.
12. BESDINE, R. W. Geriatric medicine: an overview. In: *Annual Review of Gerontology and Geriatrics.* edited by C. Eisdorfer. New York: Springer, 1979, p. 135.
13. BHAWAN, J., C. OH, R. LEW, K. NEHAL, R. LABADIE, A. TSAY, and B. A. GILCHREST. Histopathological differences in the photoaging process in facial versus arm skin. *Am. J. Dermatopathol.* 14: 224–230, 1992.
14. BIANCO, C., and V. NUSSENZWEIG. Complement receptors. *Contemp. Top. Mol. Immunol.* 6: 145–176, 1977.
15. BLACK, M. M. A modified radiographic method for measuring skin thickness. *Br. J. Derm.* 72: 67–76, 1969.
16. BRAVERMAN, I. M., and E. FONFERKO. Studies in cutaneous aging: I. The elastic fiber network. *J. Invest. Dermatol.* 78: 434–443, 1982a.
17. BRAVERMAN, I. M., and E. FONFERKO. Studies in cutaneous aging II. The microvasculature. *J. Invest. Dermatol.* 78: 444–448, 1982b.
18. BULLOUGH, W. S., and E. B. LAWRENCE. Chalones and cancer. *Nature* 220: 134–135, 1968.
19. BURKE, B. L., R. W. STEEL, and O. W. BEARD. Immune responsiveness to varicella-zoster in the aged. *Arch. Intern. Med.* 142: 291–293, 1982.
20. BURLEY-ROSSET, M., and I. JERGNON. Interleukin-1 synthesis and activity in aged mice. *Mech. Ageing Dev.* 24: 247–264, 1984.
21. CARLIZZA, L., and E. BOLOGNA. Variagioni della reativata cutana in rapporto con leta. *Bull. Soc. Ital. Biol. Sper.* 41: 344–348, 1965.
22. CAUNA, N. The effects of aging on the receptor organs of the human dermis. In: *Advances in the Biology of the Skin,* edited by W. Montagna. Oxford: Pergamon Press, 1965, vol. 6, p. 63.
23. CAWLEY, E. P., Y. T. HSU, and B. C. STURGILL. Lipofuscin ("wear and tear pigment") in human sweat glands. *J. Invest. Dermatol.* 61: 105–107, 1973.
24. CHRISTOPHERS, E., and A. M. KLIGMAN. Percutaneous absorption in aged skin. In: *Advances in the Biology of the Skin.* edited by W. Montagna. Oxford: Pergamon Press, 1965, vol. II, p. 163–175.
25. CHU, A. C., J. A. K. PATTERSON, and G. GOLDSTEIN. Thymopoetin-like substance in human skin. *J. Invest. Dermatol.* 81: 194–197, 1983.
26. CICERONE, R. J. Changes in stratopheric ozone. *Science* 237: 35–42, 1987.
27. CLARK, R. A. F. Cutaneous tissue repair: basic biological considerations. Part 1. *J. Am. Acad. Dermatol.* 13: 701–725, 1985.
28. DELO, V. A., L. DAWES, and R. JACKSON. Density of Langerhans cells (LC) in normal vs. chronic actinically damaged skin (CADS) of humans. *J. Invest. Dermatol.* 76: 330–334, 1981.
29. DUNOUY, P., and A. CARRELL. Cicatrization of wounds. *J. Exp. Biol.* 34: 339–348, 1921.
30. EAGLSTEIN, W. H. Wound healing and aging. In: *Clinics in Geriatric Medicine,* edited by B. A. Gilchrest. Philadelphia: W. B. Saunders, 1989, p. 183–187.
31. EDICK, G. F., and A. J. T. MILLIS. Fibronectin distribution on the surfaces of young and old human fibroblasts. *Mech. Ageing Dev.* 27: 249–256, 1984.
32. ENGEL, A., M. L. JOHNSON, and S. G. HAYNES. Health effects of sunlight exposure in the United States. *Arch. Dermatol.* 124: 72–79, 1988.
33. EPSTEIN, J. H. Photocarcinogenesis, skin cancer, and aging. *J. Am. Acad. Dermatol.* 9: 487–502, 1983.
34. EPSTEIN, J. H., and W. L. EPSTEIN. A study of tumor types produced by ultraviolet light in hairless and hairy mice. *J. Invest. Dermatol.* 41: 463–473, 1963.
35. EPSTEIN, J. H., K. FUKUYAMA, and W. L. EPSTEIN. UVL-induced stimulation of DNA synthesis in hairless mice epidermis. *J. Invest. Dermatol.* 51: 445–451, 1968.
36. ERSCHLER, W. G. The influence of an aging immune system on cancer incidence and progression. *J. Gerontol.* 48: B3–B7, 1993.

37. FENSKE, N. A., and C. W. LOBER. Structural and functional changes of normal aging skin. *J. Am. Acad. Dermatol.* 15: 571–585, 1986.
38. FLEISCHMAJER, R. Human dermal glycosaminoglycans and aging. *Biochim. Biophys. Acta* 279: 265–275, 1972.
39. FORSCHER, B. K., and H. C. CECIL. Some effects of age on the biochemistry of acute inflammation. *Gerontologia* 2: 174–182, 1958.
40. FRANCES, C., and L. ROBERT. Elastin and elastic fibers in normal and pathologic skin. *Int. J. Dermatol.* 23: 166–179, 1984.
41. GARMYN, M., M. YAAR, N. BOILEAU, C. BACKENDORF, and B. A. GILCHREST. Effect of aging and habitual sun exposure on the genetic response of cultured human keratinocytes to solar-simulated irradiation. *J. Invest. Dermatol.* 99: 743–748, 1992.
42. GIACOMETTI, L. The anatomy of the human scalp. In: *Advances in the Biology of the Skin.* edited by W. Montagna. Oxford: Pergamon Press, 1965, vol. 6, p. 97–104.
43. GILCHREST, B. A. Age associated changes in the skin. *J. Geriat. Soc.* 30: 139–143, 1982.
44. GILCHREST, B. A. In vitro assessment of keratinocyte aging. *J. Invest. Dermatol.* 81: 184s–189s, 1983.
45. GILCHREST, B. A. *Skin and Aging Process.* Boca Raton, FL: CRC Press, 1984, p. 124.
46. GILCHREST, B. A. Aging. *J. Am. Acad. Dermatol.* 11: 995–997, 1984.
47. GILCHREST, B. A. In vitro studies of aging human epidermis. *Rev. Biol. Res. Aging.* 4: 281–289, 1990.
48. GILCHREST, B. A. Physiology and pathophysiology of aging skin. In: *Physiology, Biochemistry and Molecular Biology of the Skin* (2nd ed.), edited by L. Goldsmith. New York: Oxford University Press, 1991, p. 1425–1442.
49. GILCHREST, B. A. The variable face of photoaging: influence of skin type. *Cosmetics Toiletries* 107: 41–42, 1992.
50. GILCHREST, B. A., and P. S. FRIEDMANN. A culture system for the study of human melanocyte physiology. In: *Structure and Function of Melanin.* edited by K. Jimbow. Sapparo, Japan: Fujishoin 1986, vol. 4, p. 1–13.
51. GILCHREST, B. A., and M. YAAR. Ageing and photoageing of the skin: observations at the cellular and molecular level. *Br. J. Dermatol.* 127 (suppl. 41: 25–30, 1992.
52. GILCHREST, B. A., F. B. BLOG, and G. SZABO. Effects of aging and chronic sun exposure on melanocytes in human skin. *J. Invest. Dermatol.* 73: 141–143, 1979.
53. GILCHREST, B. A., G. MURPHY, and N. A. SOTER. Effect of chronological aging and ultraviolet irradiation on Langerhans cells in the human epidermis. *J. Invest. Dermatol.* 79: 85–88, 1982.
54. GILCHREST, B. A., J. S. STOFF, and N. A. SOTER. Chronologic aging alters the response to UV-induced inflammation in human skin. *J. Invest. Dermatol.* 79: 11–15, 1982.
55. GILCHREST, B. A., G. SZABO, E. FLYNN, and R. M. GOLDWYN. Chronologic and actinically induced aging in human facial skin. *J. Invest. Dermatol.* 80: 81s–85s, 1983.
56. GILCHREST, B. A., M. A. VRABEL, E. S. FLYNN, and G. SZABO. Selective cultivation of human melanocytes from newborn and adult epidermis. *J. Invest. Dermatol.* 83: 370–376, 1984.
57. GILMAN, S. C., Lymphokines in immunologic aging. *Lymphokine Res.* 3: 119–123, 1984.
58. GIRARD, J. P., M. PAYCHERE, and M. CUEVAS. Cell mediated immunity in an aging population. *Clin. Exp. Immunol.* 27: 85–91, 1977.
59. GLASS, A. G., and R. N. HOOVER. The emerging epidemic of melanoma and squamous cell cancer. *JAMA* 262: 2097–2100, 1989.
60. GOLDSTEIN, S. Replicative senescence: the human fibroblast comes of age. *Science* 249: 1129–1133, 1990.

61. GOODMAN, S. A., and T. MAKINODAN. Effect of age on cell mediated immunity in long lived mice. *Clin. Exp. Immunol.* 19: 533–542, 1975.
62. GOTTESMAN, S. R. S., R. L. WALFORD, and G. J. THORNBECKE. Proliferation and cytotoxic immune functions in aging mice: II. Decreased generation of specific suppressor cells in alloreactive cultures. *J. Immunol.* 133: 1782–1787, 1984.
63. GRAHAM, J. A., and A. M. KLIGMAN. Physical attractiveness, cosmetic use, and self-perception in the elderly. *Int. J. Cosmetic Sci.* 7: 85–98, 1985.
64. GREENBERG, L. J., and E. J. YUNIS. Immunological control of aging: a possible primary event. *Gerontologica* 18: 247–266, 1977.
65. GROVE, G. L. Age related differences in healing of superficial skin wounds in humans. *Arch. Dermatol.* 272: 381–385, 1982.
66. GROVE, G. Age associated changes in the replacement rates of exfoliated corneocytes in normal human skin. In: *Cutaneous Aging,* edited by A. M. Kligman and Y. Takase. Tokyo: University of Tokyo Press, 1988, p. 185.
67. GROVE, G. L., and A. M. KLIGMAN. Age associated changes in human epidermal cell renewal. *J. Gerontol.* 38: 137–142, 1983.
68. GROVE, G. L., S. DUNCAN, and A. M. KLIGMAN. Effect of aging on the blistering of human skin with ammonium hydroxide. *Br. J. Dermatol.* 107: 393–400, 1982.
69. GROVE, G. L., R. M. LAVKER, E. HOELZLE, and A. M. KLIGMAN. Use of noninvasive tests to monitor age associated changes in human skin. *J. Soc. Cosmetic Chem.* 32: 15–26, 1981.
70. HALLGREN, H. M., C. E. BUCKLEY, and V. A. GILBERTSON. Lymphocyte phytohemagglutinin responsiveness, immunoglobulins, and autoantibodies in aging humans. *J. Immunol.* 111: 1101–1111, 1973.
71. HALLGREN, H. M., J. H. VERSEY, L. J. GREENBERG, and E. J. YUNIS. T and B cells in aging humans. *Federation Proc.* 33: 646–647, 1981.
72. HAYFLICK, L. The limited in vitro lifetime of human diploid cell strains. *Exp. Cell Res.* 37: 614–636, 1965.
73. HAYFLICK, L., and P. S. MOORHEAD. The serial cultivation of human diploid cell strains. *Exp. Cell Res.* 25: 585–621, 1961.
74. HILL, W. R., and H. MONTGOMERY. Regional changes and changes caused by age in normal skin. *J. Invest. Dermatol.* 3: 321–345, 1940.
75. HIROKOWA, K. Aging and the immune system. In: *Cutaneous Aging,* edited by A. M. Kligman and Y. Takase. Tokyo: University of Tokyo Press, 1988, p. 69.
76. HOLICK, M. F., and J. MACLAUGHLIN. Aging decreases the capacity of human skin to produce vitamin D_3. *J. Clin. Invest.* 76: 1536–1538, 1985.
77. HOLICK, M. F., J. A. MACLAUGHLIN, M. B. CLARK, J. T. POTTS, R. R. ANDERSON, I. H. BLANK, and J. A. PARRISH. Photosynthesis of previtamin D3 in human skin and the physiological consequences. *Science* 210: 203–205, 1980.
78. HOLICK, M. F., J. A. MACLAUGHLIN, and S. H. DOPPELT. Regulation of cutaneous previtamin D3 photosynthesis in man: skin pigment is not an essential regulator. *Science* 211: 501–503, 1981.
79. HOLMES, F. F., J. WILSON, K. S. BLESCH, P. R. KAESBERG, R. MILLER, and R. SPROTT. Biology of cancer and aging. *Cancer* 68: 2525–2526, 1991.
80. HOLM-PEDERSON, P., and B. ZEDERFELDT. Granulation tissue formation in subcutaneously implanted cellulose sponges in young and old rats. *Scand. J. Plast. Reconstr. Surg.* 5: 13–16, 1971.
81. HOLM-PEDERSON, P., and B. ZEDERFELDT. Respiratory gas tensions and blood flow in young and old rats. *Scand. J. Plast. Reconstr. Surg.* 7: 91–96, 1973.
82. HOLM-PEDERSON, P., A. M. FENSTAD, and L. E. A. FOLKE.

DNA, RNA, and protein synthesis in healing wounds in young and old mice. *Mech. Ageing Dev.* 3: 173–185, 1974.
83. HURLEY, J. H., and W. B. SHELLEY. *The Apocrine Sweat Gland in Health and Disease.* Springfield, IL: Charles C Thomas, 1960.
84. IPPEN, M., and H. IPPEN. Approaches to a prophylaxis of skin aging. *J. Soc. Cosmetic Chem.* 16: 305–308, 1965.
85. JACOBSON, E., J. BILLINGS, R. FRANTZ, C. KINNEY, M. STEWART, and D. DOWNING. Age related changes in sebaceous wax ester secretion rates in men and women. *J. Invest. Dermatol.* 85: 483–485, 1985.
86. JOFFE, I. Cigarette smoking and facial wrinkling. *Ann. Intern Med.* 115: 659, 1991.
87. JOHNSON, M. L. T., and J. ROBERTS. *Prevalence of Dermatological Disease among Persons 1–74 Years of Age: United States Advanced Data No. 4.* Washington: USDHEW, 1977.
88. JONES, P. G., C. A. KAUFMAN, and A. G. BERGMAN. Fever in the elderly: production of leukocyte pyrogen by monocytes from elderly persons. *Gerontology* 30: 182–187, 1984.
89. JUNG, E. G., and E. BOHNERT. Lichtbiologie der Haut. In: *Jadassohn, Handbuch der Haut-und Beschlechtskrankheiten, Vol I/4.* Berlin: Springer, 1979.
90. KADENCE, D. P., R. BURR, R. GRESS R, R. KANNER, J. LYON, and J. ZONE. Cigarette smoking: a significant risk factor for premature facial wrinkling. *Ann. Intern. Med.* 114: 840–844, 1991.
91. KAPLAN, M. M., P. GORDON, C. PAN, J. LESS, and B. A. GILCHREST. Keratinocytes convert thyroxine to triiodothyronine. *Ann. N. Y. Acad. Sci.* 548: 56–65, 1988.
92. KATO, K., S. I. KEYAMA, and M. TAKOWKI. Epithelial cell components: immunoreactants with antiserum thymic factor (FTS): possible association with intermediate filaments. *Cell* 24: 885–895, 1981.
93. KAWAMOTO, T., M. NISHI, K. TAKAHASHI, T. NISHIYAMA, J. D. SATO, and S. TANIYUCHI. Stimulation by transforming growth factor-beta of epidermal growth factor-dependent growth of aged fibroblasts: recovery of high affinity ECF receptors and growth stimulation by EGF. *In Vitro Cell Dev. Biol.* 25: 965–970, 1989.
94. KLIGMAN, A. M. Early destructive effects of sunlight on human skin. *JAMA* 210: 2377–2380, 1969.
95. KLIGMAN, A. M. Perspectives and problems in cutaneous gerontology. *J. Invest. Dermatol.* 73: 39–46, 1979.
96. KLIGMAN, A. M., and A. K. BALIN. Aging of human skin. In: *Aging and the Skin,* edited by A. K. Balin and A. M. Kligman. New York: Raven Press, 1989, p. 1–19.
97. KLIGMAN, A. M., G. L. GROVE, and A. K. BALIN. Aging of human skin. In: *Handbook of the Biology of Aging,* edited by C. E. Finch and E. L. Schneider. New York: Van Nostrand Reinhold p. 820–841, 1985.
98. KLIGMAN, L. H. Photoaging: manifestations, prevention and treatment. In: *Clinics in Geriatric Dermatology,* edited by B. A. Gilchrest. Philadelphia: WB Saunders, 1989 vol. 5, p. 235–251.
99. KLIGMAN, L. H. The ultraviolet-irradiated hairless mouse: a model for photoaging. *J. Am. Acad. Dermatol.* 21: 623–631, 1989.
100. KLIGMAN, L. H., F. J. AKIN, and A. M. KLIGMAN. The contributions of UVA and UVB to connective tissue damage in hairless mice. *J. Invest. Dermatol.* 84: 272–276, 1985.
101. LAVKER, R. M. Structural alterations in exposed and unexposed skin. *J. Invest. Dermatol.* 73: 59–66, 1979.
102. LAVKER, R. M., and A. M. KLIGMAN. Chronic heliodermatitis: a morphologic evaluation of chronic actinic damage with emphasis on the role of mast cells. *J. Invest. Dermatol.* 90: 325, 1988.
103. LAVKER, R. M., and T. T. SUN. Heterogeneity in epidermal basal keratinocyte morphological and functional correlations. *Science* 215: 1239–1241, 1982.
104. LAVKER, R. M., P. ZHENG, and G. F. DONG. Aged skin: a study by light, transmission electron, and scanning electron microscopy. *J. Invest. Dermatol.* 88: 44s–51s, 1987.
105. LAVKER, R. M., P. ZHENG, and G. F. DONG. Morphology of aged skin. In: *Geriatric Derm,* edited by B. A. Gilchrest. Philadelphia: WB Saunders, 1989, p. 53.
106. LEVIN, M. J., M. MURRAY, H. A. ROTBART, G. O. ZERBE, C. J. WHITE, and A. R. HAYWARD. Immune response of elderly individuals to a live attenuated varicella vaccine. *J. Infect. Dis.* 166: 253–259, 1992.
107. LEWIS, V. M., J. J. TWOMEY, and P. BEALMEAR. Age thymic involution and circulatory thymic hormone activity. *J. Clin. Metab.* 47: 145, 1978.
108. LIU, J. J., M. SEGRE, and D. SEGRE. Changes in suppressor, helper and B cell function in aging mice. *Cell Immunol.* 66: 372–382, 1982.
109. LOWE, N. J., A. K. VERMA, and R. K. BOUTWELL. Ultraviolet light induces ornithine decarboxylase activity. *J. Invest. Dermatol.* 71: 417–418, 1978.
110. LUGER, T. A., and T. SCHWARZ. Therapeutic use of cytokines in dermatology. *J. Am. Acad. Dermatol.* 24: 915–926, 1991.
111. MACLAUGHLIN, J. A., and M. F. HOLICK. Aging decreases the capacity of human skin to produce vitamin D3. *J. Clin. Invest.* 76: 1536–1538, 1985.
112. MAIZE, J. C., and G. FOSTER. Age related changes in melanocytic nevi. *Clin. Exp. Dermatol.* 4: 49–55, 1979.
113. MAKINODAN, T., and M. M. B. KAY. Age influence on the immune system. *Adv. Immunol.* 29: 287–330, 1980.
114. MARKS, R. Measurement of biological aging in the human epidermis. *Br. J. Dermatol.* 104: 627–633, 1981.
115. MARTIN, G. M., C. A. SPRAGUE, and C. J. EPSTEIN. Replicative lifespan of cultivated human cells: effect of donor's age, tissue, and genotype. *Lab. Invest.* 23: 86–92, 1970.
116. MENDOZA, C. B., R. W. POSTLETHWIT, and W. D. JOHNSON. Incidence of wound disruption following operation. *Arch. Surg.* 101: 396–398, 1970.
117. MODEL, D. Smoker's faces: who are the smokers? *Br. J. Med.* 291: 1755, 1985.
118. MONTAGNA, W. W. Morphology of the aging skin: cutaneous appendages. In: *Advances in the Biology of the Skin,* edited by W. Montagna. Oxford: Pergamon Press, 1965, vol. 6, p. 1–16.
119. MONTAGNA, W., and K. CARLISLE. Structural changes in aging human skin. *J. Invest. Dermatol.* 73: 47–53, 1979.
120. MURAI, A., T. MIYAHAWA, and S. SHIOZAWA. Age related variation in glycosylation of hydroxylysine in human and rat skin collagen. *Biochim. Biophys. Acta* 498: 132–142, 1977.
121. NAGEL, J. E., F. J. CHREST, and W. W. H. ADLER. Enumeration of T lymphocyte subsets by monoclonal antibodies in young and aged humans. *J. Immunol.* 127: 2086–2088, 1981.
122. NEWELL, G. R., M. R. SPITZ, and J. G. SIDER. Cancer and age. *Semin. Oncol.* 16: 3–9, 1989.
123. OBERSTE-LEHN, H. Effects of aging on the papillary body of the hair follicles and on eccrine sweat glands. In: *Advances in the Biology of the Skin,* edited by W. Montagna. Oxford: Pergamon Press, 1965, vol 6, p. 17–34.
124. O'BRIEN, D. H. The induction of ornithine decarboxylase as an early possibly obligatory event in mouse skin carcinogenesis. *Cancer Res.* 36: 2644–2653, 1976.
125. O'DELL, B. L., T. JESSEN, L. E. BECKER, R. T. JACKSON, and E. B. SMITH. Diminished immune response in sun damaged skin. *Arch. Dermatol.* 116: 559–561, 1980.
126. ORENTREICH, N., and V. J. SELMANOWITZ. Levels of biological functions with aging. *Trans. N. Y. Acad. Sci.* 231: 993–1012, 1969.

127. ORTONNE, J. P. Pigmentary changes in aging skin. *Br. J. Dermatol.* 122(suppl. 35): 21–28, 1990.
128. OWEN, D. W., and J. M. KNOX. Influence of heat, wind, and humidity on ultraviolet radiation injury. *Nat. Cancer Inst. Monogr.* 50: 161–167, 1978.
129. OWEN, D. W., J. M. KNOX, and H. T. HUDSON. Influence of wind on ultraviolet injury. *Arch. Dermatol.* 109: 200–201, 1974.
130. OWEN, D. W., J. M. KNOX, and H. T. HUDSON. Influence of humidity on ultraviolet injury. *J. Invest. Dermatol.* 64: 250–252, 1975.
131. PACHWA, S. G., R. N. PAHWA, and R. A. GOOD. Decreased in vitro humoral response in aged humans. *J. Clin. Invest.* 67: 1094, 1102, 1981.
132. PARRISH, J. A., R. R. ANDERSON, F. URBACH, and D. PITTS. *UVA: Biological Effects of Ultraviolet Radiation with Emphasis on Human Responses to Long Wave Ultraviolet.* New York: Plenum Publishing, 1978, p. 7–14, 65–73.
133. PARRISH, J. A., K. F. JAENICKE, and A. A. ANDERSON. Erythema and melanogenesis, action spectra of normal human skin. *Photochem. Photobiol.* 36: 187–191, 1982.
134. PAZMINO, N. H., and J. M. YUHAS. Senescent loss of resistance to murine sarcoma virus (moloney) in the mouse. *Cancer Res.* 33: 2668–2672, 1973.
135. PEACOCKE, M., M. YAAR, and B. A. GILCHREST. Interferon and the epidermis: implications for cellular senescence. *Exp. Gerontol.* 24: 415–421, 1989.
136. PHILLIPS, P. D., and V. J. CRISTOFALO. A review of recent research on cellular aging in culture. In: *Review of Biological Research in Aging*, edited by M. Rothstein. New York: Alan R. Liss, p. 385–415, 1987.
137. PLEWIG, G. Regional differences in cell sizes in the human stratum corneum. Part II Effects of age and sex on skin. *J. Invest. Dermatol.* 54: 19–23, 1970.
138. PLEWIG, G., and A. M. KLIGMAN. Proliferative activity of the sebaceous glands of the aged. *J. Invest. Dermatol.* 70: 314–317, 1978.
139. PLISKO, A., and B. A. GILCHREST. Growth factor responsiveness of cultured human fibroblast declines with age. *J. Gerontol.* 38: 513–518, 1983.
140. POCHI, P. E., and J. S. STRAUSS. The effect of aging on the activity of the sebaceous gland in man. In: *Advances in the Biology of the Skin,* edited by W. Montagna. Oxford: Pergamon Press Inc., 1965, vol. 6, p. 121–127.
141. POCHI, P. E., J. S. STRAUSS, and D. T. DOWNING. Age related changes in sebaceous gland activity. *J. Invest. Dermatol.* 73: 108–111, 1979.
142. POTTS, R. O., and M. L. FRANCOEUR. The influence of stratum corneum morphology on water permeability. *J. Invest. Dermatol.* 96: 495–499, 1991.
143. PRAEGER, B. In vitro studies of aging. *Dermatol. Clin.* 4: 359–369, 1986.
144. PRICE, G. B., and T. MAKINDDAN. Immunologic deficiencies in senescence. II Characterization of extrinsic deficiencies. *J. Immunol.* 108: 413–117, 1972.
145. QUEVEDO, W. C., G. SZABO, and J. VIRKS. Influence of age and UV on the populations of DOPA-positive melanocytes in human skin. *J. Invest. Dermatol.* 52: 287–290, 1969.
146. RADL, J., J. M. SEPUS, and I. SKVARIL. Immunologlobulin patterns in humans over 95 years of age. *Clin. Exp. Immunol.* 22: 84–90, 1975.
147. RASMUSSEN, D. M., K. G. WAKIM, and R. K. WINKELMANN. Effect of aging on human dermis: studies in thermal shrinkage and tension. In: *Advances in the Biology of the Skin,* edited by W. Montagna. Oxford: Pergamon Press, 1965, vol. 6, p. 151–162.

148. REED, B. R., and R. A. F. CLARK. Cutaneous tissue repair: practical implications of current knowledge. II. *J. Am. Acad. Dermatol.* 13: 919–936, 1985.
149. REENSTRA, W. R., M. YAAR, and B. A. GILCHREST. The effect of donor age on epidermal growth factor processing in man. *Exp. Cell Res.* (in press), 1994.
150. REES, T. D., D. M. LIVERETT, and C. L. GUY. The effect of cigarette smoking on skin-flap survival in the face lift patient. *Plast. Reconstr. Surg.* 73: 911–915, 1984.
151. REUS, W. F., M. C. ROBSON, L. ZACHERY, and J. P. HEGGERS. Acute effects of tobacco smoking on blood flow in the cutaneous micro-circulation. *Br. J. Plast. Surg.* 37: 213–215, 1984.
152. ROBERTS-THOMPSON, I. C., S. WHITTINGHAM, O. YOUNGCHAIYUD, and I. R. MACKAY. Aging, immune response and mortality. *Lancet* 2: 368–370, 1974.
153. ROSKOS, K. V., H. I. MAIBACH, and R. H. GUY. The effect of aging on percutaneous absorption in man. *J. Pharmacol. Biopharmacol.* 17: 617–630, 1989.
154. SAMS, W. M., JR., and J. G. SMITH, JR. Alterations in human dermal fibrous connective tissue with age and chronic sun damage. In: *Advances in the Biology of the Skin,* edited by W. Montagna. Oxford: Pergamon Press, 1965, vol. 6, p. 199–210.
155. SAMS, W. M., JR., J. G. SMITH, JR., and P. G. BURK. The experimental production of elastosis with ultraviolet light. *J. Invest. Dermatol.* 43: 467–471, 1964.
156. SAUDER, D. N., C. S. CARTER, and S. I. KATZ. Epidermal cell production of thymocyte activating factor (ETAF). *J. Invest. Dermatol.* 79: 34–39, 1982.
157. SAUDER, D. N., C. A. DINARELLO, and V. B. MORHENN. Langerhan cell production of Interleukin 1. *J. Invest. Dermatol.* 82: 605–607, 1984.
158. SAUDER, D. N., B. M. STANULIS-PRAGER, and B. A. GILCHREST. Autocrine growth stimulation of human keratinocytes by epidermal cell-derived thymocyte activating factor: implications for skin aging. *Arch. Dermatol. Res.* 280: 71–76, 1988.
159. SCHULDERMANN, E., and J. P. ZUBECK. Effect of age on pain sensitivity. *Percept. Mot. Skills* 14: 295, 1964.
160. SELMANOWITZ, V. J., K. L. RIZER, and N. ORENTREICH. Aging of the skin and its appendages. In: *Handbook of the Biology of Aging,* edited by C. E. Finch and L. Hayflick. New York: Van Nostrand Reinhold, 1977, p. 496.
161. SETLOW, R. B. DNA repair, aging and cancer. *Nat. Cancer Monogr.* 60: 249–55, 1982.
162. SHERMAN, E. D., and E. ROBILLARD. Sensitivity of pain in relationship to age. *J. Am. Geriatr. Soc.* 12: 1037–1040, 1964.
163. SHUSTER, S., M. M. BLACK, and E. MCVITIE. The influence of age and sex on skin thickness, skin collagen, and density. *Br. J. Dermatol.* 93: 639–643, 1975.
164. SIBERT, J. E. Mucopolysaccharides of ground substances. In: *Dermatology in General Medicine* (2nd ed.), edited by T. B. Fitzpatrick, A. Eisen, K. Wolff, I. Freedberg, K. Austin. New York: McGraw-Hill, 1979, p. 189.
165. SILVER, A. F., W. MONTAGNA, and I. KARACAN. The effect of age on human eccrine sweating. In: *Advances in the Biology of the Skin,* edited by W. Montagna. Oxford: Pergamon Press, 1965, vol. 6, p. 129–150.
166. SINGH, J., and A. K. SINGH. Age related changes in the human thymus. *Clin. Exp. Immunol.* 37: 507–511, 1979.
167. SMITH, J. G., E. A. DAVIDSON, W. M. SAMS, and R. D. CLARK. Alterations in human dermal connective tissue with age and chronic sun damage. *J. Invest. Dermatol.* 39: 347–350, 1962.
168. SNIDER, S. L., and R. R. KOHN. Effects of age and diabetes mellitus on the solubility and nonenzymatic glycosylation of human skin collagen. *J. Clin. Invest.* 67: 1630–1635, 1981.
169. SOLOMON, L. M., and C. VIRTUE. The biology of cutaneous aging. *Int. J. Dermatol.* 14: 172–181, 1975.

170. STANULIS-PRAEGER, B. M., M. YAAR, and G. REDZINIAK. An extract of bovine thymus stimulates human keratinocyte growth in vitro. *J. Invest. Dermatol.* 90: 749–754, 1988.
171. STERN, R. S., M. L. JOHNSON, and J. DELOZIER. Utilization of physician services for dermatological complaints. *Arch. Dermatol.* 113: 1062–1066, 1977.
172. STOY, P. J., B. ROITMAN-JOHNSON, and G. WALSH. Aging and serum immunoglobulin E levels, immediate skin tests, and RAST. *J. Allergy Clin. Immunol.* 68: 421–426, 1981.
173. STREILEIN, J. W. Skin-associated lymphoid tissues (SALT): origins and functions. *J. Invest. Dermatol.* 71: 167–171, 1978.
174. SULLIVAN, T. J., H. J. WEDNER, G. S. SHATZ, L. D. YECIES, and C. W. PARKER. Skin testing to detect penicillin allergy. *J. Allergy Clin. Immunol.* 68: 171–174, 1981.
175. TAGAMI, H. Functional characteristics of aged skin. *Acta Dermatol. (Kyoto)* 66: 19–21, 1972.
176. TAN, C. Y., B. STATHAM, R. MARKS, and P. A. PAYNE. Skin thickness measurement by pulsed ultrasound: its reproducibility, validation, and variability. *Br. J. Dermatol.* 106: 657–662, 1982.
177. TAYLOR, C. R., R. S. STERN, J. J. LEYDEN, and B. A. GILCHREST. Photoaging/photodamage and photoprotection. *J. Am. Acad. Dermatol.* 22: 1–15, 1990.
178. UITTO, J. A method for studying collagen biosynthesis in human skin biopsies in vitro. *Biochim. Biophys. Acta* 210: 438–445, 1970.
179. UITTO, J., M. J. FAZIO, and D. R. OLSEN. Molecular mechanisms of cutaneous aging. *J. Am. Acad. Dermatol.* 21: 614–622, 1989.
180. UITTO, J., J. HALMEE, M. HANNUKSELA, P. PELTOKALLIO, and K. I. KIVINKKO. Protocollagen proline hydroxylase activity in the skin of normal human subjects and of patients with scleroderma. *Scand. J. Clin. Lab. Invest.* 23: 241–247, 1969.
181. VILJANTO, J., and J. RAEKALLIO. Wound healing in children as assessed by the CELLSTIC method. *J. Pediatr. Surg.* 11: 43–49, 1976.
182. VOGELSTEIN, B., E. R. FEARON, S. R. HAMILTON, S. E. KERN, B. A. PREISINGER, M. LEPPERT, Y. NAKAMURAM, R. WHITE, A. M. M. SMITS, and J. L. BOS. Genetic alterations during colorectal tumor development. *N. Engl. J. Med.* 319: 525–532, 1988.
183. WALDORF, D. S., R. F. WILKENS, and J. L. DECKER. Impaired delayed hypersensitivity in an aging population. *JAMA* 203: 831–834, 1968.
184. WEI, Q., G. M. MATANOSKI, E. R. FARMER, M. A. HEDAYATI, and L. GROSSMAN. DNA repair and aging in basal cell carcinoma: a molecular epidemiology study. *Proc. Natl. Acad. Sci. U.S.A.* 90: 1614–1618, 1993.
185. WEINSTOCK, M. A. The epidemic of squamous cell carcinoma. *JAMA* 262: 2138–2140, 1989.
186. WEKSLER, M. E., J. B. INNIS, and G. GOLDSTEIN. Immunological studies of aging mice and reversal with thymopoitin. *J. Exp. Med.* 148: 996–1006, 1978.
187. WHITTON, J. T., and J. D. EVERALL. The thickness of the epidermis. *Br. J. Dermatol.* 89: 467–476, 1973.
188. WILLETT, W. C., and B. MACMAHON. Diet and cancer: an overview. *N. Engl. J. Med.* 310: 633–638, 1984.
189. WINKELMANN, R. K. Nerve changes in aging skin. In: *Advances in the Biology of the Skin,* edited by W. Montagna. Oxford: Pergamon Press, 1965, vol. 6, p. 51.
190. YAMAURA, H., and T. MATSUZAWA. Decrease in capillary growth during aging. *Exp. Gerontol.* 15: 145–150, 1979.
191. YAAR, M., A. V. PALLERONI, and B. A. GILCHREST. Normal human epidermis contains interferon like proteins. *J. Cell Biol.* 103: 1349–1354, 1986.
192. ZACHARSKI, L. R., L. R. ELVEBACK, and J. W. KINMAN. Lymphocyte counts in healthy adults. *Am. J. Clin. Pathol.* 56: 148–150, 1971.
193. ZELICKSON, A. S., J. H. MOTTAZ, B. D. ZELICKSON, and S. A. MULLER. Elastic tissue changes in skin following PUVA therapy. *J. Am. Acad. Dermatol.* 3: 186–192, 1980.

12. Human nervous system

ROBERT KATZMAN | Department of Neurosciences, School of Medicine, University of California, at San Diego, La Jolla, California

CHAPTER CONTENTS

Heterogeneity of Aging of the Nervous System: Genius and Dementia in the Ninth Decade
Changes in the Nervous System Associated with Normal Aging
    An important caveat: are changes due to differences between generations or to aging?
    Evidence that semantic knowledge is retained late into the life span
    Evidence that we become slower as we age
    Loss of episodic and working memory is a common but not inevitable accompaniment of aging
    How much does perception change with age?
        Vision and hearing
        Central perceptual processing
    Cerebral blood flow and cerebral metabolism in aging
    Gait and motor changes in the elderly
    Biological bases of changes in cognition and gait during normal aging
    Role of extrapyramidal changes
Alzheimer's Disease
    Dementing illnesses
    Neuropathology of Alzheimer's disease
        Plaques and tangles
        Selective vulnerability of the brain in Alzheimer's disease
        Degenerating neurites and abortive sprouting
    Molecular changes in Alzheimer's disease
        APP and the production of β-amyloid
        β-Amyloid, diffuse plaques, and the pathogenesis of Alzheimer's disease
        The paired helical filament and tau
    Molecular genetics of Alzheimer's disease
    Epidemiological findings strengthen the concept of Alzheimer's disease as a chronic disease
    Brain reserve, education, and the development of dementia
What Can Be Done to Accelerate Research into Normal Aging?
    Overlap of Alzheimer's disease and normal aging research
    Need for a new infrastructure for normal aging research

HETEROGENEITY OF AGING OF THE NERVOUS SYSTEM: GENIUS AND DEMENTIA IN THE NINTH DECADE

THE INTERACTION OF PHYSIOLOGICAL AND MOLECULAR APPROACHES has led to major advances in the understanding of how the brain functions. Yet our knowledge of the normal aging of the brain is fragmented; advances in understanding the neuropsychological changes that occur with normal aging have not been matched with corresponding biological advances. In contrast, research on the major age-related disorder of the human brain, Alzheimer's disease, has moved at a spectacular pace, to the point where findings may perhaps provide the needed focus for studies of normal aging.

There is perhaps no area in which the definition of "normal" aging is more difficult than the human nervous system. With the rapid growth of the very elderly segment of our population, taken here to mean those 75 yr or older (the "oldest old"), it has become commonplace to postpone retirement and continue productive, even creative, work into the late seventies, eighties, and even nineties, as shown in Table 12.1. There are even individuals who developed creative genius at very late ages, the prime example being Mary Robertson ("Grandma") Moses who began a series of "primitive" paintings in her ninth decade and who produced 25 works after she passed her 100th birthday.

For biomedical scientists, Michael Heidelberger (1888–1992) represents the epitome of "successful" aging. Heidelberger received his doctorate in organic chemistry but soon turned to biochemistry and immunology. He and his students were the first to demonstrate that antibodies are proteins and constitute the gamma-globulin component of serum. He discovered that polysaccharides and lipopolysaccharides present in the outer membrane of various bacteria and molds were antigenic. He twice received the Lasker Award. His research grant support from the National Science Foundation ended when he was 88 yr old, but he remained active in the laboratory and published peer-reviewed papers until age 99 yr. His last series of published papers, primarily single-authored, dealt in a sophisticated manner with the details of the chemical basis of the cross-reactivity between antipneumococcal and other antisera and strains of pneumococci and *Pseudomonas aeruginosa* (92). In addition, he published several fascinating autobiographical papers (89–91).

In contrast, there are three to four million individuals in the United States over the age of 65 yr who suffer from Alzheimer's disease and close to another million individuals with other dementias, the majority over the age of 75 yr. In between are individuals with very well-maintained cognitive functions, another group who

TABLE 12.1. *Creativity at Advanced Ages: A Selected List*

Those who were creative in their tenth decade
  Anna Mary Robertson ("Grandma") Moses (1860–1961): Although she had been a superb producer of needlework earlier in her eighth decade, did not begin painting until her ninth decade and produced 25 prized original works after the age of 100.
  Michael Heidelberger (1888–1991): Pioneer of the chemical basis of antibody–antigen reactions, two-time recipient of Lasker Award, continued active laboratory activity and publication to age 98.
  E. A. Holyoke (1730–1830): Physician, described gait apraxia of aging and theory of aging brain at age 98.
  Pablo Picasso (1881–1983): Continued as a creative artist into his tenth decade.
  Eubie Blake (1883–1983): Jazz pianist who was still performing in his tenth decade.
  Pablo Casals (1876–1973): Classical cellist and conductor, conducted the Marlboro (Vermont) Festival Chamber Orchestra until age 94.
  George Nathan Burn (1896–): Actor/comedian, still performing in his tenth decade.
  Frank Lloyd Wright (1867–1959): Designed the Guggenheim Museum in New York, and the Marin County (California) Civic Center, developed his first "pre-fabs," and authored the book *The Living City* in his nineties.

Those who continued creating in their ninth decade
  Konrad Adenauer (1876–1967): President of West Germany (1949–1963).
  David Ben-Gurion (1886–1973): Prime minister of Israel until 1968.
  Theodor (Dr. Seuss) Geisel (1905–1992): Produced one of his most meaningful works, *Oh, the Places You'll Go!* (1990) after age 80.
  Philip Johnson (1906–): A leading architect has launched a new, solo career, with projects in America and abroad at age 86.
  I. F. Stone (1907–1989): Learned classical Greek after he turned 70 and wrote a challenging critique of Socrates in his nineth decade.
  Georg Philipp Telemann (1681–1767): Composed his cantate "Ino" in 1766.
  Giuseppi Verdi (1813–1901): Composed the music for the opera *Falstaff* in 1897 and a religious chorale, *Quarto Pezzi Sacri*, in 1898.

clearly are at risk and perhaps are at an early stage of a dementing illness, and still others with minor alterations in memory, who are considered by most to represent normal aging. If one considers only the totality of individuals over age 65 yr, a number that approaches 30 million today, then those with dementia or significantly impaired memory problems are a minority. However, if one looks at the group over age 85 yr—and this is the segment of our population that is most rapidly growing—the situation changes. Based on available data, with the exception of the East Boston Study conducted by Evans et al. (62), we have hypothesized the following (114): at age 90 yr, approximately one-third of the population will be truly normal cognitively, one-third will have Alzheimer's disease, and the other third will be divided between those who have other dementias and those who show significant memory problems short of dementia, sometimes called "benign forgetfulness" or "age-associated memory impairment." This latter group may be at high risk of developing dementia.

CHANGES IN THE NERVOUS SYSTEM ASSOCIATED WITH NORMAL AGING

One is left with the following definition of normal aging of the nervous system: changes with aging that occur in individuals free of overt diseases of the nervous system (clinically and pathologically) (112). Under this definition, certain generalizations can be made about the psychological and biological aspects of normal aging:

1. Intellectual performance with respect to semantic knowledge—the type of knowledge that often is measured by tests of verbal ability in vocabulary, information, and comprehension—reaches a peak at age 20–30 yr and is then maintained throughout life, at least until the mid-80s, in the absence of disease.

2. Performance on timed tasks, including simple, choice, and conditional reaction time; athletic ability; ability to carry out abstractions, such as the digit symbol substitution test; and performance on other tasks requiring speed in processing information reaches a peak at about age 20 yr and then declines slowly throughout life. Although part of this decrease may be attributed to changes in motor or perceptual abilities, there is now unequivocal evidence that the speed of central processing declines with age. This change is noticed by almost all persons reaching their 70s. Yet there is still an overlap; that is, some 70-year-olds perform better than some 20-year-olds. The decline probably affects the efficiency with which older adults can perform all relatively complex cerebral tasks, regardless of their nature (thinking, perceiving, remembering, and so on).

3. Most, but not all, individuals experience changes in episodic memory, particularly in recall and in working memory, with aging.

4. To some degree there is loss of sensory functions, especially hearing and vibration sense, but also vision (in addition to changes in accommodation and lens opacity that eventually afflict all of us).

5. At advanced age, muscle strength and motor efficiency often decrease and posture and gait changes frequently develop.

6. Anatomically and biochemically, aging of the brain is characterized by loss of a minor-to-moderate percentage of nerve cells restricted to specific regions of the brain, loss of enzymes involved in the synthesis of transmitters, and a moderate but definite loss of post-synaptic receptors for specific neurotransmitters. There is now evidence that some presynaptic terminals in neocortex and hippocampus are lost in otherwise normal

brains during aging. In Alzheimer's disease, there is a strong correlation between loss of neocortical and hippocampal synapses and poor performance on a variety of measures of cognitive functioning. It has not been determined whether this relationship also holds in normal aging.

An Important Caveat: Are Changes due to Differences between Generations or to Aging?

When comparing 90-year-olds and 20-year-olds in regard to either cognitive function or biological measures, such as the volume of the brain measured on computed tomography (CT) scans or the weight of the brain as measured at autopsy, one must distinguish between changes that are generational and those that are age-related. For example, the number of years of schooling has increased throughout the century, so that a representative cohort of older individuals, in general, will have had less schooling than those who are younger, and comparison of these groups may lead to the misinterpretation of a secular change as being related to aging per se. Younger individuals in our society tend to have been better nourished and to have grown up to be taller and to have larger brains. Corsellis (34), for example, has shown that there is an artifact in many studies of changes in brain weight with aging, since the library of brains in the Institute of Neurology in London reveals that, on the average, brains of young adults in 1890 were smaller than brains of young adults of matched ages in 1970; hence, artifactually larger weight loss in brain as a function of aging would have been reported in 1970, failing to take this generational change into account. Thus cross-sectional studies comparing young and old suffer from the fact that they cannot fully take into account such generational or secular differences even when attempts are made to control for such variables as years of schooling.

Longitudinal studies avoid this type of problem. Here the evidence is clear-cut: if "intelligence" is measured by untimed tests that cover such topics as information, vocabulary, similarities, and picture arrangement and is re-assessed over decades in the same individuals, it does not change until the eighth decade (153, 163, 175), if then. Even at advanced ages these functions remain unchanged in some subjects: in a study of a group of men between ages 70 and 81 yr, volunteers in a National Institute of Mental Health (NIMH) study (78) who were followed between 1956 and 1967 actually improved their scores on two subtests of the Wechsler Adult Intelligence Scale (WAIS), vocabulary and picture arrangement, and six other subtests remained unchanged over the 11 yr period. Yet the normative data used to score these very subtests of the WAIS—normative based upon cross-sectional studies—show marked changes during aging. Longitudinal studies, however, show decrements in timed tests in the NIMH study: one timed subtest, the Digit Symbol Substitution, did show a decline, as did the Raven Matrices, also a timed test, consistent with the expected slowing during aging.

There is an important confound in longitudinal studies: individuals who develop cognitive impairment may drop out or die so that the most cognitively intact of the group are the ones who remain for subsequent follow-up; therefore, one may get a falsely secure picture of maintained function during aging. Of the 47 volunteers in the 1956 evaluation, only 19 were retested in 1967; 24 had died and 4 were unavailable for other reasons. Schaie and co-workers attempted to avoid these pitfalls (175) by carrying out both sequential cohort (longitudinal) and cross-sectional studies, and their work, described in the following section, provides useful data against which to check other information from both cross-sectional and longitudinal approaches.

Evidence That Semantic Knowledge Is Retained Late into the Life Span

In a classic study (153), Owens was able to retest individuals in 1950 and 1961 who were in their 50s and 60s and who as college freshmen had taken the Army Alpha test in 1919 at Iowa State College. On average their scores actually improved in seven of eight subtests between 1919 and 1950, the most significant improvements being in information, practical judgment, synonym–antonym, and disarranged sentences; their scores on these tests were stable between 1950 and 1961. Similar results were obtained by Schaie and colleagues (175) using both longitudinal and cross-sectional methods in a study of members of a large Puget Sound HMO. Neither the longitudinal study nor comparison in different years of independent samples born in the same period showed decrements in verbal and other abilities measured on the Primary Mental Abilities Test (with the sole exception of the timed word fluency subtest) up to the eighth decade. Cross-sectional studies not matched for date of birth showed loss of function, except in tests of semantic knowledge, in many tests with age. In regard to more advanced ages, the classical study is that carried out at the NIMH between 1956 and 1967 (78) in which a group of volunteers whose average age was 70 yr in 1956 was retested in 1967, neuropsychological tests and measures of cerebral blood flow being carried out in 1956 and 1967. The results were quite striking. Results of tests of what is now termed "semantic knowledge" or "crystallized knowledge," such as the vocabulary section of the WAIS, either remained unchanged or actually showed improvement over this 11 yr period. However, timed tasks, such as the digit symbol substitution task of the WAIS or the rate of addition or subtraction, showed marked decrements.

Evidence That We Become Slower as We Age

The evidence of slowing with aging observed in the NIMH study is found universally. Such simple measures as reaction time show changes with aging in both cross-sectional and longitudinal studies (18). Yet even here the heterogeneity of human skills and the aging process are apparent. Spirduso and colleagues (21, 186) have shown that some older men who are active in racquet sports or who are runners perform better on reaction time measurements than do younger, nonathletic, sedentary individuals. Recent studies have shown that education, general cognitive abilities, and adverse life events affect reaction time measures (60, 98, 99). Runners show a decrease in speed as they age (66). Payton Jordan, who ran the 200 m race in the 1936 Olympic trials with a time of 21.1 s, held the masters record for this distance for age 60 yr at 24.9 s (174). The record at age 70 yr for this event was 30.1 and at age 80 yr 41.2 s (31). It should be remembered that there are still individuals in their eighth decade who run the marathon under 4 hr, whereas there are many individuals in their 20s who would be unable to complete a marathon in twice that time.

The changes in motor speed among sedentary or nonathletic individuals with aging are quite striking. In cross-sectional studies, nonathletic subjects show a 30% decrease in speed between their 20s and 60s in such simple tasks as moving the arm aimed toward a target, a side-to-side movement of a lever, or tapping two targets alternately (214). In some instances, older subjects made fewer errors at the expense of speed, for example, in the tapping test, but the most important finding is that continuous exercise of a function seems to help maintain speed. For example, in measures of speed of copying digits, although most studies show that this decreases with aging in individuals as varied as professionals or laborers, employed clerks in their 60s could copy at a rate of 0.7 s per digit, essentially unchanged from their younger co-workers (130).

The slowing of reaction time with age is due in small part to the slowing of muscle response (213), peripheral nerve motor conduction rate (131), or sensory nerve conduction rate (129). Together, these factors may contribute less than 20% to the slowing of voluntary reaction time that occurs when the stimulus is a touch of the finger or foot.

The major factor in the slowing of the response to visual or auditory stimuli is the slowing of perceptual processing during aging. The effect of age on perceptual processing has been elegantly demonstrated by experiments using backward masking (95, 209). If two visual stimuli are presented milliseconds apart, the second stimulus may block perception of the first if appropriate strength and interstimulus intervals are used. The interval that will allow backward masking is increased 20%–70% (depending on stimulus variables) in subjects in their 60s and 70s compared with 20-year-olds, whether both stimuli are presented to one eye (monoptic) (121) or to different eyes (dichoptic stimulation) (207), thus assuring that the process is central and not retinal. Furthermore, it has been consistently found that the latency of late (over 100 ms) components of visual, auditory, and somatosensory evoked potentials is increased in older individuals. Even the slowing of simple reaction time with age is due in large part to the slowing of central processing (20). Also choice reaction time, which presumably requires additional time for central decision making, is increased to a greater degree in older subjects than simple reaction time (214); the more complex the task, the greater the age effect (17, 215).

The slowing of central processing is perhaps the most universal change that occurs with aging, yet there is no direct information as to its biological basis.

Loss of Episodic and Working Memory Is a Common but Not Inevitable Accompaniment of Aging

As we age, forgetfulness is a frequent complaint; in the words of B. F. Skinner: "Memoranda in place of memories." The complaint is real; most of us—there are a few exceptions—develop some degree of impairment of episodic memory as we age, especially after age 70 yr.

Tulving's classification of memory as semantic, episodic, and procedural (201) has proven useful in aging research. *Semantic memory* is one's cumulative knowledge of the world, of language, and of concepts. Such information is held for varying lengths of time, from seconds to a lifetime; semantic memory is stable or improves across the decades, whereas an age-related decline in episodic memory is widely reported. *Episodic memory* relates to personally experienced events contextually bound to time and place. Episodic memory is most sensitive to aging and has been most widely studied. *Procedural memory,* also called *implicit memory* (77), refers to enhancement of performance on perceptual-motor skills or cognitive operations by recent experience, without intention or conscious awareness by the individual being necessary. Although not extensively studied, procedural memory does not appear to show age-related differences. For example, accuracy may improve in word completion tasks or speed in identifying a word or picture through repetition, and performances of older and younger adults are equivalent (132), even when recall or recognition of test items is poorer in older subjects.

A decrement of episodic memory with aging in most

older subjects has been confirmed by a large number of cross-sectional studies, in most of which older and younger subjects are matched according to education. This decrement shows up especially in tasks in which the items to be learned and then recalled are not meaningful, for example, lists of words or digits. Both young and old will remember a list of 5–7 digits without difficulty; when the list is increased to 15 digits, younger subjects improve their scores more rapidly on repeated trials than older subjects do (56). Another typical finding is that on free recall of a 25-item word list, an older group (mean age 67.3 yr) recalled only 55% as many words as a younger (mean age 18.7 yr) group (208). It is interesting to note that these same older subjects learned and retained a set of 16 ideas as well as younger subjects.

A common observation of older individuals is that they have difficulty remembering several tasks simultaneously. This observation, first proposed by Broadbent and stated by Kinsbourne (25, 38, 120) in the 1970s and supported by evidence that performance on a memory task suffers more in old than in young when a secondary concurrent task is added (25, 38), has found a psychological basis in Baddeley's concept that *working memory* (8, 70) is affected by aging (7). Baddeley argues for the existence of a central executive function, which controls working memory and is "capable of selecting strategies and integrating information from several different sources." Involvement of the central executive function is seen by Baddeley as an origin of age effects in memory; he argues that stresses on the central executive system compromise the efficiency of working memory, which thereupon places constraints on a wide range of nonmemory tasks. Another viewpoint is that working memory is affected by the ability to process incoming information, especially when it is complex (146).

Most studies of memory have been cross-sectional, though most investigators have taken care to match subjects on educational experience and vocabulary or IQ scores to increase comparability of groups. However, the educational experience of a 20-year-old today differs from that of individuals with the same amount of schooling 50 yr earlier, so it is uncertain whether the groups are comparable. Again, longitudinal studies become important. These studies show that aging is usually accompanied by memory loss but that some individuals show no change over extended periods. Gilbert (71) retested 14 subjects who had taken the Babock-Levy Test of Mental Efficiency about 35 yr earlier, the average age at the time of retest being 65 yr. In accord with the studies described above, vocabulary scores were unchanged or showed a slight improvement, but scores on the Initial Learning subtest showed a marked decline and scores on the Retention subtest a modest but significant decline over the 35-yr period. Within the population of older individuals, decline in memory has been measurable over shorter time periods. For example, in a 6-yr longitudinal study of 30 older individuals (190) with memory complaints but without evidence of dementia or depression, there was a significant decline both in word-recall scores and in digit symbol scores, but the memory change did not correlate with the decline in digit symbol scores.

How Much Does Perception Change with Age?

Vision and Hearing. A matter of great concern in regard to measures of cognition is the question of visual and auditory perception. Presbyopia, an impairment in accommodation of the lens, often occurs in middle age. This change can be considered part of a lifelong process of lenticular development as changes in accommodation of the lens occur throughout life; accommodation amplitude changes from 7 diopters (D) at age 15, to 3 D at age 30, and 1 D at age 40 yr (19, 79, 124); it is not until the accommodation is below 1 D that a clinical threshold is reached and symptoms are noted (20). It has been suggested (223) that the loss of accommodative capacity during adult life plays a role in limiting the ability of older athletes in sports requiring eye–hand coordination. Cataracts, a loss of lucency of the lens, were a major cause of visual loss in the elderly up to the mid-1970s, but new techniques for replacement of the opaque lens with a plastic lens had a success rate between 95% and 97% by 1987 (223). As a result, in the absence of macular degeneration or glaucoma, most elderly people have vision better than 20/30 on the Snellen chart. However, visual acuity in the elderly is considerably worse than suggested by the Snellen measure in conditions of low contrast and low luminance (1, 9), a finding consistent with the reported deterioration of photoreceptors after age 20 yr (9, 67, 162, 212). An additional problem that affects visual processing during aging is constriction of the pupils. That many elderly patients have miotic, poorly reactive pupils with poor convergence was noted by Critchley (39) 60 yr ago. Cross-sectional studies of normal subjects between the third and ninth decades indicate a 20%–25% decrease in pupillary diameter under constant illumination (19, 128), with clinically apparent abnormalities in pupil size and reaction in up to 36% of the normal elderly. On the basis of pharmacological studies, it has been suggested that miosis of the elderly is related to diminished preganglionic sympathetic tone (124).

In contrast to the retention of basic visual acuity by many elderly people, loss of hearing, particularly of higher frequencies, occurs in almost all older people in the U.S., averaging 40% in those over age 75 yr (177). The major pathology that correlates with presbycusis is the loss of cochlear hair cells in the organ of Corti (11, 41). Although hearing aids can restore some of the loss, functional speech hearing and discrimination are not improved adequately in many elderly people. It is known that significant difficulty in speech discrimination may exist without a substantial deficit in auditory acuity (13, 177), especially in the presence of loud background noise (211). It is likely that central age-related impairments, particularly slowing of perception, may impair the understanding of speech, particularly if it is near threshold and rapid.

Central Perceptual Processing. One method of separating peripheral and central components of perceptual processing is to monitor brain potentials of sensory and event-related evoked responses as measured from scalp electrodes after repetitive presentation of sensory stimuli. The earliest components of these potentials are impulses related directly to sensory cortex, and later components reflect activity in appropriate association areas. During normal aging, early components (those occurring less than 100 ms after the stimulus) are often increased in amplitude, in contrast to the decrease in amplitude or absence of later components. There is minimal change of latency of these early components during aging, suggesting that the rate of conduction of sensory information in spinal cord, brain stem, or optic nerve is essentially normal, but the latency of later components is markedly increased (28, 183). Because these later components are presumed to be associated with information processing, their increased latency might be considered as evidence that the speed of processing sensory information, whether auditory, visual, or somatosensory, is reduced in normal aging.

However, the question remains as to what extent these electrophysiological changes are due to peripheral alterations affecting sensory input. For example, one widely used visual stimulus in studying evoked responses is a reversing checkerboard pattern of constant luminance; as expected, older subjects have a greater increase in latency of later potentials, consistent with a delay in central processing. At the luminance used in these experiments, the pupil in 70-year-olds is on the average one-fourth smaller in diameter than in 20-year-olds (35), resulting in only one-half as much light reaching the retina (223), and this does not take into account the decrease in light transmission due to the subclinical opacification of the lens that occurs in normal aging (173). It can be shown in 20-year-olds that the latency of 100 ms positive potential peak (P100) is increased from 102 ms at 20 log luminance units to 112 ms at a luminance of 1.0 log unit; the latency at 20 log luminance units would be 108 ms in 70-year-olds. Suprathreshold stimuli, for example a flasing stroboscopic light, can be used to avoid this problem; even so, all components of the occipital evoked response to a flashing light in older subjects, aged 56–81 yr, were delayed when compared with subjects aged 20–29 yr (58).

With almost all experimental paradigms, the later components of both visual and auditory evoked responses, believed to signal processing in association cortices, show a decrease in amplitude and an increase in latency in elderly subjects (75, 183). This is particularly true if event-related potentials (for example, P300, N400, and contingent negative variation) are used (51, 145, 154, 180). In this regard, it will be important to determine whether these delays are due to difficulty in pattern recognition during aging. There is some evidence that pattern recognition is related to a negative potential, N_A, that immediately precedes the N200, the latter reflecting discrimination and classification of data (164), and that much of the age effect is due to delay in the marker of pattern recognition. With the possibility that this perceptual process is especially vulnerable to aging—and much work needs to be done—one must be cautious in using computer displays to test other neuropsychological functions in older subjects.

Cerebral Blood Flow and Cerebral Metabolism in Aging

Cerebral metabolism and blood flow ought to be superb measures to use to mark the aging brain. Metabolic activity of the brain, measured in terms of either oxygen or glucose metabolism, reflects neuronal activity. Cerebral blood flow (CBF) measures the metabolic needs of the brain in normal circumstances (subjects must breathe normally because CBF is sensitive to fluctuations in carbon dioxide levels in the blood).

At the beginning of the NIMH longitudinal study discussed above, the rates of cerebral metabolism of oxygen, $CMRO_2$ (3.33 ± 0.08 ml/100 g/min), and CBF (57.9 ± 2.1 ml/100 g/min) obtained with the Kety nitrous oxide technique (119) were almost identical in this elderly cohort to those obtained in 15 normal young subjects, mean age 20.8 yr (45). When the older subjects were retested 11 yr later, the majority of those who had remained cognitively intact had significantly reduced CBF, indicating an increased vulnerability in the eighth decade in still healthy subjects and suggesting that during the eighth decade changes in CBF may occur in the absence of evident disease (44). In cross-sectional studies in which older individuals are selected as cognitively healthy, there appears to be no change in oxygen metabolism as measured by positron emission tomography (106).

The Kety nitrous oxide technique is the gold standard among methods of measuring CBF but is invasive, requiring sampling of arterial and jugular venous blood which provides data for hemispheric flow rather than local flow. There are numerous studies of CBF utilizing xenon-133 (^{133}Xe) inhalation with external gamma counting, a technique which gives specific regional values and estimates of gray matter flow (fast components) and white matter flow (slow component) (152). However, problems persist concerning interpretation (how much gray matter flow is cortical, how much is from basal ganglia or thalamus, and how much flow is affected by factors such as lung disease impairing absorption of ^{133}Xe). An assumption underlying the ^{133}Xe studies, using positron emission tomography and single photon emission tomography, is that the partition of the tracer between blood and brain is the same in younger and older brains. However, application of stable xenon imaging has in fact shown that the partition coefficient in cerebral cortex gray matter is not constant and that most of the presumed age change in CBF is due to a change in the partitioning of xenon as a result of greater density of neuritic elements in the atrophied brain (103). The result has been that some studies of CBF show as much as a 24% reduction in 80-year-olds compared to younger controls (210) but other studies do not (106).

Gait and Motor Changes in the Elderly

Although many elderly people are truly frail, others maintain excellent muscle strength as they age. In the only available longitudinal study, grip strength of 187 male alumni of Columbia College showed a slight increase between measurements made as undergraduates and measurements 37 yr later (average age 57.1 yr) (42). In a cross-sectional study of neurological changes in carefully selected normal volunteers aged 20–80 yr, Potvin et al. (160) found that by age 80 yr, grip strength had fallen to 77% of that of the 20-year-olds, but only a 7% loss was seen at age 60 yr. In the absence of longitudinal data continuing to age 80 yr, one can cite clinical experience; there are indeed 80-yr-old men with excellent retained muscle strength, and clinical experience has shown that among those very elderly who have not maintained their strength, cautious exercise regimes can restore this function.

The motor problem of aging was best described by Malcom Cowley, a prominent author and editor, who wrote after he turned 80 (37): "Age is not different from earlier life as long as you are sitting down." What happens when one stands up? There may be difficulty getting out of a chair and walking. Posture may be flexed, rather than erect, and there may be a decrease in mobility. Neurologists consider the motor changes that occur in normal aging akin to that characteristic of parkinsonian patients (223); similarities include the flexed posture and gait changes that occur frequently in subjects over 75 yr and the slowing of various motor processes that are a universal attribute of aging (191). Geriatricians (88) point out that flexion also occurs because of the dorsal kyphosis ("dowager's hump"), together with some loss of lumbar lordosis. In some people, anterior wedging and collapse of the intervertebral discs occurs with osteoporosis.

The challenge of walking is often a difficult one for an 80-year-old. The gait may be somewhat shuffling, resembling parkinsonism, yet no evidence of rigidity or tremor will be present. These changes may result in part from alterations that occur in the nigrostriatal dopaminergic system in normal aging. Again, Hazzard and Bierman (88) note that the development of painful osteoarthritis may also give rise to a stiff and awkward gait. Frequently the gait is unsteady in a nonspecific fashion; less often there is frank apraxia.

One of the best descriptions of this gait disorder is that in the memoirs of E. A. Holyoke written in 1828. (97). E. A. Holyoke, the son of a governor of Massachusetts for whom the town of Holyoke was named, a graduate of Harvard College, and a noted Massachusetts physician who helped introduce vaccination to that state, died in 1830 at age 100. His memoirs, written at age 98, describe one type of gait impairment often seen in the elderly; he formulates his own concept as to the etiology of his difficulty:

> I am now between 97 and 98 years old and enjoy good health ... excepting the complaint I now attempt to describe.
> About 10 or 11 years ago, I found that in walking, I was apt to lose my equilibrium and sometimes to stagger ... particularly if I looked up to see the town clock or how the wind blew, in doing which I have several times nearly fallen to the ground; this complaint gradually increased. ...
> My idea of the disease is this ... I presume that by disease or old age, the brain may be so shrunk or shriveled as to leave such a vacuity as to allow the brain to vacillate and so produce the staggering and unsteady walking, so common to persons much advanced in age.
> Memoirs of E. A. Holyoke (Holyoke, 1830 [97]). Cited by Wolfson and Katzman (222).

We do not know the age-specific frequency of gait disorder in the elderly. Certainly some people who are still creative into the tenth decade of life (see, for example, Table 12.1) have significantly impaired mobility. Many others remain free of evident motor disturbance until very advanced years.

The septuagenarians studied by Potvin et al. (160) did not have a gait problem, and tandem stepping was as brisk in the 70–80 yr cohort as in the 20–30 yr group. By age 80 yr, however, their subjects could no longer stand on one leg with eyes closed, a finding that might be associated with impairment of proprioception. It is difficult to quantitate proprioception. Vibration sense, however, is easily quantifiable and its threshold is almost universally elevated during aging (223). Vibration sense is carried from the lower extremities to the cerebellum over large-diameter myelinated dorsal root fibers whose bipolar axons extend from the toes to the medulla; similar fibers carry lower-extremity proprioceptive information. These neurons, required to maintain the metabolism of one of the longest processes in the body, may be among those most vulnerable to aging.

Biological Bases of Changes in Cognition and Gait during Normal Aging

Perhaps the most striking feature of most aging brains is shrinkage or atrophy, particularly of gray matter of the cerebrum. This is noted routinely during life on CT scans and magnetic resonance images (MRI) (107, 127, 133) as the relation of the volume of the ventricular and subarachnoid spaces to the volume of the cranium increases from 8% to 18% between ages 20–49 and 80–89 yr (223), corresponding well to the reported decline in brain weight over this period. There are also changes in white matter composition in the corpus callosum during normal aging (55), as seen on MRI, that perhaps reflect changes in myelination with aging.

There is a very wide individual variation in brain weight (from 930 to 1,350 g) reported in subjects aged 70–89 yr and considered "normal" (47, 193). It appears that this degree of variation may not be correct. Terry and Katzman (193) pointed out that published autopsy series often fail to document that cognition was truly normal prior to death. Moreover, there is no agreement among neuropathologists whether to include as normal the brains of elderly subjects with small numbers of neuritic plaques in the neocortex. In addition, there is a secular effect due to the lower brain weights of those born at the turn of the century secondary to nutritional or other environmental factors, as noted previously. Nevertheless, both radiological (225) and autopsy evidence that the brain shrinks with aging is overwhelming.

There is significant disagreement as to the cellular basis of cortical atrophy. In a pioneering investigation, Brody (26) reported a marked loss of neurons with aging. The neocortex was most severely involved, especially the superior temporal neocortex, in which over half of the neurons were lost by age 90 yr with the greatest loss in small neurons. Subsequent investigators have noted loss primarily of large neurons (93, 195). The decrease in total cortical neurons first reported by Brody (26) and confirmed by others (52, 93) contrasts with the later findings of Haug (87) and Terry et al. (195). Terry et al. (195), using a computerized-image analysis of the full cortical thickness in three neocortical association areas, including the superior temporal cortex, found that the large neurons (those over 90 μm^2) decreased significantly in number but that the small neurons increased to an equal extent. As a result, there was no net loss of neocortical neurons, suggesting that some of the large neurons had shrunk.

The hippocampus, thought to play a major role in memory, is relatively spared during normal aging. In contrast to the changes observed in the pyramidal cells of association neocortex during aging, the large pyramidal cells of CA 1–4, subiculum, pre- and prosubiculum of the hippocampus do not undergo significant age-related changes, at least through age 87 yr, as shown by Davies et al. (45) and Price et al. (161). In these studies great care was taken to assure that the subjects (through age 87 yr) had been neurologically and cognitively intact prior to death. On Golgi preparations no changes in the dendritic extent of the apical and basal trees of these cells were observed (64).

In contrast to the integrity of the hippocampus itself in normal aging, neurofibrillary changes occur in the parahippocampal region, primarily in entorhinal cortex but also in the anterior olfactory nucleus, though the latter has not been studied as extensively. These neurofibrillary changes are identical to the neurofibrillary tangles (NFT) observed in Alzheimer's disease and will be discussed in detail later. What is remarkable is that studies of brains from individuals who had been truly cognitively intact prior to death invariably show the presence of at least some NFT in the entorhinal cortex in all subjects beginning in the sixth decade of life (23, 161, 185).

The perforant pathway, the major projection pathway from entorhinal cortex to the dentate gyrus, is markedly altered in Alzheimer's disease (101). In normal aging, however, it appears that changes in the large neurons in the entorhinal cortex, although obvious, produce only a small change in the number of synapses in the dentate gyrus terminal field (134), changes that are compensated for by an increase in the average area of the contact zones of remaining synapses (14).

An age-related loss of neurons is observed in such major projection nuclei as the locus ceruleus (noradrenergic) (206), substantia nigra (dopaminergic) (135, 142), and basal nucleus of Meynert (49, 136, 143), though there is controversy concerning the degree of neuronal loss in the latter structure (16, 30, 219). There is good agreement that brain stem motor and cranial nerve nuclei maintain their neuronal numbers during life (194).

One of the most important changes during normal aging is a decrease in the number of synapses (100, 140). Masliah et al. (140) determined the number of presynaptic terminals in neocortical association areas using an antibody to synaptophysin, a protein that marks presynaptic vesicles. These investigators utilized confocal microscopy and counted the presynaptic terminals in frontal cortex sections from 25 subjects without dementia, aged 16–98 yr. There was a significant inverse correlation between age and synapse counts, with an $r = -0.7$ ($P < 0.001$). The number of frontal cortical synapses in those over age 60 yr was decreased by 20% compared to those under age 60 yr.

It should be noted that the brain retains plasticity during aging. Coleman and Flood (32) found a net increase in the dendritic arbor of pyramidal cells in normal aging, suggesting that this was a regenerative response to loss of presynaptic terminals.

In regard to biochemical markers of neocortical presynaptic terminals, choline acetyltransferase (ChAT), a marker of the cholinergic system projecting from the basal forebrain, has been reported to be significantly decreased during aging, especially in the hippocampus and temporal neocortex (142, 143, 155, 156). There is no significant loss with aging of ChAT in caudate and putamen, where ChAT is primarily found in small neurons.

Role of Extrapyramidal Changes

As noted above under Gait and Motor Changes in the Elderly, some of the motor changes in normal aging resemble postural and gait changes observed in Parkinson's disease. In Parkinson's disease, the major pathology involves the dopaminergic nigrostriatal pathway, resulting in a 90% loss of dopamine in the caudate and putamen (59). In normal aging most investigators find a mild to moderate decline in the concentration of dopamine at least in the caudate (27, 76), with reduction in other parts of the brain found by some (2) but not others (137, 167). Reports by two groups that the enzymes tyrosine hydroxylase and dopa decarboxylase, important in the synthesis of dopamine and of noradrenaline, respectively, decline with age in striatum, substantia nigra, and amygdala (135, 142) were not confirmed by another group of investigators (80). The brain regions affected in aging are projection sites for dopaminergic terminals arising from cell bodies in the substantia nigra, a pigmented nucleus that undergoes an age-related loss of neurons (116).

In contrast to the loss of dopaminergic markers during aging is the increase in the enzyme monoamine oxidase-B (MAO-B) (27, 76, 167), which is involved in the catabolism of dopamine. This enzyme is primarily astrocytic in location. A relatively specific antagonist of MAO-B, L-deprenyl, has been found to delay the progression of motor symptoms in PD. Also, MAO-B is involved in the conversion of 1-methyl-4-phenyl-1,2,3,6-tetrahydropyridine (MPTP), the one toxin that produces a true parkinsonian state in humans, to its toxic form. These findings raise the possibility that the increase in MAO-B in normal aging may play a role in the etiology of some cases of Parkinson's disease, thereby providing a possible explanation for the age association of this disorder (171).

ALZHEIMER'S DISEASE

Research on Alzheimer's disease has been virtually exploding. In the early 1960s the extraordinary ultrastructure of the plaque and tangle was described; in the late 1970s the ChAT deficiency was discovered, and neurochemists and pharmacologists became interested in the disorder. Even in the early 1980s there was no solid clue as to etiology, but within that decade the molecular biology of the most important abnormal proteins in the Alzheimer's disease brain were worked out such that a number of specific genotypes have been uncovered, leading to the promise that specific interventions to prevent the disease can be developed in the future. However, these advances have also made it impossible to review the subject fully within the context of a few pages and the reader is referred to additional sources for more complete reviews (117, 197).

Demening Illnesses

Dementing illnesses are the epitome of age-dependent disorders. The use of the term "senile" to describe the very elderly has some basis in observable fact since the prevalence of dementia rises exponentially between ages 65 and 85 yr, doubling every 5 yr (110), and in one U.S. study (62) afflicted half of the population over age 85 yr. More commonly, studies find that one-fourth to one-third of those over age 85 yr are demented. Between 50% and 70% of the skilled nursing home beds are occupied by demented individuals. About 20% of the deaths of those over the age of 75 yr can be attributed to dementing illnesses. Although many 80-, 90-, and even 100-year-olds are cognitively intact, the very high prevalence of dementia in the very elderly is a source of fear for the aging.

The dementia syndrome is characterized by a decline in memory and at least one other cognitive area, leading to some impairment of social or occupational functioning (3). Although more than 70 disorders may produce this syndrome, approximately two-thirds of the cases in the U.S. are caused by Alzheimer's disease or one of its variants. Alzheimer's disease is a dementing disorder characterized clinically by an insidious onset and progressive worsening in an individual who remains alert and awake until the terminal stages of the disorder. Clinicians diagnose "probable" Alzheimer's disease when these criteria are met and other disorders have been excluded (144). The diagnosis becomes definite with neuropathological confirmation.

Clinically the cognitive impairments and behavioral changes in Alzheimer's disease reflect the areas of the brain most affected, particularly the neocortical association areas, the hippocampal and parahippocampal areas, and the amygdala (178, 194). Although memory impairment is often the first symptom, other cognitive changes reflective of functions of specific neocortical associations areas, such as aphasia, constructional apraxia, visual agnosia, and frontal lobe symptomatology, may herald the onset of the disorder (113).

In regard to memory changes, the initial memory loss, manifested by forgetfulness and repetitiveness, superficially resembles that seen in normal aging, but in normal aging, if one compares the ratio of immediate recall to that of recall after a delay, this *savings score* is relatively stable across ages (158). In Alzheimer's disease, impairment of delayed recall is one of the earliest changes that has been identified by neuropsychological testing (216).

Neuropathology of Alzheimer's Disease

There is no other central nervous system disease in which the neuropathology is as rich as in Alzheimer's disease. Alois Alzheimer first recognized the disorder in 1907 when he applied silver stains, newly developed by the burgeoning photographic chemical industry, to the brain of a 55-year-old patient who died after a 5-yr progressive course that included both cognitive decline, particularly in memory and word-finding, and delusions and paranoia. At autopsy the shrunken brain contained, within the neocortex, large numbers of remarkable structures that were intensely stained by the silver dyes, the neuritic plaque (NP) and NFT.

Plaques and Tangles. In 1947, Divry (54) first suggested that the NP contained an amyloid core. In the early 1960s, in one of the first applications of electron microscopy to human nervous system disease (192, 196), the NP was indeed shown to contain a core of amyloid fibrils surrounded by swollen, apparently degenerating nerve terminals, both pre- and postsynaptic, with astrocytes and microglial cells often present. The NFT was found to be a nerve cell body full of abnormal paired helical filaments (PHF) (221). PHF are frequently present in the degenerating neurites in NP.

The relationship of NPs and NFTs to each other and to the pathogenesis of Alzheimer's disease is unknown. The amyloid-containing NP is truly a hallmark of Alzheimer's disease in that it is not found in other neurodegenerative diseases, though small numbers of NP are often seen in the brain of cognitively intact elderly. In Alzheimer's disease, the location and number of NPs are quite variable, though neocortical association areas usually contain large numbers of these structures. In contrast, the development of NFTs follows a consistent pattern, which is now used in the neuropathological staging of Alzheimer's disease (6, 23). A few NFT in the transentorhinal pre-alpha are present in most, if not all, brains of nondemented individuals after the age of 50 yr (23, 161). This is followed by involvement of hippocampal CA1 pyramidal cells and the anterodorsal nucleus of the thalamus. In Alzheimer's disease these regions become more severely involved and NFT develop throughout neocortex, striatum, basal nucleus, amygdala, thalamus, and hypothalamus. Particular weight has been given to the involvement of the entorhinal cortex neurons in the development of dementia since they relay information to the hippocampus (101).

Selective Vulnerability of the Brain in Alzheimer's Disease. Although the ravages of Alzheimer's disease are widespread in the brain, there are many areas that are relatively spared, including most brain stem nuclei and the cerebellum. In 1976, three groups independently reported the marked loss of ChAT in neocortex and hippocampus (22, 46, 156). This finding led to the discovery of the cholinergic projection system arising in the basal forebrain nucleus of Meynert (109) and its major involvement in Alzheimer's disease (218). Levels of ChAT in the Alzheimer's disease brain correlate inversely with performance on mental status tests (157). Subsequent interest in the possible use of cholinomimetic drugs in the treatment of Alzheimer's disease has led to the approval by the FDA of one such drug, tetrahydro-aminoacridine (THA, or tacrine), but the effectiveness of this and related drugs is not as robust as the loss of ChAT. Other neurotransmitter systems undergo degeneration in Alzheimer's disease, the most notable being the cortical–cortical and hippocampal–cortical glutaminergic systems (36, 40, 65); there is also involvement of the ascending cortical projection systems, including the noradrenergic projections arising in the locus coeruleus, the serotonergic projections arising in the dorsal raphe, and, in some individuals, the dopaminergic projection arising in the substantia nigra (12, 76, 170). In this regard, it is of interest that receptor ligands that mark presynaptic receptors show greater change in Alzheimer's disease than do postsynaptic receptors (170).

Although large pyramidal neurons in association neocortices and in the hippocampus are devastated in Alzheimer's disease (199), the severity of clinical dementia correlates best with loss of presynaptic terminals in neocortical association areas, particularly frontal cortex (48, 84, 140, 198).

Degenerating Neurites and Abortive Sprouting. In the NP seen in Alzheimer's disease, the amyloid core is surrounded by degenerating neurites, both dendrites and axonal terminals—presynaptic and postsynaptic elements. As shown by Terry et al. (196), these swollen neurites contain abnormal mitochondria and abnormal lysosomes in abundance. These neurites have been found to also contain increased amounts of GAP43, a marker of sprouting neurites, as well as increased amounts of amyloid precursor protein (APP) (33, 139), consistent with the hypothesis that these aberrant neurites reflect aberrant sprouting (68, 69).

Molecular Changes in Alzheimer's Disease

APP and the Production of β-Amyloid. The molecular identity of many of the abnormal fibrillar components found in the Alzheimer's disease brain has been established. The sequence of the β-amyloid component first obtained by Glenner and Wong (72) was that of a 40–43 kd peptide, which has been found to be a component of the much larger amyloid precursor protein (111, 165) whose gene is on chromosome 21. APP is expressed in all cells; in the normal brain the primary 695 kd form is the more common, but 751 kd and 771 kd forms containing Kunitz-type serine protease inhibitor inserts also occur in significant amounts. The promoter region of the APP gene contains both heat shock and c-fos regulatory elements in addition to many GC sequences.

APP is normally cleaved at a site in the middle of the β-amyloid sequence and the long, soluble portion N terminal to the cleavage site is secreted as protease-nexin II (61, 179, 182, 205). Some APP is degraded by a different, possibly lysosomal pathway, with the intracellular production of the β-amyloid peptide (83, 181). The soluble β-amyloid peptide is secreted extracellularly. In vitro, soluble β-amyloid peptide will form insoluble β-pleated amyloid very slowly, but a variety of conditions, including changes in pH or the presence of "chaperone" proteins such as α_1-antichymotrypsin, complement, and apolipoprotein E, greatly accelerate this process (189, 222). The evidence shows that these chaperone proteins are synthesized within astrocytes (159). Complement and α_1-antichymotrypsin are sometimes termed "acute phase reactants" and are thought to be released as the result of injury or other stresses.

β-Amyloid, Diffuse Plaques, and the Pathogenesis of Alzheimer's Disease. In regard to the role of β-amyloid in the pathogenesis of Alzheimer's disease, it has been suggested that extracellular focal deposits of β-amyloid without evident reaction of neurites, so-called diffuse plaques, may be present for years before other pathological or clinical changes occur. This is particularly evident in Down syndrome (trisomy 21), in which there is triplication of the APP gene. Diffuse β-amyloid plaques appear in the brain of Down subjects in their teens; typical Alzheimer's disease pathology with neuritic plaques and NFT usually appear in the fourth decade (172). Diffuse plaques are also seen in subjects with head injury (166, 200) and coronary stenosis (184), both putative risk factors for Alzheimer's disease. According to this scenario, the diffuse plaque is toxic over time, measured in years or decades.

β-Amyloid shows toxic effects in neuronal tissue culture (226), but the soluble β-amyloid peptide promotes neuritic branching in hippocampal cultures (220). It has been suggested that the toxic effect might be due to interaction with tachykinin receptors. Alternative actions of β-amyloid include increasing the toxicity of excitotoxic amino acids (122). In addition, Arispe and colleagues (4) have shown that β-amyloid peptide forms calcium channels in bilayer membranes. It has not been conclusively proven that β-amyloid is toxic in vivo.

The most direct evidence that β-amyloid is involved in the pathogenesis of Alzheimer's disease is shown by mutations in the APP molecule. It has been found that mutations of APP, both immediately C-terminal (codon APP 717) (73) and N-terminal (codon 670/671) (150) to the β-amyloid sequence, occur in a small subset of families with early-onset Alzheimer's disease. At autopsy, the brains of individuals with the 717 mutation display the usual tau pathology (85). In vitro insertion of the 670/671 mutation into cells increases the production of β-amyloid manyfold. Thus alterations in the APP gene may be a sufficient, though not necessary, cause of Alzheimer's disease.

In a number of later-onset familial cases, there is genetic linkage to the inheritance of the apolipoprotein E-4 (Apo E-4) allele, to be described below under Molecular Genetics of Alzheimer's disease. Among its functions, Apo E-4 is a chaperone protein with high avidity for the soluble β-amyloid peptide (189, 222).

Despite the strength of this evidence, there are also findings that are inconsistent with the β-amyloid hypothesis. The distribution of the diffuse plaques does not always correspond to Alzheimer's disease pathology; for example, diffuse β-amyloid plaques are frequently found in significant numbers in the cerebellum, but NP and NFT are rare in this structure. Another cogent argument is that there is no increase in the loss of synapses in the vicinity of diffuse or neuritic plaques (141). This finding, however, would be consistent with the possibility that most of the presynaptic terminals lost are those of projecting axons, such as glutaminergic axons connecting cortical neurons as well as projecting cholinergic and noradrenergic axons arising from deep nuclei.

The Paired Helical Filament and Tau. Whether the diffuse plaque sets off the sequence of events leading to the development of PHF or whether other intracellular events are primary in Alzheimer's disease remains to be resolved, but much has been learned about the molecular development of PHF.

Brion et al. (24) first identified the presence of tau in PHF using immunocytochemical methods, a finding quickly confirmed by others (50, 81, 104, 125, 224) and subsequently confirmed by identification of the binding region (123). Tau is a microtubule-associated protein, 50–64 kd, whose site on chromosome 17 is now on the genetic linkage map (126). Tau is tightly bound to tubulin and promotes the formation and stability of microtubules. In normal adult brain it is present primarily in axons. In Alzheimer's disease, however, tau forms PHFs which accumulate in neuronal soma (86, 108). The current concept (126) is that abnormal phosphorylation of tau (10, 15, 63, 74, 85, 202) causes it to be released from tubulin (82, 123). The structure of this abnormally phosphorylated tau is such that PHFs may spontaneously form, though ubiquitination of tau fragments may play a role at this point. Specific tau kinases have been identified (57, 105). While the PHFs accumulate within the soma of nerve cells, they are also found in axonal terminals and dendrites. In addition to any destructive role that might be played by the abnormal fibrillar inclusions, the loss of tau from the microtubules would be expected to disturb the important microtubular transport function. It is interesting that, in addition to the specific tau kinases, casein kinase II accumulation precedes tau accumulation in the formation of NFTs (102, 138).

Molecular Genetics of Alzheimer's Disease

It had been known for many years that Alzheimer's disease occurs both as an inherited disorder in families and sporadically. In certain families, Alzheimer's disease appears to be inherited as an autosomal dominant (FAD) gene. Several early-onset FAD kindreds have linkage to chromosome 21 (188). In 1991, Goate and colleagues (73) identified a single-point mutation at codon 717 of the APP gene in a small group of families of British origin. Subsequently, two other mutations at the same codon were identified in other families (29, 151). In a group of Swedish families, a double mutation at codons 670/671 of the APP gene was present in affected family members (150). The 717 and 670/671 mutations flank the β-amyloid region of the APP gene, giving credence to the hypothesis that deposition of extracellular β-amyloid is the initial step in the development of Alzheimer's disease. In addition, a mutation at codon 692 within the β-amyloid sequence produces both cerebral hemorrhages (due to vascular amyloidosis) and dementia within the same family (94).

Fewer than thirty FAD kindred with mutations of the APP gene have been found out of hundreds that have been investigated. It has been found that a much more frequent linkage site in early-onset families is on chromosome 14 (149, 176, 187, 203). Although the linkage site is near that of genes known to be APP promoters (c-fos and heat shock protein) or chaperone proteins (α_1-antichymotrypsin), the mutation or mutations responsible for the inheritance of Alzheimer's disease have not yet been identified.

Over 95% of Alzheimer's disease cases begin well past the age of 50 yr. In 1990, Roses and colleagues (168) reported evidence of genetic linkage of FAD subjects with late-onset disease to a site on chromosome 19. An allele of a normally occurring protein, Apo E-4 (169, 189), appears to be responsible for this linkage in the late-onset familial cases, but this allele may also be a susceptibility factor in the majority of sporadic cases of Alzheimer's disease with onset between ages 60 and 80 yr. Its action appears to be co-dominant in that the odds ratio of developing Alzheimer's disease is increased five- to ninefold in individuals with E4/E4 alleles (fortunately only 3% of the general population) and two- to fourfold in those with E4/E3 alleles (about 23% of the general population).

Epidemiological Findings Strengthen the Concept of Alzheimer's Disease as a Chronic Disease

In regard to the picture of Alzheimer's Disease as a chronic disease, as shown in Figure 12.1, there is some evidence from epidemiological research to support the role of amyloid as an initiating factor in Alzheimer's disease. The three major risk factors for Alzheimer's disease are age, a history of Alzheimer's disease in a first-degree relative, and a history of head trauma. As previously noted, the prevalence of Alzheimer's disease rises exponentially with age, doubling every 5 yr between ages 65 and 85 yr (110). A history of Alzheimer's disease in a first-degree relative increases the risk of acquiring the disease about fourfold (204). A collaborative reanalysis of 11 case-control studies established head injury with unconsciousness as an important risk factor; a history of head trauma with unconsciousness increases the odds of acquiring Alzheimer's disease about twofold (148). About one-third of the cases of severe head trauma develop diffuse plaques. A history of myocardial infarction has been found to be a risk factor for Alzheimer's disease in elderly women (5). Sparks et al. (184) found a very significant increase in diffuse and neuritic plaques in presumably normal elderly people, with critical stenosis of one or more coronary arteries. These findings add support for, but certainly do not make conclusive, the hypothesis that

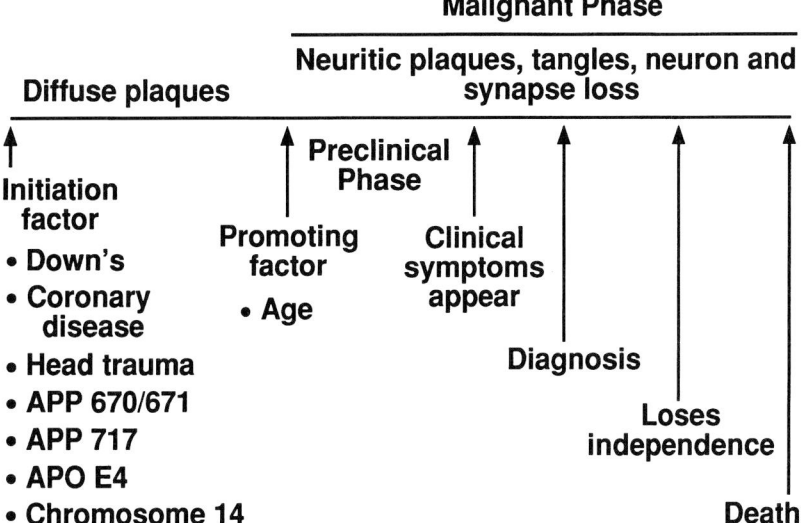

FIG. 12.1. Alzheimer's disease as a chronic disease. [Modified from Fig. 4 in Katzman and Kawas (115a).]

release of amyloid is a causative factor in Alzheimer's disease. Determining whether the diffuse amyloid plaque is indeed a critical causative factor is important because it should, at least in theory, be possible to develop drugs that would inhibit the formation of β-amyloid plaques, thereby preventing the development of Alzheimer's disease, if this hypothesis is correct.

Brain Reserve, Education, and the Development of Dementia. In most organs, one must lose a rather considerable amount of tissue or tissue function before a threshold is reached in which symptoms occur, a concept known as *functional reserve* (171). The evidence for functional reserve in regard to the human brain is strongest in terms of the nigrostriatal dopaminergic system, in which at least 80% of neurons need to be impaired before parkinsonian extrapyramidal symptoms occur. We (118) identified a subset of nondemented elderly with sufficient plaques in the neocortex to meet the criteria for a pathological diagnosis of Alzheimer's disease, who had a greater number of large (cross-sectional area ≥ 90 μm^2) neurons, especially in parietal neocortex, and a greater brain weight as compared to brains of nondemented controls of the same age without Alzheimer's disease findings, suggesting a brain reserve with numerous plaques in this subset of nondemented elderly.

Mortimer (147) predicted that "psychosocial risk factors will have their strongest associations in late-onset DAT [dementia of Alzheimer's type] of mild to moderate severity," based on a hypothesis of decline in brain reserve with normal aging reaching a threshold region within which education would be protective against decline into dementia. In studies carried out in Shanghai (96, 227) and Bordeaux (43), the risk of developing dementia was increased two- to threefold (based on multivariate analysis) in those with no education compared to those with secondary school or greater education (115). White and associates (217) similarly found that low education increased the risk for decline in mental function in a longitudinal study carried out in East Boston, New Haven, and rural counties in Iowa. The latter study also found a protective effect of higher-status occupations (professional vs. laborer) in its multivariate analysis. We have interpreted these studies as suggesting that education early in life and perhaps the cognitive demands of higher-status occupations later in life increase brain reserve, delaying the onset of symptoms associated with Alzheimer's disease by as much as 5 yr. We have hypothesized that this brain reserve is related to the number of neocortical synapses. The possibilities that brain reserve might be altered during normal aging and that "use it or lose it" might apply to brain function are speculative extrapolations from the existing data and remain unproven.

WHAT CAN BE DONE TO ACCELERATE RESEARCH INTO NORMAL AGING?

Overlap of Alzheimer's Disease and Normal Aging Research

The emerging picture of Alzheimer's Disease is that of a chronic disease in which multiple etiologies appear to be able to trigger a malignant process that, once begun, is progressive, is characterized by a common pathology, and leads to a shortened life expectancy. The multiple etiologies can be conceptualized in terms of initiation factors and a long preclinical stage. Since Alzheimer's disease is so common, a significant number of normal elderly might be supposed to be in the preclinical stage. It would be reasonable to expect that the presence of these early pathological changes might account for the mild memory loss and other cognitive changes seen in a subset of normal elderly. However, Dickson et al. (53), correlating pathological and cognitive measures in a cohort of volunteers who underwent intensive annual neuropsychological testing, did not find any relationship between the presence of plaques and performance on the cognitive measures. Thus quite different explanations may be needed to account for the variability of the effect of aging on cognitive functioning.

Need for a New Infrastructure for Normal Aging Research

It is apparent that research on normal aging has not kept pace with research on Alzheimer's disease. To understand the effect of normal aging on cognitive and other functions it will be necessary to carry out the same exhaustive clinical and pathological correlations, both qualitative and quantitative, as do Alzheimer's disease investigators. It is clear that the startling advances in understanding Alzheimer's disease required the development of an infrastructure of teams of clinicians and neuropathologists who not only provide tissue from well-defined cases but who are able to quickly correlate qualitative and quantitative measures of cognitive function during life with state-of-the-art findings in regard to structural, biochemical, and molecular aspects of Alzheimer's disease. A similar infrastructure needs to be developed for research on normal aging to succeed.

REFERENCES

1. ADAMS, A. J., L. S. WONG, L. WONG, and B. GOULD. Visual acuity changes with age: some new perspectives. *Am. J. Optom. Physiol. Optics* 65: 403–406, 1988.
2. ADOLFSSON, R., C. G. GOTTFRIES, B. E. ROOS, and B. WINBLAD. Post-mortem distribution of dopamine and homovanillic acid in human brain, variations related to age, and a review of the literature. *J. Neural Transm.* 45: 81–105, 1979.
3. American Psychiatric Association. *American Psychiatric Association Task Force on Nomenclature and Statistics: Diagnostic and Statistical Manual of Mental Disorders (DSM-III).* Washington, D.C.: American Psychiatric Association, 1980.
4. ARISPE, N., E. ROJAS, and H. B. POLLARD. Alzheimer disease amyloid β protein forms calcium channels in bilayer membranes: blockade by tromethamine and aluminum. *Proc. Natl. Acad. Sci. U.S.A.* 90: 567–571, 1993.
5. ARONSON, M. K., W. L. OOI, H. MORGENSTERN, A. HAFNER, D. MASUR, H. CRYSTAL, W. H. FRISHMAN, D. FISHER, and R. KATZMAN. Women, myocardial infarction and dementia in the very old. *Neurology* 40: 1102–1106, 1990.
6. ARRIAGADA, P., J. GROWDON, E. HEDLEY-WHYTE, and B. HYMAN. Neurofibrillary tangles but not senile plaques parallel duration and severity of Alzheimer's disease. *Neurology* 42: 631–639, 1992.
7. BADDELEY, A. D. *Working Memory.* Oxford: Oxford University Press, 1986.
8. BADDELEY, A. D., and G. J. HITCH. Working memory. In: *Recent Advances in Learning and Motivation,* edited by G. Bower. New York: Academic Press, 1974, p. 47–90.
9. BAGOLINI, B., V. PORCIATTI, B. FALSINI, G. SCALIA, M. NERONI, and G. MORETTI. Macular electroretinogram as a function of age of subjects. *Doc. Ophthalmol.* 70: 37–43, 1988.
10. BANCHER, C., C. BRUNNER, H. LASSMANN, H. BUDKA, K. JELLINGER, G. WICHE, F. SEITELBERGER, I. GRUNDKE-IQBAL, K. IQBAL, and H. M. WISNIEWSKI. Accumulation of abnormally phosphorylated tau precedes the formation of neurofibrillary tangles in Alzheimer's disease. *Brain Res.* 477: 90–99, 1989.
11. BELAL, A. The ageing ear. A clinico-pathological classification. *J. Laryngol. Otol.* 101: 1131–1135, 1987.
12. BENTON, J. S., D. M. BOWEN, S. J. ALLEN, E. A. HAAN, D. NEARY, A. N. DAVISON, R. P. MURPHY, and J. S. SNOWDEN. Alzheimer's disease as a disorder of isodendritic core. *Lancet* 1: 456, 1982.
13. BERGMAN, M. Central disorders of hearing in the elderly. In: *Hearing and Balance in the Elderly,* edited by R. Hinchcliffe. London: Churchill Livingstone, 1983, p. 145–158.
14. BERTONI-FREDDARI, C., P. FATTORETTI, T. CASOLI, W. MEIER-RUGE, and J. ULRICH. Morphological adaptive response of the synaptic junctional zones in the human denate gyrus during aging and Alzheimer's disease. *Brain Res.* 517: 69–75, 1990.
15. BIERNAT, J., E.-M. MANDELKOW, C. SCHROTER, B. LICHTENBERG-KRAAG, B. SSTEINER, B. BERLING, H. MEYER, M. MERCKEN, A. VANDERMEEREN, and M. GOEDERT. The switch of tau protein to an Alzheimer-like state includes phosphorylation of two serine proline motifs upstream of the microtubule binding region. *EMBO J.* 11: 1593–1597, 1992.
16. BIGL, V., T. ARENDT, S. FISCHER, M. WERNER, and A. ARENDT. The cholinergic system in aging. *Gerontology* 33: 172–180, 1987.
17. BIRREN, J. E. Translations in gerontology—from lab to life. Psychophysiology and speed of response. *Am. Psychol.* 29: 808–815, 1974.
18. BIRREN, J. E., and J. BOTWINICK. Age differences in finger, jaw and foot reaction time to auditory stimuli. *J. Gerontol.* 10: 429–432, 1955.
19. BIRREN, J. E., R. C. CAPERSON, and J. BOTWINICK. Age changes in pupil size. *J. Gerontol.* 5: 216–221, 1950.
20. BITO, L. Z. Presbyopia. *Arch. Ophthalmol.* 106: 1526–1527, 1988.
21. BOTWINICK, J., and L. W. THOMPSON. Age difference in reaction time: an artifact? *Gerontologist* 8: 25–28, 1968.
22. BOWEN, D. M., C. B. SMITH, P. WHITE, and A. N. DAVISON. Neurotransmitter-related enzymes and indices of hypoxia in senile dementia and other abiotrophies. *Brain* 99: 459–496, 1976.
23. BRAAK, H., and E. BRAAK. Neuropathological staging of Alzheimer-related changes. *Acta Neuropathol. (Berl.)* 82: 239–259, 1991.
24. BRION, J. P., H. PASSAREIRO, J. NUNEZ, and J. FLAMENT-DURAND. Mise en evidence immunologique de la proteine tau au niveau des lesions de degenerescence neurofibrillaire de la maladie d'Alzheimer. *Arch. Biol. (Brussels)* 95: 229–235, 1985.
25. BROADBENT, D. E., and A. HERON. Effects of a subsidiary task

on performance involving immediate memory in younger and older men. *Br. J. Psychol.* 53: 189–198, 1962.
26. BRODY, H. Organization of the cerebral cortex. III. A study of aging in the human cerebral cortex. *J. Comp. Neurol.* 102: 511–556, 1955.
27. CARLSSON, A., R. ADOLFSSON, S. M. AQUILONIUS, C. G. GOTTFRIES, L. ORELAND, L. SVENNERHOLM, and B. WINBLAD. Biogenic amines in human brain in normal aging, senile dementia, and chronic alcoholism. In: *Ergot Compounds and Brain Function: Neuroendocrine and Neuropsychiatric Aspects,* edited by M. Goldstein, A. Lieberman, D. B. Caine and H. O. Thorner. New York: Raven Press, 1980, p. 295–304.
28. CELESIA, G. G., and R. F. DALY. Effects of aging on visual evoked responses. *Arch. Neurol.* 34: 403–407, 1977.
29. CHARTIER-HARLIN, M.-C., F. CRAWFORD, H. HOULDEN, A. WARREN, D. HUGES, L. FIDANI, A. GOATE, M. ROSSOR, P. ROQUES, J. HARDY, and M. MULLAN. Early-onset Alzheimer's disease caused by mutations at codon 717 of the β-amyloid precursor protein gene. *Nature* 353: 844–846, 1991.
30. CHUI, H. C., W. BONDAREFF, C. ZAROW, and U. SLAGER. Stability of neuronal number in the human nucleus basalis of Meynert with age. *Neurobiol. Aging* 5: 83–88, 1984.
31. CLARK, T. The masters movement; age conquers some, but it doesn't conquer all. *Runner's World* 80, 1979.
32. COLEMAN, P. D., and D. G. FLOOD. Neuron numbers and dendritic extent in normal aging and Alzheimer's disease. *Neurobiol. Aging* 8: 521–545, 1987.
33. COLEMAN, P. D., K. E. ROGERS, and D. G. FLOOD. The neuropil and GAP-43/B-50 in normally aging and Alzheimer's disease human brain. *Prog. Brain Res.* 89: 263–269, 1991.
34. CORSELLIS, J. A. N. Discussion. In: *Alzheimer's Disease: Senile Dementia and Related Disorders,* edited by R. Katzman, R. D. Terry, and K. L. Bick. New York: Raven Press, 1978, p. 397.
35. CORSO, J. F. Sensory processes and age effects in normal adults. *J. Gerontol.* 26: 90–105, 1971.
36. COWBURN, R., J. HARDY, P. ROBERTS, and R. BRIGGS. Presynaptic and postsynaptic glutamatergic function in Alzheimer's disease. *Neurosci. Lett.* 86: 109–113, 1988.
37. COWLEY, M. *The View from 80.* New York: Viking Press, 1976.
38. CRAIK, F. I. M. Age differences in human memory. In: *Handbook of the Psychology of Aging,* edited by J. E. Birren and K. W. Schaie. New York: Van Nostrand Reinhold, 1977, p. 384–420.
39. CRITCHLEY, M. Neurologic changes in the aged. *J. Chron. Dis.* 3: 459–476, 1956.
40. CROSS, A. J., P. SLATER, J. M. CANDY, E. K. PERRY, and R. H. PERRY. Glutamate deficits in Alzheimer's disease. *J. Neurol. Neurosurg. Psychiatry* 50: 357–358, 1986.
41. CROWE, S., S. GUILD, and L. POLVOGT. Observations on the pathology of high tone deafness. *Bull. Johns Hopkins Hosp.* 54: 315–379, 1934.
42. DAMON, A. Discrepancies between findings of longitudinal and cross-sectional studies in adult life: physique and physiology. *Hum. Dev.* 8: 16–22, 1965.
43. DARTIGUES, J. F., M. GAGNON, P. BARBERGER-GATEAU, J. M. MAZAUX, D. COMMENGES, and L. LETENNEUR. Occupation during life and memory performance in the elderly: results of the Paquid Program. *Neurology* 41(suppl. 1): 1–322, 1991.
44. DASTUR, D. K., M. H. LANE, D. B. HANSEN, S. S. KETY, R. N. BUTLER, S. PERLIN, L. SOKOLOFF, and J. E. BIRREN. Effects of aging on cerebral circulation and metabolism in man. In: *Human Aging—Biological and Behavioral Study,* edited by J. E. Birren, R. N. Butler, S. W. Greenhouse, L. Sokoloff, and M. R. Yarrow. Washington, DC: U.S. Department of Health, Education, and Welfare, Public Health Service, National Institutes of Health, 1963, p. 59–76.
45. DAVIES, D. C., N. HORWOOD, S. L. ISAACS, and D. M. A. MANN. The effect of age and Alzheimer's disease on pyramidal neuron density in the individual fields of the hippocampal formation. *Acta Neuropathol.* 83: 510–517, 1992.
46. DAVIES, P., and A. J. R. MALONEY. Selective loss of central cholinergic neurons in Alzheimer's disease. *Lancet* 2: 1403, 1976.
47. DEKABAN, A. S., and D. SADOWSKY. Changes in brain weights during the span of human life: relation of brain weights to body heights and body weights. *Ann. Neurol.* 4: 345–356, 1978.
48. DEKOSKY, S. T., and S. W. SCHEFF. Synapse loss in frontal cortex biopsies in Alzheimer's disease: correlation with cognitive severity. *Ann. Neurol.* 27: 457–464, 1990.
49. DE LACALLE, S., I. IRAIZOZ, and L. MA GONZALO. Differential changes in cell size and number in topographic subdivisions of human basal nucleus in normal aging. *Neuroscience* 43: 445–456, 1991.
50. DELACOURTE, A., and A. DEFOSSEZ. Alzheimer's disease: tau proteins, the promoting factors of microtubule assembly, are major components of paired helical filaments. *J. Neurosci.* 76: 173–186, 1986.
51. DESMEDT, J. E., and J. DEBECKER. Wave form and neural mechanism of the decision P350 elicited without pre-stimulus CNV or readiness potential in random sequences of near-threshold auditory clicks and finger stimuli. *Electroencephalogr. Clin. Neurophysiol.* 47: 648–670, 1979.
52. DEVANEY, K. O., and H. A. JOHNSON. Neuron loss in the aging visual cortex of man. *J. Gerontol.* 35: 836–841, 1980.
53. DICKSON, D. W., H. A. CRYSTAL, L. A. MATTIACE, D. M. MASUR, A. D. BLAU, P. DAVIES, S.-H. YEN, and M. K. ARONSON. Identification of normal and pathological aging in prospectively studied nondemented elderly humans. *Neurobiol. Aging* 13: 179–189, 1991.
54. DIVRY, P. Cerebral ageing. *J. Belge Neurol. Psychiatry* 47: 65–81, 1947.
55. DORAISWAMY, P. M., G. S. FIGIEL, M. M. HUSAIN, W. M. MCDONALD, S. A. SHAH, O. B. BOYKO, E. H. ELLINWOOD, and K. R. R. KRISHNAN. Aging of the human corpus callosum: magnetic resonance imaging in normal volunteers. *J. Neuropsychiatry* 3: 392–397, 1991.
56. DRACHMAN, D. A., and M. S. ZAKS. The "memory cliff" beyond span in immediate recall. *Psychol. Rep.* 21: 105–112, 1967.
57. DREWES, G., B. LICHTENBERG-KRAAG, F. DORING, E.-M. MANDELKOW, J. BIERNAT, J. GORIS, M. DORÉE, and E. MANDELKOW. Mitogen activated protein (MAP) kinase transforms tau protein into an Alzheimer-like state. *EMBO J.* 11: 2131–2138, 1992.
58. DUSTMAN, R. E., and E. C. BECK. The effects of maturation and aging on the wave form of visually evoked potentials. *Electroencephalogr. Clin. Neurophysiol.* 26: 2–11, 1969.
59. EHRINGER, H., and O. HORNYKIEWICZ. Verteilung von Noradrenalin im Dopamin (3-hydroxytyramin) im Gehirn des Menschen und ihre Verhalten bei Erkrankungen des extrapyramidalen Systems. *Klin. Wochenschr.* 38: 1236–1239, 1960.
60. ERA, P., J. JOKELA, and E. HEIKKINEN. Reaction and movement times in men of different ages: a population study. *Percep. Mot. Skills* 63: 111–130, 1986.
61. ESCH, F. S., P. S. KEIM, E. C. BEATTIE, R. W. BLACHER, A. R. CULWELL, T. OLTERSDORF, D. MCCLURE, and P. J. WARD. Cleavage of amyloid β peptide during constitutive processing of its precursor. *Science* 248: 1122–1124, 1990.
62. EVANS, D. A., H. FUNKENSTEIN, M. S. ALBERT, P. A. SCHERR, N. R. COOK, M. J. CHOWN, L. E. HEBERT, C. H. HENNEKENS, and J. O. TAYLOR. Prevalence of Alzheimer's disease in a community population of older persons. *JAMA* 262: 2551–2556, 1989.
63. FLAMENT, S., A. DELACOURTE, and D. M. A. MANN. Phos-

phorylation of tau proteins: a major event during the process of neurofibrillary degeneration. *Brain Res.* 516: 15–19, 1990.
64. FLOOD, D. G., and P. D. COLEMAN. Hippocampal plasticity in normal aging and decreased plasticity in Alzheimer's disease. *Prog. Brain Res.* 83: 435–443, 1990.
65. FRANCIS, P. T., A. J. CROSS, and D. M. BOWEN. Neurotransmitters and Neuropeptides. In: *Alzheimer Disease*, edited by R. D. Terry, R. Katzman, and K. L. Bick. New York: Raven Press, 1994, p. 247–262.
66. FRIES, J. F. Aging, natural death, and the compression of morbidity. *N. Engl. J. Med.* 303: 130–135, 1980.
67. GARTNER, S., and P. HENKIND. Aging and degeneration of the human macula. 1. Outer nuclear layer and photoreceptors. *Br. J. Ophthalmol.* 65: 23–28, 1981.
68. GEDDES, J. W., K. J. ANDERSON, and C. W. COTMAN. Senile plaques as aberrant sprout-stimulating structures. *Exp. Neurol.* 94: 767–776, 1986.
69. GEDDES, J. W., D. T. MONAGHAN, C. W. COTMAN, I. T. LOTT, R. C. KIM, and L. H. C. CHUI. Plasticity of hippocampal circuitry in Alzheimer's disease. *Science* 230: 1179–1181, 1985.
70. GICK, M. L., F. I. M. CRAIK, and R. G. MORRIS. Task complexity and age differences in working memory. *Mem. Cogn.* 16: 353–361, 1988.
71. GILBERT, J. G. Thirty-five year follow-up of intellectual functioning. *J. Gerontol.* 28: 68–72, 1973.
72. GLENNER, G. G., and C. W. WONG. Alzheimer's disease: initial report of the purification and characterization of a novel cerebrovascular amyloid protein. *Biochem. Biophys. Res. Commun.* 120: 885–890, 1984.
73. GOATE, A., M. C. CHARTIER-HARLIN, M. MULLAN, J. BROWN, F. CRAWFORD, L. FIDANI, L. GIUFFRA, A. HAYNES, N. IRVING, L. JAMES, R. MANT, P. NEWTON, K. ROOKE, P. ROQUES, C. TALBOT, M. PERICAK-VANCE, A. ROSES, R. WILLIAMSON, M. ROSSOR, M. OWEN, and J. HARDY. Segregation of a missense mutation in the amyloid precursor protein gene with familial Alzheimer's disease. *Nature* 349: 704–706, 1991.
74. GOEDERT, M., M. G. SPILLANTINI, N. J. CAIRNS, and R. A. CROWTHER. Tau proteins of Alzheimer paired helical filaments: abnormal phosphorylation of all six brain isoforms. *Neuron* 8: 159–168, 1992.
75. GOODIN, D. S., K. C. SQUIRES, B. H. HENDERSON, and A. STARR. Age-related variations in evoked potentials to auditory stimuli in normal human subjects. *Electroencephalogr. Clin. Neurophysiol.* 44: 447–458, 1978.
76. GOTTFRIES, C. G. Amine metabolism in normal ageing and in dementia disorders. In: *Biochemistry of Dementia*, edited by P. J. Roberts. New York: Wiley 1980, p. 213–239.
77. GRAF, P., and D. L. SCHACTER. Implicit and explicit memory for new associations in normal and amnesic subjects. *J. Exp. Psychol.* 11: 501–518, 1985.
78. GRANICK, S. Psychological test functioning. In: *Human Aging. II*, edited by S. Granick and R. D. Patterson. Rockville, MD: DHEW Publication (HSM, 71-9037), 1971.
79. GREENE, H. A., and D. J. MADDEN. Adult age differences in visual acuity, stereopsis and contrast sensitivity. *Am. J. Optom. Physiol. Optics* 64: 749–753, 1987.
80. GROTE, S. S., S. G. MOSES, E. ROBINS, R. W. HUDGEN, and A. B. CRONINGER. A study of selected catecholamine metabolizing enzymes: a comparison of depressive suicides and alcoholic suicides with controls. *J. Neurochem.* 23: 791–802, 1974.
81. GRUNDKE-IQBAL, I., K. IQBAL, M. QUINLAN, Y.-C. TUNG, M. S. ZAIDI, and H. M. WISNIEWSKI. Microtubule associated protein T: a component of Alzheimer paired helical filaments. *J. Biol. Chem.* 261: 6084–6089, 1986.
82. GUSTKE, N., B. STEINER, E. M. MAKELKOW, J. BEIRNAT, H. E. MEYER, M. GOEDERT, and E. MANDELKOW. The Alzheimer-like phosphorylation of tau protein reduces microtubule binding and involves Ser-Pro and Thr-Pro motifs. *FEBS Lett.* 307: 199–205, 1992.
83. HAASS, C., M. G. SCHLOSSMACHER, A. Y. HUNG, C. VIGO-PELFREY, A. MELLON, B. L. OSTASZEWSKI, I. LIEBERBURG, E. H. KOO, D. SCHENK, and D. B. TEPLOW. Amyloid β-peptide is produced by cultured cells during normal metabolism. *Nature* 359: 322–325, 1992.
84. HAMOS, J. E., L. J. DEGENNARO, and D. A. DRACHMAN. Synaptic loss in Alzheimer's disease and other dementias. *Neurology* 39: 355–361, 1989.
85. HANGER, D. P., J. P. BRION, J. M. GALLO, N. J. CAIRNS, P. J. LUTHERT, and B. H. ANDERTON. Tau in Alzheimer's disease and Down's syndrome is insoluble and abnormally phosphorylated. *Biochem. J.* 275: 99–104, 1991.
86. HANGER, D. P., D. M. A. MANN, D. NEARY, and B. H. ANDERTON. Tau pathology in a case of familial Alzheimer's disease with a valine to glycine mutation at position 717 in the amyloid precursor protein. *Neurosci. Lett.* 145: 178–180, 1992.
87. HAUG, H. Are neurons of the human cerebral cortex really lost during aging? A morphometric examination. In: *Senile Dementia of the Alzheimer Type*, edited by J. Traber and W. H. Gispen. Berlin: Springer-Verlag, 1985, p. 150–163.
88. HAZZARD, W. R., and E. L. BIERMAN. Old age. In: *Biological Ages of Man from Conception Through Old Age* (2nd ed.), edited by D. Smith and E. L. Bierman. Philadelphia: Saunders, 1978, p. 229–253.
89. HEIDELBERGER, M. A "pure" organic chemist's downward path. *Annu. Rev. Microbiol.* 31: 1–12, 1977.
90. HEIDELBERGER, M. Michael Heidelberger. *Int. Arch. Allergy Appl. Immunol.* 57: 97–100, 1978.
91. HEIDELBERGER, M. Reminiscences. *Immunol. Rev.* 82: 7–19, 1984.
92. HEIDELBERGER, M., D. HORDON, and T. H. HASKELL. Cross reactions of lipopolysaccharides of *Pseudomonas aeruginosa* in antipneumococcal and other antisera. *Infect. Immunol.* 54: 928–930, 1986.
93. HENDERSON, G., B. E. TOMLINSON, and P. H. GIBSON. Cell counts in human cerebral cortex in normal adults throughout life using an image analysing computer. *J. Neurol. Sci.* 46: 113–136, 1980.
94. HENDRIKS, L., C. M. VAN DUIJN, P. CRAS, M. CRUTS, V. W. HUL, F. VAN HARSKAMP, A. WARREN, M. G. MCINNIS, S. E. ANTONARAKIS, J.-J. MARTIN, A. HOFMAN, and C. VAN BROECKHOVEN. Presenile dementia and cerebral haemorrhage linked to a mutation at codon 692 of the β-amyloid precursor protein gene. *Nat. Genet.* 1: 218–221, 1992.
95. HERTZOG, C. K., M. V. WILLIAMS, and D. A. WALSH. The effect of practice on age differences in central perceptual processing. *J. Gerontol.* 31: 428–443, 1976.
96. HILL, L. R., M. KLAUBER, R. KATZMAN, D. P. SALMON, E. YU, W. T. LIU, and M. ZHANG. Functional status, education, and the diagnosis of dementia in the Shanghai survey. *Neurology* 43: 138–145, 1993.
97. HOLYOKE, E. A. *Memoirs of E. A. Holyoke*. Massachusetts: Essex County Medical Society, 1830.
98. HOUX, P. J., and J. JOLLES. Age-related decline of psychomotor speed: effects of age, brain health, sex, and education. *Percept. Mot. Skills* 76: 195–211, 1993.
99. HOUX, P. J., F. W. VREELING, and J. JOLLES. Rigorous health screening reduces age effect on memory scanning task. *Brain Cogn.* 5: 246–260, 1991.
100. HUTTENLOCHER, P. R. Synaptic density in human frontal cortex—developmental changes and effects of aging. *Brain Res.* 163: 195–205, 1979.
101. HYMAN, B. T., G. W. VAN HOESEN, A. R. DAMASIO, and C. L. BARNES. Alzheimer's disease: cell-specific pathology isolates the hippocampal formation. *Science* 225: 1168–1170, 1984.

102. IIMOTO, D., E. MASLIAH, R. DETERESA, R. D. TERRY, and T. SAITOH. Aberrant casein kinase II in Alzheimer's disease. *Brain Res.* 507: 273–280, 1990.
103. IMAI, A., J. S. MEYER, M. KOBARI, M. ICHIJO, T. SHINOHARA, and W. T. ORAVEZ. LCBF values decline while Lγ values increase during normal human aging measured by stable xenon-enhanced computed tomography. *Neuroradiology* 30: 463–472, 1988.
104. IQBAL, K., I. GRUNDKE-IQBAL, A. J. SMITH, L. GEORGE, Y.-C. TUNG, and T. ZAIDI. Identification and localization of a τ peptide to paired helical filaments of Alzheimer disease. *Proc. Natl. Acad. Sci. U.S.A.* 86: 5646–5650, 1989.
105. ISHIGURO, K., M. TAKAMATSU, K. TOMIZAWA, A. OMORI, M. TAKAHASHI, M. ARIOKA, T. UCHIDA, and K. IMAHORI. Tau protein kinase I converts normal tau protein into A68-like component of paired helical filaments. *J. Biol. Chem.* 267: 10897–10901, 1992.
106. ITOH, M., J. HATAZAWA, H. MIYAZAWA, H. MATSUI, K. MEGURO, K. YANAI, K. KUBOTA, S. WATANUKI, T. IDO, and T. MATSUZAWA. Stability of cerebral blood flow and oxygen metabolism during normal aging. *Gerontology* 36: 43–48, 1990.
107. JERNIGAN, T. L., G. A. PRESS, and J. R. HESSELINK. Methods for measuring brain morphologic features on magnetic resonance images. *Arch. Neurol.* 47: 27–32, 1990.
108. JOACHIM, C. L., J. H. MORRIS, D. J. SELKOE, and K. S. KOSIK. Tau epitopes are incorporated into a range of lesions in Alzheimer's disease. *J. Neuropathol. Exp. Neurol.* 46: 611–622, 1987.
109. JOHNSTON, M. V., M. MCKINNEY, and J. R. COYLE. Evidence for a cholinergic projection to neocortex from neurons in the basal forebrain. *Proc. Natl. Acad. Sci. U.S.A.* 76: 5392–5396, 1979.
110. JORM, A. F., A. E. KORTEN, and A. S. HENDERSON. The prevalence of dementia: a quantitative integration of the literature. *Acta Psychiatr. Scand.* 76: 464–479, 1987.
111. KANG, J., H.-G. LEMAIRE, A. UNTERBECK, M. J. SALBAUM, C. L. MASTERS, K.-H. GRZESCHIK, G. MULTHAUP, K. BEYREUTHER, and B. MÜLLER-HILL. The precursor of Alzheimer's disease amyloid A4 protein resembles a cell-surface receptor. *Nature* 325: 733–736, 1987.
112. KATZMAN, R. Demography, definitions, and problems. In: *Neurology of Aging*, edited by R. Katzman and R. D. Terry. Philadelphia: Davis, 1983, p. 1–14.
113. KATZMAN, R., Clinical presentation of the course of Alzheimer's disease: the atypical patient. In: *Interdisciplinary Topics in Gerontology*, edited by H. P. von Hahn. Basel: Karger, 1985, p. 12–18.
114. KATZMAN, R. Alzheimer's disease as an age-dependent disorder. *Ciba Found. Symp.* 134: 69–85, 1988.
115. KATZMAN, R. Views and reviews: education and the prevalence of dementia and Alzheimer's disease. *Neurology* 43: 13–20, 1993.
115a. KATZMAN, R., and C. H. KAWAS. The epidemiology of dementia and Alzheimer disease. In: *Alzheimer Disease*, edited by R. D. Terry, R. Katzman, and K. L. Bick. New York: Raven Press, 1994, p. 105–122.
116. KATZMAN, R., and T. SAITOH. Advances in Alzheimer's disease. *FASEB J.* 5: 278–286, 1991.
117. KATZMAN, R., and R. D. TERRY. Normal aging of the nervous system. In: *Principles of Geriatric Neurology*, edited by R. Katzman and J. W. Rowe. Philadelphia: Davis, 1992, p. 18–58.
118. KATZMAN, R., R. D. TERRY, R. DETERESA, T. BROWN, P. DAVIES, P. FULD, X. RENBING, and A. PECK. Clinical, pathological, and neurochemical changes in dementia; a subgroup with preserved mental status and numerous neocortical plaques. *Ann. Neurol.* 23: 53–59, 1988.
119. KETY, S. S. Human cerebral blood flow and oxygen consumption as related to aging. In: *The Neurologic and Psychiatric Aspects of the Disorders of Aging*, edited by J. E. Moore, H. H. Merritt, and R. J. Masselink. Baltimore: Williams and Wilkins, 1955, p. 31–45.
120. KINSBOURNE, M. Cognitive decline with advancing age: an interpretation. In: *Aging and Dementia*, edited by W. L. Smith and M. Kinsbourne. New York: Spectrum, 1977, p. 217–235.
121. KLINE, D. W., and J. SZAFRAN. Age differences in backward monoptic visual noise masking. *J. Gerontol.* 3: 307–311, 1975.
122. KOH, J.-Y., L. L. YANG, and C. W. COTMAN. β-Amyloid protein increases the vulnerability of cultured cortical neurons to excitotoxic damage. *Brain Res.* 533: 315–320, 1990.
123. KONDO, J., T. HONEA, H. MORI, Y. HAMADA, R. MIURA, M. OGAWARA, and Y. IHARA. The carboxyl third of tau is tightly bound to paired helical filaments. *Neuron* 1: 827–828, 1988.
124. KORCZYN, A. D., N. LAOR, and P. NEMET. Sympathetic pupillary tone in old age. *Arch. Ophthalmol.* 94: 1905–1906, 1976.
125. KOSIK, K., and S. M. GREENBERG. Tau protein and Alzheimer disease. In: *Alzheimer Disease*, edited by R. D. Terry, R. Katzman, and K. L. Bick, New York: Raven Press, 1994, p. 335–344.
126. KOSIK, K. S., C. L. JOACHIM, and D. J. SELKOW. Microtubule-associated protein tau (τ) is a major antigenic component of paired helical filaments in Alzheimer's disease. *Proc. Natl. Acad. Sci. U.S.A.*, 83: 4044–4048, 1986.
127. KRISHNAN, K. R., M. M. HUSAIN, W. M. MCDONALD, P. M. DORAISWAMY, G. S. FIGIEL, O. B. BOYKO, E. H. ELLINWOOD, and C. B. NEMEROFF. In vivo stereological assessment of caudate volume in man: effect of normal aging. *Life Sci.* 47: 1325–1329, 1990.
128. KUMNICK, L. S. Pupillary psychosensory restitution and aging. *J. Optom. Soc. Am.* 44: 735, 1954.
129. LAFRATTA, C. W., and R. E. CANESTRARI. A comparison of sensory and motor nerve conduction velocities as related to age. *Arch. Phys. Med. Rehabil.* 47: 286–290, 1966.
130. LARIVIERE, J. E., and E. SIMONSON. The effect of age and occupation on speed of writing. *J. Gerontol.* 20: 415–416, 1965.
131. LAUFER, A. C., and B. SCHWEITZ. Neuromuscular response tests as predictors of sensory-motor performance in aging individuals. *Am. J. Phys. Med.* 47: 250–268, 1968.
132. LIGHT, L. L., and A. SINGH. Implicit and explicit memory in young and older adults. *J. Exp. Psychol.* 13: 531–541, 1987.
133. LIM, K. O., R. B. ZIPURSKY, M. C. WATTS, and A. PFEFFERBAUM. Decreased gray matter in normal aging: an in vivo magnetic resonance study. *J. Gerontol.* 47: 826–830, 1992.
134. LIPPA, C. F., J. E. HAMOS, D. PULASKI-SALO, L. J. DEGENNARO, and D. A. DRACHMAN. Alzheimer's disease and aging: effects on perforant pathway perikarya and synapses. *Neurobiol. Aging* 13: 405–411, 1992.
135. LLOYD, K., and O. HORNYKIEWICZ. Occurrence and distribution of L-dopa decarboxylase in the human brain. *Brain Res.* 22: 426–428, 1970.
136. LOWES-HUMMEL, P., H. J. GERTZ, R. FERSZT, and J. CERVOS-NAVARRO. The basal nucleus of Meynert revised: the nerve cell number decreases with age. *Arch. Gerontol. Geriatr.* 8: 21–27, 1989.
137. MACKAY, A. V. P., C. M. YATES, A. WRIGHT, P. HAMILTON, and P. DAVIES. Regional distribution of monoamines and their metabolites in the human brain. *J. Neurochem.* 30: 841–848, 1978.
138. MASLIAH, E., D. S. IIMOTO, M. MALLORY, T. ALBRIGHT, L. A. HANSEN, and T. SAITOH. Casein kinase II alteration precedes Tau accumulation in tangle formation. *Am. J. Pathol.* 140: 263–268, 1992.
139. MASLIAH, E., M. MALLORY, L. HANSEN, M. ALFORD, R. DETERESA, R. TERRY, J. BAUDIER, and T. SAITOH. Localization of amyloid precursor protein in GAP-43 immunoreactive aberrant

sprouting neurites in Alzheimer's disease. *Brain Res.* 574: 312–316, 1992.
140. MASLIAH, E., M. MALLORY, L. HANSEN, R. DETERESA, and R. D. TERRY. Quantitative synaptic alterations in the human neocortex during normal aging. *Neurology* 43: 192–197, 1993.
141. MASLIAH, E., R. D. TERRY, M. MALLORY, M. ALFORD, and L. A. HANSEN. Diffuse plaques do not accentuate synapse loss in Alzheimer's disease. *Am. J. Pathol.* 137: 1293–1297, 1990.
142. MCGEER, E. G. Aging and neurotransmitter metabolism in the human brain. In: *Alzheimer's Disease, Senile Dementia and Related Disorders,* edited by R. Katzman, R. D. Terry, and K. L. Bick. New York: Raven Press, 1978, p. 427–440.
143. MCGEER, P. L., E. G. MCGEER, J. SUZUKI, C. E. DOLMAN, and T. NAGAI. Aging, Alzheimer's disease, and the cholinergic system of the basal forebrain. *Neurology* 34: 741–745, 1984.
144. MCKHANN, G., D. DRACHMAN, M. FOLSTEIN, R. KATZMAN, D. PROCE, and E. M. STADLAN. Clinical diagnosis of Alzheimer's disease: report of the NINCDS-ADRDA Work Groups under the auspices of Department of Health and Human Services Task Force on Alzheimer's Disease. *Neurology* 34: 939–944, 1984.
145. MICHALEWSKI, H. J., L. W. THOMPSON, D. B. D. SMITH, J. V. PATERSON, T. E. BOWMAN, D. LITZELMAN, and G. BRENT. Age differences in the contingent negative variation (CNV): reduced frontal activity in the elderly. *J. Gerontol.* 35: 542–549, 1980.
146. MORRIS, R. G., M. L. GICK, and F. I. M. CRAIK. Processing resources and age differences in working memory. *Mem. Cogn.* 16: 362–366, 1988.
147. MORTIMER, J. A. Do psychosocial risk factors contribute to Alzheimer's disease? In: *Etiology of Dementia of Alzheimer's Type,* edited by A. S. Henderson and J. H. Henderson. New York: Wiley, 1988, p. 39–52.
148. MORTIMER, J. A., C. M. VAN DUIJN, V. CHANDRA, L. FRATIGLIONI, A. B. GRAVES, A. HEYMAN, A. F. JORM, E. KOKMEN, K. KONDO, W. A. ROCCA, S. L. SHALAT, H. SOININEN, and A. HOFMAN. Head trauma as a risk factor for Alzheimer's disease: a collaborative re-analysis of case-control studies. *Int. J. Epidemiol.* 20(suppl. 2): S28–S35, 1991.
149. MULLAN, M., F. CRAWFORD, K. AXELMAN, H. HOULDEN, L. LILIUS, B. WINBLAD, and L. LANNFELT. A pathogenic mutation for probable Alzheimer's disease in the APP gene at the N-terminus of β-amyloid. *Nat. Genet.* 1: 345–347, 1992.
150. MULLAN, M., H. HOULDEN, M. WINDELSPECHT, L. FIDANI, C. LOMBARDI, P. DIAZ, M. ROSSOR, R. CROOK, J. HARDY, K. DUFF, and F. CRAWFORD. A locus for familial early-onset Alzheimer's disease on the long arm of chromosome 14, proximal to the α_1-antichymotrypsin gene. *Nat. Genet.* 2: 340–342, 1992.
151. MURRELL, J., M. FARLOW, B. GHETTI, and M. D. BENSON. A mutation in the amyloid precursor protein associated with hereditary Alzheimer's disease. *Science* 254: 97–99, 1991.
152. OBRIST, W. D. Cerebral circulatory changes in normal aging and dementia. In: *Brain Function in Old Age,* edited by F. Hoffmeister and C. Muller. Berlin: Springer-Verlag, 1979, 278–287.
153. OWENS, W. A. Age and mental abilities: a second adult follow-up. *J. Educ. Psychol.* 57: 311–325, 1966.
154. PATTERSON, J. V., H. J. MICHALEWSKI, and A. STARR. Latency variability of the components of auditory event-related potentials to infrequent stimuli in aging, Alzheimer-type dementia, and depression. *Electroencephalogr. Clin. Neurophysiol.* 71: 450–460, 1988.
155. PERRY, E. K., M. JOHNSON, J. M. KERWIN, M. A. PIGGOTT, J. A. COURT, P. J. SHAW, P. G. INCE, A. BROWN, and R. H. PERRY. Convergent cholinergic activities in aging and Alzheimer's disease. *Neurobiol. Aging* 13: 393–400, 1992.
156. PERRY, E. K., R. H. PERRY, G. BLESSED, and B. E. TOMLINSON. Necropsy evidence of central cholinergic deficits in senile dementia. *Lancet* 1: 189, 1977.
157. PERRY, E. K., B. E. TOMLINSON, G. BLESSED, K. BERGMANN, P. H. GIBSON, and R. H. PERRY. Correlation of cholinergic abnormalities with senile plaques and mental test scores in senile dementia. *Br. Med. J.* 2: 1457–1459, 1978.
158. PETERSEN, R. C., G. SMITH, E. KOKMEN, R. J. IVNIK, and E. G. TANGALOS. Memory function in normal aging. *Neurology* 42: 396–401, 1992.
159. PITAS, R. E., J. K. BOYLES, S. H. LEE, D. FOSS, and R. W. MAHLEY. Astrocytes synthesize apolipoprotein E and metabolize apolipoprotein E-containing lipoproteins. *Biochim. Biophys. Acta* 917: 148–161, 1987.
160. POTVIN, A. R., K. SYNDULKO, W. W. TOURTELLOTTE, J. A. LEMMON, and J. H. POTVIN. Human neurologic function and the aging process. *J. Am. Geriatr. Soc.* 28: 1–9, 1980.
161. PRICE, J. L., P. B. DAVIS, J. C. MORRIS, and D. L. WHITE. The distribution of tangles, plaques and related immunohistochemical markers in healthy aging and Alzheimer's disease. *Neurobiol. Aging* 12: 295–312, 1991.
162. REPKA, M. X., and H. A. QUIGLEY. The effect of age on normal human optic nerve fiber number and diameter. *Ophthalmology* 96: 26–32, 1989.
163. RIEGEL, K. F., R. M. RIEGEL, and G. MEYER. Socio-psychological factors of aging: a cohort-sequential analysis. *Hum. Dev.* 10: 27–56, 1967.
164. RITTER, W., R. SIMSON, and H. G. VAUGHAN, JR. Effects of the amount of stimulus information processed on the negative event-related potentials. *Electroencephalogr. Clin. Neurophysiol.* 69: 244–258, 1988.
165. ROBAKIS, N. K., N. RAMAKRISHNA, G. WOLFE, and H. M. WISNIEWSKI. Molecular cloning and characterization of a cDNA encoding the cerebrovascular and the neuritic plaque amyloid peptides. *Proc. Natl. Acad. Sci. U.S.A.* 84: 4190–4194, 1987.
166. ROBERTS, G. W., D. ALLSOP, and C. BRUTON. The occult aftermath of boxing. *J. Neurol. Neurosurg. Psychiatry* 53: 273–278, 1990.
167. ROBINSON, D., T. SOURKES, A. NIES, L. HARRIS, S. SPECTOR, D. BARTLETT, and I. KAYE. Monoamine metabolism in human brain. *Arch. Gen. Psychiatry* 34: 89–92, 1977.
168. ROSES, A. D., M. A. PERICAK-VANCE, C. M. CLARK, J. R. GILBERT, L. H. YAMAOKA, C. S. HAYNES, M. C. SPEER, P. C. GASKELL, W. Y. HUNG, J. A. TROFATTER, N. L. EARL, J. E. LEE, M. J. ALBERTS, D. V. DAWSON, R. J. BARTLETT, T. SIDDIQUE, J. M. VANCE, P. M. CONNEALLY, and A. L. HEYMAN. Linkage studies of late-onset familial Alzheimer's disease. *Adv. Neurol.* 51: 185–196, 1990.
169. ROSES, A. D., A. M. SAUNDERS, W. J. STRITTMATTER, M. A. PERICAK-VANCE, and D. SCHMECHEL. Association of apolipoprotein E allele E4 with late onset familial and sporadic Alzheimer's disease. *Neurology* 43(suppl. 2): A192, 1993.
170. ROSSOR, M., and L. L. IVERSEN. Non-cholinergic neurotransmitter abnormalities in Alzheimer's disease. *Br. Med. Bull.* 42: 70–74, 1986.
171. ROWE, J. W., and R. KATZMAN. Principles of geriatrics as applied to neurology. In: *Principles of Geriatric Neurology,* edited by R. Katzman and J. W. Rowe. Philadelphia: Davis, 1992, p. 1–17.
172. RUMBLE, B., R. RETALLACK, C. HILBICH, G. SIMMS, G. MULTHAUPT, R. MARTINS, A. HOCKEY, P. MONTGOMERY, K. BEYREUTHER, and C. L. MASTERS. Amyloid A4 protein and its precursor in Down's syndrome and Alzheimer's disease. *N. Engl. J. Med.* 320: 1446–1452, 1989.
173. SAID, F. S., and R. A. WEALE. The variation with age of the spectral transmissivity of the living human crystalline lens. *Gerontologia* 3: 213–231, 1959.
174. SAN FILIPPO, S. The masters movement: Payton Jordon sprints to the front. *Runner's World* : 85, 1979.

175. SCHAIE, K. W., G. V. LABOUVIE, and B. U. BUECH. Generational and cohort-specific differences in adult cognitive functioning. A fourteen-year study of independent samples. *Dev. Psychol.* 9: 151–166, 1973.
176. SCHELLENBERG, G. D., T. D. BIRD, E. M. WIJSMAN, H. T. ORR, L. ANDERSON, E. NEMENS, J. A. WHITE, L. BONNYCASTLE, J. L. WEBER, M. E. ALONSO, H. POTTER, L. L. HESTON, and G. M. MARTIN. Genetic linkage evidence for a familial Alzheimer's disease locus on chromosome 14. *Science* 258: 668–671, 1992.
177. SCHOW, R. L., J. M. CHRISTENSEN, J. M. HUTCHINSON, and M. A. NERBONNE. *Communication Disorders of the Aged*. Baltimore: University Park Press, 1978.
178. SCOTT, S. A., S. T. DEKOSKY, D. L. SPARKS, C. A. KNOW, and S. W. SCHEFF. Amygdala cell loss and atrophy in Alzheimer's disease. *Ann. Neurol.* 32: 555–563, 1992.
179. SEUBERT, P., C. VIGO-PELFREY, F. ESCH, M. LEE, H. DOVEY, D. DAVIS, S. SINHA, M. SCHLOSSMACHER, J. WHALEY, C. SWINDLEHURST, R. MCCORMACK, R. WOLFERT, D. SELKOE, I. LIEBERBURG, and D. SCHENK. Isolation and quantification of soluble Alzheimer's β-peptide from biological fluids. *Nature* 359: 325–327, 1992.
180. SHAW, N. A., and B. R. CANT. Age-dependent changes in the latency of the pattern visual evoked potential. *Electroencephalogr. Clin. Neurophysiol.* 48: 237–241, 1980.
181. SHOJI, M., T. E. GOLDE, J. GHISO, T. T. CHEUNG, S. ESTUS, L. M. SHAFFER, X. D. CAI, D. M. MCKAY, R. TINTNER, and B. FRANGIONE. Production of the Alzheimer amyloid β protein by normal proteolytic processing. *Science* 258: 126–129, 1992.
182. SISODIA, S. S., E. H. KOO, K. BEYREUTHER, A. UNTERBECK, and D. L. PRICE. Evidence that β-amyloid protein in Alzheimer's disease is not derived by normal processing. *Science* 248: 492–495, 1990.
183. SNYDER, E., and S. A. HILLYARD. Changes in visual event-related potentials in older persons. In: *Brain Function in Old Age. Bayer-Symposium VII*, edited by F. Hoffmeister and C. Muller. New York: Springer-Verlag, 1979, p. 112–125.
184. SPARKS, D. L., J. C. HUNSAKER, S. W. SCHEFF, R. F. KRYSCIC, J. L. HENSON, and W. R. MARKESBERY. Cortical senile plaques in coronary artery disease, aging and Alzheimer's disease. *Neurobiol. Aging* 11: 601–608, 1990.
185. SPARKS, D. L., H. LIU, S. W. SCHEFF, C. M. COYNE, and J. C. HUNSAKER. Temporal sequence of plaque formation in the cerebral cortex of non-demented individuals. *J. Neuropathol. Exp. Neurol.* 52: 135–142, 1993.
186. SPIRDUSO, W. W., and P. CLIFFORD. Replication of age and physical activity effects on reaction and movement time. *J. Gerontol.* 33: 26–30, 1978.
187. ST. GEORGE-HYSLOP, P., J. HAINES, E. ROGAEV, M. MORTILLA, G. VAULA, M. PERICAK-VANCE, J.-F. FONCIN, M. MONTESI, A. BRUNI, S. SORBI, L. RAINERO, L. PINESSI, D. POLLEN, R. POLINSKY, L. NEE, J. KENNEDY, F. MACCIARDI, E. ROGAEVA, Y. LIANG, N. ALEXANDROVA, W. LUKIW, K. SCHLUMPF, R. TANZI, T. TSUDA, L. FARRER, J.-M. CANTU, R. DUARA, L. AMADUCCI, L. BERGAMINI, J. GUSELLA, A. ROSES, and D. CRAPPER MCLACHLAN. Genetic evidence for a novel familial Alzheimer's disease locus on chromosome 14. *Nat. Genet.* 2: 330–334, 1992.
188. ST. GEORGE-HYSLOP, P. H., R. E. TANZI, R. J. POLINSKY, J. L. HAINES, L. NEE, P. C. WATKINS, R. H. MYERS, R. G. FELDMAN, D. POLLEN, D. DRACHMAN, J. GROWDON, A. BRUNI, J.-F. FONCIN, D. SALMON, P. FROMMELT, L. AMADUCCI, S. SORBI, S. PLACENTINI, G. D. STEWART, W. J. HOBBS, P. M. CONNEALLY, and J. F. GUSELLA. The genetic defect causing familial Alzheimer's disease maps on chromosome 21. *Science* 235: 885–890, 1987.
189. STRITTMATTER, W. J., A. M. SAUNDERS, D. SCHMECHEL, M. PERICAK-VANCE, J. ENGHILD, G. S. SALVESEN, and A. D. ROSES. Apolipoprotein E: high-avidity binding to beta-amyloid and increased frequency of type 4 allele in late-onset familial Alzheimer disease. *Proc. Natl. Acad. Sci. U.S.A.* 90: 1977–1981, 1993.
190. TAYLOR, J. L., T. P. MILLER, and J. R. TINKLENBERG. Correlates of memory decline: a 4-year longitudinal study of older adults with memory complaints. *Psychol. Aging* 7: 185–193, 1992.
191. TERÄVÄINEN, H., and D. B. CALNE. Motor system in normal aging and Parkinson's disease. In: *The Neurology of Aging*, edited by R. Katzman and R. D. Terry. Philadelphia: Davis, 1983, p. 85–109.
192. TERRY, R. D. Neurofibrillary tangles in Alzheimer's disease. *J. Neuropathol. Exp. Neurol.* 22: 629–642, 1963.
193. TERRY, R. D., and R. KATZMAN. Senile dementia of the Alzheimer type; defining a disease. In: *The Neurology of Aging*, edited by R. Katzman and R. D. Terry. Philadelphia: Davis, 1983, p. 51–84.
194. TERRY, R. D., and R. KATZMAN. Alzheimer disease and cognitive loss. In: *Principles of Geriatric Neurology*, edited by R. Katzman and J. W. Rowe. Philadelphia: Davis, 1992, p. 207–265.
195. TERRY, R. D., R. DETERESA, and L. A. HANSEN. Neocortical cell counts in normal human adult aging. *Ann. Neurol.* 21: 530–539, 1987.
196. TERRY, R. D., N. K. GONATAS, and M. WEISS. Ultrastructural studies in Alzheimer's presenile dementia. *Am. J. Pathol.* 44: 269–297, 1964.
197. TERRY, R. D., R. KATZMAN, and K. L. BICK, eds. *Alzheimer Disease*. New York: Raven Press, 1994, p. 492.
198. TERRY, R. D., E. MASLIAH, D. P. SALMON, N. BUTTERS, R. DETERESA, R. HILL, L. A. HANSEN, and R. KATZMAN. Physical basis of cognitive alterations in Alzheimer's disease: synapse loss is the major correlate of cognitive impairment. *Ann. Neurol.* 30: 572–580, 1991.
199. TERRY, R. D., A. PECK, and R. DETERESA. Some morphometric aspects of the brain in senile dementia of the Alzheimer type. *Ann. Neurol.* 10: 184–192, 1981.
200. TOKUDA, T., S. IKEDA, N. YANAGISAWA, Y. IHARA, and G. G. GLENNER. Reexamination of ex-boxers' brains using immunohistochemistry with antibodies to amyloid beta-protein and tau protein. *Acta Neuropathol. (Berl.)* 82: 280–285, 1991.
201. TULVING, E. How many memory systems are there? *Am. Psychol.* 40: 385–398, 1985.
202. UÉDA, K., E. MASLIAH, T. SAITOH, S. L. BAKALIS, H. SCOBLE, and K. S. KOSIK. Alz-50 recognizes a phosphorylated epitope of tau protein. *J. Neurosci.* 10: 3295–3304, 1990.
203. VAN BROECKHOVEN, C., H. BACKHOVENS, M. CRUTS, G. DE WINTER, M. BRUYLAND, P. CRAS, and J.-J. MATRIN. Mapping of a gene predisposing to early-onset Alzheimer's disease to chromosome 14q24.3 *Nat. Genet.* 2: 335–339, 1992.
204. VAN DUIJN, C. M., D. CLAYTON, V. CHANDRA, L. FRATIGLIONI, A. B. GRAVES, A. HEYMAN, A. F. JORM, E. KOKMEN, K. KONDO, J. A. MORTIMER, W. A. ROCCA, S. L. SHALAT, H. SOININEN, and A. HOFMAN. Familial aggregation of Alzheimer's disease and related disorders: a collaborative re-analysis of case-control studies. *Int. J. Epidemiol.* 20(suppl. 2): S13–S20, 1991.
205. VAN NOSTRAND, W. E., S. L. WAGNER, M. SUZUKI, B. H. CHOI, J. S. FARROW, J. W. GEDDES, C. W. COTMAN, and D. D. CUNNINGHAM. Protease nexin-II, a potent anti-chymotrypsin, shows identity to amyloid β protein. *Nature* 341: 546–548, 1989.
206. VIJAYASHANKAR, N., and H. BRODY. A quantitative study of the pigmented neurons in the nuclei locus coeruleus and subcoeruleus in man as related to aging. *J. Neuropathol. Exp. Neurol.* 38: 490–497, 1979.
207. WALSH, D. A. Age differences in central perceptual processing: a dichoptic backward masking investigation. *J. Gerontol.* 31: 178–185, 1976.

208. WALSH, D. A., and M. BALDWIN. Age differences in integrated semantic memory. *Dev. Psychol.* 13: 509–514, 1977.
209. WALSH, D. A., and R. E. TILL. Age differences in peripheral perceptual processing: a monoptic backward masking investigation. *J. Exp. Psychol.* 4: 232–243, 1978.
210. WANG, H. S., W. D. OBRIST, and E. W. BUSSE. Neurophysiological correlates of the intellectual function. In: *Normal Aging*, edited by E. Palmore. Durham, NC: Duke University Press, 1974, p. 115–126.
211. WARREN, L. R., J. W. WAGENER, and G. E. HERMAN. Binaural analysis in the aging auditory system. *J. Gerontol.* 33: 731–736, 1978.
212. WEALE, R. A. The aging retina. *Geriatrics* 3: 425–450, 1985.
213. WEISS, A. D. The locus of reaction time change with set, motivation, and age. *J. Gerontol.* 20: 60–64, 1965.
214. WELFORD, A. T. Motor performance. In: *Handbook of the Psychology of Aging*, edited by J. E. Birren and K. W. Schaie. New York: Van Nostrand Reinhold, 1977, p. 450–496.
215. WELFORD, A. T. Sensory, perceptual, and motor processes in older adults. In: *Handbook of Mental Health and Aging*, edited by J. E. Birren and R. B. Sloane. Englewood Cliffs, NJ: Prentice-Hall, 1980, p. 192.
216. WELSH, K. A., N. BUTTERS, J. P. HUGHES, R. C. MOHS, and A. HEYMAN. Detection and staging of dementia in Alzheimer's disease. *Arch. Neurol.* 49: 448–452, 1992.
217. WHITE, L., R. KATZMAN, K. LOSONCZY, M. SALIVE, R. WALLACE, L. BERKMAN, J. TAYLOR, G. FILLENBAUM, and R. HAVLIK. Association of education on the incidence of cognitive impairment in three established populations for epidemiologic studies of the elderly. *J. Clin. Epidemiol.* 47: 363–374, 1994.
218. WHITEHOUSE, P. J., D. L. PRICE, R. G. STRUBLE, A. W. CLARK, J. T. COYLE, and M. R. DELONG. Alzheimer's disease and senile dementia: loss of neurons in the basal forebrain. *Science* 215: 1237–1239, 1982.
219. WHITEHOUSE, P. J., I. M. PURHAD, J. C. HEDREEN, A. W. CLARK, C. L. WHITE III, R. G. STRUBLE, and D. L. PRICE. Integrity of the nucleus basalis of Meynert in normal aging. *Neurology* 33(suppl. 2): 159, 1983.
220. WHITSON, J. S., C. G. GLABE, E. SHINTANI, A. ABCAR, and C. W. COTMAN. β-Amyloid protein promotes neuritic branching in hippocampal cultures. *Neurosci. Lett.* 110: 319–324, 1990.
221. WISNIEWSKI, H. M., H. K. NARANG, and R. D. TERRY. Neurofibrillary tangles of paired helical filaments. *J. Neurol. Sci.* 27: 173–181, 1976.
222. WISNIEWSKI, T., and B. FRANGIONE. Apolipoprotein E: a pathological chaperone protein in patients with cerebral and systemic amyloid. *Neurosci. Lett.* 135: 235–238, 1992.
223. WOLFSON, L., and R. KATZMAN. The neurologic consultation at age 80. In: *Principles of Geriatric Neurology*, edited by R. Katz and J. W. Rowe. Philadelphia: Davis, 1992, p. 75–88.
224. WOOD, J. G., S. MIRRA, N. J. POLLACK, and L. I. BINDER. Neurofibrillary tangles of Alzheimer disease share antigenic determinant with the axonal microtubule-associated protein tau. *Proc. Natl. Acad. Sci. U.S.A.* 83: 4040–4043, 1986.
225. YAMAMURA, H., M. ITO, K. KUBOTA, and T. MATSUZAWA. Brain atrophy during aging: a quantitative study with computed tomography. *J. Gerontol.* 35: 492–498, 1980.
226. YANKNER, B. A., L. R. DAWES, S. FISHER, L. VILLA-KOMAROFF, M. L. OSTERGRANITE, and R. L. NEVE. Neurotoxicity of a fragment of the amyloid precursor associated with Alzheimer's disease. *Science* 245: 417–420, 1989.
227. ZHANG, M., R. KATZMAN, H. JIN, G. CAI, Z. WANG, G. QU, I. GRANT, E. YU, P. LEVY, and W. T. LIU. The prevalence of dementia and Alzheimer's disease (AD) in Shanghai, China: impact of age, gender and education. *Ann. Neurol.* 27: 428–437, 1990.

13. Maintenance and regulation in brain of neurotransmission, trophic factors, and immune responses

CARL W. COTMAN
JENNIFER S. KAHLE
ANDREW R. KOROTZER

Department of Psychobiology, University of California Irvine, Irvine, California

CHAPTER CONTENTS

The Imbalance Hypothesis of Aging
Neurotransmitter Systems
    Glutamate receptors
        NMDA receptors decline in aged rodent models
        KA and AMPA receptors in aged rodent models
        Glutamate receptor change in control elderly and Alzheimer patients
        Lesion models of Alzheimer's disease as predictors of receptor change
        Compensatory mechanisms and maintenance of glutamate function
    GABA receptors
        Changes in $GABA_A$ receptors in aged rodent models
        Reduced GABA levels with age and in neurodegenerative disease
        The depressive effect of benzodiazepines in the elderly
    Summary
Neurotrophic Factors
    Nerve growth factor
        NGF levels in aged rodents vs humans
        Neuronal activity and regulation of neurotrophic factor synthesis
        NGF in Alzheimer's disease
    Fibrolast growth factor
        FGF-1 changes with aging
        FGF-2 cell survival after axotomy
        Possible role of FGF-2 and NGF in plaque biogenesis
    Cytokines as neurotrophic factors
        IL-1 and recovery after injury
        Effect of glucocorticoids on the immune response in aged brain
The Immune System in the CNS
    The immune system and Alzheimer's disease
    Cytokines and the immune system
        The complement cascade and Alzheimer pathology
Summary and Conclusions

RECENT DISCOVERIES ABOUT THE MECHANISMS OF CELL DEATH, degeneration, and plasticity in the nervous system have increased our understanding of the aging process. The state of the aging brain is important for the maintenance of higher cognitive function, the control of movement and indeed for the overall coordination of body functions. Most of the recent progress has been made in the area of age-related neurodegenerative diseases, particularly Alzheimer's disease. However, many of the principles that have been established for such disease conditions are also relevant to the normal aging process, since the prevention of age-related degenerative conditions is essential to the maintenance of brain function.

THE IMBALANCE HYPOTHESIS OF AGING

The precise regulation of the many different processes is essential for normal cognitive function. One example is the maintenance of a balance of inhibitory and excitatory neurotransmission in normal brain function. Within a local main network, information appears to be processed and connections strengthened or weakened as a function of the excitatory input from projection neurons and local feed-forward and feedback modulatory activity that includes both inhibitory and excitatory influences. If the system becomes imbalanced and there is insufficient modulation of excitatory transmission, seizures and seizure-like activity develop. This principle is especially important in light of evidence that overexcitation can cause neuronal death. In turn, low levels of excitatory transmission may interfere with sensory processing, and learning, and other cognitive or emotional processes.

Another example of the balance of brain function is that of cell death and compensatory plasticity and regrowth mechanisms. As the brain ages and the cells degenerate, mechanisms such as the sprouting of axons from healthy neurons can replace those connections that are lost as neurons die. Various trophic factors are key to the proper maintenance of neuronal circuitry. Trophic factors enhance cell survival after injury and stimulate the regrowth of neuronal processes. Trophic factor activity can be regulated by neuronal activity, hormone levels, and levels of other trophic factors. The interplay of these processes is illustrated by evidence that increased inhibition of neurons producing prolonged inactivity can change trophic factor levels and lead to neuronal death. Thus shifts in the balance of neuronal function can in turn affect the maintenance of neuronal integrity.

In parallel with these processes, factors that regulate the activity of neurotrophic factors also become part of the balance between normal function and dysfunction. For example, some cytokines can function not only in immune responses but also in the regulation of other trophic factors, and in some cases they have direct neurotrophic roles. Thus, as directed by signals from the environment, these cytokines can participate in the overall functional state of the brain. This underlines the importance of establishing how the immune system changes in the central nervous system (CNS) with aging and how this effects other brain functions.

In this chapter we examine what can be referred to as the "imbalance hypothesis" of brain aging; that is, imbalances at one level of brain function can affect not only that level but others as well. This can initiate a series of cellular and molecular cascades that determine the onset of pathology and ultimately cannot be regulated. In parallel with such events, other mechanisms, categorized as neural plasticity, may offset functional imbalances. We begin with a discussion of two neurotransmitter systems—glutamate and GABA—as examples of the changing balance between excitatory and inhibitory neurotransmission as a function of age. Then we discuss recent research on the state of representative trophic factors in aging and neurodegenerative conditions such as Alzheimer's disease. We illustrate how it has become increasingly clear that the regulation of certain neurotrophic factors depends on the state of neurotransmitter systems as well as on that of other trophic factors. In the last section we illustrate how the state of the immune response in the aging brain and in Alzheimer's disease can influence neural systems. Since it is not the purpose of this chapter to provide an exhaustive review of the literature on brain aging studies, the reader is directed to several such reviews (3, 56, 112).

NEUROTRANSMITTER SYSTEMS

Glutamate Receptors

It is apparent that glutamate is the major excitatory transmitter in the CNS (for review see 89), and, although normally modulated by inhibitory systems, it exerts a powerful activating influence on target neurons. Overactivation of the glutamate system coupled with circuitry involving recurrent excitation can lead to seizures and seizure-like activity. Intense stimulation of glutamate receptors beyond a certain threshold can result in neuronal death via excitotoxicity mechanisms.

One subtype of glutamate receptor that has been extensively studied is the N-methyl-D-aspartate (NMDA) receptor/channel complex. The NMDA receptor/channel complex is different from other glutamate ionotropic receptors (non-NMDA receptors) in that it has a high capacity for a calcium-mediated current (for review see 17). This current is only activated with concurrent depolarization and is highly regulated by several factors, including magnesium, glycine, and zinc (Fig. 13.1) (124). Thus, while non-NMDA ionotropic receptors carry a major portion of the excitatory signal, the NMDA receptor/channel complex allows for plasticity in cellular responses, particularly those regulated by calcium.

Influx of free calcium into neurons is an essential component of many cellular processes and thus contributes to normal neuronal function. Calcium influx through the NMDA receptor has been implicated in many processes, including long-term potentiation (11), which is thought to be a correlate of learning (77). The capacity for highly regulated plastic responses that the NMDA receptor imparts to neurons, however, also allows many points of vulnerability to dysfunction. High levels of intracellular calcium can be toxic to neurons and can cause cell death through excitotoxicity (81, 89, 116).

NMDA Receptors in Aged Rodent Models. Work done in rodent models (both mouse and rat) has established that the number of NMDA receptors (B_{max}) declines with age, particularly in the hippocampus and frontal cortex, as determined by saturation binding studies (Fig. 13.2A (10, 63, 64, 101, 122). Levels of glutamate and NMDA binding also decline with age in the monkey parietal and occipital cortices (129, 130). A recent study suggests that this change may not reflect cell loss, since binding to a site inside the associated ion channel by (+)-[^{3}H]5-methyl-10,11-dihydro-5H-dibenzo[a,d]-cycloheptane-5,10-imine maleate (MK-801) is not always decreased in parallel with the decrease in NMDA binding (78). Furthermore, coupled with a decline in B_{max}, there may be a change in the affinity (K_d) of glutamate receptors. Peterson and Cotman (101) reported an increase in K_d for glutamate binding to the NMDA receptor with age in mice, whereas Cohen and Müller (10), using a different strain of aged mouse, reported a slight decrease in K_d for MK-801.

KA and AMPA Receptors in Aged Rodent Models. Several studies in aged rodent models have examined the status of the non-NMDA ionotropic glutamate receptors AMPA and KA, named for selective agonists α-

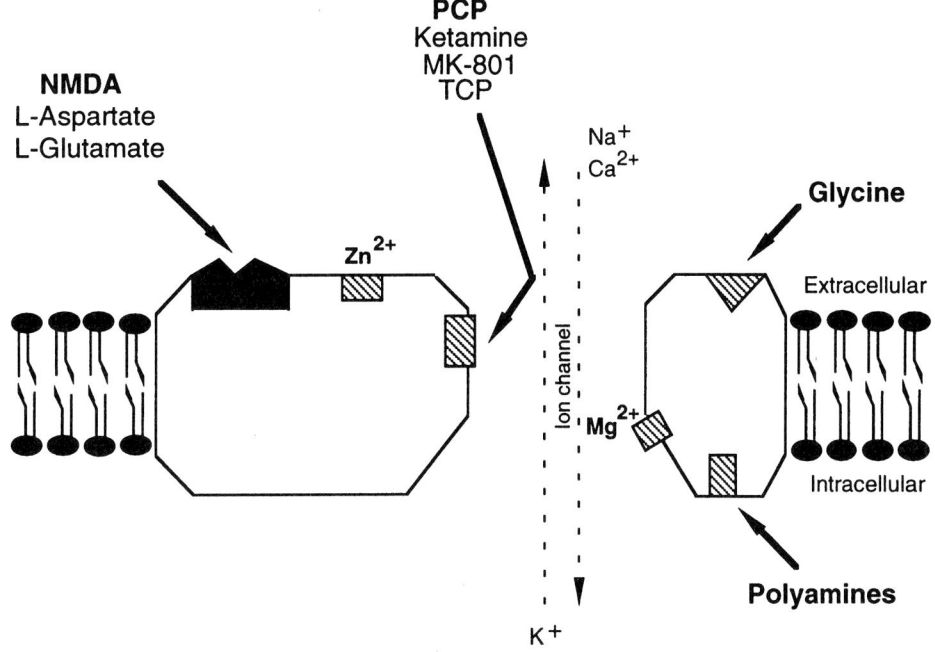

FIG. 13.1. The NMDA receptor complex. The transmitter recognition site binds agonists such as NMDA, L-glutamate, and L-aspartate. This binding opens the ion channel, allowing Na^+ and Ca^{2+} ions to flow inside the neuron and K^+ ions to flow out. The glycine site allosterically modulates receptor function, probably by increasing the frequency of agonist-induced channel opening. The NMDA-receptor complex is also regulated by polyamines and Zn^{2+} at two other modulatory sites. At resting membrane potential, Mg^{2+} blocks the ion channel in a voltage-dependent manner and this block is relieved during membrane depolarization. The ion channel also contains a phencyclidine (PCP) recognition site, which can bind PCP, ketamine, and MK-801, serving to block the open channel. [Reprinted with permission from Ulas and Cotman (124).]

amino-3-hydroxy-5-methyl-4-isoxazolepropionic acid (AMPA) and kainic acid (KA). Like NMDA receptors, AMPA receptors studied in rodent models appear to decrease in number with age (5, 9, 122). In contrast, KA receptors appear to remain stable with age (122), except for decreases in the CA1 and CA3 regions of the hippocampus and the inner frontal and parietal cortices (9, 79).

Levels of glutamate and the amount of glutamate released upon depolarization have been shown to increase with age in an accelerated aging mouse model (P/8) (63). This increase in glutamate upon depolarization may explain how a decreased number of glutamate receptors may be effectively balanced, resulting in the maintenance of function as the organism ages.

Glutamate Receptor Change in Control Elderly and Alzheimer Patients. Although not all aspects of glutamate receptor function studied in rodent models have been examined in the human, it appears that the pattern of changes in NMDA receptors observed in rodents is paralleled in the aging human brain. Recent evidence demonstrates that the number of binding sites for MK-801 declines with age (Fig. 13.2b) (102). Glutamate binding to NMDA and MK-801 receptor sites declines even further in Alzheimer brain (Fig. 13.2C) (125). Future studies examining changes in other characteristics of the NMDA receptor with aging in the human brain may indicate whether the loss of some NMDA receptors may be compensated for by an increase in efficacy of those that remain. Recent studies indicate that MK-801 binding is not blocked by zinc in the aged brain, as observed in young adult brain (102) and that glycine stimulation of MK-801 binding is reduced with age (105).

Several changes in non-NMDA receptors have been reported in aging humans and in individuals with Alzheimer's disease. Aged normal individuals show a decrease in KA-binding levels in the H_3 region of hippocampus (110). In Alzheimer's disease, it has been demonstrated that there is a significant increase in AMPA binding in the infragranular layer and, in some cases, an accompanying increase in KA binding in the outer half of the molecular layer of the dentate gyrus of the hippocampus (38). Previous reports indicate that KA binding in Alzheimer hippocampus may be increased or maintained (18, 23, 37, 98) or may be reduced in the dentate gyrus molecular layer, CA3 region, or the CA1 region (23, 98, 110).

Lesion Models of Alzheimer's Disease as Predictors of Receptor Changes. Entorhinal cortex lesions in rodents are often used to model some of the changes observed in Alzheimer's disease, and they have been used to predict specific changes in Alzheimer brain. The loss of the perforant path fiber projection from entorhinal cortex to dentate gyrus triggers a series of plasticity mechanisms, including fiber sprouting and synaptic reorganization in the molecular layer of the dentate gyrus, mechanisms that appear to compensate for the lost connections and contribute to the recovery of perforant path function (61). Similar changes have been found in Alzheimer brain (38). For example, changes in the distribution of glutamate receptors in the molecular layer reflect the remodeling processes that occur in this region, and these changes are localized to the specific laminae within the molecular layer. For example, an expansion of dense KA binding from the inner third to the inner half of the molecular layer causes an overall increase in KA binding (12). This suggests that excitatory amino acid receptor levels are precisely and specifically regulated in response to neuronal loss and that, with progressive neuronal loss observed in aging or age-related neurodegenerative disease, these changes may occur on a continual basis.

Compensatory Mechanisms and Maintenance of Glutamate Function. Taken together, these data suggest that there is a shift in the relationship between glutamate receptor number, binding affinity, and glutamate level as the organism ages. It appears that, to some degree, the functionality of the glutamate system may be maintained (108), since the decreased receptor number can be accompanied by increased glutamate levels and release. It remains to be established whether these shifts are significant enough to maintain function in the later stages of aging and in disease states, particularly in the human. Again, the natural compensatory systems may, as they become overextended, begin to contribute to neuronal death. For example, an increase in glutamate levels may be compensated for initially by a decrease in glutamate AMPA receptor number, but increased acti-

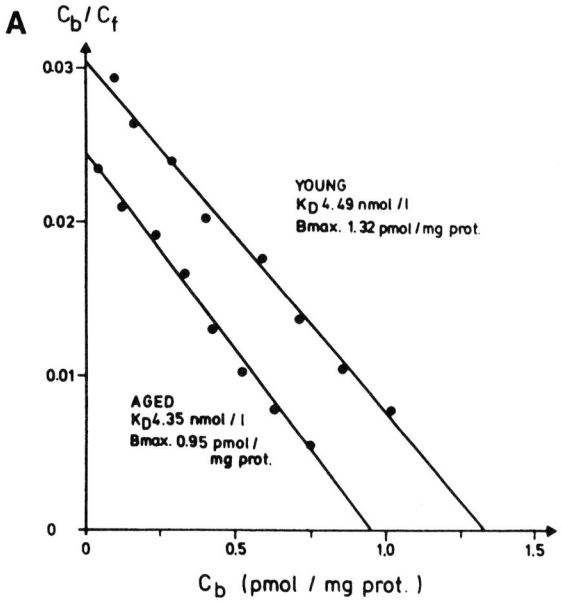
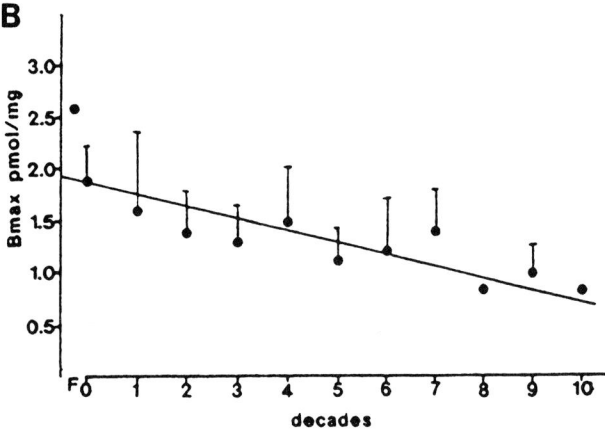
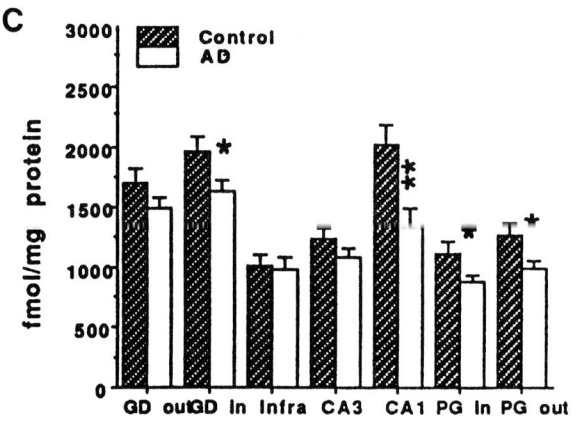

FIG. 13.2. Binding to NMDA receptors decreases with age in mice, normal human, and Alzheimer brain. **A**: Scatchard presentation of the specific binding of increasing concentrations of [^{3}H]MK-801 to forebrain homogenates of young and aged mice. **B**: Number of MK-801 binding sites (B_{max}) plotted against age shows that binding decreases with age in membranes prepared from human frontal cortex. Binding was done in the presence of glutamate and glycine. Linear correlation coefficient was $r = -0.826$, $P < 0.001$. **C**: Autoradiographical analysis showed that MK-801 binding was decreased in the anterior hippocampus and parahippocampal gyrus in Alzheimer tissue. Binding was done in the presence of glutamate and glycine. GD out, outer two-thirds of the dentate gyrus molecular layer; GD in, inner one-third of the dentate gyrus molecular layer; infra, infragranular layer; PG in, inner layer of the parahippocampal gyrus; PG out, outer layer of the parahippocampal gyrus. *$P < 0.05$, **$P < 0.01$ (one-way analysis of variance (ANOVA), Scheffe F test). [Reprinted with permission from **A**: Cohen and Müller (10); **B**: Piggott et al. (102); and **C**: Ulas et al. (125) (Pergamon Press Ltd, Headington Hill Hall, Oxford OX3 OBW, UK).]

vation of normal numbers of KA receptors may increase the incidence of NMDA-receptor activation to the point where the influx of calcium is increased to toxic levels, resulting in neuronal death. The increased activation of NMDA receptors may in turn be compensated for by a decrease in NMDA receptor number. As another example, it is possible that a decrease in receptor number, due to cell loss, for example, is compensated for in the early stages by an increase in glutamate release, but increased glutamate levels coupled with a relaxation in NMDA receptor inhibition by zinc at more advanced ages may also increase the incidence of NMDA receptor activation, resulting in toxic levels of calcium influx and neuronal death.

A recent study has shown that chronic treatment (3 wk) with phosphatidylserine was effective in normalizing the changes of the NMDA receptor with age in the mouse (10). This finding is consistent with behavioral studies showing that phosphatidylserine treatment enhances cognition. Another study has shown that treatment with acetyl-L-carnitine also normalized the decrease in the number of NMDA receptors in the frontal cortex in the aged rat and alleviated deficits in a learning task (22). Acetyl-L-carnitine is involved in the regulation of cellular metabolism. Future studies of the mechanisms underlying the effects of phosphatidylserine and acetyl-L-carnitine may indicate key points in NMDA receptor function and maintenance that are at risk in aging.

GABA Receptors

Another contributing factor to the state of excitation of the cell and susceptibility to excitotoxicity is the state of the inhibitory γ-aminobutyric acid (GABA) receptors with aging. GABA is the major inhibitory neurotransmitter in the brain, and maintenance of the balance between glutamate excitation and GABA inhibition is essential for normal CNS function. This is supported by studies that have shown that disinhibition of the glutamate system by blocking GABAergic transmission is a powerful and reliable method of inducing seizure activity. Similarly, artificially increasing glutamatergic transmission beyond levels that can be modulated by GABA also reliably produces seizure activity (for review see 128). As discussed in detail in the following sections, several lines of evidence suggest that GABA levels and binding to the GABA receptor/channel complex are reduced as a function of age, raising the possibility of a shift in the balance between GABAergic and glutamatergic activity.

Changes in GABA$_A$ Receptors in Aged Rodent Models.
In rodent models, studies have shown that although binding to GABA$_A$ receptors may not change (26, 117, 130), binding to the GABA$_A$ receptor–coupled ionophore decreases with age as the number of binding sites decreases (Fig. 13.3A) (26, 86). There is also a decrease in GABA-mediated allosteric enhancement of ligand binding to the ionophore (26). In addition, studies examining both in vitro and in vivo preparations indicate that the rate of GABA receptor turnover appears to become slower with age (87).

Reduced GABA Levels with Age and in Neurodegenerative Diseases.
Levels of GABA in cerebrospinal fluid (CSF) also appear to decrease with age. Studies in the CSF of elderly men and women show that GABA levels are markedly decreased (up to 70% at age 80 yr) in normal subjects (Fig. 13.3B) (121) and to an even greater extent in several age-related diseases: Alzheimer's, Huntington's, and Parkinson's (Fig. 13.3C) (80, 99). However, several studies suggest that GABA concentrations in Alzheimer tissue may be similar to controls, except for a reduction in the temporal lobe (75).

This decrease in levels of GABA with age and in neurodegenerative diseases does not appear to reflect a decrease in neurons that produce GABA (92, 115), a finding consistent with studies in vitro indicating that GABA neurons are significantly less vulnerable than glutamate neurons to the toxic effects of β-amyloid, an abnormally processed protein found in Alzheimer's disease (103). There is evidence of a decrease in levels of GABA synthetase with aging and in Alzheimer's disease and related disorders (82). Taken together, these results suggest that there is not a profound loss of GABA neurons but rather a reduction in the ability of these neurons to synthesize GABA.

Like the NMDA glutamate receptor, the GABA$_A$ receptor subtype is a complex structure that is highly regulated via several allosteric binding sites (sites of action of anxiolytics, hypnotics, and so-called "cage-convulsants") (7, 120). Having many points of regulation provides the possibility of a highly complex function but also many points of vulnerability to dysfunction and/or points where compensatory mechanisms may balance dysfunction. One well-characterized interaction is between GABA binding and benzodiazepine binding at the anxioloytic-binding site. Binding of benzodiazepines enhances binding of GABA to the high-affinity-binding site and vice versa.

The Depressive Effect of Benzodiazepines in the Elderly.
It has been demonstrated clinically that the depressive effect of anxiolytics increases in older populations (48, 90), but the mechanism is not fully understood. Previous research has focused on possible changes in the binding characteristics at the anxiolytic-binding site as a function of age, but no clear changes have been described. One explanation of this effect for some ben-

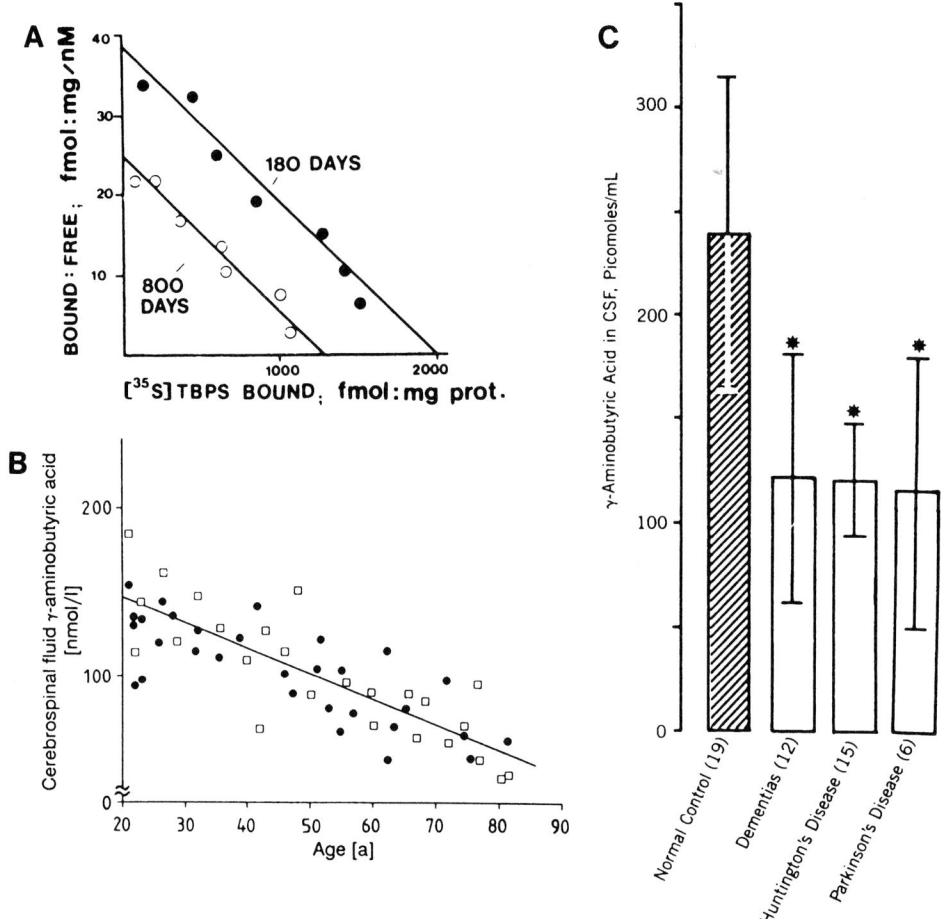

FIG. 13.3. Binding to the GABA receptor–coupled ionophore is reduced in aged rats, and CSF levels are reduced with age and in age-related diseases in the human. A: Representative Scatchard plots show saturable, single-binding components for [^{35}S]t-butyl-bicyclophosphorothionate (TBPS) in cortical membranes from adult (180-day-old) and aged (800-day-old) rats. Note that affinity of binding (slope) did not change, whereas maximal number of binding sites (intersect at the x axis) was reduced in aged animals. Data are mean values of triplicates obtained in a representative experiment. Repeated experiments gave similar results. B: Human cerebrospinal fluid GABA concentration decreases with age. *Circles* represent data from males; *squares*, from females. Linear regression analysis showed significant negative correlation ($r = -0.81$, $P < 0.01$). Significant negative correlations were also found in men ($r = -0.79$, $P < 0.01$) and in women ($r = -0.88$, $P < 0.01$). C: Levels of GABA in CSF are reduced in various neurologic disorders and controls. Height of each bar represents mean ($\pm$ SD). Numbers in parentheses represent number of cases. *$P < 0.001$ by Student's t test. [Reprinted with permission from A: Erdö and Wolff (26); B: Takayama et al. (121); and C: Manyam et al. (80) (copyright 1980, American Medical Association).]

zodiazepines is that they are not efficiently cleared in the elderly. Those benzodiazepines that are metabolized by microsomal oxidation (for example, chlordiazepoxide, diazepam, clorazepate, and prazepam) have a reduced elimination rate in older populations (48, 90). Another possibility is that there is an increase in the efficiency of the coupling between the receptor and the cellular response, rather than changes in receptor number or affinity (117). Levels of cholecystokinin binding are also reduced in the aged brain (51). Cholecystokinin is a functional antagonist for GABA effects on benzodiazepine binding, suggesting a mechanism of increasing the efficacy of GABA to balance the decrease in GABA levels.

The effects of aging on GABA receptor binding interactions and function have been examined in depth using animal models. Research in rodent models has given evidence of a shift with age in the allosteric interactions between GABA and benzodiazepine binding. For example, GABA enhancement of benzodiazepine binding has been shown to increase with age (117). In contrast, another rodent study has demonstrated that GABA enhancement of binding to the cage-convulsant site is decreased with age (26). Since benzodiazepine binding enhances GABA binding, the age-related increased binding capacity and/or decreased clearance of benzodiazepines may represent a balancing factor for the age-related reduction in GABA levels and may result in functional compensation.

Close examination of the types of receptors present in older rat brain shows that, while there may be no changes in the total number of receptors, there are shifts in the proportion of different types of receptors. For example, a recent study demonstrated an increase in the proportion of type I benzodiazepine receptor binding to hippocampal membrane preparations from aged rat (117). Type I receptors are involved in GABA enhancement of binding to the benzodiazepine receptor. In the adult animal the hippocampus is normally rich in type II receptors. An increase in the proportion of type I receptors may reflect a change in the expression of the receptor subunits, since the pharmacological properties of the benzodiazepine receptor are related to the α-subunit composition. The results of other studies suggest that there are selective age-related changes in the molecular organization of GABA receptors (26). The results of a recent study demonstrating changes in α-subunit mRNA in aged rat provide support for this hypothesis (86).

Summary

Considering the state of the glutamate and GABA systems in the aging brain, it appears likely that, although there are significant changes in levels of transmitter and receptor binding properties, the functional balance between these transmitter systems may be maintained in the aging brain. In fact, it appears that there is an overall decrease in the activity of both glutamate and GABA systems, perhaps resetting the brain state to a new level of balanced function. As the aging process continues, and especially with the introduction of neurodegenerative disease, however, the mechanisms involved in maintaining this balance may begin to contribute to the progression of cellular degeneration, as interconnecting processes are increasingly affected by the mechanistic shifts required to compensate for the initial dysfunction.

Evidence clearly shows that there are considerable changes with aging in both glutamate and GABA neurotransmitter systems. Although animal models are useful for predicting changes in the aged human brain, it is not surprising that there is considerable heterogeneity observed between species and sometimes between individuals, particularly at the level of resolution of recent studies (125). To some extent, the plasticity mechanisms of the brain and the resulting synaptic remodeling are regulated by environment, synaptic activity, and behavioral need, all of which differ depending on the species and the individual.

In this context, there is an important class of molecules, the "neurotrophic factors," which serve in the maintenance and adaptation of neuronal function. It appears that neurotrophic factors are a key link between the environment (that is, sensory input) and the regulation of brain plasticity. Age-related changes in several of these neurotrophic factors have been identified as we discuss in the next section.

NEUROTROPHIC FACTORS

Neurotrophic factors constitute a special class of endogenous signaling proteins that promote the survival, division, and growth of neurons as they regulate their differentiation and morphological plasticity (7, 74). Although it is well known that neurotrophic factors have major roles in the development of the CNS, there is increasing evidence that they are important for the function, maintenance, and long-term adjustment or plasticity of the CNS throughout life. Studies indicate that neurotrophic factors can modulate neurotransmission (133) and are in turn regulated by synaptic activity (8). This finding is consistent with the idea that they represent a signaling mechanism that operates in conjunction with neurotransmitters, but on a slower time scale.

Neurotrophic factors are pivotal in the recovery of the CNS from injury and neurodegeneration. After brain injury, extracts of both tissue and fluid around the site of injury show increased neurotrophic factor activity (95). The increase in trophic factor production and growth capabilities of cells in the CNS after cell loss is generally interpreted as a natural response of the CNS to compensate for damage. Studies suggest that neurotrophic factors can prevent neuronal degeneration as well as trigger growth of the remaining healthy neurons, a key process in the synaptic and circuit reorganizations that occur after brain injury and in neurodegenerative disease in both young and aged animals.

As an organism ages, the status of the neurotrophic factors becomes increasingly critical. As neuronal death progresses with age and in age-related neurodegenerative diseases, there is increasingly more dependence on compensatory mechanisms to maintain normal function. Through the examination of the status of neurotrophic factors in the aged brain, it is possible to gain insight into the processes of degeneration and repair and how the balance between these processes undergo changes with aging.

In this discussion of neurotrophic factors and aging, we illustrate the principles of trophic regulation of function and plasticity and how they factor into the aging process, focusing on the neurotrophin family of growth factors [for example, nerve growth factor (NGF) and brain-derived growth factor (BDNF)] and the fibroblast growth factor (FGF) family of trophic factors (for example, acidic FGF or FGF-1 and basic FGF or FGF-2). In a subsequent section, we will discuss cytokines (the interleukins IL-1 and IL-3) which are known to be both trophic factors and regulators of the immune system (for review of the status of these and other neurotrophic factors in aging see references 2 and 56).

Nerve Growth Factor

The first neurotrophic factor to be characterized was NGF (71), now included in the neurotrophin family of growth factors. Its major function in the brain appears to involve trophic actions on cholinergic neurons located primarily in the basal forebrain. Basal forebrain neurons form a significant projection to the hippocampus and have been implicated in the processes of learning and memory. It has been shown that administration of NGF can attenuate cholinergic neuron death after lesions of the fiber projection from basal forebrain to hippocampus in both young (34, 53) and aging (91) animals, and it can accelerate the recovery of memory function after lesions of the hippocampus (131, 132).

NGF Levels in Aged Rodents vs Humans. Several studies in rodent models indicate a decline with age in the levels of NGF and NGF mRNA (70) and in NGF receptor immunoreactivity in the basal forebrain (45, 65). Conversely, most studies in the aged human brain indicate that the state of NGF is unchanged. Levels of NGF and NGF receptor mRNA have been shown to be normal in human brain cortex (41, 42). Furthermore, normal NGF receptor immunoreactivity was also observed in brain cortical tissue (93). However, Hefti and Mash (54) measured an age-related decline in human NGF receptor immunoreactivity in the perinuclear area of cells in the nucleus basalis. They suggest that this may indicate a reduction in NGF receptor synthesis with age.

Neuronal Activity and Regulation of Neurotrophic Factor Synthesis. Several lines of evidence indicate that the synthesis of NGF can be regulated by neuronal activity and sensory input (35, 46, 134, 135, 136). For example, levels of NGF mRNA increase in the hippocampus due to activation of non-NMDA glutamate receptors (135). In contrast, levels of NGF mRNA are down-regulated via GABA receptors (134). These results indicate that the balance between glutamate and GABA neuronal activity is key to the regulation of NGF synthesis. This has implications for the state of NGF in the aging brain, particularly in light of the studies discussed earlier under Neurotransmitter Systems, suggesting that there are age-related changes in glutamate and GABA neurotransmission and in the balance between these neurotransmitter systems.

NGF in Alzheimer's Disease. Several studies have examined the state of NGF in Alzheimer's disease. It has been shown that levels of NGF mRNA in cortex (42) and NGF receptor mRNA in basal forebrain (41) were normal in Alzheimer tissue, whereas another study showed a decline in NGF receptor immunoreactivity in Alzheimer brain (94). It is known that basal forebrain neurons undergo progressive degeneration in Alzheimer's disease, and it has been suggested that this degeneration may underlie some of the memory deficit observed in Alzheimer's disease (6). In light of the possibility that NGF function in Alzheimer's disease may be impaired, and since NGF is a trophic factor for the cholinergic basal forebrain neurons that are involved in learning and memory, NGF has been considered for therapeutic use to preserve these neurons and thus extend normal memory function (55). Indeed, it has been demonstrated that administration of NGF improved memory function in aged rats that were previously impaired on a memory task and reduced the degree of atrophy of cholinergic neurons in rat basal forebrain structures (Fig. 13.4) (30).

Trophic factors other than NGF that influence or are modulated by hippocampal cholinergic cell function may undergo age-related changes that have an impact memory function. For example, in rat, activity of cholinergic afferents to the hippocampus has been demonstrated to regulate levels of mRNA for BDNF, another member of the neurotrophin family of growth factors (69). However, in situ hybridization and Northern blot analysis in aged rat indicate that levels or distribution of BDNF mRNA do not change in the hippocampus with age (68). Another recently identified trophic factor, insulin-like growth factor-1 (IGF-1), has been localized in the rat CNS and may be a neuromodulator of cholinergic neurotransmission in the hippocampus (4). A recent study in aged rat brain found that IGF-1 mRNA declines by 40% with age (96). Further study may clarify the therapeutic potential of IGF-1 for delaying memory decline in Alzheimer's disease.

Fibroblast Growth Factor

FGF-1 Changes with Aging. The fibroblast growth factor (FGF) family of trophic factors consists of several FGFs, including acidic FGF (FGF-1) and basic FGF (FGF-2). FGF-1 and FGF-2 exert trophic actions on astrocytes and a wide variety of neuronal cell types in the brain. FGF-1 immunoreactivity has been observed in glial cells of the optic nerve over a large age span, with no apparent changes with increasing age in

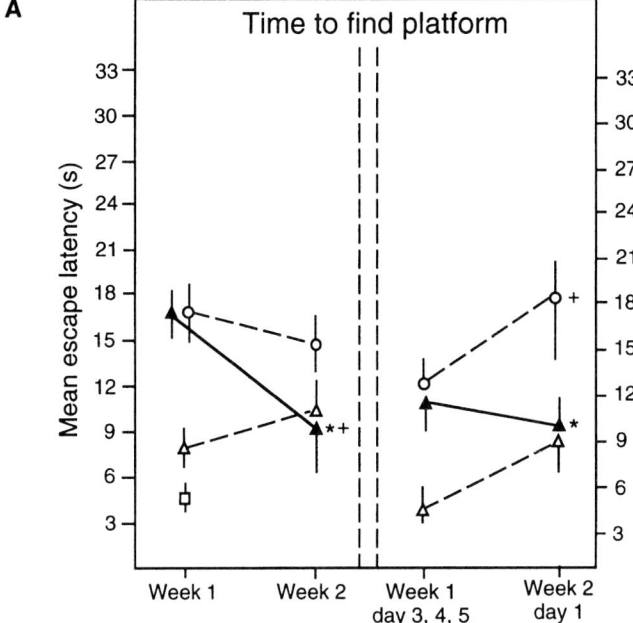

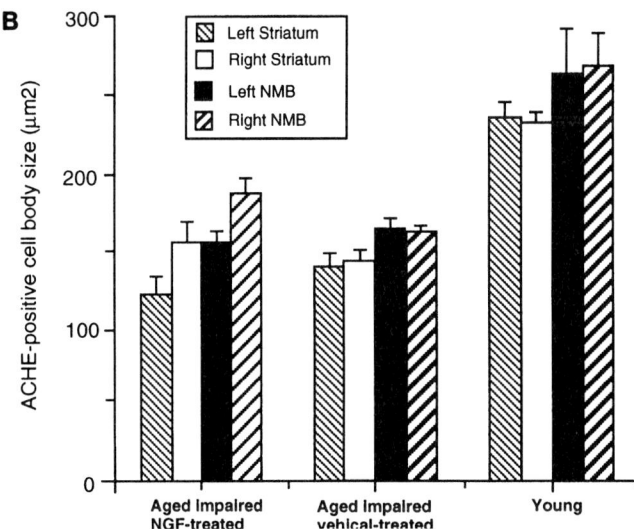

FIG. 13.4. NGF improves memory function in previously impaired aged rats on a memory task and reduces the degree of atrophy of cholinergic neurons in basal forebrain structures. **A:** Performance on a water maze test of three groups of aged rats (*open triangle*, aged nonimpaired; *circle*, aged impaired; *closed triangle*, NGF-treated aged impaired) in test weeks 1 and 2, expressed as the time to reach the hidden platform (escape latency). A group of identically tested young (3-month-old) rats (*square*) has been included for comparison. *Left panel*, mean performance ($\pm$ SEM) over all trials ($*P < 0.025$; $^+P < 0.01$). *Right panel*, memory retention expressed as difference between mean performance in last 3 days of test week 1 and first test day of test week 2 ($*P < 0.025$; $^+P < 0.025$). **B:** AChE-positive cell body size for young rats and treated and untreated aged rats. Bars represent means ($\pm$ SEM) of AChE-positive cell body size given as cross-sectional area in μm^2 from striatum and nucleus basalis magnocellularis (NBM). $*P < 0.01$ compared to the noninfused (left) side; Student's related t test. [Reprinted with permission from Fischer et al. (30), copyright (1987) Macmillan Magazines Limited.]

rat, bovine, and human tissue (29). However, in another study in mice, FGF-1 was shown to effectively increase the recovery of the density of tyrosine hydroxylase–immunopositive fibers (that is, dopaminergic axons) after methyl-phenyl-tetrahydroppyridine (MPTP)-induced lesions of dopaminergic cells in young mice, but not in aged mice (21). This suggests a deficit in the FGF-1 system in aged animals. Future studies examining specific changes in FGF-1 characteristics may clarify whether this deficit is limited to specific species and/or what aspects of the mechanisms may be at risk in aging. Immunoreactivity of FGF-1 in Alzheimer brain revealed an increase in astrocyte staining for FGF-1. The immunopositive astrocytes were often a subpopulation of astrocytes located near senile plaques (123).

FGF-2 and Cell Survival after Axotomy. Increasing evidence indicates that FGF-2 has a role in repair, regrowth, and remodeling of neuronal circuitry in the brain after injury (127). Infusion of FGF-2 has been shown to reduce cell death after axotomy in several areas of the brain. For example, infusion of FGF-2 reduced death of entorhinal cells after axotomy by knife cuts of the perforant path (Fig. 13.5) (20). Another

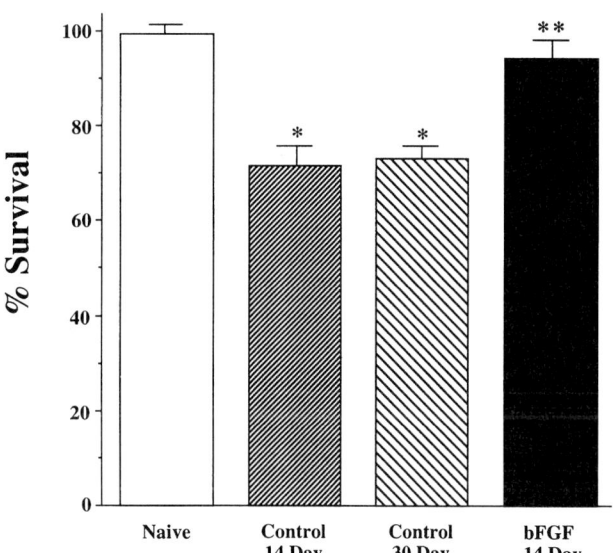

FIG. 13.5. FGF-2 (bFGF) infusion protects neurons from death after axotomy. The effect of intraventricular infusion (0.025 μg/h) of FGF-2 for 14 days on the survival of layer II stellate cells in the entorhinal cortex after axotomy. Neurons ipsilateral and contralateral to the lesion were counted in bFGF infused animals 14 days post-lesion ($n = 6$) and controls which received either saline infusion ($n = 4$) or no infusion ($n = 5$) at 14 days post-lesion and controls at 30 days post-lesion ($n = 6$). Additionally, cells in four naive unoperated animals were counted to insure there were no hemispheric differences in the entorhinal cortex. The percentage of cell survival (ipsilateral/contralateral ratios) was compared with a Student's t test. $*P \leq 0.005$ from naive group; $**P \leq 0.005$ from either control group. [Reprinted with permission from Cummings et al. (20).]

study in the rat demonstrated that infusion of FGF-2 saved cholinergic neurons from death after fimbria lesions. This property of FGF-2 is preserved in aged animals as well, although in 2-yr-old rats the effect is not as robust as in younger animals (1).

Possible Role of FGF-2 and NGF in Plaque Biogenesis. High levels of FGF-2 have been observed in neuritic plaques in Alzheimer's disease. It has been suggested that FGF-2 levels are up-regulated in response to neural degeneration in the area but then contribute to the formation of the plaque by promoting the ingrowth of sprouting fibers (Fig. 13.6) (15) and by increasing levels of amyloid precursor protein (APP) mRNA in astrocytes (47, 106). Furthermore, it has been shown that β-amyloid protein increases levels of FGF-2 (2). Thus β-amyloid and FGF-2 may contribute to a positive feedback cycle that promotes plaque growth (13).

NGF may also contribute to the formation of plaques in Alzheimer's disease. Studies have shown a transient increase in NGF levels in the hippocampus after fimbria lesions, presumably because NGF is no longer being transported away by cholinergic projections to the hippocampus (67) and its synthesis is increased, primarily in astrocytes (76). Thus, although there may not be a large, stable, easily measured increase in NGF in Alzheimer's disease as discussed above, it is possible that each time a cholinergic projection to the hippocampus degenerates there is a highly localized, transient increase in NGF. If so, such transient increases may promote axonal sprouting of remaining healthy cholinergic neurons (33). In addition, it has been reported that injection of NGF increases APP mRNA levels in neonates (88), which raises the possibility that an increase in NGF also increases APP levels in Alzheimer brain, enabling the process of plaque biogenesis to commence. If so, it would help explain why plaques form in the dentate gyrus molecular layer, particularly in light of the results of a recent study in canine brain showing that the projection field of terminals carrying APP is concentrated in the dentate gyrus molecular layer and corresponds to the projection field of neurons from the entorhinal cortex (19). Furthermore, if the effect of NGF on APP is dependent on factors found in neonatal tissue, it may

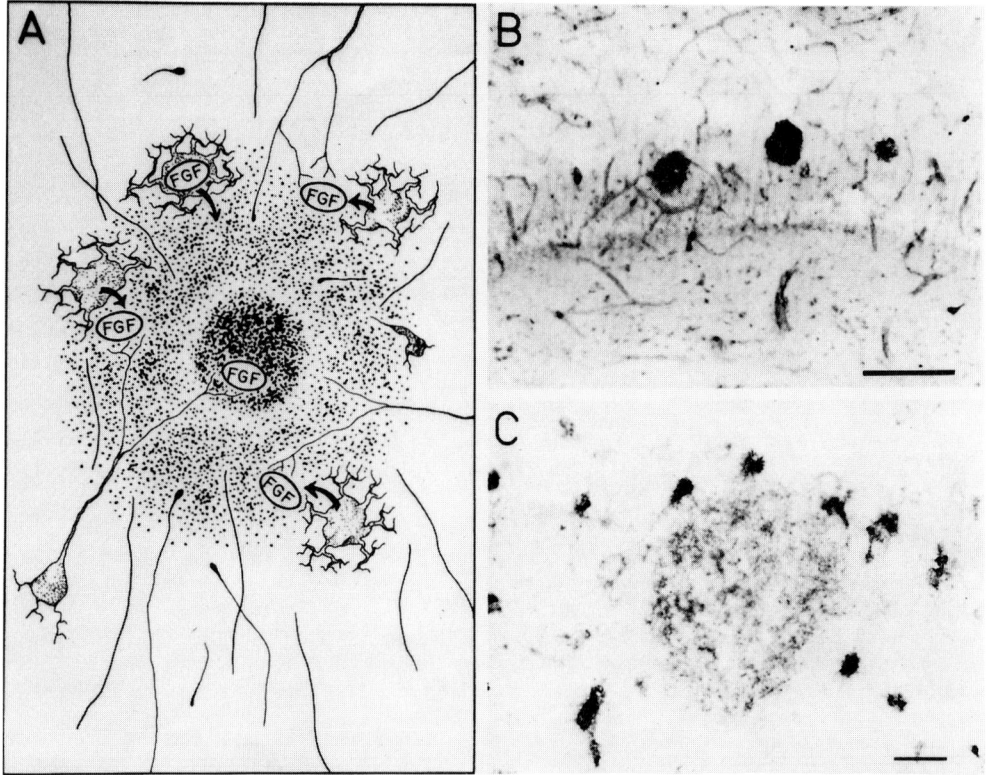

FIG. 13.6. FGF-2 is present in the senile plaque environment. **A:** Diagram illustrating potential sites of FGF-2 involvement in plaque formation and misdirected plasticity. **B:** FGF-2 immunoreactivity detects senile plaques located in dentate gyrus molecular layer of Alzheimer brain (bar = 100 μm). **C:** Photomicrograph illustrating presence of FGF-2-immunoreactive astrocytes surrounding an FGF-2-immunoreactive senile plaque (bar = 10 μm). [Reprinted with permission from Cotman et al. (15).]

be that the fibers sprouting into the dentate gyrus from entorhinal cortex may re-express neonatal factors (15) that are critical for the effect of NGF on APP levels. Thus NGF may have a modulatory effect on APP levels after entorhinal lesions and in Alzheimer's disease.

Cytokines as Neurotrophic Factors

Cytokines are factors released by leukocytes to regulate the immune response. Cytokines are also produced within the CNS and act on cells within the CNS either as trophic factors for neurons or glia or as neuromodulators. We focus on two cytokines: IL-1 and IL-3.

IL-1 and IL-3 were first described as being produced peripherally by activated macrophages and T cells, respectively, and as having many roles in the immune response, including the activation of T cells, the induction of fever, and the mediation of inflammation (24). Within the CNS, IL-1 is produced by astrocytes (72) and by microglia, resident macrophages of the CNS (39). IL-3 is produced by astrocytes and is mitogenic for microglia (32). IL-1 in turn leads to astrocytic proliferation (40), thus completing an excitatory feedback signaling loop. This molecular cascade can be triggered by neurodegeneration induced by lesions or neurodegenerative diseases.

IL-1 and Recovery after Injury. IL-1 production can be induced by lesions to the brain. Recovery of function and regrowth of connections has been well characterized in the hippocampus after lesions of the major excitatory input from the entorhinal cortex (12). Evidence indicates that the molecular cascade is triggered by the lesion and has a role in the recovery response after entorhinal lesions. Within days of this procedure, reactive microglia that are immunoreactive for IL-1 appear within the hippocampus (28). These microglia phagocytose debris from the degenerating terminals (36). Presumably in response to the IL-1 secreted by microglia, reactive astrocytes appear (28) and promote the sprouting response via up-regulation of NGF and FGF-2 (Fig. 13.7). IL-1 has been shown to increase levels of NGF mRNA (97), which promotes sprouting of cholinergic fibers into the denervated area. It appears that IL-1 helps trigger the process of repair and regrowth after injury in the CNS.

In the aged brain, however, there is an impaired ability to clear degenerating terminals from denervated hippocampus, which results in delayed reinnervation (Fig. 13.8) (57). Furthermore, accumulating evidence suggests that when compensatory mechanisms in the brain become overextended, they are capable of actually contributing to the developing pathology. This appears to be the case for IL-1. A recent report indicates that IL-1 may be involved in ischemic damage and excitotoxicity; thus high levels of IL-1 may increase the rate of degeneration (109).

Effect of Glucocorticoids on the Immune Response in Aged Brain. Like IL-1, glucocorticoid concentrations are also altered during normal aging. Aged rats have higher basal levels of these hormones and exhibit larger increases in glucocorticoids during stress than do young adult rats (118). Glucocorticoids suppress a wide variety of macrophage activities, including the release of cytokines (27).

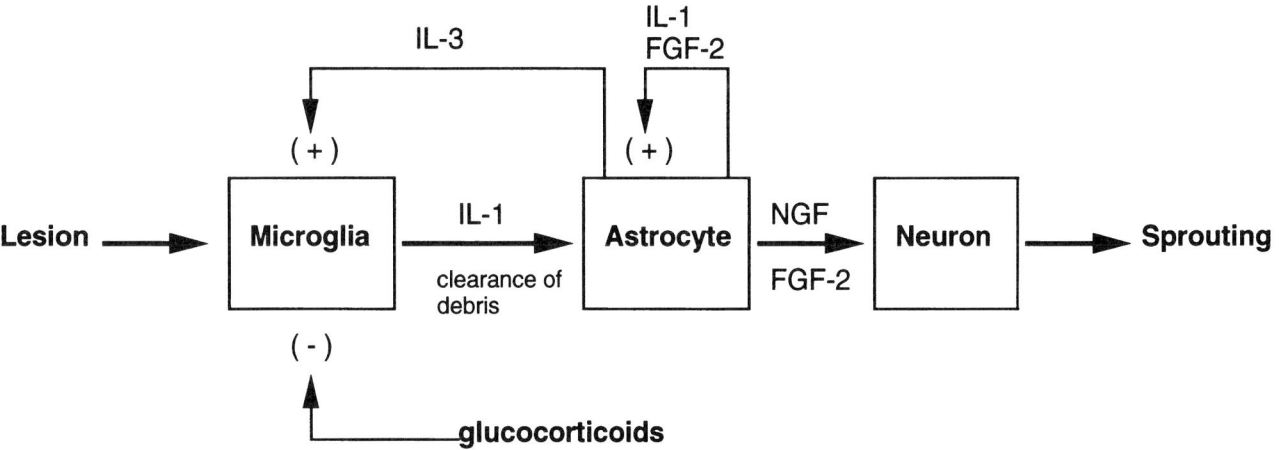

FIG. 13.7. Simplified mechanism by which cytokines may regulate neuronal plasticity following injury to CNS. Primed by the original insult, microglia start a cascade of processes leading to neuronal sprouting by the release of IL-1. Glucocorticoids from the adrenal gland can regulate the molecular cascade by inhibiting microglial function.

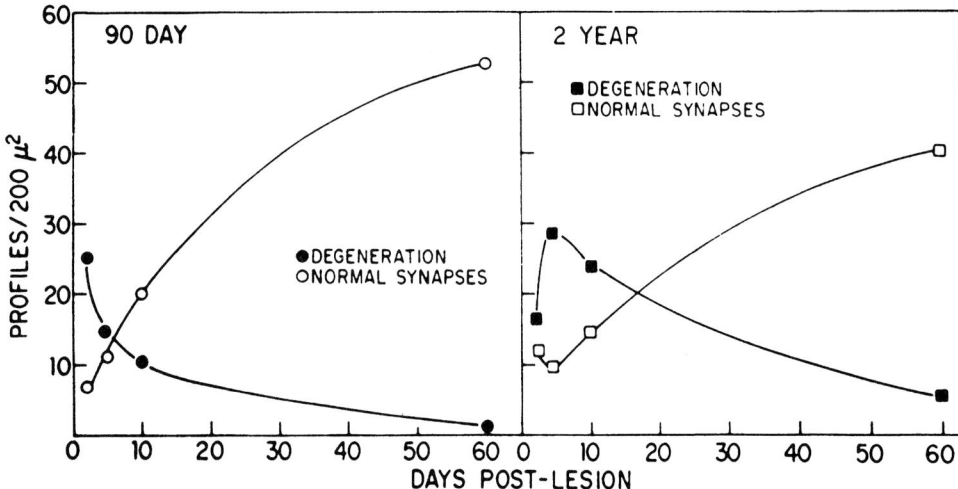

FIG. 13.8. Clearance of debris is slower and synapse replacement incomplete after lesions in aged rats. Graphs illustrate reciprocal relationship between degeneration product removal and reappearance of normal synapses in both young and aged rats. [Reprinted with permission from Hoff et al. (57).]

Glucocorticoids are known to affect the reinnervation of the hippocampus after denervation. Glucocorticoid administration to rats after lesions of projections to the dentate gyrus exhibited substantial reduction of the clearance of degenerating synaptic terminals (119) and a further reduction in the number of microglia in the dentate gyrus following the lesion (Table 13.1) (126). It has therefore been suggested that the delayed reinnervation of denervated hippocampus in the aged rat is due to the effects of changed glucocorticoid levels on the glial response to injury (57). Thus the process of aging can alter the capacity of the brain to respond to insults by reducing the efficacy of the immune response within the CNS.

TABLE 13.1. *Glucocorticoid Hydrocortisone Treatment*[a]

	Control, Nonlesion, Untreated	Untreated Lesion	Cortisol-Treated, Lesion
Astrocytes	2.65 ± 0.27 (N = 6)	3.36 ± 0.15[b,**] (N = 7)	4.40 ± 0.25[c,*] (N = 7)
Nonastrocytes	2.71 ± 0.19 (N = 6)	7.93 ± 0.50[b,*] (N = 7)	6.15 ± 0.56[c,**] (N = 7)

[a]Values are means ± SE number of glia per oil-immersion field of 0.0288-mm^2 area in the suprapyramidal denate gyrus. A total of 8–10 fields per section and four sections per animal were used to calculate the mean number of glia per field per animal. Treatment with the glucocorticoid hydrocortisone increases astrocyte number and decreases nonastrocyte cell number in the outer molecular layer of the dentate gyrus of the rat hippocampus after unilateral entorhinal lesions. [Reprinted with permission from Vijayan and Cotman (126).] [b]Comparison with control, nonlesion, untreated group. [c]Comparison with untreated, lesion group. *$P < 0.01$, **$P < 0.05$

THE IMMUNE SYSTEM IN THE CNS

Immune responses within the CNS have important implications for brain aging in at least two ways: First, changes that occur during aging affect the strength of the immune response both directly and indirectly, and immune function in turn affects normal brain function. Second, processes such as synaptic plasticity that are key to the maintenance of normal brain function during aging are regulated in part by immune responses within the CNS, as noted above under IL-1 and Recovery after Injury.

Within the CNS, it has been shown that microglia in the aged rat express some macrophage antigens that are normally down-regulated in the young adult rat. These include the major histocompatibility complex (MHC) class II antigens, which provide the ability to present foreign antigens to other leukocytes (100). The alteration of microglial responses with aging has implications for the ability of the CNS to respond to injury, as discussed earlier under IL-1 and Recovery after Injury.

The Immune System and Alzheimer's Disease

Activation of microglia has been linked to degenerative brain diseases such as Alzheimer's disease. In the Alzheimer brain, microglia are known to associate with plaques (50, 60). These microglia display morphological (60, 111) and functional indications of being in an activated or reactive state (that is, expressing MHC antigens) (84, 114).

There are several lines of evidence that an inflammatory response occurs in the Alzheimer brain. One is the finding of proteins associated with the acute phase response. The composition of serum is substantially altered during the acute phase response to include increased levels of proteins that enhance immune system functioning. These include α-1-antitrypsin and α-1-antichymotrypsin, which have been identified in association with neurofibrillary tangles (44).

Anti-brain antibodies are also associated with Alzheimer's disease. Immunoglobulins have been localized within plaques (59). Serum and CSF from Alzheimer patients contain antibodies that recognize cholinergic neurons (31) and microglia (85). These observations suggest that the loss of cholinergic neurons during the course of the disease (6) may be linked to an abnormal immune response directed specifically against these neurons. Similarly, the recent finding that β-amyloid peptides (fragments of APP protein abnormally processed in Alzheimer's disease) can cause degeneration of process-bearing microglia in culture (66) suggests that Alzheimer's disease may involve an abnormal response against microglia triggered by β-amyloid.

Cytokines and the Immune System

IL-1 levels are elevated in Alzheimer brain (49). The source of this IL-1 might be reactive microglia associated with plaques (50, 60). Activation of microglia around plaques may be in response to the dead and dying neurons in the vicinity, but it is also possible that the microglia are responding directly to the β-amyloid peptides deposited in the plaque. β1–42 will stimulate microglia in vitro to produce more IL-1 (3). IL-1 in turn has been shown to increase APP mRNA levels (43), providing a possible mechanism whereby degeneration may be actively promoted by the natural compensatory processes of the CNS.

The Complement Cascade and Alzheimer Pathology. A normal aspect of immune function is the destruction of foreign cells. In normal conditions it represents an important mechanism for the maintenance of the health of the brain. The dysfunction of this system, however, can develop into a powerful source of cell degeneration. Recent evidence suggests that serum complement, an important component of the inflammatory response, exhibits changes in Alzheimer's disease.

Complement consists of a group of proteins normally found in blood that "complement" an antibody response. The first component of complement, C1, consists of three subcomponents, C1q, C1r, and C1s. When an antigen–antibody complex binds to C1q, it causes C1r and C1s to dissociate from C1q. These fragments are active proteases, and they in turn cleave further components of complement. This cascade is known as the *classical pathway* of complement activation. It leads to the production of complement fragments with a host of biological activities. Some fragments are anaphylotoxins; these increase the permeability of blood vessels. Others are chemotactic for leukocytes, and they facilitate phagocytosis. The final outcome of the complement cascade is the formation of the membrane attack complex, in which several of the complement fragments bind together and form large pores where they insert into cell membranes. The increased membrane permeability then leads to the death of the cell under attack.

It has been known for some time that complement components are localized to plaques (25). Several such components, including C1q, have been localized specifically on the amyloid fibrils within plaques (58). The membrane attack complex itself has been localized to neurites in the vicinity of plaques (83). These observations suggest that complement factors have a role in neuritic damage.

One key factor in understanding plaque biogenesis is to ascertain when the inflammatory response is triggered in Alzheimer's disease. The β-amyloid peptides deposited in plaques have been shown to be toxic to neurons in culture (104); it is therefore probable that the degenerating neurons provide the initial signal for an inflammatory response that potentially exacerbates the damage. It is also possible that β-amyloid itself directly initiates the inflammation. C1q binds β-amyloid, which initiates the classical complement cascade (113).

In conclusion, examination of neurotrophic factors and the immune response reveals that there are age-related changes in the balance between the elements of these systems that result in altered function with age. Interestingly, not only is there extensive interaction between neurotrophic factors and the immune response, but also, completing the cycle, it has been shown that elements of the immune system can modulate neurotransmitter systems. As an illustration, IL-1 can also function as a neuromodulator and has been shown to have a direct effect on the electrical activity of neurons (133) and to inhibit long-term potentiation of synaptic responses in mouse hippocampus (62). There are examples of more long-term effects of IL-1 on neurons: increased mRNA for substance P in neurons (52), decreased acetylcholine release in rat hippocampus (107), and increased mRNA for NGF in fibroblasts (73). Thus cytokine release contributes directly to neuronal activity in the normal brain, and shifts in this regulation with age have wide repercussions in brain function.

SUMMARY AND CONCLUSIONS

Taken together, it becomes apparent that shifts in the balance of CNS activity (neurotransmitter systems, trophic factor systems, immune responses) appear relatively minor when observed in isolation but can have quite a widespread impact on the functional output of the brain when taken as a total. As we have emphasized in this chapter, there are complex interactions between and within each of these systems. The process of aging does not appear to involve single large deficits in any one biological system but a complex series of seemingly insignificant changes (losses and compensations), which slowly and progressively shift the balance between systems. The CNS has natural compensatory mechanisms that are remarkably capable of absorbing these changes on a continual basis, but it appears that as the organism ages, the process of compensation begins to have increasingly wider consequences, to the point where compensation in one system has an actively destructive impact on another system. As our understanding of the mechanisms by which the brain repairs and remodels damaged circuitry increases, it is also becoming clear that the complexity of the brain provides an opportunity for the development of interventions to help prevent degeneration, build resistance to insult, minimize damage, and regulate these mechanisms to stimulate recovery.

REFERENCES

1. ANDERSON, K. J., D. DAM, and C. W. COTMAN. Basic fibroblast growth factor prevents death of cholinergic neurons in vivo. *Nature* 332: 360–361, 1988.
2. ARAUJO, D. M., and C. W. COTMAN. β-Amyloid stimulates glial cells in vitro to produce growth factors that accumulate in senile plaques in Alzheimer's disease. *Brain Res.* 569: 141–145, 1992.
3. ARAUJO, D. M., J.-G. CHABOT, and R. QUIRION. Potential neurotrophic factors in the mammalian central nervous system: functional significance in the developing and aging brain. *Int. Rev. Neurobiol.* 32: 141–174, 1990.
4. ARAUJO, D. M., P. A. LAPCHAK COLLIER, B., J.-G. CHABOT, and R. QUIRION. Insulin-like growth factor-1 (somatomedian-C) receptors in the rat brain: distribution and interaction with the hippocampal cholinergic system. *Brain Res.* 484: 130–138, 1989.
5. BAHR, B. A., A. C. GODSHALL, R. A. HALL, and G. LYNCH. Mouse telencephalon exhibits an age-related decrease in glutamate (AMPA) receptors but no change in nerve terminal markers. *Brain Res.* 589: 320–326, 1992.
6. BARTUS, R. T., R. L. DEAN, III, B. BEER, and A. S. LIPPA. The cholinergic hypothesis of geriatric memory dysfunction. *Science* 217: 408–417, 1982.
7. BURT, D. R., and G. L. KAMATCHI. GABA$_A$ receptor subtypes: from pharmacology to molecular biology. *FASEB J.* 5: 2916–2923, 1991.
8. CASTRÉN, E., F. ZAFRA, H. THOENEN, and D. LINDHOLM. Light regulates expression of brain-derived neurotrophic factor mRNA in rat visual cortex. *Proc. Natl. Acad. Sci. USA* 89: 9444–9448, 1992.
9. CLARK, A. S., K. R. MAGNUSSON, and C. W. COTMAN. In vitro autoradiography of hippocampal excitatory amino acid binding in aged Fischer 344 rats: relationship to performance on the Morris water maze. *Behav. Neurosci.* 106: 324–335, 1992.
10. COHEN, S. A., and W. E. MÜLLER. Age-related alteration of NMDA-receptor properties in the mouse forebrain: partial restoration by chronic phosphatidylserine treatment. *Brain Res.* 584: 174–180, 1992.
11. COLLINGRIDE, G. L., and T. V. P. BLISS. NMDA receptors—their role in long-term potentiation. *Trends. Neurosci.* 10: 288–293, 1987.
12. COTMAN, C. W., and A. J. ANDERSON. Retention of function in the aged brain: the pivotal role of Aβ. In: *Proceedings of the Fifth Conference of the Center for the Neurobiology of Learning and Memory,* edited by J. McGaugh. New York: Oxford University Press (in press).
13. COTMAN, C. W., and K. J. ANDERSON. Neural plasticity and regeneration. In: *Basic Neurochemistry: Molecular, Cellular, and Medical Aspects,* edited by G. J. Siegel, B. Agranoff, R. W. Albers, and P. Molinoff. New York: Raven Press, 1989, vol. 4, p. 507–522.
14. COTMAN, C. W., and L. L. IVERSON. Excitatory amino acids in the brain—focus on NMDA receptors. *Trends Neurosci.* 10: 263–265, 1987.
15. COTMAN, C. W., B. J. CUMMINGS, and C. J. PIKE. Molecular cascades in adaptive versus pathological plasticity. In: *Neuroregeneration,* edited by A. Gorio. New York: Raven Press, 1993, p. 217–240.
16. COTMAN, C. W., J. W. GEDDES, and J. S. KAHLE. Axon sprouting in the rodent and Alzheimer's disease brain: a reactivation of developmental mechanisms? In: *Progress in Brain Research,* edited by J. Storm-Mathisen, J. Zimmer, and O. P. Ottersen. Amsterdam: Elsevier Science Publishers B. V., 1990, p. 427–434.
17. COTMAN, C. W., F. GÓMEZ-PINILLA, and J. S. KAHLE. Neural plasticity and regeneration. In: *Basic Neurochemistry: Molecular, Cellular, and Medical Aspects,* edited by G. J. Siegel, B. Agranoff, R. W. Albers, and P. Molinoff. New York: Raven Press, 1994, vol. 5, p. 607–626.
18. COWBURN, R. F., J. A. HARDY, R. S. BRIGGS, and P. J. ROBERTS. Characterization, density, and distribution of kainate receptors in normal and Alzheimer's diseased human brain. *J. Neurochem.* 52: 140–147, 1989.
19. CUMMINGS, B. J., J. H. SU, C. W. COTMAN, R. WHITE, and M. J. RUSSELL. β-Amyloid accumulation in aged canine brain: a model of early plaque formation in Alzheimer's disease. *Neurobiol. Aging* 14: 547–560, 1994.
20. CUMMINGS, B. J., G. J. YEE, and C. W. COTMAN. bFGF promotes the survival of entorhinal layer II neurons after perforant path axotomy. *Brain Res.* 591: 271–276, 1992.
21. DATE, I., M. F. D. NOTTER, S. Y. FELTEN, and D. L. FELTEN. MPTP-treated young mice but not aging mice show partial recovery of the nigrostriatal dopaminergic system by stereotaxic injection of acidic fibroblast growth factor (aFGF). *Brain Res.* 526: 156–160, 1990.
22. DAVIS, S., A. L. MARKOWSKA, G. L. WENK, and C. A. BARNES. Acetyl-L-carnitine: behavioral, electrophysiological, and neurochemical effects. *Neurobiol. Aging* 14: 107–115, 1993.
23. DEWAR, D., D. T. CHALMERS, D. I. GRAHAM, and J. McCULLOCH. Glutamate metabotropic and AMPA binding sites are reduced in Alzheimer's disease: an autoradiographic study of the hippocampus. *Brain Res.* 553: 58–64, 1991.
24. DINARELLO, C. A. Interleukin-1 and its biologically related cytokines. *Adv. Immunol.* 44: 153–205, 1989.
25. EIKELENBOOM, P., C. E. HACK, J. M. ROZEMULLER, and F. C. STAM. Complement activation in amyloid plaques in Alzheimer dementia. *Virchows Arch. [B].* 56: 259–262, 1989.
26. ERDÖ, S. L., and J. R. WOLFF. Age-related loss of t-[^{35}S] butylbicyclophosphorothionate binding to the γ-aminobutyric acid$_A$ receptor-coupled chloride ionophore in the rat cerebral cortex. *J. Neurochem.* 53: 648–651, 1989.

27. EVANS, S. W., and J. T. WHICHER. An overview of the inflammatory response. In: *Biochemistry of Inflammation,* edited by J. T. Whicher and S. W. Evans. Dordrecht: Kluwer Academic Publishers, 1992, p. 1–15.
28. FAGAN, A. M., and F. H. GAGE. Cholinergic sprouting in the hippocampus: a proposed role for IL-1. *Exp. Neurol.* 110: 105–120, 1990.
29. FAUCHEUX, B. A., S. Y. COHEN, P. DELAERE, A. TOURBAH, C. DUPUIS, M. P. HARTMANN, J. C. JEANNY, J. J. HAUW, and Y. COURTOIS. Glial cell localization of acidic fibroblast growth factor-like immunoreactivity in the optic nerve of young adult and aged mammals. *Gerontology* 38: 308–314, 1992.
30. FISHER, W., K. WICTORIN, A. BJORKLUND, L. R. WILLIAMS, S. VARON, and F. H. GAGE. Amelioration of cholinergic neuron atrophy and spatial memory impairment in aged rats by nerve growth factor. *Nature* 329: 65–68, 1987.
31. FOLEY, P., H. F. BRADFORD, M. DOCHERTY, H. FILLIT, V. N. LUINE, B. MCEWEN, G. BUCHT, B. WINBLAD, and J. HARDY. Evidence for the presence of antibodies to cholinergic neurons in the serum of patients with Alzheimer disease. *J. Neurol.* 235: 466–471, 1988.
32. FREI, K., S. BODMER, C. SWERDEL, and A. FONTANA. Astrocyte-derived interleukin 3 as a growth factor for microglia cells and peritoneal macrophages. *J. Immunol.* 137: 3521–3527, 1986.
33. GAGE, F. H., D. M. ARMSTRONG, L. R. WILLIAMS, and S. VARON. Morphological response of axotomized septal neurons to nerve growth factor. *J. Comp. Neurol.* 269: 147–155, 1988.
34. GAGE, F. H., K. S. CHEN, G. BUZSAKI, and D. ARMSTRONG. Experimental approaches to age related cognitive impairments. *Neurobiol. Aging* 9: 645–655, 1988.
35. GALL, C. M., and P. J. ISACKSON. Limbic seizures increase neuronal production of messenger RNA for nerve growth factor. *Science* 245: 758–761, 1989.
36. GALL, C. M., G. ROSE, and G. LYNCH. Proliferative and migratory activity of glial cells in the partially deafferented hippocampus. *J. Comp. Neurol.* 183: 539–548, 1979.
37. GEDDES, J. W., D. T. MONAGHAN, C. W. COTMAN, I. T. LOTT, R. C. KIM, and H. C. CHUI. Plasticity of hippocampal circuitry in Alzheimer's disease. *Science* 230: 1179–1181, 1985.
38. GEDDES, J. W., J. ULAS, L. C. BRUNNER, W. CHOE, and C. W. COTMAN. Hippocampal excitatory amino acid receptors in elderly, normal individuals and those with Alzheimer's disease: non-N-methyl-D-aspartate receptors. *Neuroscience* 50: 23–34, 1992.
39. GIULIAN, D., and T. J. BAKER. Characterization of ameboid microglia isolated from developing mammalian brain. *J. Neurosci.* 6: 2163–2178, 1986.
40. GIULIAN, D., and L. B. LACHMAN. Interleukin-1 stimulation of astroglial proliferation after brain injury. *Science* 228: 497–499, 1985.
41. GOEDERT, M., A. FINE, D. DAWBARN, G. K. WILCOCK, and M. V. CHAO. Nerve growth factor receptor mRNA distribution in human brain: normal levels in basal forebrain in Alzheimer's disease. *Mol. Brain Res.* 5: 1–7, 1989.
42. GOEDERT, M., A. FINE, S. P. HUNT, and A. ULLRICH. Nerve growth factor mRNA in peripheral and central rat tissues and in the human central nervous system: lesion effects in the rat brain and levels in Alzheimer's disease. *Mol. Brain Res.* 1: 85–92, 1986.
43. GOLDGABER, D., H. W. HARRIS, T. HLA, T. MACIAG, R. J. DONNELLY, J. S. JACOBSEN, M. P. VITEK, and D. C. GAJDUSEK. Interleukin 1 regulates synthesis of amyloid β-protein precursor mRNA in human endothelial cells. *Proc. Natl. Acad. Sci. USA* 86: 7606–7610, 1989.
44. GOLLIN, P. A., R. N. KALARIA, P. EIKELENBOOM, A. ROZEMULLER, and G. PERRY. α1-Antitrypsin and α1-antichymotrypsin are in the lesions of Alzheimer's disease. *NeuroReport* 3: 201–203, 1992.
45. GÓMEZ-PINILLA, F., C. W. COTMAN, and M. NIETO-SAMPEDRO. NGF receptor immunoreactivity in aged rat brain. *Brain Res.* 479: 255–262, 1989.
46. GÓMEZ-PINILLA, F., K. GUTHRIE, M. LEON, and M. NIETO-SAMPEDRO. NGF receptor increase in the olfactory bulb after early odor deprivation in rats. *Dev. Brain Res.* 48: 161–165, 1989.
47. GRAY, C. W., and A. J. PATEL. Induction of β-amyloid precursor protein isoform mRNA by bFGF in astrocytes. *NeuroReport* 4: 811–814, 1993.
48. GREENBLATT, D. J., R. I. SHADER, and J. S. HARMATZ. Implications of altered drug disposition in the elderly: studies of benzodiazepines. *J. Clin. Pharmacol.* 29: 866–872, 1989.
49. GRIFFIN, W. S. T., L. C. STANLEY, C. LING, L. WHITE, V. MACLEOD, L. J. PERROT, C. L. WHITE III, and C. ARAOZ. Brain interleukin 1 and S-100 immunoreactivity are elevated in Down syndrome and Alzheimer disease. *Proc. Natl. Acad. Sci. USA* 86: 7611–7615, 1989.
50. HAGA, S., K. AKAI, and T. ISHII. Demonstration of microglial cells in and around senile (neuritic) plaques in the Alzheimer brain: an immunohistochemical study using a novel monoclonal antibody. *Acta Neuropathol.* 77: 569–575, 1989.
51. HARRO, J., and L. ORELAND. Age-related differences of cholecystokinin receptor binding in the rat brain. *Prog. Neuropsychopharmacol. Biol. Psychiatry* 16: 369–375, 1992.
52. HART, R. P., A. M. SHADIACK, and G. M. JONAKAIT. Substance P gene expression is regulated by interleukin-1 in cultured sympathetic ganglia. *J. Neurosci. Res.* 29: 282–291, 1991.
53. HEFTI, F. Nerve growth factor (NGF) promotes survival of septal cholinergic neurons after fimbrial transections. *J. Neurosci.* 6: 2155–2162, 1986.
54. HEFTI, F., and D. C. MASH. Localization of nerve growth factor receptors in the normal human brain and in Alzheimer's disease. *Neurobiol. Aging* 10: 75–87, 1989.
55. HEFTI, F., and L. S. SCHNEIDER. Nerve growth factor and Alzheimer's disease. *Clin. Neuropharmacol.* 14: S62–S76, 1991.
56. HEFTI, F., J. HARTIKKA, and B. KNUSEL. Function of neurotrophic factors in the adult and aging brain and their possible use in the treatment of neurodegenerative diseases. *Neurobiol. Aging* 10: 515–533, 1989.
57. HOFF, S. F., S. W. SCHEFF, and C. W. COTMAN. Lesion-induced synaptogenesis in the dentate gyrus of aged rats: II. Demonstration of an impaired degeneration clearing response. *J. Comp. Neurol.* 205: 253–259, 1982.
58. ISHII, T., and S. HAGA. Immuno-electron-microscopic localization of complements in amyloid fibrils of senile plaques. *Acta Neuropathol.* 63: 296–300, 1984.
59. ISHII, T., S. HAGA, and F. KAMETANI. Presence of immunoglobulins and complements in the amyloid plaques in the brain of patients with Alzheimer's disease. In: *Immunology and Alzheimer's Disease,* edited by A. Pouplard-Barthelaix, J. Emile, and Y. Christen. Berlin: Springer-Verlag, 1987, p. 17–29.
60. ITAGAKI, S., P. L. MCGEER, H. AKIYAMA, S. ZHU, and D. SELKOE. Relationship of microglia and astrocytes to amyloid deposits of Alzheimer's disease. *J. Neuroimmunol.* 24: 173–182, 1989.
61. KAHLE, J. S., J. ULAS, and C. W. COTMAN. Increased sensitivity to adenosine in the rat dentate gyrus molecular layer two weeks after partial entorhinal lesions. *Brain Res.* 609: 201–210, 1993.
62. KATSUKI, H., S. NAKAI, Y. HIRAI, K. AKAJI, Y. KISO, and M. SATOH. Interleukin-1β inhibits long-term potentiation in the CA3 region of mouse hippocampal slices. *Eur. J. Pharmacol.* 181: 323–326, 1990.
63. KITAMURA, Y., X.-H. ZHAO, T. OHNUKI, M. TAKEI, and Y. NOMURA. Age-related changes in transmitter glutamate and

NMDA receptor/channels in the brain of senescence-accelerated mouse. *Neurosci. Lett.* 137: 169–172, 1992.

64. KITO, S., R. MIYOSHI, and T. NOMOTO. Influence of age on NMDA receptor complex in rat brain studied by in vitro autoradiography. *J. Histochem. Cytochem.* 38: 1725–1731, 1990.

65. KOH, S., P. CHANG, T. J. COLLIER, and R. LOY. Loss of NGF receptor immunoreactivity in basal forebrain neurons of aged rats: correlation with spatial memory impairment. *Brain Res.* 498: 397–404, 1989.

66. KOROTZER, A. R., C. J. PIKE, and C. W. COTMAN. β-Amyloid peptides induce degeneration of cultured rat microglia. *Brain Res.*, 624: 121–125, 1993.

67. KORSCHING, S., R. HEUMANN, H. THOENEN, and F. HEFTI. Cholinergic denervation of the rat hippocampus by fimbrial transection leads to a transient accumulation of nerve growth factor (NGF) without change in mRNA^{NGF} content. *Neurosci. Lett.* 66: 175–180, 1986.

68. LAPCHAK, P. A., D. M. ARAUJO, K. D. BECK, C. E. FINCH, S. A. JOHNSON, and F. HEFTI. BDNF and trkB mRNA expression in the hippocampal formation of aging rats. *Neurobiol. Aging* 14: 121–126, 1993.

69. LAPCHAK, P. A., D. M. ARAUJO, and F. HEFTI. Cholinergic regulation of hippocampal brain-derived neurotrophic factor mRNA expression: evidence from lesion and chronic cholinergic drug treatment studies. *Neuroscience* 52: 575–585, 1993.

70. LÄRKFORS, L., T. EBENDAL, S. R. WHITTEMORE, H. PERSSON, B. HOFFER, and L. OLSON. Decreased level of nerve growth factor (NGF) and its messenger RNA in the aged rat brain. *Mol. Brain Res.* 3: 55–60, 1987.

71. LEVI-MONTALCINI, R., and V. HAMBURGER. A diffusible agent of mouse sarcoma producing hyperplasia of sympathetic ganglia and hyperneurotization of viscera in the chick embryo. *J. Exp. Zool.* 123: 321–361, 1953.

72. LIEBERMAN, A. P., P. M. PITHA, H. S. SHIN, and M. L. SHIN. Production of tumor necrosis factor and other cytokines by astrocytes stimulated with lipopolysaccharide or a neurotrophic virus. *Proc. Natl. Acad. Sci. USA* 86: 6348–6352, 1989.

73. LINDHOLM, D., R. HEUMANN, B. HENGERER, and H. THOENEN. Interleukin-1 increases stability and transcription of mRNA encoding nerve growth factor in cultured rat fibroblasts. *J. Biol. Chem.* 263: 16348–16351, 1988.

74. LOUGHLIN, S. E., and J. H. FALLON (Eds). *Neurotrophic Factors.* San Diego: Academic Press, 1993.

75. LOWE, S. L., P. T. FRANCIS, A. W. PROCTER, A. M. PALMER, A. N. DAVISON, and D. M. BOWEN. Gamma-aminobutyric acid concentration in brain tissue at two stages of Alzheimer's disease. *Brain* 111: 785–799, 1988.

76. LU, B., M. YOKOYAMA, C. F. DREYFUS, and I. BLACK. NGF gene expression in actively growing brain glia. *J. Neurosci.* 11: 318–326, 1991.

77. LYNCH, G., and M. BAUDRY. The biochemistry of memory: a new and specific hypothesis. *Science* 224: 1057–1063, 1984.

78. MAGNUSSON, K. R., and C. W. COTMAN. Effects of aging on NMDA and MK801 binding sites in mice. *Brain Res.* 604: 334–337, 1993.

79. MAGNUSSON, K. R., and C. W. COTMAN. Age-related changes in excitatory amino acid receptors in two mouse strains. *Neurobiol. Aging* 14: 197–206, 1993.

80. MANYAM, N. V. B., L. KATZ, T. A. HARE, J. C. GERBER III, and M. H. GROSSMAN. Levels of γ-aminobutyric acid in cerebrospinal fluid in various neurologic disorders. *Arch. Neurol.* 37: 352–355, 1980.

81. MATTSON, M. P. Excitatory amino acids, growth factors, and calcium: a teeter-totter model for neural plasticity and degeneration. In: *Excitatory Amino Acids and Neuronal Plasticity,* edited by Y. Ben-Ari. New York: Plenum Press, 1990, p. 211–220.

82. MCGEER, P. L., and E. G. MCGEER. Enzymes associated with the metabolism of catecholamines, acetylcholine and GABA in human controls and patients with Parkinson's disease and Huntington's chorea. *J. Neurochem.* 26: 65–76, 1976.

83. MCGEER, P. L., H. AKIYAMA, S. ITAGAKI, and E. G. MCGEER. Activation of the classical complement pathway in brain tissue of Alzheimer patients. *Neurosci. Lett.* 107: 341–346, 1989.

84. MCGEER, P. L., S. ITAGAKI, H. TAGO, and E. G. MCGEER. Reactive microglia in patients with senile dementia of the Alzheimer type are positive for the histocompatibility glycoprotein HLA-DR. *Neurosci. Lett.* 79: 195–200, 1987.

85. MCRAE, A., E. A. LING, R. POLINSKY, C. G. GOTTFRIES, and A. DAHLSTROM. Antibodies in the cerebrospinal fluid of some Alzheimer's disease patients recognize ameboid microglial cells in the developing rat central nervous system. *Neuroscience* 41: 739–752, 1991.

86. MHATRE, M. C., and M. K. TICKU. Aging related alterations in $GABA_A$ receptor subunit mRNA levels in Fischer rats. *Mol. Brain Res.* 14: 71–78, 1992.

87. MILLER, L. G., M. LUMPKIN, W. R. GALPERN, D. J. GREENBLATT, and R. I. SADER. Modification of γ-aminobutyric acid$_A$ receptor binding and function by N-ethoxycarbonyl-2-ethoxy-1,2-dihydroquinoline in vitro and in vivo: effects of aging. *J. Neurochem.* 56: 1241–1247, 1991.

88. MOBLEY, W. C., R. L. NEVE, S. B. PRUSINER, and M. P. MCKINLEY. Nerve growth factor increases mRNA levels for the prion protein and the β-amyloid protein precursor in developing hamster brain. *Proc. Natl. Acad. Sci. USA* 85: 9811–9815, 1988.

89. MONAGHAN, D. T., R. J. BRIDGES, and C. W. COTMAN. The excitatory amino acid receptors: their classes, pharmacology, and distinct properties in the function of the central nervous system. *Annu. Rev. Pharmacol. Toxicol.* 29: 365–402, 1989.

90. MONTAMAT, S. C., B. J. CUSACK, and R. E. VESTAL. Management of drug therapy in the elderly. *New Engl. J. Med.* 321: 303–309, 1989.

91. MONTERO, C. N., and F. HEFTI. Intraventricular nerve growth factor administration prevents lesion-induced loss of septal cholinergic neurons in aging rats. *Neurobiol. Aging.* 10: 739–743, 1989.

92. MOUNTJOY, C. Q., M. N. ROSSOR, L. L. IVERSON, and M. ROTH. Correlation of cortical cholinergic and GABA deficits with quantitative neuropathological findings in senile dementia. *Brain* 107: 507–518, 1984.

93. MUFSON, E. J., M. BOTHWELL, L. B. HERSH, and J. H. KORDOWER. Nerve growth factor receptor immunoreactive profiles in the normal, aged human basal forebrain: colocalization with cholinergic neurons. *J. Comp. Neurol.* 285: 196–217, 1989.

94. MUFSON, E. J., M. BOTHWELL, and J. H. KORDOWER. Loss of nerve growth factor receptor-containing neurons in Alzheimer's disease: a quantitative analysis across subregions of the basal forebrain. *Exp. Neurol.* 105: 221–232, 1989.

95. NIETO-SAMPEDRO, M., and C. W. COTMAN. Growth factor induction and temporal order in central nervous system repair. In: *Synaptic Plasticity,* edited by C. W. Cotman. New York: Guilford Press, 1985, p. 407–455.

96. PARK, G. H., and D. E. BUETOW. Genes for insulin-like growth factors I and II are expressed in senescent rat tissues. *Gerontology* 37: 310–316, 1991.

97. PATTERSON, P. H., and H. NAWA. Neuronal differentiation factors/cytokines and synaptic plasticity. *Cell* 72(suppl.):123–137, 1993.

98. PENNEY, J. B., W. F. MARAGOES, J. T. GREENAMYRE, D. L. DEBOWEY, Z. HOLLINGSWORTH, and A. B. YOUNG. Excitatory

amino acid binding sites in the hippocampal region of Alzheimer's disease and other dementias. *J. Neurol. Neurosurg. Psychiatry* 53: 314–320, 1990.

99. PERRY, T. L., J. M. WRIGHT, S. HANSEN, and P. M. MACLEOD. Isoniazid therapy of Huntington disease. *Neurology* 29: 370–375, 1979.

100. PERRY, V. H., M. K. MATYSZAK, and S. FEARN. Altered antigen expression of microglia in the aged rodent CNS. *Glia* 7: 60–67, 1993.

101. PETERSON, C., and C. W. COTMAN. Strain-dependent decrease in glutamate binding to the N-methyl-D-aspartic acid receptor during aging. *Neurosci. Lett.* 104: 309–313, 1989.

102. PIGGOTT, M. A., E. K. PERRY, R. H. PERRY, and J. A. COURT. [^{3}H]MK-801 binding to the NMDA receptor complex, and its modulation in human frontal cortex during development and aging. *Brain Res.* 588: 277–286, 1992.

103. PIKE, C. J., and C. W. COTMAN. Cultured GABA-immunoreactive neurons are resistant to toxicity induced by β-amyloid. *Neuroscience* 56: 269–274, 1993.

104. PIKE, C. J., A. J. WALENCEWICZ, C. G. GLABE, and C. W. COTMAN. In vitro aging of β-amyloid protein causes peptide aggregation and neurotoxicity. *Brain Res.* 563: 311–314, 1991.

105. PROCTER, A. W., E. H. F. WONG, G. C. STRATMANN, S. L. LOWE, and D. M. BOWEN. Reduced glycine stimulation of [^{3}H]MK-801 binding in Alzheimer's disease. *J. Neurochem.* 53: 698–704, 1989.

106. QUON, D., S. CATALANO, and B. CORDELL. Fibroblast growth factor induces β-amyloid presursor mRNA in glial but not neuronal cultured cells. *Biochem. Biophys. Res. Commun.* 167: 96–102, 1990.

107. RADA, P., G. P. MARK, M. P. VITEK, R. M. MANGANO, A. J. BLUME, B. BEER, and B. G. HOEBEL. Interleukin-1β decreases acetylcholine measured by microdialysis in the hippocampus of freely moving rats. *Brain Res.* 550: 287–290, 1991.

108. RAO, G., C. A. BARNES, and B. L. MCNAUGHTON. Effects of age on L-glutamate-induced depolarization in three hippocampal subfields. *Neurobiol. Aging* 14: 27–33, 1993.

109. RELTON, J. K., and N. J. ROTHWELL. Interleukin-1 receptor antagonist inhibits ischemic and excitotoxic neuronal damage in the rat. *Brain Res. Bull.* 29: 243–246, 1992.

110. REPRESA, A., C. DUYCKAERTS, E. TREMBLAY, J. J. HAUW, and Y. BEN-ARI. Is senile dementia of the Alzheimer type associated with hippocampal plasticity? *Brain Res.* 457: 355–359, 1988.

111. RIO-HORTEGA, P. Microglia. In: *Cytology and Cellular Pathology of the Nervous System,* edited by W. Penfield. New York: Paul Hofner, 1932, p. 481–584.

112. ROGERS, J., and F. E. BLOOM. Neurotransmitter metabolism and function in the aging central nervous system. In: *Handbook of the Biology of Aging,* edited by C. E. Finch and E. L. Schneider. New York: Van Nostrand Reinhold, 1985, p. 645–691.

113. ROGERS, J., N. R. COOPER, S. WEBSTER, J. SCHULTZ, P. L. 2MCGEER, S. D. STYREN, W. H. CIVIN, L. BRACHOVA, B. BRADT, P. WARD, and I. LIEBERBURG. Complement activation by β-amyloid in Alzheimer disease. *Proc. Natl. Acad. Sci. USA* 89: 10016–10020, 1992.

114. ROGERS, J., J. LUBER-NAROD, S. D. STRYEN, and W. H. CIVIN. Expression of immune-associated antigens by cells of the human central nervous system: relationship to the pathology of Alzheimer's disease. *Neurobiol. Aging* 9: 339–349, 1988.

115. ROSSOR, M. N., N. J. GARRETT, A. L. JOHNSON, C. Q. MOUNTJOY, and M. ROTH. A post-mortem study of the cholinergic and GABA systems in senile dementia. *Brain* 105: 313–330, 1982.

116. ROTHMAN, S. M., and J. W. OLNEY. Excitotoxicity and the NMDA receptor. *Trends Neurosci.* 10: 299–302, 1987.

117. RUANO, D., J. CANO, A. MACHADO, and J. VITORICA. Pharmacological characterization of GABA$_A$/benzodiazepine receptor in rat hippocampus during aging. *J. Pharmacol. Exp. Ther.* 256: 902–908, 1991.

118. SAPOLSKY, R. M., L. C. KREY, and B. S. MCEWEN. The adrenocortical stress-response in the aged male rat: impairment of recovery from stress. *Exp. Gerontol.* 18: 55–64, 1983.

119. SCHEFF, S. W., S. F. HOFF, and K. J. ANDERSON. Altered regulation of lesion-induced synaptogenesis by adrenalectomy and corticosterone in young adult rats. *Exp. Neurol.* 93: 456–470, 1986.

120. SIEGHART, W. GABA$_A$ receptors: ligand-gated Cl$^-$ ion channels modulated by multiple drug-binding sites. *Trends Pharmacol. Sci.* 13: 446–450, 1992.

121. TAKAYAMA, H., N. OGAWA, M. YAMAMOTO, M. ASANUMA, H. HIRATA, and Z. OTA. Age-related changes in cerebrospinal fluid γ-aminobutyric acid concentration. *Eur. J. Clin. Chem. Clin. Biochem.* 30: 271–274, 1992.

122. TAMARU, M., Y. YONEDA, K. OGITA, J. SHIMIZU, and Y. NAGATA. Age-related decreases of the N-methyl-D-aspartate receptor complex in the rat cerebral cortex and hippocampus. *Brain Res.* 542: 83–90, 1991.

123. TOOYAMA, I., H. AKIYAMA, P. L. MCGEER, Y. HARA, O. YASUHARA, and H. KIMURA. Acidic fibroblast growth factor-like immunoreactivity in brain of Alzheimer patients. *Neurosci. Lett.* 121: 155–158, 1991.

124. UŁAS, J., and C. W. COTMAN. Excitatory amino acid receptors in schizophrenia. *Schizophr. Bull.* 19: 105–117, 1993.

125. UŁAS, J., L. C. BRUNNER, J. W. GEDDES, W. CHOE, and C. W. COTMAN. N-Methyl-D-aspartate receptor complex in the hippocampus of elderly, normal individuals and those with Alzheimer's disease. *Neuroscience* 49: 45–61, 1992.

126. VIJAYAN, V. K., and C. W. COTMAN. Hydrocortisone administration alters glial reaction to entorhinal lesion in the rat dentate gyrus. *Exp. Neurol.* 96: 307–320, 1987.

127. WALICKE, P. A., W. M. COWAN, N. UENO, A. BAIRD, and R. GUILLEMIN. Fibroblast growth factor promotes survival of dissociated hippocampal neurons and enhances neurite extension. *Proc. Natl. Acad. Sci. USA* 83: 3012–3016, 1986.

128. WASTERLAIN, C. Epileptic seizures. In: *Basic Neurochemistry: Molecular, Cellular, and Medical Aspects,* edited by G. J. Siegel, B. Agranoff, R. W. Albers, and P. Molinoff. New York: Raven Press, 1989, vol. 4, p. 797–810.

129. WENK, G. L., D. J. PIERCE, R. G. STRUBLE, D. L. PRICE, and L. C. CORK. Age-related changes in multiple neurotransmitter systems in the monkey brain. *Neurobiol. Aging* 10: 11–19, 1989.

130. WENK, G. L., L. C. WALKER, D. L. PRICE, and L. C. CORK. Loss of NMDA, but not GABA-A, binding in the brains of aged rats and monkeys. *Neurobiol. Aging* 12: 93–98, 1991.

131. WILL, B., and F. HEFTI. Behavioural and neurochemical effects of chronic intraventricular injections of nerve growth factor in adult rats with fimbrial lesions. *Behav. Brain Res.* 17: 17–24, 1985.

132. WILL, B., F. HEFTI, V. PALLAGE, and G. TONIOLO. Nerve growth factor. Effects on CNS neurons and on behavioral recovery from brain damage. In: *Pharmacological Approaches to the Treatment of Brain and Spinal Cord Injury,* edited by D. Stein and B. Sabel. New York: Plenum Press, 1988, p. 339–360.

133. XIN, L., and C. M. BLATTEIS. Blockade by interleukin-1 receptor antagonist of IL-1β-induced neuronal activity in guinea pig preoptic area slices. *Brain Res.* 569: 348–352, 1992.

134. ZAFRA, F., E. CASTRÉN, H. THOENEN, and D. LINDHOLM. Interplay between glutamate and γ-aminobutyric acid transmitter systems in the physiological regulation of brain-derived neuro-

trophic factor and nerve growth factor synthesis in hippocampal neurons. *Proc. Natl. Acad. Sci. USA* 88: 10037–10041, 1991.

135. ZAFRA, F., B. HENGERER, J. LEIBROCK, H. THOENEN, and D. LINDHOLM. Activity dependent regulation of BDNF and NGF nRNAs in the rat hippocampus is mediated by non-NMDA glutamate receptors. *EMBO J.* 9: 3545–3550, 1990.

136. ZAFRA, F., D. LINDHOLM, E. CASTRÉN, J. HARTIKKA, and H. THOENEN. Regulation of brain-derived neurotrophic factor and nerve growth factor mRNA in primary cultures of hippocampal neurons and astrocytes. *J. Neurosci.* 12: 4793–4799, 1992.

14. Taste and smell

LINDA BARTOSHUK | Department of Surgery, Section of Otolaryngology, Yale University School of Medicine, New Haven, Connecticut
VALERIE DUFFY | School of Allied Health Professions, University of Connecticut, Storrs, Connecticut

CHAPTER CONTENTS

Methodological Issues of Importance to Both Taste and Olfaction
    Threshold vs. suprathreshold perception
    The scaling of perceived intensity: how do we compare individuals or groups?
    Magnitude matching: another approach to comparisons across individuals or groups
Taste
    Thresholds
    Magnitude estimation with a common standard given to all subjects
    Line length with no labels
    Labeled scales
    Magnitude matching
    Consistency of taste responses
    What are appropriate inferences from the suprathreshold studies?
    Sources of taste loss
Orthonasal Olfaction
    Thresholds
    Odor identification
    Magnitude scales with no labels
    Labeled scales
    Magnitude matching
    Sources of olfactory loss
Retronasal Olfaction
    Thresholds
    Identification
    Magnitude matching
    Orthonasal vs. retronasal perception
    Sources of retronasal olfactory loss
    Summary
Conclusions

THE CHEMICAL SENSES include olfaction, taste, and trigeminal stimulation. Taste is a primitive sense, involving four basic qualitative sensations: salty, sweet, sour, and bitter. Olfaction is more complex and acts as a dual sense. Odors can stimulate the receptors (located high in the nasal cavity) by entering either the nostrils (*orthonasal route*) or the mouth (*retronasal route*). Retronasal olfactory sensation provides the major component of food flavor (41) and combines with taste, tactile, thermal, and trigeminal sensations to produce what Rozin has called "mouthsense" (P. Rozin, personal communication). The everyday usage of the term "taste" actually refers to mouthsense. Careful questioning can help correctly identify taste and/or smell complaints when the elderly state that "food just does not taste the way it used to."

The elderly probably experience many taste sensations in much the same way as the young, while other taste sensations show some loss. Olfactory experience, especially retronasal olfaction, is likely to dim with age. Because of the importance of retronasal olfaction to mouthsense, many elderly individuals live in a world of pastel food flavors. These generalizations about perception in the elderly are based on psychophysical procedures that quantify sensory experience. The procedures, while seemingly simple, rest upon some assumptions that require very careful evaluation. In this chapter, we present some of the debates over the measurement of sensation and the impact of these debates on comparisons of the sensory experiences of old and young individuals.

METHODOLOGICAL ISSUES OF IMPORTANCE TO BOTH TASTE AND OLFACTION

Rowe and Kahn (50) have underlined the importance of separating usual from successful aging in delineating the differences between older and younger cohorts. Does poorer chemosensory perception in the elderly result from aging alone or from a combination of aging with additional insults that are extrinsic to the aging process (for example, environmental, behavioral, or psychosocial factors)? Researchers often describe differences in chemosensory perception across age cohorts, by comparing a younger, more functionally homogeneous group to an older group with a large range of functional status. Researchers could improve the validity of attributing the chemosensory loss to aging by accounting for the degree of heterogeneity in the elderly. Elderly subjects need to be defined not by chronological age alone but by overall functional status and the presence of risk factors for chemosensory disorders. Including a longitudinal component in the study design helps describe the pattern of loss with aging and also diminishes the issue of reliability of sensory measures across age groups. Botwinick (9) has described variations on the traditional cross-sectional and longitudinal study designs. A cross-sequential study design, for example, includes both a cross-sectional and a longitudinal component and allows inferences about age/time effect on chemosensory function. Research in the chemical senses and aging could profit from exploration of these methodological issues in the attempt to separate usual from more successful aging.

Threshold vs. Suprathreshold Perception

Threshold methodology is rooted in the nineteenth-century work of Weber and Fechner (26a). The methodology is deceptively simple since a variety of artifacts plague the measurement of thresholds. Nonetheless, thresholds remain useful sensory investigation tools. Thresholds are easy to compare across individuals because the threshold is simply a measure of the lower limit of physical energy (for example, decibel (db) of sound, molar concentration of a taste solution, etc.) needed to evoke a sensation.

Scaling methods measure the perceived intensities of sensations across the dynamic range, that is, from nearly imperceptible to extremely intense. Stevens (66) described category and magnitude scales. In brief, a *category scale* orders stimulus intensities, while a *magnitude scale* both orders and provides ratios between stimulus intensities. For example, we might ask subjects to rate two stimuli on a 10-point category scale. If two stimuli were rated 8 and 4, this would mean only that the stimulus rated 8 was more intense than the one rated 4. However, if the two stimuli were rated 8 and 4 on a magnitude scale, this would mean that the stimulus rated 8 was twice as intense as the one rated 4. Although there is much debate about which of these approaches is superior, we agree with Pangborn's conclusions that both are useful but have limitations that must be understood by the experimenter (46). In this review, we focus not on the scaling method employed in a study but rather on a different question: How well do the studies compare sensory intensities across individuals, more particularly, across the old and the young?

Unfortunately, since we cannot share another person's experience directly, there is no absolutely valid method of comparing perceived intensities across individuals or groups. However, scaling methods in the hands of sophisticated practitioners can still lead to important inferences about the sensory experience of the old vs. that of the young. Confusion over the proper use of scaling methods is responsible for most of the controversy that exists on the effects of age on taste and smell. For this reason, we discuss efforts to make legitimate comparisons across individuals and then assess the impact of these on studies of the effects of age on taste and smell.

The Scaling of Perceived Intensity: How Do We Compare Individuals or Groups?

Adjectives describing intensity are easily applied to category scales. For example, with the Natick 9-point category scale (32) subjects apply numbers to sensations such that 1 = very weak, 5 = medium, and 9 = very strong. If two people label a stimulus "strong" and experience the same absolute intensity, then these labels would provide a way to compare intensities across individuals. Needless to say, we cannot ever determine with certainty whether or not the labels signify the same experience to different people. However, labeling of this sort may prove useful when we assume that the subjects to be compared have had many similar sensory experiences. For example, if we assume that most individuals have experienced a range of "weak" to "strong" intensities in a variety of senses, then a loss in one sense might be reflected by unexpected judgments of "weak" for that sense.

In magnitude estimation (67), we instruct subjects to judge intensity such that if one stimulus is twice as strong as another, it is assigned a number twice as large. The legitimate uses of magnitude estimate functions are often misunderstood. The most important feature to understand is that magnitude estimation only provides information about *relative* intensities among stimuli. That is, if a person estimates the intensity of one stimulus to be 8 and that of another stimulus to be 4, we know that the first stimulus is twice as intense as the second but we do not know the absolute intensity of either. This means that magnitude estimation cannot be used to make comparisons across subjects or groups. It can be used to make comparisons within one subject (for example comparisons before and after some experimental manipulation).

Magnitude estimation experiments are typically run in one of two ways. First, experimenters may allow the subjects to use any numbers they choose. Then the experimenter "normalizes" the data to remove variation due to the size of the numbers chosen by individual subjects in the following way. The experimenter selects the condition that is to be considered the standard. For example, the experimenter might select 0.3 M NaCl, then calculate a normalization factor, F, for each subject; F = 10/subject's estimate for 0.3 M NaCl (10 is an arbitrary choice). Then the experimenter would multiply all of the subject's responses by F. Note that multiplying the numbers by a common factor does not change the ratios among them, the ratios being the only meaningful part of the data. In the normalized data, all of the subject's responses to 0.3 M NaCl will then equal

10. It is important to remember that this does not mean that all of the subjects experience the same intensity from 0.3 M NaCl. It should be noted that some investigators have compared raw magnitude estimates across groups, but there is no evidence that this provides meaningful comparisons.

The second way in which magnitude estimation experiments are run is for the experimenter to provide a number that is intended to describe a particular stimulus (the standard) and ask the subject to estimate all other stimuli relative to that number. For example, the experimenter might give each subject a solution of 0.3 M NaCl to taste and ask each one to call that intensity 10. Then, if another solution tasted twice as strong, it should be called 20, etc. Again, this does not mean that all subjects experience the same intensity from the standard.

Figure 14.1 shows how incorrect inferences can be drawn from magnitude estimate data. Suppose that an experimenter used the method described above and asked each subject to call 0.1 M NaCl 10. Let us also suppose that the experimenter tested both young and old subjects with a concentration series of NaCl. The functions produced by the elderly and young subjects might look like those in the leftmost panel. They would intersect at 0.1 M NaCl. The point at which the functions intercept the y axis provides a measure of the vertical positions of the two functions. If we were to assume that the leftmost panel could be used to directly compare elderly and young subjects, we would conclude that for low concentrations, the elderly subjects perceived more intense tastes than the young and for high concentrations, the elderly subjects perceived less intense tastes than the young. This is not, however, what the data mean. Only the shapes of the functions are meaningful. We have artificially linked the elderly and young functions by asking all subjects to rate 0.1 M NaCl as 10. If the subjects followed instructions, the functions had to intersect at that point. In reality we have no way to know how the two functions relate to each other. The truth might be as suggested in the middle panel: the elderly and young subjects perceive strong stimuli equally but the elderly show elevated responses to the weak stimuli. However, the truth might also be as suggested in the rightmost panel: the elderly perceive stimuli as less intense than the young and the discrepancy grows with concentration. It should be clear that magnitude estimation by itself cannot be used to compare individuals or groups of individuals.

Moskowitz (40) developed a procedure by which adjectives can be added to a magnitude estimate function. At the end of the session, subjects are asked to provide the estimates they would have used to describe a stimulus that was "weak," "strong," etc. This very cleverly adds potential power to the magnitude estimation procedure. To the extent that adjectives prove a useful way to permit comparisons across individuals, that power can be added to magnitude estimation. The fundamental problem remaining, as noted above, is that the conditions under which adjectives really allow comparisons across individuals are still under study.

A variety of procedures direct the subject to mark a length on a line that corresponds to the intensity of a sensation. Interestingly such a line can produce data equivalent to magnitude scaling or category scaling, depending on the way in which it is labeled. For example, a line marked off into nine intervals with "nothing" on one end and "very strong" on the other is much like the Natick 9-point category scale. However, a line marked "nothing" on one end and "very strong" at a

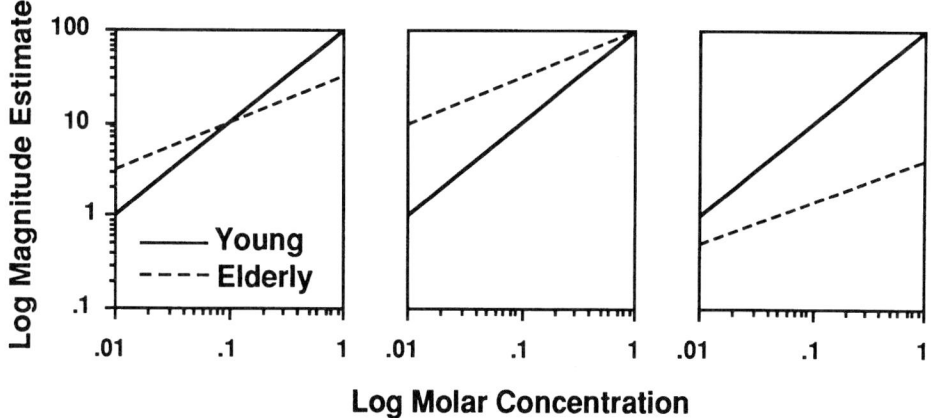

FIG. 14.1. Illustration of the logical error involved when magnitude estimation data are used to draw conclusions about absolute intensity. The leftmost panel shows how data might look if both old and young subjects were asked to call a 0.1M solution 10. Only the slopes of the data are meaningful. The vertical positions of the functions are caused by the standard given to the subjects and so are meaningless. The panels in the middle and on the right are examples of what the actual perceived intensities might be.

point about two-thirds of the way from "nothing" produces data close to those obtained with magnitude estimation (35). One variant of this procedure that has been used in aging research is a tape-pull method (71). The subject pulls the tape to a length commensurate with the perceived intensity of a stimulus. Like any line-length method, the measures that can be generated are limited to the length of the line (3 m in the case of the tape). Thus any line method has an implied limit that the subject presumably treats as the top of the intensity scale. However, just as with adjectives, we cannot be certain that the top of the scale represents equivalent sensory intensity across individuals.

Magnitude Matching: Another Approach to Comparisons Across Individuals or Groups

In an effort to provide a more satisfying solution to the problem of comparing perceived intensities across individuals or groups, Marks and Stevens developed the *magnitude matching* method (38, 62). Although Marks and Stevens based the method on magnitude estimation, the same logic can be applied to any method of scaling suprathreshold intensities. In theory, the method is simplicity itself. We treat some stimulus as a standard and assume that everyone experiences the same intensity experience from it. Including the standard in each experiment allows us to express all sensations in terms relative to it. We need only assume that subjects can always make precise estimates of perceived intensity across stimuli that vary in intensity and quality. Then, expressing all of these estimates in terms of our standard, we can make comparisons across subjects with ease.

Marks has explored the validity of the assumption that subjects can make accurate relative judgments across various stimuli. He has found that there are some limitations to our abilities to make such judgments (see 36). In particular, there are context effects. For example, in one study (36), Marks asked subjects to listen to low-frequency sounds, from very soft (30 db) to loud (86 db). Between the sounds, the subjects tasted salt solutions. In some sessions the salt solutions were relatively weak but in other sessions they were relatively strong. Both series of salt solutions contained two concentrations (0.18 and 0.32 M NaCl) that fell in the middle of the series. Those salt solutions matched different sounds, depending on the series. For example, 0.32 M NaCl matched a sound of about 82 db when it was in the weak series but it matched a sound of about 62 db when it was in the strong series. In spite of this context effect, individual subjects were consistent in their judgments. We can hope that further study will suggest ways to minimize context, but, in any case, the effects of context can be assessed. For example, Marks's studies suggest that context effects are smallest when the two sensory domains are similar (37).

Finding a standard that we can assume is equally intense to all subjects is a harder task. In fact, it is virtually impossible. However, we often need not find a perfect standard. For example, to study age we need only find a standard that is not systematically different between old and young subjects. Is this possible?

The following discussion of studies on the effects of age on taste and olfaction illustrates how investigators have used (or sometimes misused) these psychophysical methods.

TASTE

Thresholds

Many studies using various methodologies support the conclusion that taste thresholds tend to rise with age (see 43, 70). Of special interest, the effects of age are quality-specific. For example, sucrose thresholds are remarkably stable, while NaCl thresholds clearly rise with age (70). In the early years of taste research, this decrease in sensitivity was interpreted to mean that the taste world dimmed with age. We now know that changes at threshold need not predict changes in the perception of more concentrated stimuli. In the sense of taste, in particular, thresholds are sometimes dramatically dissociated from suprathreshold function. Figure 14.2 shows examples of this dissociation. Panel A shows the effects of exposing the tongue to the detergent in toothpaste, sodium laurel sulfate (20). Each NaCl concentration is reduced by a constant proportion. In log-log coordinates, this simply shifts the vertical position of the NaCl function. In this case, the threshold is elevated and the suprathreshold perceived intensity is reduced for each stimulus. Panel B shows the effects of adaptation, in this case simply the normal adaptation produced by salt in saliva (stimulated by chewing) (2). Here, the threshold is elevated to a point just above the adaptation concentration, but the psychophysical function shows a steep rise so that it quickly joins the unadapted function. This illustrates why, even though we are always adapted to the salt in saliva, this adaptation has little effect on tasting salt in foods. Panel C shows the effects of radiation therapy on a patient with cancer of the neck (2). Taste was initially totally abolished, but 2 months after therapy, the patient's thresholds had returned to normal. However, her psychophysical functions were flattened; that is, she lived in a pastel taste world. Panel D compares NaCl functions for two age groups (7). We discuss it further later in this review.

The growing realization that elevated taste thresholds do not invariably predict reduced perceived intensities

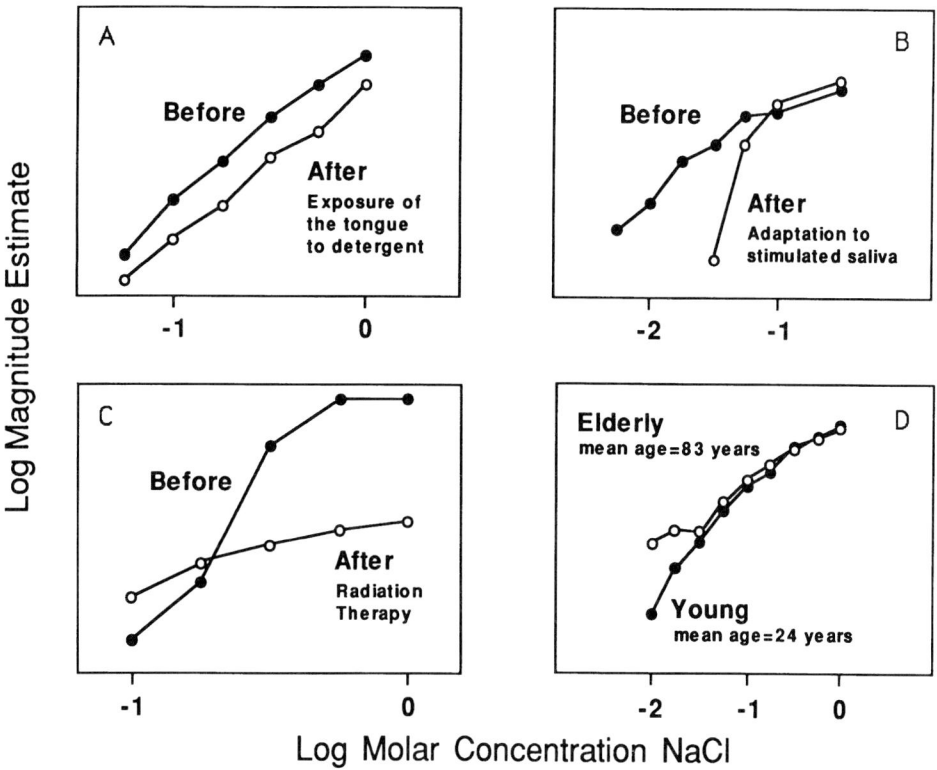

FIG. 14.2. Examples from taste showing that the threshold does not predict the suprathreshold function. See text under the heading "Thresholds" for explanation.

at higher concentrations led to studies utilizing measures of suprathreshold function, since without these we cannot hope to understand the taste world of the elderly. Since the suprathreshold studies lead to contradictory conclusions about the effects of age on taste, we treat them in some detail. The studies on suprathreshold taste are organized into groups in a slightly unconventional way. Rather than group them by method, we group them by the logic used to compare old and young.

Magnitude Estimation with a Common Standard Given to all Subjects

When the experimenter gives a particular stimulus to old and young subjects, the resulting data cannot provide information about absolute differences in perceived intensity even if the differences exist. Enns and co-workers (27) asked their subjects to assign the number "10" to the sweetness produced by 0.18 M sucrose and to assign proportional numbers to the sweetnesses of a concentration series of sucrose. Although fifth-grade students produced somewhat steeper functions than college undergraduates and elderly subjects, the most noteworthy result was that the college undergraduates and the elderly subjects (about 70 yr) produced virtually identical functions. The authors interpreted this as evidence that there is no loss in the ability to taste sweetness with age. However, the apparent similarity of functions for the undergraduates and the elderly subjects is illusory. As we showed in Figure 14.1, the elderly function might actually lie considerably below or above the undergraduate function.

Schiffman and colleagues (55) tested a variety of sweeteners on undergraduates and elderly subjects (mean age 78 yr), who were somewhat older than those in the study by Enns et al. They also gave each subject a particular stimulus and assigned it a specific value. Schiffman et al. found that the psychophysical functions for the elderly subjects were flatter than those for the undergraduates. A similar study with amino acids (54) showed the same empirical results: magnitude estimate functions were flatter for elderly subjects. The authors were careful to note that only the slopes of the functions were meaningful (55). The absolute positions of the functions are not determined with this procedure, so the flattened functions do not indicate decreased perceived taste intensities with age.

Chauhan and Hawrysh (16) provided a reference sample [0.012 M citric acid (CA)] and instructed subjects to call it 10 and to judge other stimuli relative to it. Subjects in three age groups (20–29 yr, 70–79 yr, and 80–99 yr) then judged the intensities of a series of CA solutions (including 0.012 M, the standard). Not surprisingly, the resulting psychophysical functions intersected at 0.012 M CA, the standard. The function for the 70–79-yr group was flatter than those of the other two groups, which led the authors to conclude that that group perceived more sourness at low concentrations and less at high concentrations than the other groups. In fact, as in the example in Figure 14.1, there is no way to tell how the three functions should be located vertically.

Little and Brinner (34) used a 10 cm line rather than magnitude estimation, but their study illustrates the same principle. The line was labeled "least salty" and "most salty" at the ends. Subjects were given tomato juice with no added NaCl as a standard for "least salty" and 1.5% NaCl in tomato juice as a standard for "most salty." Old (55–88 yr) and young (20–40 yr) subjects then rated a variety of concentrations of NaCl in tomato juice for saltiness. Just as with the previous study, if there were genuine differences between old and young in perceived saltiness, this method could not reveal them. This study also illustrates another complication that arises when the experimenter asks all subjects to assign a particular value to a particular stimulus. The experiment was designed to examine the possibility that CA would add saltiness to tomato juice. The experimenters tested combinations of 0–1.5% NaCl and 0–0.9% CA in tomato juice. The subjects were told that 1.5% NaCl in tomato juice was to be rated at the extreme end of the line labeled "most salty" (that is, 10 cm). However, acids taste somewhat salty themselves (see 1, 39). Thus adding CA to NaCl could be expected to produce at least some mixtures of NaCl and CA that would be saltier than the NaCl alone. What were the subjects to do? If both groups had followed instructions, they would have judged 1.5% NaCl/juice as "most salty," or 10 cm, and there would have been no room for judgments of the saltier mixtures. Not surprisingly, the subjects spread their judgments and used values close to the maximum of 10 cm for the saltiest NaCl–CA/juice mixtures and lower values for the less salty NaCl/juice stimuli. The younger subjects rated the 1.5% NaCl/juice at 7.3 cm and the older subjects rated it at 5.8 cm. This might mean that older subjects perceive NaCl to be less salty, but it also might mean something quite different. Suppose CA is saltier to older subjects. Then the NaCl–CA/juice might have been placed near the top of the scale and the NaCl/juice pushed further down in comparison.

Line Length with no Labels

Dye and Koziatek (26) looked at the effects of age on the sweet taste of sucrose with a line-length variant. Subjects were presented with a board divided in the middle, the left side labeled "less sweet" and the right side "more sweet." A wire that could be moved to either side designated the subject's judgment of length. There was little difference between subjects under 65 yr and those over 65 yr. Note that although a label of sorts was supplied, it really only indicated directionality. No points on the line were labeled with adjectives. In this case, the old and young subjects' judgments were not anchored to the same stimulus. Thus it is theoretically possible that old and young could reveal sensory differences with this method. However, we have no way to be certain that they do.

Weiffenbach et al. (71) asked subjects to pull a tape measure to a length commensurate with the intensity of the tastes of sucrose, NaCl, CA, and quinine solutions. The psychophysical functions for subjects age 40 yr and older were very similar to one another. However, the functions for subjects from 22 to 39 yr were steeper for CA and quinine but not for sucrose and NaCl. If we accept tape pull as an absolute measure of perceived intensity, then the results would imply that younger subjects perceived more intense sour and bitter sensations at the higher concentrations. Can we assume then that the young and elderly subjects have the same intensity experiences from a given size tape pull?

In another study with the tape-pull method, Cowart (19) found similar results: no age effects with sucrose and NaCl, but with CA and quinine the older group produced shorter tape pulls for sour and bitter stimuli.

These methods could work if subjects implicitly used the available length to represent the entire range of perceived sensory intensities. Assuming that not all sensations dim with age or that subjects can remember earlier, more intense experiences accurately, the methods could measure genuine differences between old and young.

Labeled Scales

Placing a label on a scale is intended to provide a measure of absolute perceived intensity. If we assume that a given label indicates the same perceived intensity in old and young subjects, this method permits the measurement of differences between them. In two studies, Hyde and his colleagues (30, 31) asked subjects to judge taste intensities on a 100-mm line labeled "no taste" at one end and "extreme" at the other end, with "extreme" defined as "the most intensely perceived sensation ever experienced." Both studies showed similar results. Sucrose and NaCl showed no age effects but CA and quinine produced weaker judgments in the older subjects.

Zallen and co-workers (74) used a 9-point labeled

scale with 1 = "least salty" and 9 = "most salty" and found no age effects on the judgments of the saltiness of samples of mashed potatoes and chicken soup containing from 0.3% to 0.9% NaCl.

In a study of various sensory attributes of foods, Stevens and Lawless (58) used a 15-cm line with labels "not at all salty" or "not at all bitter," etc. at one end and "extremely salty" or "extremely bitter," etc. at the other end. Judgments of bitterness decreased with age.

The Natick 9-point scale was used to devise a screening test for patients who might have suffered damage to the taste system (4, 5). With this procedure, highly concentrated taste stimuli were "painted" with cotton-tipped applicators (long-handled cotton swabs) onto three loci: the front and rear edges of the tongue and the palate. In addition, to compare taste intensities on these spatially localized areas to those evoked when all of the receptors were stimulated, subjects sipped and swallowed small amounts of the stimuli. Using this procedure with normal controls of varying ages (3), there were no significant age effects. However, when this procedure was used with weaker concentrations in an experiment with old (mean = 74 yr) and young (mean = 28 yr) subjects, some age effects were revealed (3, 4, 29). Responses to quinine and NaCl were reduced on some loci and responses to CA were reduced on all three loci for the older subjects. For the whole mouth, sucrose and NaCl produced similar judgments from old (mean = 74 yr) and young (mean = 28 yr) subjects, while CA and quinine produced reduced judgments at some concentrations.

In Cowart's tape-pull study (18), subjects were asked to rate the same stimuli with a labeled category scale as well. The two methods produced results similar in some respects but different in others. For both methods, there was no age effect with sucrose and little with NaCl. However, both methods produced significant age effects with CA and quinine, but the effects were not the same, particularly with CA. The labeled category scale showed weaker judgments from the oldest subjects (65–79 yr), while the young (19–35 yr) and middle (45–59 yr) groups overlapped at stronger judgments. The tape-pull scale showed weaker overlapping judgments from both the middle and the oldest subjects, while the young group showed stronger judgments. The two methods are clearly not completely equivalent.

Magnitude Matching

Cowart (18) used the tape-pull method in conjunction with lifted weights. This study, actually done earlier than the other tape-pull studies, offers some important insights into the tape-pull method. Cowart found no statistically significant effects of age on the lifted weights. If we assume that the experience of lifting weights is roughly equivalent across individuals, then this means that the tape-pulls would provide a measure of perceived intensity that is meaningful across subjects. The older subjects tended to produce flatter taste functions, particularly for quinine, and shorter tape pulls for all of the taste stimuli. Thus Cowart concluded that the older subjects experienced weaker taste sensations for all stimuli. One could argue that, although there were no statistically significant effects of age on the lifted-weight data, the tape pulls for the weights tended to be shorter for the older subjects. If Cowart had normalized the data to the weights, the apparent taste loss would have been reduced. However, the major question is whether or not lifted weights can provide a reasonable sensory experience to use as a standard. Can we assume that a young and an elderly person have the same intensity experiences when lifting a given weight?

We can gain some insights into this from an experiment by Murphy and Gilmore (44), who used auditory stimuli (1,000-hertz (Hz) tones) and lifted weights as standards in a magnitude matching experiment to assess the effects of age with NaCl, sucrose, CA and caffeine. They found that the lifted weights and the tones behaved equivalently as standards. This suggests that the lifted weights in Cowart's study (18) probably produced results much like auditory stimuli would have. Murphy and Gilmore (44) found no effect of age with NaCl or sucrose and a slight effect with CA but a greater effect with caffeine.

Magnitude matching with an auditory standard produces conclusions similar to those above (6, 7, 47). Panel D in Figure 14.2 shows NaCl functions for elderly (mean age 83 yr) and young (mean age 24 yr) subjects. These functions were obtained by asking the subjects to judge the intensities of NaCl solutions and sounds on the same intensity scale. The use of a sound standard in an experiment with age might seem unwise because we expect to find hearing loss in many elderly subjects. However, we know that age takes its greatest toll on high-frequency, low-intensity sounds. Thus we used a low-frequency band of noise at relatively high intensities for the standard stimuli. Note that for the higher concentrations of NaCl, the elderly and young functions virtually overlap. Note also that the function for the elderly subjects was flatter than that for the younger subjects, but it was flatter because of an elevation at the lower concentrations and not a reduction at the higher concentrations. We suggest that the elevation at the lower concentrations might be due to a mild dysgeusia that adds to the taste of the solutions. The other solutions tested (sucrose, CA, and quinine) showed similar results for the weakest concentrations. Like NaCl, sucrose functions overlapped for the higher concentrations, but CA and quinine functions showed reductions at the highest concentrations. We have assumed that we could, with care, select sounds that were equally loud to young and old subjects. Can we be absolutely certain that we have succeeded? The answer is no.

Consistency of Taste Responses

Weiffenbach (69) has noted that "neither chemosensory functioning nor aging are unitary processes," so we should not be surprised to find that aging takes a toll on some attributes of sensation and not on others. Weiffenbach et al. (71) measured the consistency of responses to suprathreshold taste stimuli with the ICC (intraclass correlation coefficient) and found clear age effects. This measure is high when repeated tests with the same stimulus evoke similar ratings and low when the ratings vary. ICCs stayed high across age for sucrose and diminished the most for quinine.

What Are Appropriate Inferences from the Suprathreshold Studies?

Even if comparisons of absolute intensity are unwarranted in a particular study, relative comparisons are valid. For example, several studies found no effects of age with sucrose or NaCl but did find effects with CA and bitter substances. Thus we can conclude that age takes a greater toll on the detection of CA and quinine than of sucrose and NaCl.

Can we come to any conclusion about whether or not sucrose and NaCl intensities dim with age? If we look at the studies that logically could show this (the labeled category and the magnitude matching studies), we see little evidence that these intensities dim with age.

Sources of Taste Loss

Although there are many disorders that can take a toll on taste (21), two of the most common etiologies for taste loss are head trauma and upper respiratory infection. There is some evidence to suggest that these two disorders take a greater toll on bitterness than on other qualities (57, 68). This is particularly interesting in light of the evidence reviewed above, that bitter losses do occur with age. This raises again the issue of whether there is a genuine aging effect or whether older individuals simply have had more time to encounter taste disorders.

ORTHONASAL OLFACTION

The majority of studies support the conclusion that olfactory thresholds rise with age and perceived odor intensities are substantially reduced with age (see 14 for review). The studies that led to this conclusion with olfaction are discussed below.

Older individuals show a range of function from total loss (*anosmia*) to diminished perception (*hyposmia*) to that equal to younger cohorts (*normosmia*). Individuals may suffer from a precipitous olfactory loss, as with a head trauma and the severing of the olfactory nerves as they pass through the cribriform plate of the ethmoid bone (17). The lack of longitudinal data makes it difficult to determine age-related olfactory loss. The general assumption is that a gradual loss of smell associates with aging, whereas a more precipitous loss suggests some environmental insult in combination with age-related declines (see 14 for review).

Olfactory stimuli delivered through the nostrils produce different perceptual experiences from those delivered via the mouth (51). Differences in perceived intensity between orthonasal and retronasal olfaction may depend on the effectiveness of the delivery system. For example, a higher perceived intensity of orthonasal stimuli could result if sniffing concentrated the odorant and diminished losses through adsorption to the walls of the nares. Most studies of olfactory function observe only orthonasal olfaction and simply assume that if the perception of odors by this route is blunted, then retronasal olfaction will be blunted to the same degree. However, if aging were to interfere with odor transmission via the mouth, then retronasal olfaction might show losses even when orthonasal olfaction is normal. Because the effects of age could affect orthonasal and retronasal olfaction in different ways, we discuss these two kinds of olfaction separately.

There are other issues relevant to olfaction that are of less concern with taste. Qualitative variation across odorants is one of these. The qualities sweet, salty, sour, and bitter describe most (if not all) taste sensations. The number of distinct olfactory qualities that can be perceived is vast in comparison. This provides not only an experimental dilemma (which odorants should we test?) but also an important question for aging research. Do all olfactory qualities dim with age or does age diminish some and spare others? Another concern with measuring suprathreshold function in olfaction is the state of odor adaptation and the ability of some odorants to stimulate trigeminal as well as olfactory sensations.

Thresholds

Olfactory thresholds show considerable variability (64). This variability makes repeated threshold measurements advisable so as to diminish the threshold errors to an acceptable level (13). In spite of this variability, there is a body of evidence supporting the conclusion that, like taste, olfactory thresholds rise with age (see 43 for review).

Odor Identification

Olfactory identification requires the detection of the odorant, the retrieval of the odor name from long-term memory (assuming that the odor is familiar), and the correct naming of the odor through the formation of odor–word relationships. Thus memory loss with aging (as reviewed by Katzman in Chapter 12 of this volume) and the difficulty of the elderly to attach names to unfamiliar odors (72) become issues to consider. Researchers attempt to separate olfactory identification from these confounds by providing a list of odors to counteract the difficulty in naming odors (33, 45), providing feedback (12), and screening their subjects for cognitive difficulties prior to testing.

Two large-scale epidemiological studies support the conclusion that odor identification decreases as a function of age, starting in early adulthood. Both studies used encapsulated odorants of the "scratch and sniff" variety. Doty et al. combined 40 such odorants into the University of Pennsylvania Smell Identification Test (23). Each odorant is presented with a list of four object names and the subject is asked to select the one that the odor most resembles. Doty and colleagues concluded, from cross-sectional data on 1,955 persons ranging in age from 5 to 99 yr, that 50% of individuals over the age of 65 yr suffer from major olfactory impairment (22). Wysocki and Gilbert provided a scratch and sniff test for the readers of National Geographic (73). Responses to six odorants were obtained from 1.2 million U.S. residents aged 10 yr or older. The percent correctly identified declined for the elderly. Of special interest, the decline was greater for some odorants than for others, the "sweet" odor perception being the most vulnerable to age-related loss (52).

Magnitude Scales with no Labels

Rovee and colleagues (49) used a device that permitted subjects to move an indicator along a track (a yard in length) to select lengths that reflected the perceived intensities of a series of concentrations of *n*-propanol. Subjects from 6 to 94 yr produced similar psychophysical functions. The authors concluded that the perceived intensities of odors did not diminish with age. However, just as we discussed with taste, the similarities may be illusory, since the vertical position of the functions is undetermined with suprathreshold scaling procedures that do not use labels or some comparison continuum.

Labeled Scales

The *National Geographic* survey also asked respondents to estimate the intensities of the odorants on a 5-point scale (1 = weak, 5 = strong). The intensities declined with age and the pattern of decline varied across the odorants. The convergence of the identification and intensity measures strengthens confidence in the conclusion that age takes a significant toll on suprathreshold olfaction, but the same logical limitations apply to the category scaling of olfactory intensity as applied to scaling of taste intensity. We cannot be certain that the labels reflect the same intensity experiences in the old and young subjects.

Magnitude Matching

Stevens and co-workers (65) were the first to find evidence of substantial olfactory losses with age using magnitude matching with an auditory standard. As noted above, taste showed few losses when evaluated with a similar auditory standard (6, 7, 47). Thus if magnitude matching is providing a close approximation to absolute comparisons of intensity, then olfaction should show a loss when compared directly to taste. In a direct comparison of olfaction with the taste of NaCl, olfactory intensities were diminished compared to taste (63). Further magnitude matching studies of six odorants, chosen for structural diversity, showed substantial losses for all of them (60). Three of these odorants were tested in a subsequent study that also included threshold measures and odor identification. Again, substantial losses occurred for the elderly with the magnitude matching measure. Substantial losses also occurred for the threshold and identification measures. Contrary to taste, the association between threshold and perceived intensity in these data for olfaction resembled panel A in Figure 14.2.

As part of a comprehensive study of the effects of age on both taste and smell (19), Cowart scaled pyridine and phenyl ethyl alcohol with the tape-pull method. She found only a slight suggestion of any age effect on the scaling of either odorant. This appears to disagree with the magnitude matching results of Stevens and his colleagues discussed above. One of the reasons for the differences may be that Stevens's elderly subjects tended to be older (70–90 yr) than those Cowart's (65–79 yr). However, differences in assumptions made about the methodology may also play a role. Stevens and Cowart both find that the elderly subjects tend to rate blanks (solvent only with no odorant present) as greater than zero. The reason for this is not clear. Stevens and his colleagues correct their data by subtracting the rating of the blanks from the other ratings, assuming that the ratings given to the blanks are some kind of cognitive artifact. Cowart did not subtract the blanks in her data. If she had done so, the ratings of the elderly would have diminished. The meaning of the responses to the blank stimuli deserves additional study. Botwinick has drawn attention to the conservatism shown by elderly subjects (8). This has an impact on psychophysical tests in which both old and young must make decisions. Botwinick described the reluctance of elderly subjects to report a faint sound in an auditory test. This reluctance made the elderly subjects appear to have more hearing loss than they did. Could the elderly subjects in olfactory experiments be reluctant to report smelling nothing? We should be open to the possibility that elderly subjects may have olfactory experiences even when sniffing a blank stimulus. In that case, the responses given to the blanks should not be subtracted.

Sources of Olfactory Loss

In individuals without major systemic disease (for example, chronic kidney failure, diabetes mellitus), premature chemosensory loss can occur from insults such as medication, head trauma, and upper respiratory tract infection (21). In olfaction, these factors may diminish acuity by interfering with the odor reaching the olfactory neuroepithelium (transport loss; for example, allergic rhinitis, nasal polyposis), injuring the cells that receive and transduce the olfactory stimulus (sensory loss; for example, viral infections, head radiation), or damaging peripheral or central neurophysiological systems (neural loss; for example, head trauma, damage to the cribriform plate, central losses caused by a neoplasm) (21). The probability of encountering one of these diseases or environmental toxins may increase with age so that it is difficult to separate out age-related losses from the combination of aging with pathology; however, this is a laudable goal. For example, Ship and Weiffenbach (56) find a lower incidence of olfactory dysfunction in a successfully aging population from the Baltimore Longitudinal Study of Aging (221 males, 166 females) and attribute this finding to the overall healthy status of the population.

RETRONASAL OLFACTION

Thresholds

Cain et al. (11) found that the amount of olfactory spice in a published recipe was not sufficient to allow middle-aged and elderly individuals to recognize a difference between samples with and without the spice. In their study, participants (young, middle-aged, and older cohorts) discriminated between a cold carrot soup with or without the spice marjoram in a forced-choice procedure. Additional studies on mixtures (61) led to the suggestion that the elderly show reduced ability to detect specific stimuli in mixtures.

Identification

Schiffman (53) showed that the elderly were less able than the young to identify orally sampled foods. In this study, young (n = 27) and elderly (n = 29) subjects were blindfolded and sampled blended food items (thus removing nonolfactory cues for identification). Schiffman included some pure taste stimuli (NaCl and sucrose blended with cornstarch so they would resemble the other stimuli). Interestingly, these stimuli were recognized about as well by the elderly as by the young, supporting the conclusion that age takes its greatest toll on olfaction. However, it is important to note that olfactory identification tasks may overestimate true sensory loss in the elderly because a correct response relies on the combination of cognitive and sensory abilities. Murphy, in a later study (42), minimized the influence of cognitive difficulties in identifying blended foods. Even with feedback and practice, the elderly were still less able than the young to correctly identify the foods. Murphy also found that any advantage that the young had in food identification was negated when the olfactory cues were removed. In other words, young and elderly performed equally well on identification with only taste input.

Magnitude Matching

Stevens and Cain (59) concluded that the elderly have a diminished perception of odors presented to the receptors from inside the oral cavity (as during chewing and swallowing). Young and elderly subjects orally sampled and judged the intensity of ethyl butyrate with the nose open (allowing full retronasal perception) or pinched (preventing the volatiles from reaching the olfactory receptors). Intensity ratings were normalized to those of NaCl. The younger subjects consistently gave stronger intensity ratings to the ethyl butyrate solutions when sampled with the nose open. The elderly did not notice a difference between the overall intensity of either test situation.

Orthonasal vs. Retronasal Perception

Duffy and colleagues found that retronasal impairment may exceed orthonasal impairment (24). In this study, 76 free-living, high-functioning women [overall functional status assessed with the Older Americans Resources and Services (OARS) Multideminsional Functional Assessment Questionnaire (28)] participated in a clinical measure of olfactory dysfunction [butanol threshold, 7-odor identification task, 1 trigeminal stimulus (15)] and retronasal flavor threshold. The flavor threshold stimulus was developed to model the perception of a real food item. The gelatin served to hold the olfactory volatiles until manipulated in the oral cavity and the sugar background to conceal any primary taste components of the flavoring. Subjects orally sampled the flavored gelatin and were asked to identify the sample with the orange flavoring from the blank (sweetened gelatin only) in a two-alternative, forced-choice procedure with an ascending method of limits. The test, therefore, measured the threshold of the flavoring in the gelatin–sugar background. The orthonasal and retronasal measures correlated only modestly ($r = 0.45$) and appeared to measure different functions (24). Most remarkable was that a statistically equal frequency of subjects who had orthonasal normosmia displayed low, moderate, and high functions on the flavor threshold (25). For example, some subjects with orthonasal normosmia were unable to distinguish the strongest flavor sample from the blank. The reverse pattern was not true; all subjects with orthonasal anosmia had poor retronasal olfactory perception.

Sources of Retronasal Olfactory Loss

Retronasal dysfunction may exceed that of orthonasal dysfunction if the olfactory volatiles are not completely released in the oral cavity. In a process analogous to the sniffing action in orthonasal olfaction, the movements of the tongue, cheek, and throat work together to concentrate the volatiles from food for retronasal delivery to the olfactory receptors. Burdach and Doty (10) hypothesize that the elderly are able neither to release food volatiles effectively nor to generate enough active turbulent airflow to transport these released volatiles to the olfactory cleft. Poor oral health, limited natural dentition, improperly fitting dentures, or a decline of saliva production are all factors that could lead to poor retronasal olfaction. Duffy et al. (25) found that complete dentures increased the risk of poor retronasal perception. In this study subjects with complete dentures had significantly lower retronasal perception and the effect of dentures was statistically independent of the influence of orthonasal olfaction.

A recent study of Rolls and McDermott (48) demonstrates the need to study retronasal olfaction further. The investigators hypothesized that a decline in olfactory function would result in lower sensory-specific satiety response; that is, as you eat a food, the pleasantness of its flavor decreases, while the pleasantness of other foods, smelled but not consumed, decreases much less or remains constant. Four age cohorts (adolescent, young adult, older adult, and elderly) participated in sensory-specific satiety measures and a standard measure of orthonasal olfaction (UPSIT-University of Pennsylvania Smell Identification test) (23). For the sensory-specific satiety measures, subjects rated the sensory appeal and the desire to eat a number of foods (tuna salad, sesame cracker, low-fat strawberry yogurt, raw carrot, pretzel) and then consumed low-fat strawberry yogurt. The elderly did not show satiety to a second serving of yogurt as did the younger cohort. They rated pleasantness and desire to eat the yogurt the same as the first serving. Although the elderly had lower olfactory function, no significant relationship existed between olfactory function and sensory-specific satiety.

The lack of association between the olfactory measure and the sensory-specific satiety response in the Rolls and McDermott study (48) could stem from a combination of orthonasal and retronasal olfactory difficulties. The elderly had the yogurt in their mouths for the shortest amount of time, thus limiting the release of the olfactory food volatiles. The elderly with dentures also did not report a decline in the pleasantness rating as they consumed the yogurt. The limited time exposure and the presence of dentures could have diminished retronasal olfaction and blunted the sensory-specific satiety response.

Summary

In this review, we have emphasized the importance of tempering conclusions about changes in the perceived intensity of stimuli with age since comparisons of young and old subjects depend on many assumptions. Nonetheless, taken as a whole, the studies above suggest that elderly subjects experience a loss in olfaction that manifests itself as elevated thresholds and reduced perceived intensities over a range of stimuli. However, we cannot assume that testing an individual via the nostrils will represent the olfactory abilities of stimuli presented in the oral cavity. Losses of retronasal olfaction may exceed those of orthonasal olfaction.

CONCLUSIONS

The distinction between usual and successful aging is crucial to an understanding of the effects of age on the taste and olfactory worlds of the elderly.

There are serious problems with the measurement of taste and smell losses. Thresholds are the easiest to measure, but they have limited application to the real world. What we most want to measure is the intensity of everyday sensations like those produced by foods and beverages. We have described the scales devised to do this and their logical limitations. Of particular concern, some of the most sweeping conclusions about sensory losses in the elderly have come from studies using invalid or suspect methodologies.

Given the data at hand, the severity of losses with age orders as follows: retronasal olfaction, orthonasal olfaction, taste. Within the taste sense, sucrose appears to be the most robust, followed by NaCl, with CA and quinine the most likely substances to show loss.

The term "taste" used in common conversation refers to a combination of primarily true taste and retronasal olfaction. Because of the significant reduction in retronasal olfaction in elderly persons, many may believe their taste function is decreased. Rather, it is their "mouthsense" that is altered.

REFERENCES

1. BARTOSHUK, L. M. Taste mixtures: is mixture suppression related to compression? *Physiol. Behav.* 14: 643–649, 1975.
2. BARTOSHUK, L. M. The psychophysics of taste. *Am. J. Clin. Nutr.* 31: 1068–1077, 1978.
3. BARTOSHUK, L. M. Taste: robust across the age span? In: *Nutrition and the Chemical Senses in Aging: Recent Advances and Current Research Needs*, edited by C. Murphy, W. S. Cain, and D. M. Hegsted. New York: The New York Academy of Sciences, 1989, vol. 561, p. 65–75.
4. BARTOSHUK, L. M., S. DESNOYERS, C. HUDSON, L. MARKS, M. O'BRIEN, F. CATALANOTTO, J. GENT, D. WILLIAMS, and K. M. ÖSTRUM. Tasting on localized areas. In: *Olfaction and Taste*, edited by S. Roper and J. Atema. New York: The New York Academy of Sciences, 1987, vol. IX, p. 166–168.
5. BARTOSHUK, L. M., S. DESNOYERS, M. O'BRIEN, J. F. GENT, and F. A. CATALANOTTO. Taste stimulation of localized tongue areas: the Q-tip test [Abstract]. *Chem. Senses* 10: 453, 1985.
6. BARTOSHUK, L. M., L. M. MARKS, J. C. STEVENS, and B. RIFKIN. Taste and aging. Paper presented at the VIth Annual Meeting of the Association for Chemoreception Sciences, Sarasota, FL, 1984 (Abstr. 15).
7. BARTOSHUK, L. M., B. RIFKIN, L. E. MARKS, and P. BARS. Taste and aging. *J. Gerontol.* 41: 51–57, 1986.
8. BOTWINICK, J. *Aging and Behavior*. New York: Springer Publishing, 1973.
9. BOTWINICK, J. *Aging and Behavior* (3rd ed.), New York: Springer Publishing, 1984.
10. BURDACH, K., and R. DOTY. The effects of mouth movements, swallowing and spitting on retronasal odor perception. *Physiol. Behav.* 41: 353–356, 1987.
11. CAIN, W., F. REID, and J. STEVENS. Missing ingredients: aging and the discrimination of flavor. *J. Nutr. Eld.* 9: 3–15, 1990.
12. CAIN, W. S. Olfaction. In: *Stevens Handbook of Experimental Psychology*, edited by R. C. Atkinson, R. J. Herrnstein, G. Lindzey, and R. D. Luce. New York: John Wiley and Sons, 1988, p. 409–459.
13. CAIN, W. S., and J. F. GENT. Olfactory sensitivity: reliability, generality, and association with aging. *J. Exp. Psychol. [Hum. Percept.]* 17: 382–391, 1991.
14. CAIN, W. S., and J. C. STEVENS. Uniformity of olfactory loss in aging. In: *Nutrition and the Chemical Senses in Aging: Recent Advances and Current Research Needs*, edited by C. Murphy, W. S. Cain, and D. M. Hegsted. New York: The New York Academy of Sciences, 1989, vol. 561, p. 29–38.
15. CAIN, W. S., J. F. GENT, R. B. GOODSPEED, and G. LEONARD. Evaluation of olfactory dysfunction in the Connecticut Chemosensory Clinical Research Center. *Laryngoscope* 98: 83–88, 1988.
16. CHAUHAN, J., and Z. J. HAWRYSH. Suprathreshold sour taste intensity and pleasantness perception with age. *Physiol. Behav.* 43: 601–607, 1988.
17. COSTANZO, R. M., and N. D. ZASLER. Head trauma. In: *Smell and Taste in Health and Disease*, edited by T. Getchell, R. L. Doty, L. M. Bartoshuk, and J. B. Snow. New York: Raven Press, 1991, p. 711–730.
18. COWART, B. J. Direct scaling of the intensity of basic tastes: a life span study. Paper presented at the Vth Annual Meeting of the Association for Chemoreception Sciences, Sarasota, FL, 1983 (Abstr. 24).
19. COWART, B. J. Relationships between taste and smell across the adult life span. In: *Nutrition and the Chemical Senses in Aging: Recent Advances and Current Research Needs*, edited by C. Murphy, W. S. Cain, and D. M. Hegsted. New York: The New York Academy of Sciences, 1989, vol. 561, p. 39–55.
20. DESIMONE, J. A., G. L. HECK, and L. M. BARTOSHUK. Surface active taste modifiers: a comparison of the physical and psychophysical properties of gymnemic acid and sodium lauryl sulfate. *Chem. Senses* 5: 317–330, 1980.
21. DOTY, R., L. BARTOSHUK, and J. SNOW. Causes of olfactory and gustatory disorders. In: *Smell and Taste in Health and Disease*, edited by T. V. Getchell, R. L. Doty, L. M. Bartoshuk, and J. B. Snow. New York: Raven Press, 1991, p. 449–462.
22. DOTY, R. L., P. SHAMAN, S. L. APPLEBAUM, R. GIBERSON, L. SIKORSKI, and L. ROSENBERG. Smell identification ability: changes with age. *Science* 226: 1441–1443, 1984.
23. DOTY, R. L., P. SHANNON, and M. DANN. Development of the University of Pennsylvania Smell Identification Test: a standardized microencapsulated test of olfactory function. *Physiol. Behav.* 34: 489–502, 1984.
24. DUFFY, V. B., W. S. CAIN, J. C. STEVENS, and A. M. FERRIS. A test of flavor sensitivity. *Chem. Senses* 16: 516–517, 1991.
25. DUFFY, V. B., A. M. FERRIS. Lower olfactory functioning associates with nutritional risk in elderly women. *Chem. Senses* 18: 549, 1993.
26. DYE, C. J., and D. A. KOZIATEK. Age and diabetes effects on threshold and hedonic perception of sucrose solutions. *J. Gerontol.* 36: 310–315, 1981.
26a. ENGEN, T. Psychophysics I. Discrimination and detection. In: *Woodworth & Schlosberg's Experimental Psychology, Vol. I: Sensation and Perception*. New York: Holt, Rinehart and Winston, 1972, p. 11–46.
27. ENNS, M. P., T. B. VAN ITALLIE, and J. GRINKER. Contributions of age, sex and degree of fatness on preferences and magnitude estimations for sucrose in humans. *Physiol. Behav.* 22: 999–1003, 1979.
28. FILLENBAUM, G. *Multidimensional Functional Assessment of Older Adults: The Duke Older Americans Resources and Services Procedures*. Hillsdale, N.J.: Lawrence Erlbaum, 1988.
29. HUDSON, C. A. Taste perceptions: a comparison of the elderly and the young. Senior thesis, Yale University, 1985.
30. HYDE, R. J., and R. P. FELLER. Age and sex effects on taste of sucrose, NaCl, citric acid and caffeine. *Neurobiol. Aging* 2: 315–318, 1981.
31. HYDE, R. J., R. P. FELLER, and I. M. SHARON. Tongue brushing, dentifrice, and age effects on taste and smell. *J. Dent. Res.* 60: 1730–1734, 1981.
32. KAMEN, J. M., F. J. PILGRIM, N. J. GUTMAN, and B. J. KROLL. Interactions of suprathreshold taste stimuli. *J. Exp. Psychol.* 62: 348–356, 1961.
33. LAWLESS, H. T. and T. ENGEN. Associations to odors: interface, mnemonics and verbal labeling. *J. Exp. Psychol. [Hum. Learn. Mem.]* 3: 52–59, 1977.

34. LITTLE, A. C., and L. BRINNER. Taste responses to saltiness of experimentally prepared tomato juice samples. *J. Dietet. Assoc.* 84: 1022–1027, 1984.
35. MARKS, L. E. Sensory and cognitive factors in judgments of loudness. *J. Exp. Psychol.* 5: 426–443, 1979.
36. MARKS, L. E. Magnitude estimation and sensory matching. *Percept. Psychophys.* 43: 511–525, 1988.
37. MARKS, L. E. On the relativity of chemosensory perception. *Chem. Senses* 18: 596, 1993.
38. MARKS, L. E., and J. C. STEVENS. Measuring sensation in the aged. In: *Aging in the 1980's: Psychological Issues,* edited by L. W. Poon. Washington D.C.: American Psychological Association, 1980, p. 592–598.
39. MCBURNEY, D. H., and L. M. BARTOSHUK. Interactions between stimuli with different taste qualities. *Physiol. Behav.* 10: 1101–1106, 1973.
40. MOSKOWITZ, H. R. Magnitude estimation: notes on what, how, when, and why to use it. *J. Food Qual.* 1: 195–228, 1977.
41. MOZELL, M., B. SMITH, L. SULLIVAN, and P. SWENDER. Nasal chemoreception in flavor identification. *Arch. Otolaryngol.* 90: 367–373, 1969.
42. MURPHY, C. Cognitive and chemosensory influences on age-related changes in the ability to identify blended foods. *J. Gerontol.* 40: 47–52, 1985.
43. MURPHY, C. Taste and smell in the elderly. In: *Clinical measurement of Taste and Smell,* edited by H. L. Meiselman and R. S. Rivlin. New York: Macmillan, 1986, p. 343–371.
44. MURPHY, C., and M. M. GILMORE. Quality-specific effects of aging on the human taste system. *Percept. Psychophys.* 45: 121–128, 1989.
45. MURPHY, C., W. S. CAIN, M. M. GILMORE, and R. B. SKINNER. Sensory and semantic factors in recognition memory for odors and graphic stimuli: elderly versus young persons. *Am. J. Psychol.* 104: 161–192, 1991.
46. PANGBORN, R. M. Selected factors influencing sensory perception of sweetness. In: *Sweetness,* edited by J. Dobbing. New York: Springer-Verlag, 1987, p. 49–66.
47. RIFKIN, B., and L. M. BARTOSHUK. Taste in aging. Paper presented at the 88th Annual Meeting of the American Psychological Association. 1980, p. 17–18.
48. ROLLS, B., and T. MCDERMOTT. Effects of age on sensory-specific satiety. *Am. J. Clin. Nutr.* 54: 988–996, 1991.
49. ROVEE, C. K., R. Y. COHEN, and W. SHLAPACK. Life-span stability in olfactory sensitivity. *Dev. Psychol.* 11: 311–318, 1975.
50. ROWE, J., and R. KAHN. Human aging: usual and successful. *Science* 237: 143–149, 1987.
51. ROZIN, P. "Taste-smell confusions" and the duality of the olfactory sense. *Percept. Psychophys.* 31: 397–401, 1982.
52. RUSSELL, M. J., B. J. CUMMINGS, B. F. PROFITT, C. J. WYSOCKI, A. N. GILBERT, and C. W. COTMAN. Life span changes in the verbal characterization of odors. *J. Gerontol.* 48: P49–P53, 1993.
53. SCHIFFMAN, S. S. Food recognition by the elderly. *J. Gerontol.* 32: 586–592, 1977.
54. SCHIFFMAN, S. S., and T. B. CLARK. Magnitude estimates of amino acids for young and elderly subjects. *Neurobiol. Aging* 1: 81–91, 1980.
55. SCHIFFMAN, S. S., M. G. LINDLEY, T. B. CLARK, and C. MAKINO. Molecular mechanism of sweet taste: relationship of hydrogen bonding to taste sensitivity for both young and elderly. *Neurobiol. Aging* 2: 173–185, 1981.
56. SHIP, J., and J. WEIFFENBACH. Age, gender, medical treatment and medication effects on smell identification. *J. Gerontol.* 48: M26–M32, 1993.
57. SOLOMON, G. M., F. CATALANOTTO, A. SCOTT, and L. M. BARTOSHUK. Patterns of taste loss in clinic patients with histories of head trauma, nasal symptoms, or upper respiratory infection. *Yale J. Biol. Med.* 64: 280, 1991.
58. STEVENS, D. A. and H. T. LAWLESS. Age-related changes in flavor perception. *Appetite* 2: 127–136, 1981.
59. STEVENS, J., and W. CAIN. Smelling via the mouth: effect of aging. *Percept. Psychophys.* 40: 142–146, 1986.
60. STEVENS, J. C., and W. S. CAIN. Age-related deficiency in the perceived strength of six odorants. *Chem. Senses* 10: 517–529, 1985.
61. STEVENS, J. C., and W. S. CAIN. Changes in taste and flavor in aging. *Crit. Rev. Food. Sci. Nutr.* 33: 27–37, 1993.
62. STEVENS, J. C., and L. E. MARKS. Cross-modality matching functions generated by magnitude estimation. *Percept. Psychophys.* 27: 379–389, 1980.
63. STEVENS, J. C., L. M. BARTOSHUK, and W. S. CAIN. Chemical senses and aging: taste versus smell. *Chem. Senses* 9: 167–179, 1984.
64. STEVENS, J. C., W. S. CAIN, and R. J. BURKE. Variability of olfactory thresholds. *Chem. Senses* 13: 643–653, 1988.
65. STEVENS, J. C., A. PLANTINGA, and W. S. CAIN. Reduction of odor and nasal pungency associated with aging. *Neurobiol. Aging* 3: 125–132, 1982.
66. STEVENS, S. S. The psychophysics of sensory function. In: *Sensory Communication,* edited by W. A. Rosenblith. Cambridge, MA: The M.I.T. Press, 1961, p. 1–33.
67. STEVENS, S. S. Sensory scales of taste intensity. *Percept. Psychophys.* 6: 302–308, 1969.
68. SUMNER, D. Post traumatic ageusia. *Brain* 90: 187–202, 1967.
69. WEIFFENBACH, J. M. Assessment of chemosensory functioning in aging. In: *Nutrition and the Chemical Senses in Aging: Recent Advances and Current Research Needs,* edited by C. Murphy, W. S. Cain, and D. M. Hegsted. New York: The New York Academy of Sciences, 1989, vol. 561, p. 56–64.
70. WEIFFENBACH, J. M., B. J. BAUM, and R. BURGHAUSER. Taste thresholds: quality specific variation with human aging. *J. Gerontol.* 37: 372–377, 1982.
71. WEIFFENBACH, J. M., B. J. COWART, and B. J. BAUM. Taste intensity perception in aging. *J. Gerontol.* 41: 460–468, 1986.
72. WOOD, J. B., and S. W. HARKINS. Effects of age, stimulus selection, and retrieval environment on odor identification. *J. Gerontol.* 42: 584–588, 1987.
73. WYSOCKI, C. J., and A. N. GILBERT. National Geographic smell survey: effects of age are heterogeneous. In: *Nutrition and the Chemical Senses in Aging: Recent Advances and Current Research Needs,* edited by C. Murphy, W. S. Cain, and D. M. Hegsted. New York: The New York Academy of Science, 1989, vol. 561, p. 12–28.
74. ZALLEN, E. M., L. B. HOOKS, and K. O'BRIEN. Salt taste preferences and perceptions of elderly and young adults. *J. Am. Diet. Assoc.* 90: 947–950, 1990.

15. The potential role of selected endocrine systems in aging processes

JAMES F. NELSON | Department of Physiology, The University of Texas Health Science Center, San Antonio, Texas

CHAPTER CONTENTS

Hormones and Aging: An Overview
Hormonal Alterations during Aging
    Gonadal steroids
        Ovarian steroids
        Testicular steroids
    Adrenal steroids
        Glucocorticoids
        Mineralocorticoids
        Adrenal androgens
    Growth Hormone
        Humans
        Laboratory rodents and other species
        Growth hormone and the aging phenotype
Summary

HORMONES AND AGING: AN OVERVIEW

THE NOTION THAT HORMONES PLAY A ROLE IN THE AGING PROCESS has had proponents since at least the nineteenth century when Brown-Sequard (19) attempted to rejuvenate elderly men with extracts from the testicles of guinea pigs and dogs. The prescience of Brown-Sequard is only now being realized as we see that age-related changes in both the levels of and the sensitivity to hormones are significant in some endocrine systems and that the physiological consequences of these changes can be partly ameliorated by hormonal replacement. Hormone replacement therapy has been part of the clinical armamentarium for postmenopausal estrogen deficiency for several decades (68), and studies are underway to determine whether hormone replacement can maintain or restore physiological function in other endocrine systems. The current debate centers not on whether endocrine systems contribute to the aging process but on how and to what extent they contribute.

The view that hormone deficiency contributes to the aging phenotype is but one of several hypotheses concerning the role of endocrine systems in senescence. This chapter focuses on a range of hypotheses about the role played by hormones in aging and examines the evidence relevant to these hypotheses. Such a focus is both practical and novel. An exhaustive review of the endocrinology of aging is beyond the scope of this chapter, thus it is necessary to narrow the coverage of this extensively studied topic. This chapter concentrates on the effects of age on the major classes of steroid hormones and on growth hormone, emphasizing changes observed in humans and laboratory rodents, which have been the most widely studied species. The physiological significance of these changes is also discussed, since many unanswered questions remain concerning the role of hormones in aging and in therapeutic interventions to ameliorate the effects of aging. Steroid hormones and growth hormone have been chosen primarily because they are under greatest scrutiny with regard to aging. These hormones represent, of course, only a subset of the major mammalian hormones. Prolactin has received considerable attention in studies of reproductive aging in laboratory rodents, both because prolactin adenomas are frequent concomitants of aging in the strains most commonly studied (233), and because prolactin can have profound influences on reproductive physiology. However, neither hyper- nor hypoprolactinemia is a hallmark of human aging, and therefore prolactin is not discussed in this chapter. Insulin and thyroid hormone are discussed in Chapters 6 and 7. This chapter stresses the nature of the hormonal changes associated with aging and the impact of those changes on the aging phenotype, rather than the mechanisms responsible for those changes. Helpful discussions of mechanisms underlying hormonal changes are found in several recent review articles (for example, 35, 51, 52, 233).

HORMONAL ALTERATIONS DURING AGING

Brown-Sequard's experiments were based on the view that aging is associated with a deficiency in hormone secretion and that, since a similar defiency in young adults mimics the aging phenotype, replacement of that deficiency should rejuvenate the aged organism. In retrospect, this view is an oversimplification. As discussed below, the extent of change during aging in circulating concentrations of the various hormones varies markedly. Only some hormones decrease with age; others change minimally, and some may increase in concentration. Moreover, endocrine changes other than altered concentrations of hormones characterize and may be important to the aging phenotype, including altered patterns and ratios. These changes, along with the evidence of their physiological significance, are reviewed below.

Gonadal Steroids

In humans, there are marked differences between the sexes in the pattern and magnitude of change in circulating concentrations of gonadal steroids with age. In general, changes in women occur universally and more rapidly and are greater than those in men. This largely reflects the fact that the source of gonadal steroids in females, the follicular reserve, is nonrenewable and is steadily depleted with advancing age. (Fig. 15.1; 54, 163). By contrast, Leydig cells, the source of testicular androgens, generally remain in substantial numbers throughout the life span of males (46, 129, 231, 233). Less is known about the changes in gonadal steroids in nonhuman primates, although estradiol levels are reduced in females of some species (see later, under Ovarian Steroids: Nonhuman Primates and Laboratory Rodents). Laboratory mice and rats have been the most extensively studied of the nonhuman mammals in terms of reproductive aging. Differences between the sexes in the decline of gonadal steroids are generally similar to those in humans, although the detailed patterns may differ from those in humans, as will be described.

Ovarian Steroids. After menopause, estradiol levels plummet to values less than 10% of those in women before menopause (68). Progestin and androgen levels also fall markedly (68). The reduced levels of estrogen underlie centrally mediated hot flushes, atrophy of reproductive tissues, and age-related changes in nonreproductive tissues that are estrogen-sensitive, including bone, skin, and the central nervous system (CNS) (68, 233).

The human female: ovarian failure and maximal life span. Early natural menopause is associated with increased risk for cardiovascular disease and stroke and all other causes of death except cancer (200). Although the postmenopausal decline in estrogen might be expected to be a major factor, it remains to be demonstrated. Indeed, Snowdon and co-workers (199, 200) found no evidence that estrogen depletion was related

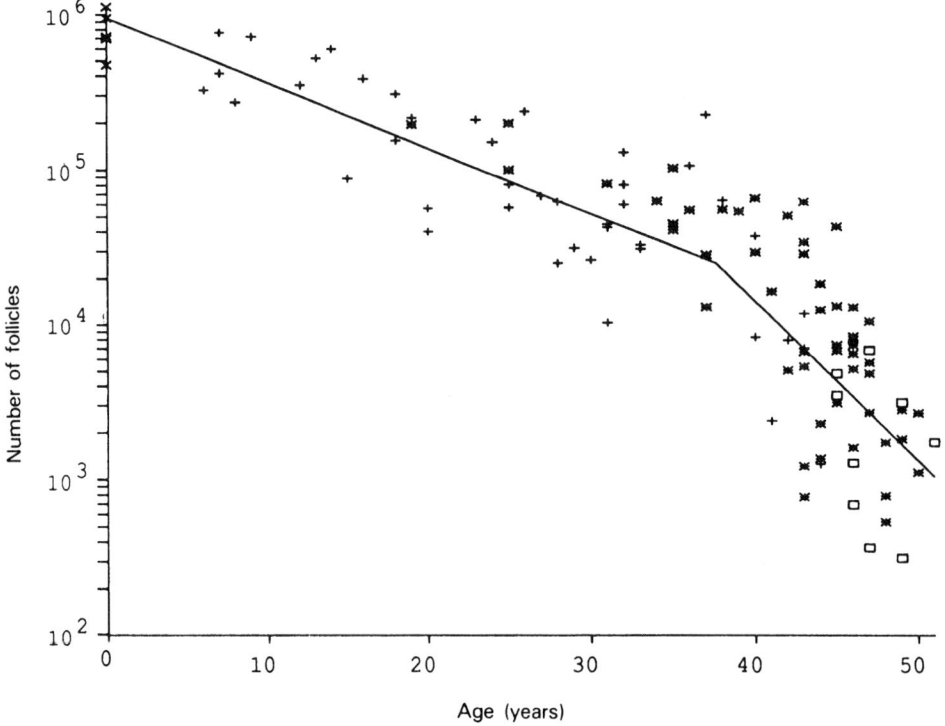

FIG. 15.1. Declining follicle numbers in pairs of human ovaries from neonatal age to 51 yr. [Redrawn from Faddy et al. (54) with permission.] Data were obtained from the studies of Block (13a) (+), Richardson et al (155) (□) and Gougeon (unpublished) (*).

to all-cause mortality. Although early age at natural menopause increased mortality risk, early age at surgical menopause was weakly associated with a reduced rather than an increased rate of all-cause mortality in a study of several thousand Seventh Day Adventist women (200). These data suggest that factors associated with menopause other than hormonal withdrawal may be involved in influencing the age-related increase in mortality. A caveat to these studies is that they are not demographically and racially representative. Further evidence against a major role for postmenopausal sex steroid loss in limiting the maximal human life span is the absence of a change in the slope of the log-transformed rate of increase in age-specific mortality before and after 50 yr, the mean age of menopause (53, 128; S. Austad, personal communication).

The lack of marked effect of ovarian hormonal withdrawal on maximal life span negates neither the beneficial effects nor the risks of estrogen replacement on postmenopausal health. Estrogen-replacement in postmenopausal women ameliorates most of the effects ascribable to estrogen-depletion: these include atrophy of estrogen-supported tissues, vasomotor instability, and accelerated trabecular bone loss (68, 233). Epidimiological study indicates reduction in all-cause mortality among postmenopausal users of estrogen replacement (21). Nevertheless, there are established as well as potential risks of estrogen replacement. Endometrial carcinoma is more likely in postmenopausal women on unopposed estrogen replacement, although combining estrogen with progesterone, an antagonist of estrogen action in the endometrium, can eliminate this risk (68, 77). Some studies have indicated an increased risk for thromboembolisms and gallbladder disease (14, 68), and concern remains about the possibility of increased risk for breast carcinoma. Given the mitogenic potential of these steroids, concern about their carcinogenic potential is justified, and the need for establishing minimal therapeutic dosages is underscored. In rodents, chronic exposure to estrogens can disrupt neuronal architecture (16, 45) and neuroendocrine function (124) as well as estrogenic responsiveness of peripheral target tissues (1). Whether estrogens exert similar effects in humans and nonhuman primates is unknown but of obvious import given the prevalence of estrogen replacement therapy in postmenopausal women.

Nonhuman primates and laboratory rodents. There is some evidence for decreased plasma estradiol in aging rhesus (242), bonnet (93), and pigtailed macaques (69, 194), but the universality of ovarian failure is not known, largely because few animals have been examined at advanced ages (233). Female laboratory mice and rats exhibit varying patterns of ovarian hormonal change during aging, and these changes usually end in the virtual cessation of ovarian hormonal secretory activity akin to that of human menopause. Before this state appears, however, there is usually a transition period characterized by markedly altered hormone patterns relative to those associated with the preceding period of regular ovulatory cyclicity (9, 133, 135, 233). Many strains exhibit periods of persistently elevated plasma concentrations of estradiol. Other strains exhibit repeated cycles of estradiol and progesterone similar to those associated with the first half of pregnancy. Women also show periods of irregular estrogen and progesterone secretion during the transitional period between regular menstrual cyclicity and menopause (192), although this period, as a fraction of the life span, is usually much shorter in women than in laboratory rodents (224, 225).

Several investigators have proposed that the irregular patterns of hormonal secretion associated with reproductive aging in females may also contribute to the aging phenotype (133, 233). Fugo and Butcher (63) demonstrated that the prolonged cycles of aged rats are associated with a 20–40% decrease in implantations and a twofold increase in abnormal embryos when compared to age-matched 4–5-day cycles. Page and Butcher (147) later demonstrated that these prolonged cycles were characterized by a prolonged elevation of preovulatory estradiol and suggested that this elevation might be a factor in the decreased fertility of the aging rat. Further evidence that the hormonal milieu associated with the transition between regular cyclicity and menopause is particularly deleterious was provided by a study showing that the persistent estrous condition was more deleterious to the subsequent potential for estrous cyclicity of C57BL/6J mice than was the regularly cycling state (134).

Testicular Steroids. The Leydig cell is the principal site of steroidogenesis in the testis. In terms of potency and concentration, testosterone is the major product of the Leydig cell, although smaller quantities of dihydrotestosterone, estradiol, and weaker sex steroids are also produced. Until recently, there was debate over whether testosterone levels declined with age in human males. Large-scale studies have established a marked decline in serum testosterone during aging. The physiological significance of this decline, however, is not known. The majority of serum dihydrotestosterone and estradiol are produced peripherally by 5-alpha reduction and aromatization, respectively, of circulating testosterone. Effects of aging on these processes are not well described and are not discussed in this chapter.

The human male. The effect of age on plasma testosterone levels is less marked in men than are the changes in ovarian steroids in women. Indeed, until recently, studies were divided over whether there was an effect of age on circulating testosterone (decrease: 39, 41, 46,

127, 155, 171, 201, 211, 232, 250; no decrease: 22, 79, 129, 130, 208, 226). All of these studies were limited by sampling and, especially, by small sample sizes. More recently, several large epidemiological surveys (38, 70, 195) have measured testosterone during aging. Each of these has involved more than 1,000 men and each has shown significant reductions in total testosterone with age (Fig. 15.2). It is noteworthy that in each of the three studies the greatest decrement in plasma testosterone occurred in the first 5- to 10-year period examined. For example, Dabbs (38; Fig. 15.2) found a decrease of about 70 ng/dl in men between the ages of 32 and 37 yr. Levels of plasma testosterone fell only about 25 ng/dl between the ages of 37 and 44 yr, the oldest age studied. This apparent deceleration in the rate of decline of plasma testosterone during midlife could explain the failure of some of the earlier studies to detect an age-related change in testosterone, either by not including young men or by grouping young with middle-aged men and thereby losing age-resolution.

The majority of circulating testosterone is bound to sex hormone–binding globulin and other proteins (64). The unbound or free fraction is believed to be the bioavailable fraction that is readily accessible to target cell receptors. Bioavailable or free testosterone generally declines at a greater rate during aging than total testosterone (41, 126, 157, 162, 170, 211, 229, 232). For example, Gray et al. (70) found that free testosterone fell at a rate of 1.3% per annum compared to 0.4% for total testosterone, resulting in a net reduction in free testosterone of 30% between 40 and 70 yr of age.

Testosterone levels vary markedly among individuals. Age-matched individuals within the normal range of androgen concentration show levels of free and total testosterone over a range of nearly one order of magnitude (70). The basis and physiological significance of this variation is not well understood. Since the range of variation within age groups is several times that accounted for by aging, it is understandable how studies with relatively small samples could have missed the 20%–40% age-related decline in testosterone levels that have been found in the epidemiological studies.

Health status is another possible contributor to the variable outcomes of studies of testosterone in aging men (79, 136). However, although less healthy men have lower levels of testosterone than healthier men, the rate of decline with advancing age appears to be similar for both groups (70). Another cause of the variable outcomes of earlier aging studies could be variation in the time of sampling. Plasma concentrations of testosterone exhibit a circadian rhythm. The rhythms of both total (17) and free (157) testosterone diminish with advancing age, mainly as a consequence of a reduction in peak levels of hormone during the day. Change in the circadian rhythms of hormones is a recurring and potentially important theme in the endocrinology of aging (245, 246).

Another factor that may influence the hormonal status of the aged male is the concentration of serum estrogens. Generally, estradiol levels decrease less than testosterone levels during aging in men (41, 70, 109, 156, 171, 195, 229, 250). As a consequence, the estradiol:testosterone ratio may increase with age. A change in this ratio, even in the absence of change in the level of estrogen, may shift the balance toward more estrogenic activity during aging. This shift could be important in some of the pathophysiological sequelae of aging in men. For example, benign prostatic hyperplasia is correlated positively with plasma estradiol level (150, 215) as well as with the estradiol:testosterone ratio (215).

In summary, both free and total serum testosterone levels decline with advancing age in men. However, because of the large degree of variability in testosterone levels and the absence of longitudinal data, the variability among men in timing and rate of age-related decline is unknown. Indeed, the possibility remains that some men show little or no change in serum testosterone with age.

Nonhuman primates and laboratory rodents. Little is known about changes in testicular androgens in aging nonhuman primates. Two independent studies report a decrease in the nocturnal elevation of serum testosterone in aging male rhesus macaques (25, 101), but these changes have not always been observed (24, 26, 154), perhaps because of small sample size or time of sampling. In laboratory rodents, the extent of change in plasma testosterone concentration is variable, ranging

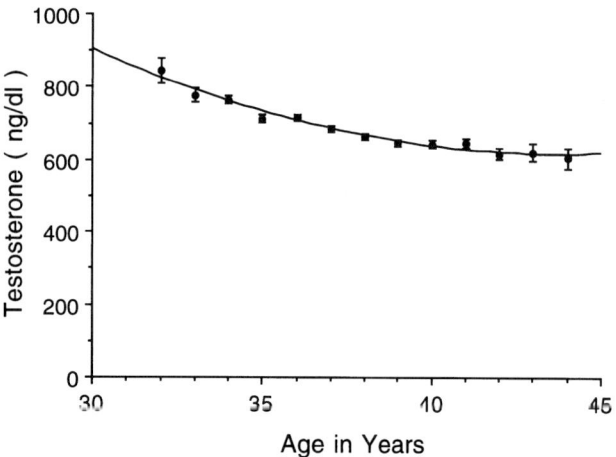

FIG. 15.2. Effect of age on plasma testosterone concentrations in men (total N = 4,462) ranging from 32 to 44 yr of age. [Redrawn from Dabbs (38) with permission.]

from no change to marked reduction. In several strains of rat (27, 28, 65, 71, 72, 107, 115, 123, 156, 164, 198) and mouse (18, 30, 34), testosterone levels decline significantly with age. By contrast, no significant loss of plasma testosterone was observed in aging C57BL/6J (50, 136), or Cr1:CD-1 (ICR) BR (190) mice or in Syrian hamsters (144), unless animals were diseased or near death.

Androgens and the aging phenotype. The contribution of reduced androgens to physiological changes during aging and to life span are far from clear. As anabolic steroids, they may be implicated in the loss of muscle and bone that accompanies aging in humans and some rodent species (216). They may also play a role in changes in sexual as well as other hormonally mediated neural processes (41). For example, in the testosterone-deficient aged Fischer 344 rat, testosterone replacement restored vasopressin mRNA levels in the bed nucleus of the stria terminalis to values observed in young rats (47). Testosterone treatment also partially restored reduced vasopressin-binding sites in the kidney of aging rats (82). A 3-month period of testosterone supplementation of a small group of older men with low serum testosterone levels increased lean body mass and reduced urinary hydroxyproline excretion (220). This regimen also increased hematocrit, reduced total and low-density lipoprotein cholesterol, and increased serum prostate-specific antigen levels, changes which indicate potential risks of androgen replacement. Larger-scale studies are underway to extend these observations.

Clearly, certain diseases of aging, notably prostate hyperplasia and carcinoma, are androgen-dependent, and androgens may also contribute to the higher incidence of cardiovascular disease in men (5, 216). As with postmenopausal estrogen replacement, there are likely risks as well as benefits to replacement, and determining the balance will require careful study.

The life span of men is significantly less than that of women (234, 244), but the role played by androgens, directly or indirectly, in this difference is not well established. Some evidence indicates that a major component of the difference is not genetically, and hence not hormonally, determined but is due to differences in such life-style variables as smoking and alcohol consumption (234). Studies in a number of species have shown that castration extends life span (75, 76, 131). It is particularly noteworthy that prepubertal but not postpubertal castration of male rats extended life span in one study (210). Prepubertal castration also attenuated the age-related decline in locomotion, motor coordination, and circadian activity rhythms of male rats (153). Although the data are limited, they indicate that testosterone influences a wide range of aging variables and, therefore, that studies aimed at determining the balance of risk and benefit to the age-related decline in testosterone in men should be fruitful.

Adrenal Steroids

The adrenal cortex synthesizes three major classes of steroid hormone: glucocorticoids, mineralocorticoids, and androgens. In humans, age-related changes among these three classes vary markedly. Changes in cortisol, the principal glucocorticoid, and aldosterone, the principal mineralocorticoid, are relatively small and not always observed. By contrast, changes in the weak but abundant androgen dehydroepiandrosterone (DHEA) and its sulfate are among the greatest of all hormone changes seen during aging.

Glucocorticoids. In humans as well as other animals, the debate centers not on whether there is a deficiency of circulating glucocorticoid during aging but on whether there is an increase and, if so, the physiological significance of that increase. A major focus of interest has been whether the presumptive elevation of glucocorticoids during aging contributes to the decreased lean body mass, osteoporosis, immune deficiencies, and cognitive impairments of aging (112, 113, 181, 212). Glucocorticoids can produce such effects in young adults when present in pathophysiologically elevated levels (110).

Humans. Cortisol is the principal glucorticoid in humans. It exhibits a circadian rhythm, reaching peak values in the morning (64). Most studies of healthy humans show no increase in total plasma cortisol with age. These include studies of samples taken only during the morning (4, 12, 61, 94) as well as 24-h samples to assess effects of age on circadian parameters of this hormone (11, 33, 43, 166, 167, 193, 223, 235). Two studies showed age-related reductions in plasma (191) and salivary (15) cortisol. Others, however, have shown increased cortisol with aging in men but not women (249) and a trend toward increased evening cortisol (152, 183). There are few data on free, or bioavailable, cortisol. One report revealed a marked (25%–50%) increase in plasma free cortisol in a small group of demented and nondemented individuals in their eighties (222). By contrast, in a much larger study, unstimulated morning salivary (presumably free) cortisol concentrations in 767 adults were negatively correlated with age in women decreasing 30% between the ages of 35 and 65 yr (15). By contrast, levels in men were unchanged with age. One possible explanation for these divergent data is that levels of cortisol do not show significant increases until the ninth decade of life.

In summary, increased plasma levels of total cortisol are not commonly found in aging individuals, and when present, the increases are relatively small. However, the observation that free cortisol decreases significantly in some older women and is substantially higher in some very old individuals merits further study. Lacking at present are large-scale epidemiological surveys of free and total cortisol, which, as in the case of testosterone, may provide more definitive answers to these questions.

Laboratory rodents and other species. There is a similar lack of agreement in the literature on glucocorticoids and aging in other species. This lack of agreement may reflect genetic as well as environmental differences. Sampling procedures may also contribute to the divergence of the reports. In a recent survey, Sapolsky (179) observed that age-related increases in plasma corticosterone in laboratory rats were most frequently observed in studies reporting basal corticosterone levels (that is, daytime) below 100 ng/ml, which, he posited, most closely reflect unperturbed values (Fig. 15.3). He argued that the absence of an age-related increase in plasma corticosterone levels in studies with higher basal levels might be the consequence of the masking of differences in unperturbed animals by elevated corticosterone levels due to a presumably stressed state. However, at least one study in Brown Norway rats with basal levels around 40–50 ng/ml showed no increase in corticosterone with age (228), while another in female Sprague-Dawley rats with basal levels around 200 ng/ml showed a marked increase in corticosterone levels with age (236). Most studies have only made measurements at one time of day and thus do not allow a complete assessment of the effect of aging on the overall profile of corticosterone, which varies markedly during the day. However, those studies that have measured the diurnal pattern generally show increases, at least in old age, in corticosterone levels both at the trough and peak of the profile (146, 175, 217, 236).

A study of aging Syrian hamsters showed an increase in plasma cortisol but a decrease in corticosterone in late middle age, and by old age cortisol levels had returned to young values (145). Two studies of aging dogs revealed elevated levels of total cortisol (148, 169). Wild, freely ranging yellow baboons (*Papio cynocephalus*) in the oldest quartile had significantly higher cortisol levels than younger baboons in blood obtained following immobilization by anesthesia (179).

Free glucocorticoid levels in plasma, presumably more biologically relevant than total levels, have not been measured directly during aging in any nonhuman species but have been measured indirectly in two species. Cortisol excreted into urine, a reflection of the freely filtrable fraction in the plasma, was more than twofold higher in old compared to young dogs (169). Mean 24-h free corticosterone, calculated by mass action principles from total corticosterone and corticosterone-binding globulin concentrations, was 70% higher in Fischer 344 rats over 15 months of age (175). These are substantial increases that are potentially biologically significant and therefore should be verified by independent, direct measurement.

In summary, only some animals exhibit moderate increases in plasma concentrations of total glucocorticoids during aging. There is also evidence that concentrations of free corticosteroids are elevated in some older animals. Additional detailed diurnal measurements of unperturbed glucocorticoid levels, particularly plasma free concentrations, are needed to establish the prevalence and magnitude of altered glucocorticoid concentrations in aging mammals.

Glucocorticoids and the aging phenotype. The physiological significance of the elevated glucocorticoid levels observed in some older humans and other animals is not established. Although most investigators have focused on possible deleterious effects of glucocorticoids (44, 112, 177, 189, 212, 239), it has not been discounted that elevated glucocorticoids may represent an adaptive response that, on balance, is beneficial to the aging organism.

Potentiation of Aging Processes. On the side of a deleterious effect, correlational experiments suggest that the elevated glucocorticoids could play a role in age-related cognitive impairment. When aged Long-Evans rats were grouped into cognitively impaired and unimpaired subgroups based on spatial memory, the impaired group displayed increased basal concentrations of adrenocorticotropic hormone (ACTH) and corticosterone compared to both the unimpaired aged and

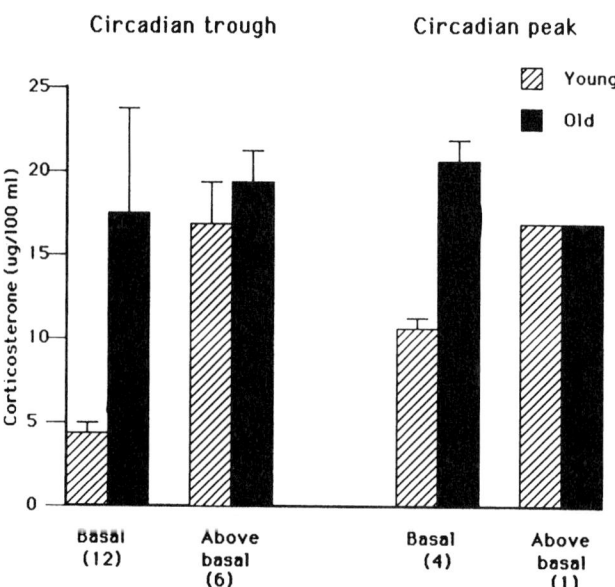

FIG. 15.3. Age-related increases in rat plasma corticosterone are observed only in studies in which basal corticosterone concentrations of young subjects were in the basal range (under 100 ng/ml). [Redrawn from Sapolsky (180) with permission.]

young animals (92). However, whether the activated hypothalamic–pituitary–adrenal axis was causally related to this impairment remains conjectural. Pyramidal cell loss was also greater in the hippocampus of the cognitively impaired subpopulation, and this loss could be a factor in the impaired cognitive performance. Previous studies have shown that adrenalectomy can protect against age-related loss of pyramidal cells in hippocampi of rats (113). However, whether this neuronal loss is a consequence of elevated levels of corticosteroids has not been established, even though severe stress and exposure to exogenous corticosterone can promote death of hippocampal neurons (103, 180). Alternative explanations for pyramidal cell loss include long-term exposure to (1) to young adult (as contrasted to elevated old) levels of corticosterone and (2) other adrenal hormones. Moreover, although adrenalectomy retards age-related pyramidal cell loss in the rodent hippocampus, it can promote loss of other neuronal cell types (196, 197). Thus, even for age-related changes in neuronal architecture, the balance between potentially positive and negative effects of glucocorticoid exposure remains unclear.

Retardation of Aging Processes. Although the hypothesis that chronic glucocorticoid exposure contributes to such age-related phenomena as impaired immune function, loss of lean body mass, osteoporosis, and increase in mortality is attractive, there is little direct evidence to support this notion. Indeed, some evidence favors the contrasting view that glucocorticoids, even at slightly elevated levels, on balance promote homeostasis and retard aging processes.

For example, in a prospective study men with morning plasma cortisol concentrations 1 standard deviation below the mean experienced a markedly increased rate of decline in pulmonary function, measured as forced expiratory volume, compared to men with cortisol concentrations 1 standard deviation above the mean (209). This difference was similar to that observed between current smokers and men who had never smoked. The authors propose that moderately elevated cortisol levels may retard the rate of decline in pulmonary function by reducing peripheral airway inflammatory processes.

Chronically food-restricted rats and mice, which live significantly longer than ad libitum–fed animals (247), exhibit higher levels of total corticosterone in early life than ad libitum–fed animals (108, 175, 213). Moreover, apparent free corticosterone levels of food-restricted rats are higher throughout life than those of ad libitum–fed rats (132, 175). This observation suggests that chronic exposure to glucocorticoids, even when moderately elevated, does not play a major role in age-related mortality and, indeed, may contribute to successful aging and life span extension by dietary restriction (132).

Although plasma corticosterone is elevated in food-restricted rodents, target-tissue sensitivity to glucocorticoids could be concomitantly reduced, since glucocorticoids can down-regulate their receptors (210). Reduced tissue sensitivity could attenuate the effect of elevated blood corticosterone in the food-restricted animal. However, a number of hormonal, biochemical, and physiological endpoints are shifted in food-restricted rodents in directions consistent with enhanced glucocorticoid activity. Plasma and pituitary levels of ACTH are suppressed in food-restricted rodents (78). Concentrations of hypothalamic pro-opiomelanocortin (POMC) (132) and neuropeptide Y (136a) mRNA are reduced and increased, respectively, in food-restricted rats. Adrenal and thymic weights, normalized to body weight, are increased and decreased, respectively, in food-restricted rats, relative to ad libitum–fed controls (108, 213). Finally, footpad edema, an inflammatory response to carrageenan injection, is attenuated in food-restricted mice (108) and rats (111). This latter observation is noteworthy, since inflammatory processes are implicated in several age-related pathologies, including arthritis, cardiovascular disease (240), colorectal cancer (221), and Alzheimer's disease (121). Heightened resistance to inflammation could be one of the mechanisms involved in the delay of age-related diseases and mortality in the food-restricted rodent.

Although suppressed inflammation and other changes are consistent with enhanced glucocorticoid activity, manipulation of the corticosterone milieu is required to determine unequivocally whether the elevated corticosterone of food-restricted rodents underlies these changes. The closest approach to this type of intervention was a study showing that the reduced tumorigenesis of food-restricted mice following carcinogenic insult was lost when mice were adrenalectomized (151).

Available data do not allow a straightforward conclusion about the long-term effect of glucocorticoids and stress on aging. Some effects of elevated glucocorticoids and stress appear deleterious, while others appear beneficial. As with estrogens, glucocorticoids appear to carry both risks and benefits and the balance of these determines their net effect on the aging organism. In this equation, the level of glucocorticoid exposure appears to be a critical variable. Although long-term exposure to severe stress or pharmacological levels of glucocorticoids is clearly deleterious (149, 165, 178, 181, 189, 238, 239), moderate stress or chronic exposure to slight elevations of glucocorticoids may have either little impact or promote health and extend the life span (132, 176). Chronic treatment with prednisolone phosphate, a synthetic glucocorticoid, increased the life span of a short-lived mouse strain (7), although no effect was observed in the longer-lived DBA/2J (59) or the C57BL/6J (88) mouse. Chronic treatment of *Drosophila melanogaster* with hydrocortisone acetate increased mean survival 20%–40% in both sexes (86, 87). Long-term exposure to moderate stress, which presumably elevates glucocorticoid levels, has also been shown to lengthen life. Mice chronically subjected to daily electric shock, intermittent exposure to a cool environment, or to a combination of these treatments lived nearly 40 days longer than controls (140). Some of these stressors also reduced the increase in mortality due to irradiation (140). Studies of rats forced to exercise daily (which may transiently activate the adrenocortical system) also are consistent with the view that chronic exposure to transient stress can extend the life span. Rats forced to run (48) had significantly lower mortality than controls. Similarly, rats immersed for 4 h a day in cool water from 6 months of age onward had 60% fewer neoplasms and lived on average over 1 month longer than controls, despite consuming 44% more calories (89). Although glucocorticoids were not measured in these studies, it is likely that they were increased. It is noteworthy that earlier studies using chronic, rather than intermittent, cold stress uniformly reported shortened life span (81, 95, 105, 106). These results have been interpreted to indicate that the intensity of a stressor can have a profound influence on the direction of change during aging (89).

As with the debate over the long-term effects of glucocorticoids on aging processes, there is no clear answer yet to the significance of the elevation in glucocorticoids that is sometimes observed in aging organisms. It appears that, in most cases, the elevations are substantially lower than those seen in Cushing's syndrome or following severe stress. Thus whether these moderate increases are deleterious to the organism or provide some benefit is an open question. The balance between benefits and risks of long-term exposure to normal levels of glucocorticoids during adulthood, and even possibly to elevated levels which may occur with advancing age, is not yet resolved.

Mineralocorticoids. Aldosterone is the principal mineralocorticoid, secreted primarily by the adrenal reticularis and acting principally on the kidney to maintain salt balance (64). There have been no large-scale population studies of plasma aldosterone during aging. Reports from numerous clinical studies of relatively small numbers of individuals give results that range from marked decreases to significant increases of plasma aldosterone concentrations in aging individuals. In one recent report, men in their eighties had plasma aldosterone concentrations that were more than 60% lower than those of men in their twenties (74). Higuchi and colleagues (83) reported a "tendency" of plasma aldosterone to decrease in older men, but the difference was not significant. Other groups have also reported no change in aldosterone levels during aging (4, 158), while others have observed an increase in 24-h mean plasma aldosterone levels (37). Even in the cases where plasma concentrations do not appear to change during aging, this lack of change does not necessarily indicate that production rates are unaltered. Pratt and colleagues (158) inferred from a 50% reduction in urinary excretion of the acid-hydrolyzable glucuronide conjugate of aldosterone that production of aldosterone was markedly reduced in elderly individuals. The finding that plasma levels of aldosterone were unaffected in the same individuals led those authors to conclude that clearance of the hormone was reduced in proportion to the reduction in its production.

Plasma aldosterone concentrations exhibit a circadian variation. Some of the discrepancies among studies may therefore be the consequence of sampling at different times, since many of the studies obtained samples at only one time of day. However, even studies that collected samples over a 24-h period report divergent effects of aging. For example, in a recent report, Cugini and colleagues (37) reported a 40% increase in 24-h mean plasma aldosterone levels, whereas in an earlier study the same laboratory reported a slight decrease in the mesor and amplitude of aldosterone (37a).

Plasma concentrations of aldosterone are also reported to decrease in aging rats (62, 161). In vitro perifusion of adrenal capsules from male Fischer 344 rats showed a progressive decrease in basal aldosterone secretion correlated with a decreased threshold sensitivity as well as maximal responsiveness to KCl and ACTH, indicating that the decrease in plasma aldosterone is in part attributable to adrenal hyporesponsiveness to secretagogues (161).

Adrenal Androgens. DHEA, a weak androgen, and its sulfate are produced in large amounts by the human adrenal, and the levels of these two products decline markedly with advancing age in both men (141, 142) and women (Fig. 15.4; 114, 141). Other than postmenopausal estrogen loss, this is the greatest age-related change in a steroid hormone that has been reported. Little is known about the changes in DHEA during age in other species. One study of rhesus monkeys reported an age-related decline similar to that in humans (143). Among a wild population of baboons (*Papio cynocephalus*), DHEA levels decreased 30%–50% during adolescence but showed no further decrease thereafter (182). DHEA concentrations were also reported to decline to undetectable levels in middle-aged mice (190).

The decline in plasma DHEA may contribute to age-related pathophysiology. Prospective studies indicate that plasma concentrations of DHEA are inversely related to risk for breast cancer (20), cardiovascular disease (6), and all-cause mortality (6) independent of age.

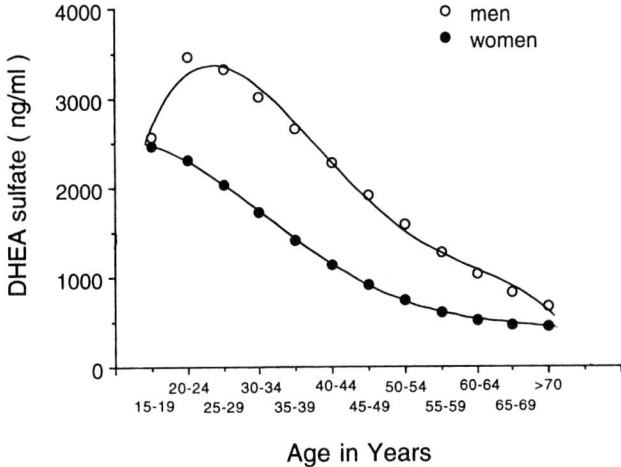

FIG. 15.4. Age-related decline in plasma concentrations of DHEA sulfate in men and women. [Redrawn from Orentreich et al. (142) with permission.]

Several studies have shown that administration of DHEA can ameliorate diabetic states (32) and reduce spontaneous as well as chemically induced carcinogenesis in rodents (184, 186, 187). DHEA administration can also reduce atherosclerotic plaques potentiated by intimal injury of the aorta in hypercholesterolemic rabbits (67) as well as their spontaneous occurrence (3). DHEA has also been shown to reduce autoimmune-related mortality in an autoimmune-prone mouse strain (119) and to improve memory in old mice (56).

Because DHEA treatment can decrease body weight and reduce food intake (31, 138, 238), the question arises as to what extent the observed effects of DHEA are independent of its effects on caloric utilization, since comparable effects are observed in food-restricted animals. In studies that specifically addressed this question, pair-fed controls often exhibited a similar effect to DHEA-treated animals (139, 237). In humans, a carefully controlled study found no relation between obesity or body mass index and plasma DHEA sulfate concentrations (6), although others have reported that both weight loss (80) and a low-fat vegetarian diet (84) are associated with increased blood levels of DHEA sulfate. However, none of these studies assessed directly the effect of caloric intake on DHEA sulfate levels.

DHEA appears to have a number of cellular and biochemical effects that could explain its ability to inhibit age-related pathogenesis. These include its role as a noncompetitive inhibitor of glucose-6-phosphate dehydrogenase, the rate-limiting enzyme of the pentose cycle responsible for the extramitochondrial production of reduced nicotinamide adenine dinucleotide phosphate (NADPH) (117, 139). One hypothesis is that relative abundance of NADPH in individuals with low levels of DHEA could increase obesity and atherosclerosis, since NADPH is an important coenzyme in the synthesis of fatty acids and cholesterol (202). NADPH-potentiated oxidative reactions could be a source of mutagens that might also be suppressed by DHEA (185). However, the relative importance of these effects of DHEA compared to its potential action on caloric intake remains to be determined.

Growth Hormone

Growth hormone is synthesized and secreted from somatotropes in the anterior pituitary gland. Growth hormone is essential for normal growth during childhood and adolescence and is also necessary for maintenance of the adult phenotype (64). In children as well as adults, growth hormone deficiency is associated with reduced lean body and bone mass, increased fat mass, and reduced protein synthesis (29, 35, 98). Reduced extracellular fluid volume and skin thickness also are characteristic of individuals with growth hormone deficiency (98). In addition, psychosocial performance appears to be affected by growth hormone deficiency. For example, in one carefully controlled study, growth hormone–deficient adults perceived themselves as being less energetic and more anxious and as having less self-control than matched controls (120). Because many of the characteristics of growth hormone deficiency are hallmarks of the aging phenotype, several investigators have hypothesized that the age-related decline in the circulating concentration of growth hormone contributes to these potentially important changes of aging (35, 122, 172). The hormone replacement studies described in the following section indicate that injection of growth hormone in older humans with reduced growth hormone levels can at least partially reverse some of the changes in body composition that are associated with growth hormone deficiency.

Humans. Growth hormone is secreted in discrete pulses, and, in young adults, the serum concentrations of growth hormone are relatively low during the daytime and high during sleep (227, 243). The 24-h integrated secretion of growth hormone declines progressively with advancing age (23, 36, 55, 85, 90, 160, 174, 230, 248). This is a robust observation; virtually every study has observed a decrease in growth hormone with age, even those with relatively small samples. The magnitude of the decrease, however, is less certain, with studies reporting reductions between 20% and 80%. This may reflect the small sample sizes, the absence of longitudinal data, and the fact that many factors, including exercise (73), obesity (49, 90, 241), and hyperglycemia (118, 159), influence growth hormone secretion. It is noteworthy that growth hormone levels are reduced as early as middle-age and that a significant fraction of the elderly have levels below normal for young adults. In a study of healthy, nonobese individuals between 21 and 71 yr of age, steady decrements in growth-hormone production rate and half-life were observed by deconvolution analysis with each successive decade of life (90).

Growth hormone has both direct and indirect effects on target tissues. Many indirect actions of growth hormone are mediated through insulin-like growth factor I (IGF-1) (40). IGF-1 is synthesized in liver and many other target tissues of growth hormone (40). IGF-1 synthesis and secretion is positively regulated by growth hormone (40, 91). When secreted from the liver into the bloodstream, IGF-1 subserves a classical endocrine role, whereas it acts primarily in a paracrine fashion when secreted within other tissues (40, 91). Most of the IGF-1 in the serum is secreted from the liver under the control of growth hormone. Serum levels of IGF-1 decline with age, paralleling the decline in growth hormone. Virtually all studies have observed a decrease in plasma IGF-1 with age in both men (85, 152, 173, 230) and women (60, 174), and the decrement between the ages of 20 and 80 yr ranges between 30 and 50%.

Laboratory Rodents and Other Species. Growth-hormone levels show marked age-related declines in laboratory rats (204, 206, 207). As in humans, these changes are evident as early as midlife (217). Detailed studies have revealed that the decrease is associated with both decrements in the frequency and the amplitude of growth-hormone pulses in male (204, 207) and female (217) rats. These studies have been limited to Long-Evans and Fischer 344 rats, and little is known about the effect of age on growth hormone secretion in other strains or mammalian species. A decrease in the nocturnal elevation of growth hormone has also been observed in aging male rhesus in captivity (100), and a study of free-ranging rhesus also revealed an age-related decline in males but no decrease in females (188).

As in humans, decreased growth hormone in aging rats is associated with decreased plasma concentrations of IGF-1 (57, 58). A decline in IGF-1 has also been observed in aging mice (206). Data on other species are not available.

Growth Hormone and the Aging Phenotype. The hypothesis that the reduced levels of growth hormone play a causal role in the development of the aging phenotype is attractive and, with the advent of recombinant human growth hormone, has become readily testable. As noted earlier, growth hormone deficiency in young adults is associated with many of the sequelae of aging, ranging from changes in body composition to alterations in psychosocial traits (96). Initial studies were conducted in relatively young growth hormone–deficient adults and showed that treatment with recombinant human growth hormone partially reversed many of the changes that accompanied growth hormone deficiency. Growth-hormone replacement therapy increased lean body mass, decreased fat mass, and increased muscle mass, strength, and exercise capacity (96). It also resulted in increased cardiac performance and normalization of kidney function (97).

Several short-term studies have examined the effects of growth-hormone replacement in aging humans. Rudman and colleagues (173) treated 21 healthy men over 60 yr of age with recombinant human growth hormone for 6 months. These men were selected because their levels of IGF-1 fell below 350 U/l of serum, which has been shown to be associated with an absence of detectable pulsatile secretion of growth hormone (85). The replacement dose of growth hormone was designed to restore IGF-1 levels to the normal range of young adults. No adverse reactions were observed during the 6-month duration of treatment. Men treated with growth hormone showed a 9% increase in lean body mass, a 14% decrease in adipose tissue mass, and a 1.6% increase in lumbar vertebral bone density, as well as a 7% increase in skin thickness. Other, smaller-scale, shorter-term studies of growth hormone treatment in older individuals have shown evidence of improved nitrogen balance and IGF-1 levels, as well as increased protein synthesis, although most of the individuals in these studies were malnourished or in postoperative or perioperative states (10, 99, 116, 214). No studies in elderly people have yet examined the effect of growth hormone replacement on functional endpoints, such as muscle strength, exercise capacity, glomerular filtration, or psychological well-being.

Studies of growth hormone replacement in aging laboratory rodents and other mammals have examined a broader range of endpoints. Sonntag and colleagues (205) observed increased protein synthesis in the skeletal muscle of aged rats receiving exogenous growth hormone. Surgical implantation of a growth hormone–secreting pituitary adenoma increased thymus weight and improved several measures of immune function in old rats (42, 102). Growth hormone treatment also enhanced thymic activity in old dogs (66). Biweekly injections of human growth hormone into 18-month-old BALB/c mice for 13 wk reduced mortality and increased the mitogenic response of splenocytes to pokeweed but not concanavalin A (104). IL-1 and -2 and TNF production were also increased, although total IgG production was reduced in growth hormone–treated mice affecting several immune parameters (104).

In summary, evidence in both rodents and humans indicates that a number of biological endpoints of growth hormone remain responsive in older individuals and that some age-related changes of potential importance to the maintenance of organismic homeostasis can be at least partially reversed or delayed in onset by growth hormone treatment. At least one potential complication, carpal tunnel syndrome, has occurred in individuals on prolonged growth hormone therapy (35), and this adverse response underscores the ever-present potential for deleterious effects of intervention. More serious effects, such as malignancy, hyperglycemia, and cardiovascular complications, remain a concern given the evidence that acromegaly (2, 8, 125) and experimental elevation of growth hormone (218) may increase the risk of developing these pathological states. In this regard, it is noteworthy that growth hormone appears to be reduced in at least the early stages of food restriction, which delay most aging processes (206). Whether reduced exposure to growth hormone plays a role in the life-extending actions of food restriction is unknown, but the question raises at least a caveat that chronic exposure to young adult levels of growth hormone may have deleterious effects.

SUMMARY

The pattern of change in hormones during aging is nonuniform among animal species, individuals, and hormonal classes. Given the relative ease of measurement, knowledge about these changes remains surprisingly incomplete for most hormones in both humans and other animals. The data are least equivocal for the hormones with the most dramatic changes: estradiol and its decreased plasma concentrations in postmenopausal women; and growth hormone, DHEA and its sulfate, which are decreased markedly in both men and women. That testosterone levels diminish substantially in most men as early as middle age is an emerging finding with potentially important implications for the age-related changes in the musculoskeletal as well as other systems. The picture for glucocorticoids and mineralocorticoids remains less clear, largely because of an absence of large-scale population studies. Some studies suggest that levels may increase, while others indicate they may decline. Genetic and/or gender differences may account for part of these discrepant findings. The evidence that chronic exposure to elevated glucocorticoids may be deleterious for some systems but beneficial for others is sufficiently compelling to encourage further study to establish the dosage domains of these effects and the balance of risk and benefit of exogenous treatment.

The question remains as to the importance of hormonal changes to the aging phenotype. These changes are correlated with, and thus may contribute to, important dysfunctional changes in the musculoskeletal, cardiovascular, and immune systems, as well as the nervous system. Classical endocrine experimentation, that is, hormonal replacement, is required to establish their role in the etiology of aging. Studies of estrogen replacement in postmenopausal women have led the way in this regard, and replacement studies with other hormones have been and are being initiated. Estrogen replacement, supplemented with progestins, is now widely accepted as a beneficial treatment for the pathophysiological sequelae of estrogen withdrawal in postmenopausal women, provided the women are carefully monitored and without history of or identified risk for estrogen-dependent neoplasms. At least two types of important knowledge can be anticipated to emanate from hormone-replacement studies. First, knowledge of the changes affected by hormone replacement will provide insight into the basis of the aging phenotype and be of potentially significant clinical import. Equally important will be the discovery of age-related changes that are independent of hormonal changes, for it will direct inquiry to other mechanisms and areas of investigation.

One reason hormone replacement may not always restore a youthful phenotype is that the hormonal signal in the plasma only constitutes the first component in the pathway that leads to altered cell and physiological function. Many age-related changes distal to the hormone may occur that can modify the impact, negatively or positively, of the altered plasma concentration of hormone on the cellular response. In humans, however, there are scant data on the effect of aging on either the bioavailability of these hormones to cells or the intracellular machinery that transduces these signals into biochemical and cellular actions. Obtaining this knowledge is an important complement for current studies of the effect of hormone replacement on aging processes. Hormone replacement may be ineffective if target tissues have attenuated responses to hormones in the aged individual. The importance of this information is underscored by studies in animals which show a wide range of effects of aging on target tissue responsiveness to hormones (168, 233).

REFERENCES

1. ADLER, A. J., and J. F. NELSON. Aging and chronic estradiol exposure impair estradiol-induced cornification but not proliferation of vaginal epithelium in C57BL/6J mice. *Biol. Reprod.* 38: 175–182, 1988.
2. ALEXANDER, L., D. APPLETON, R. HALL, W. M. ROSS, and R. WILKINSON. Epidemiology of acromegaly in the Newcastle region. *Clin. Endocrinol.* 12: 71–79, 1980.
3. ARAD, Y., J. J. BADIMON, L. BADIMON, W. C. HEMBREE, and H. N. GINSBERG. Dehydroepiandrosterone feeding prevents aortic fatty streak formation and cholesterol accumulation in cholesterol-fed rabbit. *Arteriosclerosis* 9: 159–166.
4. ARMANINI, D., I. KARBOWIAK, M. SCALI, E. ORLANDINI, V. ZAMPOLLO, and G. VITTADELLO. Corticosteroid receptors and lymphocyte subsets in mononuclear leukocytes in aging. *Am. J. Physiol.* 262: E464–E466, 1992.
5. BARRETT-CONNOR, E., and K.-T. KHAW. Endogenous sex hor-

mones and cardiovascular diseases in men: a prospective population-based study. *Circulation* 78: 539–545, 1988.
6. BARRETT-CONNER, E., K.-T. KHAW, and S. S. C. YEN. A prospective study of dehydroepiandrosterone sulfate, mortality, and cardiovascular disease. *N. Engl. J. Med.* 315: 1519–1524, 1986.
7. BELLAMY, D. Long-term action of prednisolone phosphate on a strain of short-lived mice. *Exp. Gerontol.* 3: 327–333, 1968.
8. BENGTSSON, B. A., S. EDEN, I. ERNEST, A. ODEN, and B. SJOGREN. Epidemiology and long-term survival in acromegaly. *Acta Med. Scand.* 223: 327–335, 1988.
9. BESTETTI, G. E., M. J. REYMOND, F. BLANC, C. E. BOUJON, F. FURRER, and G. L. ROSSI. Functional and morphological changes in the hypothalamo–pituitary–gonadal axis of aged female rats. *Biol. Reprod.* 45: 221–228, 1991.
10. BINNERTS, A., J. H. P. WILSON, and S. W. J. LAMBERTS. The effects of human growth hormone administration in elderly adults with recent weight loss. *J. Clin. Endocrinol. Metab.* 67: 1312–1316, 1988.
11. BLICHERT-TOFT, M. Assessment of serum corticotropin concentration and its nyctohemeral rhythm in the aging. *Gerontol. Clin.* 13: 215–220, 1975.
12. BLICHERT-TOFT, M., B. BLICHERT-TOFT, and H. KAALUND-JENSEN. Pituitary-adrenocortical stimulation in the aged as reflected in levels of plasma cortisol and compound S. *Acta Chir. Scand.* 136: 665–670, 1970.
13. BLOCK, E. Quantitative morphological investigations of the follicular system in women. Variations at different ages. *Acta Anat.* 14: 108–123, 1952.
14. Boston Collaborative Drug Surveillance Program. Surgically confirmed gallbladder disease, venous thromboembolism, and breast tumours in relation to postmenopausal estrogen therapy. *N. Engl. J. Med.* 290: 15–19, 1974.
15. BRANDTSTADTER, J., B. BALTES-GOTZ, C. KIRSCHBAUM, and D. HELLHAMMER. Developmental and personality correlates of adrenocortical activity as indexed by salivary cortisol: observations in the age range of 35 to 65 years. *J. Psychosom. Res.* 35: 173–185, 1991.
16. BRAWER, J. R., H. SCHIPPER, and B. ROBAIRE. Effects of long-term androgen and estradiol exposure on the hypothalamus. *Endocrinology* 112: 194–199, 1983.
17. BREMNER, W. F., M. V. VITIELLO, and P. N. PRINZ. Loss of circadian rhythmicity in blood testosterone levels with aging in normal men. *J. Clin. Endocrinol. Metab.* 56: 1278–1281, 1983.
18. BRONSON, F. H., and C. DESJARDINS. Reproductive failure in aged CBF1 male mice: interrelationships between pituitary gonadotropic hormones, testicular function, and mating success. *Endocrinology* 101: 939–945, 1977.
19. BROWN-SEQUARD, C. E. Des effects produits chez l'homme par des injections sous-cutanées d'un liquide retiré des testicules frais de cobayes et de chiens. *Comptes Rend. Soc. Biol.* 41: 415–422, 1889.
20. BULBROOK, R. D., J. L. HAYWARD, and C. C. SPICER. Relation between urinary androgen and corticoid excretion and subsequent breast cancer. *Lancet* 2: 395–398, 1971.
21. BUSH, T. L., L. D. COWAN, E. BARRETT-CONNER, M. H. CRIQUI, J. M. KARON, R. B. WALLACE, A. TYROLER, and B. M. RIFKIND. Estrogen use and all-cause mortality: preliminary results from the Lipid Research Clinics Program Follow-up Study. *JAMA* 249: 903–906, 1983.
22. CARANI, C., V. MONTANINI, G. F. BARAGHINI, D. ZINI, M. F. CELANI, and P. MARRAMS. Il quadro ormonal nell'uomo anziano. *Sessuologia* 1: 78, 1982.
23. CARLSON, H. E., J. C. GILLIN, P. GORDEN, and F. SNYDER. Absence of sleep-related growth hormone peaks in aged normal subjects and in acromegaly. *J. Clin. Endocrinol. Metab.* 34: 1102–1105, 1972.
24. CHAMBERS, K. C., and C. H. PHOENIX. Diurnal patterns of testosterone, dihydrotestosterone, estradiol, and cortisol in serum of rhesus males: relationship to sexual behavior in aging males. *Horm. Behav.* 15: 416–426, 1981.
25. CHAMBERS, K. C., and C. H. PHOENIX. Sexual behavior and serum levels of prolactin, testosterone and estradiol in young and old rhesus males. *Physiol. Behav.* 52: 13–16, 1992.
26. CHAMBERS, K. C., J. A. RESKO, and C. H. PHOENIX. Correlation of diurnal changes in hormones with sexual behavior and age in male rhesus macaques. *Neurobiol. Aging* 3: 37–42, 1982.
27. CHAMBERS, K. C., J. E. THORNTON, and C. E. ROSELLI. Age-related deficits in brain androgen binding and metabolism, testosterone, and sexual behavior of male rats. *Neurobiol. Aging* 12: 123–130, 1991.
28. CHAN, S. W. C., J. H. LEATHEM, and T. ESASHI. Testicular metabolism and serum testosterone in aging male rats. *Endocrinology* 101: 128–133, 1977.
29. CHRISTIANSEN, J. S., and J. O. L. JORGENSEN. Beneficial effects of GH replacement therapy in adults. *Acta Endocrinol. (Copenh.)* 125: 7–13, 1991.
30. CHUBB, C., and C. DESJARDINS. Testicular function and sexual activity in senescent mice. *Am. J. Physiol.* 247: 569–573, 1984.
31. CLEARY, M. P., N. FOX, B. LAZIN, and J. BILLHEIMER. A comparison of the effects of dehydroepiandrosterone treatment to ad libitum and pair-feeding in the obese Zucker rat. *Nutr. Res.* 5: 1247–1257, 1985.
32. COLEMAN, D. L., R. W. SCHWIZER, and E. H. LEITER. Effect of genetic background on the therapeutic effects of dehydroepiandrosterone (DHEA) in diabetes-obesity mutants and in aged normal mice. *Diabetes* 33: 26–32, 1984.
33. COLUCCI, C. F., B. D'ALESSANDRO, A. BELLASTELLA, and N. MONTALBETTI. Circadian rhythm of plasma cortisol in the aged (cosinor method). *Gerontol. Clin.* 17: 89–95, 1975.
34. COQUELIN, A., and C. DESJARDINS. Luteinizing hormone and testosterone secretion in young and old male mice. *Am. J. Physiol.* 243: 257–263, 1982.
35. CORPAS, E., S. M. HARMAN, and M. R. BLACKMAN. Human growth hormone and human aging. *Endocrine Rev.* 14: 20–39, 1993.
36. CORPAS, E., S. M. HARMAN, M. A. PINEYRO, R. ROBERSON, and M. R. BLACKMAN. GHRH 1–29 twice daily reverses the decreased GH and IGF-1 levels in old men. *J. Clin. Endocrinol. Metab.* 65: 530–535, 1992.
37. CUGINI, P., P. LUCIA, L. DIPALMA, M. RE, R. CANOVA, L. GASBARRONE, and A. CIANETTI. Effect of aging on circadian rhythm of atrail natriuretic peptide, plasma renin activity, and plasma aldosterone. *J. Gerontol.* 47: B214–B219, 1992.
37a. CUGINI, P., G. MURANO, P. LUCIA, C. LETIZIA, D. SCARO, F. HALBERG, and H. SCHRAMM. The gerontological decline of the renin-aldosterone system: A chronobiological approach extended to essential hypertension. *J. Gerontol.* 42: 461–465, 1987.
38. DABBS, J. M., JR. Age and seasonal variation in serum testosterone concentration among men. *Chronobiol. Int.* 7: 245–249, 1990.
39. DAI, W. S., L. H. KULLER, R. E. LAPORTE, J. P. GUTAI, L. FALVO-GERARD, and A. CAGGIULA. The epidemiology of plasma testosterone levels in middle-aged men. *Am. J. Epidemiol.* 114: 804–816, 1981.
40. DAUGHADAY, W. H. A personal history of the origins of the somatomedin hypothesis and recent challenges to its validity. *Perspect. Biol. Med.* 32: 194–211, 1989.
41. DAVIDSON, J. M., J. J. CHEN, L. CRAPO, G. D. GRAY, W. J.

GREENLEAF, and J. A. CATANIA. Hormonal changes and sexual function in aging men. *J. Clin. Endocrinol. Metab.* 57: 71–77, 1983.

42. DAVILA, D. R., S. BRIEF, J. SIMON, R. E. HAMMER, R. L. BRINSTER, and K. W. KELLEY. Role of growth hormone in regulating T-dependent immune events in aged, nude and transgenic rodents. *J. Neurosci. Res.* 18: 108–116, 1987.

43. DEAN, S., and S. P. FELTON. Circadian rhythm in the elderly: a study using a cortisol specific radioimmunoassay. *Age Aging* 8: 243–245, 1979.

44. DE KOSKY, S., S. SCHEFF, and C. COTMAN. Elevated corticosterone levels: a mechanism for impaired sprouting in the aged hippocampus. *Neuroendocrinology* 38: 33–40, 1984.

45. DESJARDINS, G. C., J. R. BRAWER, and A. BEAUDET. Estradiol is selectively neurotoxic to hypothalamic β-endorphin neurons. *Endocrinology* 132: 86–93, 1993.

46. DESLYPERE, J. P., and A. VERMEULEN. Leydig cell function in normal men: effect of age, lifestyle, residence, diet, and activity. *J. Clin. Endocrinol. Metab.* 59: 955–962, 1984.

47. DOBIE, D. J., M. A. MILLER, M. A. RASKIND, and D. M. DORSA. Testosterone reverses a senescent decline in extrahypothalamic vasopressin mRNA. *Brain Res.* 583: 247–252, 1992.

48. EDINGTON, D. W., A. C. COSMAS, and W. B. MCCAFFERTY. Exercise and longevity: evidence for a threshold age. *J. Gerontol.* 27: 341–343, 1972.

49. ELAHI, D., D. C. MULLER, S. P. ZANKOFF, R. ANDRES, and J. D. TOBIN. Effect of age and obesity on fasting levels of glucose, insulin, glucagon, and growth hormone in men. *J. Gerontol.* 37: 385–391, 1982.

50. ELEFTHERIOU, B. E., and L. A. LUCAS. Age-related changes in testes, seminal vesicles and plasma testosterone levels in male mice. *Gerontologia* 20: 231–238, 1974.

51. EVERETT, A. V., and J. R. WALTON (Eds). *Regulation of Neuroendocrine Aging.* Basel: Karger, 1988.

52. EVERITT, J. C., and J. MEITES. Anti-aging effects of hormones. *J. Gerontol.* 44: B130–B147, 1989.

53. FABER, J. F. *Life Tables for the United States: 1900–2050.* Actuarial study no. 87, SSA pub. no. 11-11534, Washington: Office of the Actuary, Social Security Administration, 1982.

54. FADDY, M. J., R. G. GOSDEN, A. GOUGEON, S. J. RICHARDSON, and J. F. NELSON. Accelerated disappearance of ovarian follicles in mid-life: implications for forecasting menopause. *Hum. Reprod.* 7: 1342–1346, 1992.

55. FINKELSTEIN, J., H. ROFFWARG, P. BOYAR, J. KREAM, and L. HELLMAN. Age-related changes in the twenty-four hour spontaneous secretion of growth hormone in normal individuals. *J. Clin. Endocrinol. Metab.* 35: 665–670, 1972.

56. FLOOD, J. F., and E. ROBERTS. Dehydroepiandrosterone sulfate improves memory in aging mice. *Brain Res.* 448: 178–181, 1988.

57. FLORINI, J., and S. ROBERTS. Effects of rat age on blood levels of somatomedin-like growth factor. *J. Gerontol.* 35: 23–30, 1979.

58. FLORINI, J., J. HARNED, R. RICHMAN, and J. WEISS. Effect of rat age on serum levels of growth hormone and somatomedins. *Mech. Ageing Dev.* 15: 165–176, 1981.

59. FORBES, W. F. The effect of prednisolone phosphate on the life span of DBA/2J mice. *Exp. Gerontol.* 10: 27–29, 1975.

60. FRANCHIMONT, P., D. URBAIN-CHOFFRAY, P. LABELIN, M. A. FONTAINE, G. FRANGIN, and J. Y. REGINSTER. Effects of repetitive administration of growth hormone-releasing hormone on growth hormone secretion, insulin-like growth factor I, and bone metabolism in post-menopausal women. *Acta Endocrinol. (Copenh)* 120: 121–128, 1989.

61. FRIEDMAN, M., M. F. GREEN, and D. E. SHARLAND. Assessment of hypothalamic–pituitary–adrenal function in the geriatric age group. *J. Gerontol.* 24: 292–297, 1969.

62. FROLKIS, V. V., N. S. VERKHRATSKY, and L. V. MAGDICH. Regulation of aldosterone secretion in old rats. *Gerontology* 31: 84–94, 1985.

63. FUGO, N. W., and R. L. BUTCHER. Effect of prolonged estrous cycles on reproduction in aged rats. *Fertil. Steril.* 22: 98–101, 1971.

64. GANONG, W. F. *Review of Medical Physiology.* East Norwalk, CT: Appleton and Lange, 1987, p. 317–320.

65. GHANADIAN, R., J. G. LEWIS, and G. D. CHISHOLM. Serum testosterone and dihydrotestosterone changes with age in the rat. *Steroids* 25: 753–762, 1975.

66. GOFF, B. L., J. A. ROTH, L. H. ARP, and G. S. INCEFY. Growth hormone treatment stimulates thymulin production in aged dogs. *Clin. Exp. Immunol.* 68: 580–586, 1987.

67. GORDON, G. B., D. E. BUSH, and H. F. WEISMAN. Reduction of atherosclerosis by administration of dehydroepiandrosterone. A study in the hypercholesterolemic New Zealand white rabbit with aortic intimal injury. *J. Clin. Invest.* 82: 712–720, 1988.

68. GOSDEN, R. G. *Biology of Menopause.* New York: Academic Press, 1985.

69. GRAHAM, C. E., O. R. KLING, and R. A. STEINER. Reproductive senescence in female nonhuman primates. In: *Aging in Nonhuman Primates,* edited by D. M. Bowden. New York: Van Nostrand Reinhold, 1979, p. 183–202.

70. GRAY, A., H. A. FELDMAN, J. B. MCKINLAY, and C. LONGCOPE. Age, disease, and changing sex hormone levels in middle-aged men: results of the Massachusetts male aging study. *J. Clin. Endocrinol. Metab.* 73: 1016–1025, 1991.

71. GRAY, G. D. Changes in the levels of luteinizing hormone and testosterone in the circulation of aging male rats. *J. Endocrinol.* 76: 551–552, 1978.

72. GRUENEWALD, D. A., D. L. HESS, C. W. WILKINSON, and A. M. MATSUMOTO. Excessive testicular progesterone secretion in aged male Fischer 344 rats: a potential cause of age-related gonadotropin suppression and confounding variable in aging studies. *J. Gerontol.* 47: B164–B170, 1992.

73. HAGBERG, J. M., D. R. SEALS, J. E. YERG, J. GAVIN, R. GINGERICH, P. BHARTUR, and J. HOLLOSZY. Metabolic response to exercise in young and old athletes and sedentary men. *J. Appl. Physiol.* 65: 900–908, 1988.

74. HALLENGREN, B., S. ELMSTAHL, H. GALVARD, P. JERNTORP, P. MANHEM, H. PESSAH-RASMUSSEN, and L. STAVENOW. 80-year old men have elevated plasma concentrations of catecholamines but decreased plasma renin activity and aldosterone as compared to young men. *Aging* 4: 341–345, 1992.

75. HAMILTON, J. B., and G. E. MESTLER. Mortality and survival: comparison of eunuchs with intact men and women in a mentally retarded population. *J. Gerontol.* 24: 395–411, 1969.

76. HAMILTON, J. F. The role of testicular secretions as indicated by the effects of castration in man and by studies of pathological conditions and the short life span associated with maleness. *Recent Prog. Horm. Res.* 3: 257–322, 1948.

77. HAMMOND, C. B., F. R. JELOVSEK, K. L. LEE, W. T. CREASMAN, and R. T. PARKER. Effects of long-term estrogen replacement therapy. II. Neoplasia. *Am. J. Obstet. Gynecol.* 133: 537–547, 1979.

78. HAN, E-S., N. LEVIN, B. BERGANI, J. R. ROBERTS, Y-S. SUH, and J. F. NELSON. Food restriction-induced hyperadrenocorticism in the male F344 rat: reduced plasma and pituitary adrenocorticotropic hormone without reduced pituitary proopiomelanocortin RNA. [*Abstracts: Society for Neuroscience*], p. 1743, 1993.

79. HARMAN, S. M., and P. D. TSITOURAS. Reproductive hormones

in aging men. I. Measurement of sex steroids, basal luteinizing hormone, and Leydig cell response to human chorionic gonadotropin. *J. Clin. Endocrinol. Metab.* 51: 35–40, 1980.
80. HENDRIKX, A., W. HEYNS, and P. DE MOOR. Influence of a low-calorie diet and fasting on the metabolism of dehydroepiandrosterone sulfate in adult obese subjects. *J. Clin. Endocrinol. Metab.* 28: 1525–1533, 1968.
81. HEROUX, O., and J. S. CAMPBELL. A study of the pathology and life span of 6°C- and 30°C-acclimated rats. *Lab. Invest.* 9: 305–315, 1960.
82. HERZBERG, N. H., E. GOUDSMIT, J. KRUISBRINK, and G. J. BOER. Testosterone treatment restores reduced vasopressin-binding sites in the kidney of the ageing rat. *J. Endocrinol.* 123: 59–63, 1989.
83. HIGUCHI, K., A. OGO, T. MAKI, M. HAJI, R. TAKAYANAGI, M. OHASHI, H. NAWATA, K. KATO, and H. IBAYASHI. Evidence for age-related change in plasma 19-hydroxyandrostenedione. *Endocrinol. Jpn.* 36: 881–885, 1989.
84. HILL, P. B., and E. L. WYNDER. Effect of a vegetarian diet and dexamethasone on plasma prolactin, testosterone and dehydroepiandrosterone in men and women. *Cancer Lett.* 7: 273–282, 1979.
85. HO, K. Y., W. S. EVANS, R. M. BLIZZARD, J. D. VELDHUIS, G. R. MERRIAM, E. SOMOJLIK, R. FURLANETTO, A. D. ROGOL, D. L. KAISER, and M. O. THORNER. Effects of sex and age on 24-hour profile of growth hormone secretion in men: importance of endogenous estradiol concentrations. *J. Clin. Endocrinol. Metab.* 64: 51–58, 1987.
86. HOCHSCHILD, R. Effect of membrane stabilizing drugs on mortality in *Drosophila melanogaster*. *Exp. Gerontol.* 6: 133–151, 1971a.
87. HOCHSCHILD, R. Lysosomes, membranes and aging. *Exp. Gerontol.* 6: 153–166, 1971b.
88. HOCHSCHILD, R. Effects of various drugs on longevity in female C57BL/6J mice. *Gerontologia* 19: 271–280, 1973.
89. HOLLOSZY, J. O., and E. K. SMITH. Longevity of cold-exposed rats: a reevaluation of the "rate-of-living theory." *J. Appl. Physiol.* 61: 1656–1660, 1986.
90. IRANMANESH, A., G. LIZARRALDE, and J. D. VELDHUIS. Age and relative adiposity are specific negative determinants of the frequency and amplitude of growth hormone (GH) secretory bursts and the half-life of endogenous GH in healthy men. *J. Clin. Endocrinol. Metab.* 73: 1081–1088, 1991.
91. ISAKSSON, O. G., A. LINDAHL, A. NILSSON, and J. ISGAARD. Action of growth hormone: current views. *Acta Paediatr. Scand.* 343: 12–18, 1988.
92. ISSA, A. M., W. ROWE, S. GAUTHIER, and M. J. MEANEY. Hypothalamic–pituitary–adrenal activity in aged, cognitively impaired and cognitively unimpaired rats. *J. Neurosci.* 10: 3247–3254, 1990.
93. JENSEN, G. D., E. N. SASSENRATH, and F. L. BLANTON. Sociosexual and hormonal changes in aging female bonnet macaques. *J. Gerontol.* 37: 450–453, 1982.
94. JENSEN, J. K., and M. BLICHERT-TOFT. Serum corticotropin, plasma cortisol and urinary excretion of 17-ketogenic steroids in the elderly (age group: 66–94 years). *Acta Endocrinol. (Copenh.)* 66: 25–34, 1971.
95. JOHNSON, H. D., L. D. KINTNER, and H. H. KIBLER. Effects of 48°F (8.9°C) and 83°F (28.4°C) on longevity and pathology of male rats. *J. Gerontol.* 18: 29–36, 1963.
96. JORGENSEN, J. O. L. Human growth hormone replacement therapy: pharmacological and clinical aspects. *Endocrine Rev.* 12: 189–207, 1991.
97. JORGENSEN, J. O. L., S. A. PEDERSEN, and L. THUESEN. Beneficial effects of growth hormone treatment in GH-deficient adults. *Lancet* 1: 1221–1225, 1989.
98. JORGENSEN, J. O. L., S. A. PEDERSEN, L. THUESEN, J. JORGENSEN, J. MOLLER, J. MULLER, N. E. SKAKKEBAEK, and J. S. CHRISTIANSEN. Long-term growth hormone treatment in growth hormone deficient adults. *Acta Endocrinol.* 125: 449–453, 1991.
99. KAISER, F. E., A. J. SILVER, and J. E. MORLEY. The effect of recombinant human growth hormone on malnourished older individuals. *J. Am. Geriatr. Soc.* 39: 235–240, 1991.
100. KALER, L. W., P. GLIESSMAN, J. CRAVEN, J. HILL, and V. CRITCHLOW. Loss of enhanced nocturnal growth hormone secretion in aging rhesus males. *Endocrinology* 119: 1281–1284, 1986.
101. KALER, L. W., P. GLIESSMAN, D. L. HESS, and J. HILL. The androgen status of aging male rhesus macaques. *Endocrinology* 119: 566–571, 1986.
102. KELLEY, K., S. BRIEF, H. WESTLY, J. NOVAKOFSKI, P. BECHTEL, J. SIMON, and E. WALKER. GH3 pituitary adenoma cells can reverse thymic aging in rats. *Proc. Natl. Acad. Sci. U.S.A.* 83: 5663–5667, 1986.
103. KERR, D., L. CAMPBELL, M. APPLEGATE, A. BRODISH, and P. LANDFIELD. Chronic stress-induced acceleration of electrophysiologic and morphometric biomarkers of hippocampal aging. *J. Neurosci.* 11: 1316–1321, 1991.
104. KHANSARI, D. N., and T. GUSTAD. Effects of long-term, low-dose growth hormone therapy on immune function and life expectancy of mice. *Mech. Ageing Dev.* 57: 87–100, 1991.
105. KIBLER, H. H., and H. D. JOHNSON. Metabolic rate and aging in rats during exposure to cold. *J. Gerontol.* 16: 13–16, 1961.
106. KIBLER, H. H., H. D. SILSBY, and H. D. JOHNSON. Metabolic trends and life span of rats living at 9°C and 28°C. *J. Gerontol.* 18: 235–239, 1963.
107. KINOSHITA, Y., Y. HIGASHI, S. J. WINTER, H. OSHIMA, and P. TROEN. An analysis of the age-related decline in testicular steroidogenesis in the rat. *Biol. Reprod.* 32: 309–314, 1985.
108. KLEBANOV, S., S. DIAIS, W. STAVINOHA, Y. SUH, and J. F. NELSON. Hyperadrenocorticism, attenuated inflammation and the life-prolonging action of food restriction in mice. *J. Gerontol.* (in press), 1995.
109. KLEY, H. K., E. NIESCHLAG, W. WIEGELMANN, and H. L. KRUSKEMPER. Sexual hormone beim alternden Mann. *Aktuel Gerontol.* 6: 61, 1976.
110. KRIEGER, D. T. Cushing's syndrome. *Monogr. Endocrinol.* 22: 1–142, 1982.
111. LAKSHMI, R., A. V. LAKSHMI, P. V. DIVAN, and M. S. BAMJI. Effect of riboflavin or pyridoxine deficiency on inflammatory response. *Indian J. Biochem. Biophys.* 28: 481–484, 1991.
112. LANDFIELD, P. W., and C. J. ELDRIDGE. The glucocorticoid hypothesis of brain aging and neurodegeneration: recent modifications. *Acta Endocrinol. (Copenh.)* 125: 54–64, 1991.
113. LANDFIELD, P. W., J. C. WAYMIRE, and G. LYNCH. Hippocampal aging and adrenocorticoids: quantitative correlations. *Science* 72: 1098–1102, 1978.
114. LIU, C. H., G. A. LAUGHLIN, U. G. FISCHER, and S. S. YEN. Marked attenuation of ultradian and circadian rhythms of dehydroepiandrosterone in postmenopausal women: evidence for a reduced 17,20-desmolase enzymatic activity. *J. Clin. Endocrinol. Metab.* 71: 900–906, 1990.
115. LUPO-DI PRISCO, C., and F. DESSI-FULGHERI. Endocrine and behavioral modifications in aging male rats. *Hormone Res.* 12: 149–160, 1980.
116. MARCUS, R., G. BUTTERFIELD, L. HOLLOWAY, L. GILLILAND, D. J. BAYLINK, R. L. HINTZ, and B. M. SHERMAN. Effects of short term administration of recombinant human growth hormone to elderly people. *J. Clin. Endocrinol. Metab.* 70: 519–527, 1990.
117. MARKS, P. H., and J. BANKS. Inhibition of mammalian glucose-

6-phosphate dehydrogenase by steroids. *Proc. Natl. Acad Sci. U.S.A.* 46: 445–452, 1960.

118. MASUDA, A., T. SHIBASAKI, M. NAKAHARA, T. IMAKI, Y. KIYOSAWA, K. JIBIKI, H. DEMURA, K. SHIZUME, and N. LING. The effect of glucose on growth hormone (GH) releasing hormone–mediated GH secretion in man. *J. Clin. Endocrinol. Metab.* 60: 523–526, 1985.

119. MATSUNAGA, A., B. MILLER, and G. COTTAM. Dehydroepiandrosterone prevention of autoimmune disease in NZB/WF1 mice: lack of an effect on associated immunological abnormalities. *Biochim. Biophys. Acta* 992: 265–272, 1989.

120. MCGAULEY, G. A., R. C. CUNEO, F. SALOMON, and P. H. SONKSEN. Psychological well-being before and after growth hormone treatment in adults with growth hormone deficiency. *Horm. Res.* 33(suppl. 4): 52–54, 1990.

121. MCGEER, P. L., E. MCGEER, J. ROGERS, and J. SIBLEY. Antiinflammatory drugs and Alzheimer's disease. *Lancet* 335: 1037, 1990.

122. MEITES, J. Neuroendocrine biomarkers of aging in the rat. *Exp. Gerontol.* 23: 349–358, 1988.

123. MERRY, B. J., and A. M. HOLEHAN. Serum profiles of LH, FSH, testosterone and 5 alpha-DHT from 21 to 1000 days of age in ad libitum fed and dietary restricted rats. *Exp. Gerontol.* 16: 431–444, 1981.

124. MOBBS, C. V., K. FLURKEY, D. GEE, K. YAMAMOTO, Y. SINHA, and C. E. FINCH. Estradiol-induced anovulatory syndrome in female C57BL/6J mice: age-like neuroendocrine, but not ovarian, impairments. *Biol. Reprod.* 30: 556–563, 1984.

125. NABARRO, J. D. Acromegaly. *Clin. Endocrinol.* 26: 481–512, 1987.

126. NAHOUL, K., and M. ROGER. Age-related decline of plasma bioavailable testosterone in adult men. *J. Steroid Biochem.* 35: 293–299, 1990.

127. NANKIN, J. R., and J. H. CALKINS. Decreased bioavailable testosterone in aging normal and impotent men. *J. Clin. Endocrinol. Metab.* 63: 1418–1420, 1986.

128. National Center for Health Statistics. Advance report of final mortality statistics, 1980. Monthly vital statistics report, vol. 32, no. 4, suppl. Washington: National Center for Health Statistics, 1983.

129. NEAVES, W. B., L. JOHNSON, J. C. PORTER, C. R. PARKER, and C. S. PETTY. Leydig cell numbers, daily sperm production, and serum gonadotropin levels in aging men. *J. Clin. Endocrinol. Metab.* 59: 756–763, 1984.

130. NEISCHLAG, E., U. LAMMER, C. W. FREISCHEM, K. LANGER, and E. J. WICKINGS. Reproductive functions in young fathers and grandfathers. *J. Clin. Endocrinol. Metab.* 55: 675–681, 1982.

131. NELSON, J. F. Puberty, gonadal steroids and fertility: potential reproductive markers of aging. *Exp. Gerontol.* 23: 359–367, 1988.

132. NELSON, J. F. The potential role of endocrine systems in the retardation of aging by caloric restriction. *Age Nutr.* 3: 171–178, 1992.

133. NELSON, J. F., and L. S. FELICIO. Reproductive aging in the female: an etiological perspective. *Rev. Biol. Res. Aging* 2: 251–314, 1985.

134. NELSON, J. F., and L. S. FELICIO. Radical ovarian resection advances the onset of persistent vaginal cornification but only transiently disrupts hypothalamic–pituitary regulation of cyclicity in C57BL/6J mice. *Biol. Reprod.* 35: 957–964, 1986.

135. NELSON, J. F., and L. S. FELICIO. Reproductive aging in the female: an etiological perspective updated. *Rev. Biol. Res. Aging* 3: 359–381, 1987.

136. NELSON, J. F., K. R. LATHAM, and C. E. FINCH. Plasma testosterone levels in C57BL/6J male mice: effects of age and disease. *Acta Endocrinol.* 80: 744–752, 1975.

136a. NELSON, J. F., N. LEVIN, K. KARELUS, J. ROBERTS, and B. BROOKS. Effects of aging and food restriction on hypothalamic neuropeptide Y (NPY) and corticotrophin releasing hormone (CRH) mRNAs in Fischer 344 rats. *Abstracts: Society for Neuroscience*, p. 897, 1993.

137. NICHOLS, N., C. E. FINCH, and J. F. NELSON. Effects of aging and food restriction on hypothalamic glial acidic fibrillary protein. *Abstracts: Society for Neuroscience* p. 1742, 1993.

138. NYCE, J. W., P. N. MAGEE, G. C. HARD, and A. G. SCHWARTZ. Inhibition of 1,2-dimethylhydrazine-induced colon tumorigenesis in Balb/c mice by dehydroepiandrosterone. *Carcinogenesis* 5: 57–62, 1984.

139. OERTEL, G. W., and P. BENES. The effects of steroids on glucose-6-phosphate dehydrogenase. *J. Steroid Biochem.* 3: 493–496, 1972.

140. ORDY, J. M., T. SAMORAJSKI, W. ZEMAN, and H. J. CURTIS. Interaction effects of environmental stress and deuteron irradiation of the brain on mortality and longevity of C57BL/10 mice. *Proc. Soc. Exp. Biol. Med.* 126: 184–190, 1967.

141. ORENTREICH, N., J. L. BRIND, R. L. RIZER, and J. H. VOGELMAN. Age changes and sex differences in serum dehydroepiandrosterone sulfate concentrations throughout adulthood. *J. Clin. Endocrinol. Metab.* 59: 551–555, 1984.

142. ORENTREICH, N., J. L. BRIND, J. H. VOGELMAN, R. ANDRES, and H. BALDWIN. Long-term longitudinal measurements of plasma dehydroepiandrosterone sulfate in normal men. *J. Clin. Endocrinol. Metab.* 75: 1002–1004, 1992.

143. Orentreich Foundation for Advancement of Science. Annual report. New York, 1987.

144. OTTENWELLER, J. E., C. D. TAPP, and B. H. NATELSON. Aging, stress and chronic disease interact to suppress plasma testosterone in syrian hamsters. *J. Gerontol.* 43: M175–M180, 1988.

145. OTTENWELLER, J. E., W. N. TAPP, D. L. PITMAN, and B. H. NATELSON. Interactions among the effects of aging, chronic disease and stress on adrenocortical function in Syrian hamsters. *Endocrinology* 126: 102–109, 1990.

146. OXENKRUG, G., I. MCINTYRE, and M. GERSHON. Effects of pinealectomy and aging on the serum corticosterone circadian rhythm in rats. *J. Pineal Res.* 1: 181–186, 1984.

147. PAGE, R. D., and R. L. BUTCHER. Follicular and plasma patterns of steroids in young and old rats during normal and prolonged estrous cycles. *Biol. Reprod.* 27: 383–392, 1982.

148. PALAZZOLO, D. L., and S. K. QUADRI. The effects of aging on the circadian rhythm of serum cortisol in the dog. *Exp. Gerontol.* 22: 379–387, 1987.

149. PARE, P. D. The effect of chronic environmental stress on premature aging in the rat. *J. Gerontol.* 20: 78–84, 1965.

150. PARTIN, A. W., J. E. OESTERLING, J. I. EPSTEIN, R. HORTON, and P. C. WALSH. Influence of age and endocrine factors on the volume of benign prostatic hyperplasia. *J. Urol.* 145: 405–409, 1991.

151. PASHKO, L. L., and A. G. SCHWARTZ. Reversal of food restriction–induced inhibition of mouse skin tumor promotion by adrenalectomy. *Carcinogenesis* 13: 1925–1928, 1992.

152. PAVLOV, E. P., S. M. HARMAN, G. P. CHROUSOS, D. L. LORIAUX, and M. R. BLACKMAN. Responses of plasma adrenocorticotropin, cortisol, and dehydroepiandrosterone to ovine corticotropin–releasing hormone in healthy aging men. *J. Clin. Endocrinol. Metab.* 62: 767–772, 1986.

153. PEREZ, J., E. BURUNAT, R. M. AREVALO, and M. RODRIGUEZ. Gonadal influences on behavioral deterioration with aging of male rats. *Horm. Behav.* 23: 457–465, 1989.

154. PHOENIX, C. H., and K. C. CHAMBERS. Sexual deprivation and

its influence on testosterone levels and sexual behavior of old and middle-aged rhesus males. *Biol. Reprod.* 31: 480–486, 1984.
155. PIKE, K. N., and P. DOERR. Age-related changes and interrelationships between plasma testosterone, estradiol and testosterone-binding globulin in normal adult males. *Acta Endocrinol.* 74: 792–800, 1973.
156. PIRKE, K. M., H.-J. VOGT, and M. GEISS. In vitro and in vivo studies on Leydig cell function in old rats. *Acta Endocrinol.* 89: 393–403, 1978.
157. PLYMATE, S. R., J. S. TENOVER, and W. J. BREMNER. Circadian variation in testosterone, sex hormone–binding globulin, and calculated non-sex hormone–binding globulin bound testosterone in healthy young and elderly men. *J. Androl.* 10: 366–371, 1989.
158. PRATT, J. H., J. J. HAWTHORNE, and D. J. DEBONO. Reduced urinary aldosterone excretion rates with normal plasma concentrations of aldosterone in the very elderly. *Steroids* 51: 163–171, 1988.
159. PRESS, M., W. V. TAMBORLANE, M. O. THORNER, W. VALE, J. RIVIER, J. M. GERTNER, and R. S. SHERWIN. Pituitary responses to growth hormone releasing factor in diabetes: failure of glucose-mediated suppression. *Diabetes* 33: 804–806, 1984.
160. PRINZ, P. N., E. D. WEITZMAN, G. R. CUNNINGHAM, and I. KARACAN. Plasma growth hormone during sleep in young and aged men. *J. Gerontol.* 38: 519–524, 1983.
161. RADKE, K. J. Age-related impairment of K(+)- and ACTH-stimulated aldosterone secretion by rat adrenal capsules. *Am. J. Physiol.* 264: E82–E89, 1993.
162. READ, G. F., and R. F. WALKER. Variation of salivary testosterone with age in men. In: *Immunoassays of Steroids in Saliva*, edited by G. G. Read, D. Riad-Fahmy, R. F. Walker, and K. Griffiths. Cardiff, UK: Alpha Omega, 1984.
163. RICHARDSON, S. J., V. SENIKAS, and J. F. NELSON. Follicular depletion during the menopausal transition: evidence for accelerated loss and ultimate exhaustion. *J. Clin. Endocrinol. Metab.* 65: 1231–1237, 1987.
164. RIEGLE, G. D., and A. E. MILLER. Aging effects on the hypothalamic–hypophyseal–gonadal control system in the rat. In: *The Aging Reproductive System*, edited by E. L. Schneider, New York: Raven Press, 1978, vol. 4. p. 159–192.
165. RILEY, V. Psychoneuroendocrine influences on immunocompetence and neoplasia. *Science* 212: 1100, 1981.
166. ROLANDI, E., R. FRANCESCHINI, A. MARABINI, V. MESSINA, A. CATALDI, M. SALVEMINI, and T. BARRECA. Twenty-four-hour beta-endorphin secretory pattern in the elderly. *Acta Endocrinol. (Copenh.)* 115: 441–446, 1987.
167. ROSENTHAL, M. J., and W. F. WOODSIDE. Nocturnal regulation of free fatty acids in healthy young and elderly men. *Metabolism* 37: 645–648, 1988.
168. ROTH, G. S. Mechanisms of altered hormone-neurotransmitter action during aging: from receptors to calcium mobilization. *Ann. Rev. Gerontol. Geriatr.* 10: 132–146, 1990.
169. ROTHUIZEN, J., J. M. H. M. REUL, F. J. VAN SLUIJS, J. A. MOL, A. RIJNBERK, and E. R. DE KLOET. Increased neuroendocrine reactivity and decreased brain mineralocorticoid receptor–binding capacity in aged dogs. *Endocrinology* 132: 161–168, 1993.
170. ROYER, G. L., C. E. SECKMAN, J. H. SCHWARTZ, K. P. BENNETT, and J. W. HENDRIX. Relationship between age and levels of total, free, and bound testosterone in healthy subjects. *Ther. Res.* 35: 345–353, 1984.
171. RUBENS, R., M. DHONT, and A. VERMEULEN. Further studies on Leydig cell function in old age. *J. Clin. Endocrinol. Metab.* 39: 40–45, 1974.
172. RUDMAN, D. Growth hormone, body composition, and aging. *J. Am. Geriatr. Soc.* 33: 800–807, 1985.
173. RUDMAN, D., A. G. FELLER, H. S. NAGRAJ, G. A. GERGANS, P. Y. LALITHA, A. F. GOLDBERG, R. A. SCHLENKER, L. COHN, I. W. RUDMAN, and D. E. MATTSON. Effects of human growth hormone in men over 60 years old. *N. Engl. J. Med.* 323: 1–6, 1990.
174. RUDMAN, D., M. H. VINTNER, C. M. ROGERS, M. F. LUBIN, G. H. FLEMING, and P. B. RAYMOND. Impaired growth hormone secretion in the adult population. Relation to age and adiposity. *J. Clin. Invest.* 67: 1361–1407, 1981.
175. SABATINO, F., E. J. MASORO, C. A. MCMAHAN, and R. W. KUHN. Assessment of the role of the glucocorticoid system in aging processes and in the action of food restriction. *J. Gerontol.* 46: B171–B179, 1991.
176. SACHER, G. A. Life table modification and life prolongation. In: *Handbook of the Biology of Aging*, edited by C. E. Finch and L. Hayflick. New York: Van Nostrand Reinhold, 1977, p. 582–638.
177. SAPOLSKY, R. M. Do glucocorticoid concentrations rise with age in the rat? *Neurobiol. Aging* 13: 171–174, 1992a.
178. SAPOLSKY, R. *Stress, the Aging Brain and the Mechanisms of Neuron Death.* Boston: MIT Press, 1992b.
179. SAPOLSKY, R. M., and J. ALTMANN. Incidence of hypercortisolism and dexamethasone resistance increases with age among wild baboons. *Biol. Psych.* 30: 1008–1016, 1991.
180. SAPOLSKY, R., L. KREY, and B. MCEWEN. Prolonged glucocorticoid exposure reduces hippocampal neuron number: implications for aging. *J. Neurosci.* 5: 1221–1228, 1985.
181. SAPOLSKY, R. M., L. C. KREY, and B. S. MCEWEN. The neuroendocrinology of stress and aging: the glucocorticoid cascade hypothesis. *Endocr. Rev.* 7: 284–301, 1986.
182. SAPOLSKY, R. M., J. H. VOGELMAN, N. ORENTREICH, and J. ALTMANN. Senescent decline in serum dehydroepiandrosterone sulfate concentrations in a population of wild baboons. *J. Gerontol.* 48: B196–B200, 1993.
183. SARATO, T., A. SUZUKI, M. HAYASHI, T. YASUI, T. EGUCHI, and E. KATO. Mechanism of age-related changes in renin and adrenocortical steroids. *J. Am. Geriatr. Soc.* 28: 210–214, 1980.
184. SCHWARTZ, A. Inhibition of spontaneous breast cancer formation in female C3H (Avy/a) mice by long-term treatment with dehydroepiandrosterone. *Cancer* 39: 1129–1132, 1979.
185. SCHWARTZ, A. The effects of dehydroepiandrosterone on the rate of development of cancer and autoimmune processes in laboratory rodents. *Basic Life Sci.* 35: 181–191, 1985.
186. SCHWARTZ, A. G., and R. H. TANNEN. Inhibition of 7,12-dimethylbenz(a)-anthracene and urethan-induced lung tumor formation in A/J mice by long-term treatment with dehydroepiandrosterone. *Carcinogenesis* 2: 1335–1337, 1981.
187. SCHWARTZ, A. G., D. K. FIARMAN, M. POLANSKY, M. L. LEWBART, and L. L. PASHKO. Inhibition of 7,12-dimethylbenz(alpha)anthracene-initiated and tetradecanoylphorbol-13-acetate-promoted skin papilloma formation in mice by dehydroepiandrosterone and two synthetic analogs. *Carcinogenesis* 10: 1809–1813, 1989.
188. SCHWARTZ, S. M., and J. W. KEMNITZ. Age- and gender-related changes in body size, adiposity, and endocrine and metabolic parameters in free-ranging rhesus macaques. *Am. J. Phys. Anthropol.* 89: 109–121, 1992.
189. SELYE, H., and B. TUCHWEBER. Stress in relation to aging and disease. In: *Hypothalamus, Pituitary and Aging*, edited by A. Everitt and J. Burgess. Springfield, IL: Charles C. Thomas, 1976, p. 557–573.
190. SHAPIRO, B. H., T. M. NIEDERMEYER, and G. O. BABALOLA. Serum androgen levels in senescent Cr1:CD-1 (ICR)BR mice:

effects of castration and testosterone treatment. *J. Gerontol.* 44: B15–B19, 1989.

191. SHARMA, M., J. PGALACIOS-BOIS, G. SCHWARTZ, H. ISKANDAR, M. THAKUR, R. QUIRION, and N. P. NAIR. Circadian rhythms of melatonin and cortisol in aging. *Biol. Psychiatry* 25: 305–319, 1989.

192. SHERMAN, B. M., and S. G. KORENMAN. Hormonal characteristics of the human menstrual cycle throughout reproductive life. *J. Clin. Invest.* 55: 699–706, 1975.

193. SHERMAN, B., C. WYSHAM, and B. PFOHL. Age-related changes in the circadian rhythm of plasma cortisol in man. *J. Clin. Endocrinol. Metab.* 61: 439–443, 1985.

194. SHORT, R., N. ENGLAND, W. E. BRIDSON, and D. M. BOWDEN. Ovarian cyclicity, hormones, and behavior as markers of aging in female pigtailed macaques (*Macaca nemestrina*). *J. Gerontol.* 44: B131–B138, 1989.

195. SIMON, D., P. PREZIOSI, E. BARRETT-CONNOR, M. ROGER, M. SAINT-PAUL, K. NAHOUL, and L. PAPOZ. The influence of aging on plasma sex hormones in men: the Telecom Study. *Am. J. Epidemiol.* 135: 783–791, 1992.

196. SLOVITER, R. S., A. L. SOLLAS, E. DEAN, and S. NEUBORT. Adrenalectomy-induced granule cell degeneration in the rat hippocampal dentate gyrus: characterization of an in vivo model of controlled neuronal death. *J. Comp. Neurol.* 330: 324–336, 1993.

197. SLOVITER, R. S., G. VALIQUETTE, G. M. ABRAMS, E. C. RONK, A. L. SOLLAS, L. A. PAUL, and S. NEUBORT. Selective loss of hippocampal granule cells in the mature rat brain after adrenalectomy. *Science* 243: 535–538, 1989.

198. SMITH, E. R., M. L. STEFANICK, J. T. CLARK, and J. M. DAVIDSON. Hormones and sexual behavior in relationship to aging in male rats. *Horm. Behav.* 26: 110–135, 1992.

199. SNOWDON, D. A. Early natural menopause and the duration of postmenopausal life. Findings from a mathematical model of life expectancy. *J. Am. Geriatr. Soc.* 38: 402–408, 1990.

200. SNOWDON, D. A., R. L. KANE, W. L. BERSON, G. L. BURKE, M. SPRAFKA, J. POTTER, H. ISO, D. R. JACOBS, JR., and R. L. PHILLIPS. Is early natural menopause a biologic marker of health and aging? *Am. J. Public Health* 79: 709–714, 1989.

201. SNYDER, P. J., J. F. REITANO, and R. D. UTIGER. Serum LH and FSH responses to synthetic gonadotropin-releasing hormone in normal men. *J. Clin. Endocrinol. Metab.* 41: 938–945, 1975.

202. SONKA, J., and I. GREGOROVA. Effect regulateur de la deshydroepiandrosterone sur le metabolisme. *J. Physiol. (Lond.)* 56: 650–651, 1964.

203. SONNTAG, W. E., and J. MEITES. Decline in growth hormone secretion in aging animals and man. *Interdiscipl. Topics Gerontol.* 24: 111–124, 1988.

204. SONNTAG, W. E., L. J. FORMAN, N. MIKI, J. M. TRAPP, P. E. GOTTSCHALL, and J. MEITES. L-DOPA restores amplitude of growth hormone pulses in old male rats to that observed in young male rats. *Neuroendocrinology* 34: 163–168, 1982.

205. SONNTAG, W., V. HYLKA, and J. MEITES. Growth hormone restores protein synthesis in skeletal muscle of old male rats. *J. Gerontol.* 40: 689–694, 1984.

206. SONNTAG, W. E., J. E. LENHAM, and R. L. INGRAM. Effects of aging and dietary restriction on tissue protein synthesis: relationship to plasma insulin-like growth factor-1. *J. Gerontol.* 47: B159–B163, 1992.

207. SONNTAG, W. E., R. W. STEGER, L. J. FORMAN, and J. MEITES. Decreased pulsatile release of growth hormone in old male rats. *Endocrinology* 107: 1875–1879, 1980.

208. SPARROW, D., R. BOSSE, and J. W. ROWE. The influence of age, alcohol consumption, and body build on gonadal function in men. *J. Clin. Endocrinol. Metab.* 51: 508–512, 1981.

209. SPARROW, D., G. T. O'CONNOR, B. ROSNER, D. DEMOLLES, and S. T. WEISS. A longitudinal study of plasma cortisol concentration and pulmonary function decline in men. The Normative Aging Study. *Am. Rev. Respir. Dis.* 147: 1345–1348, 1993.

210. SPENCER, R. L., A. H. MILLER, M. STEIN, and B. S. MCEWEN. Corticosterone regulation of type I and type II adrenal steroid receptors in brain, pituitary and immune tissue. *Brain Res.* 549: 236–246, 1991.

211. STEARNS, E. L., J. A. MACDONNEL, B. J. KAUFMAN, R. PADUA, T. S. LUCMAN, J. S. D. WINTER, and C. FAIRNAN. Declining testicular function with age, hormonal and clinical correlates. *Am. J. Med.* 57: 761–766, 1974.

212. STEIN-BEHRENS, B. A., and R. M. SAPOLSKY. Stress, glucocorticoids and aging. *Aging* 4: 197–210, 1992.

213. STEWART, J., M. J. MEANEY, D. AITKEN, L. JENSEN, and N. KALANT. The effects of acute and life-long food restriction on basal and stress-induced serum corticosterone levels in young and aged rat. *Endocrinology* 123: 1934–1941, 1988.

214. SUCHNER, U., M. M. ROTHKOPF, G. STANISLAUS, D. H. ELWYN, V. KVETAN, and J. ASKANAZI. Growth hormone and pulmonary disease. Metabolic effects in patients receiving parenteral nutrition. *Arch. Intern. Med.* 150: 1225–1230, 1990.

215. SUZUKI, K., S. INABA, H. TAKEUCHI, Y. TAKEZAWA, Y. FUKABORI, T. SUZUKI, K. IMAI, H. YAMANAKA, and S. HONMA. Endocrine environment of benign prostatic hyperpasia—relationship of sex steroid hormone levels with age and the size of the prostate. *Nippon Hinyokika Gakkai Zasshi* 83: 664–671, 1992.

216. SWERDLOFF, R. S., C. WANG, M. HINES, and R. GORSKI. Effect of androgens on the brain and other organs during development and aging. *Psychoneuroendocrinology* 17: 375–383, 1992.

217. TAKAHASHI, S., P. GOTTSCHALL, K. QUIGLEY, R. GOYA, and J. MEITES. Growth hormone secretory patterns in young, middle-aged, and old female rats. *Neuroendocrinology* 46: 137–142, 1987.

218. TAKUKARA, K., H. YAMADA, and V. P. HOLLANDER. The effect of growth hormone on development of plasma cell tumour lymphosarcoma. *Cancer Res.* 27: 2034–2038, 1967.

219. TALBERT, G. B., and J. B. HAMILTON. Duration of life in Lewis strain of rats after gonadectomy at birth and at older ages. *J. Gerontol.* 20: 489–491, 1965.

220. TENOVER, J. S. Effects of testosterone supplementation in the aging male. *J. Clin. Endocrinol. Metab.* 75: 1092–1098, 1992.

221. THUN, M. J., M. M. NAMBOODIRI, and C. W. HEATH. Aspirin use and reduced risk of fatal colon cancer. *N. Engl. J. Med.* 325: 1593–1596, 1991.

222. TOUITOU, Y., J. SULON, A. BOGDAN, A. REINBERG, J.-C. SODOYEZ, and E. DEMEY-PONSART. Adrenocortical hormones, ageing and mental condition: seasonal and circadian rhythms of plasma 18-hydroxy-11-deoxycorticosterone, total and free cortisol and urinary corticosteroids. *J. Endocrinol.* 96: 53–64, 1983.

223. TOUITOU, J. SULON, A. BOGDAN, C. TOUITOU, A. REINBERG, H. BECK, J. C. SODOYEZ, E. DMEY-PONSART, and H. VAN CAUWENBERG. Adrenal circadian system in young and elderly human subjects; a comparative study. *J. Endocrinol.* 93: 201–210, 1982.

224. TRELOAR, A. E. Menstrual cyclicity and the pre-menopause. *Maturitas* 3: 249–264, 1981.

225. TRELOAR, A. E., R. E. BOYNTON, B. G. BEHN, and B. W. BROWN. Variation of the human menstrual cycle through reproductive life. *Int. J. Fertil.* 12: 77–126, 1970.

226. TSITOURAS, P. D., C. E. MARTIN, and S. M. HARMAN. Relationship of serum testosterone to sexual activity in healthy elderly men. *J. Gerontol.* 37: 288–293, 1982.
227. VANCE, M. L., D. L. KAISER, W. S. EVANS, R. FURLANETTO, W. VALE, J. RIVIER, and M. O. THORNER. Pulsatile growth hormone secretion in normal man during a continuous 24-hour infusion of human growth hormone releasing factor (1–40). Evidence for intermittent somatostatin secretion. *J. Clin. Invest.* 74: 1584–1590.
228. VAN EEKELEN, J. A. M., N. Y. ROTS, W. SUTANTO, and E. R. DEKLOET. The effect of aging on stress responsiveness and central corticosteroid receptors in the Brown Norway rat. *Neurobiol. Aging* 13: 159–170, 1992.
229. VELDHUIS, J. D., R. J. URBAN, G. LIZARRALDE, M. L. JOHNSON, and A. IRANMANESH. Attenuation of luteinizing hormone secretory burst amplitude as a proximate basis for the hypoandrogenism of healthy aging in men. *J. Clin. Endocrinol. Metab.* 75: 707–713, 1992.
230. VERMEULEN, A. Nyctohemoral growth hormone profiles in young and aged men: correlations with somatomedin-C levels. *J. Clin. Endocrinol. Metab.* 64: 884–888, 1987.
231. VERMEULEN, A. Clinical review 24: androgens in the aging male. *J. Clin. Endocrinol. Metab.* 63: 221–224, 1991.
232. VERMEULEN, A., R. RUBENS, and L. VERDONCK. Testosterone secretion and metabolism in male senescence. *J. Clin. Endocrinol. Metab.* 34: 730–735, 1972.
233. VOM SAAL, F. S., C. E. FINCH, and J. F. NELSON. Natural history and mechanisms of reproductive aging in humans, laboratory rodents, and other selected vertebrates. In: *The Physiology of Reproduction* (2nd ed.), edited by E. Knobil and J. Neill. New York: Raven Press, 1994, p. 927–965.
234. WALDRON, I. Sex differences in human mortality: the role of genetic factors. *Soc. Sci. Med.* 17: 321–333, 1983.
235. WALTMAN, C., M. R. BLACKMAN, G. P. CHROUSOS, C. RIEMANN, and S. M. HARMAN. Spontaneous and glucocorticoid-inhibited adrenocorticotropic hormone and cortisol secretion are similar in healthy young and old men. *J. Clin. Endocrinol. Metab.* 73: 945–502, 1992.
236. WEILAND, N. G., K. SCARBOROUGH, and P. M. WISE. Aging abolishes the estradiol-induced suppression and diurnal rhythm of proopiomelanocortin gene expression in the arcuate nucleus. *Endocrinology* 131: 2959–2964, 1992.
237. WEINDRUCH, R. H., G. MCFEETERS, and R. L. WALFORD. Food intake reduction and immunologic alterations in mice fed dehydroepiandrosterone. *Exp. Gerontol.* 19: 297–394, 1984.
238. WEXLER, B. C. Spontaneous arteriosclerosis in repeatedly bred male and female rats. *J. Atherosclerosis Res.* 45: 613–631, 1964.
239. WEXLER, B. C. Comparative aspects of hyperadrenocorticism and aging. In: *Hypothalamus, Pituitary and Aging*, edited by A. V. Everitt and J. A. Burgess. Springfield, IL: Charles C. Thomas, 1976, p. 333–361.
240. WILLARD, J. E., R. A. LANGE, and L. D. HILLIS. Review article: the use of aspirin in ischemic heart disease. *N. Engl. J. Med.* 327: 175–181, 1990.
241. WILLIAMS, T., M. BERELOWITZ, S. N. JOFFE, M. O. THORNER, J. RIVIER, W. VALE, and L. A. FROHMAN. Impaired growth hormone responses to growth hormone-releasing factor in obesity. *N. Engl. J. Med.* 211: 1403–1407, 1984.
242. WILSON, M. E., T. P. GORDON, and D. C. COLLINS. Age differences in copulatory behavior and serum 17β-estradiol in female rhesus monkeys. *Physiol. Behav.* 28: 733–737, 1982.
243. WINER, L. M., M. A. SHAW, and G. BAUMAN. Basal plasma growth hormone levels in man: new evidence for rhythmicity of growth hormone secretion. *J. Clin. Endocrinol. Metab.* 70: 1678–1686, 1990.
244. WINGARD, D. L. The sex differential in morbidity, mortality and lifestyle. *Annu. Rev. Public Health* 5: 433–458, 1984.
245. WISE, P. M., R. C. WALOVITCH, I. R. COHEN, N. G. WEILAND, and E. D. LONDON. Diurnal rhythmicity and hypothalamic deficits in glucose utilization in aged ovariectomized rats. *J. Neurosci.* 7: 3469–3473, 1987.
246. WISE, P. M., N. G. WEILAND, K. SCARBOROUGH, G. H. LARSON, and J. M. LLOYD. Contribution of changing rhythmicity of hypothalamic neurotransmitter function to female reproductive aging. *Ann. N. Y. Acad. Sci.* 592: 31–43, 1990.
247. YU, B. P., E. J. MASORO, and C. A. MCMAHAN. Nutritional influences on aging of Fischer 344 rats. 1. Physical, metabolic and longevity characteristics. *J. Gerontol.* 40: 657–670, 1985.
248. ZADIK, Z., S. A. CHALEW, R. J. MCCARTER, M. MEISTAS, and A. A. KOWARSKI. The influence of age on the 24-hour integrated concentration of growth hormone in normal individuals. *J. Clin. Endocrinol. Metab.* 60: 513–516, 1985.
249. ZUMOFF, B., D. K. FUKUSHIMA, E. D. WEITZMAN, J. KREAM, and L. HELLMAN. The sex difference in plasma cortisol concentration in men. *J. Clin. Endocrinol. Metab.* 39: 805–812, 1974.
250. ZUMOFF, B., G. W. STRAIN, J. KREAM, J. O'CONNOR, R. S. ROSENFELD, J. LEVIN, and D. K. FUKUSHIMA. Age variation of the 24-hour mean plasma concentration of androgens, estrogens, and gonadotropins in normal adult men. *J. Clin. Endocrinol. Metab.* 54: 534–538, 1982.

16. Bone

DIKE N. KALU | *Department of Physiology, University of Texas Health Science Center, San Antonio, Texas*

CHAPTER CONTENTS

Bone Composition
Bone Cells
Bone Remodeling
Bone Loss as a Major Occurrence during Aging
Osteoporosis
Parathyroid Hormone, 1,25(OH)$_2$Vitamin D, and Calcitonin
Altered Calcium Homeostatic Control Hypotheses
Rat Model of Postmenopausal Bone Loss
Altered Hematopoiesis and Local Factor Hypothesis
Risk Factors for Age-Related Bone Loss
    Peak bone mass
    Exercise
    Nutrition
    Smoking, alcohol, and caffeine
Estrogen Receptors in Intestinal Cells

THE STRONG INTEREST IN RESEARCH ON BONE AND MINERAL METABOLISM relates in large part to the need for an understanding of the etiology of age-related bone loss. The hope is that such an understanding will lead to effective strategies for preventing bone loss and for managing the bone disease osteoporosis. Although these goals have yet to be achieved, the past decade has witnessed significant advances in the understanding of bone and mineral metabolism. The state-of-the-art reviews in *Bone and Mineral Research* (133) are an excellent resource for the interested reader. This chapter examines bone loss as a major occurrence during aging; following a brief review of bone composition and remodeling, it explores the factors underlying bone loss.

BONE COMPOSITION

The skeleton supports the body, permits locomotion, and protects vital organs. It contains 99% of the body calcium and is a potential source of calcium for maintaining extracellular calcium homeostasis when exogenous calcium is deficient. Tight regulation of calcium homeostasis is of great importance because the calcium ion is critical to many vital physiological process, including muscle contraction, neuromuscular excitability, cardiac rhythmicity, membrane permeability, exocytotic secretion of macromolecules, blood clotting, mitotic activity, and many enzyme reactions (86). The structure of bone is well suited to its many functions. Bone is a specialized connective tissue composed of an extracellular organic matrix impregnated with an inorganic component. The combination of mineral and organic material accounts for the great strength of bone and for its ability to withstand stress. These attributes become compromised with aging as bone-forming activities begin to lag behind bone resorption.

The inorganic component accounts for about 65% of the dry weight of bone and is made up primarily of calcium phosphate crystals similar to crystalline hydroxyapatite and some amorphous calcium phosphate salts. Organic compounds make up the remaining 35% of the dry weight of bone. About 90% of the organic matrix is collagen, which is the most common form of extracellular matrix protein. Collagen consists of three polypeptides that form an extremely stable triple-helical molecule. About ten types of collagen have been recognized (105). Bone contains mainly type 1 collagen, a heteropolymer consisting of two $\alpha 1(l)$ chains and one $\alpha 2(l)$ chain. Hydroxyproline, a marker for collagen, is measured in biological fluids as a useful, though nonspecific, index of bone collagen turnover, because, although 57% of body collagen is in bone, tissues other than bone contain collagen. Type 1 collagen is rich in glycosylated hydroxylysines that are excreted in urine and appear more resistant to degradation than hydroxyproline. The determination of these hydroxylysine glycosides in urine provides useful information on both the level and the origin of collagen breakdown (26). Recent reports indicate that the pyridinium cross-links of collagen, pyridinoline (Pyr) and deoxypyridinoline (dPyr), are released during bone degradation and can be measured in urine as specific indices of the rate of bone resorption (27).

The remaining 10% of the organic matrix of bone contains noncollagen proteins. About 25% of these are adsorbed to bone matrix from circulating proteins, such as serum albumin and platelet-derived growth factor (PDGF). While the latter may have a role in bone regeneration, the function of albumin in bone is unknown (173). The other noncollagen proteins in bone matrix are *(1)* proteins that facilitate cell attachment, such as fibronectin, thrombospondin, osteopontin, and bone sialoprotein; *(2)* proteoglycans, such as chondroitin and heparin sulfate, whose functions remain unclear; *(3)* growth-related proteins, such as transforming growth factor (TGF)-β and insulin-like growth factors (IGF)-I and II; and *(4)* vitamin K–dependent, gamma-carboxylated (gla) proteins, such as osteocalcin (bone-gla-protein) and matrix-gla-protein, which have calcium-binding properties (174). Osteocalcin is of particular interest because it makes up 15%–20% of noncollagenous bone protein and appears to be present almost exclusively in bone (62, 135). Although its role in bone physiology remains undefined, it is measured in biological fluids as a specific marker of the rate of bone turnover (58, 136, 161).

BONE CELLS

There are three principal types of bone cell: osteoblasts, osteocytes and osteoclasts. Osteoblasts are mononucleated cells with a basophilic cytoplasm and the fine structure of cells actively involved in protein synthesis and secretion (76). They are rich in alkaline phosphatase. Their origin is unclear but appears to involve stromal stem cells in marrow (125). Mature osteoblasts synthesize the wide variety of bone matrix proteins previously described, and they are the source of matrix vesicles, which appear to be involved in the mineralization of bone (3). Osteoblasts also synthesize collagenase (71, 124) and prostaglandin E (151) in response to stimulators of bone resorption. Osteoblasts that are no longer actively secreting bone matrix eventually become encased in calcified bone. These are the osteocytes, and they are the most abundant bone cell type. Osteocytes have long protoplasmic canaliculi with which they contact neighboring osteocytes. Their role in bone biology is uncertain. Some believe that osteocytes resorb bone and respond to parathyroid hormone (PTH) (10) and that by virtue of their large number they play an important role in the regulation of calcium homeostasis (141). Others cannot find convincing evidence that osteocytes engage in metabolic activities that result in osteocytic osteolysis (13, 159). Osteocytes also make contact by means of their canaliculi with the lining cells that separate bone from the extracellular fluid (ECF). It has been postulated that PTH acts on these lining cells to regulate the supply of calcium from the bone fluid compartment to the ECF by a mechanism that does not involve osteolysis (170).

The main resorbing cells in bone are the osteoclasts. They are large, multinucleated cells characterized by a ruffled border in the region in contact with bone undergoing resorption. Accumulating evidence supports the notion that osteoclasts are hematopoietic in origin and derive from the fusion of mononuclear cells from bone marrow (117, 179). They appear to arise from colony-forming units for the granulocyte-macrophage series (CFU-GM) (115, 117). An opposing view is that their lineage, beyond their origin in hematopoietic tissue, is completely unknown (20). Osteoclasts are found in sites of bone undergoing resorption. They resorb bone by producing H^+ ions which decalcify the surrounding bone and provide an optimum acid pH for the lysosomal enzymes they secrete to degrade the exposed bone matrix.

BONE REMODELING

Mature bone is continuously undergoing resorption and reformation by a process known as *bone remodeling*. Although the exact function of bone remodeling is not known, there are four possibilities: Maintaining the mechanical competence of bone by renewing its components and by preventing or removing fatigue and microdamage within bone, maintaining the microscopic structure and the macroscopic shape of bone, determining the net amount of bone present at any time, and providing mineral to maintain extracellular fluid calcium.

Remodeling is initiated by the appearance in bone of osteoclasts at the site to be remodeled, such as the cortical–endosteal surface, the trabecular–endosteal surface, or the interior of cortical bone (44). The osteoclasts resorb a quantum amount of bone. After a brief period the cavity formed by osteoclasts is lined by osteoblasts that act to refill the hollow with new bone which they lay down in concentric layers. The newly formed resorption cavities and those in the process of being refilled with bone are termed "basic multicellular units" (BMUs) (45). When the refilling is complete, the resultant new bone is the bone structural unit (BSU), haversian system, or osteon. Thus bone remodeling occurs in an orderly sequence involving an initiation phase, a resorption phase, and a formation phase, with a reversal phase between resorption and formation (8, 130). In humans, the resorption phase lasts for about 21 days, and the formation phase is completed in several months (142). In the young adult, the coupling of formation to resorption is balanced such that there is no net loss of bone as a result of remodeling. However, defects in this balance occur with advancing age.

Defects in bone remodeling can be expressed in several ways: the resorption cavities could become too large; there could be too many of them; and their refilling with new bone could be delayed, slowed, or incomplete. Any one of these or any combination of them can result in less bone. Currently, it is not clear what initiates the activation of BMUs or what controls their birth rate, number, and life span at any instant; nor is it known how osteoclasts or their precursors are attracted to sites destined to be resorbed. The signals for terminating osteoclastic resorption and initiating osteoblastic bone formation are equally unknown, as is the subsequent fate of osteoclasts. The clarification of these uncertainties about bone remodeling is crucial and remains the subject of intense research, because the bone loss that occurs with aging in humans likely results from remodeling defects in which resorption exceeds formation (160).

BONE LOSS AS A MAJOR OCCURRENCE DURING AGING

In their classification of aging as "usual" or "successful," bone loss was included in the "usual" class by Rowe and Kahn (153) because every population that has been studied exhibits a decline in bone mass with aging. As such, age-related bone loss appears to be an inevitable consequence of aging. Nearly all bones of the skeleton are affected to varying degrees, with loss being greater in women than in men. Although there is a consensus that age-related bone loss is a universal occurrence, there is lack of agreement on the age at which it begins. The onset and magnitude of bone loss depend on gender and the type of bone. Some reports indicate that in women vertebral bone loss begins as early as the third decade and continues linearly with aging, while loss of appendicular bone does not begin until about 51 yr of age (146). In comparison to women, normal men start to lose bone at a much later age, and for some bones, the degree of loss is trivial (146). By far the most consistent observation is that bone loss accelerates following menopause and contributes importantly to the high prevalence of osteoporosis in postmenopausal women.

OSTEOPOROSIS

Osteoporosis is characterized by low bone mass and increased susceptibility of fracture from minor trauma. It afflicts 15–20 million Americans and accounts for 1.3 million fractures annually in people aged 45 yr and older (4). The cost to society of the management of osteoporosis and its consequences in the U.S.A. is about 7 billion dollars (75). This is likely to rise as the demographic shift to a more aged population continues, unless methods are developed to detect those patients at risk and preventive therapeutic measures initiated (6).

Osteoporosis is classified as primary or secondary (110). Secondary osteoporosis is usually associated with a recognizable disease or medical therapy and accounts for about 10% of osteoporotic conditions. The majority of osteoporotic patients belong to the primary subclass, which includes idiopathic osteoporosis in children and young adults and involutional osteoporosis in adult and aging individuals. The main forms of involutional osteoporosis are postmenopausal and senile osteoporosis (2), also designated type I and type II osteoporosis, respectively (110). Type I osteoporosis is by far the most common form of age-related bone loss. In type I osteoporosis cancellous bone is mainly affected, and the accelerated bone loss is usually associated with fractures of the vertebrae and distal radius in individuals 51–75 yr of age; the main predisposing factor is menopause. Men also suffer from age-related bone loss that has the characteristics of type 1 osteoporosis; however, in type I osteoporosis women outnumber men 6:1. The lower incidence of type I osteoporosis in men has been attributed to higher peak bone mass, shorter life expectancy, and the absence of a clear-cut equivalent to menopause associated with accelerated bone loss (80). Type II osteoporosis is seen mostly in people 70 yr and older, with a ratio of about 2:1 between women and men; the bone loss involves both cancellous and cortical bone and results mainly in vertebral wedge and hip fractures. The main predisposing factor appears to be a decrease in bone formation due simply to aging (110).

Because bone loss associated with menopause is the most common form and predisposes to osteoporosis, it has attracted a great deal of attention and continues to be intensely studied. Menopause is characterized by an initial period of rapid bone loss followed by a slower rate (47, 131). The first phase occurs within the first 10 yr following the cessation of menses or therapeutic ovariectomy and is the result of increased bone turnover in which osteoclastic bone resorption exceeds formation. Both bone matrix and mineral are lost and the net effect is too little bone, the remainder being essentially normal. In one study in which surgically ovariectomized women were followed for 12 yr after ovariectomy, cortical and cancellous bone losses were 2.8% and 8.0%, respectively, in the first year; subsequently, the rate of loss decreased exponentially (165). Low serum estrogen has been implicated in bone loss, especially during the rapid phase (2, 102, 149, 160). Evidence of increased bone formation and resorption, with resorption exceeding formation, comes from radiocalcium kinetics studies (69, 70) and from increased biochemical indices of bone turnover (28, 51, 83). This was well demonstrated in a longitudinal study in which biochemical and other parameters related to skeletal remodeling were measured in 36 premenopausal women who underwent bilateral ovariectomy (40). Increases in the urinary hydroxyproline:creatinine ratio, serum calcium, phosphate, and alkaline phosphatase were seen at 6 wk after surgery; serum bone gla protein (osteocalcin) and whole-body retention of ^{99m}Tc-HEDP were elevated at 3 months, and the urinary calcium:creatinine ratio became significantly elevated at 6 months. At 18 months many of these parameters remained elevated, but by 24 months most parameters were falling toward baseline.

Although the pathogenesis of postmenopausal bone loss is related to ovarian hormone deficiency, the exact mechanism by which loss of ovarian hormones results in osteoporosis continues to be elusive. For a long time, much attention was focused on the calcium-regulating hormones, which are known to be major regulators of bone metabolism as well. It has also long been appreciated that extracellular calcium homeostasis is very tightly controlled on account of the important role of the calcium ion in the regulation of diverse cellular functions. With most of the body calcium in bone, it was reasonable to consider that defects in the hormonal regulation of calcium homeostasis may be involved in the age-related loss of bone calcium. For instance, with the age- related decrease in calcium availability, due to low dietary intake or intestinal malabsorption, the calcium-regulating hormones would mobilize calcium from bone to maintain extracellular calcium homeostasis and continue to do so as long as the deficit persists, even at the expense of the structural and mechanical functions of bone. This implication of calcium deficiency in aging bone loss is supported by the documentation that the diet of the average woman is relatively deficient in calcium (69, 122), dietary calcium intake decreases with aging, and at any age most women, who are known to lose more bone than men with aging, also ingest less calcium than men (1). Nevertheless, the role of dietary calcium in human aging bone loss is controversial. We will return to the subject later, following a brief review of the calcium-regulating hormones PTH, 1,25(OH)$_2$vitamin D, and calcitonin.

PARATHYROID HORMONE, 1,25(OH)$_2$VITAMIN D, AND CALCITONIN

The chief cells of the parathyroid glands secrete one major hormonal product, parathyroid hormone (PTH), which is initially synthesized as a high-molecular-weight precursor protein called "preproparathyroid hormone." The latter is converted to PTH intracellularly by a sequential removal of peptide fragments from the amino terminal end, first to ProPTH and then to PTH with 84 amino acid residues (60). The biological activity of PTH resides in the amino terminal part of the molecule, with the 1–34 fragment being as active as the native 1–84PTH, while the carboxyl-terminal portion is biologically inactive (59). PTH provides calcium to the ECF by stimulating calcium release from bone, enhancing renal tubular reabsorption of calcium, and promoting the activity of renal 1α- hydroxylase, which catalyzes the conversion of 25(OH)vitamin D to 1,25(OH)$_2$vitamin D (43, 52). PTH also prevents an excessive increase in plasma phosphate by inhibiting proximal renal tubular reabsorption of phosphate, thereby ensuring that calcium is retained in the ECF and not deposited in tissues as calcium phosphate salt. PTH promotes an increase in osteoclastic number and activity and thereby plays a central role in bone modeling and remodeling. Osteoblasts, but not osteoclasts, contain receptors for PTH (157), and the presence of osteoblasts appears to be required for the expression of the osteoclastic activity of PTH. These findings led to the notion that PTH induces osteoblasts to secrete a factor(s) that activates osteoclastic activity (150). Although PTH resorbs bone and inhibits bone matrix synthesis acutely, when given intermittently it has a paradoxical bone anabolic action (94).

Vitamin D, also called cholecalciferol, is a steroid derivative. It can be ingested in the diet as a vitamin or formed from 7- dehydrocholesterol by irradiation of the skin with ultraviolet light from the sun. Normal individuals who have sufficient daily exposure to sunlight synthesize enough endogenous vitamin D$_3$ to meet their requirements. Vitamin D$_3$ itself is biologically inactive. It is hydroxylated in the liver to 25-hydroxycholecalciferol [25(OH)vitamin D$_3$], which is the main circulating form of vitamin D$_3$ (134). In the kidney, 25(OH)vitamin D$_3$ is hydroxylated to form 24,25-dihydroxycholecalciferol, whose hormonal function has been disputed (30, 140), and 1,25-dihydroxycholecalciferol [1,25(OH)$_2$vitamin D$_3$], believed to be the definitive hormonal and most active form of the vitamin D$_3$ metabolites (43, 52). Like PTH, 1,25(OH)$_2$vitamin D$_3$ increases the number and activity of osteoclasts by mechanisms that involve enhanced differentiation and fusion of osteoclast progenitors to form osteoclasts (117). 1,25(OH)$_2$vitamin D$_3$ is also the major hormonal regulator of intestinal absorption of calcium and phosphate and maintains the concentrations of these ions at levels in plasma that are compatible with optimum mineralization of bone (29, 30). Whether or not 1,25(OH)$_2$vitamin D$_3$ also acts directly on bone to stimulate mineralization is uncertain. In vivo it may act in concert with PTH to regulate bone resorption and remodeling. Receptors for active 1,25(OH)$_2$vitamin D$_3$ have been localized in the intestine, in bone lining cells, and in osteoblasts (122).

The third of the classical calcium-regulating hormones is calcitonin, which is secreted by the C cells of the thyroid in mammals, including humans (23, 41, 73). Calcitonin is a single-chain polypeptide consisting of 32 amino acid residues with a carboxyl-terminal proline amide and an N-terminal 1–7 disulphide ring that are essential for optimum biological activity. Higher-molecular-weight, immunoreactive, calcitonin-like molecules that appear to be aggregates of calcitonin circulate in plasma (158). Calcitonin has potent hypocalcemic and hypophosphatemic properties. Its physiological significance in the regulation of calcium homeostasis is, however, in doubt because calcitonin deficiency or excess does not compromise plasma calcium levels in humans. However, in lower animals, calcitonin appears to have a role in controlling postprandial hypercalcemia (57), and its deficiency in fasted rats causes an immediate but transient hypercalcemia, indicating some role in the maintenance of normocalcemia as well (91). In contrast to PTH, calcitonin decreases the size, number, and motility of osteoclasts and acts directly on these cells, which have calcitonin receptors, to inhibit their activity. Consequently, like PTH, calcitonin may be important in the physiological regulation of bone resorption and remodeling.

ALTERED CALCIUM HOMEOSTATIC CONTROL HYPOTHESES

Having described the classical calcium-regulating hormones, a discussion of their implication in age-related bone loss follows. There has been a long association of the calcium-regulating hormones with bone loss due to ovarian hormone deficiency in women following menopause. The various hypotheses that have been proposed to account for bone loss share the idea of the linkage of ovarian hormone deficiency with alterations in the levels or activities of the calcium-regulating hormones, but with differing emphases on the relative contributions of PTH, calcitonin, and 1,25(OH)$_2$vitamin D or their deficiency to the imbalance in bone turnover that results in bone loss. In view of the linkage of these hypotheses to alterations in the calcium-regulating hormones and their actions, we have put them in a group designated the "altered calcium homeostatic control hypotheses" of postmenopausal bone loss. Figure 16.1 is a composite of these hypotheses, which were developed over many years with contributions from numerous investigators (14, 49, 63–65, 84, 144, 166, 184). According to the best known of the hypotheses, the loss of estrogen at menopause removes the inhibitory influence of the sex steroids on the osteolytic action of PTH, with a resultant increase in bone dissolution. This would result in a rise in plasma calcium and a feedback inhibition of PTH secretion, in the face of increased sensitivity of bone to the resorbing action of the hormone. The lowering of circulating PTH would decrease the activation of 25-(OH)D-1α-hydroxylase, resulting in a fall in the renal conversion of 25(OH)vitamin D$_3$ to 1,25-

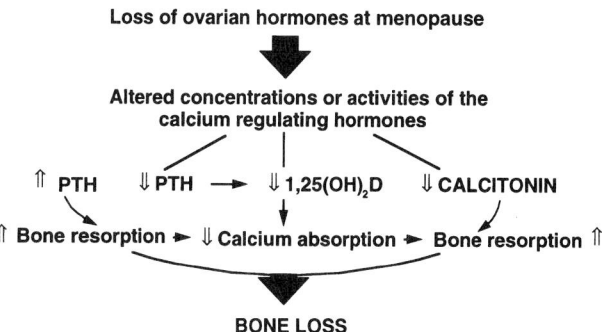

FIG. 16.1. The altered calcium homeostatic control hypotheses for the pathogenesis of postmenopausal bone loss.

(OH)$_2$vitamin D$_3$ and a decrease in intestinal absorption of calcium. The net result is a decrease in bone mass as bone calcium mobilization is increased to maintain extracellular calcium homeostasis. Support for this hypothesis comes from the observation that in some postmenopausal osteoporotic women, serum 1,25-(OH)$_2$vitamin D and intestinal absorption of calcium are low (49). Treatment of such women with estrogen has been reported to lower their serum calcium and increase their circulating PTH (145, 184). Furthermore, therapeutic ovariectomy in premenopausal women has been reported to result in increased plasma and urinary calcium (129, 183), as would be expected if estrogen normally antagonized the osteolytic action of PTH.

However, not all the available data are in line with the altered calcium homeostatic control hypotheses for the pathogenesis of postmenopausal bone loss. First, the hypotheses predict low circulating PTH in postmenopausal women in response to ovarian hormone deficiency–induced bone calcium dissolution. Actual measurements indicate that plasma PTH increases with age, and in postmenopausal osteoporotics it is high, low, or normal (11, 21, 50, 172, 180). Second, early postmenopausal bone loss does not appear to be associated with a decrease in the circulating level of 1,25(OH)$_2$vitamin D as would occur secondary to the postulated decrease in PTH-mediated hydroxylation of 25(OH)vitamin D (38). Furthermore, in a recent study of a subset of healthy, active men and women aged 20–96 yr from the Baltimore Longitudinal Study of Aging, serum 25(OH)vitamin D and 1,25(OH)$_2$vitamin D did not change with age in either sex. Total and ionized calcium remained constant women, while serum intact PTH increased significantly over the age span in both sexes. The investigators concluded that it is unlikely that the greater bone loss with aging in females than in males can be explained by alteration in vitamin D status or the circulating levels of the bone mineral regulating hormones (156). Similarly, in another a recent report, the bone mineral density of women who underwent therapeutic oophorectomy was lower than that of female controls of the same age. In contrast, the levels of the calcium-regulating hormones were not significantly different in the two groups (123).

Another aspect of the altered calcium homeostatic control hypotheses is the linkage of age-related bone loss due to menopause to calcitonin deficiency (166). Since calcitonin inhibits osteoclastic bone resorption, its withdrawal at menopause can explain the subsequent increase in bone loss as PTH-mediated bone resorption will then proceed unopposed. The implications of the calcitonin deficiency hypothesis are that some relationship exists between ovarian hormones and the secretion of calcitonin and that the latter falls with the cessation of menses. Several observations support this hypothesis. Basal circulating calcitonin levels and calcitonin secretory response to calcium challenge are lower in women than in men and decrease with aging (25); women on the estrogen–progestogen contraceptive pill have elevated calcitonin levels (72); in some studies serum calcitonin is reported to be lower in postmenopausal osteoporotics than in age-matched controls (111); and therapeutic ablation of the thyroid source of calcitonin has been associated with decreased bone mass (108). Other findings are not as supportive of the calcitonin deficiency hypothesis. For instance, calcitonin-deficient subjects and patients secreting excessive amounts of calcitonin were not found to be at greater risk of osteoporosis than normal individuals (37, 78). Furthermore, stable levels of circulating calcitonin have been observed with aging (12) in spite of the loss of bone that occurs with aging. Because there is a heterogeneity in the circulating forms of calcitonin, differences in the serum calcitonin species being measured could account in part for the apparent conflicts in the reports from various laboratories of the influence of aging on calcitonin levels. Nevertheless, from the foregoing observations it seems unlikely that alterations in the actions of the classical calcium-regulating hormones play the primary etiological role in the pathogenesis of postmenopausal bone loss.

RAT MODEL OF POSTMENOPAUSAL BONE LOSS

Rats can be ovariectomized to make them sex hormone–deficient and to simulate the accelerated loss of bone that occurs in women following menopause. Ovariectomy-induced bone loss in the rat and postmenopausal bone loss share many similar characteristics (46, 88, 181) (Table 16.1). These include increased rate of bone turnover, with resorption exceeding formation; an initial rapid phase of bone loss followed by a much slower phase; greater loss of cancellous bone than cortical bone; decreased intestinal absorption of calcium; some

TABLE 16.1. *Comparison of Postmenopausal Bone Loss with the Ovariectomized Rat Bone Loss Model*

Parameters	Postmenopausal Bone Loss	Ovariectomized Rat Bone Loss Model
Ovarian hormones	↓	↓
Bone mass	↓	↓
Rate of bone turnover	↑	↑
Resorption > Formation	Yes	Yes
Biochemical indices of bone turnover	↑	↑
Cancellous bone loss > Cortical bone loss	Yes	Yes
Bone loss involves BMUs	Yes	Yes
Bones respond similarly to identical therapies	Yes	Yes
Intestinal calcium absorption	↓	↓
Calcium-regulating hormones	↔ ↓	↔ ↓
Primary involvement of the calcium-regulating hormones	Unlikely	Unlikely
Involvement of the hematopoietic system	Likely	Likely
Involvement of cytokines	Likely	Likely

↓, decreased; ↑, increased; ↔, unchanged.

protection against bone loss by obesity; and similar skeletal response to therapy with estrogen, tamoxifen, bisphosphonates, PTH, calcitonin, and exercise. Furthermore, bone remodeling based on BMUs occurs in humans as in rats and becomes impaired following ovarian hormone deficiency in both species. These wide-ranging similarities are strong evidence that the ovariectomized rat model is suitable for studying problems relevant to postmenopausal bone loss (46, 88, 181). It is also of note that observations from the ovariectomized rat model agree with many human studies, indicating that a change in the circulating levels of the calcium-regulating hormones appears not to be obligatory for the bone loss that occurs in ovarian hormone deficiency (88, 92).

In spite of the foregoing, the rat was not always considered appropriate for studying age-related bone loss in humans. A major hindrance to the acceptance of the rat model was the notion that "human osteoporosis is a disease of BMU-based remodeling, and that rats and mice lack useful amounts of BMUs, and so cannot provide good models of the human disease or its treatment" (46). However, the evidence that has accumulated in recent years makes this view no longer tenable, according to H. M. Frost, the original protagonist of the inappropriateness of the rat for studying human bone loss. In a recent review (46) Frost and Jee argued that:

The idea that rats cannot model human osteopenias errs. The same mechanisms control gains in bone mass (longitudinal bone growth and modeling drifts) and losses (BMU-based modeling) in young and aged rats and humans. Furthermore, they respond similarly in rats and man to mechanical influences, hormones, drugs and other agents.... The rat can provide a very useful model of human osteopenias and of some other currently important human skeletal problems. The opinion that it would not stemmed from incomplete knowledge and it errs.

It is clear from the foregoing and from recent reviews (88, 181) that we are witnessing the beginning of the demise of the stigma associated with the use of the rat model for studying problems related to human bone loss. This development is of the utmost importance since it is evident that the study of any disease will profit from the availability of a well-characterized and generally accepted animal model. An appropriate animal model will, in particular, facilitate the exploration of new hypotheses for the etiological mechanisms underlying the pathogenesis of age-related bone loss, which have remained unknown.

ALTERED HEMATOPOIESIS AND LOCAL FACTOR HYPOTHESIS

If the altered calcium homeostatic control hypotheses involving systemic calcium-regulating hormones do not adequately explain the etiological basis for the pathogenesis of postmenopausal bone loss due to ovarian hormone deficiency, are there alternative hypotheses? Accumulating evidence indicates that the answer to this question is in the affirmative and may focus on factors that act within bone in an autocrine/paracrine fashion (114, 137). For instance, it has been known for some time that in postmenopausal osteoporosis all bones are not usually equally affected and that the major sites of bone loss are cancellous bone in the vertebrae and distal radius (147). If only systemic factors were primarily involved, the increased bone resorption would occur randomly on all bones (8). Therefore, the regional nature of aging bone loss points to local defects in the regulatory processes that control and integrate the precisely coordinated activities of key cells involved in bone remodeling. Also, the coupling of bone formation to resorption during remodeling is likely mediated locally by paracrine factors released from bone in the process of resorption (35, 77, 114). Candidate coupling factors may come from bone, bone cells, and marrow and include bone TGF-β and IGF-I and II, which are present in bone and known to stimulate osteoblastic activity (35, 77, 114). In fact, it is now clear that bone and related cells from marrow synthesize a plethora of growth factors and cytokines that most likely act locally to modify the replication or the differentiated function of cells of the osteoclast and osteoblast lineages. In addition to TGF-β and the IGFs, these growth factors include β_2 microglobulin (β_{2m}), fibroblast growth factors (FGFs), PDGF, interleukin 1 (IL-1), tumor necrosis factor α (TNF-α), gamma interferon, prostaglandins, and bone morphometric proteins (15, 16, 114). Many observations, mostly from in vitro studies, indicate that these factors influence bone metabolism and consequently may play important roles in the local regulation of bone physiology that may be impaired with aging, although what their exact roles are remains to be established.

The other significant development in line with potential roles for local factors and cytokines in bone remodeling and age-related bone loss involves the recent advances being made in our understanding of the relationship of hematopoietic cells to the origin of osteoclasts, the bone resorbing cells. A large body of recent evidence indicates that osteoclasts derive from hematopoietic mononuclear cells in bone marrow (109, 152, 169, 179). The progenitor cells appear to be pluripotent stem cells that have the same lineage as monocytes and granulocytes. Under appropriate stimuli, a derivative of the stem cell, most likely a CFU-GM, gives rise to precursors that fuse and differentiate into osteoclasts (115, 117). Since these cells resorb bone, age-related bone loss due to increased osteoclastic bone resorption could, therefore, result not only from the stimulation of the activity of mature osteoclasts but also from enhanced proliferation of osteoclast progenitors and increased differentiation of committed precursors into mature osteoclasts.

Recently, attention has turned to the exploration of the implications of all the new knowledge about marrow and related cells, local factors in bone, cytokines, and the hematopoietic origin of osteoclasts to age-related bone loss due to ovarian hormone deficiency in women following menopause. In one study it was hypothesized that ovarian hormone deficiency enhances the expansion of a pool of marrow-derived progenitors of osteoclasts (87). This hypothesis was first tested in mice, where the protocol for demonstrating the marrow origin of osteoclasts had been worked out by Takahashi et al. (169). These investigators demonstrated that marrow cells from mice cultured in the presence of 1,25(OH)$_2$vitamin D or PTH differentiated into tartrate-resistant acid phosphatase (TRAP) positive, multinucleated cells with the characteristics of authentic osteoclasts. When Kalu (87) cultured bone marrow cells from ovariectomized and sham-operated mice in the presence of 1,25(OH)$_2$vitamin D, the cells also gave rise in culture to TRAP-positive multinucleated cells that mostly aggregated in circumscribed areas or colonies, with some scattered randomly in the culture. The colonies contained 66% and 50% of the total number of TRAP-positive multinucleated cells in cultures derived from ovariectomized animals and sham-operated controls, respectively. The effect of ovarian hormone deficiency on the number of TRAP-positive multinucleated cells was unequivocal. Compared with the sham-operated controls, there was about a fivefold increase in the number of TRAP-positive multinucleated cells in the cultures derived from marrow cells of ovariectomized animals (Fig. 16.2A). The number of colonies, the number of TRAP-positive multinucleated cells in the colonies, and the number of these cells outside the colonies were also significantly higher in the ovariectomized animals than in controls (Fig. 16.2B–D). When the marrow cells were cultured in the presence of PTH, the findings were qualitatively similar to those observed in cultures treated with 1,25(OH)$_2$vitamin D. The total number of TRAP-positive multinucleated cells, the number of colonies of these cells, the number of TRAP-positive multinucleated cells within the colonies, and the number not in the colonies were all significantly higher in cultures from ovariectomized mice than from control mice. However, there was a quantitative difference between the responses to 1,25(OH)$_2$vitamin D and PTH, with the 1,25(OH)$_2$vitamin D–treated cultures containing three- to fourfold more TRAP- positive multinucleated cells.

The above studies have been extended to the ovariectomized rat bone loss model with similar observations (90). Furthermore, the ovariectomy-induced increase in TRAP-positive multinucleated cells in ex vivo marrow cultures was partially suppressed by estradiol administration (95). One explanation for these findings is that ovarian hormones directly or indirectly modulate the activity of a hematopoietic growth factor(s) that commits pluripotent stem cells in the marrow to the osteoclast lineage. Consequently, ovarian hormone deficiency expands the pool of marrow-derived progenitors that differentiate into osteoclasts and tip the balance of bone remodeling in favor of bone loss (87, 90, 95). These conclusions have been confirmed and extended in recent studies in which the increased osteoclastogenesis due to estrogen lack in mice was attributed to increased stimulatory action of IL-6 (56, 82). In addition, others have reported that ovariectomy not only enhanced the proliferation of bone marrow cells but also increased the number of osteoblast-like cells estimated by fibroblast colony-forming unit (FCFU) efficiency and cell counting (36). Therefore, increased proliferation of marrow-derived osteoblast progenitors is, most likely, also a component of the mechanism for the enhanced bone turnover observed early in ovarian hormone deficiency. These findings await replication in humans.

Other studies have specifically explored the implica-

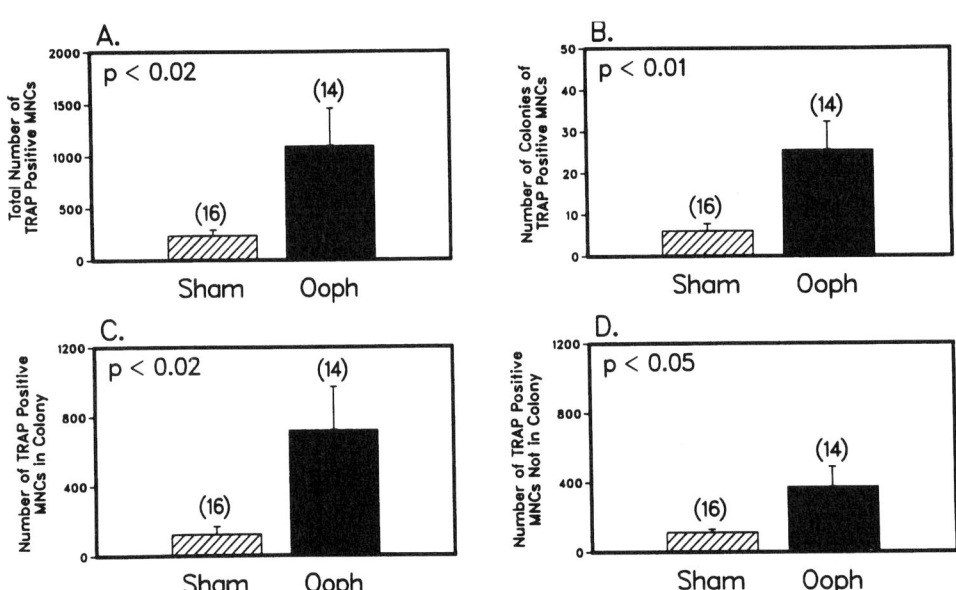

FIG. 16.2. Effect of ovariectomy on the formation of TRAP-positive multinucleated cells (MNCs) from mononuclear bone marrow cells treated with 1,25(OH)$_2$vitamin D in culture. Female ICR mice were ovariectomized (OOPH) or sham-operated (SHAM). Two weeks later bone marrow from the femurs and tibias was harvested and cultured in a medium containing $10^{-8}M$ 1,25(OH)$_2$vitamin D. TRAP-positive MNCs with three or more nuclei were counted. Each bar is mean ± SE. P values denote difference between SHAM and corresponding OOPH, and $P \leq 0.05$ is considered statistically significant. Numbers in parentheses denote the number of animals per group. [Reproduced from Kalu (87) with permission.]

tion of cytokines in age-related bone loss in humans. The focus of the human studies has been on the secretion of the cytokines, IL-1, TNF-α, and granulocyte-macrophage colony-stimulating factor (GM-CSF) by peripheral blood monocytes. Since IL-1 and TNF-α induce bone resorption and IL-1 and GM-CSF are involved in osteoclast formation (116), these cytokines may play a role in the increased bone turnover that results in bone loss, especially following menopause (126). In one study, Pacifici et al. (128) measured the spontaneous secretion of IL-1 by cultured monocytes isolated from blood and observed that monocytes from osteoporotic patients with a high rate of bone turnover produced more IL-1 activity than monocytes from control subjects (128). In another study, these investigators observed that IL-1 activity in the culture medium of peripheral blood monocytes derived from untreated postmenopausal women was higher than in medium from cultured monocytes derived from untreated premenopausal or estrogen/progesterone-treated postmenopausal women (127). The investigators also observed that oophorectomy-induced increase in the secretion of IL-1, TNFα, and GM-CSF by cultured blood monocytes was suppressed by estrogen therapy (126), and they concluded that alterations in monocyte cytokine secretion may underlie bone loss due to high bone turnover and its modulation by estrogen. Although this conclusion is based on studies with peripheral blood monocytes, it has been speculated that the increase in cytokine secretion would occur locally in marrow due to bone matrix–monocyte interaction since signs of "acute phase reaction" are not characteristic of oophorectomy (32, 126). It should be mentioned that in one report the secretion of TNF, IL-1β, and prostaglandin E_2 (PGE_2) by peripheral blood mononuclear cells was similar in postmenopausal women with and without osteoporosis (185), in contrast to the findings of Pacifici et al. (126–128). However, the experimental protocols were not exactly comparable: there were very large individual variations in cytokine secretion; the osteoporotic patients had normal biochemical indices of the rate of bone turnover; and the authors did not rule out a role for monocyte cytokines in a subset of osteoporotics with high bone turnover rate. Other investigators have also failed to observe an increase in IL-1 production by peripheral monocytes from postmenopausal women (79, 167, 168). In addition, since unstimulated monocytes do not normally secrete measurable amounts of IL-1 spontaneously, the meaning of the increased IL-1 that Pacifici et al. (126–128) observed using plastic culture plates, which can induce the expression of IL-1, has been questioned (104a). Nevertheless, the observation in a recent study that the number of marrow monocytes is increased in the ovariectomized rat bone loss model raises the possibility of an increase in the local concentration of IL-1 in bone marrow that is secondary in part to increased marrow cellularity (95).

So far, the conclusion that cytokines may be involved in the etiology of age-related bone loss due to ovarian hormone deficiency is based mainly on correlative data. The hypothesis is being explored more directly. If IL-1 is involved in inducing osteoporotic bone loss, blocking its action with IL-1 receptor antagonist (IL-1ra) would likely modulate the progression of the bone loss. Two studies have been carried out to examine this hypothesis (95, 98). In one of these studies, it was observed that long-term administration of IL-1 receptor antagonist to ovariectomized rats partially prevented the progression of the resultant bone loss (98). This finding supports the IL-1 hypothesis; because the bone loss was not inhibited completely, the study also indicates that additional factors besides IL-1 are most likely involved in the pathogenesis of the bone loss due to ovarian hormone deficiency. However, in another report, IL-1 receptor antagonist did not have a significant effect on the prevention of bone loss following ovariectomy (95). Others have assigned a major role for increased IL-6 in the etiology of bone loss due to ovarian hormone deficiency and have proposed that it is the inhibition of IL-6 production by osteoblastic and marrow stromal cells that is responsible for the protective effect of sex steroids against excessive osteoclastic bone resorption (56, 82). These investigators observed that the administration of IL-6 antibody to ovariectomized mice prevented the usual increase in the number of trabecular osteoclasts and inhibited osteoclast-like cell formation in ex vivo cultures of marrow (82), indicating an important role for the cytokine in the increased osteoclastogenesis due to ovarian hormone deficiency. It is presently unknown whether a similar IL-6 antibody therapy will also prevent ovariectomy-induced bone loss, and others could not demonstrate that estrogen regulates the secretion of IL-6 by cultured human osteoblast-like cells (22). Only continued investigations will eventually clarify these issues.

Further support for the notion that local factors within bone are involved in the pathogenesis of age-related bone loss comes from studies of the skeletal effects of PGs, which are secreted by many cell types including bone cells. The actions of PGs on bone are complex: they stimulate osteoclastic bone resorption in bone organ culture and mouse calvaria (99, 171) and they enhance bone collagen synthesis (138, 139). Several cytokines, growth factors, PTH, and mechanical factors that modulate bone metabolism increase PG production within bone (137). As a result of their extreme lability to inactivating enzymes present in virtually all tissues, PGs are believed to act mainly locally. In vivo, PGE_2 administration to young adult dogs has marked effects on bone, activating both cancellous and cortical bone remodeling characterized by increased bone resorption and formation, in favor of bone formation (101). It is notable that in the young adult rats in which the cortex is normally dormant, PG administration activates intracortical bone remodeling characterized by activation, resorption, reversal, and formation (A→R→F), creating a porous cortex with concentric lamellae that have the characteristics of Harvesian systems present in adult human skeletons (81). PGE_2 production has been shown to be increased in bones from ovariectomized rats and decreased in bones from rats given estradiol (39). All these findings suggest that alterations in local production of PG in bone may contribute to the enhanced bone turnover that results in bone loss due to ovarian hormone deficiency and its modulation by estrogen therapy. However, this has not been confirmed directly.

In summary, recent findings support the association of altered bone metabolism with elements of the hematopoietic system and their cytokines and form the basis of the altered hematopoeisis–local factor hypothesis for the pathogenesis of bone loss due to ovarian hormone deficiency. According to the hypothesis, ovarian hormones have a pleiotropic effect on the hematopoietic system. Consequently, deficiency of these hormones following menopause or ovariectomy results in alterations in the populations and/or the activities of bone-related blood cells and their cytokines especially in bone marrow; these alterations, by themselves or through their interactions with bone cells, alter the balance of bone turnover in favor of bone loss (95).

RISK FACTORS FOR AGE-RELATED BONE LOSS

Although all women lose bone as a result of ovarian hormone deficiency following menopause, not all postmenopausal women progress to the clinical expression of the osteoporotic syndrome characterized by the collapse of vertebral bodies and the liability of fracture of certain long bones. Therefore, factors extrinsic to ovarian hormone deficiency contribute to the clinical expression of the disease. These are usually described as risk factors and include being a white or Asian women, being thin-boned or petite, having low peak bone mass at maturity, a family history of osteoporosis, premature or surgically induced menopause, alcohol abuse, cigarette smoking, sedentary life-style, and poor dietary habits such as inadequate calcium intake (89, 132). These so-called risk factors are distinguished by their loose associations with osteoporosis. The largely extrinsic nature of many of them makes one wonder about the inevitability of osteoporosis if all the risk factors are eliminated. However, there is still the likelihood that the bone mass of long-lived individuals, free of risk factors, would eventually fall below the fracture threshold as a result of "normal" aging bone loss. The risk factors warrant a brief comment.

Peak Bone Mass

Since bone loss is an inevitable consequence of aging, it is now generally considered that a good predictor of the likelihood that an individual will have a fracture as a result of aging bone loss is the amount of the individual's peak bone mass at maturity and the subsequent rate of bone loss (118). The greater the peak bone mass, the less likely that bone mass will fall below a conceptual fracture threshold as a result of loss with aging. At maturity, women have about 20% lower peak bone mass than men, and this difference has been suggested to contribute to the greater incidence of fractures in elderly women than in men. Peak bone mass and aging bone loss are in part under genetic control. For instance, black women have larger peak bone mass than white women and they are correspondingly less prone to fractures due to aging bone loss (53). The physiological basis for the racial and sex differences in peak bone mass is presently unclear.

Exercise

It is likely that the achievement of an individual's peak bone mass potential is determined in part by the degree of physical activity during the growing period. Young white women with a history of high physical activity and high dietary calcium intake were found to have greater peak bone mineral density than a similar, less active group on lower calcium intake (96). The implication is that the incidence of osteoporosis can be reduced if people, especially females, adopt life-style patterns during the growing period that permit them to achieve, at maturity, a peak bone mass that is not likely to fall below the fracture threshold as a result of loss due to aging.

Several observations indicate that even after the growing period, bone mass is influenced by physical activity. For instance, limb immobilization and paralysis lead to accelerated loss of bone in adults, while continuous bed rest results in an increase in urinary calcium and hydroxyproline excretion due to enhanced dissolution of bone mineral and bone matrix (33). Loss of bone due to lack of mechanical stress also results from prolonged weightlessness in space (104), and animal experiments indicate that disuse bone atrophy is due to the suppression of bone formation with enhanced or unaltered osteoclastic bone resorption (112). These observations and the more sedentary life-style of elderly people further suggest that a decrease in physical activity may contribute to an increase in the rate of bone loss that occurs with aging in humans. Recent findings indicate that exposing bone to strain changes that are well within the limits of normal activity, such as walking, can augment skeletal mass and thereby render the skeleton more resistant to aging bone loss (154). Although substantial evidence indicates that bone mass will benefit from physical activity, there are uncertainties with respect to type of exercise, its frequency, duration, and intensity (34). Furthermore, it should be emphasized that there is no evidence that exercise can maintain bone mass at the premenopausal level or serve effectively as an alternative for hormone replacement therapy at menopause (34).

Nutrition

It has long been suspected that nutrition might play an etiological role in age-related bone loss (143). Proteins, calcium, and phosphorus, the main building blocks of bone, have received the most attention. Purified proteins enhance urinary excretion of calcium. However, in humans, a protein-rich diet causes only a transient or no loss of calcium in urine (163), probably because meat is high in phosphorus, which has been shown to decrease urinary calcium excretion (164). The habitual intake of a diet rich in phosphates has been considered a pathogenetic factor in aging bone loss because of the ability of phosphate to bind dietary calcium and render it unavailable for absorption. However, in humans, high phosphate intake was not found to compromise intestinal calcium absorption (162, 164). Dietary calcium intake and its absorption decrease with aging, and a low-calcium diet causes negative calcium balance in humans and bone loss in animals (49, 61, 69, 85). Since the dietary calcium intake of most adult Americans is well below the recommended daily allowance, inadequate availability of calcium from dietary sources could be a pathogenetic factor in aging bone loss in humans.

However, there is a lack of consensus on the level of dietary calcium required for optimum bone health (67, 97). The recommended daily allowance (RDA) for calcium varies from about 400 to about 1,500 mg in different countries (177), and dietary calcium requirements vary according to age and physiological need (67). In the U.S., where the average woman consumes about 500 mg of calcium per day, the current RDA for adults is 800 mg. Many believe that this RDA is too low and should be upgraded to about 1,000 mg for adults and 1,500 mg for postmenopausal women (67). The controversy about the importance of calcium in osteoporosis relates in part to the observation that in the first few years of menopause, a period characterized by accelerated loss of bone calcium, increased dietary calcium intake had little or no effect on the progression of bone loss (148). However, increased calcium intake has been shown by meta-analysis to promote the preservation of bone mass after menopause (24) and to modulate bone loss in premenopausal women in other studies (7, 120). Nevertheless, a lack of consensus exists within the scientific community regarding the necessity for an upward adjustment of the RDA for dietary calcium as a way to promote bone health and retard age-related bone loss. The reasons for the lack of consensus are severalfold (67, 97). First, the cause of osteoporosis is multifaceted, with the possibility that calcium deficiency is only one part. This makes it difficult to establish the exact contribution of dietary calcium in bone health. Second, the level of dietary calcium intake varies in different countries. Therefore, dietary calcium supplementation will be most important in those countries where women are already on marginal calcium intake and may appear unimportant in countries in which dietary calcium is adequate. Third, several (107, 119) but not all (54, 178) epidemiological studies show a correlation between the level of lifelong dietary calcium intake and bone mineral density or the risk of fracture in women. Fourth, epidemiological studies that indicate the beneficial effect of calcium intake to bone mass and fracture rate rarely take into account the contributive effects of increased energy intake and physical activity to that of dietary calcium. Fifth, difficulties in accurate assessment of calcium intake are underestimated. Sixth, studies based on calcium intake alone cannot easily factor in absorption efficiency and urinary excretory levels which determine the real amount of useful calcium.

Smoking, Alcohol, and Caffeine

Epidemiological studies indicate that smoking, alcohol, and caffeine are risk factors in aging bone loss (66, 155). Alcohol may mediate its effect in part by increasing urinary loss of calcium, but its role in osteoporosis must be complex because it has toxic effects on cells, and alcoholics are predisposed to malnutrition. In one study, smokers were found to have 10% to 30% less bone mineral content than nonsmokers, and other studies indicate that caffeine, which is present in coffee, tea, and cola beverages, increases the loss of calcium in urine. Although the increase is small (a cup of coffee leads to a loss of only about 8 mg more calcium in urine), this can add up to a significant amount in an individual who is on a marginal dietary calcium intake but consumes large quantities of caffeine-containing beverages. Furthermore, a recent study indicates that caffeine can stimulate calcium release from bone by potentiating the action of bone resorptive agents that act via the adenylate cyclase–cyclic AMP system (100). Nevertheless, there are conflicting reports on the role of caffeine-containing beverages as risk factors for osteoporosis (106). Some report a significant negative association between caffeine intake and bone mineral content (182), while others do not find significant relative risks for hip fractures with caffeine consumption (74). Part of the reason for the conflicting reports is that the effect of caffeine may be confounded by other factors that also have effects on bone, such as cigarette smoking, diet, and calcium; epidemiological studies do not adequately account for these other variables (106). As mentioned, the kidney and the gastrointestinal tract may be involved in the deleterious action of caffeine on bone. For instance, in one study caffeine consumption was associated with both increased urinary calcium excretion and enhanced intestinal calcium secretion, although no change in calcium balance was observed when adjustments were made for calcium intake (68). Recently, Massey (106) stated that the expression of the deleterious effect of caffeine consumption on bone is dependent on age and level of dietary calcium intake, with older individuals on low dietary calcium intake being more vulnerable.

ESTROGEN RECEPTORS IN INTESTINAL CELLS

Osteoporosis is often associated with intestinal calcium malabsorption, which is believed to aggravate the negative calcium balance that occurs with aging and to contribute importantly to bone loss in postmenopausal women (47–49, 69). The decrease in calcium absorption is due to ovarian hormone deficiency and is corrected by estrogen therapy (17, 19, 47–49, 69), but the mechanism of this estrogen action is unclear. The focus of attention in the past has been mainly on the relationship of estrogen to $1,25(OH)_2$vitamin D (47–49, 69), a proven stimulator of intestinal calcium absorption. Because estrogen administration was found to increase blood levels of $1,25(OH)_2$vitamin D in some patients (48, 103, 167) and the hydroxylation of $25(OH)$vitamin D in lower species (9, 18), it has been suggested that estrogen promotes calcium absorption indirectly by stimulating renal synthesis of the bioactive vitamin D metabolite and that estrogen deficiency at menopause results in low $1,25()H)_2$vitamin D and the resultant intestinal calcium malabsorption (48). The other suggestion that has been proposed is that the calcium malabsorption that occurs in postmenopausal osteoporosis is related to intestinal resistance to calcium absorption due to estrogen deficiency (42, 55, 113). The nature of this resistance has yet to be defined. It is, however, possible that estrogen itself acts directly on the intestine to stimulate calcium absorption rather than through $1,25()H)_2$vitamin D. At least four observations support this latter notion. First, intestinal calcium absorption was found to be impaired in women within 6 months after ovariectomy, with no decrease in $1,25()H)_2$vitamin D levels (55). Second, several investigators failed to observe any correlation between serum $1,25()H)_2$vitamin D levels and the rate of calcium absorption in postmenopausal and osteoporotic women (31, 49). Third, in the rat model of postmenopausal bone loss, ovariectomy lowered blood estrogen levels and reduced intestinal calcium absorption but did not alter blood levels of $1,25(OH)_2$vitamin D (92). Fourth, estrogen administration to rats increased blood-ionized calcium and urinary calcium levels with no effect on $1,25(OH)_2$vitamin D concentrations (93, 176).

Based on the above considerations, we hypothesize that estrogen acts directly on the intestinal mucosal cells through estrogen receptors to promote calcium absorption and that the loss of this estrogen action is directly responsible, at least in part, for the intestinal calcium malabsorption associated with postmenopausal osteoporosis. The studies we carried out to test this hypothesis demonstrated that the intestinal mucosal cells contain estrogen receptor immunoreactivity, express the mRNA for estrogen receptors, and respond directly to 17β-estradiol with enhanced calcium transport that is suppressed by gene transcription and protein synthesis inhibitors (5). These findings are novel and suggest that estrogen has a direct physiological role in the regulation of intestinal calcium absorption. Consequently, its deficiency following menopause or therapeutic ovariectomy may result directly in the calcium malabsorption that is believed to be an important factor in the bone loss that occurs in these conditions.

Thomas et al. (175) have also reported the presence of estrogen receptors in intestinal and IEC-6 cells, a nontransformed line of cells initially isolated from intestinal crypts. Scatchard analysis indicated that the IEC-6 cells contain high-affinity binding sites for estrogen and that these cells and segments of rat intestine contained estrogen receptor mRNA. Exposure of the IEC-6 cells to 17β-estradiol resulted in a rapid and transient increase in the steady-state pool of c-fos mRNA. The investigators concluded that estrogen may regulate intestinal epithelial functions by influencing cell proliferation and differentiation of intestinal crypt cells. Our findings (5) and those of Thomas et al. (175) are in remarkable agreement about the presence of hitherto unrecognized functional estrogen receptors in intestinal cells. Further studies are required to determine the pathophysiological implications of these receptors, especially in regard to the intestinal calcium malabsorption and age-related bone loss that occur in hypoestrogenic conditions.

REFERENCES

1. ABRAHAM, S. *Dietary Intake Findings, United States, 1971–1974.* National Health Survey, Vital and Health Statistics Series 11, No. 102, Publication (HRA) 77-1647. Washington DC: US Department of Health, Education and Welfare, Public Health Services.
2. ALBRIGHT, F. P. H., SMITH, and A. M. RICHARDSON. Postmenopausal osteoporosis: its clinical features. *J. Am. Med. Wom. Assoc.* 116: 2465–2474, 1941.
3. ANDERSON, H. C. Matrix calcification: review and update. In: *Bone and Mineral Research,* edited by W. A. Peck, Amsterdam: Elsevier, vol. 3, 1985, p. 109–149.
4. Anonymous. Osteoporosis: consensus conference. *JAMA* 252: 799–802, 1984.
5. ARJMANDI B. H., M A. SALIH, D. C. HERBERT, D. H. SIMS, and D. N. KALU. Evidence for estrogen receptor-linked calcium transport in the intestine. *Bone Miner.* 21: 63–74, 1993.
6. AVIOLI L. V. Osteoporosis. In: *Bone and Mineral Research,* edited by W. A. Peck, Amsterdam: Elsevier, vol. 1, 1983, p. 280–318.
7. BARAN D., A. SORENSEN, J. GRIMES, R. LEW, A. KARELLAS, B. JOHNSON, and J. ROCHE. Dietary modification with dairy products for preventing vertebral bone loss in pre-menopausal women: a three-year prospective study. *J. Clin. Endocrinol. Metab.* 70: 264–270, 1989.
8. BARON B., A. VIGNERY, and M. HOROWITZ. Lymphocytes, macrophages and the regulation of bone remodeling. In: *Bone and Mineral Research,* edited by W. A. Peck. Amsterdam: Elsevier, 1984, vol. 2, p. 175–243.
9. BASKI, S. N., A. D. KENNY. Acute effect of estradiol on the renal vitamin D hydroxylases in Japanese quail. *Biochem. Pharmacol.* 27: 2765–2768, 1978.
10. BELANGER, L. F. Ostocytic osteolysis. *Calif. Tissue Res.* 4: 1–12, 1969.
11. BERLYNE, G. M., J. BEN-ARI, A. JUSHELEVSKY, A. IDELMAN, D. GALINSKY, M. HIRSCH, R. SHAINKIN, R. YAGIL, and M. ZLOTNIK. Aetiology of senile osteoporosis: secondary hyperparathyroidism due to renal failure. *Q. J. Med.* 44: 505–521, 1975.
12. BODY, J. J., and H. HEALTH III. Estimates of circulating monomeric calcitonin: physiological studies in normal and thyroidectomized man. *J. Clin. Endocrinol. Metab.* 57: 897–903, 1983.
13. BOYDE A., E. MACONNACHIE, S. A. REID, G. DELLING, and G. R. MUNDY. Scanning electron microscopy in bone pathology: review of methods. Potential and application. *Scanning Microsc.* 4: 1537–1554, 1986.
14. BUCHANAN, J. R., S. W. CAUFFMAN, and R. B. CIREER, III. Relation of calcium regulating hormones to the pathogenesis of postmenopausal osteoporosis. In: *Osteoporosis 1,* edited by C. Christiansen, C. D. Arnand, B. E. C. Nordin, A. M. Parfitt, W. A. Peck, and B. L. Riggs. Glostrup: Aalborg Stifsbogtrykkeri, 1984, p. 275–280.
15. CANALIS, E. Regulation of bone remodeling. In: *Primer on the Metabolic Bone Diseases and Disorders of Mineral Metabolism,* edited by M. J. Favus. Richmond, VA: William Byrd Press, 1990, p. 23–26.
16. CANALIS, E., T. MCCARTHY, and M. CENTRELLA. Growth factors and the regulation of bone remodeling. *J. Clin. Invest.* 81: 277–281, 1988.
17. CANIGGIA, A., C. GENNASI, G. BORELLA, M. BENANT, L. PAGGI, and C. ESCOBAR. Intestinal absorption of calcium-47 after treatment with oral estrogen and gestagen in senile osteoporosis. *Br. Med. J.* 4: 30–32, 1970.
18. CASTILLO L., Y. TANAKA, H. F. DELUCA, and M. L. SUNDE. The stimulation of 25-hydroxyvitamin D_3-1α-hydroxylase by estrogen. *Arch. Biochem. Biophys.* 179: 211–217, 1977.
19. CIVITELLI, R., D. AGNUSDEI, P. NARDI, F. ZACCHEI, L. V. AVIOLI, and C. GENNARI. Effects of one-year treatment with estrogens on bone mass, intestinal calcium absorption, and 25-hydroxyvitamin D-1α-hydroxylase reserve in postmenopausal osteoporosis. *Calcif. Tissue Int.* 42: 77–86, 1988.
20. CHAMBERS, J. J. The origin of the osteoclast. In: *Bone and Mineral Research,* edited by W. A. Peck. Amsterdam: Elsevier, 1989, vol. 6, p. 1–25.
21. CHAPUY M. C., F. DURR, and P. CHAPUY. Age-related changes in parathyroid hormone and 25-hydroxycholecalciferol levels. *J. Gerontol.* 38: 19–22, 1983.
22. CHAUDHARY, L. R., T. C. SPELSBERG, and B. L. RIGGS. Production of various cytokines by normal human osteoblast-like cells in response to interleukin-1β and tumor necrosis factor-α: lack of regulation by 17β-estradiol. *Endocrinology* 130: 2528–2534, 1992.
23. COPP, D. H., E. C. CAMERON, B. A. CHENEY, A. G. F. DAVIDSON, and K. G. HENZE. Evidence for calcitonin—a new hormone from the parathyroid that lowers blood calcium. *Endocrinology* 70: 638–649, 1962.
24. CUMMING R. G. Calcium intake and bone mass: a quantitative review of the evidence. *Calcif. Tissue Int.* 47: 194–210, 1990.
25. DEFTOS L. J., M. H. WEISMAN, G. W. WILLIAMS, D. B. KARPF, A. M. FRUMAR, B. H. DAVIDSON, J. G. PARTHEMORE, and H. L. JUDD. Influence of age and sex on plasma calcitonin in human beings. *N. Engl. J. Med.* 302: 1351–1353, 1980.
26. DELMAS P. D. Biochemical markers of bone turnover osteoporosis. In: *Osteoporosis,* edited by B. L. Riggs and L. J. Melton, III. New York: Raven Press, 1988, p. 297–316.
27. DELMAS P. Biochemical markers of bone turnover for the clinical assessment of metabolic bone disease. *Endocrinol. Metab. Clin. North. Am.* 19: 1–18, 1990.
28. DELMAS P. D., D. STENNER, H. W. WAHNER, K. G. MANN, and B. L. RIGGS. Increase in serum bone γ-carboxyglutamic acid protein with aging in women. Implications for the mechanism of age-related bone loss. *J. Clin. Invest.* 71: 1316–1321, 1983.
29. DELUCA, H. F. Mechanism of action and metabolic fate of vitamin D. *Vitam. Horm.* 25: 315–367, 1967.
30. DELUCA, H. F. The cardinal role of 1,25-dihydroxy- vitamin D_2 in mineral homeostasis. In: *Clinical Disorders of Bone and Mineral Metabolism,* edited by B. Frame and J. T. Potts, Jr. Amsterdam: Excerpta Medica, 1983, p. 78–81.
31. DEVINE A., R. L. PRINCE, D. A. KERR, I. M. DICK, R. A. CRIDDLE, G. N. KENT, R. I. PRICE, and P. G. WEBB. Correlates of intestinal calcium absorption in women 10 years past the menopause. *Calcif. Tissue Int.* 52: 358–360, 1993.
32. DINARELLO, C. A. Biology of interleukin 1. *FASEB J.* 2: 108–115, 1988.
33. DONALDSON, C. L., S. B. HULLEY, J. M. VOGEL, R. S. HATTNER, J. H. BAYER, and D. E. MCMILLAN. Effect of prolonged bed rest on bone mineral. *Metabolism* 19: 1071–1084, 1970.
34. DRINKWATER, B. L. Preserving strong bones: the young adult female. In: *Clinical Disorders of Bone and Mineral Metabolism.* edited by M. Kleerekoper and S. M. Krane. New York: Mary Ann Liebert, 1989, p. 173–178.
35. DRIVDAHL, R. H., G. A. HOWARD, and D. J. BAYLINK. Extracts of bone contain a potent regulator of bone formation. *Biochim. Biophys. Acta.* 714: 26–33, 1982.
36. EGRISE, D., D. MARTIN, P. NEVE, A. VIENNE, M. VERHAS, and A. SCHOUTENS. Bone blood flow and in vitro proliferation of bone marrow and trabecular bone osteoblast-like cells in ovariectomized rats. *Calcif. Tissue Int.* 50: 336–341, 1992.

37. EMMERSTON, K., F. MELSEN, L. MOSEKIDLE, B. LUND, B. LUND, O. H. SORESEN, H. E. NIELSON, H. SOLLING, and H. H. HANSEN. Altered vitamin D metabolism and bone remodeling in patients with medullary carcinoma and hypercalcitoninemia. *Metab. Bone Dis. Relat. Res.* 4: 17–23, 1981.
38. FALCH, J. A., H. OFTEBRO, and E. HANG. Early postmenopausal bone loss is not associated with a decrease in circulating levels of 25-hydroxy-vitamin D, 1,25-dihydroxyvitamin D or vitamin D binding proteins. *J. Clin. Endocrinol. Metab.* 64: 836–841, 1987.
39. FEYEN, J. H. M., and L. G. RAISZ. Prostaglandin production by calvariae from sham operated and oophorectomized rats: effects of 17β-estradiol in vivo. *Endocrinology* 121: 819–821, 1987.
40. FOGELMAN, I., J. W. POSER, M. L. SMITH, D. M. HART, and J. A. BEVAN. Alterations in skeletal metabolism following oophorectomy. In: *Osteoporosis*, edited by C. Christiansen, C. D. Arnand, B. E. C. Nordin, A. M. Parfitt, W. A. Peck, and B. L. Riggs. Glostrup: Aalborg Stiftsbogtrykkeri, 1984, p. 519–522.
41. FOSTER, G. V., A. BAGHDIANTZ, M. A. KUMAR, E. SLACK, H. A. SOLIMAN, and I. MACINTYRE. Thyroid origin of calcitonin. *Nature* 202: 1303–1305, 1964.
42. FRANCIS, R. M., M. PEACOCK, G. A. TAYLOR, J. H. STORER, and B. E. NORDIN. Calcium malabsorption in elderly women with vertebral fractures: evidence for resistance to the action of vitamin D metabolites on the bowel. *Clin. Sci.* 66: 103–107, 1984.
43. FRASER, D. R., and E. KODICEK. Unique biosynthesis by kidney of a biologically active vitamin D metabolite. *Nature* 228: 764–766, 1970.
44. FROST, H. M. *Mathematical Elements of Bone Remodeling*. Springfield, IL: Charles C. Thomas, 1964.
45. FROST, H. M. Tetracycline based histologic analysis of bone remodeling. *Calcif. Tissue Res.* 3: 211–237, 1969.
46. FROST H. M., and W. S. S. JEE. On the rat model of human osteopenias and osteoporoses. *Bone Miner.* 18: 227–236, 1992.
47. GALLAGHER, J. C. The pathogenesis of osteoporosis. *Bone Miner.* 9: 215–227, 1990.
48. GALLAGHER, J. C., B. L. RIGGS, and H. F. DELUCA. Effect of estrogen on calcium absorption and serum vitamin D metabolites in postmenopausal osteoporosis. *J. Clin. Endocrinol. Metab.* 51: 1359–1364, 1980.
49. GALLAGHER, J. C., B. L. RIGGS, J. EISMAN, A. HANSTRA, S. B. ARNAUD, and H. F. DELUCA. Intestinal calcium absorption and serum vitamin D metabolites in normal subjects and osteoporotic patients. Effect of age and dietary calcium. *J. Clin. Invest.* 64: 729–736, 1979.
50. GALLAGHER, J.C., B. L. RIGGS, C. M. JERBAK, and C. D. ARNAUD. The effect of age in serum immunoreactive parathyroid hormone in normal and osteoporotic women. *J. Lab. Clin. Med.* 95: 373–385, 1980.
51. GALLAGHER, J. C., M. N. YOUNG, and B. E. C. NORDIN. Effects of artificial menopause on plasma and urine calcium and phosphate. *Clin. Endocrinol.* 1: 57–64, 1972.
52. GARABEDIAN, M., M. F. HOLICK, H. F. DELUCA and I .T. BOYLE. Control of 25-hydroxycholecalciferol metabolism by parathyroid hormone. *Proc. Natl. Acad. Sci. U.S.A.* 69: 1673–1676, 1972.
53. GARN, S. M. Bone loss and aging. In: *Physiological and Pathology of Human Aging*, edited by R. Goldman and M. Rockstein. New York: Academic Press, 1975, p. 39–57.
54. GARN, S. M., C. G. ROHOMAN, B. WAGNER, G. H. DAVILA, and W. ASCOLI. Population similarities in the onset and rate of adult endosteal bone loss. *Clin. Orthop.* 65: 51–60, 1969.
55. GENNARI C., D. AGNUSDEI, P. NARDI, and R. CIVITELLI. Estrogen preserves a normal intestinal responsiveness to 1,25-dihydroxyvitamin D_3 in oophorectomized women. *J. Clin. Endocrinol. Metab.* 71: 1288–1293, 1990.
56. GIRASOLE G., R. L. JILKA, G. PASSERI, S. BOSWELL, G. BODER, D. C. WILLIAMS, and S. C. MANOLAGAS. 17 beta-estradiol inhibits interleukin-6 production by bone marrow derived stromal cells and osteoblasts in vitro—a potential mechanism for the antiosteoporotic effect of estrogens. *J. Clin. Invest.* 89: 883–891, 1992.
57. GRAY, T. K., and P. L. MUNSON. Thyrocalcitonin: evidence for physiological function. *Science* 166: 512–513, 1969.
58. GUNBERG, C. M., J. M. LIAN, P. M. GALLOP, and J. J. STEINBERG. Urinary γ-carboxyglutamic acid and serum osteoclacin as bone markers: studies in osteoporosis and Paget's disease. *J. Clin. Endocrinol. Metab.* 57: 1221–1225, 1983.
59. HABENER, J. F., and J. T. POTTS, JR. Chemistry, biosynthesis, secretion and metabolism of parathyroid hormone. In: *Handbook of Physiology, Endocrinology, Section 7*, edited by G. D. Aurbach. Washington, DC: American Physiological Society, 1976, p. 313–342.
60. HABENER, J. F., M. ROSENBLATT, B. KEMPER, H. M. KRONENBERG, A. RICH, and J. T. POTTS, JR. Pre-proparathyroid hormone: amino acid sequence, chemical synthesis, and some biological studies of the precursor region. *Proc. Natl. Acad. Sci. U.S.A.* 75: 2616–2620, 1978.
61. HARRISON, M., and R. FRASER. Bone structure and metabolism in calcium deficient rats. *J. Endocrinol.* 21: 197–205, 1960.
62. HAUSCHKA, P. V., J. B. LIAN, and P. M. GALLOP. Direct identification of the calcium binding amino acid, γ-carboxyglutamate, in mineralized tissue. *Proc. Natl. Acad. Sci. U.S.A.* 72: 3925–3929, 1975.
63. HEANEY, R. P. A unified concept of osteoporosis. *Am. J. Med.* 39: 877–880, 1965.
64. HEANEY, R. P. A unified concept of osteoporosis: a second look. In: *Osteoporosis*, edited by U. S. Barzel. New York: Grune & Stratton, 1969, p. 257–265.
65. HEANEY, R. P. Pathophysiology of osteoporosis: implications for treatment. *Tex. Med.* 70: 37–45, 1974.
66. HEANEY, R. P. Calcium intake, bone health and aging. In: *Nutrition, Aging and Health,* edited by E. A. Young. New York: Alan R. Liss, 1986, p. 165–186.
67. HEANEY, R. P. Lifelong calcium intake and prevention of bone fragility in the aged. *Calcif. Tissue Int.* 49: S42–S45, 1991.
68. HEANEY, R. P., and R. R. RECKER. Effects of nitrogen, phosphorus, and caffeine on calcium balance in women. *J. Lab. Clin. Med.* 99: 46–55, 1982.
69. HEANEY, R. P., R. R. RECKER, and P. D. SAVILLE. Menopausal changes in calcium balance performance. *J. Lab. Clin. Med.* 92: 953–963, 1978.
70. HEANEY, R. P., R. R. RECKER, and P. D. SAVILLE. Menopausal changes in bone remodeling. *J. Lab. Clin. Med.* 92: 964–970, 1978.
71. HEATH, J. K., S. J. AITKINSON, M. C. MEIKLE, and J. J. REYNOLDS. Mouse osteoblast synthesize collagenase in response to bone resorbing agents. *Biochem. Biophys. Acta* 802: 151–154, 1984.
72. HILLYARD, C. J., J. C. STEVENSON, and I. MACINTYRE. Relative deficiency of plasma calcitonin in normal women. *Lancet* 1: 961–962, 1978.
73. HIRSCH, P. F., G. F. GAUTHIER, and P. L. MUNSON. Thyroid hypocalcemic principle and recurrent laryngeal nerve injury as factors affecting the response to parathyroidectomy in rats. *Endocrinology* 73: 244–252, 1963.
74. HOLBROOK, T. L., E. BARRETT-CONNOR, and D. L. WINGARD. Dietary calcium and risk of hip fracture: 14-year prospective population study. *Lancet* 2: 1046–1049, 1988.

75. HOLBROOK, T. L., K. GRAZIER, J. L. KELSEY, and R. N. STAUFFER. *The Frequency of Occurrence, Impact and Cost of Selected Musculoskeletal Conditions in the United States.* Chicago: American Academy of Orthopedic Surgeons, 1984.
76. HOLTROP, M. E. The ultrastructure of bone. *Ann. Clin. Lab. Sci.* 5: 264–271, 1975.
77. HOWARD, G. A., B. L. BOTTEMILLER, R. T. TURNER, J. H. RADER, and D. J. BAYLINK. Parathyroid hormone stimulates bone formation and resorption in organ culture: evidence for a coupling mechanism. *Proc. Natl. Acad. Sci. U.S.A.* 78: 3204–3208, 1981.
78. HURLEY, D. L., R. D. TIEGS, H. W. WAHNER, and H. HEATH III. Does prolonged calcitonin excess or deficiency affect bone mineral density in women? *J. Bone Miner. Res.* 1 (suppl. 1): 240, 1986.
79. HUSTMYER, F. G., E. WALKER, X.-P. YU, G. GIRASOLE, Y. SAKAGAMI, M. PEACOCK, and S. C. MANOLAGAS. Cytokine production and surface antigen expression by peripheral blood mononuclear cells in postmenopausal osteoporosis. *J. Bone Miner. Res.* 8: 51–59, 1993.
80. JACKSON, J. A. Osteoporosis in men. In: *Primer on Metabolic Bone Diseases and Disorders of Mineral Metabolism.* edited by M. J. Favus. Richmond, VA: William Byrd Press, 1990, p. 162–164.
81. JEE, W. S. S., S. MORI, X. J. LI, and S. CHAN. Prostaglandin E_2 enhances cortical bone mass and activates bone remodeling in intact and ovariectomized female rats. *Bone* 11: 253–266, 1990.
82. JILKA, R. L., G. HANGOC, G. GIRASOLE, G. PASSERI, D. C. WILLIAMS, J. S. ABRAMS, B. BOYCE, H. BROXMEYER, and S. C. MANOLAGAS. Increased osteoclast development after estrogen loss: mediation by interleukin-6. *Science* 257: 88–91, 1992.
83. JOHANSEN, J. S., K. THOMSEN, and C. CHRISTIANSEN. Plasma bone gla protein concentrations in healthy adults. Dependence on sex, age and glomerular filtration. *Scand. J. Clin. Lab. Invest.* 47: 345–350, 1987.
84. JOHNSON, C. C., JR., and S. EPSTEIN. The endocrinology of osteoporosis. In: *Endocrinology of Calcium Metabolism,* edited by J. A. Parsons. New York: Raven Press, 1982, p. 467–484.
85. JOWSEY, J., and J. GERSHON-COHEN. Effect of dietary calcium levels on production and reversal of experimental osteoporosis in cats. *Proc. Soc. Exp. Biol. Med.* 116: 437, 1964.
86. KALU, D. N. Calcium and skeletal metabolism and aging bone loss. In: *Handbook of Endocrinology,* edited by G. H. Gass and H. Kaplan. Boca Raton, FL: CRC Press, 1987, p. 43–83.
87. KALU, D. N. Proliferation of tartrate-resistant acid phosphatase positive multinucleated cells in ovariectomized animals. *Proc. Soc. Exp. Biol. Med.* 195: 70–74, 1990.
88. KALU, D. N. The ovariectomized rat model of postmenopausal bone loss. *Bone Miner.* 15: 175–192, 1991.
89. KALU, D. N., and E. J. MASORO. The biology of aging, with particular reference to the musculoskeletal system. *Clin. Geriatr. Med.* 4: 257–267, 1988.
90. KALU, D. N., R. ECHON, and B. W. HOLLIS. Modulation of ovariectomy-related bone loss by parathyroid hormone in rats. *Mech. Ageing Dev.* 56: 49–62, 1990.
91. KALU, D. N., A. HADJI-GEORGOPOULOS, and G. V. FOSTER. Evidence for physiological importance of calcitonin in the regulation of plasma calcium in rats. *J. Clin. Invest.* 55: 722–727, 1975.
92. KALU, D. N., C. C. LIU, R. R. HARDIN, and B. W. HOLLIS. The aged rat model of ovarian hormone deficiency bone loss. *Endocrinology* 124: 7–16, 1989.
93. KALU, D. N., C. C. LIU, E. SALERNO, B. W. HOLLIS, R. M. ECHON, and M. RAY. Skeletal response of ovariectomized rats to low and high doses of 17β-estradiol. *Bone Miner.* 14: 175–188, 1991.
94. KALU, D. N., J. PENNOCK, F. H. DOYLE, and G. V. FOSTER. Parathyroid hormone and experimental osteosclerosis. *Lancet* 1: 1363–1366, 1970.
95. KALU, D. N., E. SALERNO, C. C. LIU, F. FERARRO, B. H. ARJMANDI, and M. A. SALIH. Ovariectomy induced bone loss and the hematopoietic system. *Bone Miner.* 23: 145–161, 1993.
96. KANDERS, B., R. LINDSAY, D. DEMPSTER, L. MARKHARD, and G. VALIQUETTE. Determinants of bone mass in young healthy women. In: *Osteoporosis 1,* edited by C. Christiansen, C. D. Arnaud, B. E. C. Nordin, A. M. Parfitt, W. A. Peck, and B. L. Riggs. Glostrup: Aalborg Stiftsbogtrykkeri, 1984, p. 337–340.
97. KANIS, J. A. Calcium requirements for optimal skeletal health in women. *Calcif. Tissue Int.* 49: S33–S41, 1991.
98. KIMBLE, R. B., J. L. VANNICE, D. C. BLOEDOW, R. C. THOMPSON, and R. PACIFICI. Infusion of IL-1 receptor antagonist prevents bone loss in ovariectomized rats. *J. Bone Miner. Res.* 7(suppl. 1): S116, 1992.
99. KLEIN, D. C., and L. G. RAISZ. Prostaglandins: stimulation of bone resorption in tissue culture. *Endocrinology* 86: 1436–1440, 1970.
100. LERNER, U. H., and D. MELLSTROM. Caffeine has the capacity to stimulate calcium release in organ culture of neonatal mouse calvaria. *Calcif. Tissue Int.* 51: 424–428, 1992.
101. LI, X. J., W. S. S. JEE, Y. L. LI, and P. PATTERSON-BUCKENDAHL. Transient effects of subcutaneously administered prostaglandin E_2 on cancellous and cortical bone in young adult dogs. *Bone* 11: 353–364, 1990.
102. LINDSAY, R. Sex steroids in the pathogenesis and prevention of osteoporosis. In: *Osteoporosis: Etiology, Diagnosis and Management,* edited by B. L. Riggs and L. J. Melton, III. New York: Raven Press, 1988, p. 333–358.
103. LUND, B., H. SORENSEN, B. LUND, and E. AGNER. Serum 1,25-dihydroxyvitamin D in normal subjects and in patients with postmenopausal osteopenia. Influence of age, renal function and oestrogen therapy. *Horm. Metab. Res.* 14: 271–274, 1982.
104. MACK, P. B., P. A. LACHANGE, G. P. VOSE, and F. B. VOGT. Bone demineralization of foot and hand of Gemini-Titan IV, V and VII astronauts during orbital flight. *Am. J. Roentgenol.* 100: 503–511, 1967.
104a. MANOLAGAS, S. C., F. G. HUTSMYER, G. GIRASOLE, and X-P YU. Cytokine production and surface antigen expression by peripheral blood mononuclear cells in postmenopausal osteoporosis. *J. Bone Mineral. Res.* 8: 777–778, 1993.
105. MARTIN, G. R., R. TIMPL, P. K. MILLER, and K. KUHN. The genetically distinct collagens. *Trends Biochem. Sci.* 10: 285–287, 1985.
106. MASSEY, L. A. Caffeine and bone: directions for research. *Calcif. Tissue Int.* 6: 1149–1151, 1991.
107. MATKOVIC, V., K. KOSTIAL, I. SIMONOVIC, R. BUZINA, A. BRODEREC, and B. E. C. NORDIN. Bone status and fracture rates in two regions of Yugoslavia. *Am. J. Clin. Nutr.* 32: 540–549, 1979.
108. MCDERMOTT, M. T., G. S. KIDD, P. BLUE, V. GHAED, and F. D. HOFELDT. Reduced bone mineral content in totally thyroidectomized patients: possible effect of calcitonin deficiency. *J. Clin. Endocrinol. Metab.* 56: 936–937, 1983.
109. MCDONALD, B., N. TAKAHASHI, L. MCMANUS, J. HOLAHAN, G. MUNDY, and G. ROODMAN. Formation of multinucleated cells that respond to osteotropic hormones in long-term human bone marrow cultures. *Endocrinology* 120: 2326–2333, 1987.
110. MELTON, L. J., III, and B. L. RIGGS. Clinical spectrum. In: *Osteoporosis: Etiology, Diagnosis and Management.* edited by

B. L. Riggs and L. J. Melton, III. New York: Raven Press, 1988, p. 155–179.

111. MILHAUD, G. M., M. BENEZECH-LEFEVRE, and M. S. MOUKHTAR. Deficiency of calcitonin in age-related osteoporosis. *Biomedicine* 29: 272–276, 1978.

112. MOREY-HOLTON, E. R., and S. B. ARNAUD. Spaceflight and calcium metabolism. Proceedings of the Seventh Annual Meeting of the IUPS Commission on Gravitational Physiology. *Physiologist* 28(suppl.): 9–12, 1985.

113. MORRIS, H. A., A. G. NEED, M. HOROQITZ, P. D. O'LOUGHLIN, and B. E. C. NORDIN. Calcium absorption in normal and osteoporotic postmenopausal women. *Calcif. Tissue Int.* 49: 240–243, 1991.

114. MUNDY, G. R. Identifying mechanisms for increasing bone mass. *J. N.I.H. Res.* 1: 65–68, 1989.

115. MUNDY, G. R. Bone resorbing cells. In: *Primer of the Metabolic Bone Diseases and Disorders of Mineral Metabolism,* edited by M. J. Favus. Richmond VA: William Byrd Press, 1990, p. 18–22.

116. MUNDY, G. R. Local factors regulating osteoclast function. In: *Biology and Physiology of the Osteoclast,* edited by B. R. Rifkin and C. V. Gay. Boca Raton, FL: CRC Press, 1992, p. 171–185.

117. MUNDY, G. R., and G. D. ROODMAN. Osteoclast ontogeny and function. In: *Bone and Mineral Research,* edited by W. A. Peck. Amsterdam: Elsevier, 1987, vol. 5, p. 209–279.

118. NEWTON-JOHN, H. F., and D. B. MORGAN. Osteoporosis: disease or senescence? *Lancet* 1: 232–233, 1968.

119. NORDIN, B. E. C. International patterns of osteoporosis. *Clin. Orthop.* 45: 17–30, 1966.

120. NORDIN, B. E. C., and K. J. POLLEY. The Adelaide bone loss risk factor survey. *Calcif. Tissue Int.* 41: S1–S59, 1987.

121. NORDIN, B. E. C., A. HORSMAN, and D. H. MARSHALL. Calcium requirement and calcium therapy. *Clin. Orthop.* 140: 216–239, 1979.

122. NORMAN, A. W., J. ROTH, and L. ORCI. The vitamin D endocrine system: steroid metabolism, hormone receptors, and biological response (calcium binding proteins). *Endocr. Rev.* 3: 313–366, 1982.

123. OHTA, H., K. MAKITA, Y. SUDA, T. IKEDA, T. MASUZAWA, and S. NOZAWA. Influence of oophorectomy on serum levels of sex steroids and bone metabolism and assessment of bone mineral density in lumbar trabecular bone by QCT-C value. *J. Bone Miner. Res.* 7: 659–665, 1992.

124. OTSUKA, K., J. SODEK, and H. F. LIMEBACK. Collagenase synthesis by osteoblast-like cells. *Calcif. Tissue Int.* 36: 722–724, 1984.

125. OWEN, M. Lineage of osteogenic cells and their relationship to the stromal system. In: *Bone and Mineral Research,* edited by W. A. Peck. Amsterdam: Elsevier, 1985, vol. 3, p. 1–25.

126. PACIFICI, R., C. BROWN, E. PUSCHECK, E. FRIEDRICH, E. SLATOPOLSKY, D. MAGGIO, R. MCCRACKEN, and L. V. AVIOLI. Effect of surgical menopause and estrogen replacement on cytokine release from human blood mononuclear cells. *Proc. Natl. Acad. Sci. U.S.A.* 88: 5134–5138, 1991.

127. PACIFICI, R., L. RIFAS, R. MCCRACKEN, I. VERED, C. MCMURTRY, L. V. AVIOLI, and W. A. PECK. Ovarian steroid treatment blocks a postmenopausal increase in blood monocyte interleukin release. *Proc. Natl. Acad. Sci. U.S.A.* 86: 2398–2402, 1988.

128. PACIFICI, R., L. RIFAS, S. TEITELBAUM, E. SLATOPOLSKY, R. MCCRACKEN, M. BERGFELD, W. LEE, L. W. AVIOLI, and W. A. PECK. Spontaneous release of interleukin-1 from blood monocytes reflects bone formation in idiopathic osteoporosis. *Proc. Natl. Acad. Sci. U.S.A.* 84: 4616–4620, 1987.

129. PANSISI, F., S. BETTOECHI, JR., C. BERGAMINI, A. BIANCHI, R. AMBROSECCHIA, B. BAGNI, and G. MOLLICA. Influence of acute estrogenic withdrawal on blood calcitonin. *Gynecol. Obstet. Invest.* 18: 21–26, 1984.

130. PARFITT, A. M. The cellular basis of bone remodeling: the quantum concept reexamined in light of recent advances in the cell biology of bone. *Calcif. Tissue Int.* 36: S37–S45, 1986.

131. PARFITT, A. M., C. H. E. MATHEWS, A. R. VILLANUEVA, M. KLEEREKOPER, B. FRAME, and D. S. RAO. Relationships between surface, volume, and thickness of iliac trabecular bone in aging and in osteoporosis. Implications for the microanatomic and cellular mechanisms of bone loss. *J. Clin. Invest.* 72: 1396–1409, 1983.

132. PECK, W. A. Diagnosis and treatment of osteoporosis. In: *Endocrine Function and Aging,* edited by H. J. Armbrecht and N. Wongsurawat. New York: Springer-Verlag, 1988, p. 67–78.

133. PECK, W. A. (Ed.) *Bone and Mineral Research.* Amsterdam: Elsevier, vol. 1–7, 1983–1990.

134. PONCHON, G., A. L. KENNAN, and H. F. DELUCA. Activation of vitamin D by the liver. *J. Clin. Invest.* 48: 2032–2037, 1969.

135. PRICE, P. A., A. S. OTSUKA, J. W. POSER, J. KRISTAPONIS, and N. RAMAN. Characterization of a γ-carboxyglutamic acid containing protein from bone. *Proc. Natl. Acad. Sci. U.S.A.* 73: 1447–1451, 1976.

136. PRICE, P. A., J. G. PARTHEMORE, and L. G. DEFTOS. New biochemical marker for bone metabolism. *J. Clin. Invest.* 66: 878–883, 1980.

137. RAISZ, L. G. Local and systemic factors in the pathogenesis of osteoporosis. *N. Engl. J. Med.* 318: 818–828, 1988.

138. RAISZ, L. G., and B. E. KREAM. Regulation of bone formation. *N. Engl. J. Med.* 309: 29–35, 1983a.

139. RAISZ, L. G., and B. E. KREAM. Regulation of bone formation. *N. Engl. J. Med.* 309: 83–89, 1983b.

140. RASMUSSEN, H. The role of $1,25(OH)_2D_3$ in the pathogenesis of osteomalacia. In: *Clinical Disorders of Bone and Mineral Metabolism,* edited by B. Frame and J. T. Potts, Jr. Amsterdam: Excerpta Medica, 1983, p. 82–89.

141. RASMUSSEN, H., and P. BORDIER. *The Physiological and Cellular Basis of Metabolic Bone Disease.* Baltimore: Williams and Wilkins, 1974.

142. RECKER, R. R., D. B. KIMMEL, A. M. PARFITT, K. M. DAVIS, N. KESHAWARZ, and S. HINDERS. Static and tetracycline based bone histomorphometric data from 34 normal postmenopausal females. *J. Bone Miner. Res.* 3: 133–144, 1988.

143. RIGGS, B. L. Nutritional factors in age-related osteoporosis. In: *Nutrition and Aging,* edited by M. L. Hutchinson and H. N. Munro. New York: Academic Press, 1986, p. 207–216.

144. RIGGS, B. L., and L. J. MELTON, III. Evidence for two distinct syndromes of involutional osteoporosis. *Am. J. Med.* 75: 899–901, 1983.

145. RIGGS, B. L., J. JOWSEY, R. S. GOLDSMITH, P. J. KELLY, D. L. HOFFMAN, and C. D. ARNAUD. Short and long-term effects of estrogen and synthetic anabolic hormone in postmenopausal osteoporosis. *J. Clin. Invest.* 51: 1659–1663, 1972.

146. RIGGS, B. L., H. W. WAHNER, W. L. DUNN, R. B. MAZESS, K. P. OFFORD, and L. J. MELTON, III. Differential changes in bone mineral density of the appendicular and axial skeleton with aging. Relationship to spinal osteoporosis. *J. Clin. Invest.* 67: 328–335, 1981.

147. RIGGS, B. L., H. W. WAHNER, L. J. MELTON, III, L. S. RICHELSON, H. L. JUDD, and K. P. OFFORD. Rates of bone loss in appendicular and axial skeletons of women: evidence of substantial vertebral bone loss before menopause. *J. Clin. Invest.* 77: 1487–1491, 1986.

148. RIIS, B., K. THOMSEN, and C. CHRISTIANSEN. Does calcium supplementation prevent postmenopausal bone loss and frac-

tures? A double-blind, controlled clinical study. *N. Engl. J. Med.* 316: 173–177, 1987.
149. RIIS, B. J., C. CHRISTIANSEN, L. J. DEFTOS, and B. D. CATHERWOOD. The role of serum concentrations of estrogens in postmenopausal osteoporosis and bone turnover. In: *Osteoporosis*, edited by C. Christiansen, C. D. Arnaud, B. E. C. Nordin, A. M. Parfitt, W. A. Peck, and B. L. Riggs. Glostrup: Aalborg Stiftsbogtrykkeri, 1984, p. 333–336.
150. RODAN, G. A., and T. J. MARTIN. Role of osteoblasts in hormonal control of resorption—a hypothesis. *Calcif. Tissue Int.* 33: 349–351, 1981.
151. RODAN, S. B., G. A. RODAN, H. A. SIMMONS, R. W. WALENGA, M. B. FEINSTEIN, and L. G. RAISZ. Bone resorptive factor produced by osteosarcoma cells with osteoblast features is PGE_2. *Biochem. Biophys. Res. Commun.* 102: 1358–1365, 1981.
152. ROODMAN, G., K. IBBOTSON, B. MCDONALD, T. KUEHL, and G. MUNDY. 1,25-dihydroxyvitamin D_3 causes formation of multinucleated cells with several osteoclast characteristics in cultures of primate marrow. *Proc. Natl. Acad. Sci. U.S.A.* 82: 8123–8317, 1985.
153. ROWE, J. W., and R. L. KAHN. Human aging: usual and successful. *Science* 237: 143–149, 1987.
154. SANDLER, R. B., R. LAPORTE, D. SASHIN, J. CAULEY, C. BAYLES, C. SLEMENDA, A. PETRINI, and M. SCHRAMM. The epidemiology of physical activity and postmenopausal bone loss. First year of clinical trial. In: *Osteoporosis I*, edited by C. Christiansen, C. D. Arnaud, B. E. C. Nordin, A. M. Parfitt, W. A. Peck, and B. L. Riggs. Glostrup: Aalborg Stiftsbogtrykkeri, 1984, p. 317–322.
155. SEEMAN, E., L. J. MELTON III, W. M. O'FALLON, and B. L. RIGGS. Risk factors for spinal osteoporosis in men. *Am. J. Med.* 75: 977–983, 1983.
156. SHERMAN, S. S., B. W. HOLLIS, and J. D. TOBIN. Vitamin D status and related parameters in a healthy population: the effects of age health and season. *J. Clin. Endocrinol. Metab.* 71: 405–413, 1990.
157. SILVE, C. M., G. T. HRADEK, A. L. JONES, and C. D. ARNAUD. Parathyroid hormone receptors in intact embryonic chicken bone: characterization and cellular localization. *J. Cell Biol.* 94: 379–386, 1982.
158. SINGER, F. R., and J. F. HABENER. Multiple immunoreactive forms of calcitonin in human plasma. *Biochem. Biophys. Res. Commun.* 61: 710–716, 1974.
159. SISSONS, H. A., G. L. KELMAN, and G. MAROTTI. Mechanisms of bone resorption in calcium deficient rats. *Calcif. Tissue Int.* 36: 711–721, 1984.
160. SLEMENDA, C., S. L. HUI, C. LONGCOPE, and C. C. JOHNSTON. Sex steroids and bone mass: a study of changes about the time of menopause. *J. Clin. Invest.* 80: 1261–1269, 1987.
161. SLOVIK, D. M., C. M. GUNBERG, R. M. NEER, and J. B. LIAN. Clinical evaluation of bone turnover by serum osteocalcin measurements in a hospital setting. *J. Clin. Endocrinol. Metab.* 59: 228–230, 1984.
162. SPENCER, H., L. KRAMER, and D. OSIS. Factors contributing to calcium loss in aging. *Am. J. Clin. Nutr.* 36: 776–787, 1982.
163. SPENCER, H., L. KRAMER, D. OSIS, and C. NORRIS. Effect of a high protein (meat) intake on calcium metabolism in man. *Am. J. Clin. Nutr.* 31: 2167–2180, 1978a.
164. SPENCER, H., L. KRAMER, D. OSIS, and C. NORRIS. Effect of phosphorus on the absorption of calcium and on the calcium balance in man. *J. Nutr.* 108: 447–457, 1978b.
165. STEPHAN, J. J., J. POSPICHAL, J. PRESL, and V. PACOVSKY. Bone loss and biochemical indices of bone remodeling in surgically induced postmenopausal women. *Bone* 8: 279–284, 1987.
166. STEVENSON, J. C. Differential effects of aging and menopause on CT secretion. In: *Calcitonin*, edited by A. Pecile. Amsterdam: Excerpta Medica, 1985, p. 145–152.
167. STOCK, J. L., J. A. CODERRE, and L. E. MALLETTE. Effects of a short course of estrogen on mineral metabolism in postmenopausal women. *J. Clin. Endocrinol. Metab.* 61: 595–600, 1985.
168. STOCK, J. L., J. A. CODERRE, B. MCDONALD, and L. J. ROSENWASSER. Effects of estrogen in vivo and in vitro on spontaneous interleukin-1 release by monocytes from postmenopausal women. *J. Clin. Endocrinol. Metab.* 48: 364–368, 1989.
169. TAKAHASHI, N., H. YAMANA, S. YOSHIKI, G. D. ROODMAN, G. R. MUNDY, D. J. JONES, and A. BOYDE. Osteoclast-like cell formation and its regulation by osteotropic hormones in mouse bone marrow cultures. *Endocrinology* 122: 1373–1382, 1988.
170. TALMAGE, R. V., and R. A. MEYER. Physiological role of parathyroid hormone. In: *Handbook of Physiology. Section 7. Endocrinology. Volume VII. Parathyroid Gland*, edited by R. Greep and E. B. Astwood. Baltimore: Waverly Press, 1976, p. 343–351.
171. TASHJIAN, A. H., E. F. VOELKEL, L. LEVINE, and P. GOLDHABER. Evidence that the bone resorption-stimulating factor produced by mouse fibrosarcoma cells is prostaglandin E_2: a new model for hypercalcemia of cancer. *J. Exp. Med.* 136: 1329–1343, 1972.
172. TEITELBAUM, S. L., E. M. ROSENBERG, C. A. RICHARDSON, and L. AVIOLI. Histologic studies of bone from normacalcemic postmenopausal osteoporotic patients with increased circulating parathyroid hormone. *J. Clin. Endocrinol. Metab.* 42: 537–543, 1976.
173. TERMINE, J. D. Noncollagen proteins in bone. In: *Cell and Molecular Biology of Vertebrate Hard Tissues, Ciba Foundation Symposium 136*, edited by D. Evered and S. Harnett. Chichester: John Wiley and Sons, 1988, p. 178–190.
174. TERMINE, J. D. Bone matrix proteins and the mineralization process. In: *Primer on the Metabolic Bone Diseases and Disorders of Mineral Metabolism*, edited by M. J. Favur. Richmond, VA: William Byrd Press, 1990, p. 16–18.
175. THOMAS, M. L., X. XU, A. M. NORFLEET, and C. S. WATSON. The presence of functional estrogen receptors in intestinal epithelial cells. *Endocrinology* 132: 426–430, 1993.
176. TOBIAS, J. H., J. CHOW, K. W. COLSTON, and T. J. CHAMBERS. High concentrations of 17β-estradiol stimulate trabecular bone formation in adult female rats. *Endocrinology* 128: 408–412, 1991.
177. TRUSWELL, A. S., T. IRWIN, G. H. BEATON, R. SUZUE, H. HAENEL, S. HEJDA, X. C. HOU, G. LEVEILLE, E. MORAVA, J. PEDERSON, and J. M. L. STEPHEN. Recommended dietary intake around the world. *Nutr. Abstr. Rev.* 53: 939–1015, 1983.
178. VAN BERESTEIJN, E. C. H., M. A. VAN T'HOF, H. DE WAARD, J. A. RAYMAKERS, and S. A. DUURSMA. Relation of axial bone mass to habitual calcium intake and to cortical bone loss in healthy early postmenopausal women. *Bone* 11: 7–13, 1990.
179. WALKER, D. G. Control of bone resorption by hematopoietic tissue. The induction and reversal of congenital osteopetrosis in mice through the use of bone marrow mononuclear phagocytes. *J. Exp. Med.* 156: 1604–1614, 1975.
180. WISKE, P. S., S. EPSTEIN, N. H. BELL, S. F. QUEENER, J. EDMONDSON, and C. C. JOHNSON, JR. Increase in immunoreactive parathyroid hormone in normal and osteoporotic women. *N. Engl. J. Med.* 300: 1419–1421, 1979.
181. WRONSKI, T. J., and C. F. YEN. The ovariectomized rat as an animal model for postmenopausal bone loss. *Cells Materials* 1(suppl.): 69–74, 1991.
182. YANO, K., L. K. HEIBRUN, R. D. WASNICH, J. H. HANKIN, and J. M. VOGEL. The relationship between diet and bone mineral content of multiple skeletal sites in elderly Japanese-American

men and women living in Hawaii. *Am. J. Clin. Nutr.* 42: 877–888, 1985.
183. YOUNG, M. M., and B. E. C. NORDIN. Effects of natural and artificial menopause on plasma and urinary calcium and phosphorus. *Lancet* 2: 118–120, 1967.
184. YOUNG, M. M., C. JASANI, D. A. SMITH, and B. E. C. NORDIN. Some effects of ethinyl oestradiol on calcium and phosphorus metabolism in osteoporosis. *Clin. Sci.* 34: 411–417, 1968.
185. ZARRABEITIA, M. T., J. A. RIANCHO, J. A. AMADO, J. NAPAL, and J. GONZALEZ-MACIA. Cytokine production by peripheral blood cells in postmenopausal osteoporosis. *Bone Miner.* 14: 161–167, 1991.

17. Cardiovascular system

EDWARD G. LAKATTA

Laboratory of Cardiovascular Science, Gerontology Research Center, National Institute on Aging, National Institutes of Health, Baltimore, Maryland

CHAPTER CONTENTS

Cardiovascular Structure in Younger and Older Humans
    Arterial structure and mechanical properties
        Arterial stiffness and pressure
        Peripheral vascular resistance
        Arterial impedance
    Cardiac structure
    Ventricular–vascular coupling
Myocardial and Cardiac Pump Function at Rest
    Integrated regulation of cardiac function
    Cardiac filling (diastolic) properties
    Cardiac volumes and ejection fraction
    Myocardial contractile properties
    Heart rate and rhythm
    Cardiac output
Cardiovascular Reserve
    Postural reflexes
        Arterial pressure and peripheral vascular resistance
        Heart rate and cardiac volumes
    Isometric exercise
    Dynamic exercise
        Aerobic capacity
        Arterial pressure, vascular resistance, and impedance
        End-diastolic and end-systolic volumes
        Myocardial contractile reserve
        Heart rate, stroke volume, and cardiac output
Sympathetic Modulation of Cardiovascular Function
    Intact organisms
        β-Adrenergic modulation of cardiac volumes and heart rate during exercise
        Neurotransmitter elaboration during stress
        Cardiovascular target organ response to β-adrenergic stimulation with aging
        β-adrenergic receptor response in the healthy aging heart resembles that in chronic heart failure
    Isolated tissue or cells
        Vascular responses
        Cardiac responses
        β-AR
        G-protein and adenylate cyclase activity
        cAMP, protein kinase activation, and intracellular phosphorylation
        Desensitization of the β-adrenoceptor system
Parasympathetic Modulation of Cardiovascular Function
Cardiovascular Structure and Function in Younger and Older Animals
    Cardiac structure
    Myocardial stiffness
        Passive stiffness
        Active stiffness
    Regulation of the cardiac contraction
        The cardiac excitation–contraction process
        Cardiac muscle and myocyte changes with adult aging
        Similar effects of aging and experimental pressure overload on cardiac regulatory mechanisms and gene expression
        Possible mechanisms of altered cardiac gene regulation with aging
        Response of older rat heart to chronic hemodynamic overload
        Coronary blood flow, oxygen consumption, and oxidative metabolism
Effect of Chronic Physical Conditioning on Cardiovascular Performance in Older Humans and Animals
    Studies in humans
    Studies in rodents
Summary

DIFFERENCES IN CARDIOVASCULAR FUNCTION between older and younger individuals have been extensively described in the literature. However, confusion often arises in the interpretation of these differences because of a failure to acknowledge, or to control for, interactions among age, disease, and life-style. Although recent studies have used more rigorous screening techniques to separate older individuals with clinical or occult disease—for example, coronary artery disease—from those without disease, the perfect aging study (one that completely controls for both disease and life-style variations) has yet to emerge. Even in the absence of the confounding influences of disease and life-style, the rate of "true" aging of an organ system, such as the cardiovascular system, may vary from one individual to the next. Thus even when experimental measurements differ among younger and older individuals, age per se does not usually account for all or even most of the total variance in the data.

Various aspects of study design also complicate the interpretation of measurements of the impact of age on cardiovascular regulatory mechanisms. Cross-sectional studies (those in which different individuals of varying ages are compared) neither quantify nor control for life-long habits of nutrition, exercise, or other birth cohort effects. While a longitudinal study design (see chapter 2 for a discussion of the design of aging studies) intuitively appears to be superior to the cross-sectional approach, the advantage is more often apparent than real: the development of occult disease or changes in life-style, for example, due to popular education regarding dietary lipids, body weight or smoking, still confound the longitudinal characterization of the results of aging.

Alterations in some cardiovascular regulatory mechanisms occurring over certain parts of the age spectrum (fetal, postpartum, neonatal, maturational, adult, and senescent periods) may differ from those occurring over other parts of the spectrum; still other aspects of cardiovascular function may change progressively across the entire age span. Furthermore, cellular mechanisms underlying altered function at one age may not be the same as those at another period of the life cycle. "Aging" is a rather nonspecific term that is applied to the spectrum of life periods. Statements about the effects of age on a given aspect of cardiovascular structure or function, without strict qualification as to the specific range investigated, have caused confusion. The definition of age-related effects on cardiovascular regulation also requires that a broad age range be studied. If a sufficient adult age range is not sampled, erroneous or incomplete generalizations about an "age effect" may be made. Extrapolating findings of an age effect to groups younger or older than those studied is not warranted. Finally, it is noteworthy that very few data are available regarding cardiovascular regulatory mechanisms in individuals older than 80 yr who are healthy and maintain a reasonable level of physical activity.

Because the cardiovascular system at rest functions at only a fraction of its capacity, studies at rest do not adequately characterize this system or its regulatory mechanisms. Subtle signs of age-associated differences in cardiovascular function between younger and older individuals become manifest, in particular, during stress, for example, during acute exercise. In this regard, while most older individuals have a lower aerobic capacity than most younger ones, it has not usually been emphasized that the amount of physical work performed dictates the level of cardiovascular performance achieved or vice versa. In older individuals, noncardiovascular factors often limit the amount of physical work that can be achieved. In these individuals, parameters of cardiovascular performance at termination of exercise will be reduced, but maximum cardiovascular performance will not have been sampled. Finally, whether age-associated differences in noncardiac or cardiac factors that may limit aerobic work capacity are due to aging per se or in part to the sedentary life-style that accompanies aging cannot easily be sorted out, as aging and the assumption of a more sedentary behavior are interdependent covariants with time.

Studies of cardiovascular regulatory mechanisms in humans are, of necessity, relatively descriptive in nature. Use of animal models permits mechanistic studies not achievable in humans. The rat is by far the most popular animal model employed in studies of cardiovascular aging. While the problem of coronary artery disease is obviated in this species, the major issue of physical deconditioning with age of rats in captivity may be even more severe than in humans. Additionally, with increasing age senescent rats usually exhibit renal disease, which may complicate the interpretation of certain measurements. While the applicability of research findings in animal models to humans is often questioned, this potential constraint is a relatively minor one since studies that address the nature of aging in any model, regardless of direct applicability to humans, have merit in their own right.

Attempts such as the present one to integrate the information contained in the literature need to proceed cautiously. Yet despite the aforementioned problems in the design and interpretation of studies that have addressed the issue of how aging affects the cardiovascular system, when the data of many studies are considered collectively, a pattern of change in cardiovascular regulatory mechanisms with age does emerge.

CARDIOVASCULAR STRUCTURE IN YOUNGER AND OLDER HUMANS

Arterial Structure and Mechanical Properties

Arterial Stiffness and Pressure. Table 17.1 summarizes the changes in arterial structural and functional properties with aging in humans. Both in vitro and in vivo studies have indicated that the stiffness of large arteries increases with age (13, 21, 25, 29, 46, 110, 160, 180, 197, 207, 284, 303, 359, 406, 407, 414, 480, 558). Vascular stiffness can be quantified in terms of an elastic modulus. Both in vivo and in vitro studies indicate that the pressure–strain modules of large arteries increases with age (29, 180, 304, 407, 411).

Changes in arterial stiffness with aging are accompanied by an increase in arterial diameter and wall thickness in both humans and rats (78, 553). In rats the average number of nuclei in the aortic wall decreases with aging (78), much like that in the myocardium in humans (see below, under Cardiac Structure). The mean systolic internal radius of the ascending aorta in humans increases 9% per decade over the age range 20–60 yr (363). It has been estimated that the thoracic aorta provides about one-half the total blood volume buffering capacity of the arterial system (29), that is, one-half the stroke volume (SV) is stored in the aorta. Up to the age of 60 yr the aortic buffering capacity is not markedly decreased by the increased aortic wall stiffness because the concomitant increase in aortic volume accommodates a given volume ejected into it with less change in radius (480). Thus the *volume elasticity* (change in pressure for a given volume change) measured in vitro shows

TABLE 17.1. *Arterial Changes with Aging**

Changes in arterial geometry and structure with aging
Dilatation of the aorta and large arteries
Increase in arterial wall thickness
Increase in number of collagen fibers in the arterial wall
Decreased glycoprotein content and increased mineralization (Ca, PO$_4$) of elastin

Functional changes in arteries
Increased arterial stiffness, manifest as an increased elastic modulus of the arteries and increased arterial pulse wave velocity
Increased arterial wall tension
Increased peripheral resistance

Alterations in arterial pressure and impedance
Increase in systolic pulse pressure
Increased mean arterial pressure
Increase in absolute amplitude of wave reflections
Decreased amplification of the pressure pulse between the ascending aorta and the peripheral arteries, due in part to reflected pulse waves
Alteration in aortic input impedance spectra
  Increase in characteristic impedance
  Increase in maximum–minimum impedance moduli
  Shift of impedance modulus minimum and phase crossover to higher frequencies
Mismatch between aortic input impedance and energy of LV ejection wave
Increased systolic pressure time index

*Modified from Nichols et al. (365) with permission.

no age-associated changes up to about 60 yr, likely reflecting the large increases in aortic volume up to that age (29). However, beyond that age the volume elasticity markedly decreases (29). As the aorta stiffens with age, less diastolic aortic recoil also occurs, resulting in a change in the distribution of blood flow throughout the cardiac cycle.

Age-associated changes also occur in the more peripheral vessels (53, 65, 301, 414), though the increase in diameter of these vessels with age is less and the increase in wall thickness with age is greater than that of the aorta (414). In individuals who have no symptoms of peripheral vascular disease, the pressure–strain elastic modulus of the femoral artery, measured noninvasively via an ultrasonic tracking system and auscultatory pressure, increases greater than twofold with aging over several decades (351), though considerable variation occurs within and among age groups.

Age-associated increases in arterial stiffness, wall thickness, and diameter are thought to result from a diffuse process in the vessel wall and cannot readily be explained on the basis of atherosclerosis, a highly prevalent vascular disease in older individuals (110, 163, 207, 303, 359). The alterations in stress–strain curves of aged vessels in vitro have been interpreted to be consistent with a relative decrease of elastin and an increase of collagen (414), and chemical analyses indicate that this is the case (129). A change in the distribution of unstretched collagen may also occur with age, and it has been proposed that age-associated changes involve a decrease in the coiling and twisting of molecular chains and a reduction in effective chain length (204, 257). While the total mucopolysaccharide content (ground substance of the interstitial matrix) is unaltered with aging, chondroitin sulfate β and heparin sulfate increase and the hyaluronate and chondroitin content decrease (243). With maturation and aging, the glycoprotein component of elastic fibrils decreases and eventually disappears (415), elastin (in rats) becomes frayed (553), and Ca^{2+} content increases (303). The increased mineralization (Ca^{2+}, phosphorus) of elastin with increasing age is associated with an increase in the content of more polar amino acids (457).

In addition to structural properties, arterial stiffness in vivo is determined by vascular smooth muscle cell (VSMC) contractile tonus, which is controlled in part by neurohumoral factors, for example, catecholamines and angiotensin (386, 405, 428, 465, 517). Vascular tonus is regulated in part by VSMC Ca^{2+} balance. That the increased arterial stiffness in older patients with heart disease can be reduced by vasodilators and that this effect is greater than that in younger individuals (64) suggest that a component of the increased in vivo arterial stiffening with aging may be due to augmented VSMC tone.

The age-associated increase in arterial stiffening is reflected in an increase in the pulse wave velocity (Fig. 17.1A) with aging (24, 46, 147, 160, 207, 528, 558). It has been suggested that an increased aortic pulse wave velocity with aging (due to increased aortic stiffness) causes waves reflected from peripheral sites to the ascending aorta at an earlier time, that is, during the ventricular ejection period (pulse waves are reflected to the aorta after closure of the aortic valve in younger adults). Reflected pulse waves merge (or sum) with the incident (or forward) waves generated by left ventricular (LV) ejection and influence the contour of measured pressure and flow waves (348, 356, 357, 363, 365, 380). Characteristic changes of the pressure pulse contour with age have been widely described (110, 160, 250, 356, 357, 363, 381, 527) and include a large secondary systolic wave in older individuals (Fig. 17.1B) and disappearance of the diastolic pressure wave (381). The duration of the dicrotic wave, which is also related to arterial stiffness and correlated with the pulse wave velocity, as measured from a piezogram of the carotid pulse, also decreases with age (284). It has recently been shown that, in a healthy sedentary study population of a broad age range, arterial stiffness varies inversely with aerobic capacity. This inverse relationship occurs over

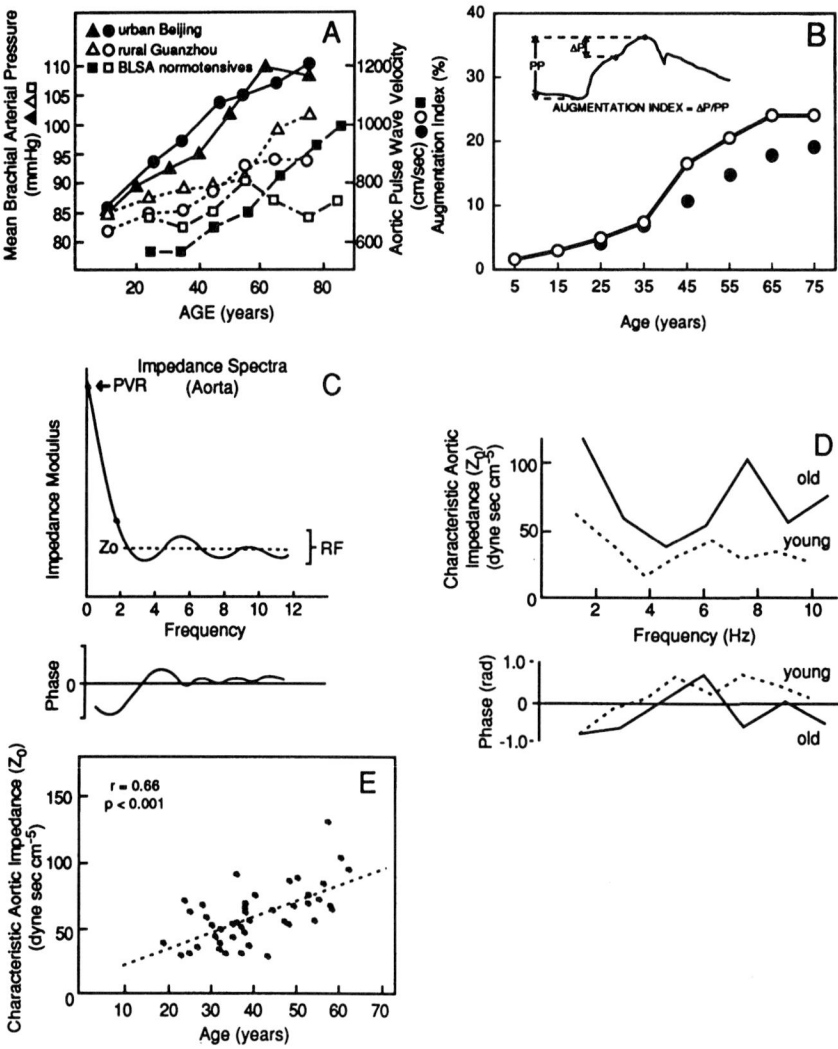

FIG. 17.1. **A**: Mean brachial arterial aortic pressure and aortic pulse wave velocity in two Chinese populations (25) selected without respect to arterial pressure (clinically hypertensive subjects included) and in a North American study population, the Baltimore Longitudinal Study of Aging (BLSA), in which hypertensive subjects (blood pressure greater than 140/90 mm Hg) were excluded from analysis (527). **B**: Augmentation index of the carotid artery pressure pulse in healthy individuals, measured in an applanation tonometry. The augmentation index is defined as the ratio of $\Delta P/PP\%$; ΔP is the pressure difference from the shoulder to peak; PP is pulse pressure. The ○ population included mildly hypertensive subjects. [From Kelly et al. (250) with permission]; the ● population (BLSA) excluded clinically hypertensive subjects (blood pressure greater than 140/90 mm Hg). [From Vaitkevicius et al. (527) with permission.] **C**: Hypothetical aortic input impedance spectra. Upper tracing, impedance modulus values decline from a high value at 0 Hz (the PVR) to a minimum at approximately 3.5 Hz. This is approximately the same frequency at which phase crosses zero (lower tracing). Negative phase values indicate that flow harmonics lead pressure harmonics; positive phase values indicate that flow harmonics lag pressure harmonics. Impedance moduli oscillate around a characteristic value (Z_0 average of moduli > 2 Hz) because of wave reflections. A wave reflection index can be calculated as the difference between maximum and minimum impedance moduli. [From Nichols et al. (365) with permission.] **D**: Aortic input impedance spectra and flow modulus vs. frequency in a young subject and an elderly subject. [From Nichols et al. (363) with permission.] **E**: Characteristic aortic impedance increase with age. [From Nichols et al. (363) with permission.]

and above the effects of age to increase the arterial stiffness and to decrease aerobic capacity (527). The Na dependence of arterial pressure also increases with aging (186, 256, 546). The altered features of the central arterial pulse pressure with aging have been attributed to early reflected pulse waves (380). Thus early reflected pulse waves are the primary determinant for the long recognized increase in systolic (Fig. 17.1A) and pulse pressures with aging (242, 343, 356, 357, 380, 565).

In summary, central arteries increase in diameter and wall thickness with aging, and these changes are associated with an increase in arterial wall stiffness, a reduction in volume elasticity, and an increase in systolic arterial pressure. The extent to which these changes occur with aging appears to be modified by diet (NaCl intake) and aerobic capacity.

Peripheral Vascular Resistance. It has been suggested that changes in the pressure pulse contour of central arteries are related not only to the stiffness properties of the large vessels but apparently to the properties of the small vessels which determine the total peripheral vascular resistance (PVR) (140, 251).

The stiffening of the large arteries, with a concomitant increase in pulse wave velocity and a late increase in systolic pressure due to earlier reflected pulse waves, ought to lead to a reduction in diastolic pressure. This is so because the reflected pulse wave usually returns after aortic valve closure and contributes to the diastolic pressure (381). As this has not routinely been observed, it has been suggested that total PVR increases with age. In individuals with clinical hypertension it has indeed been well established in both cross-sectional and longitudinal studies that PVR increases with age (248, 326, 344, 345). However, a great deal of heterogeneity in PVR is observed among normotensive individuals with aging (47, 147, 238). In healthy, sedentary men PVR, calculated in the sitting position at rest, does not increase with age (see Fig. 17.6G).

Mechanisms that underlie the heterogeneity in the extent to which PVR is increased in older individuals are not presently well defined but include wide variations of basal cardiac output (see below, under Arterial Impedance) and heterogeneities among older individuals in the age-associated decreases in skeletal muscle mass and capillary density. Although renal blood flow per gram decreases progressively after the fourth decade (cortical flow decreases to a greater extent that medullary flow) (316), the decline is due to selective renal vasoconstriction (91). While the nature of this increase in renal vascular resistance with aging is not completely understood, there is presently no conclusive evidence that renal ischemia is a cause of the age-associated changes in renal structure or of the increase in PVR in some elderly normotensive subjects. Age-associated differences in blood flow to the skin and its regulation during heat stress have also been identified (211, 253, 254, 412, 511).

Arterial Impedance. The relationship between the steady and the pulsatile components of flow and the resulting pressure wave in the aorta defines the aortic input impedance. The impedance modulus (the ratio of oscillatory pressure and flow) is usually considered in the frequency domain, that is, as the power spectrum of the pressure–flow relationship (Fig. 17.1C). The phase relationship between flow and pressure waves varies with frequency. The zero frequency impedance modulus (total PVR) is the opposition to steady flow, and the average of impedance moduli of the frequency-dependent terms above those that encompass the heart rate, referred to as the characteristic aorta impedance (Z_0), is the opposition to pulsatile flow (380, 381). Fluctuations of the impedance modulus about mean level (Fig. 17.1C) are caused by reflected pulse waves. Aging is associated with an increase in the characteristic aortic impedance (Fig. 17.1E), greater fluctuations about the mean value (Fig. 17.1D), and a shift of the characteristic impedance spectrum with the minimum impedance modulus and the pressure–flow phase crossover occurring at higher frequencies (363, 365, 381). An increase in the PVR (the zero frequency impedance term) occurs in some, but not all, study populations with aging (see Fig. 17.6G). It is noteworthy, in this regard, that increases in aortic stiffness and characteristic aortic impedance can exist in the absence of a substantial increase in PVR (64, 142, 364, 421).

Cardiac Structure

Autopsy data from several thousand human hearts, unselected for health or disease status, showed that in subjects aged 30–90 yr, the heart increases in mass by an average of 1 g/yr in men and 1.5 g/yr in women. During this time the ratio of heart weight to body weight also increases (317). More recent autopsy analyses of hearts without coronary artery disease have found an increase with age in heart mass indexed to body mass only in women (260). In both sexes the interventricular septal thickness increases more with aging than does the LV free wall thickness (260). Left ventricular mass may decrease in the very old (80–100 yr of age) (541), perhaps because the extremely sedentary life-style of individuals surviving to this age is accompanied by regression of cardiac mass; alternatively, an increase in LV mass may never have accompanied aging in these long-lived individuals.

During the life span, the effect of age on heart size and mass has been assessed by chest X-ray, echocardiography, and gated blood-pool scans. In cross-sectional studies the cardiothoracic ratio, assessed from the chest X-ray, has been found either to increase or not to change with age (494). An increase in the cardiothoracic ratio in men is due to an increase in cardiac diameter and in women to a reduction in thoracic diameter. In contrast, longitudinal studies consistently report that heart size on chest X-ray increases with age in men between 60 and 98 yr (125, 396). Some cross-sectional studies of sedentary volunteer subjects without disease

(Fig. 17.2) indicate that both the end-diastolic and the end-systolic LV wall thicknesses and the estimated LV mass, measured via M-mode (one-dimensional) echocardiography, increase progressively with age in both sexes (170, 172, 471, 477, 506). Other studies using M-mode echocardiography have found only a minor increase in LV mass with age in healthy women and no change in healthy men (89). It should be noted that M-mode echocardiography samples only a single small area of the LV posterior wall or the ventricular septum and extrapolates this to represent the global LV thickness; LV mass is then estimated, assuming a constant ventricular geometry at all ages. The LV cavity size at end-diastole and end-systole, measured in the semisupine position by 2-D echocardiography or in the sitting position by gated cardiac blood-pool scans of technetium-labeled red cells (see Fig. 17.6), increases moderately with age in healthy, normotensive, sedentary men but does not vary with age in women (147, 421, 528). A marked reduction in LV cavity volume observed in a small minority of older individuals, particular women (244, 522), and likely associated with clinical arterial hypertension, is thus an exception to the rule (236).

When an increase in heart mass occurs with aging, for the most part it is due to an increase in the average myocyte size (526). In some older, apparently healthy hospitalized patients in whom LV mass decreased with age (375), cardiac myocyte enlargement occurred concurrently with an estimated decrease in myocyte number. An increase in the amount and a change in the physical properties of collagen (due to altered cross-linking) also occurs within the myocardium with aging (for review see 173). However, the cardiac muscle to collagen ratio either remains constant or increases in the older heart (375). Myocardial lipofuscin increases with aging (501), but this is of no known functional significance. Additionally, some forms of amyloid protein can be found in the hearts of about half of individuals over 70 yr of age, the frequency increasing sharply with increasing age (297). About half the cases have only minor quantities of amyloid, confined to the atria. Whether the cardiac form of amyloid can strictly be considered a feature of "normal" aging is debatable, since it is not an invariable finding even in centenarians. The type of amyloid accumulation in primary cardiac amyloidosis (that associated with atrophy of the myofibers and a firm, large, waxy heart) is not a feature of cardiac amyloid deposition in healthy older individuals (297).

In summary, aging between 20 and 80 yr appears to be associated with a modest increase in LV wall thickness, due mainly to an increase in the size of cardiac myocytes. The resting LV end-diastolic (LVED) diameter increases moderately with age in men but not in women. Increases in heart mass with aging are exaggerated by coexisting diseases (coronary artery or hypertension) and are substantially influenced by life-style (physical fitness).

Ventricular–Vascular Coupling

The interplay of age-associated cardiac and vascular changes is depicted in Figure 17.3. Age-associated changes in the structure, size, and reactivity of the arterial bed affect myocardial performance by contributing to the vascular impedance of LV ejection. Since pulsatile ascending aortic pressure and flow fluctuate around mean values, the total arterial load the LV must overcome to eject blood includes several components: frequency-dependent, *dynamic elastic* components related to the characteristic aortic impedance (Fig. 17.1D), *reflective* components related to reflected pulse waves (Fig. 17.1B, E), and frequency-independent, *static resistive* components determined by PVR (365). In other words, the LV load is affected not only by aortic distensibility and arteriolar tone but also by reflected waves from arterial reflecting sites. Changes in these components individually or in any combination affect ventricular ejection and function (123, 362, 366, 503). Properties intrinsic to the aorta minimize the characteristic aortic impedance over a range of frequencies (about 3–7 Hz) (Fig. 17.1C) in which the energy of the flow wave is greatest, and this favorable matching permits pulsatile ejection of blood at a minimal energy expenditure, that is, only about 10% of total ventricular work (381). Chronic abnormalities in aortic distensibility, such as those associated with advancing age, as described above, under Cardiac Structure, create a chronic mismatch between ventricular ejection and aortic flow energies (380). It has been suggested that earlier wave reflection in older individuals, caused by an increase in pulse wave velocity due to arterial stiffening (381), would increase the LV hydraulic load more than would an increase in characteristic impedance alone (365, 379, 381). In any event, increases in arterial stiffness and PVR, when they occur (363), and the consequent change in the aortic impedance spectrum result in an age-associated increase in vascular loading of the heart (363, 365). The increased vascular loading of the myocardium with aging appears to be a major cause of the increase in cardiac myocyte size (375, 526) that leads, in some older individuals, to an increase in LV wall thickness (170, 172, 471). When measurements from normotensive and hypertensive subjects of a given age range are analyzed concurrently, the aortic elastic modulus and the cardiac mass index are highly correlated (225). Additionally, the reduction in arterial distensibility in hypertensive subjects correlates with the increase in LV mass to volume ratio, that is, to an

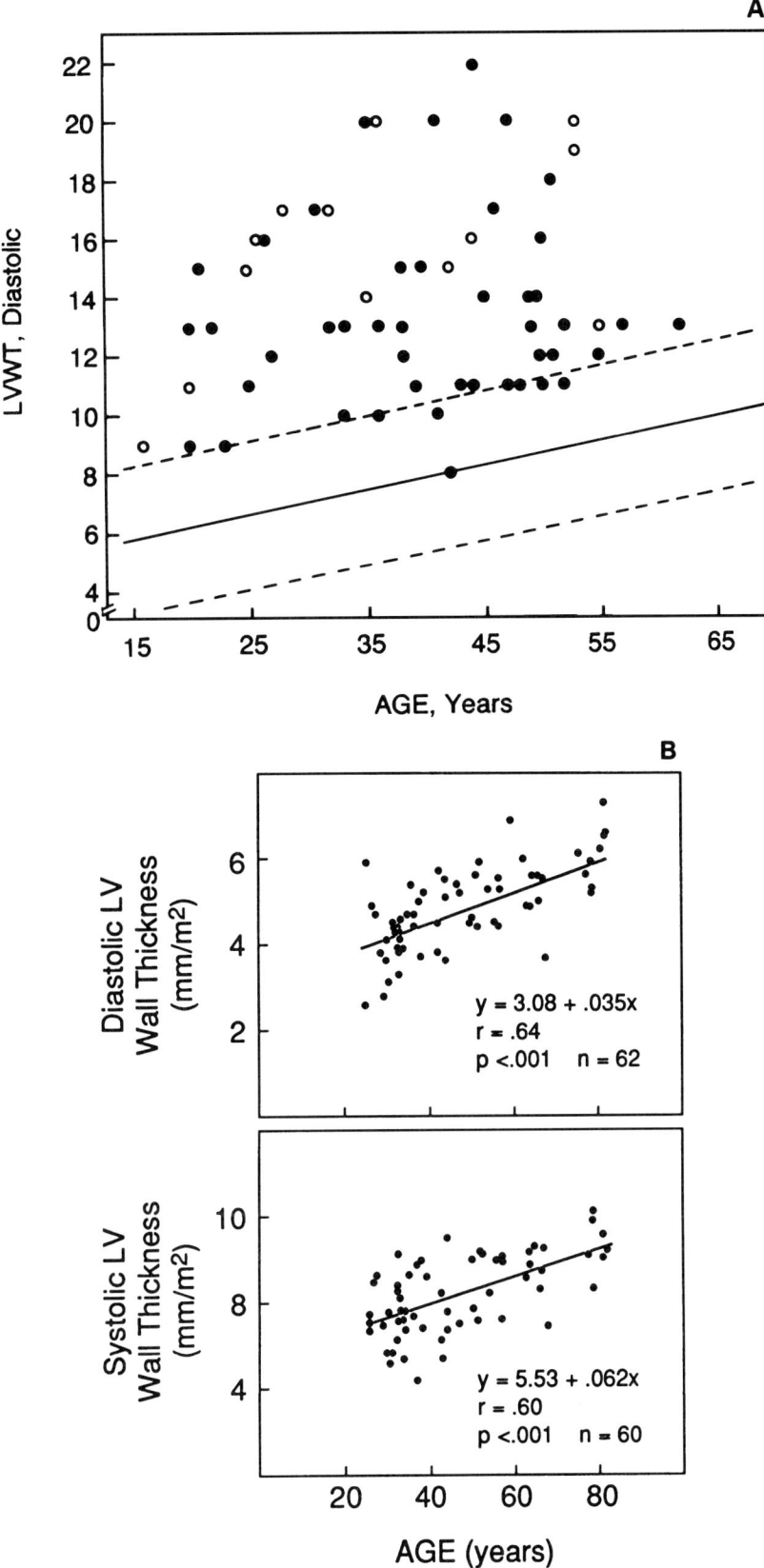

FIG. 17.2. **A:** Least-squares linear regression of left ventricular end-diastolic wall thickness (LVWT) on age (*solid line* = mean; *dashed lines* = ± 2 standard deviations of the mean) in healthy men and women as measured by echocardiography. *Circles* indicate LVWT in patients with aortic valve disease. [From Sjögren (471) with permission.] **B:** LVWT at end-diastole (top) and at end-systole (lower) measured via M-mode echocardiography in healthy men participating in the BLSA (From reference 172, with permission).

CARDIAC ADAPTATIONS TO ARTERIAL STIFFENING DURING AGING

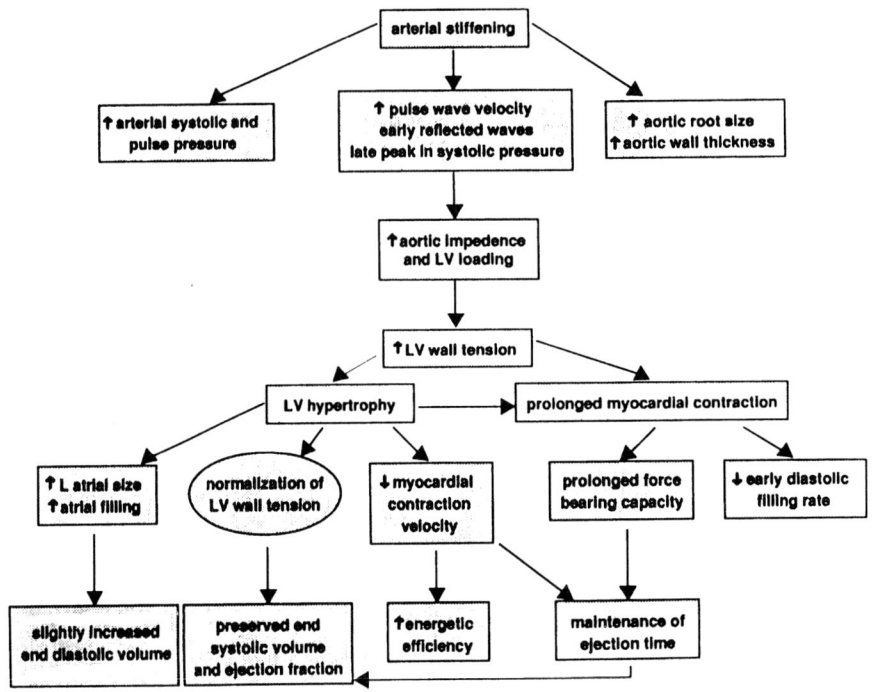

FIG. 17.3. Arterial and cardiac changes that occur with aging in normotensive subjects and at any age in hypertensive subjects. One interpretation of the constellation (flow of arrows) is that vascular changes lead to cardiac structural and functional alterations that maintain cardiac function. [Modified from Lakatta (288) with permission.]

increase in ventricular wall thickness (45, 428). LV cardiac mass estimates via ultrasound are more closely related to arterial pressures recorded in the patient's natural setting during normal activity or exercise, whether measured by portable recorder or home monitor, than to blood pressures measured by a physician (100). In pondering the association between arterial pressure and heart mass, which is influenced by aortic pressure, it is important to recall that the amplification of arterial pressure from the aorta to peripheral arterial sites that normally occurs in younger individuals does not occur, or is markedly blunted, in older individuals (365, 380). Hence, identical brachial arterial pressures (Fig. 17.1A, F) measured in a younger and an older individual may indicate a higher aortic pressure in the older individual.

Theoretically, an acute increase in vascular impedance is accompanied by an acute reduction in SV, and this has also been observed experimentally (381). A chronic reduction in SV has also been observed in some older vs. younger patients in whom aortic impedance has been quantified (363). In contrast, other studies in which arterial stiffness, pulse wave velocity, and systolic arterial pressure (and presumably aortic impedance) increase with age (Figs. 17.1A, B, F) indicate that resting SV is preserved in healthy older men, as is the ejection fraction (EF) (Fig. 17.6A, C). Thus a normal SV and EF (at rest) can be maintained in the presence of aortic stiffening in healthy older men. Preservation of SV is enabled by chronic myocardial adaptations, which include a mild augmentation of cardiac size at end-diastole (Fig. 17.6A). It is important to note that an increased LV size prior to and during the myocardiac contraction places a greater load on cardiac fibers and that this constitutes a "cardiac" component of afterload (Fig. 17.4) via the law of LaPlace. However, modest myocardial wall thickening (Fig. 17.2) which reduces wall stress (and the cardiac component of afterload) and prolonged Ca^{2+} activation of the myofilaments (see below, under Regulation of Cardiac Contraction) occurs with aging. Thus in male members of a healthy, community-dwelling population (142, 421), both the LV wall thickness (170) and the end-diastolic volume index (EDVI) increase with age (see below, under Cardiac Volume and Ejection Fraction), suggesting that the expected increase in LV wall stress based on both LV

REGULATION OF CARDIAC OUTPUT

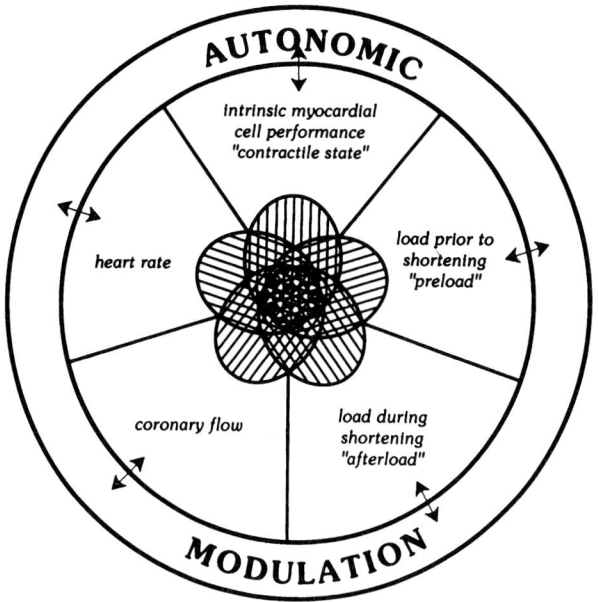

FIG. 17.4. Multiple interdependent factors regulate cardiac output. [From Lakatta (285) with permission.]

dilatation and increased arterial stiffness is minimized. Still, the stroke work index (SWI) at rest, measured as the product of arterial pressure and the stroke volume index (SVI), increases with age in normotensive men (147, 421) due largely to the increase in systolic pressure but also in part to an increase in SVI (see Figs. 17.6A, F, 17.7A). In females, neither EDVI, SVI, nor SWI increase with age (Figs. 17.6A, 17.7B). Since the LV wall thickness increases with aging in women to the same extent as in men, the lack of an increase in EDVI with aging in women suggests that older women may function at a reduced LV wall tension. This may be a factor for the age-associated tendency for end-systolic volume index (ESVI) to decrease and for EF to increase at rest in women.

While the cardiac changes in the scheme in Figure 17.3 are depicted as resulting from increased vascular loading of the heart, a decrease in effective β-adrenergic stimulation of both the heart and the vasculature occurs with aging and in hypertension (see below, under Sympathetic Modulation of the Cardiovascular System) and may be implicated in the associated myocardial changes in part via a reduction in the heart rate at rest in the sitting position and during stress, for example, routine activities of daily life or exercise. In addition, possible age-associated changes in the level or activity of other growth factors that influence the size and structure of myocardial or vascular cells or their matrices may have a role in the schema depicted in Figure 17.3.

MYOCARDIAL AND CARDIAC PUMP FUNCTION AT REST

Integrated Regulation of Cardiac Function

An understanding of the mechanisms that regulate cardiovascular function is tantamount to addressing the issue of how these mechanisms are affected by age. Cardiac output is regulated by multiple mechanisms, the macroscopic descriptors of which include the heart rate and factors that affect SV, that is, the quantity of blood that fills the heart prior to excitation *(preload)*, the mechanical load encountered following the onset of contraction *(afterload)*, the intrinsic myocardial contractile properties *(contractile* or *inotropic* state or level of effectiveness of excitation–contraction coupling), and coronary flow (Fig. 17.4).

When physiologists began to discover these factors they were often described as independent determinants of cardiovascular function, but, as indicated in Figure 17.4, these factors are highly interdependent. Additionally, each of these factors is subject to autonomic modulation, which forms the basis of many cardiovascular reflexes. Each of the factors in Figure 17.4 has determinants at multiple levels (Table 17.2). For example, determinants of afterload at the cardiovascular system level are vascular and blood properties; at the ventricular level are cardiac pressures and volumes; at the muscle level are fiber length and load; at the myocyte level are sarcomere length and load; and at the molecular level are the conformation of the contractile proteins and the extent of Ca^{2+} binding to the myofilaments during contraction. Thus the changing face of the categories in Figure 17.4 must be kept in mind when utilizing these simplified terms (293).

Cardiac Filling (Diastolic) Properties

Early LV filling begins as ventricular pressure decreases below that in the atrium and continues during the cardiac diastole with a further evolution of the atrioventricular (AV) pressure gradient. The stiffness of the ventricular myocardium is a determinant of the ventricular pressure and thus of the AV pressure gradient. The initial ventricular pressure reduction is due to relaxation of myocardial fibers from the prior systole. While this relaxation begins prior to ventricular filling, that is, during the isovolumic relaxation period, it continues to occur following opening of the mitral valve (during the early LV filling period). Thus while ventricular stiffness (more often referred to as "compliance," that is, the inverse of stiffness) is often thought to reflect the passive (structural) properties of the myocardial during the early filling period, it is due, in large part, to the extent of the declining Ca^{2+}-dependent myofilament interac-

TABLE 17.2. *Some Determinants of Cardiovascular Performance*

Cardiovascular system properties	Cardiac muscle properties
Ventricular properties	Myocyte properties
Pericardial properties	Nonmyocyte properties
Arterial properties	Nutrient supply and waste removal
Venous properties	Cell length and pre- and (postexcitation)
Blood properties (i.e., volume and rheologic properties, including viscosity)	Collagen strain
Body position	**Cardiac myocyte properties**
Intrathoracic pressure	Myofilament properties
Heart rate	Excitation properties
Cardiac ventricular properties	Myofilament activation
Myocardial properties, length dependent (i.e., preload- and afterload-dependent fiber orientation)	Sarcomere length
	Crossbridge number
Activation sequence	Crossbridge activation
Coronary vascular properties: preload system, autonomic system, and afterload	Intracellular skeleton
Afterload system properties: arterial properties, ventricular size and blood density	Organelle phosphorylation (e.g., protein kinase or calmodulin kinase)
Preload system properties: blood volume, body position, autonomic tone, and intrathoracic pressure	Oxygen and substrate supply
Valves: preload and afterload	ATP production
Intrachamber communication: loading, activation, autonomic and fiber orientation	

A quantitative description of cardiovascular function would require a polynomial equation with at least as many terms as the number of factors listed above (293). Simultaneous measurements of these factors would be required to define the contribution of each at a given moment and under many diverse physiological and pathological conditions. Adapted from Lakatta and Maughan (293) with permission.

tion. Thus both active, that is, Ca^{2+}-dependent, and structural mechanisms likely regulate the rates of ventricular pressure decay and early filling. Ventricular stiffness or compliance is most often measured as the end-diastolic pressure–volume relation. Despite the popular notion that LV compliance decreases with aging, this parameter, in fact, has not been measured in healthy humans, as simultaneous measurements of pressure and volume have not been made. Whether the atrial or LV pressure during the early filling period or at end-diastole differ in healthy younger and older individuals is also presently unknown.

The time course of isovolumic myocardial relaxation (the time between aortic valve closure and mitral valve opening) becomes prolonged (40% increase) with aging in both men and women (205, 325, 484) (Fig. 17.5A). The LVED is influenced by the pattern of LV filling following the opening of the mitral valve. The peak rate at which the LV fills with blood during early diastole is markedly (50%) reduced with aging between 20 and 80 yr in healthy men and women, as shown by multiple studies utilizing echocardiography, and echo-Doppler or radionuclide techniques (20, 43, 75, 172, 261, 269, 276, 345, 478, 484, 507, 536) (Fig. 17.5B). Asynchrony of relengthening among ventricular segments increases with aging and contributes to the reduction in filling rate (42). In hypertensive subjects, the decrease in the early ventricular filling rate varies directly with the isovolumic relaxation time (479). Following Ca^{2+} channel blocker treatment in older hypertensive subjects, increases in LV peak filling rate were accompanied by reductions in LV mass (449). In a small study sample, in which neither systolic arterial pressure nor LV wall thickness increased with age, the pulmonary capillary wedge pressure, an index of the LVED filling pressure, still increased with age and a marked reduction of early filling rate occurred in the older individuals (261). This suggests that the early LV filling deficit that accompanies aging may not be directly related to an increase in LV wall thickness. Life-style variables, for example, physical activity and ethanol, affect the LV filling rate measured via Doppler techniques in younger individuals (536). However, the peak LV early filling rate measured by radionuclide imaging or echo-Doppler techniques does not differ between older endurance-trained athletes and age-matched, sedentary controls (151, 157, 448).

Regardless of the uncertainties and the likely multifactorial nature of the reduction in the LV early diastolic filling rate with aging, the LVED volume (LVEDV) at rest is not reduced in healthy older individuals (147, 298, 420, 421); in fact, it increases with age in men and is unchanged in women (Figs. 17.6A and 17.8; also see below under Cardiac Volumes and Ejection Fraction). The reduction in early filling rate does not result in a reduced EDV in part because greater filling occurs later in diastole, particularly during the atrial contraction (20, 75, 279, 352, 484, 507). The enhanced atrial contribution to ventricular filling with advancing age is

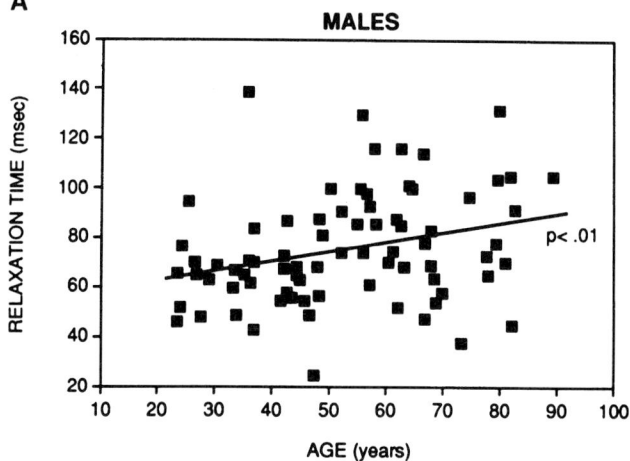

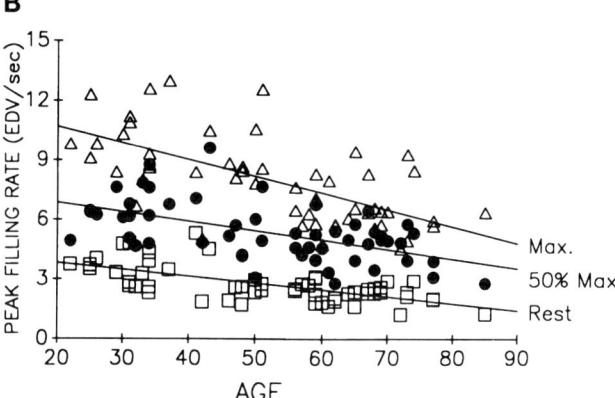

FIG. 17.5. **A:** Isovolumic relaxation time at rest measured from the closure of the aortic valve to the opening of the mitral valve in healthy male participants of the BLSA (Lakatta, E. G., and Fleg, J. L., unpublished results). **B:** Relationships between age and peak filling rate obtained at rest, at 50% of maximal workload, and at maximal workload. For each of these workloads, there was a significant inverse correlation between age and peak filling rate, r = −0.64 (rest), −0.53 (50% maximal workload), and −0.64 (maximal workload). The slopes of the three lines did not differ with a decrease in peak filling rate from 6% to 7% per decade (448).

associated with left atrial enlargement (170, 172) and is the basis of an audible fourth heart sound in most healthy older individuals (143).

Cardiac Volumes and Ejection Fraction

While blood volume in healthy men does not appear to change with age (493), the EDVI (EDV normalized for body size) in the sitting position at rest is moderately increased in healthy older vs. younger sedentary me (Figs. 17.7A, 17.8) (147). An increase in the resting heart size with aging has also been observed in the supine position in some (181, 529), but not all (331), other studies. As we have seen, the increases in myocyte size and LV wall thickness appear to ameliorate the increase in LV wall tension that would occur due to the increase in LVEDVI, increases in arterial impedance, and the increase in peak LV systolic pressure with aging. The resting end-systolic volume index (ESVI) does not increase significantly with aging in healthy men (Fig. 17.6A) (147). In the absence of hypertension, the SVI at rest in the sitting position has been found to not decrease with age in many studies of highly screened subjects of a broad age range (147, 216, 398, 421, 544, 569), in contrast to some prior studies (47, 363 and see 171 for review). In fact, as noted above, the resting, sitting SVI increases slightly with aging in men (Fig. 17.6A) (133), and this is attributable to the increase in EDVI with age (Fig. 17.6A), as EDVI and SVI are highly correlated in healthy individuals of any age (408). Thus in a study of young and middle-aged men in whom EDVI was found to not increase with age at rest in the sitting position (216), no increase in SVI with age was observed. In contrast to men, in healthy women neither the resting EDVI nor the SVI increases with age, the ESVI tends to decrease slightly, and the EF tends to increase slightly (Figs. 17.6A, 17.7). The gender differences in cardiac EDVI, ESVI, EF, and SVI among healthy sedentary individuals (Fig. 17.6) may be attributable in part to differences in fitness level even between sedentary men and women, as these effects are abolished when the fitness influence is controlled for in multiple regression statistical analyses (147) or by a priori matching of younger and older study subjects for a common exercise capacity (298).

In contrast to findings in normotensive men, in hypertensive men SVI has been found to decrease with aging in both cross-sectional and longitudinal studies (130, 326, 345, 346). An age-associated reduction in EDVI in older hypertensive men would be a plausible mechanism for the decrease in SVI in these individuals, but no data are available in this regard. However, in support of this notion, it has been observed that the reduction in SVI with age in some hypertensive men in the supine position is abolished when a sitting position is assumed (130).

The overall systolic function of the heart as a pump is best judged from measurement of the EF [(EDV−ESV)/EDV]. The EF is not altered with aging in healthy men or women at rest (147, 421) (Fig. 17.6C).

Myocardial Contractile Properties

Because of the interaction of factors that regulate cardiac performance (Fig. 17.4), the intrinsic contractile behavior of myocardial fibers cannot be determined satisfactorily in situ. Several noninvasive indices that have been proposed to characterize myocardial contractility have essentially fallen by the wayside due to their non-

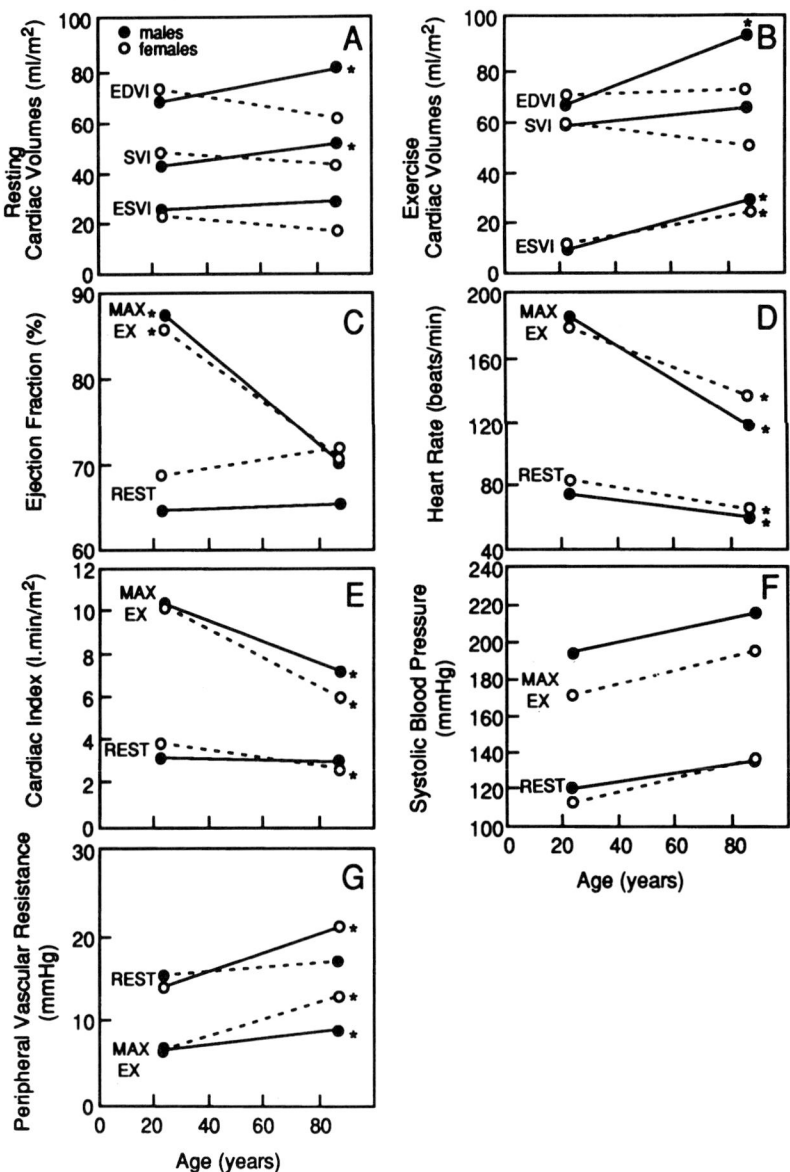

FIG. 17.6. Linear regression on age of cardiac volume indices (**A**, at rest; **B**, during exercise) and ejection fraction (**C**), heart rate (**D**), cardiac index (**E**), systolic arterial pressure (**F**), and peripheral vascular resistance (**G**) at rest and during maximal cycle ergometry in the upright position. Study participants were healthy, sedentary male (n = 95, closed symbols) and female (n = 50, open symbols), community-dwelling volunteers from the BLSA who had been rigorously screened to exclude clinical hypertension and occult coronary artery disease (147). Cardiac volumes were measured via gated blood-pool scans (421). *Linear regression on age within sex is statistically significant. Age–gender interactions are described in Fleg et al. (147).

specificity or lack of sensitivity. The index of myocardial contractility that is presently considered superior to others (although under some conditions it is "preload-dependent") is the trajectory of ESV vs. mean arterial pressure, sometimes referred to as "E_{max}," derived from a series of pressure–volume loops measured over a range of cardiac volumes (428, 429, 430). In noninvasive studies, a crude index of this trajectory, that is, the ratio of end-systolic arterial pressure to ESV, is not reduced at rest with age in either healthy men (Fig. 17.8A) or women (148).

The relationship of SWI to EDVI is also a measure of cardiac pump function. Figure 17.7A indicates that both LV SWI and EDVI at rest shift with age in men, that is,

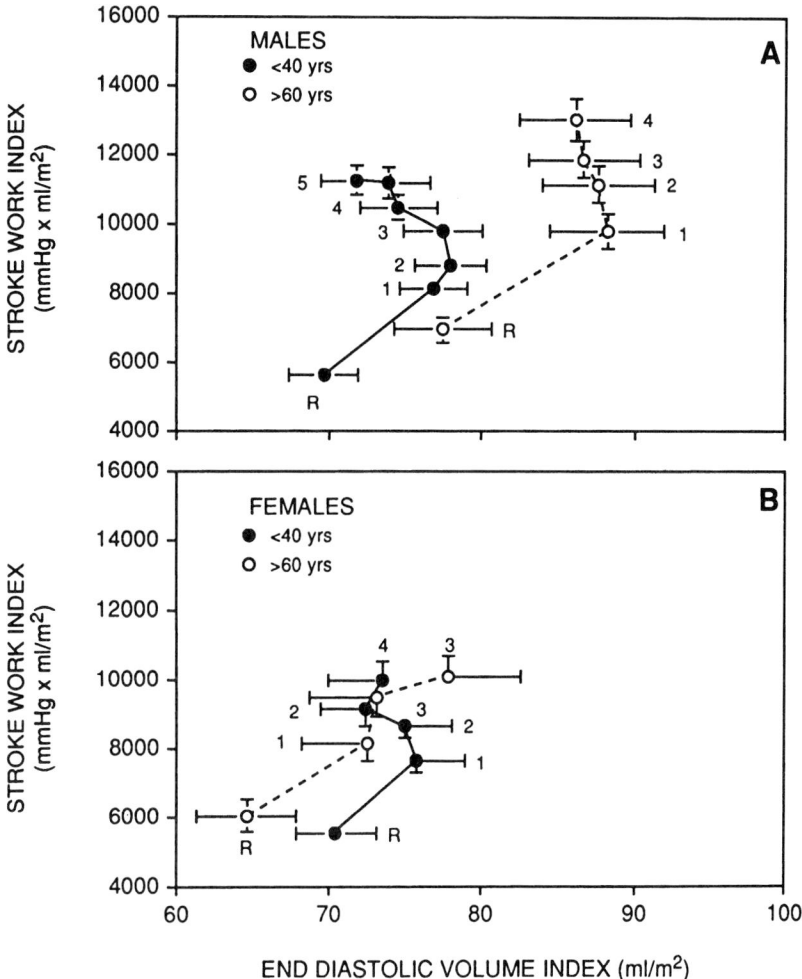

FIG. 17.7. Left ventricular SWI measured as the product of SVI and brachial systolic pressure at rest and during graded exercise in younger (< 40 yr) and older (> 60 yr) men (top), and women (bottom) of the study population depicted in Figure 17.7. [From Fleg et al. (147) with permission.]

a greater resting SWI is achieved from a greater EDVI. In contrast, an age-associated shift in resting SWI is not apparent in women (Fig. 17.7B).

Heart Rate and Rhythm

Beginning by age 60 yr there is a pronounced decrease in the number of pacemaker cells in the sinoatrial (SA) node, and by age 75 yr less than 10% of the cell number found in the young adult remains (see 145 for review). With advancing age, there is an increase in elastic and collagenous tissue in all parts of the conduction system, as well as of fat around the SA node. A variable degree of calcification of the left side of the cardiac fibrous skeleton, which includes the aortic and mitral annuli, the central fibrous body, and the summit of the interventricular septum, occurs. Because of their proximity to these structures, the AV node, the AV bundle, bifurcation, and proximal left and right bundle branches may be affected by this process, resulting in so-called "primary" or "idiopathic" heart block. A modest prolongation of the P-R interval within the normal range (< 20 ms) occurs with aging in healthy individuals and is localized to the proximal P-R segment, probably reflecting delay within the AV junction (144). An increase in both supraventricular and ventricular premature beats occurs in older healthy men and women compared to their younger counterparts, but this does not appear to be of clinical significance (142, 144).

Most cross-sectional studies have indicated that the supine basal heart rate does not differ among younger and older individuals (144, 147, 435, 449). Studies of a large number of rigorously screened, healthy individuals, however, indicate that in the sitting position, heart

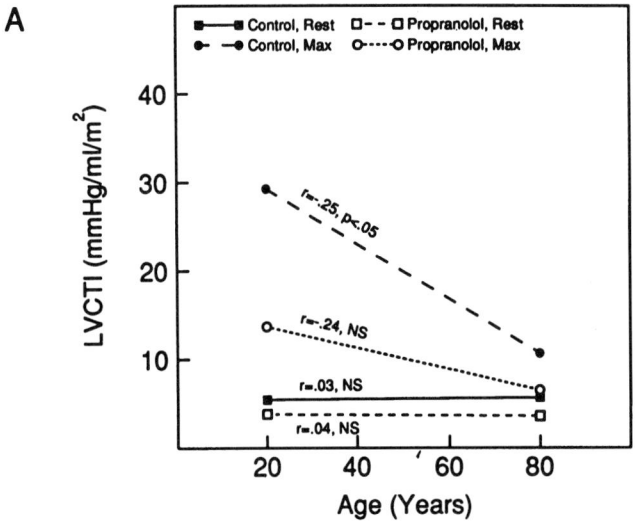

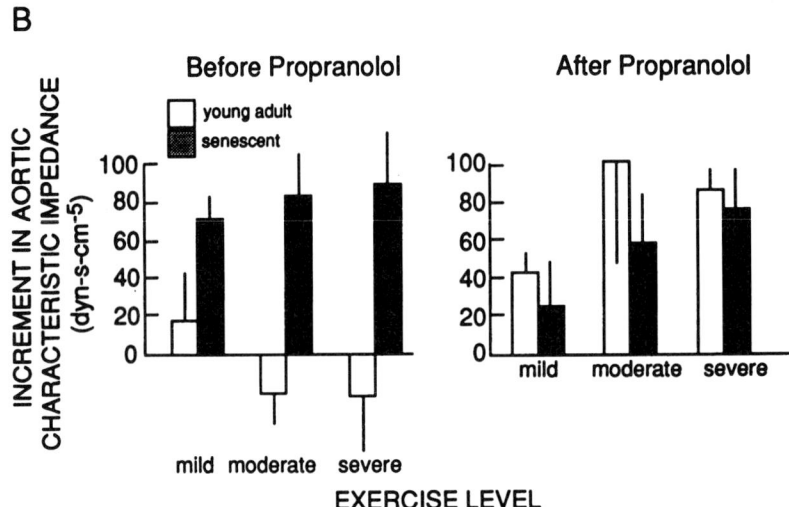

FIG. 17.8. **A:** Left ventricular contractility index (LVCTI) measured as the ratio of end-systolic arterial pressure and ESVI. Lines are the best fit, linear regressions at rest and during exercise in the presence and absence of β-adrenergic blockade with propranolol. [From Fleg et al. (150) with permission.] **B:** The effect of exercise on characteristic aortic impedance during graded treadmill exercise in the presence and absence of β-adrenergic blockade (propranolol) in healthy adult □ and senescent ■ beagle dogs. In the absence of β-adrenergic blockade, exercise increased impedance in senescent but not in younger dogs. In contrast, during β-blockade impedance was increased during exercise in dogs of both ages. [From Yin et al. (567) with permission.]

rate decreases with age in both males and females (147, 451, 466) (Fig. 17.6D). In a longitudinal study, a decrease in resting heart rate (81–60 bpm) occurred over 30 yr (20).

Resting heart rate is modulated in part by the balance of sympathetic and parasympathetic tones, with the latter predominating. The interaction of age and posture on heart rate as noted above suggests that age-associated changes occur in mechanisms that regulate heart rate (see below under Postural Reflexes). The respiratory variation of the heart rate, which is also determined largely by autonomic tone, is diminished with advancing age (93), as is the spontaneous variation in heart rate measured over a 24-h period via Holter monitoring (248, 269, 389) or spectral analysis (267, 451, 466). In the latter studies the decreased variation in heart rate with aging was thought to result from reduction in both parasympathetic and sympathetic modulation. The intrinsic sinus node rate, that is, in the presence of both sympathetic and parasympathetic blockade, is significantly diminished with age: at 20 yr the average intrinsic heart rate is 104 bpm as compared with 92 bpm in at

45–55 yr (237). No data are presently available for older individuals. Heart rate may be influenced by levels of circulatory catecholamines. Plasma levels of norepinephrine and epinephrine at rest have been found to increase with age in many (128, 134, 248, 424), but not all (152), studies. Blocking only the sympathetic system at rest with propranolol does not produce a differential effect with age on supine heart rate or LV hemodynamics in healthy men at supine rest (561).

Cardiac Output

Resting cardiac output (the product of SV and heart rate) and cardiac index (CI) (cardiac output normalized for body surface area) have been found to be markedly reduced (47, 85), mildly reduced (80, 238, 312, 344, 495, 496), or unchanged (Fig. 17.6E) in older vs. younger individuals (148, 215, 420, 421). The variability of results among these studies can be attributed largely to differences in the criteria employed for selecting individuals for study, number of individuals selected, body position during study, body composition, and measurement methods employed. Cardiac output is influenced by the basal metabolic rate and body composition, both of which change substantially with age (see below, under Dynamic Exercise). Age-associated declines in basal metabolic rate are abolished when O_2 consumption is normalized to an index of lean muscle mass (525). Age range also influenced the outcome of cardiac function studies at rest. Close inspection of the data of one study reporting a marked age-associated decline in resting cardiac output and EF (277) indicates that most of the age effect occurred between the ages of 6 and 20 yr. In the highly screened population of 95 men depicted in Figure 17.6, the resting CI (Fig. 17.6E) does not change with age because an increase in SVI, due to an increase in the EDVI, compensates for the age-associated reduction in heart rate (Fig. 17.6E). In women in the same study, however, the resting sitting CI was found to decrease slightly with age, in part due to the absence of cardiac dilatation at end-diastole and its accompanying increase in SVI (Fig. 17.6A). In older hypertensive men, that is, those in whom arterial pressure exceeds the clinically defined upper limits of normal (140/90 mm Hg), CI at rest is less than in younger hypertensive men and is associated with a diminution of SVI (326, 344, 345). Part of the difference in age-associated changes, or the lack of change, of CI in normotensive and hypertensive men may be due to a greater CI in young hypertensive than in young normotensive individuals.

For simplicity, blood flow from the heart is sometimes considered a steady rather than a pulsatile phenomenon, and PVR is derived from cardiac output (flow) and mean arterial pressure (Ohm's law applied to the circulation). Arterial pressure and PVR in the sitting position in healthy, sedentary men and women of a broad range are depicted in Figure 17.6F and G. Systolic brachial arterial pressure increases with age at rest in both sexes; mean arterial pressure increases mildly with age. PVR at rest in the sitting position is not altered by age in healthy men but increases with age in women in the same study population.

The age-associated changes, or the lack thereof, in several aspects of cardiovascular function at rest in men are integrated in the lower part of Figure 17.3. A prolonged myocardial contraction time in older individuals maintains a normal ejection time in the presence of the late augmentation of aortic impedance due to early reflected pulse waves. The prolonged contraction also contributes to the maintenance of SV, ESV, and EF at rest. Thus in healthy humans, systolic cardiac function at rest is not much altered by age, even though the arterial tree stiffens and imposes an increased afterload on the heart. The down side of prolonged contractile activation is that myocardial relaxation time is prolonged in older individuals and at the time of the mitral valve opening some contractile activation persists. This is one factor that causes the early LV filling rate to be reduced in older individuals. Structural changes and functional heterogeneity occurring within the LV with aging may also contribute to this reduction in peak LV filling rate. However, a concomitant adaptation (left atrial enlargement and an enhanced atrial contribution to ventricular filling) compensates for the reduced early filling and in part maintains an increased LVEDV in men and prevents a decrease in LVEDV in women.

In individuals with hypertension, the same vascular and cardiac changes observed with aging in normotensive individuals occur at a younger age and in some instances are exaggerated. The similarities between aging and hypertension are so striking that aging has been referred to as "muted hypertension" and hypertension has been referred to as "accelerated aging" (390, 553). According to the perspective depicted in Figure 17.3, changes in the large arteries, cardiac mass, myocardial relaxation, and filling parameters in both normotensive and hypertensive individuals at any age form a continuum. In this regard, a clinical distinction between normotensive and hypertensive subjects may be somewhat artificial but clinically useful with regard to risk for cardiovascular morbidity and mortality (393). However, some changes occur with aging in hypertensive subjects that are not observed in normotensive subjects. In hypertensive men PVR increases substantially with aging, in contrast to normotensive men in whom no change is observed (Fig. 17.7G). Thus in hypertensive subjects an increase in PVR elevated diastolic and mean arterial pressures and plays a greater role in vascular loading of the heart than in normotensive subjects. Also, in older hypertensive men, resting SVI and CI are not maintained at the levels measured in younger hypertensive men.

CARDIOVASCULAR RESERVE

Cardiovascular reflex mechanisms become operative in response to perturbations from the supine basal state and partially mediate the utilization of cardiovascular reserve functions. The end result of these reflex mechanisms is enhanced blood flow within selected body organs and preservation of arterial pressure. A change in blood flow from the heart depends upon the product of changes in heart rate and SV, the latter being determined by the changes in EDV and ESV (Fig. 17.4). Changes in EDV are determined in part by changes in venous return, which depend upon the ability of the blood to flow through the vascular system.

Postural Reflexes

Arterial Pressure and Peripheral Vascular Resistance. Several studies suggest a general tendency toward either maintenance or augmentation of PVR during orthostatic stress in subjects (mostly male) up to 60–70 yr. In general, in healthy, community-dwelling older individuals the arterial pressure change with posture is also maintained (230, 457, 459, 472), and postural hypotension or acute orthostatic intolerance, that is, dizziness or fainting when assuming an upright from a supine position or during a passive tile, thus does not occur (472). In contrast to healthy, community-dwelling volunteer subjects, orthostatic intolerance is common in older (>70 yr), debilitated, chronically institutionalized individuals. (318). The likelihood for orthostatic intolerance is increased in individuals who, prior to orthostatic stress, exhibit marked reductions in peak LV filling rate, EDV, and SV in the supine position (319). In studies of this sort, however, the effects of very advanced age cannot be dissociated from those of a very sedentary life-style.

Heart Rate and Cardiac Volumes. The acute heart rate increase caused by orthostatic stress decreases in magnitude with age and takes longer to achieve. The immediate heart rate responses to sudden increments of neck suction and neck pressure also change with aging: a lesser tachycardia during decreases in carotid transmural pressure and lesser bradycardia during increases in transmural pressure occur with aging in both women (395) and men (473). During spontaneous breathing, age-associated differences in heart rate with postural movements have been attributed in part to decreases in β-adrenergic responses, while differences during standing metronome breathing have been attributed to both reduced parasympathetic withdrawal and β-adrenergic activation (451). The decreased variability of heart rate observed in older vs. younger individuals in the upright vs. the supine position has been attributed to a diminished recruitment of baroreceptor sensitivity, that is, the slope of the relationship of the change in heart rate vs. the change in arterial pressure is negatively correlated with increasing age and increased resting arterial pressure (116, 183, 248, 400, 461, 559). In beagle dogs the baroreflex control of renal sympathetic nerve activity and arterial pressure, in addition to heart rate, declines with age (195, 196). The basal sympathetic nerve activity to muscles in humans increases with age (195, 196). The basal sympathetic nerve activity to muscles in humans increases with age (116, 559) in both normotensive and hypertensive individuals. However, the baroreceptor control of sympathetic outflow to skeletal muscle can be well maintained in healthy individuals even into the seventh decade (116). The low-pressure baroreceptor, or cardiopulmonary reflex, also decreases with age in normotensive (77, 195) but not in hypertensive individuals (481). The sensitivity of the chemoreceptor reflex also appears to decline with aging, as the increase in heart rate in healthy men (aged 64–73 yr) is less than that in young men (aged 22–30 yr) following exposure to hypoxia (11 vs. 34% increase) or to hypercarbia (0% vs. 15%) (275). The apparent age-associated reduction in the effectiveness of autonomic nervous system–mediated reflexes during postural maneuvers occurs in the presence of age-associated increases in plasma catecholamine levels (see above and below). The reduction in baroreceptor function and the increase in muscle sympathetic nerve activity with aging may be related to the age-associated increase in plasma catecholamines (461, 559).

The SV reduction with postural stress tends to be less in healthy older than in younger individuals; thus the postural change in cardiac output does not vary significantly with age because the lesser increase in heart rate in older individuals is balanced by a lesser reduction in SV (420). This leads to the profile of heart rate and SVI observed in healthy older individuals in the sitting position at rest shown in Figure 17.6. Even in studies that have found cardiac output to be reduced with aging in the supine position (on the basis of a reduced SV in older vs. younger men), this age effect was abolished in the sitting position due to lesser reduction in SV in older men upon assumption of the upright position (130, 182). As with a change to an upright position in response to gradual tilt or graded lower-body negative pressure (LBNP), SV and cardiac output decrease less in older than in younger individuals (115, 161, 328), although the heart rate increase is blunted in these older individuals (115). A lesser reduction in SV in older vs. younger individuals following a postural stress implies either less of a reduction of LVEDV or more of a reduction in LVESV in older individuals. Cardiac volumes (measured by equilibrium-gated cardiac blood-pool scans) and heart rate have been measured in the steady-state in supine and sitting positions in male volunteer subjects (aged 25–80 yr) who had been rigorously screened to exclude cardiovascular disease (420). Following assumption of the sitting position from the supine, changes in cardiac output with posture in older vs. younger individuals depend more on changes in LVEDV and SV and less on changes in heart rate (420).

Although the cardiac filling rate during early diastole is less in older than in younger individuals and an apparent age-associated decrease in ventricular compliance is manifest during postural maneuvers (367), filling volume deficits, in fact, do not occur in healthy older individuals either at rest or during orthostatic stress. Rather, LVEDV and SV in the sitting position at rest are preserved or even enhanced (Fig. 17.6) in sedentary, healthy, older vs. younger individuals (331, 420, 421, 445, 458, 569). A reduced venous compliance in older vs. younger individuals, advanced as a mechanism to account for less of a peripheral fluid shift during orthostatic maneuvers (115, 513), could be a mechanism that preserves cardiac filling volume and maintains SV in the upright position in healthy elderly individuals. A reduction in the venous response to β-adrenergic stimulation (relaxation) with preservation of the α-adrenergic (constrictor) response (see below, under Sympathetic Modulation of Cardiovascular Function), resulting in a greater relative venoconstriction in older individuals, may contribute to a reduced venous compliance with aging.

In contrast to the above observations, when old (74 ± 2 yr) were compared to young (27 ± 3 yr) individuals, the SV decline with tilt was found to be greater in the former than in the latter and was attributed not to differences in EDV response but to a relative inability of older individuals to reduce ESV (458). In this study, a substantial PVR increase in the older group occurred with tilt and was sufficient to maintain arterial pressure, whereas an increase in PVR did not occur in the younger group. Intriguingly, age-associated differences in the ESV response to postural stress were lessened after a Ca^{2+} channel blocker (458), perhaps associated with a reduction in Ca^{2+}-dependent determinants of arterial impedance (see above, under Cardiac Filling (Diastolic Properties)).

In summary, in response to orthostatic stress, maintenance of total PVR does not decline with aging. The heart rate increase is blunted in older vs. younger individuals. The expected LVEDV reduction is less in older vs. younger individuals, and SV is better preserved.

Isometric Exercise

Sustained isometric handgrip increases both arterial pressure and heart rate and the response varies in magnitude in proportion to the relative level and duration of effort (334). After 30 s of maximal handgrip heart rate was observed to increase 50 bpm in young (aged 23–31 yr) vs. 12 bpm in older (aged 54–78 yr) healthy men (258). Heart rates prior to handgrip were not age-related. During sustained isometric handgrip at 40% of maximum, held to fatigue, the heart rate increase in healthy men was found to diminish over a narrow (20–50 yr) age range (387).

Another type of pressor stress, that induced pharmacologically, has also been used to assess the intrinsic myocardial reserve capacity. In response to a 30-mmHg increase in systolic blood pressure induced by phenylephrine infusion (in the presence of β-adrenergic blockade), significant LV dilatation was noted in healthy older (60–68 yr), but not in younger (18–34 yr), men; the cardiac dilatation, measured via M-mode echocardiography, in older men occurred even in the presence of a smaller reduction of the heart rate (561). Thus because of an apparent age-associated decrease in the intrinsic myocardial contractile reserve response to an increase in afterload, the senescent heart dilates and contracts from a greater preload than does the young heart. The cardiac response to a pressor stress is also diminished in senescent rats, whereas the response to a volume stress is unimpaired (308).

Dynamic Exercise

Aerobic Capacity. The maximum oxygen consumption ($\dot{V}O_{2max}$) achieved during exercise is about ninefold greater than the basal level of O_2 consumption. In addition to a four-to-fivefold increase in cardiac output, the O_2 extraction by working tissues increases and causes the arteriovenous O_2 difference, $(AV)O_2$, to increase up to twofold during strenuous exercise. This results in part from an increase (up to 15-fold) in the relative proportion of cardiac output delivered to working muscles (76). The cardiopulmonary factors that underlie total body O_2 consumption or aerobic capacity have been traditionally referred to as "central circulatory," while local tissue O_2 delivery, extraction, and utilization are referred to as "peripheral" factors.

It has been well documented that $\dot{V}O_{2max}$, adjusted

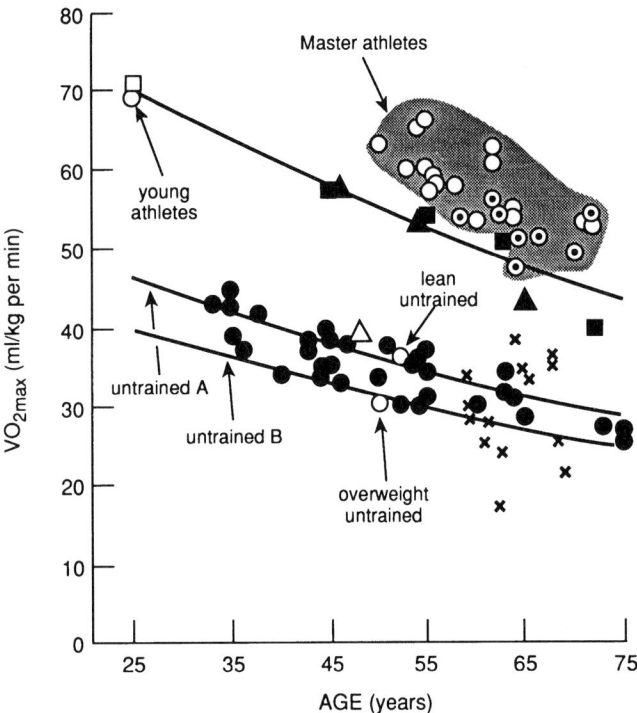

FIG. 17.9. $\dot{V}O_{2max}$ as a function of age as measured in males of varying age, fitness, and body composition. [Modified from Heath et al. (208) with permission.] Points are average $\dot{V}O_{2max}$ values for groups of men of different ages from reports in the literature for young athletes, master athletes, lean untrained, and overweight untrained men (14,23,33,39,52,92,96,102,184,350,392,416,417). Champion young athletes, ○, Heath et al. (208) and □ Dill et al. (102); ex-champion athletes, △, Dill et al. (102) and Robinson et al. (417); cross-country runners, ▲, Grimby and Saltin (184); runners ■, Pollock et al. (392): groups of untrained men from 9 studies, ● and X; master athletes ○ and ●. [From Heath et al. (208) and Fleg et al. (149), respectively, with permission.]

for body weight, declines with age (Fig. 17.9). The extent of this decline varies among studies, relating in part to uncontrolled population truncation due to cross-sectional sampling and changes in body weight, composition, and fitness levels among the individuals studied. Longitudinal studies report a more pronounced age-associated decline in $\dot{V}O_{2max}$ than do cross-sectional studies (95). Whether or not the same factors that regulate $\dot{V}O_{2max}$ are limiting the $\dot{V}O_{2max}$ in individuals of different ages is not known (401). The maximum cardiac output may be lower in older than in younger individuals due to the age-associated reduction in maximum heart rate (see below, under Cardiovascular Reserve).

Whether or not a measured reduction in cardiac output (compared to younger individuals) at exhaustion actually limits treadmill exercise capacity and therefore $\dot{V}O_{2max}$ in older individuals is difficult ascertain. Treadmill exercise is usually limited by dyspnea (shortness of breath). However, a reduction in respiratory muscle reserve function in older individuals, due to an age-associated reduction in the number of muscle fibers or to a reduction in the muscle utilization of O_2 per muscle unit (due to aging or to a sedentary disposition), might contribute to the age-associated limitation of work capacity, even though arterial PO_2 is maintained. A concomitant reduction in cardiac output would be expected to accompany a reduced work capacity. Thus a reduction in cardiac output measured at exhaustion cannot ipso facto be implicated as the cause of reduced work capacity and $\dot{V}O_{2max}$. Indeed, some studies during graded upright cycle exercise have been interpreted to indicate that the cardiac response for the work performed ($\dot{V}O_{2max}$ achieved) in older subjects is as adequate as that in younger subjects (182, 238). Is is of note, however, that during cycle ergometry, the peak O_2 consumption in a given individual averages about 80% of that during treadmill exercise (147), and the factor limiting the duration of the exercise is usually leg fatigue. While this difference in peak O_2 consumption between the two modes of aerobic exercise is not age-related (147), it still may preclude extrapolation of the maximum cardiac output and $\dot{V}O_{2max}$ measurements during cycle ergometry to cardiac output and $\dot{V}O_{2max}$ achieved during maximum treadmill exercise in a given individual.

Other noncardiac factors leading to a reduction in peak (A-V)O_2, for example age-associated changes in body composition and muscle mass (44, 59, 143, 167, 168, 313, 414, 525), also appear to be involved in $\dot{V}O_{2max}$ reduction with aging. In spite of a decline in skeletal muscle mass with aging, total body mass remains constant because of an increase in body fat, not only subcutaneously but also intraperitoneally and intramuscularly (44, 167, 168). Normalization of peak $\dot{V}O_2$ to an index of muscle mass, creatinine excretion, markedly reduces the magnitude of the apparent age-related decline in $\dot{V}O_2$ normalized for body mass (kg wt), that is, the routine normalization procedure utilized in most studies (143, 222). Changed in muscle strength and work capacity with aging in sedentary individuals likely reflect changes in the number of functional motor units and the presence of neuromuscular dysfunction or loss of muscle fibers in some older individuals (59, 314).

The metabolism of skeletal muscle (flexor digitorum superficialis) in younger and older healthy humans has been studies in vivo by ^{31}P nuclear magnetic resonance, and, in contrast to the morphological changes noted above, neither at rest nor during exercise were age differences noted in intracellular pH or concentrations of adenosine triphosphate (ATP), phosphocreatine, or inorganic phosphate (P_i) (514). Thus aging does not affect the metabolic ability of human hand skeletal muscles, at least, to respond to exercise, and morphological changes found in superficial hand muscles of the elderly are not accompanied by alterations in energy metabolism (514). Similar conclusions have been reached from measurements of mitochondrial volumes and various enzyme activities in vastus lateralis biopsies from men 22–65 yr of age (378). Still, decreases in total skeletal muscle mass or in neuromuscular function with aging, if these do indeed occur, would have severe functional implications.

Arterial Pressure, Vascular Resistance, and Impedance. During cycle exercise, unlike treadmill exercise, the diastolic pressure shows a modest increase due, possibly in part, to some degree of involuntary isometric contraction and to increased force generation by the legs of the subject during this procedure. The age-associated increases in brachial systolic arterial pressure at rest persist at a similar magnitude during cycle exercise (Fig. 17.6F); in some instances systolic pressure at maximum exercise increases more than it does at rest in older vs. younger individuals (147, 238, 349). (With respect to the arterial load on the LV, it is important to recall that the relationship between brachial and aortic systolic pressure in young individuals differs from that in older ones due to the early return of reflected pulse waves in the later. Specifically, when brachial arterial pressures are of equal magnitude in younger and older individuals the aortic pressure is greater in older individuals.)

The extent to which PVR becomes reduced and arterial pressure and impedance increase during exercise depends on the maximum work capacity, which depends in part on the physical fitness and other noncardiac neuroendocrine and metabolic factors. In some studies the reduction in PVR during exercise was less in older than in younger individuals (238), while in others (Fig. 17.6G) the age effect was minimal in men but substantial in women (147, 421).

During exercise in young humans, aortic input impedance does not appear to increase, probably due to an increase in the aortic diameter (357). In older individuals, were a further increase in aortic impedance to occur during exercise than noted at rest, it could explain, in part at least, the observed age-associated differences in the pattern of ventricular ejection during exercise. The effect of age on vascular impedance during exercise has not been studied in humans. However, in the canine model it has been observed that aortic impedance, which does not vary with age at rest (567), increases over a wide range of exercise stresses in 10–12-yr-old beagle dogs but not in 1–3-yr-old dogs (Fig. 17.8B). Although changes in the passive stiffness characteristics of the aorta in both dogs (563) and humans are an apparent cause of increased aortic impedance, age differences in autonomic modulation might also play a role. Thus in the presence of β-adrenergic blockade effected by propranolol, aortic impedance increased during exercise in younger dogs and the age-associated differences in impedance seen during exercise in the absence of propranolol were abolished (567).

End-Diastolic and End-Systolic Volumes. Augmentation of LVEDV during exercise (as in the case of postural maneuvers) is one mechanism through which SV may be maintained or augmented during exercise stress. In instances where cardiac volumes in a sufficient number of healthy individuals of a sufficiently broad age range have been measured during upright cycle exercise, the peak diastolic filling rate increased in both older and younger individuals (448) and no deficit in LVEDVI during upright cycle exercise was observed (147, 421). In these healthy, sedentary older men (147, 421) the LVEDVI at exhaustion during upright cycle exercise was increased compared to younger men (Fig. 17.6); however, an age-associated increase in LVEDVI during exercise was not present in women (147). The age–gender interaction in LVEDVI regulation during exercise, largely due to age–gender differences in LVEDVI at rest (Fig. 17.6), confounds the interpretation of studies that compare, without respect to age, cardiac volume responses during exercise in men and women across a broad age range (215, 502). A greater end-diastolic dilatation during supine exercise in older vs. younger individuals has also been observed (182, 331, 445, 529). In contrast, a study in which the age range of subjects was truncated (20–50 yr) failed to detect this age-associated increase in LVEDVI (216, 217); in this latter study, however, LVEDVI at rest in the sitting position decreased with age, that is, older men had smaller hearts (Fig. 17.6).

Enhanced LVEDVI during exercise in some older men, even in the absence of ventricular compliance changes, may be accompanied by enhanced filling pressure. This may explain the observation that in older individuals in whom filling pressure increased the most during exercise, SV also increased the most (182). However, an increase in LV diastolic filling pressure is associated with an increase in pulmonary venous pressure, which enhances the likelihood for pulmonary congestion. This may predispose older individuals to a lower threshold for dyspnea (shortness of breath) during exercise. Additionally, because the generation of a given ventricular pressure requires a greater ventricular wall stress (force/unit cross-sectional area) if the ventricular radius is increased, a greater level of myocardial contractility and energy consumption per stroke is required by the dilated aged heart. The age-associated increase in ventricular wall thickness, as noted above (see Cardiac Structure), reduces the magnitude of the increased LV stress due to ventricular dilatation.

While LVEDVI is preserved or enhanced during exercise in healthy, sedentary, older individuals relative to younger ones, the reduction in LVESVI during exercise (Fig. 17.6) is blunted in both healthy older men and women (147, 331, 421, 445, 448). This may be attributed in part to an apparent coupling that has been observed between the change in LVEDV and LVESV in the transition from rest to exercise in individuals of any age (408). Alternatively, the increase in LVESVI during exercise in older individuals may exceed that expected on the basis of the increase in LVEDVI and may reflect a relative reduction in myocardial contractile reserve or a relatively greater increase in impedance of LV ejection with aging during exercise. The failure of SVI at peak exercise (Fig. 17.6B) to remain higher in older than in younger men, as it is at rest, appears to be related to the failure of LVESVI to decrease in older men to the extent that it does in younger men. Because the augmentation of EF during exercise depends on the extent to which the LVESV is reduced (408), EF also increases less during exercise in older than in younger men and women (Fig. 17.6C) (147, 394, 421). As both maximum myocardial contractile reserve and regulation of vascular impedance during exercise (567) depend in part on the response to β-adrenergic stimulation, a deficit in the effectiveness of the latter with aging (see below, under Cardiovascular Target Organ Response . . .) could account for the failure of ESVI to decrease and for EF to increase during exercise in older individuals to the extent that it does in younger ones.

As we know interactions of age, disease, and life-style (for example, fitness) confound the interpretation of measures of cardiovascular performance, particularly during stress. Significant occult obstructive coronary disease can largely be eliminated noninvasively by the combination of electrocardiogram (ECG) and thallium imaging during exercise stress (383). In older individuals with occult coronary artery disease the age-associated trends for LVED dilatation, reduced LVESV, and reduced EF during exercise are exaggerated (146, 148, 394).

Myocardial Contractile Reserve. The LV contractility index increases to a lesser extent during exercise in older men (Fig. 17.8A). this age difference is markedly attenuated during exercise in the presence of β-adrenergic blockade, suggesting a diminution in the effectiveness of β-adrenergic modulation of myocardial contractility with aging (see below, under Cardiovascular Target Organ Response . . .).

Heart Rate, Stroke Volume, and Cardiac Output. It has long been known that, relative to younger individuals, a deficit in the increase in heart rate during vigorous treadmill or upright cycle exercise (Fig. 17.6D) occurs in older individuals (see 171 for review). The decrease in the maximum heart rate achieved during exercise in older individuals is not attributable to disease or sedentary left-style, as a deficit of similar magnitude occurs in both healthy, sedentary men and women and in older athletes (121, 149, 208). It is of interest that during exercise, extrasystoles, including short runs of ventricular tachycardia, are more commonly observed in healthy older than in younger individuals but have no prognostic significance with respect to 5-yr cardiac morbidity or mortality (54, 141).

In some studies, a reduced SVI during vigorous exercise has also been observed in older vs. younger individuals (238, 277), while in other studies, SVI during vigorous exercise is equivalent in younger and older individuals (147, 216, 217, 569) or greater in some older individuals (181, 331, 421, 495). The heterogeneity of the SVI measurements among older individuals is in part the cause of variable CI results observed during upright cycle exercise among older individuals in various studies (31, 147, 181, 182, 216, 238, 277, 331, 421). This heterogeneity results from differences in the extent to which occult coronary artery disease was present among older study subjects or from differences in fitness status, heart size, and body composition. A cross-sectional study of 145 healthy, sedentary individuals of a broad age range indicates that the maximum CI during cycle ergometry declines modestly with age due to a smaller heart rate increment in older individuals (Fig. 17.6E), whereas SVI during exercise does not decline with age in either men or women (Fig. 17.6B). It is noteworthy, however, that during peak exercise, despite persistent end-diastolic dilatation in older men, SVI is not greater than in younger men as it is at rest. Thus some age-associated factors limit SV during exercise (see below, under Dynamic Exercise). In other studies, the age-associated decline in CI during maximum cycle exercise in the sitting position has been noted to be more marked than that reported by older individuals in these studies vs. the former (147) study. The SVI achieved during exercise in the healthy, older, sedentary, normotensive men and women in Figure 17.6B is determined in part by their respective heart volumes at rest (Fig. 17.6A). The larger hearts at rest (due to an increase in LVEDVI) in healthy older men deliver larger SVIs at rest than the smaller hearts of younger men. As we have seen peak exercise SVI in healthy younger men equals that in healthy older men in spite of an augmented LVEDVI in the latter, because the LVESVI decreases to a greater extent in the former than in the latter. The relationship between SWI and LVEDVI during exercise is often used as an index of cardiac reserve pump function. Figure 17.7 depicts this relationship for the healthy men and women described in Figure 17.6. During exercise, LVSWI is similar in healthy older and younger men but in older men occurs from a larger LVEDV. Thus the LVSWI–LVEDVI relationship for older men is shifted rightward of that for younger men. This suggests a decrease in LV pump functional reserve with age in men. In contrast, there is no evidence for a decrease in exercise LV pump function in women as the relationship of stroke work to LVEDVI is similar in older and younger women. In studies in which SVI during dynamic exercise has been reported to be reduced in older vs. younger individuals (238, 277), LVEDVI and LVESVI have not been measured and SVI has been calculated from the measured O_2 consumption, heart rate, and CI. Thus from these studies it is not known whether the failure of SVI to increase in older individuals to the extent that it did in younger ones is attributable to a relative reduction in venous return and LVEDVI, perhaps due in part to a markedly diminished myocardial compliance, or from failure of the LVESVI to decrease to the same extent in elderly vs. younger individuals. In contrast to healthy, normotensive men (Fig. 17.6), both cross-sectional and longitudinal studies in hypertensive men report that exercise SVI declines with aging (130, 326), an effect that may be related in part to age-associated deficits in LVEDVI, LVESV, SVI, and CI at rest in older hypertensives (326).

Variation in heart rate and cardiac volume during exercise may relate to differences in fitness among individuals when comparing study populations. Fitness levels among younger and older individuals can be quantified by measurements of $\dot{V}O_{2max}$. Although there is a statistically significant decline of the latter with aging (see below, under Aerobic Capacity), wide variations occur in the exercise capacity and $\dot{V}O_{2max}$ among sedentary individuals of a given age. This variability in aerobic capacity among sedentary individuals is sometimes interpreted as a genetic effect, as opposed to a training effect. When younger and older sedentary men are matched for maximum work capacity (and therefore for maximum CI), *(1)* the maximum heart rate still decreases with age; *(2)* SVI at maximum exercise, due to substantial end-diastolic dilatation, increases in older men, offsetting the heart rate deficit; *(3)* LVESVI still fails to decrease to the same extent in older men as it does in younger ones and both the reduction LVESVI and the increase in EF are reduced in the older individuals to the same extent as observed in a general, healthy, sedentary population (292). A similar picture with respect to age-associated differences in LV cardiac volumes emerges when sedentary younger and older individuals who vary in $\dot{V}O_{2max}$ are studied (as in Fig. 17.6) and fitness is controlled for via statistical multiple regression techniques (147). Thus these age-associated changes in heart rate and cardiac volumes during exercise are not solely attributable to the physical deconditioning that may accompany aging in many individuals.

SYMPATHETIC MODULATION OF CARDIOVASCULAR FUNCTION

Intact Organisms

β-Adrenergic Modulation of Cardiac Volumes and Heart Rate during Exercise.

Each of the factors that determines cardiac output (Fig. 17.4) is influenced by autonomic nervous control. During maximum exercise, and sympathetic (β-adrenergic) component is the major autonomic modulator and a marked increase in catecholamine secretion occurs. β-Adrenergic receptor (AR) stimulation has two modulatory effects on myocardial contraction: it enhances contractile strength and decreases the contraction duration. This latter effect is particularly necessary in the intact circulation, because the heart rate increases dramatically in response to β-stimulation and the contraction time must be briefer to permit myocardial relaxation and proper filling of the ventricle during a shorter diastole. The precise impact of β-adrenergic modulation of heart rate and cardiac volume during exercise can be determined when exercise is performed in the presence of β-adrenergic blockade. In young individuals the same cardiac output is achieved during upright cycle exercise in the presence of acute β-blockade with propranolol as in the absence of β-blockade, but the hemodynamic profile differs: the increment in heart rate and the reduction in ESV are markedly less in the presence of β-blockade, but during β-blockade the EDV increases substantially, permitting a larger SV than in the absence of β-blockade (409). The rate of early LV filling and the myocardial contractility index are reduced. This altered hemodynamic pattern during acute β-blockade is indicative of the interaction among parameters (Fig. 17.4) which maintain cardiac output when a deficit in adrenergic modulation is present: cardiac dilatation at end-diastole (or the use of the Frank-Starling mechanism) augments SV, which compensates for a reduction in heart rate.

An age-associated diminution in the effectiveness of sympathetic modulation of the cardiovascular response to exercise could contribute to many of the changes identified in the cardiovascular response to exercise in healthy older humans (Fig. 17.6, 17.7): the decline in maximum heart rate, the increases in LVEDVI and LVESVI, and decreased EF. A recent study, in fact, has demonstrated that the age-associated changes in LVEDVI and SVI during upright cycle exercise do not occur in the presence of propranolol and that the age-associated reduction in heart rate is markedly attenuated, due to a greater effect of β-adrenergic blockade to decrease heart rate and increase heart size in younger than in older subjects (150). Age differences in the early diastolic filling rate and the LV contractility index (Fig.

17.8A) during exercise have also been found to be reduced or abolished when exercise was performed during β-adrenergic blockade (81, 448).

Neurotransmitter Elaboration during Stress. One possible explanation for an apparent diminution in the effectiveness of β-adrenergic modulation of cardiovascular performance during exercise in older individuals is that the secretion of high levels of norepinephrine or epinephrine during exercise stress, as reflected in plasma levels, may decline with advancing age. However, during exercise or under other circumstances that require an adjustment in the performance of the variables in Figure 17.4 from their basal levels, plasma concentrations of norepinephrine and epinephrine are increased rather than decreased in older vs. younger subjects (133, 152, 179, 389, 397, 424, 425, 482). Although clearance of plasma catecholamines appears to be reduced in older individuals (128, 134), excessive spillover into the plasma also occurs, and this, rather than a diminished clearance rate, best correlates with the increased plasma levels (134). The lack of evidence for a reduced secretion of catecholamines during exercise in older individuals suggests that if a decline in tissue catecholamine content occurs in humans, as it does with adult aging in animal models (see below, under Sympathetic Modulation of Cardiovascular Function), it appears to be of little functional importance, at least for maintenance of neurotransmitter levels during short-term stress. It is noteworthy that older (average 66 yr) endurance-trained individuals (cyclists) at a given submaximal workload also appear to have higher adrenaline and noradrenaline levels than younger (average 25 yr) ones. However, when expressed at the same relative workload, no apparent age difference emerges (310). In contrast, in sedentary subjects, the age-associated increase in plasma norepinephrine at rest persists at all relative and absolute workloads, including the maximum workload (152). (In this regard, the observed similarities and differences in the hemodynamic pattern between younger and older individuals at maximum exercise [Fig. 17.5] also pertain to a common exercise workload, for example, at 50% maximum [147].) Thus a most obvious explanation for the apparent age-associated reduction in adrenergic modulation of cardiovascular function is that neurotransmitters are not as effective at the level of the target organs.

Cardiovascular Target Organ Response to β-Adrenergic Stimulation with Aging.

Cardiovascular response in humans. One method to assess the postsynaptic response to neurotransmitters is to infuse these substances at rest. β-Adrenergic modulation of pacemaker cells accounts in part for the increase in heart rate during exercise. Bolus infusions of β-adrenergic agonists in humans (Fig. 17.10A) have been found to elicit a diminished heart rate response in older vs. younger individuals (280, 323, 500, 533, 564, 568). In humans, isoproterenol infusion also elicits a greater increase in the LVEF (500) and CI (280, 500) in younger vs. older individuals (Fig. 17.10B).

Vascular responsiveness to adrenergic stimuli modulates the redistribution of cardiac output during exercise. Arterial impedance due to dilation of large arteries may also be affected by adrenergic stimuli. The dilatation of the forearm arteries in response to infusions of isoproterenol (Fig. 17.10C) is less in elderly than in younger men (539). [In contrast, the decrease in calf vascular resistance in response to isoproterenol has been found to not differ with age (262)]. The vascular responses to prostaglandin E or to nitroglycerin are not reduced with aging (218, 244). A deficient β-adrenergic relaxant effect is, in part at least, a cause for the increase in characteristic aortic impedance during exercise in the older beagle dog (Fig. 17.6B). The ability of catecholamines to modulate venous capacitance is a major circulatory adjustment to exercise. The ability of β-stimulation to relax veins decreases with aging (Fig. 17.10D), but the constrictor response to α_1-adrenergic agonists remains intact (383). Increased neural sympathetic discharge has been implicated in a greater constriction of forearm resistance vessel (an α-adrenergic response) in older vs. younger men (515) (c.f. also above section titled Postural Reflexes).

In summary, there is indeed a large body of convincing evidence to indicate that the heart rate, vascular smooth muscle cell (VSMC), and myocardial contractile response to β-adrenergic stimulation decline with age.

Cardiovascular responses in intact animals. Isoproterenol infusions into intact rats, as in humans, also elicit a diminished increase in heart rate with aging (2, 305, 368, 562). The major age-associated deficit in some studies, however, has been found with maturation rather than with senescence. Infusion of epinephrine and norepinephrine into intact adult and senescent rats, or into young and adult cats and rabbits, has elicited a variety of complex changes in other aspects of cardiovascular function (164, 165). While the specific adrenergic cardiovascular effects cannot be ascertained from such studies, some data suggest a lower threshold or a supersensitivity in the total cardiovascular response in the senescent animal, while the response to high agonist concentrations is diminished (163). Supersensitivity of the heart to catecholamines has been described following depletion of tissue catecholamine content (83). It is well documented that myocardial catecholamine concentration in the senescent rate is reduced by 25%–50% compared to that in younger adult rats (175, 274, 296). However, it is unlikely that a depletion of cardiac catecholamine content could explain the lower threshold

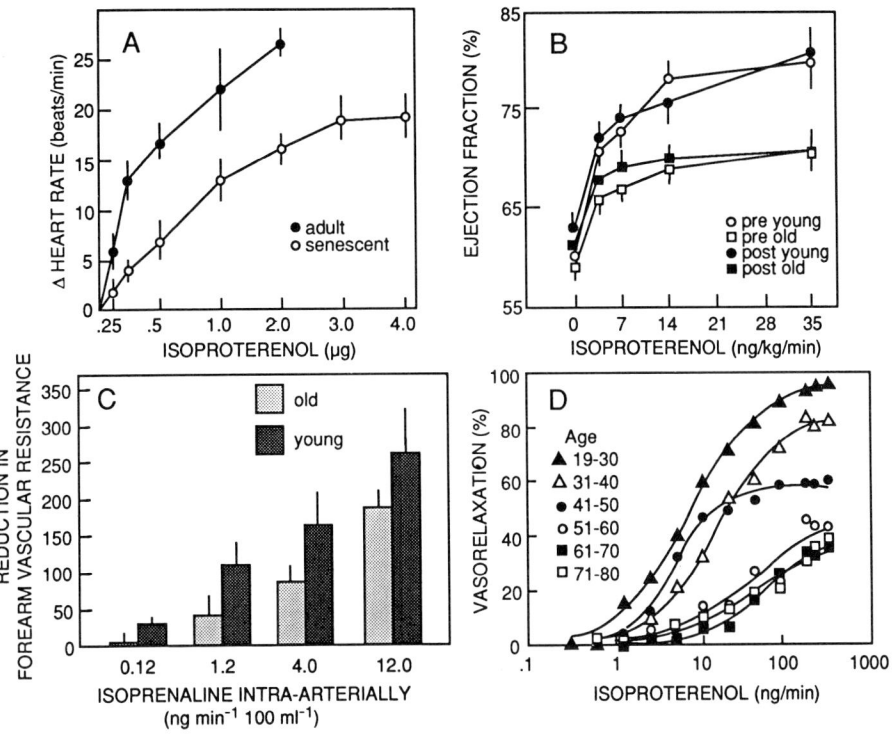
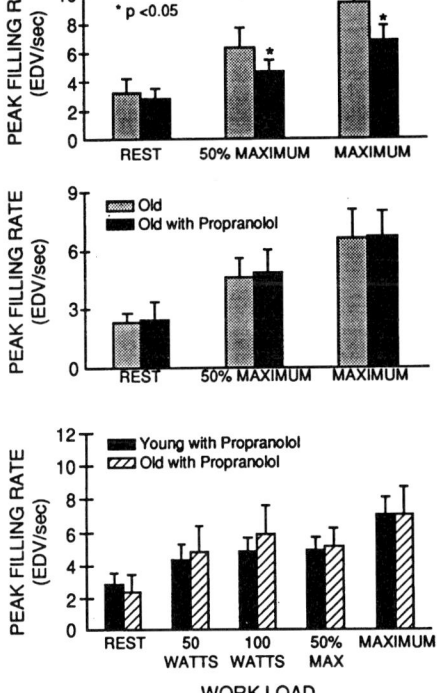

FIG. 17.10. **A:** The effect of a bolus I.V. isoproterenol infusion to increase heart rate in healthy young and older men at rest. [From Yin et al. (564) with permission.] **B:** Isoproterenol increases the LV ejection fraction in younger and older healthy men in the supine position prior to (pre) and following (post) chronic endurance training. Endurance training had no effect on this index of cardiac pump function or on its response to isoproterenol. [From Stratton et al. (500) with permission.] **C:** Intraarterial isoproterenol (isoprenaline) infusions decrease the forearm vascular resistance in healthy younger and older men. [From van Brummelin et al. (528) with permission.] **D:** I.V. arterial infusion of isoproterenol relaxes dorsal hand veins previously constricted by phenylephrine in men of varying ages. [From Pan et al. (383) with permission.] **E:** *Top:* Peak LV filling rates at rest and during exercise for young β-blocked subjects and age-matched non-β-blocked subjects. Peak filling rate was significantly less in those young subjects pretreated with propranolol at both relative and absolute workloads of 50% of maximal and maximal workloads (left) and 50 and 100 watts (right), respectively. *Middle:* Peak filling rates at rest and exercise for the older β-blocked subjects and age-matched non-β-blocked subjects. Peak filling rates were similar between the two groups both at relative workloads of 50% of maximal and maximal workloads (left) and absolute workloads of 50 and 100 watts (right). *Lower:* Peak filling rates at rest and exercise for young and old subjects pretreated with propranolol. Age differences noted during exercise in the absence of β-blockade are no longer seen during exercise in the presence of β-blockade. [From Schulman et al. (448) with permission.]

for the cardiovascular response to infused catecholamines in the senscent organism. No comparable evidence for supersensitivity to catecholamines has been found in isolated cardiac muscle from the senescent rate (see below) or in humans (499).

While age-associated differences in the extent of parasympathetic tone affect the interpretation of most studies that have infused β-adrenergic agonists into young and old humans or animals (and vice versa for infusion of parasympathetic agonists), it has been demonstrated in senescent vs. younger adult beagle dogs that the maximum heart rate increase in response to isoproterenol infusion in the presence of full vagal blockade with atropine decreases with age (562). In contrast, the maximum heart rate that could be elicited by external electrical pacing, which was far in excess of that elicited by isoproterenol infusion, was not age-related. A deficient β-adrenergic relaxant effect on aortic smooth muscle during exercise in the senescent beagle dog is, in part at least, a cause for the increase in characteristic aortic impedance (Fig. 17.8B). Regarding the α-adrenergic modulation of arterial tone in the intact organism, a greater voltage stimulation of the paravertebral sympathetic chain is necessary to evoke a pressor response in the leg vessels in the senescent, as compared to the adult, rate (164). Redistribution of blood flow to various organs during isoproterenol infusion, including skeletal muscle, decreases in senescent rats (305).

β-Adrenergic Receptor Response in the Healthy Aging Heart Resembles That in Chronic Heart Failure.

In severe, chronic heart failure due to a variety of causes, an increase in the activity of the sympathetic nervous system in response to reduced cardiac output is a general adaptive mechanism to maintain the pressure and flow requirements of the organism. Studies in patients suffering from heart failure have demonstrated that plasma norepinephrine levels are elevated and that myocardial catecholamines become depleted (18, 413, 546). Although this increased sympathetic activity may be initially helpful for the chronically failing heart, it can simultaneously lead to a desensitization of β-ARs. In experimental models of heart failure, induced by pressure-overloading or pacing-overdrive, it has recently been reported that the total β-AR number is decreased (58, 131, 550). In heart failure in humans, the number of cardiac β-ARs is also decreased, especially that of $β_1$-AR (48, 50), and it has been speculated that this preferential $β_1$-AR decrease might be caused by high levels of plasma norepinephrine, which is a rather selective $β_1$-AR agonist. It has also been noted that in failing human hearts there is a selective decline in the high-affinity β-ARs, as well as a decrease in the coupling of receptors with the G_s-protein (337). When these changes in the β-AR system in heart failure patients are compared to the characteristic of age-associated alterations in β-modulation of cardiac function, the similarities become very evident. As we know, in old vs. young animals or humans, the plasma catecholamine concentration is increased. Although most studies have shown that the β-AR density does not change with aging, the affinity of the receptor for agonists and the coupling of the receptor to the catalytic subunits decrease (see below, under G-Protein and Adenylate Cyclase Activity). In both healthy aged humans and those with chronic heart failure, reductions in the effectiveness of β-adrenergic modulation of heart rate, vascular relaxation, and myocardial contractility occur. It has been suggested that age may be the dominant variable in the reduced β-adrenergic augmentation in cardiac cells isolated from the failing human heart (204). The kinetics of myocardial Ca^{2+} cycling are also altered in chronic heart failure (290), and many strikingly similar changes in excitation–contraction mechanisms occur in the healthy aged and chronically failing heart. Thus the aging heart in health and the chronically failing heart exhibit many common biochemical features; nevertheless, in the former, overall cardiac performance is remarkably preserved, while in the latter it is severely reduced.

Isolated Tissue or Cells

Vascular Responses. Adrenergic modulation of isolated blood vessels, particularly β-adrenergic-mediated vasodilatation, has been found in decrease with age in most (126, 153–155, 178, 224, 370–372, 518, 524), but not all (12, 329, 476), studies. Some studies report aging effects that represent changes during development (113, 153). Other studies suggest that different β-AR or α-adrenergic subtypes are differentially regulated by aging (107, 372, 373). Stimulation of presynaptic β-AR, the majority of which are $β_2$, facilitates the release of noradrenaline (302, 488), while stimulation of presynaptic α-receptor, predominantly of the $α_2$ subtype (108, 302, 488), has an opposite effect on norepinephrine release (135, 263, 530). The $α_2$-AR mediated responsiveness appears to be selectively reduced with age in human saphenous vein (107, 108), rat vasculature (109), and human platelets (504, 505). In contrast, no significant correlation between aging and $α_1$ receptor responses has been observed (114, 329, 453). However, in large and medium coronary arteries of beagle dogs $α_1$-adrenoceptor-mediated responses may increase with age (518). Studies in which the relaxation response of the aged aorta is more significantly reduced than that of the pulmonary artery (370–372) have concluded that age affects $β_2$-AR stimulation responses more than $β_1$-AR, since the aorta has more $β_2$-AR than the pulmonary artery, although additional interpretations of the data are plausible.

In summary, data in tissues isolated from many species, including humans, demonstrate that autonomic modulation of the vasculature changes with age, and in particular, that the response to β-adrenoceptor vascular dilatation is impaired. Additional studies, however, are required to further characterize age-associated changes in specific adrenoceptor subtypes and their interactions.

Cardiac Responses. In isolated rat hearts a progressive age-associated reduction in heart rate response to norepinephrine has been observed (273). Intracellular mechanisms that mediate the AR stimulation within cardiovascular cells have been probed with respect to age-associated changes. Considering that norepinephrine is the physiological neurotransmitter and that α- and β-ARs are stimulated simultaneously, the roles of both α- and β-adrenergic effects on contractility need to be discriminated. The direct effect of α-AR stimulation of the myocardium in response to norepinephrine is inconsequential relative to the β-adrenergic effect: α-adrenergic stimulation does not enhance cardiac relaxation and its strengthening effect on contraction is about an order of magnitude less than that of the β-adrenergic system. The effects of adult aging in the $α_1$-adrenergic-mediated increase in myocardial contractility have not been studied.

The immediate cause of the increase in cardiac muscle performance by β-receptor stimulation in an increase in the amplitude of the Ca_i transient that follows excitation. While the contractile responsiveness of the myofilaments to Ca^{2+} does not change with aging (37, 187, 295), studies in isolated LV muscle (Fig. 17.11A) and in individual rat ventricular cardiocytes (Fig. 17.11B) indicate that a reduced contractile response to β-AR stimulation occurs with aging. This is due, at least in part, to a failure of the Ca_i transient to increase in senescent heart cells to the same extent to which it increase in younger adult heart cells (556) (Fig. 17.11C). The blunted increase in the Ca^{2+} transient in cells from the aged heart is attributed to a decrease in the ability of β-AR stimulation to increase L-type sarcolemmal Ca^{2+} channel availability in cells from senescent vs. younger adult hearts (556) (Fig. 17.11D).

β-AR. One possible mechanism for the observed decrease in the responsiveness of β-AR-mediated action on the heart and vasculature with aging would be an age-associated decrease in cellular β-adrenoceptor density. This possibility has been extensively studied in a variety of tissues, including myocardium (4, 72, 187, 282, 361, 434), VSMC (524), and lymphocytes (2, 3, 111, 137) of humans and animals. In humans, lymphocytes have been commonly used as a model to study the effect of aging on AR function because other human tissues are not readily available. Such studies have found no significant changes in the β-AR density with age. This may indicate that β-adrenergic responsiveness of the cardiovascular system is impaired in aging at levels other than the β-AR per se but may involve distal intracellular steps. However, the β-ARs of lymphocytes are of the $β_2$ subtype (32,49) and the aforementioned studies do not provide information about β-AR subpopulations with age. Additionally, it has not been established that changes in β-AR properties and responsiveness of lymphocytes with aging reflect similar changes of β-AR in cardiovascular tissues with aging.

While rat myocardial β-AR density has not been found to change with aging in most studies, agonist binding properties of the receptor do appear to change with aging. The β-AR affinity for agonist binding is decreased three- to twentyfold with aging (361, 434–436, 438). A reduction in β-AR affinity has also been found in rat lung (437). In contrast, there is no correlation between age and β-AR antagonist affinity (4, 136, 187). The decreased β-AR agonist affinity correlates with the decrease in the ability to form the high-affinity binding complex, that is, the percent of receptors in the high-affinity state decreases with age (136, 434, 438, 439). In addition, the high-affinity receptor state become less stable with aging (136, 434, 438, 439). Recently, an age-associated increase in the extent of β-AR sequestration in light-density membrane vesicles isolated from lung has been observed (439). Since light-density membrane particles (vesicles), when isolated, are devoid of adenylate cyclase activity and G_s-protein (464, 495, 499). it has been suggested that a functional receptor down-regulation occurs in the aged rat lung (439). It has yet to be determined whether with aging both $β_1$- and $β_2$-AR subtypes undergo the same qualitative and quantitative changes in affinity or sequestration.

G-Protein and Adenylate Cyclase Activity. G-proteins and the adenylate cyclase catalytic subunit are important components of the β-AR–adenylate cyclase enzyme complex (176). G-proteins act as coupling factors to transduce the signal from the receptor to the catalytic subunit of adenylate cyclase. A number of studies suggest that G_S-protein activity is diminished with aging (271, 272, 282, 369, 434, 435, 438). Both the G_S-protein activity and the adenylate cyclase activity are simultaneously altered with aging in the rat myocardium (282, 361, 369), human lymphocytes (271, 272), and rat lung (439). In some tissues it has been demonstrated that the G_S-protein is present in excess of the adenylate cyclase catalytic subunit (369, 419). While the G_S-protein activity is unchanged in human lymphocytes of older donors, the catalytic subunit activity is lower than that in lymphocytes from younger individuals (3, 4). Thus a reduction in adenylate cyclase catalytic subunit

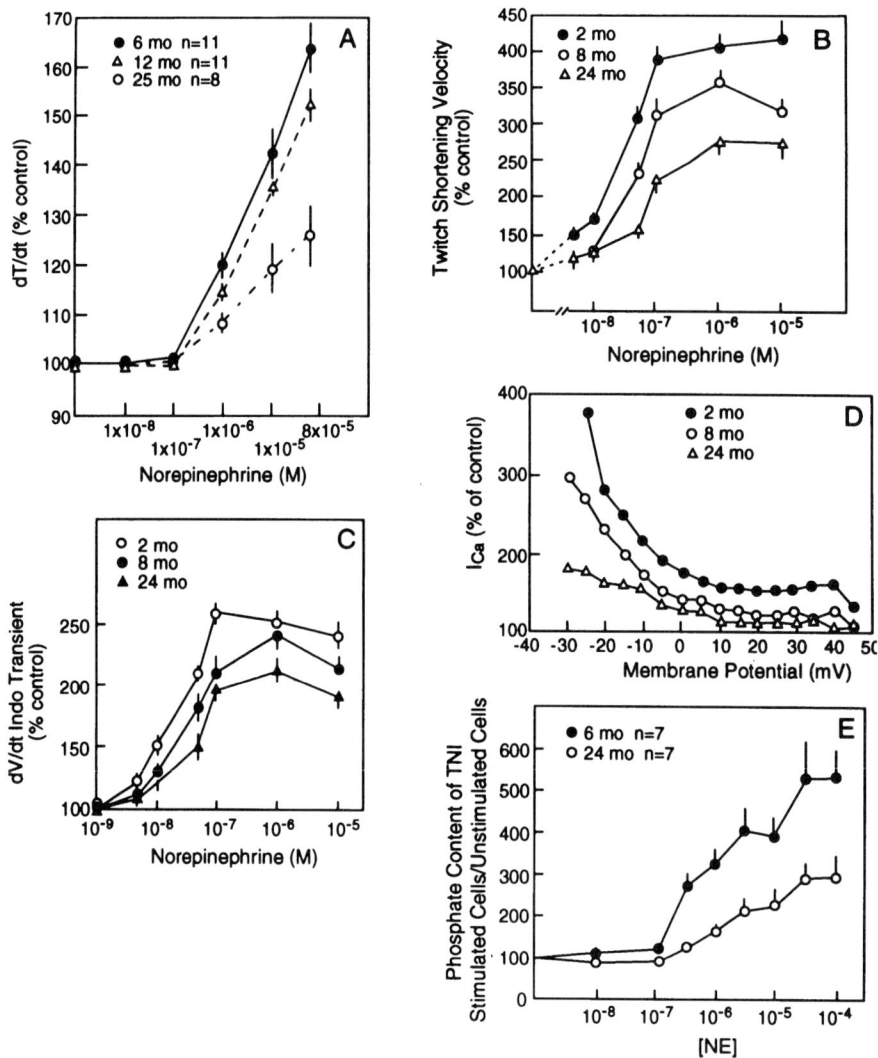

FIG. 17.11. **A**: The effect of norepinephrine on the maximum rate of isometric tension development in isolated trabeculae from hearts of varying ages. [From Lakatta et al. (295) with permission.] **B**: Velocity of cell shortening and **C** maximum rate of increase of the Indo-1 fluorescence transient, an index of sarcoplasmic reticulum Ca^{2+} release into the cytosol, during electrically stimulated twitch in single cardiac myocytes isolated from the hearts of rats of varying ages and loaded with the fluorescent probe Indo-1. [From Xiao et al. (557) with permission.] **D**: Norepinephrine increases the L-type sarcolemmal channel current (I_{Ca}) measured via whole-cell patch clamp technique in single cells isolated as in *B* and *C*. [From Xiao et al. (557) with permission.] **E**: Norepinephrine increases phosphorylation of troponin I (TNI) in suspensions of heart cells isolated from hearts of rats of varying ages as in above panels. [From Sakai et al. (431) with permission.] In *B–E* norepinephrine stimulated β-receptors, because prazosin and α_1-AR antagonist had no effect on the results.

activity may play a more important role in the age-associated alteration of the β-AR cascade than does a reduction of G_s-protein activity. However, most studies have not differentiated changes in G_s-protein with aging from those in the catalytic subunit of adenylate cyclase.

Cyclic AMP, Protein Kinase Activation, and Intracellular Phosphorylation. The increase of adenylate cyclase activity or cAMP stimulated by catecholamines, NaF, or forskolin is diminished with aging in human lymphocytes (3, 104, 271, 272, 434), rat heart (139, 282, 368, 434), and other tissues (131, 493). In aortic tissue, the isoproterenol-induced relaxation and increase in intracellular cAMP binding decreases with age (between 5 wk and 11 months), accompanied by a reduced activation of cAMP-dependent protein kinase (PKA) (74, 97). In contrast, these responses to forskolin or to dibutyryl cAMP are not affected by age over this range (74, 97). The deficit in cAMP of the old rat aorta is reduced by phosphodiesterase inhibition, suggesting that an increase in phosphodiesterase could be responsible for the diminished isoproterenol-induced cAMP accumulation and relaxation (446). Other studies in a variety of tissues have not found that cAMP production is reduced following β-AR stimulation of these tissues from older animals (187, 240, 270, 273). An additional study has observed that neither basal nor stimulated activities of ventricular muscle PKA are altered during adult aging (187). Interpretation of how subcellular biochemical measurements relate to the functional effect of β-AR stimulation is complicated by compartmentation of increases in cell cAMP and PKA activity (1, 57, 84, 138, 206) and by variable contributions of different cell types in tissue studies. In the heart, PKA has different distributions between cytosolic and particulate fractions. The amount of cAMP in the particulate fraction appears to be the important factor for regulation of contraction and relaxation of the myocardium (1). While some aging studies have addressed the compartmentation issue per se (187), additional studies controlling for a shift in the amount of cAMP within compartments following β-stimulation seem warranted.

There is evidence that steps distal to protein kinase activation are also affected by aging. The extent of phosphorylation of the myofilament proteins troponin-I (TNI) and C-protein effected by β-AR stimulation induced by norepinephrine in rat myocytes decreases with age (431) (Fig. 17.11E). This decrease may be caused by age-associated changes at more than one locus, for example, less effective β-AR coupling to the adenylate cyclase complex, increased phosphodiesterase activity, or acceleration of protein dephosphorylation. In the above study (431), it was observed that the age-associated differences in TNI (and C-protein) phosphorylation were abolished by the cAMP phosphodiesterase inhibitor IBMX (isobutyl methyl xanthine), and no evidence for increased protein phosphatase activity was observed, suggesting that the age difference in the phosphorylation of these two myofilament proteins resulted from a reduction in the net production of cAMP in cells of the old rat heart. In sarcoplasmic reticulum (SR) vesicles isolated from rat hearts, the ability of phospholamban, a protein in the membrane of SR which modulates the activity of the SR Ca^{2+} pump, to undergo cAMP-mediated phosphorylation and the relative responsiveness of SR Ca^{2+} pump to phospholamban phosphorylation are not appreciably altered with aging (235, 239). There are presently no data regarding whether the sarcolemmal voltage-dependent Ca^{2+} channel proteins (88, 221) or other contractile proteins (6, 552) are phosphorylated to a different extent following β-AR stimulation in younger and older cardiac tissues or cells. However, the relative inability of β-AR stimulation to augment the Ca^{2+} channel current amplitude in cells from older rat hearts (Fig. 17.11D) may indicate that phosphorylation of this channel protein by PKA is reduced with aging, but this, like the decreased phosphorylation of TNI, could be due to a reduction in the net increase in cAMP production with aging. Alternatively, age-associated differences in direct Ca^{2+} channel modulation by G_s (51) could be involved and this requires further study.

Interactions between various aspects of α- and β-receptor modulation of cell Ca^{2+} homeostasis have become the focus of recent studies (56, 90), and α–β-AR interactions, which are not completely characterized at present, may indeed affect the β-adrenergic response (90). In addition to $α_1$-adrenergic agonists, adenosine, opioid peptides, and cholinergic agonists can modulate the effects of β-AR stimulation on heart contraction. The precise role of an interaction among α- and β-adrenergic and cholinergic agonists and these other peptide-linked modulating effects on the age-associated decline in the cardiac response to β-AR stimulation are presently not well understood. However, it has recently been demonstrated that the negative contractile and chronotropic responses to exogenous adenosine are increased with age in guinea pigs (94). Adenosine release from aged (12–22 months) rat hearts is greater than that from younger (3–5 months) rat hearts (106). Since adenosine has an antiadrenergic action—that is, it reduces the β-adrenoceptor-induced increase in cAMP and the subsequent increase in PKA, Ca^{2+} current, and contractility (105, 137, 300, 418, 447)—enhanced adenosine levels in aged myocardium may be responsible in part for the diminished contractile responsiveness of the older adult heart to β-AR stimulation (106). However, it is unlikely that age-associated changes in adenosine metabolism can directly account for the age-associated differences in the β-AR of isolated cardiocytes (Fig. 17.11B–E).

Desensitization of the β-Adrenoceptor System. It has long been recognized that prolonged exposure of myocardial tissue to β-AR agonists modifies β-AR responsiveness. As we have seen, in humans and animals plasma catecholamines, especially plasma norepinephrine, are increased in older vs. younger organisms during perturbations from the basal state (128, 132, 152, 179, 295, 390, 397, 425, 482). Chronic elevations of plasma catecholamines in older individuals, due to excessive neural discharge and/or reduced clearance, might induce β-AR desensitization. Desensitization of β-AR stimulation occurs via modifications of both receptor and postreceptor events (34, 246, 309, 311, 320, 403, 404, 497, 498). A comparison of such β-AR desensitization and the reduced efficacy of β-AR stimulation with aging (Table 17.3) suggests that the age-associated alterations may be caused, at least in part, by a desensitization of the β-AR adenylate cyclase system.

The acute elevation in humans of endogenous plasma catecholamines associated with assumption of the

TABLE 17.3. *Comparison of β-AR Desensitization and Alterations in β-Adrenergic Response with Aging*

Characteristics	Aging	Desensitization Homologous	Desensitization Heterologous	Possible Mechanisms
Plasma catecholamines	↑	↑	↑	Spillover ↑ or clearance ↓ or both, good correlation between spillover and increased plasma norepinephrine concentration with aging.
Receptor density	↔ (heart and vessels) ↓ (liver and brain)	↓	↓	Phosphorylation of receptor by PKA and cAMP-independent β-AR kinase. β-AR kinase effects may involve arresting-like protein (barrestin).
Receptor sequestration	↑	↑	↑	Unknown, but phosphorylation may not be the trigger. Residues 222–229 of the β_2 receptor are important for sequestration.
Catecholamine or NaF-stimulated adenylate cyclase	↓ ↓	↓ ↔	↓ ↓	Receptor coupling ↓, alteration of G_s, G_i, G_s/G_i, and catalytic subunit. Modification of the G-protein may be induced by PKA or PKC.
Forskolin-stimulated adenylate cyclase	↓	↔	↓	A cyclase catalytic subunit ↓ by PKA.

↑ Increased; ↓ decreased; ↔ no change.
Reprinted from Xiao and Lakatta (555) with permission.

upright posture decreases the proportion of high-affinity β-AR in lymphocytes (due to desensitization) in younger, but not in older, individuals (136). A desensitization of β-AR mechanisms in older individuals in the supine position, prior to the postural change, could explain in part this result. In this regard, it has been noted that catecholamine desensitization of the rat myocardium induced by the chronic in vivo administration of a β-adrenergic agonist, occurs to a lesser extent in senescent than in younger rat hearts; this has also been interpreted to indicate that the β-AR system of aged rat myocardium had been partially desensitized prior to study (438). Additional studies indicated that, while NaF-stimulated adenylate cyclase activity is less in untreated older vs. younger rats, it is unaffected by chronic β-adrenergic treatment, suggesting that desensitization may not be fully responsible for the diminution of the β-AR response with age (435, 438). Also, in older humans the impaired augmentation of the heart rate and venous relaxation by isoproterenol is not reversed by chronic administration of a β-adrenergic antagonist. The results of these studies suggest that impaired stimulation of heart rate by isoproterenol in older individuals is probably not due to desensitization of β-receptors since this difference between young and older subjects could not be reversed by treatment with a β-adrenergic antagonist (156).

In summary, an age-associated reduction in the postsynaptic response of the cardiovascular system to β-AR stimulation in human and animal tissues and cells has been richly documented and appears to be due to multiple changes in molecular and biochemical receptor coupling and post receptor mechanisms rather than to a major modification of a single rate-limiting step, as might occur, for example, in a genetic defect. The most remarkable change within the β-AR system is the decrease in the receptor affinity for agonists without substantial changes in β-AR density. However, there is little information regarding changes of β-AR subtype density, affinity, or functional regulation in aging. The postreceptor changes with aging include decreases in the activities of G_s-protein and the adenylate cyclase catalytic unit, as well as a decrease in PKA-induced protein phosphorylation. Quantitative differences in G-protein or adenylate cyclase catalytic subunit activities with age have not been measured nor have specific functional changes resulting from their altered activities been defined. The striking similarities between the decreased effectiveness of β-adrenergic stimulation with age and the phenomenon of desensitization of β-AR by chronic β-AR agonist exposure at younger age suggest that the age-associated changes, especially the reduced receptor-to-catalytic subunit coupling, may occur in part via desensitization mechanisms.

PARASYMPATHETIC MODULATION OF CARDIOVASCULAR FUNCTION

There is some evidence that parasympathetic control of cardiovascular function changes with age, but it is conflicting. Some studies in rats suggest a more efficient cholinergic modulation with aging. The threshold of the negative chronotropic effects of vagus nerve stimulation and concentrations of acetylcholine required to cause changes in myocardial contractility are decreased with advancing age in rats (164, 165). Additionally, significantly greater increases in cyclic GMP in response to submaximal doses of acetylcholine have been observed in hearts of 24–26-month-old rats compared to 6–8-month-old rats. This difference persisted in the presence of acetyl-cholinesterase blockade, suggesting that the mechanisms of the age-associated differences are at or distal to the receptor (278). Other studies have observed an enhanced sensitivity to the direct chronotropic action of acetylcholine in right atria isolated from aged vs. younger Fischer 344 rats but have attributed this to an age-associated reduction in cholinesterase activity (252). In contrast, other observations indicate an age-associated reduction in the response to parasympathetic agonists. In one such study, a decrease in heart rate reduction in old rats to both vagal nerve stimulation and bolus injections of methacholine was observed (249). More recent studies have indicated that the number of cholinergic receptors in the LV decreases with age in rats, as does the response to acetylcholine (72). Finally, a marked reduction in acetylcholine content of atrial tissue from senescent rats has been demonstrated (532). In humans, a decrease in heart rate variability at rest or in response to a postural stress in older individuals has been attributed in part to a reduction in parasympathetic tone with aging.

CARDIOVASCULAR STRUCTURE AND FUNCTION IN YOUNGER AND OLDER ANIMALS

Cardiac Structure

The vast majority of studies of age-related changes in the myocardium have employed the rat model (294), the most commonly studied strains being Wistar, Fischer 344, and Sprague-Dawley. Two-year-old rats housed in cages are commonly referred to as "senescent," because at approximately that age 50% colony mortality occurs (294). Similarities and differences with respect to morphological changes that accompany aging in these strains have been noted.

The senescent Wistar rat heart exhibits moderate (25%) LV hypertrophy compared to hearts from young and middle-aged animals (565, 566). This occurs in the absence of arterial hypertension (423). The increase in LV mass with aging in the rat differs from that in humans in that the LV cavity size is enlarged, while the estimated LV wall thickness does not increase (463). Fluctuations in body weight and composition with aging in rats make body weight an unreliable reference for normalizing heart weight for comparisons across age (as for V_{O_2}). An alternative index of body size (tibial length) appears to be more appropriate for normalization of heart mass (565). The majority of the increase in cardiac mass with aging in the Wistar rat, however, is due to myocardial cell enlargement (as in humans). In individual myocytes isolated from Wistar rats of 2, 6–9, and 24–26 months of age, the average myocyte length increases from 133 μm at 2 months to 146 μm at 6–9 months to 162 μm at 24–26 months, but the average slack sarcomere length does not change with age (159). The average volume of individual cells, measured via Coulter counter techniques, approximately doubles between 2 and 24 months (Fig. 17.13F). In Wistar-Kyoto rats, there is some evidence to indicate that a reduction in the volume fraction of cardiac myocytes in myocardial tissue decreases with age between 6 and 24 months (124). Myocyte enlargement also occurs with aging in the Wistar-Kyoto strain. While no prominent changes in the ultrastructural appearance of the myofibers are observed in the hearts of aging Wistar rats, an increase in lipofuscin occurs (523), as in humans. In rats older than 19 months, increased numbers of residual bodies among the mitochondria in the nuclear pole zone and in the mitochondrial rows separating the myofilament masses have also been observed, as have signs of increased lysosomal activity, particularly prominent in the mitochondrial regions (523). The functional significance of such changes, however, is unknown.

In hearts of male Fischer 344 rats, LV collagen increases from 5.5% of total protein at 1–4 months to approximately 12%–16% at 22 and 26 months (16, 119); in the right ventricle (RV), collagen increases from 7%–8% at 1 month to approximately 19.5%–22% at 22–26 months (16, 119). Collagen accumulates in intrinsic collagenous structures, including perimysial weaves, coiled perimysial fibers, and struts, where the preexisting fibers are thickened and are more extensive. Regions of fibrosis also increase in size and volume in older animals, with predominant subendocardial localization (16, 119). Papillary muscles of the LV become fibrosed to a greater extent than in the RV of Fischer rats with advancing age (17). In Fischer 344 rats, an apparent (19%) reduction in the number of cardiac myocytes (reminiscent of the case in some skeletal muscle) has been estimated in both ventricles between 4 and 12 months of age (16). While at 20 months this reduction in cell number persists in the LV, it is reversed in the RV. Moreover, from 20 to 29 months, an apparent 59% increase in the number of cells has been inferred in the RV, with only a 3% increase estimated in the LV (16). While this has been interpreted to indicate cardiac myocyte hyperplasia, that is, an increase in the number of cardiac myocytes, more direct evidence of cell hyperplasia is required to substantiate this provocative notion.

In Sprague-Dawley rats, an age-associated increase in the extent of myocardial fibrosis, involving 60% of rats at the time of spontaneous death, has been observed (549). This fibrosis is dispersed rather widely within the myocardium, with greater concentrations in the subendocardial and subepicardial regions. In male Sprague-Dawley rats between 3 months and 10–12 months of age, the mean myocyte cell volume per nucleus increases 53% and 26% in the LV and RV, respectively. The total number of myocyte nuclei remains constant in both ventricles. By 19–20 months, a further (39%) cellular hypertrophy of the LV occurs in association with an apparent (18%) loss of cell number. LV cell loss is accompanied by discrete areas of interstitial and replacement fibrosis in the subendocardium (15). In contrast to the LV, no focal myocardial damage is observed in the RV, and the measured additional 35% enlargement of RV myocytes occurs without an apparent change in cell number. Thus the aged LV of this rat strain, similar to that of the Fischer 344 strain, appears to be composed of a smaller number of hypertrophied cells. The cellular changes with aging in this rat strain occur in the absence of an increase in the ratio of heart weight to body weight. The Sprague-Dawley strain, like the Wistar strain, does not become hypertensive with aging, the stimuli for cell loss and hypertrophy of the remaining cells with aging being unknown. In the Sprague-Dawley strain, the myofibers of senescent hearts appear irregular and often small, with tapering projections, and foci of dense mitochondrial accumulations are observed (521). This contrasts with other species and other types of muscle, in which there is an apparent decrease in mitochondrial density with aging. Older Sprague-Dawley hearts also contain autophagic vacuoles that are rarely noted in the myocardium of young animals.

In summary, in the normotensive rat, cardiac fibrosis increases with age, the number of myocytes decreases, and myocyte size increases. Variable degrees of LV hypertrophy occur, depending upon the strain, and this is due to ventricular dilatation, with apparent preservation of a normal ventricular wall thickness.

Myocardial Stiffness

Passive Stiffness. Data arising from studies in animal models are often cited as being indicative of a change in *passive* mechanical myocardial properties with advancing age. Passive mechanical properties of myocardial cells and tissue, that is, those properties determined by the amount and composition of matrix (interstitial) proteins (for example, collagen and cytoskeletal proteins), affect the contraction amplitude and relaxation of cardiac muscle and the filling properties of the cardiac ventricle. One way of assessing passive muscle properties is to examine the passive length–tension curve. However, it is difficult to directly compare the results of different studies that examined the length–tension relationship as a function of age (see 294 for review). An estimation of the elastic or viscoelastic modulus is a more meaningful method of assessing passive muscle properties than measurement of the passive length–tension curve (349). In isolated, unstimulated rat trabecular carneae, using small sinusoidal length perturbations across a range of muscle lengths, several studies have failed to demonstrate an age-associated alteration in the passive viscoelastic stiffness modulus (486, 487, 566). In contrast, no generalization can be made from studies of the intact, isolated heart as the passive viscoelastic modulus was found to increase in the beagle dog (516), to remain unchanged in the hamster (241), and to decrease in the rat (232) with age.

In addition to the variable results of different studies, more fundamental considerations underlie the ambiguity of the effect of age on passive myocardial properties, among which is the assumption of classic muscle mechanics that Ca^{2+} activation of myofilaments (see below, under Regulation of the Cardiac Contraction) does not contribute to passive force, that is, force measured in the absence of electrical stimulation. In isolated cardiac cells from rats, and from other species as well, a tonic, Ca^{2+}-dependent myofilament interaction is also present at rest and modulates the resting cell length in the absence of external loading (571). Additionally, in the rat, the passive force in the isolated heart and cardiac muscle may indeed be influenced by asynchronous spontaneous cytosolic Ca^{2+} oscillations among myocardial cells that occur even when the bathing milieu contains Ca^{2+} in the range of 2.5 mM or less, that is, over the range where most mechanical measurements have been made (268, 293, 492).

Active Stiffness. *Active dynamic* stiffness, that is, the force change in response to sinusoidal changes in muscle length made during Ca^{2+} activation of the myofilaments, has been experimentally found to increase as force increases with time during cardiac muscle contraction, making active stiffness a linear function of the force. In muscle from senescent rat hearts, the slope coefficient of the linear active stiffness vs. the force relationship during contraction increases, but the intercept of the relationship does not change, relative to measurements in muscle from younger rats (486, 487, 566). The time to peak stiffness and to half-relaxation of peak stiffness are also prolonged in senescent vs. young adult cardiac muscle (486, 487, 566). As just noted, age differences in passive viscoelastic properties do not affect stiffness, as measured by this technique (486, 487, 566), and thus cannot account for the increased dynamic stiffness during contraction in senescent muscle. Prolongation of the force transient and the prolonged time course of active stiffness in senescent muscle appear to result, in part at least, from the prolonged Ca_i transient with aging.

Regulation of the Cardiac Contraction

The Cardiac Excitation–Contraction Process. The cardiac cycle is initiated as Ca^{2+} influx via voltage-gated sarcolemmal Ca^{2+} channels that become activated by membrane depolarization during an action potential (AP), triggering Ca^{2+} release from the SR (Fig. 17.12). Following its abrupt increase after excitation, the Ca_i concentration is then reduced, in large measure via SR pumping and in part via Na–Ca exchange. Following each cycle, some of the excitation–contraction coupling mechanisms, for example, sarcolemmal ionic conductances and SR Ca^{2+} recycling, require a restitution time for optimal operation following a subsequent excitation.

The myofilaments (actin, myosin, troponin, tropomyosin) within each myofibril are arranged in serial units referred to as "sarcomeres," which can vary in length from about 1.9 to 2.4 μm in the unstimulated state and from about 1.6 to 2.2 μm following excitation. Ca^{2+} binding to troponin C following excitation results in actin–myosin interaction (formation of *crossbridges*) followed by stiffening of the myofilament lattice *(force production)* and displacement of actin relative to myosin *(sarcomere shortening)*. The extent and duration of Ca^{2+} binding to troponin C is a major determinant of the velocity and extent of sarcomere shortening following excitation. The extent of Ca^{2+} binding to troponin C following excitation depends upon the magnitude of the Ca^{2+} release from the SR and on the resting myofilament or sarcomere length (233, 234). The extent to which Ca^{2+} remains bound during contraction depends in part on the velocity and extent of sarcomere shortening during a given contraction (283). Thus the duration of Ca^{2+} myofilament activation is regulated by sarcomere length prior to excitation and by sarcomere shortening during contraction (see 291 for review).

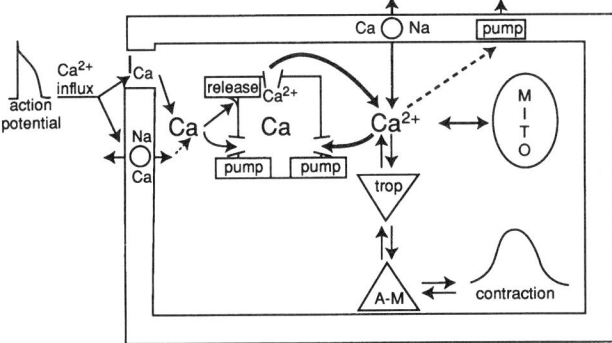

FIG. 17.12. Simplified schematic of excitation–contraction coupling mechanisms in cardiac muscle. Ca^{2+} influx (I_{Ca}) via L-type sarcolemmal Ca^{2+} channels, activated by depolarization during an action potential, triggers the release of Ca^{2+} from the sarcoplasmic reticulum to increase the cytosolic $[Ca^{2+}]$. The binding of Ca^{2+} to troponin (TROP) enables actomyosin (AM) interaction, resulting in myofilament force production and shortening. Cytoplasmic $[Ca^{2+}]$ is then lowered and relaxation ensues (Mito, mitochondria).

In addition to the extent of Ca^{2+} activation of myofilaments, the rate and extent of sarcomere shortening following excitation and the resultant increases in myofilament, cellular and myocardial stiffness, and force production are dependent on the ambient forces within the tissue, sometimes referred to as the "load" borne by these structures. The sarcomere load depends in part on the length of the sarcomeres and other cytoskeletal structures to which sarcomeres are attached within cells and in part the fibrous connections of myocytes to matrix collagen (see above, under Passive Stiffness). When sarcomeres shorten during contraction, their myofilament Ca^{2+} activation, length, and load are each important determinants of the cardiac contraction; these factors are highly interdependent and cannot be considered to be completely independent of each other (291). Additional factors that determine the sarcomere dynamics following excitation are the myosin heavy chain (MHC) isoform composition, the extent of phosphorylation of myofilament components (as determined by receptor-mediated second messengers, for example), and the local concentrations of ATP, ADP, P_i, H^+, and Mg^{2+}. Sarcomere relengthening and relaxation of force, in addition to a dependence on the removal of Ca^{2+} from troponin C, depends on the mechanical loading factors discussed above.

Cardiac Muscle and Myocyte Changes with Adult Aging.

Cardiac muscle function has been studied with respect to aging in thin trabeculae, papillary muscles, and isolated cardiac myocytes that have been removed from the heart and superfused in physiological saline. Several of the steps in the excitation–contraction cascade discussed above differ in cardiac muscle or cells isolated from senescent rat hearts vs. those from younger adult hearts. In general, the kinetics of many of these steps are reduced in the senescent vs. the younger adult muscle (Fig. 17.13).

Action potential and membrane currents. The heart beat represents the synchronized cellular Ca^{2+} oscillations and cyclic contractions of myocardial cells. For an organized Ca^{2+} oscillation to occur within and among myocardial cells, several cellular mechanisms must act in concert. In isolated muscle preparations, several aspects of the heart beat can be simulated as a twitch contraction elicited by an AP that occurs in response to external electrical stimulation. Representative examples of AP, contraction, and the Ca_i transient in muscle isolated from adult and senescent male rats are illustrated in Figure 17.13A–C. While the resting membrane potential is unaltered with adult aging (60, 539, 545, 557), the repolarization of the membrane potential in senescent muscle is strikingly (about twofold) prolonged (Fig. 17.13A). This has been observed in separate studies using different rat strains (Wistar and Fischer 344) in

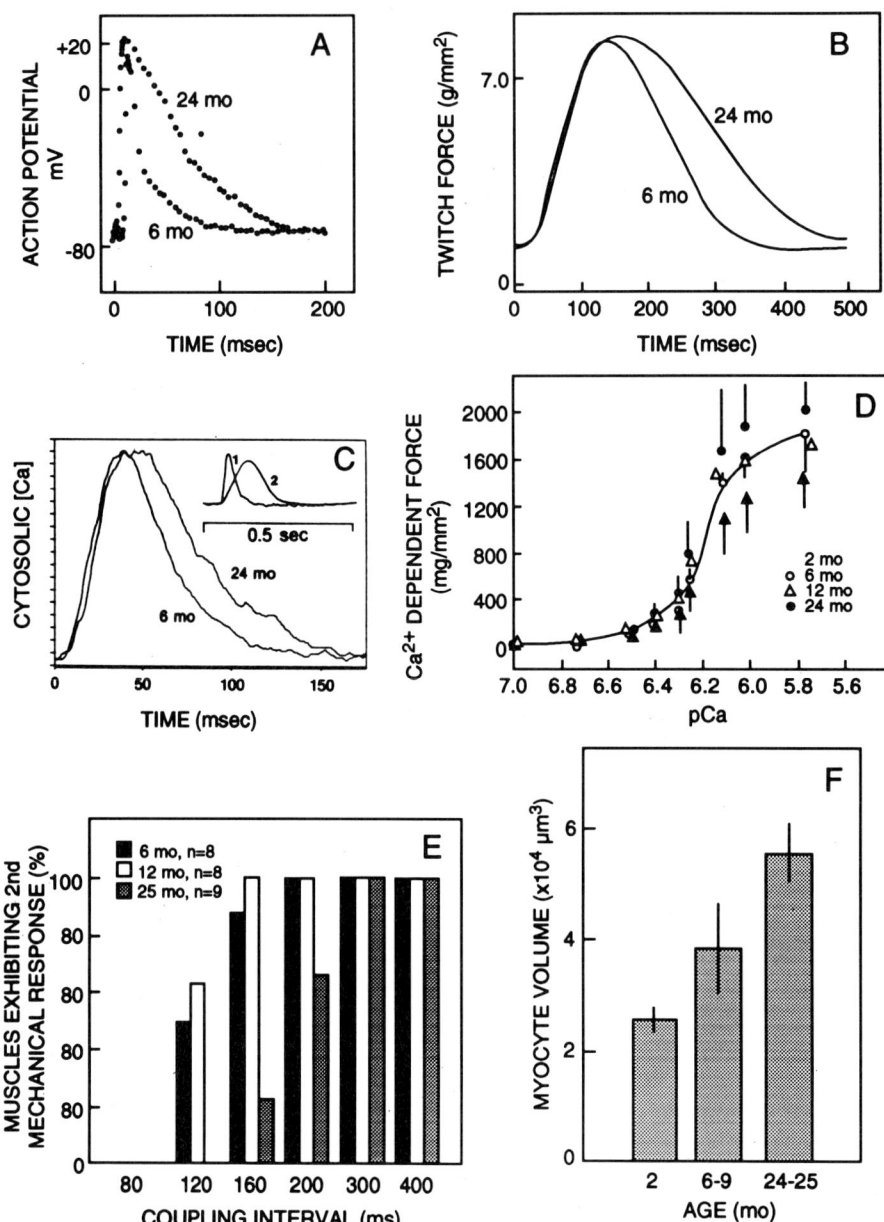

FIG. 17.13. Action potential (**A**), isometric twitch (**B**), and Ca_i transient (**C**) measured via aequorin luminescence in isometric right ventricular papillar muscles isolated form the hearts of young adult and senescent Wistar rats. Inset in C indicates the time course of the Ca_i transient (trace 1) relative to that of the contraction (trace 2). [A and B from Wei et al. (545); C from Orchard and Lakatta (377) with permission.] **D**: The force–pCa relationship in cardiac muscle in which membranes have been destroyed by detergent (Triton X) treatment does not vary with age. [From Bhatnagar et al. (37) with permission.] **E**: The ability of left ventricular trabeculae carneae to respond, via a detectable twitch contraction, to paired stimulation decreases with age as the coupling interval of the paired stimuli decreases. [From Lakatta et al. (296) with permission.] **F**: Left ventricular cell volume (single cells isolated via collagenase digestion of hearts), measured via Coulter counter technique, increases with age. [From Fraticelli et al. (159) with permission.]

"pseudoisometric" (auxotonic) RV (545) and LV (59) papillary muscle and in isolated LV myocytes (539). An age-related increase in the AP duration of isolated human atrial fibers has been reported (127); however, the ages compared were 10 months and 55 years. The AP amplitude above zero millivolts *(overshoot)* in rat cardiac muscle is Ca^{2+}-dependent; in the Wistar strain, the AP amplitude is greater in senescent than in adult muscle in both high- and low-Ca^{2+} loading conditions (545). The dramatic prolongation of the AP observed in isometric contractions in the senescent heart depicted in Figure 17.13 has not been observed in nonworking intact heart preparations (291), suggesting that the age differences observed in the AP in working myocardial tissue in part involve an age difference in response to stretch. However, recent evidence indicates that the AP is prolonged in unloaded, single (and thus unstretched) LV myocytes isolated from senescent hearts compared to that in cells from younger hearts (539).

Recent studies have begun to address the ionic basis of the AP prolongation with aging. The peak L-type Ca^{2+} current (measured via the whole-cell patch clamp) normalized for cell capacitative area does not change with aging, suggesting that the density of this Ca^{2+} channel is not markedly altered in myocytes from older hearts (539). However, a reduction in the inactivation rate of the Ca^{2+} current has been observed with aging (537) and an age-associated decrease in the magnitude of I_{To} (an outwardly-directed K current) contributes to the prolonged AP with aging (540). The magnitude of the "inward going rectifier" K current does not change with age (540). Prolongation of the AP duration with aging may also relate to a prolonged Ca_i transient (see the following section), as Ca^{2+} extrusion via the Na^+–Ca^p exchanger during the AP repolarization produces an inward current and prolongs AP duration of rat cells (112).

Cytosolic $[Ca^{2+}]$, contraction, and relaxation. The Ca_i transient that follows sarcolemmal depolarization in isolated cardiac muscle has been monitored by injecting the chemiluminescent protein aequorin into multiple cells of that tissue and measuring the light transient that ensues following the AP (377). The amplitude of the aequorin luminescence transient triggered by excitation is not altered by age when the $[Ca^{2+}]$ in the superfusate is in the physiological range and the rate of stimulation is low (Fig. 17.13C). Studies in which cell and organelle membranes within thin papillary muscle have been solubilized by detergent (Triton X-100) treatment to permit the buffering of $[Ca^{2+}]$ within the myofilament space indicate that neither the maximum force nor the shape of the relationship between force and $[Ca^{2+}]$ differ with age (38) (Fig. 17.13D).

Peak contraction amplitude of isolated, isometric (auxotonic) cardiac muscle at relatively low rates of stimulation (6–48 min^{-1}) does not differ with age (Fig. 17.13) when measured across a broad range of bathing $[Ca^{2+}]$ or resting lengths, that is, preloads (10, 60, 163, 187, 294–296, 545). (It should be noted that the relatively low rates of stimulation, and usually low temperatures, required for isolated cardiac muscle (30°C) studies do not permit assessment of the extent of Ca^{2+} release at cycling rates approaching those in the rat in vivo, for example, 5 Hz and above.) More recent studies show that the twitch contraction amplitude in single cardiac myocytes (which in some ways is analogous to the extent of shortening in the isotonic muscle), when normalized to myocyte length during stimulation at either 0.5 or 1.0 Hz at either 29° or 37°C, does not differ with age (159, 432, 557).

Increasing the stimulation rate or varying the stimulation pattern places a stress upon excitation–contraction mechanisms. In rat muscles bathed in physiological $[Ca^+]$ in the absence of drugs, the amplitude of the twitch force and the Ca_i transient decline as the stimulation frequency is increased, but the magnitude of this decline does not differ with age (377). In contrast, in higher bathing $[Ca^{2+}]$, which increases the net myocardial cell Ca^{2+} load, muscles from younger adults are able to maintain the amplitude of twitch force and of Ca_i transient as the stimulation frequency increases but senescent muscles cannot (377). The postextrasystolic potentiation of contraction amplitude during continual paired stimulation at low rates is also preserved in senescent muscles bathed in a medium of low $[Ca^{2+}]$ and stimulated at 24 pairs/min (174). However, when the coupling interval of paired stimuli is decreased from 200 to 100 ms, senescent, but not adult, muscles fail to generate a twitch response to the second stimulus (Fig. 17.13E). Additionally, muscles from senescent rats show a greater likelihood to exhibit contractions of alternating amplitude at high frequencies of stimulation (166). Thus under the experimental stress of altered stimulation patterns during which restitution time is decreased, the reduced kinetics of ionic channel restitution or of Ca^{2+} cycling in the senescent myocardium produce contractions of smaller amplitude.

The time courses of both the Ca_i transient and the simultaneously measured isometric contraction are prolonged with advancing age (Fig. 17.13B, C). At times during the contraction when force is still increasing and Ca_i concentration is decreasing (see Fig. 17.13C, inset), the latter remains higher in senescent than in young adult muscles. This may result in a relative increase in the Ca^{2+}–myofilament interaction in senescent muscles at later times following excitation and would be expected to prolong the time course of active stiffness (see below, under Myofilament Proteins) and force-

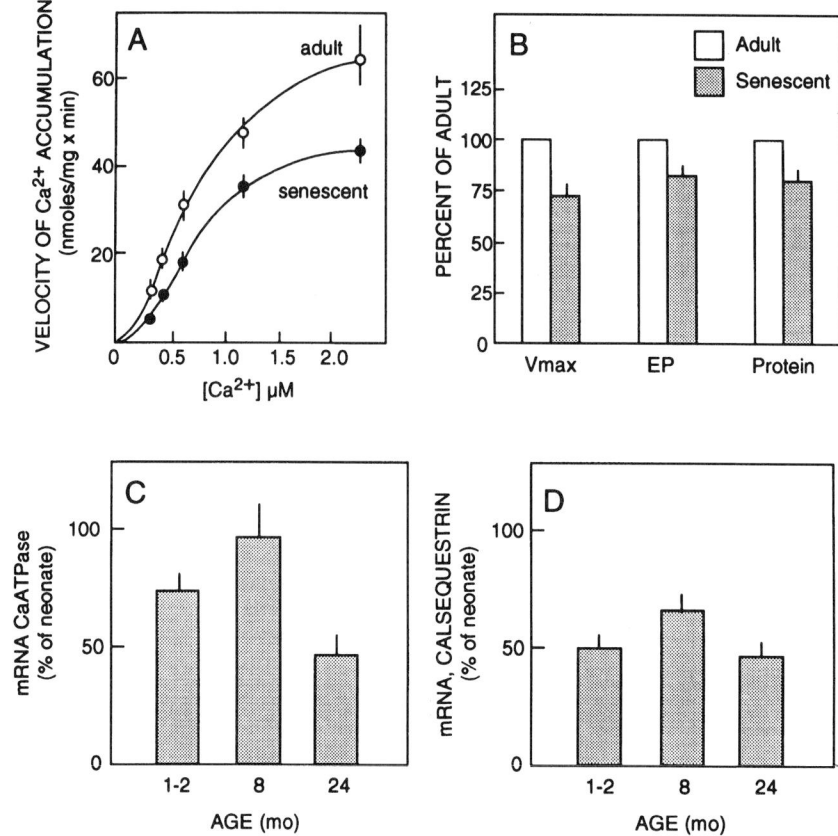

FIG. 17.14. **A**: The effect of age on Ca^{2+} accumulation velocity by sarcoplasmic reticulum (SR) isolated from senescent and adult Wistar rat hearts. [From Froehlich et al. (163) with permission.] **B**: The effect of age on SR isolated from adult and senescent Fischer 344 rat hearts. Left, V$_{max}$ for Ca^{2+}-ATPase activity in isolated SR vesicles; middle, formation of phosphoenzyme product; right, concentration of SR Ca^{2+} pump protein. [From Tate et al. (512) with permission.] The effect of age on steady-state mRNA levels for SR calsequestrin (**D**) Ca^{2+}-ATPase (**C**) in adult senescent Wistar rat hearts. [From Lompre et al. (321) with permission.]

bearing capacity. Stated alternatively, the prolonged Ca$_i$ transient is a cause of the prolonged relaxation of force of cardiac muscle of the older heart. Recall that the isovolumic relaxation period is prolonged in the human heart with aging; the basis for this could be prolonged contractile protein activation due to a prolonged Ca$_i$ transient. While the reduction rate of Ca$_i$ concentration decreases with age, there are no data to indicate that the diastolic Ca$_i$ concentration changes with age (the Ca^{2+} indicator aequorin is not sufficiently sensitive to report changes in Ca$_i$ at the diastolic level).

The load-dependent aspects of relaxation, that is, those purported to be independent of Ca$_i$ concentration and Ca^{2+} activation of the myofilaments but dependent on mechanical displacement of crossbridges by loading factors, of posterior papillary muscle relaxation from the LV and rV of Fischer 344 and Sprague-Dawley rats have been studied at 4, 10, and 20 months of age (62). In the Fischer 344 strain, the relaxation of RV muscle from young animals was found to be completely load-independent, that is dependent on Ca$_i$, whereas the LV muscle was fully load-dependent at all physiological afterloads. With aging, the load dependence of LV muscle relaxation decreased (and thus the Ca$_i$ dependence increased). In contrast, no aging effects on the load dependence of relaxation were observed in muscles from Sprague-Dawley rats (62).

SR function. Although any mechanism that can alter the flux of Ca^{2+} into or out of the myoplasmic space might affect the duration of the Ca$_i$ transient, its decay is thought to largely depend upon the rate of Ca^{2+} removal by the SR Ca^{2+} pump (377). The prolongation of the Ca$_i$ transient in senescent muscle may be related in part to a diminished SR Ca^{2+} pumping rate. Early studies (Fig. 17.14A) have demonstrated that the rate of Ca^{2+} uptake into SR vesicles isolated from senescent Wistar rat hearts is less than that from younger adult hearts (163). The net Ca^{2+} uptake in studies of this sort depends on the Ca^{2+} pumped into vesicles and any Ca^{2+} efflux that may occur during the experiment. The latter can result from a passive, nonspecific leak or from an efflux via Ca^{2+} channels (ryanodine receptors), through which Ca^{2+} release is thought to occur following excitation. The passive leaking of Ca^{2+} of cardiac homogenate membrane preparations has been found to not differ with age (360). The rate of Ca^{2+} pumping into the SR depends on the Ca_i concentrations (or in isolated vesicles, on the $[Ca^{2+}]$ of the medium bathing the vesicles; Fig. 17.14A). The reduction in the SR Ca^{2+} uptake rate with aging applies to the entire range of Ca_i concentrations that occur in cardiac cells from diastole to systole (Fig. 17.14A). More recent studies in SR isolated from other rat strains (Fischer 344 and Sprague-Dawley) have produced results very similar (214, 239, 360, 512) to those in the Wistar strain, as depicted in Figure 17.14A. In the Fischer 344 strain, the diminished SR Ca^{2+} uptake rate persisted in the presence of added calmodulin (214). A decrease in constitutive levels of phosphorylation of phospholamban, an SR protein membrane that modulates the Ca^{2+} pump activity, has also been reported in native cardiac microsomes obtained from senescent rats (259). As unphosphorylated phospholamban inhibits Ca^{2+} uptake by the Ca^{2+} ATPase pump of the cardiac SR, it is possible that lower levels of phosphorylated phospholamban factor into the decreased rate of Ca^{2+} uptake by cardiac SR from older animals observed in the absence of cAMP-dependent stimulation in the above studies (163, 239, 360, 509, 512). In one study in isolated membrane preparations from senescent Fischer 344 rats, although the Ca^{2+} uptake rate was found to be depressed, Ca^{2+}-induced stimulation of SR pump enzyme (that is, the SR Ca^{2+}-ATPase) was not found to be reduced by aging (360). Accordingly, it was suggested that there is an age difference in the efficiency of coupling between ATP splitting and Ca^{2+} pumping (360). In contrast, another study in SR isolated from Fischer 344 rat hearts (509) observed about a 25% age-associated reduction in the maximum rate of SR Ca^{2+}-ATPase activity (Fig. 17.14B), which accompanied reductions of similar magnitude in the formation of acylphosphate and in Ca^{2+} uptake in SR vesicles from senescent vs. young adult hearts (509). Thus the reduction in the rate of Ca^{2+} pumped into the SR is likely due to a reduction in the total SR pump protein (Ca^{2+}-ATPase) activity. The diminished Ca^{2+}-ATPase activity and the rate at which SR from senescent hearts pumps Ca^{2+} may be related to a reduction in mRNA coding for the SR Ca^{2+}-ATPase (Fig. 17.14C) observed in some (321, 328), but not all (55), studies, possibly reflecting a decrease in the relative density of SR pump sites with age (Fig. 17.14C). This conclusion is further supported by the observation that gel electrophoresis shows a 40% reduction in the SR Ca^{2+}-ATPase protein (Fig. 17.14B) without a concomitant reduction in calsequestrin, a Ca^{2+}-binding protein within SR (509). The mRNA levels for calsequestrin (Fig. 17.14D) do not decline with adult aging (321).

Spontaneous sarcoplasmic reticulum Ca^{2+} oscillations and their functional sequelae. As noted, the heartbeat is essentially an organized cycling of Ca^{2+} from the SR to the cytosol and back. In a machine of this design, the potential for spontaneous Ca^{2+} oscillations (S-CaOs) is ever present. The probability of S-CaOs varies with the extent to which the cytosol and the SR become Ca^{2+}-loaded (287). Aggregate alterations in cytosolic Ca^{2+}, Na^+–Ca^+ exchanger, Na^+/K^+-pump, and SR Ca^{2+} pump, possibly in conjunction with nonspecific changes in sarcolemmal membrane ionic permeabilities, may predispose myocardium to altered cell Ca^{2+} homeostasis. Spontaneous SR Ca^{2+} release, unlike that triggered by an AP, occurs focally and sporadically within cardiac cells and asynchronously among cells comprising myocardial tissue. At a given instant, one or multiple loci of increases in Ca_i due to S-CaOs can be present within a cell. The local increase of cytosolic $[Ca^{2+}]$ due to S-CaOs can be as high as that triggered by an AP during systole. Recent experimental results indicate that acute perturbations that result in S-CaOs occurrence can produce the triad of manifestations common to chronic heart failure of various etiologies, that is, abnormal diastolic tonus, limited systolic function, and a high probability of arrhythmias (287). Intriguingly, the aged myocardium and that chronically exposed to pressure overload (see below, under Similar Effects of Aging and Experimental Pressure Overload . . .) are more susceptible to Ca^{2+} overload and S-CaOs (200, 289). When cell Ca^{2+} loading is enhanced, the myocardium of such hearts demonstrates diastolic after-depolarization. The threshold for ventricular fibrillation, which is preceded by an increase in SCaOs, is reduced during Ca^{2+} overload in the senescent heart (200).

Na^+ regulation. The cytosolic $[Na^+]$ regulates the cell Ca^{2+} load by affecting Ca^{2+} flux through the Na^+–Ca^+ exchanger (Fig. 17.12). It has been suggested that the Na^+–Ca^+ exchanger is more active in ejecting Ca^{2+} from cells of older vs. younger hearts during diastole (213, 360). Cytosolic $[Na^+]$ is primarily regulated by the Na^+/K^+-pump. While N^+a/K^+–ATPase activity has been reported to decrease with age, the cytosolic $[Na^+]$ measured via Na^+-selective microelectrodes does not appear to change with age, either at rest or during rapid stimulation (426). In this regard, it is of interest to note that an age-associated decline in the contractile response to digitalis glycosides, which act via Na^+/K^+-pump inhibition, occurs in the absence of an age difference in the relative extent of glycoside-induced Na^+–K^+-ATPase inhibition in both rat and beagle dog models (174, 188).

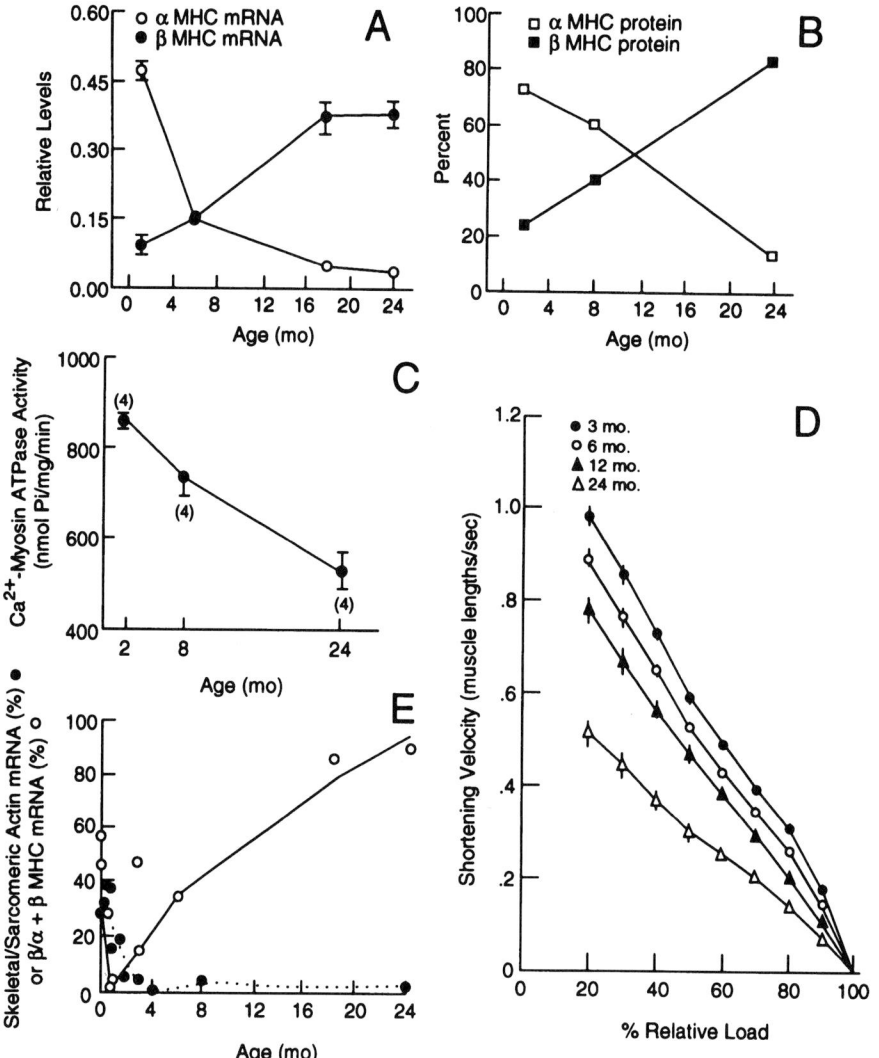

FIG. 17.15. **A:** Average values for α and β myosin heavy chain (MHC) mRNA/mRNA18S of individual Wistar rat hearts measured by dot blot analysis (n = 11, 6, 10, and 10 for ages 6 wk, 6, 18, and 24 months, respectively). [From O'Neill et al. (376) with permission.] **B:** The α and β MHC proteins (V_1 and V_3 isoforms) of hearts of the same rat strain. [From Effron et al. (118) with permission.] **C:** Ca^{2+}-activated myosin ATPase activity of Wistar rat hearts decreases with age. [From Effron et al. (118) with permission.] **D:** The velocity of shortening during lightly loaded isotonic contractions in isolated cardiac muscle from younger and older rats decreases with aging. [From Capasso et al. (60) with permission.] **E:** Left ventricular actin isoforms (cardiac or skeletal) do not change with aging as do the MHC isoforms in the Wistar rat. [From Carrier et al. (63) with permission.]

Myofilament proteins. In addition to the extent of Ca^{2+} binding to troponin C, the ATPase activity of myofilament proteins is a determinant of contraction. Myofibrillar ATPase activity, in preparations using detergents, exhibits the identical Ca^{2+} dependence (K_m 0.6 μm and Hill coefficient of approximately 4.5) as does force (see Fig. 17.13D) (37). Although the Ca^{2+} sensitivity of myofibrillar ATPase activity does not change with adult age, the maximum ATPase activity declines during maturation and then remains stable from 6 months through senescence (37, 294). The Ca^{2+}-activated ATPase activity in actomyosin preparations (that is, actin plus myosin in the absence of troponin and tropomyosin) declines during maturation but also shows a further decline with age (61, 69, 132).

The Ca^{2+}-activated ATPase activity of purified isolated myosin preparations (Fig. 17.15C) declines progressively in the rat throughout the age range of 1–24 months (36, 61, 118, 512). This ATPase activity is modulated in part by the muscle MHC isoform composition (220). The content of the αMHC isoform (often referred to as the "V_1" isoform), which has a rapid ATPase activ-

TABLE 17.4. *Myocardial Changes with Adult Aging in Rats*

Structural Δ	Functional Δ	Ionic Biophysical/Biochemical Mechanisms	Molecular Mechanisms
↑ Myocyte size*	Prolonged contraction duration	Prolonged cytosolic Ca^{2+} transient	↓ SR Ca^{2+} pump mRNA
↓ Myocyte number*		↓ SR Ca^{2+} pumping rate	Calsequestrin mRNA no Δ
		↓ Pump site density	
	Prolonged action potential duration	↓ I_{Ca} inactivation	
		↓ I_{To} density	
	Diminished contraction velocity	↓ αMHC protein	↓ αMHC mRNA
		↑ βMHC protein	↑ βMHC mRNA
		↓ Myosin ATPase activity	Actin mRNA
			Cardiac no Δ
			Skeletal no Δ
	Diminished β-adrenergic contractile response	? ↓ Coupling βAR-acyclase	
		↓ Ca_i transient augmentation	
		↓ TNI phosphorylation	
↑ Matrix collagen	↑ Myocardial stiffness		
			↑ ANF mRNA*
			↑ Proenkephalin mRNA

* ↑, increase; ↓, decrease.

ity, decreases progressively with age (Fig. 17.15B). The lower level of the αMHC protein in preparations isolated from senescent hearts (55, 61, 118, 132, 450) appears to be a major factor underlying the decreased myosin ATPase activity. The mRNA coding for αMHC also declines with age in the myocardium of Wistar (Fig. 17.15A) and Fischer 344 rats (55, 376, 450), and the diminished expression of this gene with aging may account in large part for the reduction in the αMHC content with aging (Fig. 17.15B). Conversely, with aging, the mRNA coding for the βMHC isoform (which has a lower ATPase activity than the αMHC and is sometimes referred to as the "V_3" isoform) exhibits a severalfold increase (55, 376, 450) (Fig. 17.15A) and is the apparent mechanism for an increase in the βMHC protein (Fig. 17.15B).

The switching of the MHC genes with advancing adult age may in part underlie the decline in the velocity of shortening in lightly loaded isotonic contractions (Fig. 17.15D) (10, 61) and may also be related to the prolonged time to peak tension in isometric contractions (Fig. 17.12B) and the prolonged time to peak shortening in isotonic contractions in cardiac muscle from adult vs. older animals (60, 61). It is noteworthy that the βMHC isoform is energy-efficient in that a given level of tension development in hearts with predominantly the βMHC (V_3) isoform produces less heat than in hearts with mixed or predominantly the αMHC (V_1) isoform (8). The pattern of expression of MHC genes in the senescent heart resembles that around the time of birth (376). In this regard, a marked increase in mRNA coding for atrial natriuretic factor (ANF) occurs in the LV with advancing adult age (40). In contrast, the expression of genes coding for actin isoforms (that is, cardiac and skeletal) does not shift with aging (Fig. 17.15E) and thus does not resemble the fetal pattern (63). A marked increase in the expression of the preproenkephalin gene occurs with aging (41), but the functional significance of this is presently not defined.

A summary of the structural, functional, biophysical/biochemical, pharmacological, and molecular changes that occur in the rat heart with aging is presented in Table 17.4. Coordinated changes in several key steps of excitation–contraction coupling occur with aging. These biochemical, biophysical, and molecular changes result in a prolonged Ca^{2+} transient and a prolonged contraction. The resultant altered Ca^{2+} homeostasis renders the older heart more prone to S-CaOs and Ca^{2+}-dependent arrhythmias.

Similar Effects of Aging and Experimental Pressure Overload on Cardiac Regulatory Mechanisms and Gene Expression

The multiple changes in cardiac excitation, myofilament activation, and contraction mechanisms that occur with aging (Fig. 17.13–15 and Table 17.4) are interrelated. Many of these changes can be interpreted as adaptive in nature, since they also occur in the hypertrophied myocardium of younger animals that have adapted to experimentally induced chronic hypertension (7, 8, 11, 28, 40, 55, 60, 61, 67, 71, 98, 105, 117, 171, 187, 189, 199, 210, 212, 223, 229, 265, 286, cf289 for review, 294, 299, 306, 307, 322, 333, 338, 339, 341, 358, 379,

381, 427, 433, 442, 452, 462, 466, 470, 508, 531, 551, 554, 560).

In addition to these changes, the electrical manifestation of S-CaOs, that is, diastolic after-depolarization, is observed in cardiac muscle of pressure-loaded hearts under conditions in which it is not observed in normal myocardia of younger rats (19, 209). A predisposition to pacing-induced ventricular arrhythmias in aortic banded cats has also been reported (460). Hypertrophied hearts due to renal hypertension also show an enhanced likelihood for voltage oscillations on the AP plateau. In contrast to diastolic membrane potential oscillations, these early afterdepolarizations on the AP plateau appear to be due to the removal of inactivation of Ca^{2+} channels during the long AP plateau (231), and the resultant cytosolic Ca^{2+} transients are driven by the oscillations in I_{Ca} (485). The greater likelihood for plateau oscillations may lead to an enhanced susceptibility for arrhythmias under some circumstances in the pressure-hypertrophied heart (534).

Because similar reductions in the cellular ribonucleic acid (RNA) concentration and in the rate of protein synthesis have been observed with aging and chronic myocardial overload in the rat model, it has been suggested that the latter (which is usually accompanied by myocardial hypertrophy) represents accelerated aging (340). The initial myocardial hypertrophy in pressure overload is a manifestation of an enhanced net protein synthesis due to enlargement of a relatively constant number of cardiac myocytes and reflects global activation of cardiac genes at the translational and posttranslational levels (452).

There is evidence that one signal involved in the transduction enhanced pressure load stress is mechanical, that is, stretch or tension (30, 82, 255, 264, 332, 354, 467, 543, 560). In this regard, the relationship of an increase in protein synthesis and force (both systolic and diastolic) is described by a single linear function (82). This tension effect may be mediated in part by enhanced coronary flow (30) or hormonal stimulation (245, 353, 467, 468, 535, 543). Interactions occur between stretch and cell-surface-receptor-mediated intracellular signal transduction mechanisms, for example, increases in cAMP or in PKC activity (245, 353, 468, 535, 543) or changes in ion flux [for example, Na^+ (255) or Ca^{2+}] possibly related to stretch-induced activation of ionic channels (85, 86). Reorganization of intracellular matrix proteins, for example, desmin and tubulin, may also mediate the stretch response (542). Additionally, stretch of extracellular matrix and ventricular and cardiac endothelium may lead to the production of growth factors which can initiate protein synthesis and regulate gene expression (442).

The initial events in response to increased aortic pressure occur rapidly (within 30 min) and mimic the normal stress and growth responses, including the transient induction of heat shock proteins (99, 198, 199, 468), protooncogenes (228, 355, 360, 469), and other early growth response genes (73). There is also an induction of proteins that are usually present in ventricular myocardium during the fetal period, for example, α skeletal actin (228) and β-tropomyosin (228), or proteins that are usually present only in the atria of adult hearts, for example, ANF (94, 456). Subsequently, shifts in the expression of genes coding myofilament, ion channel, or membrane pump proteins occur. Initially at least, substantial spatio-temporal heterogeneity exists in the increase in mRNA encoding these various proteins (400, 443). This could be due in part to a heterogeneity of the specific factors stimulating the initial growth response. The phenotype of the stable, adapted hypertensive heart in some cases is due to differential expression of multigene families of contractile proteins, for example, the shift of the MHC isoform, and in other instances involves differential activation of single genes, for example, the coding for the SR Ca^{2+}-ATPase protein.

A similar pattern of altered gene expression occurs in both hypertension in young animals and aging in normotensive animals (290) and in neonatal heart cells exposed to growth factors (444). It is tempting to speculate that, because a nearly identical pattern of change in cell mechanisms occurs in both experimental pressure overload and aging (and after growth factors in neonatal heart cells), this pattern may reflect a "logic" within the genome, that is, that a common set of transcription factors regulates the expression of multiple genes resulting in cellular adaptation. This particular constellation of shifts in gene expression appears to be adaptive in that it allows for an energy-efficient and prolonged contraction. In the hypertensive rodent heart it can be inferred that these changes in gene expression permit functional adaptations in response to an increased vascular afterload.

Possible Mechanisms of Altered Cardiac Gene Regulation with Aging

If the changes depicted in Figures 17.13–15 and Table 17.4 were to occur in normal human myocardium with aging, they could easily be construed as adaptations to the stiffer arterial system and to an increase in arterial pressure and impedance, as discussed earlier, under Ventricular-Vascular Coupling. However, with aging in the normotensive rat, whether the similar changes that occur with hypertension in younger rats are adaptive or degenerative is uncertain because the stimuli for these changes with normotensive aging remain to be identified. There are presently few data to indicate that arterial stiffening or enhanced arterial impedance occurs with aging in rats up to 24 months of age at least.

Although peripheral resistance increases with age in rats, it appears to plateau at 10–12 months and cannot directly be related to the changes shown in Figures 17.13–15, which are progressive with advancing age (534). Additionally, as noted above (see Similar Effects of Aging and Experimental Pressure Overload . . .), the changes depicted in Figures 17.13–15 and Table 17.4 have been described in two strains of rat that do not become hypertensive with aging.

Unlike the hypertensive heart, the increased LV mass with aging in the Wistar rat strain is largely due to an increase in LV cavity size, that is, the wall thickness appears to remain normal with aging (463). However, as in the young hypertensive rat, cardiac myocytes become enlarged in the senescent heart. It may be argued that the mechanical or hormonal stimuli that initiate and maintain the cardiac hypertrophic response in the hypertensive heart are also present in the aging heart. It has been hypothesized that the apparent "dropout" of some myocardial cells with aging (15, 16) leads to augmented stretch upon the remaining cells, this being the stimulus of cellular hypertrophy and of the accompanying changes in gene expression and biophysical mechanisms that lead to a prolonged contraction. Nevertheless, prolonged contraction in older hearts persists when these hearts are transplanted, mechanically unloaded, and atrophied (266). Also, prolonged AP, Ca_i transient, and contraction occur with aging in RV muscle (486, 545) in which the ventricular myocyte number may not be reduced in senescence (15). Additionally, unlike the LV, the RV does not hypertrophy with age in the Wistar rat strain (565).

Alterations of thyroid status can produce alterations in the variables depicted in Figures 17.13–15 and Table 17.4. In this regard, the changes observed in the aging heart mimic to some extent those observed in the hypothyroid state (9, 66, 103, 219, 220, 227, 450). Whether or not a relative hypothyroid state accompanies aging is uncertain. An age-associated decline in plasma levels of thyroid hormones (T_3 or T_4) occurs in at least two rat strains (55, 66, 118, 328), but the magnitude of the decline is small. Still, it has been reported that replacement of sufficient thyroxine to restore plasma levels in older rats to those found in younger rats can abolish the age-associated decline in myosin ATPase activity (66); however, complete reversal of the MHC isoform profile did not occur with small doses of thyroxine (66). Very high doses of T_4 administered for a short period of time have been noted to increase the myosin αMHC content of senescent hearts, but they do not fully restore this level to that in the younger heart (118). Administration of T_3 or T_4 to senescent rats also decreases the βMHC protein content (118, 450) and the βMHC and mRNA levels (449). Still, a failure of myocardial cells to respond to thyroxine (for example, due to deficits in nuclear thyroid receptors or changes of the binding properties of thyroid regulatory elements on the MHC and other genes) may occur with aging and in part underlie the pattern of change depicted in Figures 17.13–15 and Table 17.4.

Glucose intolerance has been observed in aged rats (402) and could possibly relate to some of the changes noted above. In insulin-deficient diabetic rats, marked shifts occur in the MHC isoform pattern (increases in βMHC isoform) and in myofilament ATPase activities (104, 330). Additionally, the SR Ca^{2+}-ATPase activity and the Ca^{2+} uptake of isolated SR are depressed in insulin-deficient diabetic hearts (169, 324, 385), and the contraction time is prolonged (135). In noninsulin-dependent diabetes, the type more typically associated with aging, the SR Ca^{2+} pumping rate and the ATPase activity are also reduced (441), and a shift to the βMHC isoform occurs. A diminished β-adrenergic response also occurs in this form of diabetes (440).

Finally, a reduction of physical activity occurs with aging even rats in captivity (384, 570). Because many of the changes in the cardiac mechanisms depicted in Figures 17.13–15 and Table 17.4 can be modulated by physical conditioning, which in older animals has been shown to modify some of these changes, physical deconditioning with aging (or lifelong residence in cages) may have a role in effecting some of these changes.

Response of Older Rat Heart to Chronic Hemodynamic Overload

The extent to which MHC isoform composition, myosin ATPase activity, and AP and contraction durations become altered following pressure overload appears to be correlated with the extent of hypertrophy, regardless of age (61). The response to mechanical stresses that evoke substantial myocardial hypertrophy, for example, pressure or volume overload, appears, in some instances, to be reduced in the senescent heart. For example, the extent of ventricular hypertrophy following aortic (226) or pulmonary artery banding (281) volume overload or the creation of renal hypertension (61) is reduced in senescent vs. younger rats. Although in the latter study the significance of this is unclear because of four age groups tested, one younger age group also showed a reduction in the extent of hypertrophy. Additionally, a subsequent study utilizing the same pressure loading model in the same rat strain observed that the hypertrophic response of the senescent heart was not decreased (54). The induction of early-response genes (protooncogenes) following aortic banding becomes blunted with age (510). The hypertrophic response to chronic AV block, which causes a 50% reduction in heart rate, decreases with age and is accompanied by reduced functional adaptations in isolated cardiac muscle (538). Furthermore, the contractile response to stressful conditions (high pacing rate and high bathing $[Ca^{2+}]$) is reduced in senescent hearts that have responded to mild aortic banding with an appropriate degree of hypertrophy (42). Thus it may be argued that the adaptive reserve capacity, that is, an increase in cardiac mass or cardiac muscle function, may become diminished with advancing age. This may indicate that some cardiac adaptations, for example, an increased myocyte or heart size, become utilized during normal aging and that a further utilization of these cannot occur in response to these experimental stresses. In other words, the reserve capacity of the aged heart to respond to these stressful situations appears to be diminished. This could be related in part to cardiac myocyte cell death and fibrosis that may occur due to, for example, an excessive increase in myocyte cell size, relative ischemia, or inadequacy of cell ionic homeostasis or of energy balance for reasons not related to blood flow. In a spontaneously hypertensive rat strain, advanced age and chronic hypertension are accompanied by deterioration of hemodynamic function (388), evidence for impaired myocardial force production, increases in myocardial collagen, and clinical signs of severe congestive heart failure (38).

Coronary Blood Flow, Oxygen Consumption, and Oxidative Metabolism

Excitation, contraction, and relaxation mechanisms of cardiac muscle, which determine myocardial performance, require ATP to maintain cytosolic $[Na^+]$ and Ca_i concentrations at levels far removed from their thermodynamic equilibria to maintain ionic homeostasis and to permit Ca_i transients and cyclic Ca^{2+}-actomyosin interactions. Thus an understanding of how aging affects cardiac contractile regulation requires not only specific studies of the effects of intrinsic myofilament function, cell organelles, or ion pumps but also a delineation of whether or not O_2 delivery (coronary flow) and energy metabolism change with aging.

Myocardial cell enlargement (Fig. 17.13F), interstitial fibrosis, and chronic changes in myocardial function that have been noted in the isolated working heart from rats of advanced age (5, 162, 308, 489, 490) may affect the adequacy of coronary flow. In senescent vs. adult hearts in vitro, coronary blood flow per gram heart is diminished, and the magnitude of this decrement is approximately 15% (5, 548). In unrestrained, male Fischer 344 rats of 4, 12, and 20 months of age, maximal coronary blood flow per 100 g tissue decreases by 43% in the LV at both 12 and 20 months vs. 4 months and by 44% and 47% in RV at the same time intervals (192). Minimal coronary vascular resistance per 100 g of myocardium (measured after maximal vasodilatation) increased with age by 56% and 36% in the LV and by 48% and 44% in the RV at 12 and 20 months, respectively. Maximal coronary blood flow to the endocardium was depressed more than epicardial flow at 20 months. In isolated, working Wistar-Kyoto rat hearts, coronary blood flow varied threefold (depending on the prevailing afterload); at any given afterload, coronary flow was 25% less in hearts from 19-month-old vs. 4-month-old rats (162). In isolated, senescent Wistar rat hearts, maximum coronary flow, that is, elicited by hypoxia, was found to be approximately 70–80 ml/g dry weight in the mature adult and approximately 65 ml/g dry weight in the senescent heart (548). Thus coronary flow per unit heart mass decreases with age in three different rat strains.

These changes in coronary blood flow associated with maturation and aging are comparable with those seen in pressure overload hypertrophy in younger rats and may predispose to an increased vulnerability of the myocardium to ischemic episodes during stress, particularly of the subendocardial region of the LV. Since macroscopic structural alterations in the large, medium, or small coronary vessels are not present in these hearts, the age-associated reduction in coronary flow reserve and myocardial O_2 consumption may result from a change in vascular reactivity or from a failure of the coronary bed to enlarge commensurate with the increase in heart mass that occurs with senescence. Earlier studies have documented a decrease in the number of capillaries in 26–27-month-old compared with 4-month-old rat hearts and in increase in fiber to capillary ratio (399, 519). This diminution in coronary blood flow and capillary density might indicate that the aged heart is chronically hypoxic. However, it should be emphasized that the capillary density in the aged heart is not fixed but can be enhanced by chronic exercise (519, 520). Thus it appears unlikely that chronic anoxia has any significant role in whatever anatomical or functional alterations may occur in the senescent rat heart. In contrast, the reduction in coronary flow with aging, in conjunction with the marked shift in MHC isoform toward the βMHC type may down-regulate (hibernate) myocardial function and thus energy consumption in aged hearts (see below).

Whereas the most instructive studies of excitation-contraction mechanisms with aging have been implemented in isolated cardiac muscles or cells, similar studies of energy metabolism have been conducted in intact hearts and isolated mitochondria. The maximum myocardial substrate oxidation rates in working heart preparations from Sprague-Dawley rats decline about 20% from adulthood to senescence (5). However, energy production rates are appropriate for the reduced work performed by older hearts (for reviews see 202, 294). More recent studies in isolate, working hearts from Fischer 344 rats found cardiac work and efficiency to decline with age, particularly at high aortic pressures (489, 490). This latter study, in which the workload on the heart was twofold greater than in prior studies (5), clearly shows that the capacity for energy production in the heart of the Fischer 344 rat does not decline from adulthood to advanced old age (489). This is indicated by the lack of an age-associated decline in maximum activities of rate-limiting enzymes in both the glycolytic pathway and the Krebs cycle or in the concentration of cytochromes in the mitochondrial respiratory chain. In this study (489), appropriate measurements, which allowed for the calculation of the free energy of ATP hydrolysis (ΔG_{atp}), indicated that ΔG_{ATP} was not affected by aging under conditions where heart pumping performance had declined, strongly suggesting that the capacity of the aged heart to pump blood is not limited by bioenergetic factors. An additional observation of this study was that, while chronic exercise conditioning did not affect maximum aerobic energy production capacity, it did enhance other performance measurements of the isolated hearts of aged animals (489, 490). This dissociation of performance and energetics also indicates that nonenergetic mechanisms (perhaps a primary decrease in coronary blood flow or a shift in MHC isoform types) determine performance of the senescent heart by chronic exercise training.

In contrast to the aforementioned studies in intact hearts, those in isolated mitochondria have observed that oxidation of certain substrates is diminished in senescent vs. adult rat hearts (68, 201, 202). ADP-stimulated (state 3) respiration of myocardial mitochondria was diminished in Fischer 344 rats aged 20–24 months vs. 12–16 months when glutamate–pyruvate, glutamate–malate, and palmitylcarnitine were used as substrates. However, no age-associated differences were observed when succinate and ascorbate were employed as substrates (68). In mitochondria isolated from hearts of Wistar rats, a 40% decline in palmitylcarnitine oxidation was also observed between 6 and 24 months of age (201); further studies showed that the mitochondria from aged hearts retained less carnitine than that from young ones and that this limited the rate of translocation and thus the rate of palmitate oxidation in the senescent mitochondria. In addition to these findings, it was observed that, as in the study of the intact working heart of the Fischer 344 rat (5), tissue concentrations of both carnitine and acetylcarnitine are reduced in the senescent vs. the adult myocardium (201). However, why isolated mitochondria show declines in oxidation rates with aging, whereas isolated heart preparations do not, remains an enigma. An explanation usually offered by "mitochondriacs" to explain this enigma is that the maximum energy demand of isolated cardiac preparations is insufficient to stress the maximum energy production rates in situ.

EFFECT OF CHRONIC PHYSICAL CONDITIONING ON CARDIOVASCULAR PERFORMANCE IN OLDER HUMANS AND ANIMALS

Studies in Humans

There is mounting evidence that age-associated increases in arterial stiffness and pressure can be modified by life-style and diet. NaCl dependence of arterial pressure increases with age (186, 257, 546). The rate at which the aorta stiffens with age, manifested by the pulse wave velocity increase, differs in two Chinese populations (27) that differ in exercise and dietary habits, particularly with reference to the amount of NaCl ingested (Fig. 17.1A). In a study population advised to ingest low quantities of NaCl (44 mmol/24 h) for an average period of 2 yr the expected age-associated increases in aortic, arm, and leg pulse velocities did not occur (26). Age-associated increases in pulse wave velocity or carotid pressure pulse late augmentation are blunted in exercise-trained, older athletes (191, 527).

Endurance training younger men blunts the baroreceptor response, measured as the change in heart rate over that of arterial pressure during phenylephrine infusion or during lower body negative pressure (LBNP) (475). In healthy, rigorously screened sedentary, middle-aged and older men, strenuous and prolonged endurance training, sufficient to elicit large increases in maximal exercise capacity and small reductions in heart rate at rest, appears to increase cardiac vagal tone at rest and does not alter arterial baroreflex control of heart rate but does result in a diminished forearm vasoconstrictor response to reductions in baroreflex sympathoinhibition (454). During LBNP in endurance-trained, older (60–80 yr) individuals, LVEDV, SV, and arterial pressure are better preserved compared to age-matched controls (158). This contrasts with a reduction in SV during LBNP in young, endurance-trained vs. young, sedentary individuals (474).

In younger individuals, endurance training enhances $\dot{V}O_2$ by augmentation in both central and peripheral mechanisms (77, 88). Maximum cardiac output is augmented following endurance training in younger individuals via cardiac dilatation, increase in cardiac mass (347), and enhanced circulating blood volume (87, 335, 410). Cardiac enlargement occurs at both end-diastole and end-systole; the former change is greater than the latter, resulting in an augmentation of SVI (177). Ejection fraction may decrease or remain unchanged. Increased SVI at rest and during submaximal exercise is accompanied by a reduced heart rate; cardiac output for a given external workload may be even less in conditioned vs. sedentary individuals due to concomitant augmentation of O_2 delivery–extraction–utilization induced by training. In healthy, sedentary, older men, moderate cardiac dilatation, bradycardia, and augmented SVI occur at both end-diastole and end-systole in the sitting position at rest and during exercise (Fig. 17.8). Thus some of the macroscopic cardiac adaptations induced by endurance training in younger adults occur with aging in sedentary individuals.

To determine the interaction of physical conditioning status and age on cardiorespiratory performance, young, middle-aged (184, 185), and old individuals who remain competitive in sports (master athletes) have often been compared to their sedentary counterparts. Master athletes (149, 208, 247, 391, 422) have a lesser accumulation of subcutaneous fat, a better preservation of muscle mass and lean tissue, an increased peripheral O_2 utilization, a greater work performance at a given target heart rate, and nearly twice the aerobic capacity of sedentary older individuals (Fig. 17.9). Master athletes exhibit type I skeletal muscle fiber hypertrophy and augmentation of glycolytic and oxidative enzymes of gastrocnemius muscle compared to younger runners (80). While in highly trained middle-aged (52–59 yr) men leg blood flow during cycle exercise increased less than in younger (25–30 yr) men, equivalent O_2 consumption occurred in the older men due to a greater increase in $(A-V)O_2$ (537).

In cross-sectional studies, cardiac status, measured in older master athletes, has been compared to that in sedentary controls. Maximum heart rate during cycle or treadmill exercise does not differ between master athletes and sedentary older individuals (149, 193). During treadmill exercise, it has been estimated that the cardiac output (assuming that the SV measured at submaximum exercise is the same as that at maximum exercise) is increased in master athletes vs. sedentary, age-matched controls (193). Estimation of the maximum SV during exercise as the O_2 pulse, that is, $\dot{V}O_2$/heart rate, also suggests that SV in master athletes is increased compared to their sedentary counterparts (208). Another cross-sectional report indicates that about 85% of the nearly twofold increase in peak $\dot{V}O_2$ achieved during upright cycle exercise in master athletes is due to increases in both $(A-V)O_2$ and SVI, the latter being due to an increase in EDVI (150). Results employing the acetylene rebreathing technique to measure SV during treadmill exercise suggest that the nearly twofold greater $\dot{V}O_{2max}$ in master athletes (63 yr of age) than in sedentary, age-matched controls is accompanied by both an increase in cardiac output, due to an increase in estimated SV, and an increase in maximum $(A-V)O_2$ (374).

Longitudinal assessment has been made of the factors underlying changes in $\dot{V}O_{2max}$ with aging in endurance-trained individuals. In 74 habitually physically active men and women over a 21-yr period during which age increased from 25–33 to 41–54 yr, a 20% decrease in $\dot{V}O_{2max}$ was accompanied by a 9% reduction in heart rate. There was no correlation between the decline in maximum heart rate and the decline in $\dot{V}O_{2max}$ among given individuals (22). Thus a decrease in the efficiency of peripheral factors that underlie O_2 utilization must have occurred with aging. However, a decline in training status during the course of longitudinal and most other long-term studies confounds the interpretation regarding longitudinal reductions in aerobic capacity. In master athletes who continue to train during aging, it has been observed that the maximum aerobic capacity and O_2 pulse can be maintained (391) or can decline less (422) over an 8–10-year period compared to sedentary controls or athletes who decrease their training intensity (391). During a 10-year follow-up study, in which the $\dot{V}O_{2max}$ of master athletes who continued to train during the test interval did not decline, the expected age-associated decline in heart rate did occur despite continued training. This suggests that compensatory cardiac or peripheral adaptations maintained the enhanced aerobic capacity (391).

In another type of longitudinal study design, measurements of factors that determine aerobic capacity have been made prior to and following endurance training of sedentary middle-aged and older individuals. *Middle-aging* in sedentary individuals is accompanied by increased body fat, decreased muscle mass, lower maximal O_2 uptake, and lower energy intake. In both young and middle-aged men who complete a training program at 65%–80% maximal O_2 uptake, changes in body composition and energy requirements, as well as aerobic capacity, are observed when compared to sedentary men (342). A 7-month endurance-training program, sufficient to increase $\dot{V}O_{2max}$ 18% (from 35.8 to 40 ml/kg/min), for sedentary middle-aged (46–51 yr) men was accompanied by a decrease in cardiac output at rest and during vigorous exercise for a given O_2 uptake, indicating more efficient peripheral O_2 extraction and utilization (203). This suggests that the physical deconditioning that accompanies middle-aging, or the middle-aging process per se, is associated with a decrease in peripheral O_2 delivery–transport–utilization mechanisms, which can be restored by fitness training. SVI and ventricular ejection rates are also increased by training during middle age (203). Additionally, swim training of middle-aged men increased both peripheral and central factors, which increased $\dot{V}O_2$ from 29.2 to 34.7% (336).

Longitudinal studies of the effects of endurance training have demonstrated that regular exercise conditioning also enhances aerobic capacity in older individuals (101, 120, 139, 191, 194, 247, 401). The magnitude of the $\dot{V}O_{2max}$ augmentation and the underlying mechanisms vary with relative fitness prior to training, with intensity and duration of training (120, 247, 401), and with the experimental paradigm in which performance is measured (401). It is clear that the reduction in maximum heart rate in older individuals is not affected by physical conditioning, regardless of duration or intensity. Changes in both central and peripheral mechanisms have been found with endurance training of older individuals (121, 374, 444). After high-intensity training of older (60–69 yr) individuals for 10 months to 1 yr, $\dot{V}O_{2max}$ increased by about 20% (25.4 to 32.9 ml/kg/min); this was achieved primarily by an increase in estimated (A-V)O_2, with little increase in estimated maximum cardiac output (453). The results of a study employing the acetylene rebreathing method show that SV at peak treadmill exercise increases by 15% in older (64 yr) men following 12 months of endurance training (483). This was accompanied by a 7% increase in (A-V)O_2. In contrast, a similar training regimen in women increased $\dot{V}O_{2max}$ exclusively via an augmentation of (A-V)O_2, with no demonstrable changes in cardiac function (455) as neither peak SV nor maximum heart rate increased. In another study, similarly aged individuals (60–70 yr), who increased their $\dot{V}O_{2max}$ by about 25% (29.6–37.2 ml/kg/min) following training, had an 18% increase in maximum cardiac output during supine cycle exercise (121). This increase in cardiac output following chronic endurance training was achieved by an increase in SV due to an increase in EDV. Following training, a greater reduction in ESV during exercise augmented the EF achieved during exercise. Since arterial pressure during supine exercise testing was not affected by conditioning, the enhanced EF and reduced ESV after conditioning have been interpreted (121) to reflect an increase in myocardial contractility induced by conditioning. A peculiarity of this study is that the estimated (A-V)O_2 did not increase following exercise, in contrast to other observations using similar training paradigms (455). This may relate to the supine body position during exercise in this more recent study (121). In contrast to the above study, less intense exercise paradigms in older individuals do not enhance cardiac performance (increased EF or reduced ESV) during cycle ergometry (445; see also Fig. 17.10B).

Marked changes have been observed in skeletal muscle following endurance training of older individuals (79, 168, 342). Short-term (2 wk), endurance training at 70% maximum effort, which had no effect on weight or body composition in either age group, increased $\dot{V}O_{2max}$ to the same extent (5.5–6 ml/kg/min) in both young (23 yr) and older 65 yr) individuals (338). Prior to training, older subjects had more adipose tissue and less muscle mass than younger subjects. Muscle biopsies taken at rest before training showed that muscle glycogen stores were 61% higher in younger subjects. Following training, glycogen stores and muscle O_2 utilization increased significantly (by 25% and 28%) in older, but not in younger, individuals. In another study, a 30% increase in $\dot{V}O_{2max}$ effected by intense endurance training of older (65 yr) men for 9–12 months was accompanied by a 50% increase in the number of type IIa gastrocnemius muscle fibers, a 13% increase in fiber area, a 25% increase in capillary/fiber ratio, and a 30%–50% increase in succinate dehydrogenase, citrate synthase, and β-hydroxyacyl CoA-dehydrogenase activities (79). These skeletal muscle adaptations likely have a role in augmented peripheral utilization of O_2 and in the enhanced work capacity and $\dot{V}O_{2max}$ after endurance training in older individuals. Strength training also enhances muscle structure and function in older individuals (168). Leg strength (isometric) training of knee extensors in healthy older (60–73 yr) individuals increases the $\dot{V}O_{2max}$ of the exercised muscles and is accompanied by increases in muscle strength, as with endurance training (166). It has been observed that, following leg strength training, the mean vastus lateralis fiber area increased in these older individuals by 28% (both types I and II fibers), the fiber/capillary ratio by 15%, and citrate synthase by 38%. In contrast, resistance training (one set of 8–12 repetitions on Nautilus machines) in older individuals had no effect on cardiovascular responses to submaximal or maximal treadmill exercise (194).

In summary, it is quite clear that the aerobic capacity of both middle-aged and older individuals can increase following endurance training and that this is mediated by adaptations in peripheral, and in some cases (depending on the intensity of exercise and the baseline $\dot{V}O_{2max}$) cardiac, mechanisms. These adaptations also explain, in part at least, differences in $\dot{V}O_{2max}$ measured in cross-sectional comparisons in younger and older sedentary individuals and between master athletes and their sedentary counterparts.

Studies in Rodents

Chronic exercise in senescent rats abolishes prolonged isometric contraction (Fig. 17.16A) in isolated LV trabeculae measured across a range of [Ca^{2+}] and reduces active dynamic stiffness (486). This chronic (5-month), mild wheel exercise protocol was insufficient to alter the body or heart weights in adult (6–9 month) and senescent (24–26 month) rats at time of death and did not alter the twitch amplitude at any age. In the younger animals, this exercise protocol was ineffective in altering the duration of contraction (Fig. 17.16A) or dynamic stiffness measured during contraction in muscles. The reduction in both the slope stiffness coefficient and the duration of contraction (Fig. 17.16A) would be consistent with an effect of exercise to reduce the duration of the Ca_i transient. Indeed, subsequent studies show that the duration of the Ca_i transient in senescent cardiac muscle is reduced following chronic exercise (190). The AP prolongation in isolated muscle of senescent hearts is not reversed by exercise, however (190). The reduced rate of SR Ca^{2+} sequestration (Fig. 17.16B) and SR Ca^{2+} ATPase and mRNA levels in the senescent heart (509, 512) can also be reversed by chronic physical conditioning. The progressive decline in myocardial Ca^{2+}-activated actomyosin ATPase activity, that begins during maturation (after 1 month in the rat) and progresses with advancing adult age, can be retarded by a chronic (3-month) period of exercise, but the beneficial effects of exercise are relatively small throughout 12–15 months (70). Moreover, in older animals that began exercise at 17–22 months and were sacrificed at 20–25 months, a decline in actomyosin ATPase occurred (70). The altered MHC isoform profile with aging (Fig. 16C) or myosin or myosin ATPase activities (Fig. 16D) in the senescent heart are not affected by chronic physical conditioning (35, 132, 512).

A greater relative effect of chronic exercise on aspects of cardiac biochemistry that relate to metabolism has also been observed in senescent vs. young adult rat myocardium. Although chronic exercise does not usually augment cytochrome c oxidase activity in cardiac muscle of younger animals as it does in skeletal muscle (382), a modest augmentation of this enzyme has been observed in hearts of senescent animals (382, 512). This is accompanied by exercise-induced increases in rates of glutamate, palmitylcarnitine, and succinate oxidation in

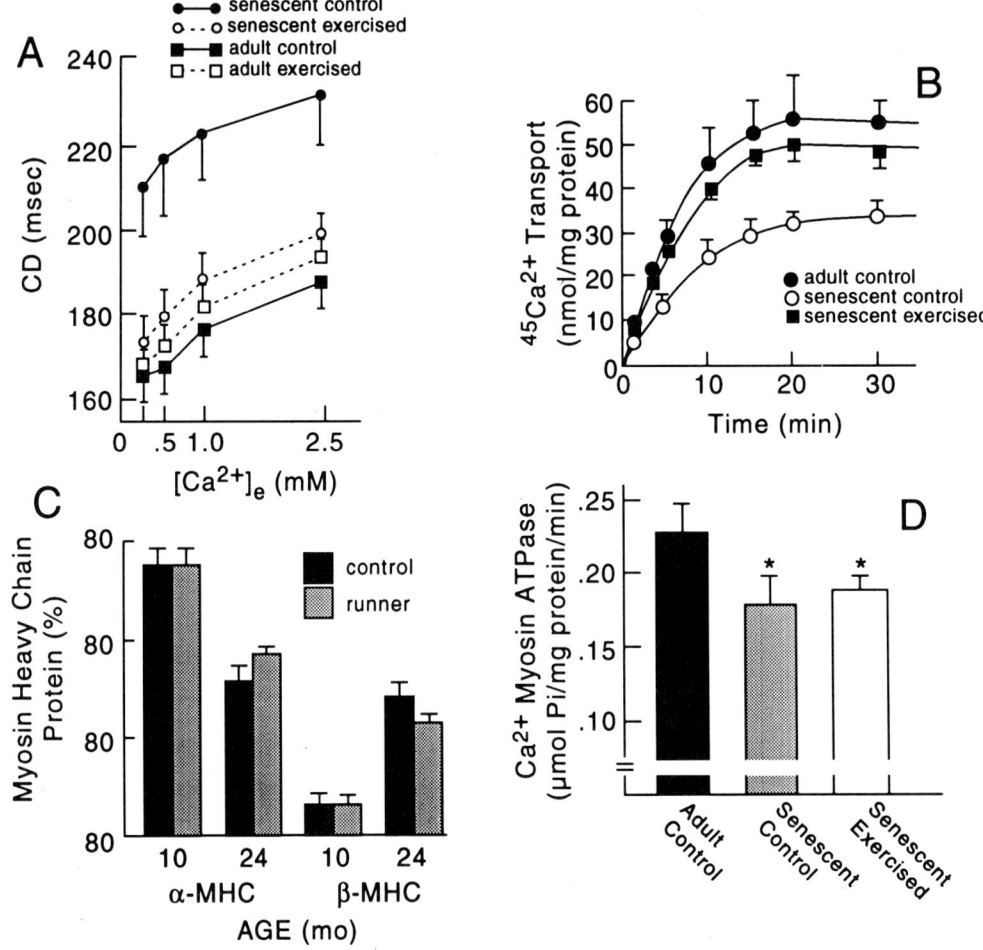

FIG. 17.16. Chronic exercise training decreases the isometric contraction duration in isolated right ventricular papillary muscles of older Wistar rats (A) and the velocity of Ca^{2+} accumulation in sarcoplasmic reticulum isolated from Fischer 344 rats (B). In contrast, chronic exercise alters neither age-associated decreases in the MHC isoform content (C) nor age-associated changes in myosin ATPase activity (D). [A from Spurgeon et al. (486); B and D from Tate et al. (512); C from Farrar et al. (132) with permission.]

isolated mitochondria (382). Thus exercise can partially reverse the declines in oxidation rates of these substrates and in cytochrome c activity that occur with aging in rats (490). In mice the marked age-associated declines in cardiac aldolase and superoxide dismutase activities between 9 and 27 months are also prevented by chronic exercise that began at 6 months of age and continued into old age (491). Finally, the response of senescent cardiac muscle to reoxygenation following hypoxia (315, 544) and insulin resistance of the aging rat are also ameliorated by chronic exercise (402).

In summary, chronic exercise in older animals reverses some of the alterations in cardiac function (prolonged contraction, reduced SR function) that occur with aging. Other aspects of cardiac function that change with aging (prolonged AP, altered myosin isoform expression) are not affected by chronic exercise.

SUMMARY

Age-associated changes in cardiovascular structure and function in healthy individuals have been defined. Arteries increase in diameter and wall thickness with aging and these changes are associated with an increase in arterial wall stiffness, a reduction in volume elasticity, and an increase in systolic arterial pressure. The extent to which these changes occur with aging appears to be modified by diet (reduced NaCl intake) and aerobic capacity. PVR, in contrast, does not markedly increase with aging in healthy, normotensive individuals. Aging between 20 and 80 yr is associated with a modest increase in LV wall thickness, due mainly to an increase in the size of cardiac myocytes. The resting LVED diameter increases moderately with age in men but not in women. Increases in heart mass with aging are exaggerated by coexisting disease (coronary artery disease or hypertension) and are substantially influenced by lifestyle (physical fitness).

A prolonged myocardial contraction time in older individuals maintains a normal ejection time in the presence of the late augmentation of aortic impedance due to early reflected pulse waves. The prolonged contraction also contributes to the maintenance of LVSV, LVESV, and LVEF at rest. Thus in healthy humans, systolic cardiac function at rest is not much altered by age even though the arterial tree stiffens and imposes an increased afterload on the heart. The down side of prolonged contractile activation in older individuals is that myocardial relaxation time is prolonged and at the time of the mitral valve opening some contractile activation persists. This is one factor that causes the early LV filling rate to be reduced in older individuals. Structural changes and functional heterogeneity within the LV with aging may also contribute to this reduction in peak LV filling rate. However, concomitant adaptation, left atrial enlargement, and enhanced atrial contribution to ventricular filling compensate for the reduced early filling and in part maintain increased LVEDV in men and prevent a decrease in LVEDV in women.

In response to orthostatic stress, maintenance of PVR does not decline with aging but the heart rate increase is blunted in older vs. younger individuals. The expected LVEDV reduction is less in older vs. younger individuals and LVSV is better preserved. Although there is a decrease in the maximum aerobic work capacity in most healthy older individuals, it has become clear that this limitation may not be due to solely to limitations of the central circulation. Rather, the limitations of exercise ability in the aged individual are, in part at least, related to peripheral factors that determine O_2 utilization, particularly in women. Peripheral factors that appear to be involved in the age-associated decline in the $\dot{V}O_{2max}$ include a decline in skeletal muscle mass with aging. In spite of this muscle mass decline, body mass may remain constant due to an increase in body fat, not only subcutaneously but also intraperitoneally and intramuscularly.

During high levels of physical exertion, heart rate is substantially lower in healthy elderly vs. younger individuals. The peak rate of LV filling increases in both younger and older individuals during exercise but a diminished rate of filling of similar magnitude (about a 50% reduction), is still observed in older individuals during exercise, as at rest. However, cardiac dilatation at end-diastole and end-systole still occurs during vigorous exercise in older men. Thus healthy older individuals do not exhibit a compromised LVEDV due to a "stiff heart," either at rest or during exercise. During vigorous exercise the LVSV is not reduced in healthy older individuals. Maximum CI is moderately decreased with age in healthy men, on the basis of a reduction in heart rate. In contrast, in older women, LVSV during exercise is not maintained as well as it is in older men, due to a relatively smaller LVEDV during exercise in older women than in men. The inability of healthy older individuals of both genders to reduce the LVESV during vigorous exercise accounts for a smaller increase in LVEF during exercise compared to younger individuals. This can result from an age-associated decrease in the myocardial contractile reserve or the failure of ventricular afterload to sufficiently decrease. In this regard, while the pulsatile determinants of ventricular afterload during exercise have not been characterized with respect to age, PVR is mildly increased in older vs. younger men during vigorous exercise. The slope of the LVESV/systolic blood pressure relationship, an index of myocardial contractility, is not age-associated at rest but decreases with age during vigorous exercise. In response to an increase in arterial pressure at rest elicited by infusions of a vasopressor, the older heart dilates and contracts from a greater preload than the younger heart. This also suggests an apparent age-associated decrease in the intrinsic myocardial contractile reserve.

It is quite clear that the aerobic capacity of both middle-aged and older individuals can increase following endurance exercise training and that this is mediated by adaptations in peripheral, and in some cases (depending on the intensity of exercise and the baseline $\dot{V}O_{2max}$) in cardiac, mechanisms. These adaptations also explain, in part at least, differences in $\dot{V}O_{2max}$ measured in cross-sectional comparisons in younger and older sedentary individuals and between older endurance-trained individuals and their sedentary counterparts.

An age-associated reduction in the postsynaptic response of the cardiovascular system to β-AR stimulation in human and in animal tissues and cells has been richly documented and appears to be due to multiple changes in molecular and biochemical receptor coupling and postreceptor mechanisms, rather than to a major modification of a single rate-limiting step, as might occur, for example, in a genetic defect. Cellular and molecular mechanisms that account for age-associated changes in myocardial performance can be studied in animal models. The most remarkable change within the β-AR system is the decrease in the receptor affinity for agonists, without substantial changes in β-AR density. Postreceptor changes with aging include decreases in the activities of G_s-protein, the adenylate cyclase catalytic unit, and PKA-induced protein phosphorylation and a diminution in the augmentation of the Ca^{2+} current, Ca_i transient, and contraction amplitudes. The striking similarities between the decreased effectiveness of β-adrenergic stimulation with age and the phenomenon of desensitization of β-AR by chronic β-AR agonist exposure at younger age suggest that the age-associated changes may occur in part via desensitization mechanisms.

In the normotensive rat, cardiac fibrosis increases, the number of myocytes decreases, and myocyte size increases with aging. Variable degrees of LV hypertrophy occur, depending upon strain, due to ventricular dilatation with apparent preservation of a normal ventricular wall thickness. Functional, biophysical/biochemical, pharmacological, and molecular changes have been noted in the rat heart with aging. There are coordinated changes in several key steps of excitation–contraction coupling which result in a prolonged Ca_i transient and a prolonged contraction. The transmembrane AP is prolonged by about twofold in cardiac muscle isolated from senescent (24-month-old compared to younger adult, (6–8-month-old) rats. The L-type sarcolemmal Ca^{2+} current is not substantially increased in magnitude but inactivates more slowly and could possibly account in part for the prolonged transmembrane AP. However, it is likely that changes in outward currents substantially contribute to the transmembrane AP prolongation. The cytosolic Ca^{2+} transient following excitation is prolonged in senescent rats. The rate of Ca^{2+} sequestration by the SR decreases in senescent rats and can explain in part the prolonged Ca_i transient. A reduction in the mRNA coding for the SR Ca^{2+} ATPase suggests that the diminished Ca^{2+} accumulation rate in senescent rats could in part be secondary to a decrease in the SR pump site density. The steady myofilament force response to Ca^{2+} is not altered by age. However, marked shifts occur in the MHC, that is, the β or V_3 isozyme becomes predominant in senescent rat (85% β vs. 15% α). Steady-state messenger RNA levels for α- and αMHC parallel the age-associated changes in the MHC proteins V_1 and V_3, and thus the isozyme shift appears to be transcriptionally regulated. The myosin Ca^{2+} ATPase activity declines with the decline in V_1 content. The altered cellular profile, which results in a contraction that exhibits a reduced velocity and a prolonged time course, can be considered adaptive rather than degenerative in nature because the reduced velocity is energy-efficient and prolonged contraction permits continued ejection for a prolonged period. A strikingly similar pattern of phenotypic and molecular changes that occur with advancing age in normotensive rats is induced in young animals within weeks following chronic pressure loading. The resultant altered Ca^{2+} homeostasis renders the older (and hypertensive younger) heart more prone to S-CaOs and Ca^{2+}-dependent arrhythmias. Chronic exercise in older animals reverses some of the alterations in cardiac function (prolonged contraction, reduced SR function) that occur with aging. Other aspects of cardiac function that change with aging (prolonged AP, altered myosin isoform expression) are not affected by chronic exercise.

REFERENCES

1. AASS, H., T. SKOMEDAL, and J.-B. OSNES. Increase of cyclic AMP in subcellular fractions of heart muscle after β-adrenergic stimulation: prenalterol and isoprenaline caused different distribution of bound cyclic AMP. *J. Mol. Cell. Cardiol.* 20: 847–860, 1988.
2. ABRASS, I. B., and P. J. SCARPACE. Human lymphocyte beta-adrenergic receptors are unaltered with age. *J. Gerontol.* 36: 298–301, 1981.
3. ABRASS, I. B., and P. J. SCARPACE. Catalytic unit of adenylate cyclase: reduced activity in aged-human lymphocytes. *J. Clin. Endocrinol. Metab.* 55: 1026–1028, 1982.
4. ABRASS, I. B., J. L. DAVIS, and P. J. SCARPACE. Isoproterenol responsiveness and myocardial β-adrenergic receptors in young and old rats. *J. Gerontol.* 37: 156–160, 1982.
5. ABU-ERREISH, G. M., J. R. NEELY, J. T. WHITMER, V. WHITMAN, and D. R. SANADI. Fatty acid oxidation by isolated perfused working hearts of aged rats. *Am. J. Physiol.* 232 (*Endocrinol. Metab. Gastrointest. Physiol.* 1): E258–E252, 1977.
6. ADELSTEIN, R. S., and E. EISENBERG. Regulation and kinetics of

the actin-myosin-ATP interaction. *Annu. Rev. Biochem.* 49: 921–956, 1980.
7. AFFLITTO, J. J., and M. A. INCHIOSA, JR. Decrease in rat cardiac myosin ATPase with aortic constriction: prevention by thyroxine treatment. *Life Sci.* 25: 353–364, 1979.
8. ALPERT, N. R., and L. A. MULIERI. Increased myothermal economy of isometric force generation in compensated cardiac hypertrophy induced by pulmonary artery constriction in the rabbit. A characterization of heat liberation in normal and hypertrophied right ventricular papillary muscles. *Circ. Res.* 50: 491–500, 1982.
9. ALPERT, N. R., E. M. BLANCHARD, and L. A. MULIERI. The quantity and rate of Ca^{2+} uptake in normal and hypertrophied hearts. In: *Pathophysiology of Heart Disease,* edited by N. Dhalla, P. Singel, and R. E. Beamish. New York: Raven, 1983.
10. ALPERT, N. R., H. H. GALE, and N. TAYLOR. The effect of age on contractile protein ATPase activity and the velocity of shortening. In: *Factors Influencing Myocardial Contractility,* edited by R. D. Tanz, F. Kavaler, and J. Roberts. New York: Academic, 1967, p. 127–133.
11. ALPERT, N. R., L. A. MULIERI, and R. Z. LITTEN. Functional significance of altered myosin adenosine triphosphatase activity in enlarged hearts. *Am. J. Cardiol.* 44: 946–953, 1979.
12. ALTURA, B. M., and B. T. ALTURA. Some physiological factors in vascular reactivity. I. Aging in vascular smooth muscle and its influence on reactivity. In: *Factors Influencing Vascular Reactivity,* edited by O. Carrier, Jr., and S. Shibata. Tokyo: Igaku-Shoin, 1977, p. 169–188.
13. AMERY, A., H. BOSSAERT, and M. VERSTRAETE. Muscle blood flow in normal and hypertensive subjects. Influence of age, exercise, and body position. *Am. Heart J.* 78: 211–216, 1969.
14. ANDERSEN, K. L., and L. HERMANSEN. Aerobic work capacity in middle-aged Norwegian men. *J. Appl. Physiol.* 20: 432–436, 1965.
15. ANVERSA, P., B. HILER, R. RICCI, G. GUIDERI, and G. OLIVETTI. Myocyte cell loss and myocyte hypertrophy in the aging rat heart. *J. Am. Coll. Cardiol.* 8: 1441–1448, 1986.
16. ANVERSA, P., T. PALACKAL, E. H. SONNENBLICK, G. OLIVETTI, L. G. MEGGS, and J. M. CAPASSO. Myocyte cell loss and myocyte cellular hyperplasia in the hypertrophied aging rat heart. *Circ. Res.* 67: 871–885, 1990.
17. ANVERSA, P., E. PUNTILLO, P. NIKITIN, G. OLIVETTI, J. M. CAPASSO, and E. H. SONNENBLICK. Effects of age on mechanical and structural properties of myocardium of Fischer 344 rats. *Am. J. Physiol.* 256 (*Heart Circ. Physiol.* 25): H1440–H1449, 1989.
18. ARMSTRONG, P. W., T. P. STOPPS, S. E. FORD, and A. J. DE BOLD. Rapid ventricular pacing in the dog: pathophysiologic studies of heart failure. *Circulation* 74: 1075–1084, 1986.
19. ARONSON, R. S. Afterpotentials and triggered activity in hypertrophied myocardium from rats with renal hypertension. *Circ. Res.* 48: 720–727, 1981.
20. ARORA, R. R., J. MACHAC, M. E. GOLDMAN, R. N. BUTLER, R. GORLIN, and S. F. HOROWITZ. Atrial kinetics and left ventricular diastolic filling in the healthy elderly. *J. Am. Coll. Cardiol.* 9: 1255–1260, 1987.
21. ASCHOFF, L. *Lectures in Pathology.* New York: Paul Hoeber, 1924, p. 131.
22. ASMUSSEN, E., K. FRUENSGAARD, and S. NORGAARD. A follow-up longitudinal study of selected physiologic functions in former physical education students after forty years. *J. Am. Geriatr. Soc.* 23: 442–450, 1975.
23. ASTRAND, I. Aerobic work capacity in men and women with special reference to age. *Acta Physiol. Scand. Suppl.* 169: 1–92, 1960.
24. ASTRAND, I., P. O. ASTRAND, I. HALLBACK, and A. KILBOM. Reduction in maximal oxygen uptake with age. *J. Appl. Physiol.* 35: 649–654, 1973.
25. AVOLIO, A. P., S. G. CHEN, R. P. WANG, C. L. ZHANG, M. F. LI, and M. F. O'ROURKE. Effects of aging on changing arterial compliance and left ventricular load in a northern Chinese urban community. *Circulation* 68: 50–58, 1983.
26. AVOLIO, A. P., K. M. CLYDE, T. C. BEARD, H. M. COOKE, K. K. HO, and M. F. O'ROURKE. Improved arterial distensibility in normotensive subjects on a low salt diet. *Arteriosclerosis* 6: 166–169, 1986.
27. AVOLIO, A. P., F. Q. DENG, W. Q. LI, Y. F. LUO, Z. D. HUANG, L. F. XING, and M. F. O'ROURKE. Effects of aging on arterial distensibility in populations with high and low prevalence of hypertension: comparison between urban and rural communities in China. *Circulation* 71: 202–210, 1985.
28. AYOBE, H. M., and R. C. TARAZI. Reversal of changes in myocardial β-receptors and inotropic responsiveness with regression of cardiac hypertrophy in renal hypertensive rats (RHR). *Circ. Res.* 54: 125–134, 1984.
29. BADER, H. Dependence of wall stress in the human thoracic aorta on age and pressure. *Circ. Res.* 20: 354–361, 1967.
30. BAUTERS, C., J. M. MOALIC, J. BERCOVICI, C. MOUAS, R. EMANOIL-RAVIER, S. SCHIAFFINO, and B. SWYNGHEDAUW. Coronary flow as a determinant of c-myc and c-fos proto-oncogene expression in an isolated adult rat heart. *J. Mol. Cell. Cardiol.* 20: 97–101, 1988.
31. BECKLAKE, M. R., H. FRANK, G. R. DAGENAIS, G. L. OSTIGUY, and C. A. GUZMAN. Influence of age and sex on exercise cardiac output. *J. Appl. Physiol.* 20: 938–947, 1965.
32. BEER, M., S. HACKER, J. POAT, and S. M. STAHL. Independent regulation of $β_1$ and $β_2$-adrenoceptors. *Br. J. Pharmacol.* 92: 827–834, 1987.
33. BENESTAD, A. M. Trainability of old men. *Acta Med. Scand.* 178: 321–327, 1965.
34. BENOVIC, J. L., M. BOUVIER, M. G. CARON, and R. J. LEFKOWITZ. Regulation of adenylyl cyclase-coupled β-adrenergic receptors. *Annu. Rev. Cell Biol.* 4: 405–428, 1988.
35. BHAN, A. K., and J. SCHEUER. Effects of physical training on cardiac myosin ATPase activity. *Am. J. Physiol.* 228: 1178–1182, 1975.
36. BHATNAGAR, G. M., M. B. EFFRON, G. RUANO-ARROYO, H. A. SPURGEON, and E. G. LAKATTA. Dissociation of myosin Ca^{2+}-ATPase activity from myosin isoenzymes and contractile function in rat myocardium [Abstract]. *Fed. Proc.* 44: 826, 1985.
37. BHATNAGAR, G. M., G. D. WALFORD, E. S. BEARD, S. HUMPHREYS, and E. G. LAKATTA. ATPase activity and force production in myofibrils and twitch characteristics in intact muscle from neonatal, adult, and senescent rat myocardium. *J. Mol. Coll. Cardiol.* 16: 203–218, 1984.
38. BING, O. H. L., W. W. BROOKS, C. H. CONRAD, S. SEN, C. L. PERREAULT, and J. P. MORGAN. Intracellular calcium transient in myocardium from spontaneously hypertensive rats during the transition to heart failure. *Circ. Res.* 68: 1390–1400, 1991.
39. BINKHORST, R. A., J. POOL, P. VAN LEEUWEN, and A. BOUHUYS. Maximum O_2 uptake in healthy nonathletic males. *Int. Z. Angew. Physiol. Einschl. Arbeitsphysiol.* 22: 10–18, 1966.
40. BOLUYT, M. O., L. O'NEILL, E. G. LAKATTA, and M. T. CROW. Progressive elevation of atrial natriuretic factor mRNAs in rat heart with advancing age [Abstract]. *J. Mol. Cell. Cardiol.* 24(Suppl. III): S.35, 1992.
41. BOLUYT, M. O., A. YOUNES, J. L. CAFFREY, L. O'NEILL, B. A. BARRON, M. T. CROW, and E. G. LAKATTA. Age-associated increase in rat cardiac opioid production. *Am. J. Physiol.* 265: H212–H218, 1993.
42. BOLUYT, M. O., J. A. OPITECK, K. A. ESSER, and T. P. WHITE. Cardiac adaptations to aortic-constriction in adult and aged

rats. *Am. J. Physiol.* 257 (*Heart Circ. Physiol.* 26): H643–H648, 1989.
43. BONOW, R. O., D. F. VITALE, S. L. BACHARACH, B. J. MARON, and M. V. GREEN. Effects of aging on asynchronous left ventricular regional function and global ventricular filling in normal human subjects. *J. Am. Coll. Cardiol.* 11: 50–58, 1988.
44. BORKAN, G. A., D. E. HULTS, S. G. GERZOF, A. H. ROBBINS, and C. K. SILBERT. Age changes in body composition revealed by computed tomography. *J. Gerontol.* 38: 673–677, 1983.
45. BOUTHIER, J. D., N. DE LUCA, M. E. SAFAR, and A. C. SIMON. Cardiac hypertrophy and arterial distensibility in essential hypertension. *Am. Heart J.* 109: 1345–1352, 1985.
46. BRAMWELL, J. C., and A. V. HILL. The velocity of the pulse wave in man. *Proc. R. Soc. Lond. B Biol. Sci.* 93: 298–306, 1922.
47. BRANDFONBRENER, M., M. LANDOWNE, and N. W. SHOCK. Changes in cardiac output with age. *Circulation* 12: 557–566, 1955.
48. BRISTOW, M. R., R. E. HERSHBERGER, J. D. PORT, W. MINOBE, and R. RASMUSSEN. Beta 1- and beta 2-adrenergic receptor-mediated adenylate cyclase stimulation in nonfailing and failing human ventricular myocardium. *Mol. Pharmacol.* 35: 295–303, 1989.
49. BRODDE, O.-E., A. DAUL, A. WELLSTEIN, D. PALM, M. C. MICHEL, and J. J. BECKERINGH. Differentiation in β_1- and β_2-adrenoceptor-mediated effects in humans. *Am. J. Physiol.* 254 (*Heart Circ. Physiol.* 23): H199–H206, 1988.
50. BRODDE, O.-E., H-R. ZERKOWSKI, N. DOETSCH, S. MOTOMURA, M. KHAMSSI, and M. C. MICHEL. Myocardial beta-adrenoceptor changes in heart failure: concomitant reduction in beta 1- and 2-adrenoceptor function related to the degree of heart failure in patients with mitral valve disease. *J. Am. Coll. Cardiol.* 14: 323–331, 1989.
51. BROWN, A. M. Regulation of heartbeat by G protein-coupled ion channels. *Am. J. Physiol.* 259 (*Heart Circ. Physiol.* 28): H1621–H1628, 1990.
52. BRUCE, R. A., and T. R. HORNSTEN. Exercise stress testing in evaluation of patients with ischemic heart disease. *Prog. Cardiovasc. Dis.* 11: 371–390, 1969.
53. BUSBY, D. E., and A. C. BURTON. The effect of age on the elasticity of the major brain arteries. *Can. J. Physiol. Pharmacol.* 43: 185–202, 1965.
54. BUSBY, M., E. A. SHEFRIN, and J. L. FLEG. Prevalence and long-term significance of exercise-induced frequent or repetitive ventricular ectopic beats in apparently healthy volunteers. *J. Am. Coll. Cardiol.* 14: 1659–1665, 1989.
55. BUTTRICK, P., A. MALHOTRA, S. FACTOR, D. GREENEN, L. LEINWAND, and J. SCHEUER. Effect of aging and hypertension on myosin biochemistry and gene expression in the rat heart. *Circ. Res.* 68: 645–652, 1991.
56. BUXTON, I. L. O., and L. L. BRUNTON. Action of the cardiac α_1-adrenergic receptor. Activation of cyclic AMP degradation. *J. Biol. Chem.* 260: 6733–6737, 1985.
57. BUXTON, I. L. O., and L. L. BRUNTON. Compartments of cyclic AMP and protein kinase in mammalian cardiomyoctes. *J. Biol. Chem.* 258: 10233–10239, 1983.
58. CALDERONE, A., M. BOUVIER, K. LI, C. JUNEAU, J. DE CHAMPLAIN, and J. L. ROULEAU. Dysfunction of the beta- and alpha-adrenergic systems in a model of congestive heart failure. The pacing-overdrive dog. *Circ. Res.* 69: 332–343, 1991.
59. CAMPBELL, M. J., A. J. MCCOMAS, and F. PETITO. Physiological changes in ageing muscles. *J. Neurol. Neurosurg. Psychiatry* 36: 174–182, 1973.
60. CAPASSO, J. M., A. MALHOTRA, R. M. REMILY, J. SCHEUER, and E. H. SONNENBLICK. Effects of age on mechanical and electrical performance of rat myocardium. *Am. J. Physiol.* 245 (*Heart Circ. Physiol.* 14): H72–H81, 1983.
61. CAPASSO, J. M., A. MALHOTRA, J. SCHEUER, and E. H. SONNENBLICK. Myocardial biochemical, contractile and electrical performance after imposition of hypertension in young and old rats. *Circ. Res.* 58: 445–460, 1986.
62. CAPASSO, J. M., E. PUNTILLO, G. OLIVETTI, and P. ANVERSA. Differences in load dependence of relaxation between the left and right ventricular myocardium as a function of age in rats. *Circ. Res.* 65: 1499–1507, 1989.
63. CARRIER, L., K. R. BOHELER, C. CHASSAGNE, D. DE LA BASTIE, C. WISNEWSKY, E. G. LAKATTA, and K. SCHWARTZ. Expression of the sarcomeric actin isogenes in the rat heart with development and senescence. *Circ. Res.* 70: 999–1005, 1992.
64. CARROLL, J. D., S. SHROFF, P. WIRTH, M. HALSTED, and S. I. RAJFER. Arterial mechanical properties in dilated cardiomyopathy. Aging and the response to nitroprusside. *J. Clin. Invest.* 87: 1002–1009, 1991.
65. CARTER, S. A. In vivo estimation of elastic characteristics of the arteries in the lower extremities of man. *Can. J. Physiol. Pharmacol.* 42: 309–413, 1964.
66. CARTER, W. J., W. F. KELLY, F. H. FAAS, M. E. LYNCH, and C. A. PERRY. Effect of graded doses of tri-iodothyronine on ventricular myosin ATPase activity and isomyosin profile in young and old rats. *Biochem. J.* 247: 329–334, 1987.
67. CHARLEMAGNE, D., J.-M. MAIXENT, M. PRETESEILLE, and L. G. LELIEVRE. Ouabain binding sites and (Na^+,K^+)-ATPase activity in rat cardiac hypertrophy. Expression of the neonatal forms. *J. Biol. Chem.* 261: 185–189, 1986.
68. CHEN, J. C., J. B. WWARSHAW, and D. R. SANADI. Regulation of mitochondrial respiration in senescence. *J. Cell. Physiol.* 80: 141–148, 1972.
69. CHESKY, J. A., and M. ROCKSTEIN. Reduced myocardial actomyosin adenosine triphosphatase activity in the ageing male Fischer rat. *Cardiovasc. Res.* 11: 242–246, 1977.
70. CHESKY, J. A., S. LaFOLLETTE, M. TRAVIS, and C. FORTADO. Effects of physical training on myocardial enzyme activities in aging rats. *J. Appl. Physiol.* 55: 1349–1353, 1983.
71. CHEVALIER, B., P. MANSIER, F. CALLENS-EL AMRANI, and B. SWYNGHEDAUW. β-Adrenergic system is modified in compensatory pressure cardiac overload in rats: physiological and biochemical evidence. *J. Cardiol. Pharmacol.* 13: 412–420, 1989.
72. CHEVALIER, B., P. MANSIER, E. TEIGER, F. CALLENS-EL AMRANI, and B. SWYNGHEDAUW. Alterations in β adrenergic and muscarinic receptors in aged rat heart. Effects of chronic administration of propranolol and atropine. *Mech. Ageing Dev.* 60: 215–224, 1991.
73. CHIEN, K. R., K. U. KNOWLTON, H. ZHU, and S. CHIEN. Regulation of cardiac gene expression during myocardial growth and hypertrophy: molecular studies of an adaptive physiologic response. *FASEB J.* 5: 3037–3046, 1991.
74. CHIN, J. H., and B. B. HOFFMAN. Age-related deficit in beta receptor stimulation of cAMP binding in blood vessels. *Mech. Ageing Dev.* 53: 111–125, 1990.
75. CHOU, H.-T., Y. YOKOTA, and H. FUKUZAKI. Left ventricular reserve of the hypertrophied heart in patients with systemic hypertension and hypertrophic cardiomyopathy—relation to age and left ventricular relative wall thickness. *Jap. Circ. J.* 54: 373–382, 1990.
76. CLAUSEN, J. P. Effects of physical conditioning. A hypothesis concerning circulatory adjustment to exercise. *Scand. J. Clin. Lab. Invest.* 24: 305–313, 1969.
77. CLÉROUX, J., C. GIANNATTASIO, G. BOLLA, C. CUSPIDI, G. GRASSI, C. MAZZOLA, L. SAMPIERI, G. SERAVALLE, M. VALSECCHI, and G. MANCIA. Decreased cardiopulmonary reflexes with aging in normotensive humans. *Am. J. Physiol.* 257 (*Heart Circ. Physiol.* 26): H961–H968, 1989.

78. CLIFF, W. J. The aortic tunica media in aging rats. *Exp. Mol. Pathol.* 13: 172–189, 1970.
79. COGGAN, A., R. J. SPINA, D. S. KING, M. A. ROGERS, M. BROWN, and P. M. NEMETH. Skeletal muscle adaptations to endurance training in 60 to 70-yr old men and women. *J. Appl. Physiol.* 72: 1780–1786, 1992.
80. COGGAN, A. R., R. J. SPINA, M. A. ROGERS, D. S. KING, M. BROWN, P. M. NEMETH, and J. O. HOLLOSZY. Histochemical and enzymatic characteristics of skeletal muscle in master athletes. *J. Appl. Physiol.* 68: 1896–1901, 1990.
81. CONWAY, J., R. WHEELER, and R. SANNERSTEDT. Sympathetic nervous activity during exercise in relation to age. *Cardiovasc. Res.* 5: 577–581, 1971.
82. COOPER, G., IV, W. E. MERCER, J. K. HOOBER, P. R. GORDON, R. L. KENT, I. K. LAUVA, and T. A. MARINO. Load regulation of the properties of adult feline cardiocytes. Role of substrate adhesion. *Circ. Res.* 58: 692–705, 1986.
83. COOPER, T. G. Surgical sympathectomy and adrenergic function. *Pharmacol. Rev.* 18: 611–618, 1966.
84. CORBIN, J. D., P. H. SUGDEN, T. M. LINCOLN, and S. L. KEELY. Compartmentalization of adenosine 3′:5′-monophosphate and adenosine 3′:5′-monophosphate-dependent protein kinase in heart tissues. *J. Biol. Chem.* 253: 3854–3861, 1977.
85. COURNAND, A., R. L. RILEY, E. S. BREED, and E. BALDWIN. Measurement of cardiac output in man using the technique of catheterization of the right auricle or ventricle. *J. Clin. Invest.* 24: 106–116, 1945.
86. CRAELIUS, W., V. CHEN, and N. EL-SHERIF. Stretch activated ion channels in ventricular myocytes. *Biosci. Rep.* 8: 407–414, 1988.
87. CRAWFORD, M. H., M. A. PETRU, and C. RABINOWITZ. Effect of isotonic exercise training on left ventricular volume during upright exercise. *Circulation* 72: 1237–1243, 1985.
88. CURTIS, B. M., and W. A. CATTERALL. Phosphorylation of the calcium antagonist receptor of the voltage-sensitive calcium channel by cAMP-dependent protein kinase. *Proc. Natl. Acad. Sci. U.S.A.* 82: 2528–2532, 1985.
89. DANNENBERG, A. L., D. LEVY, and R. J. GARRISON. Impact of age on echocardiographic left ventricular mass in a healthy population (the Framingham Study). *Am. J. Cardiol.* 64: 1066–1068, 1989.
90. DANZIGER, R. S., M. SAKAI, E. G. LAKATTA, and R. G. HANSFORD. Interactive α- and β-adrenergic actions of norepinephrine in rat cardiac myocytes. *J. Mol. Cell. Cardiol.* 22: 111–123, 1990.
91. DANZIGER, R. S., J. D. TOBIN, L. C. BECKER, E. G. LAKATTA, and J. L. FLEG. The age-associated decline in glomerular filtration in healthy normotensive volunteers: lack of relationship to cardiovascular performance. *J. Am. Geriatr. Soc.* 38: 1127–1132, 1990.
92. DAVIES, C. T. M. Limitations to the prediction of maximum O_2 intake from cardiac frequency measurements. *J. Appl. Physiol.* 24: 700–706, 1968.
93. DAVIES, H. E. F. Respiratory change in heart rate, sinus arrhythmia in the elderly. *Gerontol. Clin.* 17: 96–100, 1975.
94. DAY, M. L., D. SCHWARTZ, R. C. WIEGAND, P. T. STOCKMAN, S. R. BRUNNERT, H. E. TOLUNAY, M. G. CURRIE, D. G. STANDAERT, and P. NEEDLEMAN. Ventricular atriopeptin. Unmasking of messenger RNA and peptide synthesis by hypertrophy or dexamethasone. *Hypertension* 9: 485–491, 1987.
95. DE GARAVILLA, L., H. L. VALENTINE, J. S. SCHENDEN, W. J. KINNIER, and R. C. HANSON. Age-related cardiovascular effects of adenosine in guinea pigs. *Drug Dev. Res.* 28: 496–502, 1993.
96. DEHN, M. M., and R. A. BRUCE. Longitudinal variations in maximal oxygen intake with age and activity. *J. Appl. Physiol.* 33: 805–807, 1972.
97. DEISHER, T. A., S. MANKANI, and B. B. HOFFMAN. Role of cyclic AMP-dependent protein kinase in the diminished beta adrenergic responsiveness of vascular smooth muscle with increasing age. *J. Pharmacol. Exp. Ther.* 249: 812–819, 1989.
98. DE LA BASTIE, D., D. LEVITSKY, L. RAPPAPORT, J. J. MERCADIER, F. MAROTTE, C. WISNEWSKY, V. BROVKOVICH, K. SCHWARTZ, and A. M. LOMPRE. Function of the sarcoplasmic reticulum and expression of its Ca^{2+} ATPase gene in pressure overload-induced cardiac hypertrophy in the rat. *Circ. Res.* 66: 554–564, 1990.
99. DELCAYRE, C., J. L. SAMUEL, F. MAROTTE, M. BEST-BELPOMME, J. J. MERCADIER, and L. RAPPAPORT. Synthesis of stress proteins in rat cardiac myocytes 2–4 days after imposition of hemodynamic overload. *J. Clin. Invest.* 82: 460–468, 1988.
100. DEVEREUX, R. B., T. G. PICKERING, M. H. ALDERMAN, S. CHIEN, J. S. BORER, and J. H. LARAGH. Left ventricular hypertrophy in hypertension. Prevalence and relationship to pathophysiologic variables. *Hypertension* 9: II-53–II-60, 1987.
101. DEVRIES, H. A. Physiological effects of an exercise training regimen upon men aged 52 to 88. *J. Gerontol.* 25: 325–336, 1970.
102. DILL, D. B., S. ROBINSON, and J. C. ROSS. A longitudinal study of 16 champion runners. *J. Sports Med. Phys. Fitness* 7: 4–27, 1967.
103. DILLMANN, W. Influence of thyroid hormone administration on myosin ATPase activity and myosin isoenzyme distribution in the heart of diabetic rats. *Metabolism* 31: 199–204, 1981.
104. DILLON, N., S. CHUNG, J. KELLY, and K. O'MALLEY. Age and beta adrenoceptor-mediated function. *Clin. Pharmacol. Ther.* 27: 769–772, 1980.
105. DOBSON, J. G., JR. Mechanism of adenosine inhibition of catecholamine-induced responses in heart. *Circ. Res.* 52: 151–160, 1983.
106. DOBSON, J. G., JR., R. A. FENTON, and F. D. ROMANO. Increased myocardial adenosine production and reduction of β-adrenergic contractile response in aged hearts. *Circ. Res.* 66: 1381–1390, 1990.
107. DOCHERTY, J. R., and L. HYLAND. Aging and α-adrenoceptor function. *Trends Pharmacol. Sci.* 7: 131–132, 1986.
108. DOCHERTY, J. R., and L. HYLAND. Evidence for neuro-effector transmission through postjunctional α_2-adrenoceptors in human saphenous vein. *Br. J. Pharmacol.* 84: 573–576, 1985.
109. DOCHERTY, J. R., A. MACDONALD, and J. C. MCGRATH. Further subclassification of α-adrenoceptors in the cardiovascular system, vas deferens and anococcygeus of the rat. *Br. J. Pharmacol.* 67: 421–422, 1979.
110. DONTAS, A. S., H. C. TAYLOR, and A. KEYS. Carotid pressure plethysmograms: effects of age, diastolic pressure, relative body weight, and physical activity. *Archiv. Kreislaufforsch.* 36: 49–58, 1961.
111. DOYLE, V., K. O'MALLEY, and J. G. KELLY. Human lymphocyte beta-adrenoceptor density in relation to age and hypertension. *J. Cardiovasc. Pharmacol.* 4: 738–740, 1982.
112. DUBELL, W. H., M. R. BOYETT, H. A. SPURGEON, A. TALO, M. D. STERN, and E. G. LAKATTA. The cytosolic calcium transient modulates the action potential of rat ventricular myocytes. *J. Physiol.* 436: 347–369, 1991.
113. DUCKLES, S. P. Age-related changes in adrenergic neuronal function of rabbit vascular smooth muscle. *Neurobiol. Aging* 4: 151–156, 1983.
114. DUCKLES, S. P., B. J. CARTER, and C. L. WILLIAMS. Vascular adrenergic neuroeffector function does not decline in aged rats. *Circ. Res.* 56: 109–116, 1985.
115. EBERT, T. J., C. V. HUGHES, F. E. TRISTANI, J. A. BARNEY, and J. J. SMITH. Effect of age and coronary heart disease on the circulatory responses to graded lower body negative pressure. *Cardiovasc. Res.* 16: 663–669, 1982.
116. EBERT, T. J., B. J. MORGAN, J. A. BARNEY, T. DENAHAN, and

J. J. SMITH. Effects of aging on baroreflex regulation of sympathetic activity in humans. *Am. J. Physiol.* 263 (*Heart Circ. Physiol.* 32): H798–H803, 1992.
117. EBRECHT, G., H. RUPP, and R. JACOB. Alterations of mechanical parameters in chemically skinned preparations of rat myocardium as a function of isoenzyme pattern of myosin. *Basic Res. Cardiol.* 77: 220–234, 1982.
118. EFFRON, M. B., G. M. BHATNAGAR, H. A. SPURGEON, G. RUANO-ARROYO, and E. G. LAKATTA. Changes in myosin isoenzymes, ATPase activity, and contraction duration in rat cardiac muscle with aging can be modulated by thyroxine. *Circ. Res.* 60: 238–245, 1987.
119. EGHBALI, M., M. EGHBALI, T. F. ROBINSON, S. SEIFTER, and O. O. BLUMENFELD. Collagen accumulation in heart ventricles as a function of growth and aging. *Cardiovasc. Res.* 23: 723–729, 1989.
120. EHSANI, A. A. Cardiovascular adaptations to exercise training in the elderly. *Fed. Proc.* 46: 1840–1843, 1987.
121. EHSANI, A. A., T. OGAWA, T. R. MILLER, R. J. SPINA, and S. M. JILKA. Exercise training improves left ventricular systolic function in older men. *Circulation* 83: 96–103, 1991.
122. EICHLER, H. G., A. HIREMATH, T. F. BLASCHKE, and B. B. HOFFMAN. Absence of age-related changes in venous responsiveness to nitroglycerin in vivo in humans. *Clin. Pharmacol. Ther.* 42: 521–524, 1987.
123. ELZINGA, G., and N. WESTERHOF. Pressure and flow generated by the left ventricle against different impedances. *Circ. Res.* 32: 178–186, 1973.
124. ENGELMANN, G. L., J. C. VITULLO, and R. G. GERRITY. Morphometric analysis of cardiac hypertrophy during development, maturation, and senescence in spontaneously hypertensive rats. *Circ. Res.* 60: 487–494, 1987.
125. ENSOR, R. E., J. L. FLEG, Y. C. KIM, E. F. DE LEON, and S. M. GOLDMAN. Longitudinal chest x-ray changes in normal men. *J. Gerontol.* 38: 307–314, 1983.
126. ERICSSON, E., and L. LUNDHOLM. Adrenergic β-receptor activity and cyclic AMP metabolism in vascular smooth muscle; variations with age. *Mech. Ageing Dev.* 4: 1–6, 1975.
127. ESCANDE, D., D. LOISANCE, C. PLANCHE, and E. CORABOEUF. Age-related changes of action potential plateau shape in isolated human atrial fibers. *Am. J. Physiol.* 249 (*Heart Circ. Physiol.* 18): H843–H850, 1985.
128. ESLER, M., H. SKEWS, P. LEONARD, G. JACKMAN, A. BOBOK, and P. KORNER. Age-dependence of noradrenaline kinetics in normal subjects. *Clin. Sci.* 60: 217–219, 1981.
129. FABER, M., and G. MOLLER-HOU. The human aorta. V. Collagen and elastin in the normal and hypertensive aorta. *Acta Pathol. Microbiol. Scand.* 31: 377–382, 1952.
130. FAGARD, R., and J. STAESSEN. Relation of cardiac output at rest and during exercise to age in essential hypertension. *Am. J. Cardiol.* 67: 585–589, 1991.
131. FAN, T. H., C. S. LIANG, S. KAWASHIMA, and S. P. BANERJEE. Alterations in cardiac beta-adrenoceptor responsiveness and adenylate cyclase system by congestive heart failure in dogs. *Eur. J. Pharmacol.* 140: 123–132, 1987.
132. FARRAR, R. P., J. W. STARNES, G. D. CARTEE, P. Y. OH, and H. L. SWEENEY. Effects of exercise on cardiac myosin isozyme composition during the aging process. *J. Appl. Physiol.* 64: 880–883, 1988.
133. FEATHERSTONE, J. A., R. C. VEITH, D. FLATNESS, M. M. MURBURG, E. C. VILLACRES, and J. B. HALTER. Age and alpha-2 adrenergic regulation of plasma norepinephrine kinetics in humans. *J. Gerontol.* 42: 271–276, 1987.
134. FEATHERSTONE, J. A., R. C. VEITH, and J. B. HALTER. Effect of age and alpha-2 adrenergic stimulation on plasma norepinephrine kinetics in man [Abstract]. *Clin. Res.* 32: 69A, 1984.
135. FEIN, F. S., L. B. KORNSTEIN, J. E. STROBECK, J. M. CAPASSO, and E. H. SONNENBLICK. Altered myocardial mechanics in diabetic rats. *Circ. Res.* 47: 922–933, 1980.
136. FELDMAN, R. D., L. E. LIMBIRD, J. NADEAU, D. ROBERTSON, and A. J. WOOD. Alterations in leukocyte beta-receptor affinity with aging. A potential explanation for altered beta-adrenergic sensitivity in the elderly. *N. Engl. J. Med.* 310: 815–819, 1984.
137. FENTON, R. A., and J. G. DOBSON, JR. Adenosine and calcium alter adrenergic-induced intact heart protein phosphorylation. *Am. J. Physiol.* 246 (*Heart Circ. Physiol.* 15): H559–H565, 1984.
138. FILBURN, C. R., and E. G. LAKATTA. Aging alterations in beta-adrenergic modulation of cardiac cell function. In: *Aging and Cell Function,* edited by J. E. Johnson, Jr. New York: Plenum, 1984, p. 211–246.
139. FISCHER, A., J. PARIZKOVA, and Z. ROTH. The effect of systematic physical activity on maximal performance and functional capacity in senescent men. *Int. Z. Angew. Physiol. Einschl. Arbeitsphysiol.* 21: 269–304, 1965.
140. FITCHETT, D. H., G. J. SIMKUS, J. P. BEAUDRY, and D. G. F. MARPOLE. Reflected pressure waves in the ascending aorta: effect of glyceryl trinitrate. *Cardiovasc. Res.* 22: 494–500, 1988.
141. FLEG, J. L. Arrhythmias and conduction disorders. In: *The Merck Manual of Geriatrics,* edited by W. B. Abrams and R. Berkow. Rahway, NJ: Merck Sharp & Dohme, 1990, p. 370–380.
142. FLEG, J. L., and H. L. KENNEDY. Cardiac arrhythmias in healthy elderly population: detection by 24-hour ambulatory electrocardiography. *Chest* 81: 302–307, 1982.
143. FLEG, J. L., and E. G. LAKATTA. Role of muscle loss in the age-associated reduction in VO_{2max}. *J. Appl. Physiol.* 65: 1147–1151, 1988.
144. FLEG, J. L., D. N. DAS, J. WRIGHT, and E. G. LAKATTA. Age-associated changes in the components of atrioventricular conduction in apparently healthy volunteers. *J. Gerontol. Med. Sci.* 45: M95–M100, 1990.
145. FLEG, J. L., G. GERSTENBLITH, and E. G. LAKATTA. Pathophysiology of the aging heart and circulation. In: *Cardiovascular Disease in the Elderly* (2nd ed.), edited by F. H. Messerli. Boston: Martinus Nijhoff, 1988, p. 9–35.
146. FLEG, J., S. P. SCHULMAN, G. GERSTENBLITH, L. C. BECKER, F. C. O'CONNOR, and E. G. LAKATTA. Additive effects of age and silent myocardial ischemia on the left ventricular response to upright cycle exercise. *J. Appl. Physiol.* 75: 499–504, 1993.
147. FLEG, J. L., G. GERSTENBLITH, S. P. SCHULMAN, L. C. BECKER, F. C. O'CONNOR, and E. G. LAKATTA. Gender differences in exercise hemodynamics of older subjects: effects of conditioning status [Abstract]. *Circulation* 82: III-239, 1990b.
148. FLEG, J. L., G. GERSTENBLITH, A. B. ZONDERMAN, L. C. BECKER, M. L. WEISFELDT, P. T. COSTA, JR., and E. G. LAKATTA. Prevalence and prognostic significance of exercise-induced silent myocardial ischemia detected by thallium scintigraphy and electrocardiography in asymptomatic volunteers. *Circulation* 81: 423–436, 1990c.
149. FLEG, J. L., S. P. SCHULMAN, F. C. O'CONNOR, G. GERSTENBLITH, L. C. BECKER, S. FORTNEY, A. P. GOLDBERG, and E. G. LAKATTA. Cardiovascular response to exhaustive upright cycle exercise in highly trained older men. *J. Appl. Physiol.* 77: 1500–1506, 1994.
150. FLEG, J. L., S. SCHULMAN, F. O'CONNOR, G. GERSTENBLITH, J. F. CLULOW, D. G. RENLUND, and E. G. LAKATTA. Effect of propranolol on age-associated changes in left ventricular performance during exercise [Abstract]. *Circulation* 84: II-187, 1991.
151. FLEG, J. L., E. SHAPIRO, F. O'CONNOR', L. LAKATTA, and E. L. LAKATTA. Failure of intensive aerobic conditioning to alter the age-associated decline in diastolic left ventricular performance [Abstract]. *Circulation* 8 (suppl. I): I-377, 1992.
152. FLEG, J. L., S. P. TZANKOFF, and E. G. LAKATTA. Age-related

augmentation of plasma catecholamines during dynamic exercise in healthy males. *J. Appl. Physiol.* 59: 1033–1039, 1985.
153. FLEISCH, J. H. Age-related decrease in beta adrenoreceptor activity of the cardiovascular system. *Trends Pharmacol. Sci.* 2: 337–339, 1981.
154. FLEISCH, J. H., and C. S. HOOKER. The relationship between age and relaxation of vascular smooth muscle in the rabbit and rat. *Circ. Res.* 38: 243–249, 1976.
155. FLEISCH, J. H., H. M. MALING, and B. B. BRODIE. Beta-receptor activity in aorta; variations with age and species. *Circ. Res.* 26: 151–162, 1970.
156. FORD, G. A., B. B. HOFFMAN, and T. F. BLASCHKE. Cardiac chronotropic and vascular smooth muscle beta adrenergic responses during propranolol therapy and withdrawal in young and elderly persons. *J. Gerontol.: Med. Sci.* 47: M22–M26, 1992.
157. FORMAN, D. E., W. J. MANNING, R. HAUSER, E. V. GERVINO, W. J. EVANS, and J. Y. WEI. Enhanced left ventricular diastolic filling associated with long-term endurance training. *J. Gerontol.: Med. Sci.* 47: M56–M58, 1992.
158. FORTNEY, S., C. TANKERSLEY, J. T. LIGHTFOOT, D. DRINKWATER, J. CLULOW, F. O'CONNOR, L. BECKER, E. LAKATTA, and J. FLEG. Cardiovascular responses to lower body negative pressure in trained and untrained older men. *J. Appl. Physiol.* 73: 2693–2700, 1992.
159. FRATICELLI, A., R. JOSEPHSON, R. DANZIGER, E. LAKATTA, and H. SPURGEON. Morphological and contractile characteristics of rat cardiac myocytes from maturation to senescence. *Am. J. Physiol.* 257 (*Heart Circ. Physiol.* 26): H259–H265, 1989.
160. FREIS, E. D., W. C. HEATH, P. C. LUCHSINGER, and R. E. SNELL. Changes in the carotid pulse which occur with age and hypertension. *Am. Heart J.* 71: 757–765, 1966.
161. FREY, M. A. B., and G. W. HOFFLER. Association of sex and age with responses to lower-body negative pressure. *J. Appl. Physiol.* 65: 1752–1756, 1988.
162. FRIBERG, P., M. NORDLANDER, S. LUNDIN, and B. FOLKOW. Effects of ageing on cardiac performance and coronary flow in spontaneously hypertensive and normotensive rats. *Acta Physiol. Scand.* 125: 1–11, 1985.
163. FROEHLICH, J. P., E. G. LAKATTA, E. BEARD, H. A. SPURGEON, M. L. WEISFELDT, and G. GERSTENBLITH. Studies of sarcoplasmic reticulum function and contraction duration in young adult and aged rat myocardium. *J. Mol. Cell Cardiol.* 10: 427–438, 1978.
164. FROLKIS, V. V., V. V. BEZRUKOV, L. N. BOGATSKAYA, N. S. VERKHRATSKY, V. P. ZAMOSTIAN, V. G. SHEVTCHUK, and I. V. SHTCHEGOLVA. Catecholamines in the metabolism and function regulation in aging. *Gerontologia* 16: 129–140, 1979.
165. FROLKIS, V. V., V. V. BEZRUKOV, and V. G. SCHEVTCHUK. Hemodynamics and its regulation in old age. *Exp. Gerontol.* 10: 251–271, 1975.
166. FROLKIS, V. V., R. A. FROLKIS, L. S. MKHITARIAN, V. G. SCHEVCHUK, V. E. FRAIFELD, L. G. VAKULENKO, and I. SYROVY. Contractile function and Ca^{2+} transport system of myocardium in ageing. *Gerontology* 34: 64–74, 1988.
167. FRONTERA, W. R., C. N. MEREDITH, K. P. O'REILLY, and W. J. EVANS. Strength training and determinants of VO_2max in older men. *J. Appl. Physiol.* 68: 329–333, 1990.
168. FRONTERA, W. R., C. N. MEREDITH, K. P. O'REILLY, H. G. KNUTTGEN, and W. J. EVANS. Strength conditioning in older men: skeletal muscle hypertrophy and improved function. *J. Appl. Physiol.* 64: 1038–1044, 1988.
169. GANGULY, P. K., G. N. PIERCE, K. S. DHALLA, and N. S. DHALLA. Defective sarcoplasmic reticulum calcium transport in diabetic cardiomyopathy. *Am. J. Physiol.* 244 (*Endocrinol. Metab.* 7): E528–E535, 1983.
170. GARDIN, J. M., W. L. HENRY, D. D. SAVAGE, J. H. WARE, C. BURN, and J. S. BORER. Echocardiographic measurements in normal subjects: evaluation of an adult population without clinically apparent heart disease. *J. Clin. Ultrasound* 7: 439–447, 1979.
171. GENDE, O. A., A. MATTIAZZI, M. C. CAMILLION, P. PEDRONI, C. TAQUINI, H. GOMEZ-LLAMI, and H. E. CINGOLANI. Renal hypertension impairs inotropic isoproterenol effect without β-receptor changes. *Am. J. Physiol.* 249 (*Heart Circ. Physiol.* 18): H814–H819, 1985.
172. GERSTENBLITH, G., J. FREDERIKSEN, F. C. P. YIN, N. J. FORTUIN, E. G. LAKATTA, and M. L. WEISFELDT. Echocardiographic assessment of a normal adult aging population. *Circulation* 56: 273–278, 1977.
173. GERSTENBLITH, G., E. G. LAKATTA, and M. L. WEISFELDT. Age changes in myocardial function and exercise response. *Prog. Cardiovasc. Dis.* 19: 1–21, 1976.
174. GERSTENBLITH, G., H. A. SPURGEON, J. P. FROEHLICH, M. L. WEISEFELDT, and E. G. LAKATTA. Diminished inotropic responsiveness to ouabain in aged rat myocardium. *Circ. Res.* 44: 517–523, 1979.
175. GEY, K. P., W. P. BURKARD, and A. PLETSCHER. Variation of the norepinephrine metabolism of the rat heart with age. In: *Structure and Chemistry of the Aging Heart,* edited by K. F. Gey, W. P. Burkard, V. V. Frolkis, et al. New York: MSS Information, 1974, p. 10–19.
176. GILMAN, A. G. G-proteins: transducers of receptor-generated signals. *Annu. Rev. Biochem.* 56: 615–649, 1987.
177. GINZTON, L. E., R. CONANT, M. BRIZENDINE, and M. M. LAKS. Effect of long-term high intensity aerobic training on left ventricular volume during maximal upright exercise. *J. Am. Coll. Cardiol.* 14: 364–371, 1989.
178. GODFRAIND, T. Alternative mechanisms for the potentiation of the relaxation evoked by isoprenaline in aortae from young and aged rats. *Eur. J. Pharmacol.* 53: 273–279, 1979.
179. GOLDSTEIN, D. S., C. R. LAKE, B. CHERNOW, M. G. ZIEGLER, M. D. COLEMAN, A. A. TAYLOR, J. R. MITCHELL, I. J. KOPIN, and H. R. KEISER. Age-dependence of hypertensive-normotensive differences in plasma norepinephrine. *Hypertension* 5: 100–104, 1983.
180. GOZNA, E. R., A. E. MARBLE, A. SHAW, and J. G. HOLLAND. Age-related changes in the mechanics of the aorta and pulmonary artery of man. *J. Appl. Physiol.* 36: 407–411, 1974.
181. GRANATH, A., and T. STRANDELL. Relationships between cardiac output, stroke volume and intracardiac pressures at rest and during exercise in supine position and some anthropometric data in healthy old men. *Acta Med. Scand.* 176: 447–466, 1964.
182. GRANATH, A., B. JONSSON, and T. STRANDELL. Circulation in healthy old men studied by right heart catheterization at rest and during exercise in supine and sitting position. *Acta Med. Scand.* 176: 425–446, 1964.
183. GRIBBIN, B., T. G. PICKERING, P. SLEIGHT, and R. PETO. Effect of age and high blood pressure on baroreflex sensitivity in man. *Circ. Res.* 297: 424–431, 1971.
184. GRIMBY, G., and B. SALTIN. Physiological analysis of physically well-trained middle-aged and old athletes. *Acta Med. Scand.* 179: 513–526, 1966.
185. GRIMBY, G., N. J. NILSSON, and B. SALTIN. Cardiac output during submaximal and maximal exercise in active middle-aged athletes. *J. Appl. Physiol.* 21: 1150–1156, 1966.
186. GROBBEE, D. E., and A. HOFMAN. Does sodium restriction lower blood pressure? *Br. Med. J. Clin. Res.* 293: 27–29, 1986.
187. GUARNIERI, T., C. R. FILBURN, G. ZITNIK, G. S. ROTH, and E. G. LAKATTA. Contractile and biochemical correlates of β-adrenergic stimulation of the aged heart. *Am. J. Physiol.* 239 (*Heart Circ. Physiol.* 10): H501–H508, 1980.

188. GUARNIERI, T., H. SPURGEON, J. P. FROEHLICH, M. L. WEISFELDT, and E. G. LAKATTA. Diminished inotropic response but unaltered toxicity to acetylstrophanthidin in the senescent beagle. *Circulation* 60: 1548–1554, 1979.
189. GWATHMEY, J. K., and J. P. MORGAN. Altered calcium handling in experimental pressure-overload hypertrophy in the ferret. *Circ. Res.* 57: 836–843, 1985.
190. GWATHMEY, J. K., M. T. SLAWSKY, C. L. Perreault, G. M. BRIGGS, J. P. MORGAN, and J. Y. WEI. The effect of exercise conditioning on excitation–contraction coupling in aged rats. *J. Appl. Physiol.* 69: 1366–1371, 1990.
191. HABER, P., B. HONIGER, M. KLICPERA, and M. NIEDERBERGER. Effects in elderly people 67–76 years of age of three-month endurance training on a bicycle ergometer. *Eur. Heart J.* 5(suppl. E): 37–39, 1984.
192. HACHAMOVITCH, R., P. WICKER, J. M. CAPASSO, and P. ANVERSA. Alterations of coronary blood flow and reserve with aging in Fischer 344 rats. *Am. J. Physiol.* 256 (*Heart Circ. Physiol.* 27): H66–H73, 1989.
193. HAGBERG, J. M., W. K. ALLEN, D. R. SEALS, B. F. HURLEY, A. A. EHSANI, and J. O. HOLLOSZY. A hemodynamic comparison of young and older endurance athletes during exercise. *J. Appl. Physiol.* 58: 2041–2046, 1985.
194. HAGBERG, J. M., J. E. GRAVES, M. LIMACHER, D. R. WOODS, S. H. LEGGETT, C. CONONIE, J. J. GRUBER, and M. L. POLLOCK. Cardiovascular responses of 70- to 79-yr-old men and women to exercise training. *J. Appl. Physiol.* 66: 2589–2594, 1989.
195. HAJDUCZOK, G., M. W. CHAPLEAU, and F. M. ABBOUD. Increase in sympathetic activity with age. II. Role of impairment of cardiopulmonary baroreflexes. *Am. J. Physiol.* 260 (*Heart Circ. Physiol.* 31): H1121–H1127, 1991.
196. HAJDUCZOK, G., M. W. CHAPLEAU, S. L. JOHNSON, and F. M. ABBOUD. Increase in sympathetic activity with age. I. Role of impairment of arterial baroreflexes. *Am. J. Physiol.* 260 (*Heart Circ. Physiol.* 31): H1113–H1120, 1991.
197. HALLOCK, P. and I. C. BENSON. Studies on the elastic properties of human isolated aorta. *J. Clin. Invest.* 16: 595–602, 1937.
198. HAMMON, G. L., Y. K. LAI, and C. L. MARKERT. Diverse forms of stress lead to new patterns of gene expression through a common and essential metabolic pathway. *Proc. Natl. Acad. Sci. U.S.A.* 79: 3485–3488, 1982.
199. HANF, R., I. DRUBAIX, F. MAROTTE, and L. G. LELIEVRE. Rat cardiac hypertrophy. Altered sodium–calcium exchange activity in sarcolemma vesicles. *FEBS Lett.* 236: 145–149, 1988.
200. HANO, O., K. Y. BOGDANOV, and E. G. LAKATTA. Enhanced calcium intolerance manifest as aftercontractions and ventricular fibrillation in hearts of aged rats [Abstract]. *J. Moll. Cell. Cardiol.* 22: S.24, 1990.
201. HANSFORD, R. G. Lipid oxidation by heart mitochondria from young adult and senescent rats. *Biochem. J.* 170: 285–295, 1978.
202. HANSFORD, R. G. Metabolism and energy production. In: *Aging: The Aging Heart: Its Function and Response to Stress,* edited by M. L. Weisfeldt. New York: Raven, 1980, vol. 12, p. 25–76.
203. HANSON, J. S., B. S. TABAKIN, and A. M. LEVY. Long-term physical training and cardiovascular dynamics in middle-aged men. *Circulation* 38: 783–799, 1968.
204. HARDING, S. E., S. M. JONES, P. O'GARA, F. DEL MONTE, G. VESCOVO, and P. A. POOLE-WILSON. Isolated ventricular myocytes from failing and non failing human heart: the relation of age and clinical status of patients to isoproterenol response. *J. Mol. Cell. Cardiol.* 24: 549–564, 1992.
205. HARRISON, T. R., K. DIXON, P. O. RUSSELL, JR., P. S. BIDWAI, and H. N. COLEMAN. The relation of age to the duration of contraction, ejection, and relaxation of the normal human heart. *Am. Heart J.* 67: 189–199, 1964.
206. HAYES, J. S., L. L. BRUNTON, and S. E. MAYER. Selective activation of particulate cAMP-dependent protein kinase by isoproterenol and prostaglandin E_1. *J. Biol. Chem.* 255: 5113–5119, 1980.
207. HAYNES, F. W., L. B. ELLIS, and S. WEISS. Pulse wave velocity and arterial elasticity in arterial hypertension, arteriosclerosis and related conditions. *Am. Heart J.* 11: 385–401, 1936.
208. HEATH, G. W., J. M. HAGBERG, A. A. EHSANI, and J. O. HOLLOSZY. A physiological comparison of young and older endurance athletes. *J. Appl. Physiol.* 51: 634–640, 1981.
209. HELLER, L. J. Augmented aftercontractions in papillary muscles from rats with cardiac hypertrophy. *Am. J. Physiol.* 237 (*Heart Circ. Physiol.* 8): H649–H654, 1979.
210. HELLER, L. J., and W. V. WHITEHORN. Age-associated alterations in myocardial contractile properties. *Am. J. Physiol.* 222: 1613–1619, 1972.
211. HELLON, R. F., and A. R. LIND. The influence of age on peripheral vasodilatation in a hot environment. *J. Physiol. (Lond.)* 141: 262–272, 1958.
212. HENRY, P. D., G. G. AHUMADA, W. F. FRIEDMAN, and B. E. SOBEL. Simultaneously measured isometric tension and ATP hydrolysis in glycerinated fibers from normal and hypertrophied rabbit heart. *Circ. Res.* 31: 740–749, 1972.
213. HEYLIGER, C. E., A. R. PRAKASH, and J. H. MCNEILL. An assessment of phospholipid methylation in sarcolemma and sarcoplasmic reticulum of the aging myocardium. *Biochim. Biophys. Acta* 960: 462–465, 1988.
214. HEYLIGER, C. E., A. R. PRAKASH, and J. H. MCNEILL. Effect of calmodulin on sarcoplasmic reticular Ca^{2+}-transport in the aging heart. *Mol. Cell. Biochem.* 85: 75–79, 1989.
215. HIGGINBOTHAM, M. B., K. G. MORRIS, R. E. COLEMAN, and F. R. COBB. Sex-related differences in the normal cardiac response to upright exercise. *Circulation* 70: 357–366, 1984.
216. HIGGINBOTHAM, M. B., K. G. MORRIS, R. S. WILLIAMS, and F. R. COBB. Physiologic basis for the age-related decline in aerobic work capacity. *Am. J. Cardiol.* 57: 1374–1379, 1986.
217. HIGGINBOTHAM, M. B., K. G. MORRIS, R. S. WILLIAMS, P. A. MCHALE, R. E. COLEMAN, and F. R. COBB. Regulation of stroke volume during submaximal and maximal upright exercise in normal man. *Circ. Res.* 58: 281–291, 1986.
218. HIREMATH, A. M., R. A. PERSHE, B. B. HOFFMAN, and T. F. BLASCHKE. Comparison of age-related changes in prostaglandin E1 and beta-adrenergic responsiveness of vascular smooth muscle in adult males. *J. Gerontol. Med. Sci.* 44: M13–M17, 1989.
219. HOH, J. F. Y., and G. H. ROSSMANITH. Ventricular isomyosins and the tonic regulation of cardiac contractility. In: *Pathobiology of Cardiovascular Injury,* edited by H. L. Stone and W. B. Weglicki. Boston: Martinus Nijhoff, 1985.
220. HOH, J. F. Y., P. A. MCGRATH, and P. T. HALE. Electrophoretic analysis of multiple forms of rat cardiac myosin: effects of hypophysectomy and thyroxine replacement. *J. Mol. Cell. Cardiol.* 10: 1053–1076, 1978.
221. HOSEY, M. M., M. BORSOTTO, and M. LAZDUNSKI. Phosphorylation and dephosphorylation of dihydropyridine-sensitive voltage-dependent Ca^{2+} channel in skeletal muscle membranes by cAMP- and CA^{2+}-dependent processes. *Proc. Natl. Acad. Sci. U.S.A.* 83: 3733–3737, 1986.
222. HOSSACK, K. F., and R. A. BRUCE. Maximal cardiac function in sedentary normal men and women: comparison of age-related changes. *J. Appl. Physiol.* 53: 799–804, 1982.
223. HOUSER, S. R., A. R. FREEMAN, J. M. JAEGER, E. A. BREISCH, R. L. COULSON, R. CAREY, and J. F. SPANN. Resting potential changes associated with Na-K pump in failing heart muscle. *Am. J. Physiol.* 240 (*Heart Circ. Physiol.* 11): H168–H176, 1981.

224. IKEZONO, K., H. R. ZERKOWSKI, J. J. BECKERINGH, M. C. MICHEL, and O. E. BRODDE. Beta-2 adrenoceptor-mediated relaxation of the isolated human saphenous vein. *J. Pharmacol. Exp. Ther.* 241: 294–299, 1987.

225. ISNARD, R. N., B. M. PANNIER, S. LAURENT, G. M. LONDON, B. DIEBOLD, and M. E. SAFAR. Pulsatile diameter and elastic modulus of the aortic arch in essential hypertension: a noninvasive study. *J. Am. Coll. Cardiol.* 13: 399–405, 1989.

226. ISOYAMA, S., W. GROSSMAN, and J. Y. WEI. Effect of age on myocardial adaptation to volume overload in the rat. *J. Clin. Invest.* 81: 1850–1857, 1988.

227. IZUMO, S., B. NADAL-GINARD, and V. MAHDAVI. All members of the MHC multigene family respond to thyroid hormone in a highly tissue-specific manner. *Science* 231: 597–600, 1986.

228. IZUMO, S., B. NADAL-GINARD, and V. MAHDAVI. Protooncogene induction and reprogramming of cardiac gene expression produced by pressure overload. *Proc. Natl. Acad. Sci. U.S.A.* 85: 339–343, 1988.

229. JACOB, R., G. KISSLING, G. EBRECHT, C. HOLUBARSCH, I. MEDUGORAC, and H. RUPP. Adaptive and pathological alterations in experimental cardiac hypertrophy. In: *Advances in Myocardiology*, edited by E. Chazov, V. Saks, and G. Rona. New York: Plenum, 1983, vol. 4., p. 55–77.

230. JANSEN, R. W., J. W. M. LENDERS, T. THIEN, and W. H. L. HOEFNAGELS. The influence of age and blood pressure on the hemodynamic and humoral response to head-up tilt. *J. Am. Geriatr. Soc.* 37: 528–532, 1989.

231. JANUARY, C. T., J. M. RIDDLE, and J. J. SALATA. A model for early after-depolarizations: induction with the Ca^{2+} channel agonist Bay K 8644. *Circ. Res.* 62: 563–571, 1988.

232. JANZ, R. F., B. R. KUBERT, I. MIRSKY, B. KORECKY, and G. C. TAICHMAN. Effect of age on passive elastic stiffness of rat heart muscle. *Biophys. J.* 16: 281–290, 1976.

233. JEWELL, B. R. A reexamination of the influence of muscle length on myocardial performance. *Circ. Res.* 40: 221–230, 1977.

234. JEWELL, B. R. Activation of contration in cardiac muscle. *Mayo Clin. Proc.* 57: 6–13, 1982.

235. JIANG, M. T., and N. NARYANAN. Effects of aging on phospholamban phosphorylation and calcium transport in rat cardiac sarcoplasmic reticulum. *Mech. Ageing Dev.* 54: 87–101, 1990.

236. JOINT NATIONAL COMMITTEE. The 1984 report of the Joint National Committee on the Detection, Evaluation and Treatment of High Blood Pressure. *Arch. Intern. Med.* 144: 1045–1057, 1984.

237. JOSE, A. D. Effect of combined sympathetic and parasympathetic blockade on heart rate and cardiac function in man. *Am. J. Cardiol.* 18: 476–478, 1966.

238. JULIUS, S., A. AMERY, L. S. WHITLOCK, and J. CONWAY. Influence of age on the hemodynamic response to exercise. *Circulation* 36: 222–230, 1967.

239. KADOMA, M., B. SACKTOR, and J. P. FROEHLICH. Stimulation by cAMP and protein kinase of calcium transport in sarcoplasmic reticulum from senescent rat myocardium [Abstract]. *Fed. Proc.* 39: 2040, 1980.

240. KALISH, M. I., M. S. KATZ, M. A. PINEYRO, and R. I. GREGERMAN. Epinephrine- and glucogon-sensitive adenylate cyclases of rat liver during aging. Evidence for membrane instability associated with increased enzymatic activity. *Biochim. Biophys. Acta* 483: 452–466, 1977.

241. KANE, R. L., T. A. MCMAHON, R. L. WAGNER, and W. H. ABELMANN. Ventricular elastic modulus as a function of age in the Syrian golden hamster. *Circ. Res.* 38: 74–80, 1976.

242. KANNEL, W. B., P. A. WOLF, D. L. MCGEE, T. R. DAWBER, P. MCNAMARA, and W. P. CASTELLI. Systolic blood pressure, arterial rigidity, and risk of stroke. The Framingham study. *JAMA* 245: 1225–1229, 1981.

243. KAPLAN, D., and K. MEYER. Mucopolysaccharides of aorta at various ages. *Proc. Soc. Exp. Biol. Med.* 105: 78–81, 1960.

244. KARAM, R., H. M. LEVER, and B. P. HEALY. Hypertensive hypertrophic cardiomyopathy or hypertrophic cardiomyopathy with hypertension? A study of 78 patients. *J. Am. Coll. Cardiol.* 13: 580–584, 1989.

245. KARIYA, K., L. R. KARNS, and P. C. SIMPSON. Expression of a constitutively activated mutant of the β-isozyme of protein kinase C in cardiac myocytes stimulates the promoter of the β-myosin heavy chain isogene. *J. Biol. Chem.* 266: 10023–10026, 1991.

246. KASSIS, S., and P. H. FISHMAN. Functional alteration of the β-adrenergic receptor during desensitization of mammalian adenylyl cyclase by β-agonists. *Proc. Natl. Acad. Sci. U.S.A.* 81: 6686–6690, 1984.

247. KAVANAGH, T., and R. J. SHEPHARD. The effects of continued training on the aging process. *Ann. N.Y. Acad. Sci.* 301: 656–670, 1977.

248. KAWAMOTO, A., K. SHIMADA, K. MATSUBAYASHI, T. CHIKAMORI, O. KUZUME, H. OGURA, and T. OZAWA. Cardiovascular regulatory functions in elderly patients with hypertension. *Hypertension* 13: 401–407, 1989.

249. KELLIHER, G. J., and J. CONAHAN. Changes in vagal activity and response to muscarinic receptor agonists with age. *J. Gerontol.* 35: 842–849, 1980.

250. KELLY, R., C. HAYWARD, A. AVOLIO, and M. O'ROURKE. Noninvasive determination of age-related changes in the human arterial pulse. *Circulation* 80: 1652–1659, 1989.

251. KELLY, R. P., H. H. GIBBS, M. F. O'ROURKE, J. E. DALEY, K. MANG, J. J. MORGAN, and A. P. AVOLIO. Nitroglycerin has more favourable effects on left ventricular afterload than apparent from measurement of pressure in a peripheral artery. *Eur. Heart J.* 11: 138–144, 1990.

252. KENNEDY, R. H., and E. SEIFEN. Aging: effects of chronotropic actions of muscarinic agonists in isolated rat atria. *Mech. Ageing Dev.* 51: 81–87, 1990.

253. KENNEY, W. L. Control of heat-induced cutaneous vasodilatation in relation to age. *Eur. J. Appl. Physiol.* 57: 120–125, 1988.

254. KENNEY, W. L., C. G. TANKERSLEY, D. L. NEWSWANGER, D. E. HYDE, S. M. PUHL, and N. L. TURNER. Age and hypohydration independently influence the peripheral vascular response to heat stress. *J. Appl. Physiol.* 68: 1902–1908, 1990.

255. KENT, R. L., J. K. HOOBER, and G. COOPER, IV. Load responsiveness of protein synthesis in adult mammalian myocardium: role of cardiac deformation linked to sodium influx. *Circ. Res.* 64: 74–85, 1989.

256. KHAW, K. T., and E. BARRETT-CONONR. The association between blood pressure, age, and dietary sodium and potassium: a population study. *Circulation* 77: 53–61, 1988.

257. KING, A. L. Pressure-volume relation for cylindrical tubes with elastomeric walls: the human aorta. *J. Appl. Physics* 17: 501–505, 1946.

258. KINO, M., V. Q. LANCE, A. SHAHAMATPOUR, and D. H. SPODICK. Effects of age on responses to isometric exercise. Isometric handgrip in noninvasive screening for cardiovascular disease. *Am. Heart J.* 90: 575–581, 1975.

259. KIRCHBERGER, M. A., E. ZHEN, C. KASINATHAN, and M. A. KIRCHBERGER. Altered phospholamban phosphorylation in cardiac microsomes obtained from senescent rats [Abstract]. *Biophys. J.* 57: 504a, 1990.

260. KITZMAN, D. W., D. G. SCHOLZ, P. T. HAGEN, D. M. ILSTRUP, and W. D. EDWARDS. Age-related changes in normal human hearts during the first ten decades. Part II (Maturity): a quantitative anatomic study of 765 specimens from subjects 20 to 99 years old. *Mayo Clin. Proc.* 63: 137–146, 1988.

261. KITZMAN, D. W., K. H. SHEIKH, P. A. BEERE, J. L. PHILIPS, and

M. B. HIGGINBOTHAM. Age-related alterations of Doppler left ventricular filling indexes in normal subjects are independent of left ventricular mass, heart rate, contractility and loading conditions. *J. Am. Coll. Cardiol.* 18: 1243–1250, 1991.

262. KLEIN, C., W. R. HIATT, J. G. GERBER, and A. S. NIES. Age does not alter human vascular and nonvascular β₂-adrenergic responses to isoproterenol. *Clin. Pharmacol. Ther.* 44: 573–578, 1988.

263. KOBINGER, W. α-Adrenoceptors in cardiovascular regulation. In: *Norepinephrine*, edited by M. G. Ziegler and C. R. Lake. Baltimore: Williams and Wilkins, 1984, p. 307–326.

264. KOMURO, I., Y. KATOH, T. KAIDA, Y. SHIBAZAKI, M. KURABAYASHI, E. HOH, TAKAKU, and Y. YAZAKI. Mechanical loading stimulates cell hypertrophy and specific gene expression in cultured rat cardiac myocytes. Possible role of protein kinase C activation. *J. Biol. Chem.* 266: 1265–1268, 1991.

265. KOMURO, I., M. KURABAYASHI, Y. SHIBAZAKI, F. TAKAKU, and Y. YAZAKI. Molecular cloning and characterization of a Ca²⁺ + Mg²⁺-dependent adenosine triphosphatase from rat cardiac sarcoplasmic reticulum. Regulation of its expression by pressure overload and developmental stage. *J. Clin. Invest.* 83: 1102–1108, 1989.

266. KORCKY, B. The effects of load, internal environment and age on cardiac mechanics [Abstract]. *J. Mol. Cell. Cardiol.* 11(suppl. 1): 33, 1979.

267. KORKUSHKO, O. V., V. B. SHATILO, and J. K. KAUKENAS. Changes in heart rhythm power spectrum during human aging. *Aging* 3: 177–179, 1991.

268. KORT, A. .A, and E. G. LAKATTA. Calcium-dependent mechanical oscillations occur spontaneously in unstimulated mammalian cardiac tissues. *Circ. Res.* 54: 396–404, 1984.

269. KOSTIS, J. B., A. E. MOREYRA, M. T. AMENDO, J. DI PIETRO, N. COSGROVE, and P. T. KUO. The effect of age on heart rate in subjects free of heart disease. Studies by ambulatory electrocardiography and maximal exercise stress test. *Circulation* 65: 141–145, 1982.

270. KRAFT, C. A., and C. M. CASTLEDEN. The effect of aging on β-adrenoceptor-stimulated cyclic AMP formation in human lymphocytes. *Clin. Sci.* 60: 587–589, 1981.

271. KRALL, J. F., M. CONNELLY, and M. L. TUCK. Evidence for reversibility of age-related decrease in human lymphocyte adenylate cyclase activity. *Biochem. Biophys. Res. Commun.* 99: 1028–1034, 1981.

272. KRALL, J. F., M. CONNELLY, R. WEISBART, and M. L. TUCK. Age-related elevation of plasma catecholamine concentration and reduced responsiveness of lymphocyte adenylate cyclase. *J. Clin. Endocrinol. Metab.* 52: 863–867, 1981.

273. KRANZ, D., and A. WOLLENBERGER. Age dependence of adenylate cyclase activity and cAMP generation in aortas and femoral arteries of rats. *Z. Alternsforsch.* 32: 461–466, 1976.

274. KREIDER, M. S., P. B. GOLDBERG, and J. ROBERTS. Effect of age on adrenergic neuronal uptake in rat heart. *J. Pharmacol. Exp. Ther.* 231: 367–372, 1984.

275. KRONENBERG, R. S., and C. W. DRAGE. Attenuation of the ventilatory and heart rat responses to hypoxia and hypercapnia with aging in normal men. *J. Clin. Invest.* 52: 1812–1819, 1973.

276. KUECHERER, H., K. RUFFMANN, and W. KUEBLER. Effect of aging on Doppler echocardiographic filling parameters in normal subjects and in patients with coronary artery disease. *Clin. Cardiol.* 11: 303–306, 1988.

277. KUICKKA, J. T., and E. LANSIMIES. Effect of age on cardiac index, stroke index and left ventricular ejection fraction at rest and during exercise as studied by radiocardiography. *Acta Physiol. Scand.* 114: 339–343, 1982.

278. KULCHITSKII, O. K. Effect of acetylcholine on the cyclic GMP level in the rat heart at different ages. *Bull. Exp. Biol. Med.* 90: 1237–1239, 1980.

279. KUO, L. C., M. A. QUINONES, R. ROKEY, M. SARTORI, E. G. ABINADER, and W. A. ZOGHBI. Quantification of atrial contribution to left ventricular filling by pulsed Doppler echocardiography and the effect of age in normal and diseased hearts. *Am. J. Cardiol.* 59: 1174–1178, 1987.

280. KURAMOTO, K., S. MATSUSHITA, J. MIFUNE, M. SAKAI, and M. MURAKAMI. Electrocardiographic and hemodynamic evaluations of isoproterenol test in elderly ischemic heart disease. *Jpn. Circ. J.* 42: 955–960, 1978.

281. KUROHA, M., S. ISOYAMA, N. ITO, and T. TAKISHIMA. Effects of age on right ventricular hypertrophic response to pressure-overload in rats. *J. Mol. Cell. Cardiol.* 23: 1177–1190, 1991.

282. KUSIAK, J. W., and J. PITHA. Decreased response with age of the cardiac catecholamine sensitive adenylate cyclase system. *Life Sci.* 33: 1679–1686, 1983.

283. LAB, M. J. Contraction–excitation feedback in myocardium. Physiological basis and clinical relevance. *Circ. Res.* 40: 757–766, 1982.

284. LAGRUE, G., J. C. ANSQUER, and A. MEYER-HEINE. Peripheral action of spironolactone: improvement in arterial elasticity. *Am. J. Cardiol.* 65: 9K–11K, 1990.

285. LAKATTA, E. G. Determinants of cardiovascular performance: modification due to aging. *J. Chron. Dis.* 36: 15–30, 1983.

286. LAKATTA, E. G. Do hypertension and aging have a similar effect on the myocardium? *Circulation* 75(suppl. I): I69–I77, 1987.

287. LAKATTA, E. G. Chaotic behavior of myocardial cells: possible implications regarding the pathophysiology of heart failure. *Perspect. Biol. Med.* 32: 421–433, 1989.

288. LAKATTA, E. G. Normal changes of aging. In: *Merck Manual of Geriatrics*, edited by W. B. Abrams and R. Berkow. Rahway, NJ: Merck Sharp & Dohme, 1990, p. 310–325.

289. LAKATTA, E. G. Regulation of cardiac muscle function in the hypertensive heart. In: *Cellular and Molecular Mechanisms of Hypertension*, edited by R. H. Cox. New York: Plenum, 1991, p. 149–173.

290. LAKATTA, E. G. Excitation–contration coupling in heart failure. *Hosp. Pract.* 26: 85–88, 1991.

291. LAKATTA, E. G. Length modulation of muscle performance: Frank-Starling law of the heart. In: *The Heart and Cardiovascular System* (2nd ed.), edited by H. M. Fozzard, E. Haber, R. B. Jennings, A. M. Katz, and H. E. Morgan. New York: Raven, 1992, vol. 2, p. 1325–1351.

292. LAKATTA, E. G., and D. L. LAPPE. Diastolic scattered light fluctuation, resting force and twitch force in mammalian cardiac muscle. *J. Physiol. (Lond.)* 315: 369–394, 1981.

293. LAKATTA, E. G., and W. L. MAUGHAN. Cardiovascular function. In: *Current Concepts in Cardiovascular Physiology*, edited by O. B. Garfein. New York: Academic Press, 1990, p. 351–464.

294. LAKATTA, E. G., and F. C. P. YIN. Myocardial aging: functional alterations and related cellular mechanisms. *Am. J. Physiol.* 242 (*Heart Circ. Physiol.* 13): H927–H941, 1982.

295. LAKATTA, E. G., G. GERSTENBLITH, C. S. ANGELL, N. W. SHOCK, and M. L. WEISFELDT. Diminished inotropic response of aged myocardium to catecholamines. *Circ. Res.* 36: 262–269, 1975a.

296. LAKATTA, E. G., G. GERSTENBLITH, C. S. ANGELL, N. W. SHOCK, and M. L. WEISFELDT. Prolonged contraction duration in aged myocardium. *J. Clin. Invest.* 55: 61–68, 1975b.

297. LAKATTA, E. G., H. J. MITCHELL, A. POMERANCE, and G. G. ROWE. Human aging: changes in structure and function. *J. Am. Coll. Cardiol.* 10: 42A–47A, 1987.

298. LAKATTA, E. G., F. O'CONNOR, S. SCHULMAN, G. GERSTENBLITH, L. BECKER, and J. L. FLEG. Cardiac volumes at rest and

during cycle exercise in healthy men of a broad age range: effect of fitness matching [Abstract]. *FASEB J.* 5: A766, 1991.
299. LAMERS, J. M. J., and J. T. STINIS. Defective calcium pump in the sarcoplasmic reticulum of the hypertrophied rabbit heart. *Life Sci.* 24: 2313–2319, 1979.
300. LAMONICA, D. A., N. FROHLOFF, and J. G. DOBSON, JR. Adenosine inhibition of catecholamine-stimulated cardiac membrane adenylate cyclase. *Am. J. Physiol.* 248 (*Heart Circ. Physiol.* 19): H737–H744, 1985.
301. LANDOWNE, M. The relation between intra-arterial pressure and impact pulse wave velocity with regard to age and arteriosclerosis. *J. Gerontol.* 13: 153–161, 1958.
302. LANGER, S. Z. The role of α- and β-presynaptic receptors in the regulation of noradrenaline release elicited by nerve stimulation. *Clin. Sci. Mol. Med.* 51(suppl. 3): 423s–426s, 1976.
303. LANSING, A. I. *The Arterial Wall: Aging, Structure, and Chemistry*. Baltimore: Williams and Wilkins, 1959, p. 136–160.
304. LEAROYD, B. M., and M. G. TAYLOR. Alterations with age in the viscoelastic properties of human arterial walls. *Circ. Res.* 18: 278–292, 1966.
305. LE BLAC, P. R., and K. RAKUSAN. Effects of age and isoproterenol on the cardiac output and regional blood flow in the rat. *Can. J. Cardiol.* 3: 246–250, 1987.
306. LECARPENTIER, Y., L. B. BUGAISKY, D. CHEMLA, J. J. MERCADIER, K. SCHWARTZ, R. G. WHALEN, and J. L. MARTIN. Coordinated changes in contractility, energetics, and isomyosins after aortic stenosis. *Am. J. Physiol.* 252 (*Heart Circ. Physiol.* 23): H275–H282, 1987.
307. LECARPENTIER, Y., A. WALDENSTROM, M. CLERQUE, D. CHEMLA, P. OLIVIERO, J. L. MARTIN, and B. SWYNGHEDAUW. Major alterations in relaxation during cardiac hypertrophy induced by aortic stenosis in guinea pig. *Circ. Res.* 61: 107–116, 1987.
308. LEE, J. C., L. M. KARPELES, and S. E. DOWNING. Age-related changes of cardiac performance in male rats. *Am. J. Physiol.* 222: 432–438, 1972.
309. LEFKOWITZ, R. J., W. P. HAUSDORFF, and M. G. CARON. Role of phosphorylation in desensitization of the β-adrenoceptor. *Trends Pharmacol. Sci.* 11: 190–194, 1990.
310. LEHMANN, M., P. SCHMID, and J. KEUL. Age- and exercise-related sympathetic activity in untrained volunteers, trained athletes and patients with impaired left-ventricular contractility. *Eur. Heart J.* 5(suppl. E): 1–7, 1984.
311. LEVITZKI, A. Regulation of hormone-sensitive adenylate cyclase. *Trends Pharmacol. Sci.* 8: 299–303, 1987.
312. LEWIS, W. H. Changes with age in the cardiac output of adult men. *Am. J. Physiol.* 121: 517–527, 1938.
313. LEXELL, J., K. HENRIKSSON-LARSEN, B. WINBLAD, and M. SJÖSTRÖM. Distribution of different fiber types in human skeletal muscles: effects of aging studied in whole muscle cross sections. *Muscle Nerve* 6: 588–595, 1983.
314. LEXELL, J., C. C. TAYLOR, and M. SJÖSTRÖM. What is the cause of the ageing atrophy? Total number, size and proportion of different fiber types studied in whole vastus lateralis muscle from 15- to 83-year-old men. *J. Neurol. Sci.* 84: 275–294, 1988.
315. LI, Y. X., T. LINCOLN, D. MENDELOWITZ, W. GROSSMAN, and J. Y. WEI. Age-related differences in effect of exercise training on cardiac muscle function in rats. *Am. J. Physiol.* 251 (*Heart Circ. Physiol.* 22): H12–H18, 1986.
316. LINDEMAN, R. D., and R. GOLDMAN. Anatomic and physiologic age changes in the kidney. *Exp. Gerontol.* 21: 379–406, 1986.
317. LINZBACH, A. J., and E. AKUAMOA-BOATENG. Die alternsveranderungen des menschlichen herzens I. Das herzgewicht im alter. *Klin. Wochenschr.* 51: 156–163, 1973.
318. LIPSITZ, L. A. Orthostatic hypotension in the elderly. *N. Engl. J. Med.* 321: 952–957, 1989.
319. LITSITZ, L. A., P. V. JONSSON, B. L. MARKS, J. A. PARKER, J. D. ROYAL, and J. Y. WEI. Reduced supine cardiac volumes and diastolic filling rates in elderly patients with chronic medical conditions. *J. Am. Geriatr. Soc.* 38: 103–107, 1990.
320. LOHSE, M. J., J. L. BENOVIC, J. CODINA, M. G. CARON, and R. J. LEFKOWITZ. Barrestin—a novel protein that regulates β-adrenergic-receptor function [Abstract]. *Circulation* 82(suppl. III): III-L, 1990.
321. LOMPRES, A. M., F. LAMBERT, E. G. LAKATTA, and K. SCHWARTZ. Expression of sarcoplasmic reticulum Ca^{2+}-ATPase and calsequestrin genes in rat heart during ontogenic development and aging. *Circ. Res.* 69: 1380–1388, 1991.
322. LOMPRE, A. M., K. SCHWARTZ, A. D'ALBIS, G. LACOMBE, N. VAN THIEM, and B. SWYNGHEDAUW. Myosin isozyme redistribution in chronic heart overload. *Nature* 282: 105–107, 1979.
323. LONDON, G. M., M. E. SAFAR, Y. A. WEISS, and P. L. MILLIEZ. Isoproterenol sensitivity and total body clearance of propranolol in hypertensive patients. *J. Clin. Pharmacol.* 16: 174–183, 1976.
324. LOPASCHUK, G. D., A. G. TAHILIANI, R. V. S. V. VADLAMUDI, S. KATZ, and J. H. MCNEILL. Cardiac sarcoplasmic reticulum function in insulin- or carnitine-treated diabetic rats. *Am. J. Physiol.* 245 (*Heart Circ. Physiol.* 16): H969–H976, 1983.
325. LUISADA, A. A., K. WATANABE, P. K. BHAT, D. B. RAO, and V. KNIGHTEN. Correlates of the echocardiographic waves of the mitral valve in normal subjects of various ages. *J. Am. Geriatr. Soc.* 23: 216–223, 1975.
326. LUND-JOHANSEN, L. Twenty-year follow-up of hemodynamics in essential hypertension during rest and exercise. *Hypertension* 18: III54–III61, 1991.
327. LYE, M., nad E. VARGAS. An analysis of impedance cardiography in the elderly. *J. Med. Eng. Technol.* 5: 289–292, 1981.
328. MACIEL, L. M. Z., R. POLIKAR, D. ROHRER, B. K. POPOVICH, and W. V. DILLMANN. Age-induced decreases in the messenger RNA coding for the sarcoplasmic reticulum Ca^{2+}-ATPase of the rat heart. *Circ. Res.* 67: 230–234, 1990.
329. MACLENNAN W. J., M. R. P. HALL, and J. I. TIMOTHY. Postural hypotension in old age: is it a disorder of the nervous system or of blood vessels? *Age Ageing* 9: 25–32, 1980.
330. MALHOTRA, A., S. PENPARGKUL, F. S. FEIN, E. H. SONNENBLICK, and J. SCHEUER. The effect of streptozotocin-induced diabetes in rats on cardiac contractile proteins. *Circ. Res.* 49: 1243–1250, 1981.
331. MANN, D. L., B. S. DENENBERG, A. K. GASH, P. T. MAKLER, and A. A. BOVE. Effects of age on ventricular performance during graded supine exercise. *Am. Heart J.* 111: 108–115, 1986.
332. MANN, D. L., R. L. KENT, and G. COOPER, IV. Load regulation of the properties of adult feline cardiocytes: growth induction by cellular deformation. *Circ. Res.* 64: 1079–1090, 1989.
333. MANSIER, P., B. CHEVALIER, and B. SWYNGHEDAUW. Characterization of the beta adrenergic system in adult rat hypertrophied hearts [Abstract]. *J. Mol. Cell. Cardiol.* 21: S.17, 1989.
334. MARTIN, C. E., J. A. SHAVER, D. F. LEON, M. E. THOMPSON, P. S. REDDY, and J. J. LEONARD. Autonomic mechanisms in hemodynamic responses to isometric exercise. *J. Clin. Invest.* 54: 104–115, 1974.
335. MARTIN W. H., III, E. F. COYLE, S. A. BLOOMFIELD, and A. A. EHSANI. Effects of physical deconditioning after intense endurance training on left ventricular dimensions and stroke volume. *J. Am. Coll. Cardiol.* 7: 982–989, 1986.
336. MARTIN, W. H., III, J. MONTGOMERY, P. G. SNELL, J. R. CORBETT, J. J. SOKOLOV, J. C. BUCKEY, D. A. MALONEY, and C. G. BLOMQVIST. Cardiovascular adaptations to intense swimming training in sedentary middle-aged men and women. *Circulation* 75: 323–330, 1987.
337. MARZO, K. P., M. J. FREY, J. R. WILSON, B. T. LIANG, D. R. MANNING, V. LANOCE, and P. B. MOLINOFF. Beta-adrenergic

receptor-G protein-adenylate cyclase complex in experimental canine congestive heart failure produced by rapid ventricular pacing. *Circ. Res.* 69: 1546–1556, 1991.
338. MAUGHAN, D., E. LOW, R. LITTEN, III, J. BRAYDEN, and N. ALPERT. Calcium-activated muscle from hypertophied rabbit hearts. Mechanical and correlated biochemical changes. *Circ. Res.* 44: 279–287, 1979.
339. MAYOUX, E., F. CALLENS, B. SWYNGHEDAUW, and D. CHARLEMAGNE. Adaptational process of the cardiac Ca^{2+} channels to pressure overload: biochemical and physiological properties of the dihydropyridine receptors in normal and hypertrophied rat hearts. *J. Cardiovasc. Pharmacol.* 12: 390–396, 1988.
340. MEERSON, F. Z., M. P. JAVICH, and M. I. LEWRMAN. Decrease in the rate of RNA and protein synthesis and degradation in the myocardium under long-term compensatory hyperfunction and on aging. *J. Mol. Cell. Cardiol.* 10: 145–159, 1978.
341. MERCADIER, J.-J., A.-M. LOMPRE, C. WISNEWSKY, J.-L. SAMUEL, J. BERCOVICI, B. SWYNGHEDAUW, and K. SCHWARTZ. Myosin isoenzyme changes in several models of rat cardiac hypertrophy. *Circ. Res.* 49: 525–532, 1981.
342. MEREDITH, C. N., M. J. ZACKIN, W. R. FRONTERA, and W. J. EVANS. Body composition and aerobic capacity in young and middle-aged endurance-trained men. *Med. Sci. Sports Exerc.* 19: 557–563, 1987.
343. MERILLON, J. P., G. MOTTE, C. MASQUET, I. AZANCOT, A. GUIOMARD, and R. GOURGON. Relationship between physical properties of the arterial system and left ventricular performance in the course of aging and arterial hypertension. *Eur. Heart J.* 3(suppl. A): 95–102, 1982.
344. MESSERLI, F. H., E. D. FROHLICH, D. H. SUAREZ, E. REISIN, G. R. DRESLINSKY, F. G. DUNN, and F. E. COLE. Borderline hypertension: relationship between age, hemodynamics and circulating catecholamines. *Circulation* 64: 760–764, 1981.
345. MESSERLI, F. H., SUNDGAARD-RIISE, H. O. VENTURA, F. G. DUNN, W. OIGMAN, and E. D. FROHLICH. Clinical and hemodynamic determinants of left ventricular dimensions. *Arch. Intern. Med.* 144: 477–481 1984.
346. MILLER, T. R., S. J. GROSSMAN, K. B. SCHECTMAN, D. R. BIELLO, P. A. LUDBROOK, and A. A. EHSANI. Left ventricular diastolic filling and its association with age. *Am. J. Cardiol.* 58: 531–535, 1986.
347. MILLIKEN, M. C., J. STRAY-GUNDERSEN, R. M. PESHOCK, J. KATZ, and J. H. MITCHELL. Left ventricular mass as determined by magnetic resonance imaging in male endurance athletes. *Am. J. Cardiol.* 62: 301–305, 1988.
348. MILNOR, W. R. *Hemodynamics.* Baltimore: Williams and Wilkins, 1982.
349. MIRSKY, I., and M. M. LAKS. Time course of changes in the mechanical properties of the canine right and left ventricles during hypertrophy caused by pressure overload. *Circ. Res.* 46: 530–542, 1980.
350. MITCHELL, J. H., B. J. SPROULE nad C. B. CHAPMAN. The physiological meaning of the maximal oxygen intake test. *J. Clin. Intest.* 37: 538–547, 1958.
351. MITHOEFER, J. C., and M. S. KARETZKY. *Surgery of the Aged and Debilitated Patient.* Philadelphia: J. H. Powers, 1968, p. 765–779.
352. MIYATAKE, K., M. OKAMOTO, N. KINOSHITA, M. OWA, I. NAKASONE, H. SAKAKIBARA, and Y. NIMURA. Augmentation of atrial contribution to left ventricular inflow with aging as assessed by intracardiac Doppler flowmetry. *Am. J. Cardiol.* 53: 586–589, 1984.
353. MOCHLY-ROSEN, D., C. J. HENRICH, L. CHEEVER, H. KHANER, and P. C. SIMPSON. A protein kinase C isozyme is translocated to cytoskeletal elements on activation. *Cell Reg.* 1: 693–706, 1990.
354. MORGAN, H. E., and K. M. BAKER. Cardiac hypertrophy. Mechanical, neural, and endocrine dependence. *Circulation* 83: 13–25, 1991.
355. MULVAGH, S. L., L. H. MICHAEL, M. B. PERRYMAN, R. ROBERTS, and M. D. SCHNEIDER. A hemodynamic load in vivo induces cardiac expression of the cellular oncogene, c-myc. *Biochem. Biophys. Res. Commun.* 147: 627–636, 1987.
356. MURGO, J. P., N. WESTERHOF, J. P. GIOLMA, and S. A. ALTOBELLI. Aortic input impedance in normal man: relationship to pressure wave forms. *Circulation* 62: 105–116, 1980.
357. MURGO, J. P., N. WESTERHOF, J. P. GIOLMA, and S. A. ALTOBELLI. Effects of exercise on aortic input impedance and pressure wave forms in normal humans. *Circ. Res.* 48: 334–343, 1981.
358. NAGAI, R., A. ZARAIN-HERZBERG, C. J. BRANDL, J. FUJII, M. TADA, D. H. MACLENNAN, N. R. ALPERT, and M. PERIASAMY. Regulation of myocardial Ca^{2+}-ATPase and phospholamban mRNA expression in response to pressure overload and thyroid hormone. *Proc. Natl. Acad. Sci. U.S.A.* 86: 2966–2970, 1989.
359. NAKASHIMA, T., and J. TANIKAWA. A study of human aortic distensibility with relations to atherosclerosis and aging. *Angiology* 22: 477–490, 1971.
360. NARAYANAN, N. Differential alterations in ATP-supported calcium transport activities of sarcoplasmic reticulum and sarcolemma of aging myocardium. *Biochim. Biophys. Acta.* 678: 442–459, 1981.
361. NARAYANAN, N., and J. A. DERBY. Alterations in the properties of beta-adrenergic receptors of myocardial membranes in aging: impairment of agonist-receptor interactions and guanine nucleotide regulation accompany diminished catecholamine-responsiveness of adenylate cyclase. *Mech. Ageing Dev.* 19: 127–139, 1982.
362. NICHOLS, W. W., and C. J. PEPINE. Left ventricular afterload and aortic input impedance: implications of pulsatile blood flow. *Prog. Cardiovasc. Dis.* 24: 293–306, 1982.
363. NICHOLS, W. W., M. F. O'ROURKE, A. P. AVOLIO, T. YAGINUMA, J. P. MURGO, C. J. PEPINE, and C. R. CONTI. Effects of age on ventricular–vascular coupling. *Am. J. Cardiol.* 55: 1179–1184, 1985.
364. NICHOLS, W. W., M. F. O'ROURKE, A. P. AVOLIO, T. YAGINUMA, C. J. PEPINE, and C. R. CONTI. Ventricular/vascular interaction in patients with mild systemic hypertension and normal peripheral resistance. *Circulation* 74: 455–462, 1986.
365. NICHOLS, W. W., M. F. O'ROURKE, A. P. AVOLIO, T. YAGINUMA, J. P. MURGO, C. J. PEPINE, and C. R. CONTI. Age-related changes in left ventricular/arterial coupling. In: *Ventricular Vascular Coupling: Clinical Physiology, and Engineering Aspects,* edited by F. C. P. Yin. New York: Springer-Verlag, 1987, p. 79–114.
366. NICHOLS, W. W., C. J. PEPINE, R. L. FELDMAN, J. WHITTLE, J. H. SELBY, T. KELLY, and C. R. CONTI. Influence of changes in pulsatile components of vascular load on left ventricular function: power-load relations in patients without heart failure [Abstract]. *Circulation* 59/60: II-94, 1979.
367. NIXON, J. V., H. HALLMARK, K. PAGE, P. R. RAVEN, and J. H. MITCHELL. Ventricular performance in human hearts aged 61 to 73 years. *Am. J. Cardiol.* 56: 932–937, 1985.
368. O'CONNOR, S. W., P. J. SCARPACE, and I. B. ABRASS. Age-associated decrease of adenylate cyclase activity in rat myocardium. *Mech. Ageing Dev.* 16: 91–95, 1981.
369. O'CONNOR, S. W., P. J. SCARPACE, and I. B. ABRASS. Age-associated decrease in the catalytic unit activity of rat myocardial adenylate cyclase. *Mech. Ageing Dev.* 21: 357–363, 1983.
370. O'DONNELL, S. R., and J. C. WANSTALL. Demonstration of both β_1- and β_2-adrenoceptor mediating relaxation of isolated ring preparations of rat pulmonary artery. *Br. J. Pharmacol.* 74: 547–552, 1981.

371. O'DONNELL, S. R., and J. C. WANSTALL. Beta-1 and beta-2 adrenoceptor-mediated responses in preparations of pulmonary artery and aorta from young and aged rats. *J. Pharmacol. Exp. Ther.* 228: 733–738, 1984.

372. O'DONNELL, S. R., and J. C. WANSTALL. Thyroxine treatment of aged or young rats demonstrates that vascular responses mediated by β-adrenoceptor sybtypes can be differentially regulated. *Br. J. Pharmacol.* 88: 41–49, 1986.

373. O'DONNELL, S. R., and J. C. WANSTALL. Functional evidence for differential regulation of β-adrenoceptor subtypes. *Trends Pharmacol. Sci.* 8: 265–268, 1987.

374. OGAWA, T., R. J. SPINA, W. H. MARTIN, III, W. M. HOHRT, K. B. SCHECHTMAN, J. O. HOLLOSZY, and A. A. EHSANI. Effects of aging, sex, and physical training on cardiovascular responses to exercise. *Circulation* 86: 494–503, 1992.

375. OLIVETTI, G., M. MELISSARI, J. M. CAPASSO, and P. ANVERSA. Cardiomyopathy of the aging human heart. Myocyte loss and reactive cellular hypertrophy. *Circ. Res.* 68: 1560–1568, 1991.

376. O'NEILL, L., N. J. HOLBROOK, J. FARGNOLI, and E. G. LAKATTA. Progressive changes from young adult age to senescence in mRNA for rat cardiac myosin heavy chain genes. *Cardioscience* 2: 1–5, 1991.

377. ORCHARD, C. H., and E. G. LAKATTA. Intracellular calcium transients and developed tensions in rat heart muscle. A mechanism for the negative interval–strength relationship. *J. Gen. Physiol.* 86: 637–651, 1985.

378. ORLANDER, J., K. H. KIESSLING, L. LARSSON, J. KARLSSON, and A. ANIANSSON. Skeletal muscle metabolism and ultrastructure in relation to age in sedentary men. *Acta. Physiol. Scand.* 104: 249–261, 1978.

379. ORLOWSKI, J., and J. B. LINGREL. Differential expression of the Na,K-ATPase α_1 and α_2 subunit genes in murine myogenic cell line. Induction of the α_2 isozyme during myocyte differentiation. *J. Biol. Chem.* 263: 17817–17821, 1988.

380. O'ROURKE, M. F. *Arterial Function in Health and Disease.* New York: Churchill Livingstone, 1982, p. 275.

381. O'ROURKE, M. F. Vascular impedance in studies of arterial and cardiac function. *Physiol. Rev.* 62: 570–623, 1982.

382. OSCAI, L. B., P. A. MOLE, and J. O. HOLLOSZY. Effects of exercise on cardiac weight and mitochondria in male and female rats. *Am. J. Physiol.* 220: 1944–1948, 1971.

383. PAN, H. Y., B. B. HOFFMAN, R. A. PERSHE, and T. F. BLASCHKE. Decline in beta adrenergic receptor-mediated vascular relaxation with aging in man. *J. Pharmacol. Exp. Ther.* 239: 802–807, 1986.

384. PENG, M. T., and M. KANG. Circadian rhythms and patterns of running-wheel activity, feeding and drinking behaviors of old rats. *Physiol. Behav.* 33: 615–620, 1984.

385. PENPARGKUL, S., F. FEIN, E. H. SONNENBLICK, and J. SCHEUER. Depressed cardiac sarcoplasmic reticular function from diabetic rats. *J. Mol. Cell. Cardiol.* 13: 303–309, 1981.

386. PETERSON, L. H., R. E. JENSEN, and J. PARNELL. Mechanical properties of arteries in vivo. *Circ. Res.* 8: 622–639, 1960.

387. PETROFSKY, J. S., and A. R. LIND. Isometric strength, endurance, and the blood pressure and heart rate responses during isometric exercise in healthy men and women, with special reference to age and body fat content. *Pflugers Arch.* 360: 49–61, 1975.

388. PFEIFFER, J. M., M. A. PFEIFFER, M. C. FISHBEIN, and E. D. FROHLICH. Cardiac function and morphology with aging in the spontaneously hypertensive rat. *Am. J. Physiol.* 237 (*Heart Circ. Physiol.* 8): H461–H468, 1979.

389. PFEIFER, M. A., C. R. WEINBERG, D. COOK, J. D. BEST, A. REENAN, and J. B. HALTER. Differential changes of autonomic nervous system function with age in man. *Am. J. Med.* 75: 249–258, 1983.

390. PICKERING, G. W. *High Blood Pressure.* London: Churchill, 1955, p. 154–183.

391. POLLOCK, M. L., C. FOSTER, D. O. KNAPP, J. L. ROD, and D. H. SCHMIDT. Effect of age and training on aerobic capacity and body composition of master athletes. *J. Appl. Physiol.* 62: 725–731, 1987.

392. POLLOCK, M. L., H. S. MILLER, JR., and J. WILMORE. Physiological characteristics of champion American track athletes 40 to 75 years of age. *J. Gerontol.* 29: 645–649, 1974.

393. POOLING PROJECT RESEARCH GROUP. Relationship of blood pressure, serum cholesterol, smoking, relative weight and ECG abnormalities to incidence of major coronary events: final report of the pooling project. *J. Chron. Dis.* 31: 201–306, 1978.

394. PORT, S., F. R. COBB, R. E. COLEMAN, and R. H. JONES. Effect of age on the response of the left ventricular ejection fraction to exercise. *N. Engl. J. Med.* 303: 1113–1117, 1980.

395. PORTH, C. J., L. GROBAN, and J. J. SMITH. Carotid–cardiac baroreflex rsesponses decrease with early aging in women [Abstract]. *Physiologist* 28: 350, 1985.

396. POTTER, J. F., D. ELAHI, J. D. TOBIN, and R. ANDRES. Effect of aging on the cardiothoracic ratio of men. *J. Am. Geriatr. Soc.* 30: 404–409, 1982.

397. PRINZ, P. N., J. HALTER, C. BENEDETTI, and M. RASKIND. Circadian variation of plasma catecholamines in young and old men: relation to rapid eye movement and slow wave sleep. *J. Clin. Endocrinol. Metab.* 49: 300–304, 1979.

398. PROPER, R., and F. WALL. Left ventricular stroke volume measurements not affected by chronologic aging. *Am. Heart J.* 83: 843–845, 1972.

399. RAKUSAN, K., and O. POUPA. Capillaries and muscle fibers in the heart of old rats. *Gerontologia* 9: 107–112, 1964.

400. RANDALL, O., M. ESLER, B. CULP, S. JULIUS, and A. ZWIFLER. Determinants of baroreflex sensitivity in man. *Lab. Clin. Med.* 91: 514–519, 1978.

401. RAVEN, P. B., and J. MITCHELL. The effect of aging on the cardiovascular response to dynamic and static exercise. In: *The Aging Heart,* edited by M. L. Weisfeldt. New York: Raven Press, 1980, p. 269–296.

402. REAVEN, E. P., and G. M. REAVEN. Structure and function changes in the endocrine pancreas of aging rats with reference to the modulating effects of exercise and caloric restriction. *J. Clin. Invest.* 68: 75–84, 1981.

403. REITHMANN, C., P. GIERSCHIK, U. MÜLLER, K. WERDAN, and K. H. JAKOBS. Pseudomonas exotoxin A prevents β-adrenoceptor-induced upregulation of Gi protein α-subunits and adenylyl cyclase desensitization in rat heart muscle cells. *Mol. Pharmacol.* 37: 631–638, 1990.

404. REITHMANN, C., P. GIERSCHIK, D. SIDIROPOULOS, K. WERDAN, and K. H. JAKOBS. Mechanism of noradrenaline-induced heterologous desensitization of adenylate cyclase stimulation in rat heart muscle cells: increase in the level of inhibitory G-protein α-subunits. *Eur. J. Pharmacol.* 172: 211–221, 1989.

405. REMINGTON, J. W. The physiology of the aorta and major arteries. In: *Handbook of Physiology. Circulation II,* edited by W. F. Hamilton and P. Dow. Washington, DC: American Physiological Society, 1963, p. 808.

406. RENEMAN, R. S., T. VAN MERODE, P. HICK, and A. P. G. HOEKS. Flow velocity patterns in and distensibility of the carotid artery bulb in subjects of various ages. *Circulation* 71: 500–509, 1985.

407. RENEMAN, R. S., T. VAN MERODE, and A. P. G. HOEKS. Noninvasive assessment of arterial flow patterns and wall properties in humans. *News Physiol. Sci.* 4: 185–190, 1989.

408. RENLUND, D. G., G. GERSTENBLITH, J. L. FLEG, L. C. BECKER, and E. G. LAKATTA. Interaction between left ventricular end-diastolic and end-systolic volumes in normal humans. *Am. J. Physiol.* 258 (*Heart Circ. Physiol.* 29): H473–H481, 1990.

409. RENLUND, D. G., G. GERSTENBLITH, R. J. RODEHEFFER, J. L. FLEG, and E. K. LAKATTA. Potency of the Frank Starling reverse in normal man [Abstract]. *J. Am. Coll. Cardiol.* 5: 514, 1985.

410. RERYCH, S. K., P. M. SCHOLZ, D. C. SABISTON, JR., and R. H. JONES. Effects of exercise training on left ventricular function in normal subjects: a longitudinal study by radionuclide angiography. *Am. J. Cardiol.* 45: 244–252, 1990.

411. RICH, K. A., J. CODINA, G. FLOYD, R. SEKURA, J. D. HILDEBRANDT, and R. IYENGAR. Glucagon-induced heterologous desensitization of MDCK cell adenylyl cyclase. Increase in the apparent levels of the inhibitory regulator (Ni). *J. Biol. Chem.* 259: 7893–7901, 1984.

412. RICHARDSON, D. Effects of age on cutaneous circulatory response to direct heat on the forearm. *J. Gerontol.: Med. Sci.* 44: M189–M194, 1989.

413. RIEGGER, G. A., D. ELSNER, E. P. KROMER, C. DAFFNER, W. G. FORSSMANN, F. MUDERS, E. W. PASCHER, and K. KOCHSIEK. Atrial natriuretic peptide in congestive heart failure in the dog: plasma levels, cyclic guanosine monophosphate, ultrastructure of atrial myoendocrine cells, and hemodynamic, hormonal, and renal effects. *Circulation* 77: 398–406, 1988.

414. ROACH, M. R., and A. C. BURTON. The effect of age on the elasticity of human iliac arteries. *Can. J. Biochem. Physiol.* 37: 557–570, 1959.

415. ROBERT, L., B. ROBERT, and A. M. ROBERT. Molecular biology of elastin as related to aging and atherosclerosis. *Exp. Gerontol.* 5: 339–356, 1970.

416. ROBINSON, S. Experimental studies of physical fitness in relation to age. *Arbeitsphysiologie* 10: 251:323, 1938.

417. ROBINSON, S., D. B. DILL, R. D. ROBINSON, S. P. TZANKOFF, and J. A. WAGNER. Physiological aging of champion runners. *J. Appl. Physiol.* 41: 46–51, 1976.

418. ROCKOFF, J. B., and J. G. DOBSON, JR. Inhibition by adenosine of catecholamine-induced increase in rat atrial contractility. *Am. J. Physiol.* 239 (*Heart Circ. Physiol.* 10): H365–H370, 1980.

419. RODBELL, M. The role of hormone receptors and GTP-regulatory proteins in membrane transduction. *Nature* 284: 17–22, 1980.

420. RODEHEFFER, R. J., G. GERSTENBLITH, E. BEARD, J. L. FLEG, L. C. BECKER, M. L. WEISFELDT, and E. G. LAKATTA. Postural changes in cardiac volumes in men in relation to adult age. *Exp. Gerontol.* 21: 367–378, 1986.

421. RODEHEFFER, R. J., G. GERSTENBLITH, L. C. BECKER, J. L. FLEG, M. L. WEISFELDT, and E. G. LAKATTA. Exercise cardiac output is maintained with advancing age in healthy human subjects: cardiac dilatation and increased stroke volume compensate for a diminished heart rate. *Circulation* 69: 203–213, 1984.

422. ROGERS, M. A., J. M. HAGBERG, W. H. MARTIN, III, A. A. EHSANI, and J. O. HOLLOSZY. Decline in VO_{2max} with aging in master athletes and sedentary men. *J. Appl. Physiol.* 68: 2195–2199, 1990.

423. ROTHBAUM, D. A., D. J. SHAW, C. S. ANGELL, and N. W. SHOCK. Cardiac performance in the unanesthetized senescent male rat. *J. Gerontol.* 28: 287–292, 1973.

424. ROWE, J. W., and B. R. TROEN. Sympathetic nervous system and aging in man. *Endocr. Rev.* 1: 167–179, 1980.

425. RUBIN, P. C., P. J. SCOTT, K. MCLEAN, and J. L. REID. Noradrenaline release and clearance in relation to age and blood pressure in man. *Eur. J. Clin. Invest.* 12: 121–125, 1982.

426. RUCH, S., W.-B. IM, R. H. KENNEDY, E. SEIFEN, and T. AKERA. Aging: stimulation rate of cardiac intracellular Na^+ activity and developed tension. *Mech. Ageing Dev.* 60: 303–313, 1991.

427. RUPP, H. The adaptive changes in the isoenzyme pattern of myosin from hypertrophied rat myocardium as a result of pressure overload and physical training. *Basic Res. Cardiol.* 76: 79–88, 1981.

428. SAFAR, M. E., J. J. TOTO-MOUKOUO, J. A. BOUTHIER, R. E. ASMAR, J. A. LEVENSON, A. C. SIMON, and G. M. LONDON. Arterial dynamics, cardiac hypertrophy, and antihypertensive treatment. *Circulation* 75: I156–I161, 1987.

429. SAGAWA, K. The ventricular pressure–volume diagram revisited. *Circ. Res.* 43: 678–687, 1978.

430. SAGAWA, K. Editorial: The pressure–volume relation of the ventricle: definition, modifications and clinical use. *Circulation* 63: 1223–1227, 1981.

431. SAKAI, M., R. S. DANZIGER, J. M. STADDON, E. G. LAKATTA, and R. G. HANSFORD. Decrease with senescence in the norepinephrine-induced phosphorylation of myofilament proteins in isolated rat cardiac myocytes. *J. Mol. Cell. Cardiol.* 21: 1327–1336, 1989.

432. SAKAI, M., R. S. DANZIGER, R.-P. XIAO, H. A. SPURGEON, and E. G. LAKATTA. Contractile response of individual cardiac myocytes to norepinephrine declines with senescence. *Am. J. Physiol.* 262 (*Heart Circ. Physiol.* 33): H184–H189, 1992.

433. SCAMPS, F., E. MAYOUX, D. CHARLEMAGNE, and G. VASSORT. Calcium current in single cells isolated from normal and hypertrophied rat heart. Effect of beta-adrenergic stimulation. *Circ. Res.* 67: 199–208, 1990.

434. SCARPACE, P. J. Decreased β-adrenergic responsiveness during senescence. *Fed. Proc.* 45: 51–54, 1986.

435. SCARPACE, P. J. Decreased receptor activation with age. Can it be explained by desensitization? *J. Am. Geriatr. Soc.* 36: 1067–1071, 1988.

436. SCARPACE, P. J. Forskolin activation of adenylate cyclase in rat myocardium with age: effects of guanine nucleotide analogs. *Mech. Ageing Dev.* 52: 169–178, 1990.

437. SCARPACE, P. J., and I. B. ABRASS. Decreased beta-adrenergic agonist affinity and adenylate cyclase activity in senescent rat lung. *J. Gerontol.* 38: 143–147, 1983.

438. SCARPACE, P. J., and I. B. ABRASS. Beta-adrenergic agonist-mediated desensitization in senescent rats. *Mech. Ageing Dev.* 35: 255–264, 1986.

439. SCARPACE, P. J., and L. A. BARESI. Increased beta-adrenergic receptors in the light-density membrane fraction in lungs from senescent rats. *J. Gerontol.* 43: B163–B167, 1988.

440. SCHAFFER, S. W., S. ALLO, S. PUMMA, and T. WHITE. Defective response to cAMP-dependent protein kinase in non-insulin-dependent diabetic heart. *Am. J. Physiol.* 261 (*Endocrinol. Metab.* 24): E369–E376, 1991.

441. SCHAFFER, S. W., M. S. MOZAFFARI, M. ARTMAN, and G. L. WILSON. Basis for myocardial mechanical defects associated with non-insulin-dependent diabetes. *Am. J. Physiol.* 256 (*Endocrinol. Metab.* 19): E25–E30, 1989.

442. SCHEUER, J., A. MALHOTRA, C. HIRSCH, J. CAPASSO, and T. F. SCHAIBLE. Physiologic cardiac hypertrophy corrects contractile protein abnormalities associated with pathologic hypertrophy in rats. *J. Clin. Invest.* 70: 1300–1305, 1982.

443. SCHIAFFINO, S., J. L. SAMUEL, D. SASSOON, A. M. LOMPRE, I. GARNER, F. MAROTT, M. BUCKINGHAM, L. RAPPAPORT, and K. SCHWARTZ. Non-synchronous accumulation of α_1 skeletal actin and β-myosin heavy chain mRNAs during early stages of pressure-overload-induced cardiac hypertrophy demonstrated by in situ hybridization. *Circ. Res.* 64: 937–948, 1989.

444. SCHNEIDER, M. D., and T. G. PARKER. Cardiac myocytes as targets for the action of peptide growth factors. *Circulation* 81: 1443–1456, 1990.

445. SCHOCKEN, D. D., J. A. BLUMENTHAL, S. PORT, P. HINDLE, and R. E. COLEMAN. Physical conditioning and left ventricular performance in the elderly: assessment by radionuclide angiocardiography. *Am. J. Cardiol.* 52: 359–364, 1983.

446. SCHOEFFTER, P., and J.-C. STOCLET. Age-related differences in cyclic AMP metabolism and their consequences on relaxation induced by isoproterenol and phosphodiesterase inhibitors in rat isolated aorta. *Mech. Ageing Dev.* 54: 197–205, 1990.

447. SCHRADER, J., G. BAUMANN, and E. GERLACH. Adenosine as inhibitor of myocardial effects of catecholamines. *Pflugers Arch.* 372: 29–35, 1977.

448. SCHULMAN, S., E. G. LAKATTA, J. L. FLEG, L. LAKATTA, L. C. BECKER, and G. GERSTENBLITH. Age-related decline in left ventricular filling at rest and exercise. *Am. J. Physiol.* 263 (*Heart Circ. Physiol.* 34): H1932–H1938, 1992.

449. SCHULMAN, S. P., J. L. WEISS, L. C. BECKER, S. O. GOTTLIEB, K. M. WOODRUFF, M. L. WEISFELDT, and G. GERSTENBLITH. The effects of antihypertensive therapy on left ventricular mass in elderly patients. *N. Engl. J. Med.* 322: 1350–1356, 1990.

450. SCHUYLER, G. T., and L. R. YARBROUGH. Comparison of myosin and creatine kinase isoforms in left ventricles of young and senescent Fischer 344 rats after treatment with triiodothyronine. *Mech. Ageing Dev.* 56: 39–48, 1990.

451. SCHWARTZ, J. B., W. J. GIBB, and T. TRAN. Aging effects on heart rate variation. *J. Gerontol.: Med. Sci.* 46: M99–M106, 1991.

452. SCHWARTZ, K., A. M. LOMPRE, D. DE LA BASTIE, and J. J. MERCADIER. Mechanogenic transduction in the hypertrophied heart [Abstract]. *J. Mol. Cell. Cardiol.* 21(suppl. III): S.24, 1989.

453. SCOTT, P. J., and J. L. REID. The effect of age on the responses of human isolated arteries to noradrenaline. *Br. J. Clin. Pharmacol.* 13: 237–239, 1982.

454. SEALS, D. R., and P. B. CHASE. Influence of physical training on heart rate variability and baroreflex circulatory control. *J. Appl. Physiol.* 66: 1886–1895, 1989.

455. SEALS, D. R., J. M. HABERG, B. F. HURLEY, A. A. EHSANI, and J. O. HOLLOSZY. Endurance training in older men and women. I. Cardiovascular responses to exercise. *J. Appl. Physiol.* 57: 1024–1029, 1984.

456. SEIDMAN, C. E. Expression of atrial natriuretic factor in the normal and hypertrophied heart. *Heart Failure* 5: 130–134, 1989.

457. SELIGMAN, M., R. F. EILBERG, and L. FISHMAN. Mineralization of elastin extracted from human aortic tissues. *Calcif. Tiss. Res.* 17: 229–234, 1975.

458. SHANNON, R. P., K. A. MAHER, J. T. SANTINGA, H. D. ROYAL, and J. Y. WEI. Comparison of differences in the hemodynamic response to passive postural stress in healthy subjects > 70 years and < 30 years of age. *Am. J. Cardiol.* 67: 1110–1116, 1991.

459. SHANNON, R. P., J. Y. WEI, R. M. ROSA, F. H. EPSTEIN, and J. W. ROWE. The effect of age and sodium depletion on cardiovascular response to orthostasis. *Hypertension* 8: 438–443, 1986.

460. SHECHTER, J. A., T. D. FRIEHLING, C. UBOH, G. J. KELLIHER, K. M. O'CONNOR, and P. R. KOWEY. The effect of left ventricular hypertrophy on inducible ventricular arrhythmias [Abstract]. *Circulation* 70: II-234, 1984.

461. SHIMADA, K., T. KITAZUMI, N. SADAKANE, H. OGURA, and T. OZAWA. Age-related changes of baroreflex function, plasma norepinephrine, and blood pressure. *Hypertension* 7: 113–117, 1985.

462. SHIVERICK, C. T., B. B. HAMRELL, and N. R. ALPERT. Structural and functional properties of myosin associated with the compensatory cardiac hypertrophy in the rabbit. *J. Mol. Cell. Cardiol.* 8: 837–851, 1976.

463. SHREINER, D. P., M. L. WEISFELDT, and N. W. SHOCK. Effects of age, sex, and breeding status on the rat heart. *Am. J. Physiol.* 217: 176–180, 1969.

464. SIBLEY, D. R., and R. J. LEFKOWITZ. Molecular mechanisms of receptor desensitization using the β-adrenergic receptor-coupled adenylate cyclase system as a model. *Nature* 317: 124–129, 1985.

465. SIMON, A. C., J. A. LEVENSON, J. L. BOUTHIER, and M. E. SAFAR. Captopril-induced changes in large arteries in essential hypertension. *Am. J. Med.* 76: 71–75, 1984.

466. SIMPSON, D. M., and R. WICKS. Spectral analysis of heart rate indicated reduced baroreceptor-related heart rate variability in elderly persons. *J. Gerontol.: Med. Sci.* 43: M21–M24, 1988.

467. SIMPSON, P. Stimulation of hypertrophy of cultured neonatal rat heart cells through an α_1-adrenergic receptor interaction. Evidence for independent regulation of growth beating. *Circ. Res.* 56: 884–894, 1985.

468. SIMPSON, P. C., Molecular mechanisms in myocardial hypertrophy. *Heart Failure* 5: 113–129, 1989a.

469. SIMPSON, P. C. Proto-oncogenes and cardiac hypertrophy. *Ann. Rev. Physiol.* 51: 189–202, 1989b.

470. SIRI, F. M., J. KUREGER, C. NORDIN, Z. MING, and R. S. ARONSON. Depressed intracellular calcium transients and contraction in myocytes from hypertrophied and failing guinea pig hearts. *Am. J. Physiol.* 261 (*Heart Circ. Physiol.* 32): H514–H530, 1991.

471. SJÖGREN, A. L. Left ventricular wall thickness determined by ultrasound in 100 subjects without heart disease. *Chest* 60: 341–346, 1971.

472. SMITH, J. J., and C. J. M. PORTH. Age and response to orthostatic stress. In: *Circulatory Response to the Upright Posture*, edited by J. J. Smith. Boca Raton: FL: CRC Press, 1990, p. 1–46.

473. SMITH, J. J., J. A. BARNEY, L. GROBAN, A. STADNICKS, and T. J. EBERT. Carotid–cardiac baroreflex responses decrease with early aging in man [Abstract]. *Fed. Proc.* 44: 1887, 1985.

474. SMITH, M. L., and P. B. RAVEN. Cardiovascular responses to lower body negative pressure in endurance and static exercise-trained men. *Med. Sci. Sports Exerc.* 18: 545–550, 1986.

475. SMITH, M. L., H. M. GRAITZER, D. L. HUDSON, and P. B. RAVEN. Baroreflex function in endurance- and static exercise-trained men. *J. Appl. Physiol.* 64: 585–591, 1988.

476. SMITH, S. A., and J. J. FASLER. Age-related changes in autonomic function: relationship with postural hypotension. *Age Ageing* 12: 206–210, 1983.

477. SMITH, V. E., G. H. RUTAN, and L. H. KULLER. LV mass is best predicted by systolic ambulatory blood pressure in the elderly [Abstract]. *J. Am. Coll. Cardiol.* 17: 269A.

478. SMITH, V. E., P. SCHULMAN, M. K. KARIMEDDINI, W. B. WHITE, M. K. MEERAN, and A. M. KATZ. Rapid ventricular filling in left ventricular hypertrophy II. Pathologic hypertrophy. *J. Am. Coll. Cardiol.* 5: 869–874, 1985.

479. SMITH, V. E., W. B. WHITE, and M. K. KARMEDDINI. Echocardiographic assessment of left ventricular diastolic performance in hypertensive subjects: correlation with changes in left ventricular mass. *Hypertension* 9(suppl. 2): II81–II84, 1987.

480. SMULYAN, H., T. J. CSERMELY, S. MOOKHERJEE, and R. A. WARNER. Effect of age on arterial distensibility in asymptomatic humans. *Arteriosclerosis* 3: 199–205, 1983.

481. SOWERS, J. R., and P. K. MOHANTY. Effect of advancing age on cardiopulmonary baroreceptor function in hypertensive men. *Hypertension* 10: 274–279, 1987.

482. SOWERS, J. R., L. Z. RUBENSTEIN, and N. STERN. Plasma norepinephrine responses to posture and isometric exercise increase with age in the absence of obesity. *J. Gerontol.* 38: 315–317, 1983.

483. SPINA, R. J., R. OGAWA, W. M. KOHRT, W. H. MARTIN, III, J. O. HOLLOSZY, and A. A. EHSANI. Differences in cardiovascular adaptations to endurance exercise training between older men and women. *J. Appl. Physiol.* 75: 849–855.

484. SPIRITO, P., and B. J. MARON. Influence of aging on Doppler echocardiographic indices on left ventricular diastolic function. *Br. Heart J.* 59: 672–679, 1988.

485. SPURGEON, H. A., duBell, M. BOYETT, A. TALO, M. C. CAPOGROSSI, and E. G. LAKATTA. Cytosolic Ca^{2+} modulation of membrane potential during a heart beat: perspectives from the

single cardiac cell [Abstract]. *J. Mol. Cell. Cardiol.* 21: S.19, 1989.
486. SPURGEON, H. A., M. F. STEINBACH, and E. G. LAKATTA. Chronic exercise prevents characteristic age-related changed in rat cardiac contraction. *Am. J. Physiol.* 244 (*Heart Circ. Physiol.* 15): H513–H518, 1983.
487. SPURGEON, H. A., P. R. THORNE, F. C. P. YIN, N. W. SHOCK, and M. F. WEISFELDT. Increased dynamic stiffness of trabeculae carneae from senescent rats. *Am. J. Physiol.* 232 (*Heart Circ. Physiol.* 3): H373–380, 1977.
488. STARKE, K. Regulation of noradrenaline release by presynaptic receptor systems. *Rev. Physiol. Biochem. Pharmacol.* 77: 1–124, 1977.
489. STARNES, J. W., and W. L. RUMSEY. Cardiac energetics and performance of exercised and food-restricted rats during aging. *Am. J. Physiol.* 254 (*Heart Circ. Physiol.* 25): H599–H608, 1988.
490. STARNES, J. W., R. E. BEYER, and D. W. EDINGTON. Myocardial adaptations to endurance exercise in aged rats. *Am. J. Physiol.* 245 (*Heart Circ. Physiol.* 16): H560–H566, 1983.
491. STEINNHAGEN-THEISSEN, E., A. Z. REZNICK, and J. D. RINGE. Age dependent variations in cardiac and skeletal muscle during short and long term transmill-running of mice. *Eur. Heart J.* 5(suppl. E): 37–30, 1984.
492. STERN, M. D., A. A. KORT, G. M. BHATNAGER, and E. G. LAKATTA. Scattered-light intensity fluctuations in diastolic rat cardiac muscle caused by spontaneous Ca^{++}-dependent cellular mechanical oscillations. *J. Gen. Physiol.* 82: 119–153, 1983.
493. STESSMAN, J., R. ELIAKIM, C. CAHAN, and R. P. EBSTEIN. Deterioration of beta-receptor-adenylate cyclase function in elderly, hospitalized patients. *J. Gerontol.* 39: 667–672, 1984.
494. STRANDELL, T. Heart volume and its relation to anthropometric data in old men compared with young men. *Acta Med. Scand.* 176: 205–218, 1964a.
495. STRANDELL, T. Total haemoglobin, blood volume and haemoglobin concentration at rest and circulatory adaptation during exercise in relation to some anthropometric data in old men compared with young men. *Acta Med. Scand.* 176: 219–232, 1964b.
496. STRANDELL, T. Circulatory studies on healthy old men. With special reference to the limitation of the maximal physical working capacity. *Acta Med. Scand.* 175(414): 1–44, 1964c.
497. STRASSER, R. H., R. A. CERIONE, J. CODINA, M. G. CARON, and R. J. LEFKOWITZ. Homologous desensitization of the beta-adrenergic receptor. Functional integrity of the desensitized receptor from mammalian lung. *Mol. Pharmacol.* 28: 237–245, 1985.
498. STRASSER, R. H., D. R. SIBLEY, and R. J. LEFKOWITZ. A novel catecholamine-activated adenosine cyclic 3′,5′-phosphate independent pathway for β-adrenergic receptor phosphorylation in wild-type and mutant S_{49} lymphoma cells: mechanism of homologous desensitization of adenylate cyclase. *Biochemistry* 25: 1371–1377, 1986.
499. STRASSER, R. H., G. L. STILES, and R. J LEFKOWITZ. Translocation and uncoupling of the beta-adrenergic receptor in rat lung after catecholamine promoted desensitization in vivo. *Endocrinology* 115: 1392–1400, 1984.
500. STRATTON, J. R., M. D. CERQUERIRA, R. S. SCHWARTZ, W. C. LEVY, R. C. VEITH, S. E. KAHN, and I. B. ABRASS. Differences in cardiovascular responses to isoproterenol in relation to age and exercise training in healthy men. *Circulation* 86: 504–512, 1992.
501. STREHLER, B. L., D. D. MARK, A. S. MILDVAN, and M. V. GEE. Rate and magnitude of age pigment accumulation in the human myocardium. *J. Gerontol.* 14: 430–439, 1959.
502. SULLIVAN, M. J., F. R. COBB, and M. B. HIGGINBOTHAM. Stroke volume increases by similar mechanisms during upright exercise in normal men and women. *Am. J. Cardiol.* 67: 1405–1412, 1991.
503. SUNAGAWA, K., W. L. MAUGHAN, and K. SAGAWA. Optimal arterial resistance for the maximal stroke work studied in isolated canine left ventricle. *Circ. Res.* 56: 586–595, 1985.
504. SUPIANO, M. A., O. A. LINARES, J. B. HALTER, K. M. RENO, and S. G. ROSEN. Functional uncoupling of the platelet α_2-adrenergic receptor-adenylate cyclase complex in the elderly. *J. Clin. Endocrinol. Metab.* 64: 1160–1164, 1987.
505. SUPIANO, M. A., R. R. NEUBIG, O. A. LINARES, J. B. HALTER, and S. G. ROSEN. Effects of low-sodium diet on regulation of platelet α_2-adrenergic receptors in young and elderly humans. *Am. J. Physiol.* 256 (*Endocrinol. Metab.* 19): E399–E344, 1989.
506. SUTTON, M. S., S. N. REICHEK, J. LOVETT, J. A. KASTOR, and E. GUILIANI. Effects of age, body size and blood pressure on the normal human left ventricle [Abstract]. *Circulation* 62: III-305, 1980.
507. SWINNE, C. J., E. P. SHAPIRO, S. D. LIMA, and J. L. FLEG. Age-associated changes in left ventricular diastolic performance during isometric exercise in normal subjects. *Am. J. Cardiol.* 69: 823–826, 1992.
508. SWYNGHEDAUW, B. Remodelling of the heart in response to chronic mechanical overload. *Eur. Heart J.* 10: 935–943, 1989.
509. TAFFET, G. E., and C. A. TATE. The sarcoplasmic reticulum calcium ATPase from rat heart is decreased in senescence [Abstract]. *Gerontologist* 30: 111A, 1990.
510. TAKAHASHI, T., H. SCHUNKERT, S. ISOYAMA, J. Y. WEI, B. NADAL-GINARD, W. GROSSMAN, and S. IZUMO. Age-related differences in the expression of proto-oncogene and contractile protein genes in response to pressure overload in the rat myocardium. *J. Clin. Invest.* 89: 939–946, 1992.
511. TANKERSLEY, C. G., J. SMOLANDER, W. L. KENNEDY, and S. M. FORTNEY. Sweating and skin blood flow during exercise: effects of age and maximal oxygen uptake. *J. Appl. Physiol.* 71: 236–242, 1991.
512. TATE, C. A., G. E. TAFFET, E. K. HUDSON, S. L. BLAYLOCK, R. P. MCBRIDE, and L. H. MICHAEL. Enhanced calcium uptake of cardiac sarcoplasmic reticulum in exercise-trained old rats. *Am. J. Physiol.* 258 (*Heart Circ. Physiol.* 29): H431–H435, 1990.
513. TAWNEY, K. W., E. C. JOHNSON, and E. R. GREENE. Age-related differences in reactivity of the central circulation to head-up tilt [Abstract]. *Physiologist* 31: A130, 1988.
514. TAYLOR, D. J., M. CROWE, P. J. BORE, P. STYLES, D. L. ARNOLD, and G. K. RADDA. Examination of the energetics of aging skeletal muscle using nuclear magnetic resonance. *Gerontology* 30: 2–7, 1984.
515. TAYLOR, J. A., G. A. HAND, D. G. JOHNSON, and D. R. SEALS. Augmented forearm vasoconstriction during dynamic exercise in healthy older men. *Circulation* 86: 1789–1799, 1992.
516. TEMPLETON, G. H., M. R. PLATT, J. T. WILLERSON, and M.L. WEISFELDT. Influence of aging on left ventricular hemodynamics and stiffness in beagles. *Circ. Res.* 44: 189–194, 1979.
517. TING, C. T., K. P. BRIN, S. J. LIN, S. P. WANG, M. S. CHANG, B. N. CHIANG, and F. C. YIN. Arterial hemodynamics in human hypertension. *J. Clin. Invest.* 78: 1462–1471, 1986.
518. TODA, N., and M. MIYAZAKI. Senescent beagle coronary arteries in response to catecholamines and adrenergic nerve stimulation. *J. Gerontol.* 42: 210–218, 1987.
519. TOMANEK, R. J. Effects of age and exercise on the extent of the myocardial capillary bed. *Anat. Rec.* 167: 55–62, 1970.
520. TOMANEK, R. J., and J. M. HOVANEC. The effects of long-term pressure-overload and aging on the myocardium. *J. Mol. Cell. Cardiol.* 13: 471–488, 1981.
521. TOMANEK, R. J., and U. L. KARLSSON. Myocardial ultrastructure of young and senescent rats. *J. Ultrastruc. Res.* 42: 201–220, 1973.

522. TOPOL, E. J., T. A. TRAILL, and N. J. FORTUIN. Hypertensive hypertrophic cardiomyopathy of the elderly. *N. Engl. J. Med.* 312: 277–183, 1985.

523. TRAVIS, D. F., and A. TRAVIS. Ultrasound changes in the left ventricular rat myocardial cells with age. *J. Ultrastruct. Res.* 39: 124–148, 1972.

524. TSUJIMOTO, G., C.-H. LEE, and B. B HOFFMAN. Age-related decrease in beta adrenergic receptor-mediated vascular smooth muscle relaxation. *J. Pharmacol. Exp. Ther.* 239: 411–415, 1986.

525. TZANKOFF, S. P., and A. H. NORRIS. Effect of muscle mass decrease on age-related BMR changes. *J. Appl. Physiol.* 43: 1001–1006, 1977.

526. UNVERFERTH, D. V., J. K. FETTERS, B. J. UNVERFERTH, C. V. LEIER, R. D. MAGORIEN, A. R. ARN, and P. B. BAKER. Human myocardial histologic characteristics in congestive heart failure. *Circulation* 68: 1194–1200, 1983.

527. VAITKEVICIUS, P. V., J. L. FLEG, J. H. ENGEL, F. C. O'CONNOR, J. G. WRIGHT, L. E. LAKATTA, F. C.-P. YIN, and E. G. LAKATTA. Efects of age and aerobic capacity on arterial stiffness in healthy adults. *Circulation* 88: 1456–1462, 1993.

528. VAN BRUMMELEN, P., F. R. BUHLER, W. KIOWSKI, and F. W. AMANN. Age-related decrease in cardiac and peripheral vascular responsiveness to isoprenaline: studies in normal subjects. *Clin. Sci.* 60: 571–577, 1981.

529. VANTOSH, A., E. G. LAKATTA, J. L. FLEG, J. WEISS, C. KALLMAN, M. WEISFELDT, and G. GERSTENBLITH. Ventricular dimensional changes during submaximal exercise: effect of aging in normal man [Abstract]. *Circulation* 62: III-129, 1980.

530. VEITH, R. C., J. D. BEST, and J. B. HALTER. Dose-dependent suppression of norepinephrine appearance rate in plasma by clonidine in man. *J. Clin. Endocrinol. Metab.* 59: 151–155, 1984.

531. VENTURA-CLAPIER, R., H. MEKHFI, P. OLIVIERO, and B. SWYNGHEDAUW. Pressure overload changes cardiac skinned-fiber mechanics in rats, not in guinea pigs. *Am. J. Physiol.* 254 (*Heart Circ. Physiol.* 25): H517–524, 1988.

532. VERKHRATSKY, N. S. Acetylcholine metabolism peculiarities in aging. *Exp. Gerontol.* 5: 49–56, 1970.

533. VESTAL, R. E., A. J. H. WOOD, and D. G. SHAND. Reduced beta-adrenoreceptor sensitivity in the elderly. *Clin. Pharmacol. Ther.* 26: 181–186, 1979.

534. VIZEK, M., and I. ALBRECHT. Development of cardiac output in male rats. *Physiol. Bohemoslov.* 22: 573–580, 1973.

535. VON HARSDORF, R., R. E. LANG, M. FULLERTON, and E. A. WOODCOCK. Myocardial stretch stimulates phosphatidylinositol turnover. *Circ. Res.* 65: 494–501, 1989.

536. VOUTILAINEN, S., M. KUPARI, M. HIPPELAINEN, K. KARPPINEN, M. VENTILA, and J. HEIKKILA. Factors influencing Doppler indexes of left ventricular filling in healthy persons. *Am. J. Cardiol.* 68: 653–659, 1991.

537. WAHREN, J., B. SALTIN, L. JORFELDT, and B. PERNOW. Influence of age on the local circulatory adaptation to leg exercise. *Scand. J. Clin. Lab. Invest.* 33: 79–86, 1974.

538. WALFORD, G. D., H. A. SPURGEON, and E. G. LAKATTA. Diminished cardiac hypertrophy and muscle performance in older compared to younger adult rats with chronic atrioventricular block. *Circ. Res.* 63: 502–511, 1988.

539. WALKER K. E., and S. R. HOUSER. Intracellular calcium buffers affect age-related calcium current decay [Abstract]. *Circulation* 82: III-746, 1990.

540. WALKER, K. E., E. G. LAKATTA, and S. R. HOUSER. Age associated changes in membrane currents in rat ventricular myocytes. *Cardiovasc. Res.* 27: 1968–1977, 1993.

541. WALLER, B. F., and W. C. ROBERTS. Cardiovascular disease in the very elderly. Analysis of 40 necropsy patients ages 90 years or over. *Am. J. Cardiol.* 51: 403–421, 1983.

542. WATKINS, S. C., J. L. SAMUEL, F. MAROTTE, B. BERTIER-SAVALLE, and L. RAPPAPORT. Microtubules and desmin filaments during onset of heart hypertrophy in rat: a double immunoelectron microscope study. *Circ. Res.* 60: 327–336, 1987.

543. WATSON, P. A., T. HANEDA, and H. E. MORGAN. Effect of higher aortic pressure on ribosome formation and cAMP content in rat heart. *Am. J. Physiol.* 256 (*Cell Physiol.* 25): C1257–C1261, 1989.

544. WEI, J. Y., Y. X. LI, T. LINCOLN, W. GROSSMAN, and D. MENDELOWITZ. Chronic exercise training protects aged cardiac muscle against hypoxia. *J. Clin. Invest.* 83: 778–784, 1989.

545. WEI, J. Y., H. A. SPURGEON, and E. G. LAKATTA. Excitation–contraction in rat myocardium: alterations with adult aging. *Am. J. Physiol.* (*Heart Circ. Physiol.* 17): H784–H791, 1984.

546. WEINBERGER, M. H., and N. S. FINEBERG. Sodium and volume sensitivity of blood pressure. Age and pressure change over time. *Hypertension* 18: 67–71, 1991.

547. WEISFELDT, M. L., W. A. LOEVEN, and N. W. SHOCK. Resting and active mechanical properties of trabeculae carneae from aged male rats *Am. J. Physiol.* 220: 1921–1927, 1971.

548. WEISFELDT, M. L., J. R. WRIGHT, D. P. SHREINER, E. LAKATTA, and N. W. SHOCK. Coronary flow and oxygen extraction in the perfused heart of senescent male rats. *J. Appl. Physiol.* 30: 44–49, 1971.

549. WILENS, S. L., and E. E. SPROUL. Spontaneous cardiovascular disease in the rat. *Am. J. Pathol.* 14: 177–216, 1938.

550. WILSON, J. R., P. DOUGLAS, W. F. HICKEY, V. LANOCOE, N. FERRARO, A. MUHAMMAD, and N. REICHEK. Experimental congestive heart failure produced by rapid ventricular pacing in the dog: cardiac effects. *Circulation* 75: 857–867, 1987.

551. WISENBAUGH, T., P. ALLEN, G. COOPER, IV, W. N. O'CONNOR, L. MEZAROS, R. STRETER, A. BAHINSKI, S. HOUSER, and J. F. SPANN. Hypertrophy without contractile dysfunction after reversal of pressure overload in the cat. *Am. J. Physiol.* 247 (*Heart Circ. Physiol.* 18): H146–H154, 1984.

552. WOLF, H., and F. HOFMANN. Purification of myosin light chain kinase from bovine cardiac muscle. *Proc. Natl. Acad. Sci. U.S.A.* 77: 5852–5855, 1980.

553. WOLINSKY, H. Long-term effects of hypertension on the rat aortic wall and their relation to concurrent aging changes. Morphological and chemical studies. *Circ. Res.* 30: 301–309, 1972.

554. WOODCOCK, E. A., J. W. FUNDER, and C. I. JOHNSTON. Decreased cardiac β-adrenergic receptors in deoxycorticosterone-salt and renal hypertensive rats. *Circ. Res.* 45: 560–565, 1979.

555. XIAO, R.-P., and E. G. LAKATTA. Mechanisms of altered β-adrenergic modulation of the cardiovascular system with aging. *Rev. Clin. Gerontol.* 1: 309–322, 1991.

556. XIAO, R.-P., M. C. CAPOGROSSI, H. A. SPURGEON, and E. G. LAKATTA. Stimulation of δ opioid receptors in single heart cells blocks β-adrenergic receptor mediated increase in calcium and contraction [Abstract]. *J. Mol. Cell. Cardiol.* 23(suppl. III): S83, 1991.

557. XIAO, P.-P., H. A. SPURGEON, F. O'CONNOR, and E. G. LAKATTA. Age-associated changes in beta-adrenergic modulation on rat cardiac excitation–contraction coupling. *J. Clin. Invest.* 1994 (in press).

558. YAKOVLEV, V. M. Some data on the functional state of the arterial system in aged persons. *Kardiologiia* 11: 99–103, 1971.

559. YAMADA, Y., E. MIYAJIMA, O. TOCHIKUBO, T. MATSUKAWA, and M. ISHII. Age-related changes in muscle sympathetic nerve activity in essential hypertension. *Hypertension* 13: 870–877, 1989.

560. YAZAKI, Y., and I. KOMURO. Molecular analysis of cardiac hypertrophy due to overload [Abstract]. *J. Mol. Cell. Cardiol.* 21(suppl. III): S.29, 1989.

561. YIN, F. C. P., G. S. RAIZES, T. GUARNIERI, H. A. SPURGEON, E. G. LAKATTA, N. J. FORTUIN, and M. L. WEISFELDT. Age-associated decrease in ventricular response to haemodynamic stress during beta-adrenergic blockade. *Br. Heart J.* 40: 1349–1355, 1978.
562. YIN, F. C. P., H. A. SPURGEON, H. L. GREENE, E. G. LAKATTA, and M. L. WEISFELDT. Age-associated decrease in heart rate response to isoproterenol in dogs. *Mech. Ageing Dev.* 10: 17–25, 1979.
563. YIN, F. C. P., H. A. SPURGEON, and C. H. KALLMAN. Age-associated alterations in viscoelastic properties of canine aortic strips. *Circ. Res.* 53: 464–472, 1983.
564. YIN, F. C. P., H. A. SPURGEON, G. S. RAIZES, H. L. GREENE, M. L. WEISFELDT, and N. W. SHOCK. Age-associated decrease in chrontropic response to isoproterenol [Abstract]. *Circulation* 4(suppl. 2): II-167, 1976.
565. YIN, F. C. P., H. A. SPURGEON, K. RAKUSAN, M. L. WEISFELDT, and E. G. LAKATTA. Use of tibial length to quantify cardiac hypertrophy: application in the aging rat. *Am. J. Physiol.* 243 (*Heart Circ. Physiol.* 14): H941–H947, 1982.
566. YIN, F. C. P., H. A. SPURGEON, M. L. WEISFELDT, and E. G. LAKATTA. Mechanical properties of myocardium from hypertrophied rat hearts. A comparison between hypertrophy induced by senescence and by aortic banding. *Circ. Res.* 46: 292–300, 1980.
567. YIN, F. C. P., M. L. WEISFELDT, and W. R. MILNOR. Role of aortic input impedance in the decreased cardiovascular response to exercise with aging in dogs. *J. Clin. Invest.* 68: 28–38, 1981.
568. YOUNG, J. B., J. W. ROWE, J. A. PALLOTTA, D. SPARROW, and L. LANDSBERG. Enhanced plasma norepinephrine response to upright posture and oral glucose administration in elderly human subjects. *Metabolism* 29: 532–539, 1980.
569. YOUNIS, L. T., J. A. MELIN, A. R. ROBERT, and J. M. R. DETRY. Influence of age and sex on left ventricular volumes and ejection fraction during upright exercise in normal subjects. *Eur. Heart J.* 11: 916–924, 1990.
570. YU, B. P., E. J. MASORO, and C. A. MCMAHAN. Nutritional influences on aging of Fischer 344 rats: I. Physical, metabolic, and longevitiy characteristics. *J. Gerontol.* 40: 657–670, 1985.
571. ZIMAN, B., H. A. SPURGEON, M. D. STERN, and E. G. LAKATTA. A Ca^{2+} myofilament interaction modulates resting length of single rat ventricular myocytes [Abstract]. *Circulation* 82: III-214, 1990.

18. Respiratory system

DAVID SPARROW | *Normative Aging Study, VA Outpatient Clinic, Boston, Massachusetts*
SCOTT T. WEISS | *Channing Laboratory, Harvard Medical School, Boston, Massachusetts*

CHAPTER CONTENTS

Pulmonary Mechanics
    Respiratory muscles and chest wall
    Lung recoil
    Lung volumes
    Flow rates
Gas Exchange
Respiration
    Respiratory control
    Respiratory sensation
Exercise Capacity
Defense Mechanisms
Airway Responsiveness
Natural History of Disease

GROWTH AND DEVELOPMENT OF THE HUMAN LUNG continue until age 20. Following a variable period of stability, many parameters of pulmonary function decline steadily with advancing age. Knowledge of the normal growth and decline of pulmonary function facilitates an understanding of the effects of genetic and environmental factors, particularly cigarette smoking, that can modify normal function.

The role of normal physiological changes and epidemiological risk factors in the decline of pulmonary function with aging and the development of chronic obstructive lung disease are described in this chapter. The discussion focuses on important physiological changes in pulmonary mechanics, gas exchange, respiratory control, exercise capacity, defense mechanisms, and airway responsiveness. These physiological data are integrated with epidemiological risk factors, such as cigarette smoking, to describe aging of the respiratory system.

PULMONARY MECHANICS

Respiratory Muscles and Chest Wall

The respiratory muscles, including the diaphragm, intercostal muscles, and accessory muscles, provide the forces that move the lung and chest wall. It appears that the strength of the respiratory muscles declines moderately with age. Older individuals have both lower maximal inspiratory and expiratory pressures than younger individuals (7, 14, 18). Atrophy, decreased work capability, temporal dispersion within motor units, and increased duration of motor potentials all may influence changes in muscle strength (12, 20, 28). In addition, an age-related increase in pleural elastin may impose an increased elastic load on the respiratory muscles (58).

With advancing age, chest wall compliance also changes. The chest wall begins to stiffen after about 20 yr, and hence its natural tendency to expand outward is inhibited (23, 48). This stiffening has been attributed to age-related changes in the rib cage, particularly calcification of its articulations (64).

Lung Recoil

The lungs and chest wall are bound together by the potential pleural space and function as a bellows. At the end of quiet expiration, when the entire system is at its resting volume, the tendency of the lungs to recoil inwardly from the chest wall is balanced by the tendency of the chest wall to recoil outwardly. In contrast to the chest wall, which stiffens with advancing age, the lung parenchyma becomes more compliant.

Cross-sectional studies have shown a progressive age-related loss of lung elastic recoil after 20–25 yr that results in increased lung compliance (39, 79). This loss of elastic force cannot be accounted for by a loss of collagen or elastin in pulmonary parenchyma (30) or a decrease in the total length and diameter of elastic fibers (53). Alterations in the location and orientation of individual elastic fibers may provide some explanation for the decline in lung elasticity. It is unclear how the aging process influences this remodeling. In addition, it remains unknown how inflammatory processes in the lung, with the attendant release of oxidant and antioxidant enzymes, influences this remodeling process.

Lung Volumes

Decreasing elastic recoil and stiffening of the chest wall with age explain age-related changes in several standard lung volumes and capacities, which are defined as follows: *Total lung capacity* (TLC) is the total amount of air in the lungs following a maximum inspiration.

Residual volume (RV) is the amount of air in the lungs at the end of a maximum expiration. *Vital capacity* is the maximum amount of air expired after a maximum inspiration. The amount of air in the lungs at the end of a quiet expiration is called *functional residual capacity* (FRC).

The relationships between lung volumes and age are depicted in Figure 18.1. TLC remains essentially constant with age after adulthood. In contrast, RV increases during the adult years primarily due to airway collapse at higher lung volumes secondary to the loss of elastic recoil (36), although decreased chest wall compliance or decreased muscle strength may also contribute (45). Vital capacity, therefore, declines slightly, since it is equal to TLC minus RV. FRC represents the point at which the inward elastic recoil of the lungs is balanced by the outward elastic recoil of the chest wall. As lung recoil decreases with advancing age, FRC increases slightly.

Flow Rates

Muscular strength and elastic recoil have an important influence on the flow rate in the lungs, but their effects depend on lung volume (25). When lung volumes are large, both muscular strength and the pressure supplied by lung elastic recoil have a significant impact on flow rate. When a subject is at TLC and makes a forced expiratory maneuver, both contraction of chest wall voluntary muscles and elastic recoil of the lungs provide the force to generate flow until airway narrowing limits further expiratory flow. This phenomenon (*dynamic compression of the airways*) occurs after exhalation of only 20%–30% of the vital capacity. When dynamic compression occurs, the only force preventing further collapse is the driving pressure generated by lung elastic recoil. Age-related loss of elastic recoil may result in the collapse of peripheral airways earlier in the expiratory process. Dynamic compression of the smaller airways in older lungs, therefore, may lead to a decrease in flow at low lung volumes, generating a pattern of airflow obstruction in the small airways similar to that produced by chronic cigarette smoking.

Various indexes of airflow have been shown to decline with age, including *forced vital capacity* (FVC), *forced expiratory volume in 1 s* (FEV_1), and *forced expiratory flow*$_{25-75}$, that is, the flow between 25% and 75% of the vital capacity (FEF_{25-75}) (40). The greatest decline is seen in FEF_{25-75}, reflecting reduced flow at low lung volumes and the primacy of a decrease in elastic recoil. FEV_1 and FVC reflect flows at high lung volumes and thus depend on muscular strength more than on elastic recoil.

Pulmonary function is generally summarized using regression equations that are gender-specific and include age and height as the main independent variables (3). The fit of these regression equations can be assessed with the square of the correlation coefficient (r^2) and the standard error of the estimate (SEE). The amount of variation in the observed data explained by age and height is measured by r^2. SEE is the average standard deviation of the data around the regression line. Distributions of most pulmonary function measures tend to be normal in the middle-age (40–60 yr) range in adults but not at the extremes. Transformation or age stratification may produce more normal distributions. A lower limit of normal, generally taken to be values below the fifth percentile, can be estimated by a regression model. Ideally, reference equations will be derived from a random sample of the nonsmoking, asymptomatic population.

A variety of equations have been developed, but they are based on relatively little data from adolescents and the elderly. The clinical practice of classifying spirometric values less than 80% of predicted values as "abnormal" has no statistical basis in adults. Utilizing some reference equations, 80% of predicted value is close to the fifth percentile; however, use of such a fixed value will tend to increase misclassification of shorter, older subjects as "abnormal" and increase misclassification of taller, younger subjects as "normal."

A recent American Thoracic Society statement, "Lung Function Testing: Selection of Reference Values and Interpretative Strategies," provides a number of acceptable reference equations drawn from a variety of studies (3). No single equation is acceptable over all ages. A survey of pulmonary function laboratories (26) showed

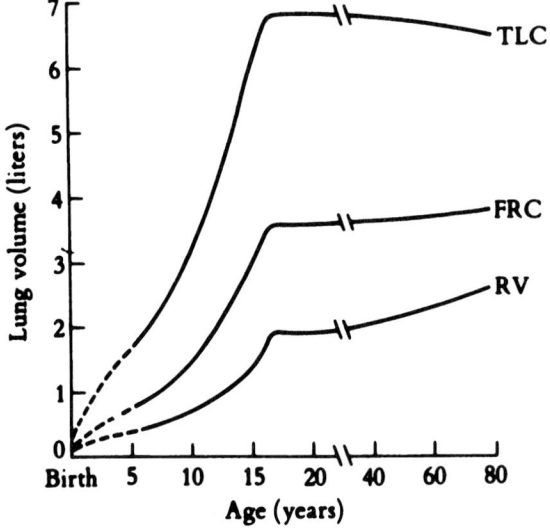

FIG. 18.1. Total lung capacity (TLC), functional residual capacity (FRC), and residual volume (RV) as functions of age from birth to 80 yr for an "average" body build. [Reproduced from Murray (50) with permission.]

TABLE 18.1. *Prediction Equations for FEV_1 and FVC*

Study	Age Range (yr)	Number Studied	FEV_1 Equation	FVC Equation
Men				
Morris et al. (49)	20–84	517	3.62 ht* − 0.032 age − 1.26	5.83 ht* − 0.025 age − 4.24
Enright et al. (19)	65–85	245	3.78 ht* − 0.027 age − 1.73	5.67 ht* − 0.021 age − 4.37
Women				
Morris et al. (49)	20–84	471	3.50 ht* − 0.025 age − 1.93	4.53 ht* − 0.024 age − 2.85
Enright et al. (19)	65–85	532	2.81 ht* − 0.032 age − 0.09	3.65 ht* − 0.033 age − 0.70

*Height measured in meters.

that the most widely used prediction equations for nonsmoking Caucasian men and women are those of Morris et al. (48) (Table 18.1). However, for the elderly, the recently developed reference values of Enright et al. (19) may be more appropriate (Table 18.1).

After accounting for age, height, and gender, 40% of the variability in pulmonary function remains unexplained (3). Racial differences may account for 10% of this variation, with the remainder being unexplained but related to environmental exposures, genetic factors, or past or present health status. Some of these factors, both host and environmental, are discussed later under NATURAL HISTORY OF DISEASE.

GAS EXCHANGE

The exchange of oxygen and carbon dioxide is the main function of the respiratory system. Adequate exchange of gas depends on the close matching of *ventilation* (the amount of air taken into the lungs) to *perfusion* (the amount of blood flow into the lungs). In the normal young lung, ventilation and perfusion are matched very closely, although there are regional variations (82). Because ventilation and, to a greater extent, perfusion increase proceeding from top to bottom in the upright lung, the ratio of ventilation to perfusion ($\dot{V}_A/\dot{Q}$) is greater than one at the apex and less than one at the base. The overall $\dot{V}_A/\dot{Q}$ ratio is close to one.

With advancing age, loss of elastic recoil causes closure of small airways in the lower regions of the lung during the normal respiratory cycle. Inspired gas appears to be preferentially distributed to the upper regions without decreasing blood flow to the lower regions (32). The importance of distributional changes in lung ventilation can be demonstrated by describing the phenomenon of closing volume (Fig. 18.2). If a subject inhales 100% oxygen to TLC and then exhales, the nitrogen concentration in expired gas can be measured (Fig. 18.2). Four separate levels of nitrogen can be identified. Initially (phase 1) the nitrogen concentration in expired gas is zero, because exhaled gas initially comes from the anatomical dead space that is a nongas-exchanging area of the lung. In phase 2, a rapidly rising nitrogen concentration is seen, as this phase represents a mixture of anatomical dead space gas and alveolar gas. In phase 3, a constant nitrogen concentration is detected, as this is pure alveolar gas without any dead space ventilation. Finally (phase 4), there is an abrupt increase in the nitrogen concentration, which signals closure of the airways at the base of the lung coupled with preferential emptying of alveoli at the lung apex, which has a relatively high nitrogen concentration. The reason that alveoli at the apex of the upright lung have a higher nitrogen concentration is that during a vital capacity breath of oxygen, these alveoli expand less, and, therefore, the nitrogen is less diluted by the inspired oxygen. The closing volume is that volume of the lung

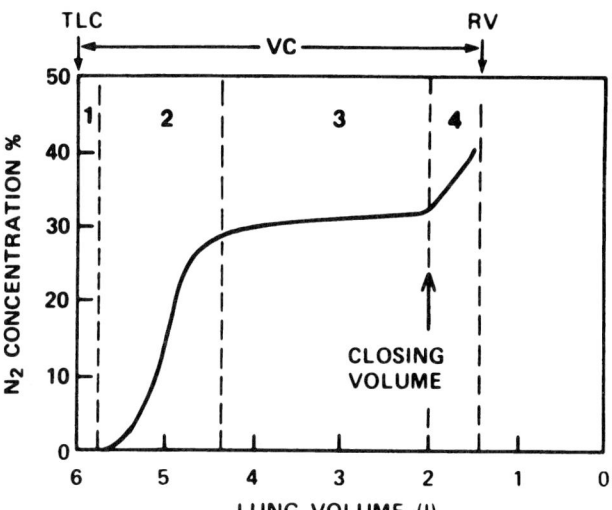

FIG. 18.2. Measurement of the closing volume. If a vital capacity inspiration of 100% O_2 is followed by a full expiration, four phases in the N_2 concentration measured at the lips can be recognized. The last is caused by preferential emptying of the apex of the lung after the lower zone airways have closed. [Reproduced from West (83) with permission.]

at which the dependent airways begin to close and the nitrogen concentration abruptly rises in phase 4.

Age-related changes in the single breath nitrogen washout (Fig. 18.2) include an increase in slope of phase 3 with increasing age, reflecting increasing unhomogeneity of lung unit emptying (9, 17, 65). After age 65 yr the increase in slope of phase 3 may be exponential (65). Closing volume increases steadily with increasing age, representing roughly 15% of the vital capacity in a 30-year-old and increasing steadily to about 30% of vital capacity by age 70 (65). In addition, the closing capacity (closing volume + RV) may exceed the FRC, indicating that closure of terminal airways occurs prior to the end of a normal tidal breath. The physiological reason for the age-related changes in slope of phase 3, closing volume, and closing capacity may be loss of elastic recoil (65). In addition to these age-related changes, there is also a significant increase in dead space ventilation with increasing age (60, 75).

These age-related changes in closing volume, dead space, and slope of phase 3 have important implications for gas exchange in aging subjects. The distributional changes in ventilation result in a further mismatch of ventilation and perfusion that has an adverse effect on arterial oxygenation in the elderly. The influence of age on arterial P_{O_2} has been examined in several studies (46, 51, 66), and results are summarized in Figure 18.3. Among adults there is a small but steady decrease in arterial P_{O_2} of approximately 4 mm Hg for each decade of age. A regression equation describing the change in arterial P_{O_2} (PaO_2) with increasing age for normal adults over age 20 is given by the following formula (E. E. Mays, unpublished observations):

$$PaO_2 = 100.1 - 0.323 \; (age)$$

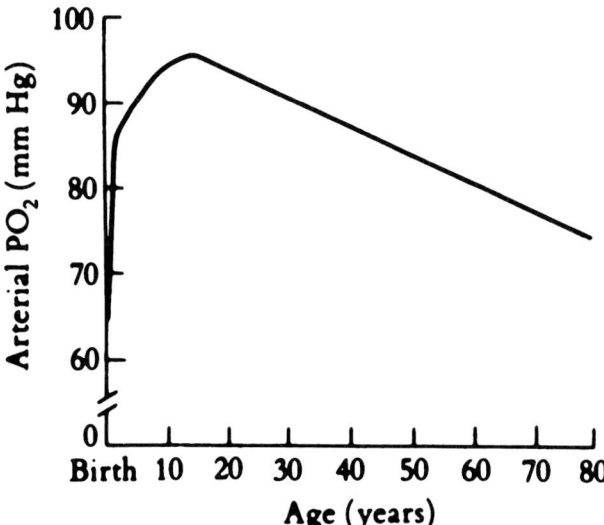

FIG. 18.3. Arterial P_{O_2} as a function of age from birth to 80 yr. [Reproduced from Murray (50) with permission.]

In contrast to arterial P_{O_2}, alveolar P_{O_2} stays constant or increases slightly with age. The most likely explanation for this age-dependent widening of the alveolar–arterial oxygen difference is the functional alteration in ventilation–perfusion dynamics described above. Other factors exacerbating ventilation–perfusion inequalities in older persons include an age-related reduction in cardiac output with a concomitant decrease in mixed venous return.

Gas exchange may also be influenced by lung size and alveolar surface area. Alveolar capillary surface area decreases with increasing age (76, 77). Alveolar septa decrease and alveolar duct diameter increases (52, 78), resulting in a smaller lung. This is confirmed by studies revealing that lung weight at autopsy is approximately 20% lighter in older vs. younger adults (42). The decrease in surface area results in a decreased diffusion capacity for carbon monoxide (29, 49), which may contribute to age-related hypoxemia.

RESPIRATION

Respiratory Control

Respiration is controlled by a complex system of sensors and effectors, with a central controller in the brain stem. The central controller coordinates the information it receives from the sensors and adjusts the activity of the respiratory muscles. The central chemoreceptor, located in the medulla, is responsible for most of the ventilatory responses to hypercapnia. The peripheral chemoreceptors, located in the carotid and aortic bodies in the neck, are responsible for the increase in ventilation that accompanies hypoxemia.

Available data indicate that the ventilatory response to hypercapnia decreases with increasing age (2, 13, 41, 56), which may reflect diminished neural output to the respiratory muscles (56) or altered mechanics of the respiratory system in the elderly (47, 61). However, the response to hypoxia in the elderly is less clear-cut. Some reports have found that the ventilatory response to hypoxia is blunted as well (41, 56), though Chapman and Cherniack (13) failed to confirm this. The reasons for these study differences are unclear but may reflect population selection, biological heterogeneity, differences in test procedure, or variables that are unknown or uncontrolled.

Respiratory Sensation

Young subjects perceive shortness of breath more intensely than older subjects. This is observed in normal subjects (8) and in subjects with asthma (35) in response to a bronchoconstrictive stimulus and is independent of lung function level. Normal older subjects also have a reduction in the capacity to perceive elastic (71) or resistive (1, 72) respiratory loads relative to younger subjects. The reasons for these relationships are unknown but may relate to a decrease in central nervous system (CNS) integrative functions with advancing age.

EXERCISE CAPACITY

Exercise performance, determined by maximal oxygen uptake ($\dot{V}O_{2max}$), reaches a peak in the late teens, is maintained until the mid-twenties, and then gradually declines with advancing age (4, 16, 34). $\dot{V}O_{2max}$ is related to cardiovascular function, muscle mass, and the ability of the muscles to extract and use oxygen. Muscle mass, whether measured by hydrodensitometry or 24-h urinary creatinine excretion, declines with age (15, 21). After adjustment for muscle mass, the age differences in $\dot{V}O_{2max}$ persisted in one study (15) but were attenuated in another (21).

There are several theoretical reasons, quite separate from changes in muscle mass, that might account for a decrease in $\dot{V}O_{2max}$ with age. Both decreased chest wall compliance and increased pleural elastin could contribute to an increased elastic load on the respiratory muscles with age and a decreased $\dot{V}O_{2max}$. An increase in airway resistance could decrease $\dot{V}O_{2max}$. Finally, a decrease in respiratory muscle strength with age could lead to an increased use of accessory muscles and thus a decrease in $\dot{V}O_{2max}$.

DEFENSE MECHANISMS

The lung has a variety of defenses against inhaled chemicals, toxic dust, and microorganisms. Local defense mechanisms involve the epiglottis and upper airway, which prevent aspiration, and the cough reflex, which expels mucus or unwanted material from the lung. Both laryngeal and cough reflexes decline with age (59). There is a marked age-related reduction in sensitivity to inhaled ammonia as a cough stimulus, with older individuals tending to cough less than younger individuals (59). The relationship of decrease in cough and laryngeal reflexes to increased aspiration is still unclear. Factors other than attenuation of reflexes may also be important. It has been observed (using radiopaque disks) that mean tracheal mucus velocity is slower in nonsmoking elderly subjects (27), although, as seen in Figure 18.4, there is considerable overlap between young and older subjects. In view of the seriousness of pneumonia in elderly populations, further effort needs to be directed toward the definition and investigation of the above changes in local defenses.

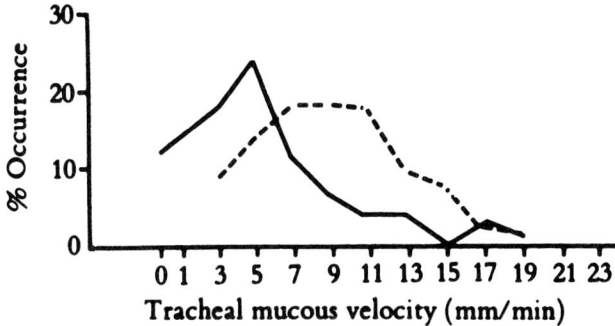

FIG. 18.4. Frequency histogram (percent of total number of analyzed disks) of individual disk velocities in young (*broken line*) and elderly (*solid line*) nonsmokers. [Reproduced from Goodman et al. (27) with permission.]

In addition to these local mechanisms, cellular and humoral immunity play an important role in defending the lung from microorganisms. Specific lung-related changes in immune system function have not been described, though the general immune system changes described in Chapter 21 would contribute to increased susceptibility to acute infection and to autoimmune diseases that accompany the aging process. What remains unknown, however, is the extent to which these immune system changes in and of themselves can account for disease development. Thus there are no data establishing a direct clinical link between these immune system changes and clinical disease.

AIRWAY RESPONSIVENESS

Airway responsiveness is an integrated physiological function that depends on airway epithelium, cells, nerves, and smooth muscle. Airway responsiveness is measured by the decline in pulmonary function from baseline, using a bronchoconstrictor agonist, usually histamine or methacholine. Several studies suggest that airway responsiveness increases after 40 yr in adults (10, 33, 63). The disadvantage of these studies is that none adjusted for the level of pulmonary function. In a recent paper (69), Sparrow and co-workers suggested that after adjustment for level of pulmonary function, smoking status modified the age–airway responsiveness relationship. Specifically, airway responsiveness increased with age only among former smokers.

NATURAL HISTORY OF DISEASE

Knowledge of the normal growth and decline of pulmonary function facilitates an understanding of natural history of disease. Figure 18.5 presents a model of the

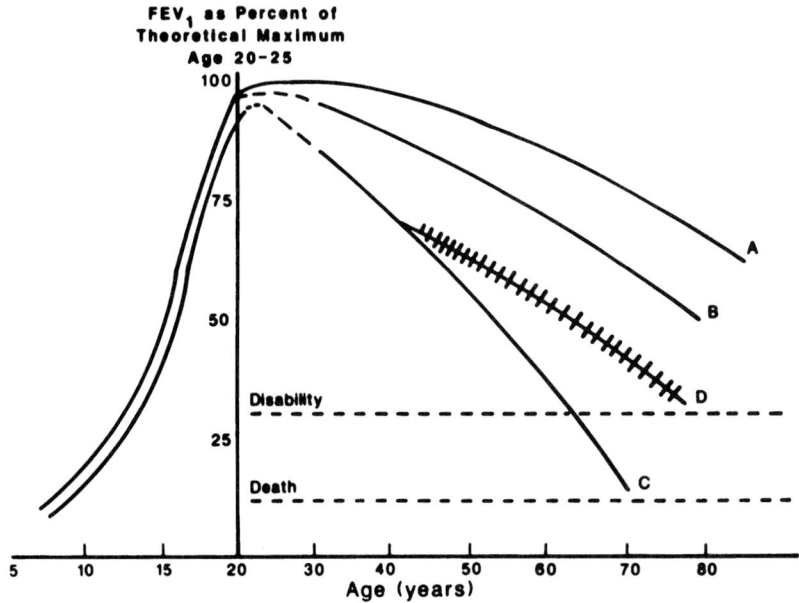

FIG. 18.5. Development and decline in forced expiratory volume in one second (FEV$_1$) plotted as percent of theoretical maximum against age. Curve A depicts a hypothetical nonsmoker. Curve B depicts a hypothetical smoker who is not susceptible to the development of chronic obstructive lung disease (COLD). Curve C depicts a hypothetical smoker with accelerated decline of FEV$_1$ suggestive of increased risk of COLD. Curve D depicts a hypothetical susceptible smoker who quit smoking. [Reproduced from Weiss and Sparrow (80).]

development and decline of FEV$_1$ and the development of chronic obstructive lung disease (COLD) that is modified from the articles of Fletcher et al. (22) and Speizer and Tager (70). This figure uses FEV$_1$ to describe the evolution of the disease, since FEV$_1$ is the measure most frequently reported in epidemiological studies and is clearly associated with clinically disabling COLD. FEV$_1$ tends to reach a maximum level by the early twenties and to decline thereafter with advancing age. According to this model, the risk of developing the disease could be increased by factors that reduce the maximal level of FEV$_1$ attained during growth and development or that accelerate the rate of decline in FEV$_1$ during adulthood. Cigarette smoking is the single most important factor in the development of COLD (22). During childhood, smoking ("active" or "passive") may inhibit the maximally attained level of pulmonary function (6, 74). During adulthood, the normal decline in FEV$_1$ is doubled or tripled in the smoker (see Fig. 18.5, curves B and C). This accelerated loss of pulmonary function markedly increases disease risk in individuals with low maximally attained levels or in those who smoke a greater amount (assuming a dose response).

A number of factors may also determine the susceptibility of a cigarette smoker to COLD. Genetic factors have a potentially important influence on susceptibility to cigarette smoke, but a definite genetic basis for the development of emphysema has been established only for the small proportion of cases caused by a genetically determined deficiency of alpha$_1$- antitrypsin in persons with the homozygous ZZ phenotype (43). Familial clustering of pulmonary function (31, 73) and obstructive airways disease (44) among those without alpha$_1$-antitrypsin deficiency suggest that other genetic or familial–environmental influences may also be important in the pathogenesis of COLD.

Prospective longitudinal data on nonspecific airway responsiveness and pulmonary function in population and occupational samples indicate that airway hyperresponsiveness is associated with accelerated longitudinal decline of pulmonary function. Methacholine airway responsiveness has been found to be related to the rate of FEV$_1$ decline in smokers (24). Similar results have also been seen with carbachol (57). In contrast, an association between histamine airway responsiveness and the rate of FEV$_1$ decline has been observed in nonsmokers as well as in smokers (62). Nonspecific airway hyperresponsiveness is a trait that may precede and predispose to the development of chronic airflow obstruction. Alternatively, both heightened nonspecific airway responsiveness and accelerated decline of lung function may result from a shared underlying cause, such as inflammation.

Occupational exposures may also play an etiological role in some cases. Epidemiological investigations have shown that firefighters (55, 67) and workers exposed to toluene-diisocyanate (54) and various types of dust (5, 37, 38) have an accelerated decline in pulmonary function.

COLD is an insidious process that develops only over many years. Current research is directed at understanding why only a minority of cigarette smokers develop this illness. Host characteristics that influence susceptibility to COLD are of great interest, both for public health considerations and for understanding the pathogenesis of this disorder. Longitudinal population studies currently under way in Boston (68, 81), Tucson (11), and the Netherlands (63) will hopefully shed new light on susceptibility to the development of COLD.

This work was supported in part by the Health Services Research and Development Service of the Department of Veteran's Affairs.

REFERENCES

1. ALTOSE, M. D., J. LEITNER, and N. S. CHERNIACK. Effects of age and respiratory efforts on the perception of resistive ventilatory loads. *J. Gerontol.* 40: 147–153, 1985.
2. ALTOSE, M. D., W. C. MCCAULEY, S. G. KELSEN, and N. S. CHERNIACK. Effects of hypercapnia and inspiratory flow-resistive loading on respiratory activity in chronic airways obstruction. *J. Clin. Invest.* 59: 500–507, 1977.
3. AMERICAN THORACIC SOCIETY. Lung function testing: selection of reference values and interpretative strategies. *Am. Rev. Respir. Dis.* 144: 1202–1218, 1991.
4. ASTRAND, I., P.-O. ASTRAND, I. HALLBACK, and A. KILBOM. Reduction in maximal oxygen uptake with age. *J. Appl. Physiol.* 35: 649–654, 1973.
5. BECKLAKE, M. R. Chronic airflow limitation: its relationship to work in dusty occupations. *Chest* 88: 608–617, 1985.
6. BERKEY, C. S., J. H. WARE, D. W. DOCKERY, B. G. FERRIS, JR., and F. E. SPEIZER. Indoor air pollution and pulmonary function growth in preadolescent children. *Am. J. Epidemiol.* 123: 250–260, 1986.
7. BLEECKER, E. R., E. F. HAPONIK, S. M. WALDEN, D. A. MEYERS, and P. L. SMITH. Relationship between aging, pulmonary mechanics, respiratory muscle function and obstructive sleep apnea [Abstract]. *Gerontologist* 24: 99, 1984.
8. BRAND, P. L. P., B. RIJCKEN, J. P. SCHOUTEN, G. H. KOETER, S. T. WEISS, and D. S. POSTMA. Perceptions of airway obstruction in a random sample. Relationship to airway hyperresponsiveness in the absence of respiratory symptoms. *Am. Rev. Respir. Dis.* 146: 396–401, 1992.
9. BUIST, A. S., H. GHEZZO, N. R. ANTHONISEN, R. M. CHERNIACK, S. DUZIC, P. T. MACKLEM, J. MANFREDA, R. R. MARTIN, D. MCCARTHY, and B. B. ROSS. Relationship between the single-breath N_2-test and age, sex and smoking habits in three North American cities. *Am. Rev. Respir. Dis.* 120: 305–318, 1979.
10. BURNEY, P. G. J., J. R. BRITTON, S. CHINN, A. E. TATTERSFIELD, A. O. PAPACOSTA, M. C. KELSON, F. ANDERSON, and D. R. CORFIELD. Descriptive epidemiology of bronchial reactivity in an adult population; results from a community study. *Thorax* 42: 38–44, 1987.
11. BURROWS, B., M. D. LEBOWITZ, R. A. BARBEE, R. J. KNUDSON, and M. HALONEN. Interactions of smoking and immunologic factors in relation to airways obstruction. *Chest* 84: 657–661, 1983.
12. CARLSON, K. E., W. ALSTON, and D. J. FELDMAN. Electromyography study of aging in skeletal muscle. *Am. J. Phys. Med.* 43: 141–145, 1964.
13. CHAPMAN, K. R., and N. S. CHERNIACK. Aging effects on the interaction of hypercapnia and hypoxia as ventilatory stimuli. *J. Gerontol.* 42: 202–209, 1987.
14. COOK, C. D., J. MEAD, and M. M. ORZALESI. Static volume-pressure characteristics of the respiratory system during maximal efforts. *J. Appl. Physiol.* 19: 1016–1022, 1964.
15. COON, P. J., E. R. BLEECKER, D. T. DRINKWATER, D. A. MEYERS, and A. P. GOLDBERG. Effects of body composition and exercise capacity on glucose tolerance, insulin, and liprotein lipids in healthy older men: a cross-sectional and longitudinal intervention study. *Metabolism* 38: 1201–1209, 1989.
16. DEHN, M. M., and R. A. BRUCE. Longitudinal variations in maximal oxygen intake with age and activity. *J. Appl. Physiol.* 33: 805–807, 1972.
17. DOSMAN, J. A., D. J. COTTON, B. L. GRAHAM, D. L. HALL, R. LI, R. FROH, and G. D. BARNETT. Sensitivity and specificity of early diagnostic tests of lung function in smokers. *Chest* 79: 6–11, 1981.
18. DUBOIS, A. B., and R. ALCALA. Airway resistance and mechanics of breathing in normal subjects 75 to 90 years of age. In: *Aging of the Lung: Perspectives,* edited by L. Cander and J. H. Moyer. New York: Grune and Stratton, 1964, p. 156–162.
19. ENRIGHT, P. L., R. A. KRONMAL, M. HIGGINS, M. SCHENKER, and E. F. HAPONIK. Spirometry reference values for women and men 65 to 85 years of age. *Am. Rev. Respir. Dis.* 147: 125–133, 1993.
20. ERMINI, M. Aging changes in mammalian skeletal muscle. *Gerontology* 22: 301–316, 1976.
21. FLEG, J. L., and E. G. LAKATTA. Role of muscle loss in the age associated reduction in VO_{2max}. *J. Appl. Physiol.* 65: 1147–1151, 1988.
22. FLETCHER, C. M., R. PETO, C. TINKER, and F. E. SPEIZER. *The Natural History of Chronic Bronchitis and Emphysema.* London: Oxford University Press, 1976.
23. FRANK, N. R., J. MEAD, and B. G. FERRIS, JR. The mechanical behavior of the lungs in healthy elderly persons. *J. Clin. Invest.* 36: 1680–1687, 1957.
24. FREW, A. J., S. M. KENNEDY, and M. CHAN-YEUNG. Methacholine responsiveness, smoking, and atopy as risk factors for accelerated FEV_1 decline in male working populations. *Am. Rev. Respir. Dis.* 146: 878–883, 1992.
25. FRY, D. L., and R. E. HYATT. Pulmonary mechanics. A unified analysis of the relationship between pressure, volume and gas flow in the lungs of normal and diseased human subjects. *Am. J. Med.* 29: 672–689, 1960.
26. GHIO, A. J., R. O. CRAPO, and C. G. ELLIOTT. Reference equations used to predict pulmonary function at institutions with respiratory disease training programs in the United States and Canada: a survey. *Chest* 97: 400–403, 1990.
27. GOODMAN, R. M., B. M. YERGIN, J. F. LANDA, M. H. GOLINVAUX, and M. A. SACKNER. Relationship of smoking history and pulmonary function tests to tracheal mucous velocity in nonsmokers, young smokers, ex-smokers, and patients with chronic bronchitis. *Am. Rev. Respir. Dis.* 117: 205–214, 1978.
28. GUTMANN, E., and V. HANZLIKOVA. Fast and slow motor units in aging. *Gerontology* 22: 280–300, 1976.
29. HAMER, N. A. The effect of age on the components of the pulmonary diffusing capacity. *J. Clin. Sci.* 23: 85–93, 1962.
30. HANCE, A. J., and R. G. CRYSTAL. The connective tissue of lung. *Am. Rev. Respir. Dis.* 112: 657–711, 1975.
31. HIGGINS, M., and J. KELLER. Familial occurrence of chronic respiratory disease and familial resemblance in ventilatory capacity. *J. Chronic Dis.* 28: 239–251, 1975.

32. HOLLAND, J., J. MILIC-EMILI, P. T. MACKLEM, and D. V. BATES. Regional distribution of pulmonary ventilation and perfusion in elderly subjects. *J. Clin. Invest.* 47: 81–92, 1968.
33. HOPP, R. J., A. BEWTRA, N. M. NAIR, and R. G. TOWNLEY. The effect of age on methacholine response. *J. Allergy Clin. Immunol.* 76: 609–613, 1985.
34. HOSSACK, K. F., and R. A. BRUCE. Maximal cardiac function in sedentary normal men and women: comparison of age-related changes. *J. Appl. Physiol.* 53: 799–804, 1982.
35. JANSON-BJERKLIE, S., S. S. RUMA, M. STULBARG, and V. K. CARRIERI. Predictors of dyspnea intensity in asthma. *Nurs. Res.* 36: 179–183, 1987.
36. JONES, R. L., T. R. OVERTON, D. M. HAMMERLINDL, and B. J. SPROULE. Effects of age on residual volume. *J. Appl. Physiol.* 44: 195–199, 1978.
37. KAUFFMANN, F., D. DROUET, L. LELLOUCH, and D. BRILLE. Occupational exposure and 12-year spirometric changes among Paris area workers. *Br. J. Ind. Med.* 39: 221–232, 1982.
38. KORN, R. J., D. W. DOCKERY, F. E. SPEIZER, J. H. WARE, and B. G. FERRIS, JR. Occupational exposures and chronic respiratory symptoms: a population-based study. *Am. Rev. Respir. Dis.* 136: 298–304, 1987.
39. KNUDSON, R. J., D. F. CLARK, T. C. KENNEDY, and D. E. KNUDSON. Effect of aging alone on mechanical properties of the normal adult human lung. *J. Appl. Physiol.* 43: 1054–1062, 1977.
40. KNUDSON, R. J., M. D. LEBOWITZ, C. J. HOLBERG, and B. BURROWS. Changes in the normal maximal expiratory flow-volume curve with growth and aging. *Am. Rev. Respir. Dis.* 127: 725–734, 1983.
41. KRONENBERG, R. S., and C. W. DRAGE. Attenuation of the ventilatory and heart rate responses to hypoxia and hypercapnia with aging in normal men. *J. Clin. Invest.* 52: 1812–1819, 1973.
42. KRUMPE, P. E., R. J. KNUDSON, G. PARSONS, and K. REISER. The aging respiratory system. *Clin. Geriatr. Med.* 1: 143–175, 1985.
43. KUEPPERS, F., and L. F. BLACK. α_1 antitrypsin and its deficiency. *Am. Rev. Respir. Dis.* 110: 176–194, 1974.
44. LARSON, R. K., M. L. BARMAN, F. KUEPPERS, and H. H. FUDENBERG. Genetic and environmental determinants of chronic obstructive pulmonary disease. *Ann. Intern. Med.* 72: 627–632, 1970.
45. LEITH, D. E., and J. MEAD. Mechanisms determining residual volume of the lungs in normal subjects. *J. Appl. Physiol.* 23: 221–227, 1967.
46. MANSELL, A., C. BRYAN, and H. LEVISON. Airway closure in children. *J. Appl. Physiol.* 33: 711–714, 1972.
47. MITTMAN, C., N. H. ENDELMAN, A. H. NORRIS, and N. W. SHOCK. Relationship between chest wall and pulmonary compliance and age. *J. Appl. Physiol.* 20: 1211–1216, 1965.
48. MORRIS, J. F., A. KOSKI, and L. C. JOHNSON. Spirometric standards for healthy nonsmoking adults. *Am. Rev. Respir. Dis.* 103: 57–67, 1971.
49. MUIESAN, G., C. A. SORBINI, and V. GRASSI. Respiratory function in the aged. *Bull. Eur. Physiopathol. Resp.* 7: 973–1009, 1971.
50. MURRAY, J. F. *The Normal Lung.* Philadelphia: Saunders, 1976.
51. NELSON, N. M. Neonatal pulmonary function *Pediatr. Clin. North Am.* 13: 769–799, 1966.
52. NIEWOEHNER, D. E., and J. KLEINERMAN. Morphologic basis of pulmonary resistance in the human lung and effects of aging. *J. Appl. Physiol.* 36: 412–418, 1974.
53. NIEWOEHNER, D. E., and J. KLEINERMAN. Morphometric study of elastic fibers in normal and emphysematous human lungs. *Am. Rev. Respir. Dis.* 115: 15–21, 1977.
54. PETERS, J. M., R. L. H. MURPHY, and B. G. FERRIS, JR. Ventilatory function in workers exposed to low levels of toluene-diisocyanate: a six month follow up. *Br. J. Ind. Med.* 26: 115–120, 1969.
55. PETERS, J. M., G. P. THERIAULT, L. J. FINE, and D. H. WEGMAN. Chronic effect of fire fighting on pulmonary function. *N. Engl. J. Med.* 291: 1320–1322, 1974.
56. PETERSON, D. D., A. I. PACK, D. A. SILAGE, and A. P. FISHMAN. Effects of aging on ventilatory and occlusion pressure responses to hypoxia and hypercapnia. *Am. Rev. Respir. Dis.* 124: 387–391, 1981.
57. PHAM, O. T., J. M. MUR, N. CHAN, M. GABIENO, J. C. HENQUEL, and D. TECULESCU. Prognostic value of acetylcholine challenge test: a prospective study. *Br. J. Ind. Med.* 41: 207–271, 1984.
58. PIERCE, J. A., and R. V. BERT. Fibrous network of the lung and its change with age. *Thorax* 20: 469–476, 1965.
59. PONTOPPIDAN, H., and H. K. BEECHER. Progressive loss of protective reflexes in the airway with the advance of age. *JAMA* 174: 2209–2213, 1960.
60. RAINE, J. M., and J. M. BISHOP. A-a difference in O_2 tension and physiological dead space in normal man. *J. Appl. Physiol.* 18: 284–288, 1963.
61. REBUCK, A. S., J. RIGG, M. KANGALEE, and L. PENGELLY. Control of tidal volume during rebreathing. *J. Appl. Physiol.* 37: 475–478, 1974.
62. RIJCKEN, B., J. P. SCHOUTEN, S. T. WEISS, M. SEGAL, F. E. SPEIZER, and R. VAN DER LENDE. Longitudinal analysis of the relationship between bronchial hyperreactivity and pulmonary function. In: *Bronchitis IV*, edited by H. J. Sluiter and R. van der Lende. Assen: Van Gorcum, 1989, p. 94–119.
63. RIJCKEN, B., J. P. SCHOUTEN, S. T. WEISS, F. E. SPEIZER, and R. VAN DER LENDE. The relationship of nonspecific bronchial responsiveness to respiratory symptoms in a random population sample. *Am. Rev. Respir. Dis.* 136: 62–68, 1987.
64. RIZZATO, G., and L. MARAZZINI. Thoracoabdominal mechanics in elderly men. *J. Appl. Physiol.* 28: 457–460, 1970.
65. SIXT, R., B. BAKE, and H. OXHOJ. The single-breath N_2-test and spirometry in healthy non-smoking males. *Eur. J. Respir. Dis.* 65: 296–304, 1984.
66. SORBINI, C. A., V. GRASSI, E. SOLINAS, and G. MUIESAN. Arterial oxygen tension in relation to age in healthy subjects. *Respiration* 25: 3–13, 1968.
67. SPARROW, D., R. BOSSÉ, B. ROSNER, and S. T. WEISS. The effect of occupational exposure on pulmonary function: a longitudinal evaluation of fire fighters and nonfire fighters. *Am. Rev. Respir. Dis.* 125: 319–322, 1982.
68. SPARROW, D., G. O'CONNOR, T. COLTON, C. L. BARRY, and S. T. WEISS. The relationship of nonspecific bronchial responsiveness to the occurrence of respiratory symptoms and decreased levels of pulmonary function. The Normative Aging Study. *Am. Rev. Respir. Dis.* 135: 1255–1260, 1987.
69. SPARROW, D., G. T. O'CONNOR, B. ROSNER, M. R. SEGAL, and S. T. WEISS. The influence of age and level of pulmonary function on nonspecific airway responsiveness. The Normative Aging Study. *Am. Rev. Respir. Dis.* 143: 978–982, 1991.
70. SPEIZER, F. E., and I. B. TAGER. Epidemiology of chronic mucus hypersecretion and obstructive airways disease. *Epidemiol. Rev.* 1: 124–142, 1979.
71. TACK, M., M. D. ALTOSE, and N. S. CHERNIACK. Effect of aging on respiratory sensations produced by elastic loads. *J. Appl. Physiol.* 50: 844–850, 1981.
72. TACK, M., M. D. ALTOSE, and N. S. CHERNIACK. Effect of aging on the perception of resistive ventilatory loads. *Am. Rev. Respir. Dis.* 126(suppl.): 463–467, 1982.
73. TAGER, I. B., B. ROSNER, P. V. TISHLER, F. E. SPEIZER, and E. H. KASS. Household aggregation of pulmonary function and

chronic bronchitis. *Am. Rev. Respir. Dis.* 114: 485–492, 1976.
74. TAGER, I. B., S. T. WEISS, A. MUNOZ, B. ROSNER, and F. E. SPEIZER. Longitudinal study of the effects of maternal smoking on pulmonary function in children. *N. Engl. J. Med.* 309: 699–703, 1983.
75. TENNEY, S. M., and R. M. MILLER. Dead space ventilation in old age. *J. Appl. Physiol.* 9: 321–327, 1956.
76. TERRY, P. B., R. J. TRAYSTMAN, H. H. NEWBALL, G. BATRA, and H. A. MENKES. Collateral ventilation in man. *N. Engl. J. Med.* 298: 10–15, 1978.
77. THURLBECK, W. M. The internal surface area of non-emphysematous lungs. *Am. Rev. Respir. Dis.* 95: 765–773, 1967.
78. THURLBECK, W. M. The effect of age on the lung. *Aging—Its Chemistry,* edited by A. A. Dietz. Washington: American Association for Clinical Chemistry, 1980, p. 88–109.
79. TURNER, J. M., J. MEAD, and M. E. WOHL. Elasticity of human lungs in relation to age. *J. Appl. Physiol.* 25: 664–671, 1968.
80. WEISS, S. T., and D. SPARROW. *Airway Responsiveness and Atopy in the Development of Chronic Lung Disease.* New York: Raven Press, 1989.
81. WEISS, S. T., I. B. TAGER, J. W. WEISS, A. MUNOZ, F. E. SPEIZER, and R. H. INGRAM, JR. The epidemiology of airways responsiveness in a population sample of adults and children. *Am. Rev. Respir. Dis.* 129: 898–902, 1984.
82. WEST, J. B. *Ventilation/Blood Flow and Gas Exchange.* Oxford: Blackwell, 1977, p. 28–29.

19. Renal and urinary tract function

ROBERT D. LINDEMAN | *Division of Geriatric Medicine, Department of Medicine, University of New Mexico School of Medicine, Albuquerque, New Mexico*

CHAPTER CONTENTS

Age-Related Changes in Kidney Function
    Cross-sectional studies
        Glomerular filtration rates
        Renal blood and plasma flow
        Maximum tubular transport capacity
        Concentrating and diluting abilities
        Excretion of hydrogen ions
        Glomerular permeability
        Correlations with renal morphology
    Modification of view of inevitable change from results of longitudinal studies
    Age-related proteinuria and glomerular lesions in rodents
    Pathophysiology of the decrease in renal function with age
Age-Related Changes in Renal Control of Fluid and Electrolyte Homeostasis
    Control of sodium balance
    Control of potassium balance
    Control of water balance and susceptibility of older individuals to dehydration (hypernatremia)
    Susceptibility of older individuals to the development of hyponatremia
Aging and Kidney Disease
    Acute renal failure
        Acute tubular necrosis
        Acute interstitial or tubulointerstitial nephritis
        Acute glomerulonephritis
        Postrenal obstruction
        Prognosis of acute renal failure in the elderly
    Glomerular disease (nephrotic syndrome)
        Primary glomerulopathies
        Nephrotic syndrome and neoplasia
        Nephrotic syndrome related to systemic disease
    Chronic renal failure
        Renal vascular disorders
        Arteriolar nephrosclerosis—benign and malignant
        Systemic vasculitis
        Polycystic renal disease
        Analgesic nephropathy
        Multiple myeloma
        Scleroderma
    Urinary tract infections
Lower Urinary Tract Dysfunction with Aging
    Anatomy and physiology of the lower urinary tract
    Effect of age on lower urinary tract
    Transient incontinence
    Established incontinence
    Pathophysiology of voiding dysfunction in benign prostatic hyperplasia
    Pathophysiology of benign prostatic hyperplasia
    Pathophysiology of the obstructed detrusor
    Other diseases of the lower urinary tract

THE ACCURACY AND SIMPLICITY WITH WHICH RENAL CLEARANCES CAN BE PERFORMED, requiring only timed urine samples and blood samples drawn at the midpoints of these collections, has made the kidney an accessible organ system for studying the changes that occur with aging. In both cross-sectional and longitudinal studies, mean values of kidney function decrease substantially with age. Most renal function decreases tend to parallel the decline in glomerular filtration rate. Results from the Baltimore Longitudinal Study on Aging (62) suggest that loss of renal function with age, however, is not inevitable and that the decreases in mean values are primarily the result of superimposed pathology (for example, undetected glomerulonephritis or interstitial nephritis secondary to infections, immunological insults, drugs, or other toxic exposures; atherosclerotic vascular occlusions with resultant ischemic injury; urinary tract infections; or urinary tract obstruction). The terms "successful" and "usual" aging have been used to distinguish between individuals who age without loss of organ function (*successful*) and the usual cross-section of any aging population where mean values are tabulated (*usual*) (93). The latter must include individuals with asymptomatic, or at least undetected, pathology.

A variety of lesions can impair renal function. These can be divided into glomerular, tubular, interstitial, and vascular pathologies. Renal disorders are best described clinically as acute renal failure, nephrotic syndrome, chronic renal failure, and urinary tract infection.

Lower urinary tract dysfunction in the aging individual introduces a number of medical concerns, which, for the most part, are not life-threatening (with the exceptions of a variety of malignancies and unrelieved obstruction) but do affect quality of life and are medically manageable. Urinary incontinence, for example, is one of the most frequent reasons elderly persons are placed in nursing homes; it occurs in more than 50% of nursing home residents. The involuntary loss of urine so severe as to cause social and hygienic problems is seen in 15%–30% of community-living elders (24). Although changes in the lower urinary tract with age may predispose one to the development of incontinence, age per se is not a cause of incontinence. Another example of lower tract disease is benign prostatic hypertrophy, which occurs in virtually all men if they live long enough.

AGE-RELATED CHANGES IN KIDNEY FUNCTION

Cross-Sectional Studies

Most data on changes in renal function with age come from cross-sectional studies, since they are easier to conduct and can be accomplished over relatively short periods of time. It must be recognized, however, that potential misinterpretations can be introduced by cohort differences and selective mortality. These can be avoided by longitudinal studies.

Glomerular Filtration Rates. Cross-sectional studies have consistently shown an age-related decline in renal function after age 30–40 yr (20, 94, 114). Wesson (114) collected data from 38 studies where individual inulin clearance and age were recorded and found an accelerating decrease in glomerular filtration rate (GFR) with increasing age in both men (Fig. 19.1) and women. The rate of decline was more rapid in men. Rowe et al. (94), reporting on results from the Baltimore Longitudinal

TABLE 19.1. *Cross-Sectional Age Difference in Creatinine Clearances, Serum Creatinine Concentrations, and 24 h Urine Creatinine Excretions*

Age, yr	No. Subjects	Creatinine Clearance, ml/min/1.73 m²	Serum Creatinine Concentration, mg/100 ml	Creatinine Excretion, mg/24 h
25–34	73	140.1	0.81	1,862
35–44	122	132.6	0.81	1,746
45–54	152	126.8	0.83	1,689
55–64	94	119.9	0.84	1,580
65–74	68	109.5	0.83	1,409
75–84	29	96.9	0.84	1,259

Adapted from Rowe et al. (94) with permission.

Study on Aging, showed a similar decline in mean creatinine clearances in normal male subjects followed over a 10 yr period.

Although mean true creatinine clearances fell from 140 cc/min/1.73 m² between 25 and 34 yr of age to 97 cc/min/1.73 m² between 75 and 84 yr of age, mean serum creatinine concentrations rose insignificantly from 0.81 to 0.84 mg/dl. This indicates that mean creatinine production falls at essentially the same rate as mean creatinine clearance, reflecting the decrease in body muscle mass with age (Table 19.1). Serum creatinine concentrations in older patients must be interpreted with this in mind when used to determine or modify dosages of drugs cleared totally (for example, the aminoglycoside antibiotics) or partially (for example, digoxin) by the kidney.

Renal Blood and Plasma Flow. The effective renal plasma flow (ERPF), generally measured by determining paraaminohippuric acid (PAH) clearance, decreases from a mean of 649 ml per min during the fourth decade to a mean of 289 ml per min during the ninth decade (20), a more rapid decrease than GFR. Since the extraction ratio (ERPF/RPF) at low arterial PAH concentrations is not influenced by age (92% in both young and old subjects), PAH clearance can be used to reflect changes in renal blood flow with age (76).

The decrease in renal blood flow with age (without a parallel decrease in blood pressure) could be explained by either intraluminal vascular pathology (atheromata, sclerosis) or increased renal vascular resistance caused by arteriolar vasoconstriction. McDonald et al. (70) reported that administration of a pyrogen produced a greater increase in ERPF percentage-wise (91% vs. 71%) in older subjects than in younger subjects, suggesting a greater resting vasoconstriction in the older subjects.

Using Xenon washout techniques, Hollenberg et al. (44) reported that perfusion of the outer cortical

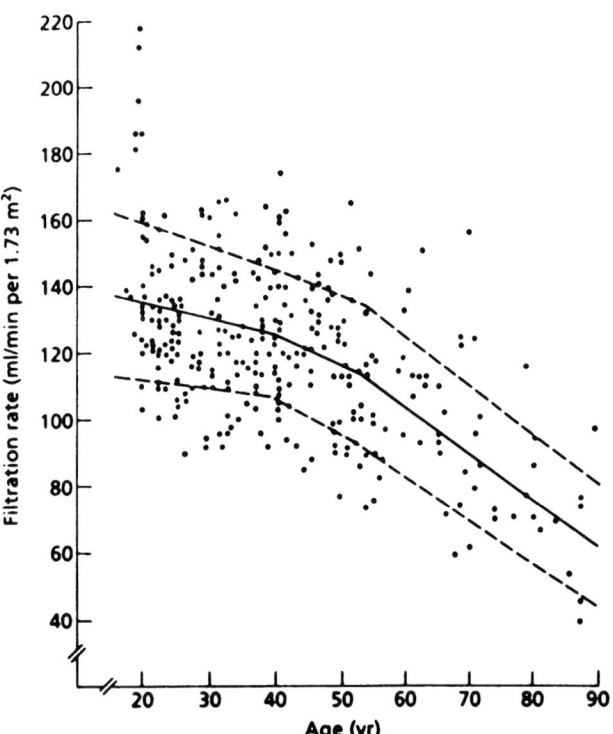

FIG. 19.1. GFR (inulin clearances) per 1.73 m² in normal male volunteers plotted against age from 38 studies. *Solid* and *broken* lines represent mean ± one standard deviation. [Reprinted from Wesson (114) with permission.]

nephrons fell more with age than perfusion of corticomedullary nephrons. Further investigations were designed to determine if this selective decrease in outer cortical nephron perfusion was due to sclerotic changes in the small arcuate arterioles or to a selective vasoconstriction of these vessels. The vasodilator acetylcholine increased renal blood flow in both young and old subjects, but the effect was much more striking in younger subjects. In contrast, the vasoconstrictor response to angiotensin was similar in young and old subjects. This study suggests that renal vasculature in the older subjects is in a relatively greater state of baseline vasodilatation compared to that of younger subjects. Since these are the only two investigations that have addressed this question directly and the results are contradictory, additional studies will be needed to resolve this issue.

Because the cortical component of renal blood flow decreases more rapidly than mean renal blood flow rate, it is felt that cortical nephrons are more severely affected by age than juxtamedullary nephrons. Since juxtamedullary nephrons have a higher filtration fraction than cortical nephrons, a selective loss of the latter might explain the increase in filtration fraction (GFR/ERPF) observed with age (20, 60, 70, 114). An alternative explanation for this is that the efferent arteriole is disproportionately vasoconstricted when compared to the afferent arteriole, thereby increasing the filtration pressure in the glomerular capillary bed.

Maximum Tubular Transport Capacity. The tubular maximum for PAH secretory transport decreases with age at a rate paralleling the decrease in inulin clearance (20, 110), as does the tubular maximum for glucose reabsorption (77).

Although reductions in the secretory and reabsorptive tubular maxima with age could be explained simply by a progressive loss of functioning nephrons, animal studies suggest that tubular cells in old compared to young kidneys have fewer energy-producing mitochondria (8), lower enzyme concentrations (8, 16, 115), lower concentrations of total or sodium–potassium-activated adenosine triphosphatase (ATPase) (9), decreased sodium extrusion and oxygen consumption (87), and decreased tubular transport capacity (8). It is difficult to be sure that these decreases are all attributable to a true decrease in renal tubular cell function and not to a higher proportion of nontubular mass in old vs. young kidneys since these studies were performed on tissue slices.

Concentrating and Diluting Abilities. A decrease in concentrating ability with age is well documented (26, 60, 63, 75, 96). Twelve hours of water deprivation increased mean urine osmolality to 1,109 mOsm/liter in young subjects (mean age 33 yr), 1,051 mOsm/liter in middle-aged subjects (mean age 49 yr), and 882 mOsm/liter in old subjects (mean age 68 yr) (96). The decrease in concentrating ability could not be related strictly to an increase in solute load in surviving functional nephrons (60, 96). Rowe et al. (96) suggested that the relative increase in medullary blood flow per nephron with age, as shown by Hollenberg et al. (44), would result in enhanced removal of medullary solute (washout) and thus decrease maximum urinary osmolality.

Maximum urine osmolality following infusions of large doses of pitressin is similarly decreased in older subjects undergoing water diuresis (75). The kidneys of elderly subjects, in contrast, respond normally to graded doses of pitressin insufficient to maximally concentrate the urine (60). This suggests that the decrease in concentrating ability of older subjects is the result of a decrease in medullary hypertonicity rather than any defect in the ability of the tubule to respond to pitressin.

Maximum diluting ability, as measured by minimum urine osmolality achieved with water loading, also decreases with age (60). However, when one compares maximum free water clearance per unit of nephron mass (GFR), there is little difference between young and old subjects, suggesting no basic defect in the ability of the individual tubule to produce a dilute urine (21, 57, 60).

Excretion of Hydrogen Ions. To maintain systemic acid-base balance, the kidney must excrete a quantity of hydrogen ion equal to the net quantity of fixed acid generated by metabolism. Under basal conditions, the blood pH, pCO_2, and bicarbonate of older persons without significant renal disease do not differ from the values observed in young subjects (2, 98). However, the decreases in blood pH and bicarbonate concentrations following ingestion of an acid load persist longer in elderly persons (2, 3). The minimum urine pH achieved after an acid load is similar in young and old subjects. A much larger percentage of the ingested acid load, as measured by total acid excretion (ammonium plus titratable acid minus bicarbonate), was excreted over an 8 h period by younger vs. older subjects. However, if total acid excretion in 8 h is factored by GFR, similar rates of excretion are obtained. Young subjects excrete a greater percentage of total acid as ammonium, presumably because older subjects have an increase in urinary buffers responsible for titratable acid, for example, phosphate or creatinine, per unit of GFR. Agarwal and Cabebe (3) subsequently reported that elderly subjects showed a small pH gradient defect and that ammonium excretion was reduced in the elderly even after correction for GFR. Adler et al. (2) reported that the administration of glutamine, the major substrate for renal ammoniagenesis, did not correct the defect in ammonium excretion in older subjects, suggesting that the defect was not due to a lack of substrate. A limitation of the kidney's ability to excrete acid may predispose to the development of, and delay recovery from, metabolic acidosis in older persons.

Glomerular Permeability. Functional studies of glomerular filtration show no changes in membrane permeability. Glomerular permeability to free hemoglobin and a spectrum of different molecular weight dextrans does not differ between young and old subjects (31, 66). This is true even though the mesangium of the individual glomerulus takes up a greater percentage of total glomerulus volume and the glomerular basement membrane thickens with age (101).

Correlations with Renal Morphology. Both kidney mass and function decrease after the third or fourth decade of life at a rate of approximately 1% per year. The loss of renal mass is principally from the cortex and is primarily vascular in origin, with the most significant changes occurring at the capillary level. The number of glomerular tufts per unit area as well as the number of glomerular and tubular cells decrease, while the size of the individual cell increases with age (39).

Normal aging is associated with sclerotic changes in the walls of the larger renal arteries, but these lesions generally do not encroach on the lumen sufficiently to produce functional changes (71, 116). Smaller vessels are relatively spared in nonhypertensive elderly subjects, with only a small percentage of senescent kidneys showing arteriolar changes. The incidence of sclerotic glomeruli increases with advancing age, from less than 5% of the total glomeruli at 40 yr to 10%–30% of the total by the eighth decade (49, 50, 72, 105). Kasiske (50) reported a strong direct correlation between the number of sclerotic glomeruli and the severity of atherosclerotic disease. He also found that when the percentage of sclerosed glomeruli was less than five, the distribution between cortex and medulla was relatively uniform, but as it exceeded this level, it became predominantly cortical.

Several investigators (65, 104) have provided detailed descriptions of ischemic obsolescence in cortical vs. juxtamedullary glomeruli. Initially, there is a progressive collapse of the glomerular tuft with wrinkling of the basement membranes, followed by a simplification and reduction in the vascular channels. Hyaline is deposited within both the residual glomerular tuft and the space of Bowman's capsule. Identifiable structures rapidly disappear. The obsolete glomerulus may be reabsorbed and disappear entirely. Reabsorption is suggested by the scantiness of the cellular response and the residual scar. This process can leave a single vessel in place of the glomerular capillary arterioles (juxtamedullary glomeruli) or atrophy can result in an abrupt termination of the arteriole (cortical glomeruli).

Modification of View of Inevitable Change from Results of Longitudinal Studies

Rowe et al. (94) initially reported results from the Baltimore Longitudinal Study of Aging that showed a decline in mean creatinine clearance in normal subjects followed over a 10 yr period similar to that described earlier in cross-sectional studies. A subsequent report from this study (62) showed that the mean decrease in creatinine clearance in 446 normal volunteers followed over a 23-yr period was 0.87 ml/min/yr, very close to that observed in cross-sectional analyses.

One-third of these subjects, however, had no decline in creatinine clearance, as illustrated by six subjects followed for 15–21 yr (bottom, Fig. 19.2). These observations suggest that the decline in renal function observed with age in cross-sectional analyses is not the result of chronic involutional changes, which occur in all persons, albeit at different rates, but more likely stems from intervening pathology, for example, undetected glomerulonephritis or interstitial nephritis secondary to infections, immunological insults, drugs, or other toxic exposures; vascular occlusions with resultant ischemic injury; urinary tract infections; or obstruction. At least one of the variables that affects the rate of decline in renal function is blood pressure, as hypertensive subjects showed a more rapid decline in renal function than normotensive subjects (61).

Age-Related Proteinuria and Glomerular Lesions in Rodents

A number of reports have described age-related chronic glomerular lesions (*glomerulosclerosis*), increasing proteinuria, and renal insufficiency in rats, hamsters, and mice. Bell et al. (10), for example, reported progressive increases in glomerular basement membrane thickness and mesangial area followed by glomerular hyalinization and sclerosis in Lewis strain rats. Tubulointerstitial inflammation and fibrosis developed later, independent of the glomerular lesions. This chronic nephropathy, which results in kidney failure in older animals, has been found to be the major terminal disease process in various rat strains (18, 67). A restriction in protein and total caloric intake delays the increase in proteinuria and the decrease in renal function (11, 47). Masoro and Yu (68) are of the opinion that caloric restriction is more important than protein restriction in preventing the development of these renal lesions with age, citing evidence that supports their position.

When the population of normal glomeruli is reduced, as with aging, by surgical ablation or infarction in the rat model, the remaining glomeruli react with an "adaptive" hyperperfusion and hyperfiltration. This glomer-

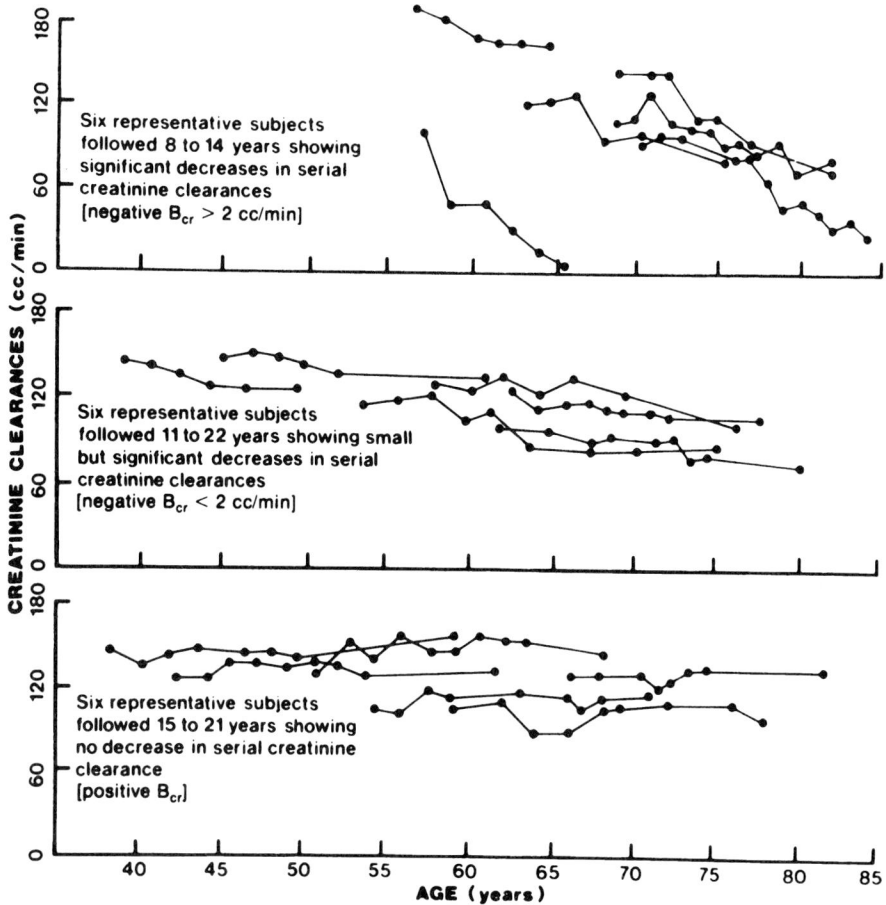

FIG. 19.2. Individual longitudinal displays of serial creatinine clearances plotted against age in years for representative subjects from the Baltimore Longitudinal Study of Aging. **A:** Six representative subjects followed 8–14 yr showing significant decreases in serial creatinine clearances (negative $B_{cr} > 2$ cc/min). **B:** Six representative subjects followed 11–22 yr showing small but significant decreases in serial creatinine clearances (negative $B_{cr} < 2$ cc/min). **C:** Six representative subjects followed 15–21 yr showing no decrease in serial creatinine clearance (positive B_{cr}). Note especially the six subjects in **C**, representative of nearly one-third of the subjects followed, who had no decrease in creatinine clearances over periods up to 21 yr. [Reprinted from Lindeman et al. (62) with permission.]

ular hyperfiltration disrupts the integrity of the capillary membrane, resulting in proteinuria, accumulation of mesangial deposits, and initiation or acceleration of renal function loss through a process of developing glomerulosclerosis. The increases in glomerular capillary pressure and plasma flow that follow uninephrectomy in the rat are accompanied by a moderate acceleration in the development of the glomerulosclerosis normally seen in the aging rat (18, 67). With the rat remnant kidney, where even greater increases in glomerular pressure and flow are created, structural changes develop even more rapidly (22, 42).

The hemodynamic changes in this renal ablation model, as in other models of renal injury where there is diffuse injury to the entire nephron population, occur soon after surgical insult and well before development of glomerulosclerosis. Urinary protein excretion increases relative to a loss of the permselective properties in the glomerulus (size and charge selectivity). In all experimental models of glomerulosclerosis, dietary (low-protein diet) and pharmacological (converting enzyme inhibitors) interventions, which alter the rate of evolution of the glomerulosclerosis, similarly affect glomerular permselective properties and urinary protein excretion.

Advances in micropuncture techniques have permitted more precise characterization of the adaptive hemodynamic changes in the remnant kidney. Single nephron glomerular filtration rate (SNGFR) is increased to almost twice that observed in controls due primarily to an increase in single nephron glomerular plasma flow (Q_A) (22). Subsequent studies in rats with more extreme renal ablation showed elevations of both Q_A and the transcapillary hydraulic pressure gradient (ΔP) (45). Early evidence of glomerular injury, for example, mesangial expansion and endothelial cell damage, was observed. Nath et al. (79) and Meyer et al. (73) studied the effects of normal vs. low protein intakes on single nephron hemodynamics in the remnant kidneys model. ΔP was the hemodynamic abnormality most closely associated with progressive glomerular injury. Even after glomerular damage was established, when glomerular hypertension was eliminated, proteinuria diminished and glomerular injury became less apparent. These observations, as discussed later under pathophysiology, may help to explain the accelerating loss of renal function observed in the elderly even in the absence of underlying renal disease.

Pathophysiology of the Decrease in Renal Function with Age

Whether the decrease in renal function with age is the result of a progressive involutional process with loss of nephron units and a decline in cellular function similar to the glomerulosclerosis described above in rodents or the result of various pathological processes, often undetected, producing acute and chronic injuries, or both, remains unresolved. While results from the Baltimore Longitudinal Study of Aging (62) showed that over one-third of the male volunteers followed, some for over 20 yr, failed to show any decrease in renal function over the period studied, pathological studies show a progressive increase in the number of sclerotic glomeruli with advancing age (50). The former data suggest that there is no inevitable progressive involutional change, at least not in all cases, and support the concept that the decrease in renal function with age observed in cross-sectional studies is the result of superimposed pathology. A number of examples of undetected pathology as potential causes of reduced renal function in the elderly have been cited and discussed elsewhere (59, 64). Friedman et al. (36), for example, utilized scanning techniques to localize defects in kidney function in elderly patients with no history of renal disease. They found abnormal scans in 25 of 35 elderly subjects (71%) with a mean age of 75 yr and mean creatinine clearance of 53 ml/min. Sixteen (46%) showed focal areas of diminished uptake which were felt to represent ischemic lesions. Significant pyuria was present in 37% of the patients; however, I.V. pyelograms were interpreted as normal in all cases. No significant proteinuria was detected in any patient. These findings are consistent with the hypothesis that focal lesions due to vascular occlusions, interstitial infection (pyelonephritis), or both contribute to the decrease in renal function observed in any aging population. An alternative explanation would be that, with any involutional change (glomerulosclerosis, tubulointerstitial scarring), there is a compensatory increase in function of the remaining nephron units, probably related to release of a variety of growth factors, for example, epidermal growth factor (EGF) or insulin-like growth factor 1 (IGF-1), as demonstrated in early insulin-dependent diabetes mellitus (46) and in subjects after unilateral nephrectomy (12).

Once a critical level of renal functional deterioration is reached in individuals with kidney injury from any cause, progression of the disease occurs, even if the initiating event or condition is resolved. This is due to a progressive glomerulosclerosis. A vast literature has been generated on the role of hyperperfusion and hyperfiltration in the progression of declining renal function in rodents, as cited above. Brenner and colleagues (5, 14) have suggested that the protein-rich diet characteristic of modern Western society itself induces chronic renal hyperperfusion and hyperfiltration, thereby contributing to the structural and functional deterioration of the aging kidney. Presumably, the high glomerular pressures and plasma flow rates created by the high protein intake contribute to the development of glomerulosclerosis, resulting in a progressive decline in renal function with age alone, as with primary renal disease, diabetes mellitus, hypertension, and renal ablation. Not all of the evidence supports this theory; long-term follow-up of patients undergoing nephrectomy for unilateral renal disease or kidney transplant donation fails to show deteriorating renal function or glomerulosclerosis (40, 74, 106, 107, 109, 112). The evidence that a high-protein diet contributes to a deterioration in renal function in the elderly is reviewed elsewhere (58), but, in conclusion, it does not appear to be a significant factor unless other pathology-diminishing renal function also exists.

Unilateral nephrectomy causes compensatory hypertrophy in the normal remaining kidney; however, the rates of enlargement and increased function are much lower in the old compared to the young. There is no increase after birth in the number of nephrons. Cellular hyperplasia is the predominant response in the young, whereas cellular hypertrophy is the chief response in the elderly (85). Even though the kidneys of older animals enlarge primarily by hypertrophy, the rate of hypertrophy is less than that observed in younger animals. The role of the growth factors mentioned above in cellular hyperplasia and hypertrophy and their impact on recovery of the kidney from injury and development of glomerulosclerosis has been the subject of a great deal of recent investigation, some of which was reviewed in a recent symposium (34). It would appear that the processes of glomerular hypertrophy and glomerulosclerosis are closely linked.

AGE-RELATED CHANGES IN RENAL CONTROL OF FLUID AND ELECTROLYTE HOMEOSTASIS

Under normal circumstances, age has no effect on serum sodium and potassium concentrations or the ability to maintain normal extracellular volumes. The extrarenal mechanisms responsible for maintaining volume and composition of the extracellular fluids, however, often become impaired in the elderly, especially when stressed by acute and/or chronic illness.

Control of Sodium Balance

Epstein and Hollenberg (30) found that older subjects failed to conserve sodium as efficiently as younger subjects. The half-time for reduction of urinary sodium excretion after rigid salt restriction was 17.6 h in the young compared to 30.9 h in older subjects. Elderly subjects consistently have lower plasma renin activities and plasma or urinary aldosterone excretions on both restricted and unrestricted salt diets and in both supine and upright positions (Table 19.2) (19, 108, 111). These decreased plasma renin activities and plasma concentrations or urinary excretions of aldosterone in the elderly may be related to the impaired responsiveness to β-adrenergic stimulation observed in the elderly since one of the effects of β-adrenergic stimulation is to increase levels of circulating renin and aldosterone. The decrease in aldosterone at least partially explains the decreased ability of the elderly to conserve sodium when challenged with a low-salt diet.

Two other factors may be operative in the relative inability to conserve salt by the elderly. First, circulating atrial natriuretic factor (ANF) levels, while very variable in the elderly, are substantially higher than those observed in healthy young adults (41, 82). These elevated levels may play a role in the salt-losing tendency of the aging kidney, both directly by its natriuretic effect and indirectly by suppressing renin and aldosterone synthesis and release. Second, as renal function decreases in the older person, assuming food and salt intake are reasonably well maintained, the solute load per residual functioning nephron increases, thus producing a relative osmotic diuresis which impairs ability to conserve sodium.

Control of Potassium Balance

The low renin and aldosterone levels also could account for the greater tendency of older individuals to develop hyperkalemia when receiving supplemental potassium. Lawson (56) reported that the incidence of hyperkalemia complicating diuretic therapy and potassium supplementation was 0.5% in persons under age 50 yr but rose to 4.0% in persons aged 50–60 yr, and was even higher in older persons. The combination of a decreased GFR and impaired renin–aldosterone response leaves older individuals at risk for the development of hyperkalemia. Because the distal nephron has such a large capacity for secreting potassium, even in patients with severely reduced renal function, hyperkalemia generally develops only when one or more additional factors, for example, oliguria, or an excess endogenous or exogenous potassium load is introduced into the body. Drugs that interfere with this aldosterone-dependent tubular secretion of potassium in the distal tubule include the potassium-sparing diuretics (spironolactone, triamterene, and amiloride), the β-adrenergic blockers, the angiotensin-converting enzyme (ACE) inhibitors, and the nonsteroidal antiinflammatory drugs. Elderly persons with interstitial nephritis, especially diabetics, develop a more pronounced hyporeninemic hypoaldosteronism referred to as "type IV renal tubular acidosis."

Control of Water Balance and Susceptibility of Older Individuals to Dehydration (Hypernatremia)

Snyder et al. (100) reported that over 1% of their hospital admissions were patients over age 60 yr who developed hypernatremia (serum sodium concentration >148 mEq/liter). Surgery, febrile illness, infirmity, and diabetes mellitus accounted for two-thirds of their cases. One-half developed hypernatremia while in the hospital. The increased tendency of the older person to lose both salt and water (concentrating defect) undoubtedly contributed to the more rapid development of dehydration and hypernatremia in this population. Yamamoto et al. (117) reported that decreases in the renin–angiotensin–aldosterone system in the elderly also may affect the development of dehydration, since hypoangiotensinemia resulted in impaired secretion of arginine vasopressin. This could be corrected by an infusion of angiotensin II. More important, however, is the impairment in the thirst mechanism that develops with age. Phillips

TABLE 19.2. *Serum Renin (ng/ml/16 h) and Aldosterone Concentrations (ng/100 ml) in Healthy Young (20–30 yr) and Elderly (62–70 yr) Volunteers under Varying Conditions of Posture and Sodium Intake*

Age Group	Sodium Intake, mEq/24 h	Supine		Upright	
		Renin	Aldosterone	Renin	Aldosterone
Young	120 × 3 days	17.7	4.2	41.1	12.6
Elderly		11.9	3.1	26.4	5.6
Young	10 × 6 days	44.3	13.8	124.3	59.7
Elderly		27.4	6.4	55.1	20.3

Adapted from Weidmann et al. (111) with permission.

et al. (84) studied the thirst response, as well as pituitary and renal responses, to 24 h of water deprivation in young vs. old subjects and showed increased serum osmolalities and plasma arginine vasopressin (AVP) levels and decreased urine osmolalities in the older group. The younger subjects, however, reported much more thirst after water restriction and, at the end of the study, rapidly drank water to restore plasma osmolality to normal, whereas the older individuals drank little water and still had not corrected the hyperosmolality after 2 h. One explanation for the hypodipsia is a decreased effectiveness of the opioid ingestive drive. If older persons had a normal thirst response to water deprivation, the inability to conserve salt and to concentrate urine would be compensated for by increased fluid intake.

Susceptibility of Older Individuals to the Development of Hyponatremia

Surveys of older persons in both acute- and chronic-care facilities show a high incidence of hypoatremia. Kleinfeld et al. (54) reported that 36 of 160 chronically ill patients (23%) had a serum sodium concentration below 132 mEq/liter (mean 120 mEq/liter). In most, the low serum sodium concentration was not readily explained except by the presence of debilitating disease and old age. In another nursing home study (78), over half of the patients had been hyponatremic on at least one occasion over the previous year, with one-third of the study population being chronically hyponatremic. The chronically hyponatremic patients, after administration of a water load, were able to achieve a mean minimum urine osmolality of only 237 mOsm/kg H_2O compared to 84 mOsm/kg H_2O in the nonhyponatremic population. Chronically hyponatremic patients excreted only 57% of the water load over a 5-h period compared to the nonhyponatremic population. Patients with intermittent hyponatremia also had a less severe, but still abnormal, response to the water load. In another geriatric unit survey (103), over 10% of patients had serum sodium concentrations below 130 mEq/liter, with administration of thiazide diuretics and hypotonic I.V. solutions most often implicated as etiological factors.

Anderson et al. (4) prospectively evaluated the prevalence, cause, and outcome of hyponatremia in an acute-care facility. Prevalence was 2.5%, with two-thirds being hospital acquired. Mean age was nearly 60 yr. The most frequent etiology was a normovolemic hyponatremia [syndrome of inappropriate antidiuretic hormone (SIADH)] seen in 34% of cases. Hypovolemia (primary salt loss), hypervolemia (dilutional hyponatremia), and hyperglycemia each accounted for 16%–19% of the cases, and renal failure with overhydration and error accounted for most of the remainder. They demonstrated that nonosmotic (baroreceptor) stimulation of vasopressin release was a major factor in this electrolyte disorder, regardless of cause.

Antidiuresis and hyponatremia have been observed postoperatively primarily in elderly patients (23). Sulfonylureas create SIADH almost exclusively in older individuals (113). Diuretic-induced hyponatremia occurs primarily in older patients (6, 33), suggesting that elderly persons may be more susceptible to the development of hyponatremia (SIADH-like picture) than their younger counterparts.

A number of studies suggest increasing antidiuretic hormone activity in the serum or plasma of elderly persons (53, 92). Rondeau and associates (92) found a significant relationship between age and morning supine AVP levels by radioimmunoassay in overnight water-deprived subjects. Regression of these values predicts a baseline serum AVP of 2.37 pg/ml, with an increase of 0.03 pg/ml per year of age.

Observations reported by Helderman et al. (43) may help to explain the increased susceptibility of older persons to the development of hyponatremia. Older subjects showed increased AVP concentrations more (twofold) after a standardized hypertonic saline infusion designed to raise serum osmolality to 306 mOsm/l than younger subjects, despite comparable baseline AVP concentrations. In contrast, ethanol infusions, known to inhibit AVP secretion, produced a more prolonged depression in serum AVP concentrations in young than in old subjects. These two observations suggest an increasing osmoreceptor sensitivity with age, with a greater release of AVP and thus more water retention in response to any given osmotic stimulus.

Rowe et al. (95) subsequently reported studies designed to determine if this represented a consistent, age-related increase in vasopressin responsiveness or was specific for osmotic stimuli. Older subjects, following periods of quiet standing, failed to increase serum AVP concentrations as much or as consistently as younger subjects. They divided subjects into those who released AVP (responders) and those who failed to release AVP (nonresponders) in response to orthostasis. Whereas fewer than 10% of young subjects were nonresponders, nearly half of the older subjects showed a failure to release AVP in response to orthostasis. Because these subjects had an intact norepinephrine response to orthostasis, the authors felt that the age-related defect was distal to the vasomotor center in the afferent limb of the baroreceptor reflex arc. They further suggested that the contrasting influence of age on the vasopressin response to osmolar and volume-pressure stimuli in some elderly subjects might be related to impaired baroreceptor input to the supraoptic nucleus, which in turn might remove constraints on the response to osmotic stimuli.

AGING AND KIDNEY DISEASE

Acute Renal Failure

The inability of the kidney to excrete, through the process of formation of a glomerular filtrate and reabsorption/secretion in the tubular system, the normal load of metabolites produced by the body can be separated into acute or chronic renal failure. When one discusses acute renal failure (ARF) (and, to a lesser extent, chronic renal failure), a further differentiation needs to be made between prerenal, renal, and postrenal azotemia. Useful in categorizing these broad groups is calculation of the blood urea nitrogen (BUN)/serum creatinine ratio. With prerenal azotemia, there is either a decrease in renal perfusion (dehydration, hypotension, congestive heart failure) or an increase in nitrogen production (blood loss into the gastrointestinal tract) so that the BUN/serum creatinine ratio increases, often into the 20 or 30 to 1 range or even higher. The decreased perfusion associated with prerenal azotemia enhances tubular urea reabsorption, thereby disproportionately raising BUN levels relative to serum creatinine concentrations. The increased hydrostatic pressure transmitted to the tubular fluid in postrenal (obstructive) azotemia also creates a disproportionate reabsorption of urea compared to creatinine, which also then increases the BUN/serum creatinine ratio.

Of the intrarenal causes of ARF, glomerular, tubulointerstitial, and/or vascular pathology may be causative. The BUN/serum creatinine ratio tends to be in the range of 14 to 1 but, on a protein-restricted diet, may fall to the range of 8 to 1.

Tubulointerstitial nephropathies are the most common causes of ARF, with acute tubular necrosis and acute interstitial nephritis being the major etiologies (86). In general, the tubulointerstitial nephropathies are characterized by, in addition to renal insufficiency, an impaired ability to concentrate the urine, to excrete potassium and hydrogen ions, and to conserve sodium so that polyuria (nocturia), hyperkalemia, metabolic acidosis, and salt wasting (dehydration) appear out of proportion to the impairment in GFR.

Acute Tubular Necrosis. Acute tubular necrosis (ATN) may be ischemic or nephrotoxic in origin. Prerenal azotemia, if severe or prolonged, may result in ischemic ATN. In a survey of 122 elderly subjects with ATN (55), renal failure was attributable to ischemic ATN in 84 patients (69%). Dehydration and electrolyte imbalance were important contributors in 48%, and major surgery accounted for 30% of cases. Other contributing factors included hypotension, cardiac failure, and postoperative fluid losses secondary to gastrointestinal pathology, drainage, and third spacing. Infection was either a causative factor or a complication of ATN in 25% of these cases, with pneumonia, wound and abdominal infections, and urinary infections leading to sepsis being the major contributors.

In a more recent study of ARF in 246 patients over age 65 yr, 45% had renal failure associated with surgical procedures and problems, including pre- and postoperative sepsis, 36% with medical illnesses (pneumonia, sepsis, ischemic heart disease, drugs, etc.), and 19% with urological and gynecological causes (91). In only 13 cases was ARF caused by drug therapy, and, surprisingly, in none of these cases were the aminoglycoside antibiotics implicated.

Pascual et al. (83) compared the causes of ARF in 152 subjects over age 70 yr with 285 subjects below that age. The most impressive finding was that in nearly half of the older patients, ARF was prerenal in origin (over half attributed to dehydration), with less than one-third of the younger patients showing this as an etiology.

Antibiotics, especially the aminoglycosides, are the predominant cause of nephrotoxic ATN. Risk factors include advanced age, existing impairment of renal function, volume contraction (dehydration), and possibly concurrent use of some cephalosporin. The monitoring of serum concentrations of the aminoglycosides has greatly reduced the incidence of ARF due to this cause, but even with careful monitoring, some cases still occur. The radiocontrast agents now used in I.V. pyelography, angiography, and computerized tomography remain as the second most common cause of nephrotoxic ATN. The principal contrast agents currently in use are the sodium and meglumine salts diatrizoate, iothalamate, metrizamide, and ioxadate. The incidence of contrast-induced ARF is less than 2% unless risk factors exist, and most are reversible. Factors that increase risk include age, diabetes mellitus, preexisting renal insufficiency, multiple myeloma, renal hypoperfusion (dehydration), hypertension, and hepatic disease. The risk in the elderly diabetic with preexisting renal insufficiency approaches 100%, much of which may be irreversible. Acute renal failure following oral cholecystography or biliary tract visualization following iopanoic acid (Telepaque®) is now rare unless excessively high doses are used. Other causes of ATN in the elderly include heavy metal exposure, cisplatinum therapy, hemoglobinuria, myoglobinuria, and exposure to fluorinated anesthetic agents (Penthrane®).

Acute Interstitial or Tubulointerstitial Nephritis. Drug-induced acute interstitial nephritis (AIN) has become an increasingly common cause of ARF in the elderly; AIN can also be seen as a complication of infectious or systemic disease (27). Over 40 drugs have been implicated as possible etiological agents, with the penicillins (penicillin G, methicillin, ampicillin, oxacillin, nafcillin), the cephalosporins, and the nonsteroidal antiinflammatory agents being the most commonly incriminated. Methicillin is the most frequently reported penicillin, at times approaching 20% of treated patients developing ARF, perhaps because higher doses are used over a long period in staphylococcal septicemia and endocarditis.

Patients with penicillin-associated AIN frequently develop fever, rash, and eosinophilia/eosinophiluria in addition to a nonoliguric, progressive azotemia. The widespread use of nonsteroidal antiinflammatory drugs (NSAIDs) has led to many reports of acute to chronic renal failure, especially in the elderly. An inhibition in the synthesis of the vasodilatory prostaglandins may contribute to the loss of renal function observed in patients placed on NSAIDs.

Acute Glomerulonephritis. Although acute glomerulonephritis is generally regarded as a disease of children and young adults, a number of papers in the literature conclude that it is more common in the elderly than generally believed (15). The essential clinical features (hematuria, proteinuria, sodium and fluid retention, decreased renal function, and hypertension) are not different in the elderly. Diagnosis may be obscured by the presence of preexisting conditions or by preconceived ideas regarding its occurrence in the elderly. Adults frequently present with a picture of cardiovascular decompensation attributed to underlying atherosclerotic or hypertensive heart disease and azotemia, which is either overlooked or attributed to prerenal causes. The diagnostic red cell casts are often overlooked because of a low index of suspicion. While many of these patients will be found to have a poststreptococcal or postinfectious acute proliferative glomerulonephritis on histological examination, it may be difficult to clinically distinguish these cases from patients with rapidly progressive (*crescentic*) glomerulonephritis or glomerulonephritis resulting from a systemic disease (for example, systemic lupus erythematosus, vasculitis, subacute bacterial endocarditis, Henoch-Schönlein purpura) (55).

Postrenal Obstruction. Postrenal obstruction is an important cause of ARF as it is common and often treatable. Prostatic hyperplasia is the most common etiology and occurs only in men. Hospitalized elderly patients on bed rest may be unable to generate the necessary pressure to void without being able to stand. The frequent use of anticholinergic drugs, particularly the tricyclic antidepressants, also may potentiate retention.

Prognosis of Acute Renal Failure in the Elderly. Pascual et al. (83) reviewed the literature on prognosis of ARF in older patients and added observations on 152 patients over 70 yr of age among their 437 patients with ARF. They cited six reports that showed that advanced age increased mortality in ARF, but they also found four studies that agreed with the finding that age did not significantly affect survival rates. They found that survival correlated more with the presence or absence of specific complications, for example, use of dialysis, level of consciousness, use of mechanical respiration, and presence of hypotension. They did agree that older patients needed more time to recover renal function and recovered less fully.

Glomerular Disease (Nephrotic Syndrome)

The nephrotic syndrome is defined by the urinary excretion of protein in excess of 3 g per day and other features that are a consequence of this continued protein loss (hypoalbuminemia, hyperlipidemia, edema, and a hypercoagulable state). Diastolic hypertension and renal failure are seen in about one-third of patients. The nephrotic syndrome can result from primary glomerular disease, neoplastic disease, or multisystem disease. The incidence of nephrotic syndrome in the elderly is poorly defined, but in one study of 100 consecutive cases 25% were over age 60 yr (32), suggesting that nephrotic syndrome is at least as common in the elderly as it is in younger age groups.

Brown (15) reviewed the histopathology from five series, with 215 patients over the age of 60 yr presenting with nephrotic syndrome. The histopathological examinations showed membranous nephropathy in 38%, minimal change nephropathy in 18%, proliferative glomerulonephritis in 13%, amyloidosis in 15%, and a variety of other lesions in the remaining 17%. The incidence of membranous nephropathy and amyloidosis was higher than in younger adult subjects, proliferative glomerulonephritis was much lower, while minimal change disease was comparable but lower than in children.

In the most recent review on this subject, Johnston et al. (48) reviewed clinicopathological findings in 317 patients over age 60 yr with nephrotic syndrome from the British Medical Research Council Glomerulonephritis Registry. They reported 36.6% with membranous nephropathy, 11% with minimal change lesions, 10.7% with amyloidosis, 11.7% with mesangiocapillary and mesangial proliferative glomerulonephritis, 10.4% with focal/segmental glomerulosclerosis, and the remaining 19.6% with a wide array of other diagnoses.

Primary Glomerulopathies. The primary glomerulopathies seen in elderly patients for the most part are not different from those seen in younger patients, though their incidence appears lower in the geriatric population. Two diagnoses did appear to be substantially less frequent in the older age group. Johnston et al. (48) reviewed their experience and that of seven other authors and found IgA nephropathy in only 19 of 1,386 patients over age 60 yr (1.4%). They also found rapidly progressive (crescentic) glomerulonephritis presenting as nephrotic syndrome in only three patients; however, another 103 elderly patients with crescentic glomerulonephritis presented with acute or chronic renal failure.

Nephrotic Syndrome and Neoplasia. Brown (15) reviewed a series of six articles that showed a high incidence of neoplasia in elderly patients with nephrotic syndrome. When she looked only at those patients with membranous glomerulopathy, 11% had an underlying malignancy.

Johnston et al. (48), in the British MRC Registry study of 317 nephrotics, found 15 cases of malignancy associated with nephrotic syndrome (4.7%). The authors provide data to suggest that this is not too different from what might be anticipated in any elderly population. In comparison, 8 of 116 patients with membranous nephropathy (6.9%) had malignancies.

Nephrotic Syndrome Related to Systemic Disease. In contrast, glomerulopathies resulting from systemic disease are more common in the elderly because of the increased incidence of such underlying diseases as diabetes mellitus, amyloidosis (dysproteinemias), vasculitis, and scleroderma. In the largest and most recent experience (48), a secondary cause for nephrotic syndrome was found in 103 of 317 patients (32%). Nephritis associated with systemic lupus erythematosus appears to be less common in the elderly than in the younger population. Diabetic nephropathy is the most frequent cause of glomerular disease associated with systemic illness in the elderly. Since many of these patients have an obvious etiology for their nephrotic syndrome, documentation in biopsy series tends to be low and to underestimate the prevalence of this lesion, especially in the elderly. All nephrotics over age 50 yr should have urine and serum electrophoresis performed, since in two large series of elderly nephrotics (51, 118), amyloidosis was the most frequent cause of secondary nephrotic syndrome, being responsible for 22 and 13% of all cases. In the British MRC Glomerulonephritis Registry, amyloidosis accounted for 34 of 317 cases (10.7%) (48).

Chronic Renal Failure

Chronic renal failure results from irreversible damage to both kidneys from a wide variety of causes. Up to 90% of kidney function may be lost without significant morbidity. Progression of the renal lesions and worsening of the condition can be prevented, or at least delayed, by managing hypertension, infection, obstructive uropathy, heart failure, and dehydration.

Discussions of some of the more common causes of chronic renal failure without preceding nephrotic syndrome follow.

Renal Vascular Disorders. Occlusive arterial disease can cause either acute or chronic renal failure. Renal arterial embolization or thrombosis may occur in patients with acute myocardial infarction, chronic atrial fibrillation, and subacute bacterial endocarditis. Renal artery stenosis (RAS) is common in the elderly and is usually due to atherosclerosis. Although it is often totally asymptomatic, it should be considered in the differential diagnosis whenever an older person suddenly develops hypertension, if a patient with well-controlled hypertension develops an accelerated course, or whenever a patient develops an unexplained increase in his blood urea nitrogen or serum creatinine, especially after treatment with an ACE inhibitor. The last suggests bilateral lesions.

Renal cholesterol embolization is a specific geriatric disorder that may occur spontaneously or in association with aortic surgery or angiography in patients with diffuse atherosclerosis (35). The clinical course is variable but most often involves a progressive renal insufficiency (86). A definitive diagnosis is difficult because it requires visualization of cholesterol crystals on biopsy and alternative diagnoses are often valid concerns (99).

Arteriolar Nephrosclerosis—Benign and Malignant. The small arteries and arterioles of the kidney are usually affected by elevations in systemic blood pressure. Patients with mild to moderate blood pressure elevations develop a benign arteriolar nephrosclerosis characterized by fibrosis and thickening of the intima of the larger arteries and by a patchy hyaline thickening of the afferent arteriolar wall, both resulting in a progressive decrease in luminal size. Chronic renal failure associated with this lesion tends to develop very slowly over a period of years.

Hypertensive cases with diastolic pressures in excess of 130 mm Hg develop an accelerated or malignant phase in which afferent arterioles and interlobular arteries show a proliferative endarteritis ("onion skin" appearance of the endothelium) and necrotizing arteriolitis (fibrinoid necrosis of media) along with a glomerulitis with necrosis. Hematuria with red cell casts, albuminuria, and loss of renal function develop.

Systemic Vasculitis. Systemic vasculitis refers to a heterogenous group of disorders having in common inflammation and necrotizing lesions of blood vessel walls. These can be either primary lesions or associated with other systemic diseases. Manifestations include fever, weight loss, arthritis, abdominal pain, polyneuritis, myopathy, and cardiac and central nervous system dysfunctions. In some instances, these can be classified into specific disorders, for example, periarteritis nodosa or Wegener's granulomatosis. Tests for antineutrophil cytoplasmic antibodies (ANCA) have been particularly helpful in identifying the latter and classifying the various systemic vasculitides. Patients over the age of 60 yr appear to comprise 30% or more of cases (97).

Polycystic Renal Disease. Although the diagnosis of autosomal dominant polycystic kidney disease is usually made before age 60 yr, a few patients are not diagnosed until later life. Family history is not always present.

Analgesic Nephropathy. The frequency of arthritis and arthralgia in the elderly increases the risk of long-term analgesic use and abuse. Phenacetin is the most frequently incriminated, but salicylate, acetaminophen, and the NSAIDs also must be implicated. These latter drugs, because they inhibit vasodilatory prostaglandins which reduce medullary blood flow and inhibit the hexose monophosphate shunt which leads to oxidative injury of medullary cells, frequently cause chronic interstitial nephritis and ultimately papillary necrosis leading to renal insufficiency, mild proteinuria, and hypertension, often severe. The lesions are dose- and duration-dependent.

Multiple Myeloma. Multiple myeloma should be ruled out in any patient with unexplained renal insufficiency. A strong relationship exists between the presence of Bence Jones proteinuria (immunoglobulin light chains) and the presence of renal insufficiency. Renal damage may result from tubular obstruction or tubular nephrotoxicity from the light chains. Other causes of renal insufficiency in myeloma include amyloidosis, hypercalcemia, and urate deposition. Myeloma patients specifically are at risk with radiocontrast dyes and antibiotics such as the aminoglycosides.

Scleroderma. The elderly patient with other manifestations consistent with scleroderma may develop hypertension, at times malignant in character, and acute to chronic renal insufficiency. Narrowing of the interlobular arteries without inflammatory infiltrates produces the renin-mediated hypertension.

Urinary Tract Infections

Pyelonephritis is a serious infection and is the most common cause of gram-negative bacteremia in elderly, hospitalized patients. *Escherichia coli* causes approximately two-thirds of the episodes of infection, with *Klebsiella, Enterobacter, Citrobacter, Enterococcus, Proteus,* and *Pseudomonas aeruginosa* accounting for most of the rest.

Acute symptomatic pyelonephritis often offers a greater diagnostic challenge in elderly than in younger patients, where the classic irritative voiding symptoms make diagnosis readily apparent. Patients with neurological disease (dementia, cerebral vascular disease, Parkinsonism) have an increased incidence of infection and often present only with altered mental status (somnolence, confusion), tachypnea, and vague abdominal pains that may suggest pneumonia, diverticulitis, or intestinal obstruction as alternative diagnoses. They may not have fever or leukocytosis.

The presence of pyuria (>10 WBC/HPF), confirmed by a clean void urine sample containing more than 10^5 colony-forming organisms per milliliter, establishes the diagnosis. Failure to obtain this number of bacteria does not exclude pyelonephritis, as one needs to consider the possibilities that (1) prior antibiotic therapy may have been administered or (2) the infection was proximal to a site of obstruction.

Bacteremia has been detected in over half of elderly men and women with acute symptomatic pyelonephritis, necessitating multiple blood cultures as a part of patient evaluation. Significant pyuria and bacteriuria with lower urinary tract symptoms are common in elderly persons, especially women, and can be due to cystitis. It is often difficult to determine whether or not infections are limited to the bladder and urethra alone or extend up to involve the kidney. High fever and back (costovertebral angle) pain and tenderness suggest the latter.

Asymptomatic bacteriuria (pyuria and bacteria in the urine greater than 10^5 organisms per ml on clean voided examination) is increasingly prevalent with advancing age, being present in one-third of patients in long-term care facilities. Although there clearly is an increased mortality in individuals with asymptomatic bacteriuria, it has been argued that it is merely a marker for severe underlying disease rather than an independent risk factor for shortened survival (81). Antibiotic therapy has been unsuccessful in prolonging survival or preventing recurrent bacteriuria or symptomatic infection in men compared to untreated controls followed over a 2-yr period (80), so it probably is best left untreated until the patient becomes symptomatic (1).

LOWER URINARY TRACT DYSFUNCTION WITH AGING

Anatomy and Physiology of the Lower Urinary Tract

The anatomy of the lower urinary tract can be divided into three components: (1) the bladder and its outlet,

(2) the local innervation, and (3) the connections to the central nervous system. The lower urinary tract is made up of the urethral outlet and a muscular storage and contractile portion known as the detrusor (bladder). The proximal portion of the urethra is surrounded by the internal urethral sphincter, which is predominantly smooth muscle, located in the region of the bladder neck, and autonomically innervated. Distal to this sphincter is the external sphincter, which is striated muscle under voluntary control.

The normal processes of urine storage and voiding are under the control of the central nervous system (Fig. 19.3) (7). The main reflex center for the bladder, the brain stem micturition center (BSMC), appears to be located in the mesencephalic-reticular formation. A less dominant center, the spinal cord micturition center (SCMC), also has some influence. Sensory, proprioceptive fibers arising in the bladder transmit impulses via the pelvic nerves and posterior columns to the BSMC. Motor fibers in the BSMC transmit impulses via the reticulospinal tracts to the detrusor motor nucleus in the sacral spinal cord. From here, parasympathetic fibers innervate the detrusor muscle, with the neurotransmitter being the cholinergic agent acetylcholine. Increased cholinergic activity increases the frequency and force of detrusor contractions, and reduced activity (atropine) has the opposite effect. Suprasacral interruption of this pathway releases the SCMC from inhibition so that a

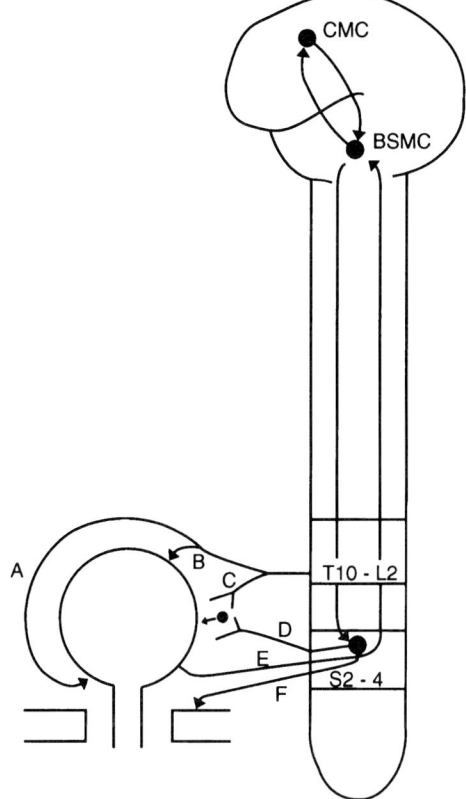

FIG. 19.3. Neural innervation of the detrusor (bladder). [Adapted from Augspurger (7) with permission.]

low-capacity bladder with unsustained, uninhibited contractions develops. Other supraspinal pathways modulate the detrusor reflex through inputs on the BSMC. The overall effect is one of inhibition of the detrusor reflex. Interruption of these pathways results in loss of voluntary control over the detrusor reflex, characterized by sustained uninhibited detrusor contraction.

Sympathetic innervation originates in the thoracolumbar spinal cord. The dome of the bladder is innervated primarily by β-adrenergic fibers, with the bladder neck innervated by α-adrenergic fibers. Stimulation of β-adrenergic fibers results in detrusor muscle relaxation, whereas stimulation of α-adrenergic fibers causes contraction and tightening of the bladder neck, both of which promote urine retention. While storage of urine is accomplished by sympathetic stimulation, voiding is under parasympathetic control. Knowledge of these effects is important in understanding the side effects of medications and the selection of appropriate medicines in the treatment of urinary incontinence.

The striate (skeletal) external sphincter is largely under voluntary control. Motor fibers originate in the cerebrum (medial aspect of the central sulcus). Suprasacral interruption of this pathway produces spasticity in the striate external sphincter. There is a reciprocal innervation between the external sphincter and the detrusor so that contraction of one produces reflex relaxation of the other and vice versa. Any lesion below the BSMC produces dyscoordination (dyssynergia) between the bladder and the external sphincter.

Effect of Age on Lower Urinary Tract

Aging affects the lower urinary tract in a number of ways, but incontinence is not a normal consequence. Bladder capacity, the ability to postpone voiding, bladder compliance, and urinary flow rate appear to decline in both sexes, and maximum urethral closure pressure and urethral length appear to decline in women (88, 89). The number of uninhibited contractions probably increases with age, and postvoiding residual volume may increase but probably to no more than 25–50 ml (88). While none of these age-related changes causes incontinence, each can predispose to incontinence, especially since older persons are prone to additional problems which increase the likelihood of incontinence.

Another age-related change that can contribute to the development of incontinence is the shift in diurnal excretion of fluid (89). Younger persons excrete a higher percentage of daily fluid load during the daytime hours; older individuals excrete more during the night. This occurs even in the healthy elderly and is accentuated in individuals with hypertension, heart failure, lower extremity venous insufficiency, and renal disease.

Transient Incontinence

A number of conditions superimposed on an elderly person can lead to the development of incontinence. Resnick (88) has used the mnemonic DIAPPERS (with the double P) to describe some of these, as shown in Table 19.3. Delirium is an acute confusional state, often precipitated by an acute medical problem, such as pneumonia or heart failure, that affects one's ability to react appropriately when the bladder becomes distended with urine. Symptomatic urinary tract infections produce a sense of urgency which precipitates voiding before the older person reaches the toilet. Atrophic vaginitis in elderly women is due to estrogen deficiency and presents with dysuria, dyspareunia, urgency, and incontinence. A number of medications are capable of causing incontinence, most notably drugs with anticholinergic properties (such as the tricyclic antidepressants, certain antipsychotic and anti-Parkinsonian agents, antispasmotics, and antidiarrheals), drugs with α-adrenergic agonist or antagonist properties (such as certain antihypertensives and decongestants), and finally calcium channel blockers.

Psychological causes of incontinence are not common in the elderly, but depression is one disturbance that can lead to incontinence. Endocrine causes of incontinence include hypercalcemia and hyperglycemia, both of which increase urine flow rates. Reduced mobility and stool impaction also can contribute to the development of incontinence. Many times in the elderly, the onset of incontinence becomes multifactorial, with confusion, drugs, and mobility all playing significant roles.

TABLE 19.3. *Common Causes of Transient Incontinence*

Mnemonic Designation	Cause
D	Delirium or confusional state
I	Infection, urinary (symptomatic)
A	Atrophic urethritis or vaginitis

P	Pharmaceuticals
	    Sedative hypnotics
	    Loop diuretics
	    Anticholinergics (antipsychotics, antidepressants, antihistamines, opiates, antiarrythmics, anti-Parkinsonism medications, α-adrenergic agonists and antagonists, calcium channel blockers)

P	Psychological disorders (depression)
E	Endocrine disorders (hypercalcemia, hypokalemia, hyperglycemia)
R	Restricted mobility
S	Stool impaction

Adapted from Resnick (88) with permission.

Established Incontinence

Table 19.4 lists the common causes of established incontinence. There are essentially four ways that the lower urinary tract may malfunction to create incontinence. The bladder either contracts when it should not (detrusor overactivity), leading to urge incontinence, or fails to contract or fails to contract as well as it should (detrusor underactivity), leading to overflow incontinence. Also, outlet resistance can be either persistently high as in obstructive lesions such as prostatism, leading to overflow incontinence, or persistently low as in the outlet incompetence seen in stress incontinence. Incontinence can also result from neurogenic causes.

Detrusor overactivity is a condition in which the bladder contracts precipitously with little warning and often empties itself completely. Detrusor hyperactivity can exist with normal contractile function or with impaired contractile function (DHIC) (90). This condition presents itself as urge incontinence. It can result from damage to the central nervous system inhibitory centers, for example, cerebrovascular accident (CVA), Parkinsonism, or Alzheimer's dementia, or it can result from local, irritative pathology, for example, cystitis, bladder carcinoma, or stone, which impairs the ability of the normal brain to inhibit bladder contraction. Both outlet obstruction and outlet incompetence can predispose to detrusor hyperactivity.

Detrusor underactivity can result from damage to the nerves supplying the bladder (disk compression, tumors) or to an autonomic neuropathy (diabetes, alcoholism, pernicious anemia, tabes dorsalis). It can also result from replacement of bladder muscle by fibrosis and connective tissue, as seen with chronic obstruction (prostatism), whereby the bladder is no longer able to empty normally.

Pathophysiology of Voiding Dysfunction in Benign Prostatic Hyperplasia

Interest in the pathogenesis and pathophysiology of obstructive voiding dysfunction has increased over the last decade; however, many questions remain. The inability of elderly men to fully empty the bladder generally involves the prostate and the mechanisms affected by hypertrophy of this gland. Perhaps equally important, however, are the hypertrophic changes observed in the obstructed detrusor which impair contraction and thereby contribute to emptying problems (90).

Pathophysiology of Benign Prostatic Hyperplasia.

Benign prostatic hyperplasia (BPH) is the most common pathological process to afflict aging men. At least 70% of men over age 70 yr have histological evidence of BPH, and more than half of these have either symptoms of bladder outflow obstruction or reduced uroflow (37). These symptoms of bladder outflow obstruction do not necessarily progress but often wax and wane. The prostate contains adrenergically innervated smooth muscle which contracts in response to norepinephrine. There are both α_1- and α_2-adrenoreceptors in prostatic smooth muscle, but the former are the most important in mediating contraction. Fluctuations in sympathetic nervous system activity may then account for variations in symptoms of prostatism and have led to the use of α_1-selective blocking agents (prazosin, doxazosin, terazosin) for the treatment of this disorder (13, 17, 52).

Surgical and medical castration produce approximately a 30% reduction in the size of the hyperplastic prostate, suggesting that high plasma testosterone levels contribute to the development of BPH. More impressively, the clinical syndrome of 5α-reductase deficiency in the prostate, producing pseudovaginal perineoscrotal hypospadias, is characterized by the absence of a palpable prostate. The intracellular 5α-reduction of testosterone to dihydrotestosterone (DHT) amplifies the androgenic signal in a variety of target tissues, most notably the prostate. Inhibition of the 5α-reductase enzyme would be expected to impair prostate growth without affecting sexual function, as is the case with androgen ablation therapy. This has led to the search for a competitive inhibitor of 5α-reductase which would suppress plasma levels of DHT without lowering testosterone. Finasteride (Proscar®) is such an agent, as it suppresses levels of DHT but has no measurable binding affinity for the androgen receptor (69). This agent produces a 10% increase in plasma gonadotropin and testosterone levels (well within normal physiological ranges) and appears to have no significant effects on

TABLE 19.4. *Common Causes of Established Incontinence*

Detrusor Overactivity (urge incontinence)
Neurogenic (stroke, Parkinsonism, Alzheimer's dementia)
Nonneurogenic (bladder carcinoma, cystitis, obstruction)

Detrusor Underactivity (overflow incontinence)
Neurogenic (disk compression, autonomic neuropathy)
Nonneurogenic (long-standing obstruction)

Outlet Incompetence (stress incontinence)
Neurogenic (rare)
Nonneurogenic (sphincter damage and pelvic floor laxity due to previous pregnancies)

Outlet Obstruction (overflow incontinence)
Neurogenic (detrusor–sphincter dyssynergia associated with spinal cord disease)
Nonneurogenic (BPH, urethral stricture, stenosis)

Adapted from Resnick (88) with permission.

other endocrine or lipid levels. It does appear to be effective in decreasing the mass of prostatic tissue (38, 69, 102).

Pathophysiology of the Obstructed Detrusor. Three integrated microstructural components, specifically smooth muscle, interstitium, and intrinsic nerves, determine the functional response of the detrusor (28, 29). The fundamental feature of the obstructed detrusor is hypertrophy. The hypertrophy pattern has three characteristic features: (1) marked separation of the detrusor muscle cells; (2) abundant collagen in the expanded spaces between individual muscle cells; and (3) big, bizarre, branched, and braided hypertrophic muscle cells (29). These features combine to limit the ability of the obstructed detrusor to mount a contraction so that one can empty the full bladder completely. Contortion of hypertrophic and braided interlocking of branched cells curtails their ability to shorten (contract). Wide separation of muscle cells, with loss of intermediate junctions, would greatly restrict or eliminate mechanical cell coupling to transmit contractions generated by one or a group of cells to coupling cells. Excessive intercellular collagen would further impede mechanical cell coupling and "stiffen" the detrusor.

Often superimposed on this hypertrophic pattern is a degenerative process characterized by widespread degeneration of muscle cells and intrinsic axons. Degenerating muscle cells would not generate a contraction even if stimulated by intrinsic nerves; degeneration of intrinsic axons would impede neural impulses.

Structural changes ("dysfunctional" pattern) in the obstructed detrusor appear to explain the detrusor overactivity (instability) that often leads to urge incontinence (29). This pattern is characterized by (1) loss or depletion of intermediate cell junctions characteristic of normal detrusor and (2) abundance of alien, distinctive protrusion junctions which have a narrow interspace comparable to that of gap junctions. Spread of contraction (cell coupling) in normal detrusor is achieved primarily by mechanical coupling. Protrusion junctions have the structural attributes of a "low-resistance pathway," imparting to the widely separated muscle cells of the obstructed detrusor the properties of a functional syncytium, through which electrical (in lieu of mechanical) cell coupling can take place. In such a "syncytium," a contractile impulse of sufficient amplitude generated in one or a few muscle cells would be transmitted readily, with negligible delay and rapidly to outlying cells, resulting, during bladder filling, in a measurable involuntary contraction. Repetition of this sequence of events would result in a succession of similar independent, involuntary contractions. This would not, however, interfere with the development of nerve-triggered, coordinated, and efficient voiding contractions.

Bladder obstruction also can lead to chronic retention and massive distension. Such bladders are characterized by excessive elastic fibers intermingled with collagen in the widely expanded spaces between individual muscle cells (29). Such excessive elastic promotes distensibility of the bladder.

Evaluation of patients suspected of having a voiding dysfunction associated with BPH should consist of a detailed neurological evaluation, a rectal examination to evaluate prostate size and to rule out prostate carcinoma, and a functional evaluation in patients suspected of having detrusor dysfunction and marginal outlet obstruction. This can start simply with a postvoid residual urine measurement and progress as indicated to uroflowmetry, detailed cystometry, assessment of bladder contractility, and evaluation of the outlet conduit (voiding cystourethrography).

Other Diseases of the Lower Urinary Tract

Malignancies and infections occur at multiple sites along the lower urinary tract. Cancer of the prostate is the most common tumor in men in the United States, with mean age at presentation being 72 yr (25). Although no specific etiological factors are known, it is hormone-dependent as DHT, the intracellularly active metabolite of testosterone, is necessary for prostatic growth and metabolism.

Prostatitis is also common in both young and elderly men. The majority of cases are not due to bacterial infection but are related to introduction of chemical irritants which cause inflammation of the prostate. These irritants include caffeine, alcohol, pharmacological agents, dietary factors, and even physical activity (25). Increased intravesical pressure generated by heavy lifting or exercise against a closed external urethral sphincter can force urine into the prostatic ducts, creating a chemical prostatitis. Anxiety, stress, and iatrogenic factors, such as introduction of indwelling catheters, also can play a role. Bacterial prostatitis can be either acute or chronic, with varying degrees of fever, chills, dysuria, frequency, nocturia, and perineal and lower back pain. It should be suspected in any elderly man with recurrent urinary tract infections and normal I.V. pyelogram and can be diagnosed on digital examination.

REFERENCES

1. ABRUTYN, E., J. A. BOSCIA, and D. KAYE. The treatment of asymptomatic bacteriuria in the elderly. *J. Am. Geriatr. Soc.* 36: 473–475, 1988.
2. ADLER, S., R. D. LINDEMAN, M. J. YIENGST, E. S. BEARD, and N. W. SHOCK. Effect of acute acid loading on urinary acid excretion by the aging human kidney. *J. Lab. Clin. Med.* 72: 278–289, 1968.

3. AGARWAL, B. H., and R. G. CABEBE. Renal acidification in elderly subjects. *Nephron* 26: 291–293, 1980.
4. ANDERSON, R. I., H. M. CHUNG, R. KLUGE, and R. W. SCHRIER. Hyponatremia: a prospective analysis of its epidemiology and the pathogenic role of vasopressin. *Ann. Intern. Med.* 102: 164–168, 1985.
5. ANDERSON, S., and B. M. BRENNER. Effects of aging on the renal glomerulus. *Am. J. Med.* 80: 435–442, 1986.
6. ASHOURI, O. S. Severe diuretic-induced hyponatremia in the elderly. *Arch. Intern. Med.* 146: 1355–1357, 1986.
7. AUGSPURGER, R. R. Urinary incontinence and catheters in the elderly male and female. In: *Geriatric Medicine,* edited by R. W. Schrier. Philadelphia: Saunders, 1990, p. 156–167.
8. BARROWS, C. H., Jr., J. A. FALZONE, Jr., and N. W. SHOCK. Age differences in the succinoxidase activity of homogenates and mitochondria from the livers and kidneys of rats. *J. Gerontol.* 1: 130–133, 1960.
9. BEAUCHENE, R. E., D. D. FANESTIL, and C. H. BARROWS, Jr. The effect of age on active transport and sodium–potassium activated ATPase activity in renal tissue of rats. *J. Gerontol.* 20: 306–310, 1965.
10. BELL, R. H., Jr., B. A. BORJESSON, P. L. WOLF, L. FERNANDEZ-CRUZ, J. E. BRIMM, S. LEE, H. J. SAYERS, and M. J. ORLOFF. Quantitative morphologic studies of aging changes in the kidney of the Lewis rat. *Renal Physiol.* 7: 176–184, 1984.
11. BERTANI, T., C. ZOJA, M. ALBATE, M. ROSSINI, and G. REMUZZI. Age-related nephropathy and proteinuria in rats with intact kidneys exposed to diets with different protein content. *Lab. Invest.* 60: 196–204, 1989.
12. BONER, G., W. D. SHELP, M. NETON, and R. E. RIESELBACH. Factors influencing the increase in glomerular filtration rate in the remaining kidney of transplant donors. *Am. J. Med.* 55: 169–174, 1973.
13. BRAWER, M., H. EPSTEIN, and G. ADAMS. Efficacy and safety of terazosin in patients with symptoms of benign prostatic hyperplasia. A new double-blind study [Abstract]. *J. Urol.* 147: 365, 1992.
14. BRENNER, B. M., T. W. MEYER, and T. H. HOSTETTER. Dietary protein intake and the progressive nature of kidney disease: the role of hemodynamically mediated glomerular injury in the pathogenesis of progressive glomerular sclerosis in aging, renal ablation and intrinsic renal disease. *N. Engl. J. Med.* 307: 652–659, 1982.
15. BROWN, W. W. Glomerulonephritis in the elderly. In: *Geriatric Nephrology,* edited by M. F. Michelis, B. B. Davis, and H. G. Preuss. New York: Field, Rich, 1986, p. 90–98.
16. BURICH, R. J. Effects of age on renal function and enzyme activity in male C57BL/6 mice. *J. Gerontol.* 30: 539–545, 1975.
17. CHAPPLE, C. R., P. CARTER, and T. J. CHRISTMAS. A three-month, double-blind, placebo-controlled trial of doxazosin as a treatment of benign prostatic hyperplasia obstruction. *Neurourol. Urodyn.* 10: 298–299, 1991.
18. COUSER, W. G., and M. M. STILMANT. Mesangial lesions and focal glomerular sclerosis in the aging rat. *Lab. Invest.* 33: 491–501, 1975.
19. CRANE, M. G., and J. J. HARRIS. Effect of aging on renin activity and aldosterone excretions. *J. Lab. Clin. Med.* 87: 947–959, 1976.
20. DAVIES, D. F., and N. W. SHOCK. Age changes in glomerular filtration rate, effective renal plasma flow, and tubular excretory capacity in adult males. *J. Clin. Invest.* 29: 496–507, 1950.
21. DAVIS, P. J., and F. B. DAVIS. Water excretion in the elderly. *Endocrinol. Metab. Clin.* 16: 867–875, 1987.
22. DEEN, W. M., D. A. MADDOX, C. R. ROBERTSON, and B. M. BRENNER. Dynamics of the glomerular ultrafiltration in the rat. VII. Response to reduced renal mass. *Am. J. Physiol.* 277: 556–562, 1974.
23. DEUTSCH, S., M. GOLDBERG, and R. D. DRIPPS. Postoperative hyponatremia with the inappropriate release of antidiuretic hormone. *Anesthesia* 27: 250–256, 1966.
24. DIOKNO, A. C., B. M. BROCK, M. B. BROWN, and A. R. HERZOG. Prevalence of urinary incontinence and other urological symptoms in the non-institutionalized elderly. *J. Urol.* 136: 1022–1025, 1986.
25. DONOHUE, R. E., M. A. DAVIS, and E. D. CRAWFORD. Diseases of the prostate. In: *Geriatric Medicine,* edited by R. W. Schrier. Philadelphia: Saunders, 1990, p. 168–178.
26. DONTAS, A. S., S. MARKETOS, and P. PAPANAYIOUTOU. Mechanism of renal tubular defects in old age. *Postgrad. Med. J.* 48: 295–303, 1972.
27. EKNOYAN, G. Tubulointerstitial nephropathies in the aged. In: *Hypertension and Renal Disease in the Elderly,* edited by M. Martinez-Maldonado. Boston: Blackwell, 1992, p. 225–241.
28. ELBADAWI, A. Neuromuscular mechanics of micturition. In: *Neurourology and Urodynamics: Principles and Practice,* edited by S. V. Yalla, E. J. McGuire, A. Elbadawi, and J. G. Blaivas. New York City: MacMillan, 1988, p. 3–35.
29. ELBADAWI, A. Pathophysiology of voiding dysfunction in benign prostatic hypertrophy. Presented at the Preconference Symposium of the American Geriatric Society, Washington, D. C., November 14, 1992.
30. EPSTEIN, M., and N. K. HOLLENBERG. Age as a determinant of renal sodium conservation in normal men. *J. Lab. Clin. Med.* 87: 411–417, 1976.
31. FAULSTICK, D., M. J. YIENGST, and D. A. OURSTER. Glomerular permeability in young and old subjects. *J. Gerontol.* 17: 40–44, 1962.
32. FAWCETT, L. W., P. J. HILTON, N. E. JONES, and A. J. WING. Nephrotic syndrome in the elderly. *Br. Med. J.* 2: 387–388, 1971.
33. FICHMAN, M. P., H. VORHERR, and C. R. KLEEMAN. Diuretic-induced hyponatremia. *Ann. Intern. Med.* 75: 853–863, 1971.
34. FINE, L. G. Proceedings from a symposium on renal growth in health and disease. *Am. J. Kidney Dis.* 17: 601–686, 1991.
35. FINE, M. J., W. KAPOOR, and V. FALENGA. Cholesterol crystal embolization: a review of 221 cases in the English literature. *Angiology* 38: 769–784, 1987.
36. FRIEDMAN, S. A., A. E. RAIZNER, H. ROSEN, N. A. SOLOMON, and W. SY. Functional defects in the aging kidney. *Ann. Intern. Med.* 76: 41–45, 1972.
37. GARRAWAY, W. M., G. M. COLLINS, and R. J. LEE. High prevalence of benign prostatic hypertrophy in the community. *Lancet* 338: 469–471, 1991.
38. GORMLEY, G. J., E. STONER, R. C. BRUSKEWITZ, J. IPERATO-MCGINLEY, P. C. WALSH, J. D. MCCONNELL, G. L. ANDRIOLE, J. GELLER, B. R. BRACKIN, J. S. TENOVER, E. D. VAUGHAN, F. PAPPAS, A. TAYLOR, B. BINKOWITZ, and J. NG. The effect of finasteride in men with benign prostatic hyperplasia. *N. Engl. J. Med.* 327: 1185–1191, 1992.
39. GOYAL, V. K. Changes with age in the human kidney. *Exp. Gerontol.* 17: 321–331, 1982.
40. HAKIM, R. M., R. C. GOLDSZER, and B. M. BRENNER. Hypertension and proteinuria: long-term sequelae of uninephrectomy in humans. *Kidney Int.* 25: 930–936, 1984.
41. HALLER, B. G., H. ZUST, S. SHAW, M. P. GNADINGER, D. E. UEHLINGER, and P. WEIDMAN. Effects of posture and aging on circulating atrial natriuretic peptide levels in man. *J. Hypertens.* 5: 551–556, 1987.
42. HAYSLETT, J. P. Functional adaptation to reduction in renal mass. *Physiol. Rev.* 59: 137–164, 1979.
43. HELDERMAN, J. H., R. E. VESTAL, J. W. ROWE, J. D. TOBIN, R. ANDRES, and G. L. ROBERTSON. The response of arginine vaso-

pressin to intravenous ethanol and hypertonic saline in man. The impact of age. *J. Gerontol.* 33: 39–47, 1978.
44. HOLLENBERG, N. K., D. F. ADAMS, H. S. SOLOMON, A. RASHID, L. A. ABRAM, and J. P. MERRILL. Senescence and the renal vasculature in normal man. *Circulation Res.* 34: 309–316, 1974.
45. HOSTETTER, T. H., J. L. OLSON, H. G. RENNKE, M. A. VENKATACHALAM, and B. M. BRENNER. Hyperfiltration in remnant nephrons: a potentially adverse response to renal ablation. *Am. J. Physiol.* 9: 85–93, 1981.
46. HOSTETTER, T. H., J. L. TROY, and B. M. BRENNER. Glomerular hemodynamics in experimental diabetes mellitus. *Kidney Int.* 19: 410–415, 1981.
47. IWASAKI, K., C. A. GLEISER, E. J. MASORO, C. A. MCMAHON, E. J. SEO, and B. P. YU. The influence of dietary protein source on longevity and age-related disease processes of Fischer rats. *J. Gerontol.* 43: B5–B12, 1988.
48. JOHNSTON, P. A., J. S. BROWN, and A. M. DAVISON. The nephrotic syndrome in the elderly: clinico-pathological correlations in 317 patients. *Geriatr. Nephrol. Urol.* 2: 85–90, 1992.
49. KAPLAN, C., B. PASTERNACK, H. SHAH, and G. GALLO. Age-related incidence of sclerotic glomeruli in human kidneys. *Am. J. Pathol.* 80: 227–234, 1975.
50. KASISKE, B. L. Relationship between vascular disease and age-associated changes in the human kidney. *Kidney Int.* 31: 1153–1159, 1987.
51. KINGSWOOD, J. C., R. A. BANKS, C. R. TRIBE, J. OWEN-JONES, and J. C. MCKENZIE. Renal biopsy in the elderly: clinicopathological correlations in 143 patients. *Clin. Nephrol.* 22: 183–187, 1984.
52. KIRBY, R. S., S. W. COPPINGER, M. O. CORCORAN, C. R. CHAPPLE, M. FLANIGAN, and E. J. G. MILROY. Prazosin in the treatment of prostatic obstruction: a placebo-controlled study. *Br. J. Urol.* 60: 136–142, 1987.
53. KIRTLAND, J., M. LYE, C. GODDARD, E. VARGAS, and I. DAVIES. Plasma arginine vasopressin in dehydrated elderly patients. *Clin. Endocrinol.* 20: 451–456, 1984.
54. KLEINFELD, M., M. CASIMIR, and S. BORRA. Hyponatremia as observed in a chronic disease facility. *J. Am. Geriatr. Soc.* 27: 156–161, 1979.
55. KUMAR, R., C. M. HILL, and M. G. MCGEOWN. Acute renal failure in the elderly. *Lancet* 1: 90–91, 1973.
56. LAWSON, D. H. Adverse reactions to potassium chloride. *Q. J. Med.* 43: 433–440, 1974.
57. LEDINGHAM, J. G., M. J. CROWE, M. L. FORSLING, P. A. PHILLIPS, and B. J. ROLLS. Effect of aging on vasopressin secretion, water excretion, and thirst in man. *Kidney Int.* 32(suppl. 21): S90–S92, 1987.
58. LINDEMAN, R. D. Is a high protein intake harmful to the aging human kidney? *Geriatr. Nephrol. Urol.* 1: 113–119, 1991.
59. LINDEMAN, R. D., and R. GOLDMAN. Anatomic and physiologic age changes in the kidney. *Exp. Gerontol.* 21: 379–406, 1986.
60. LINDEMAN, R. D., T. D. LEE, Jr., M. J. YIENGST, and N. W. SHOCK. Influence of age, renal disease, hypertension, diuretics and calcium on the antidiuretic response to suboptimal infusions of vasopressin. *J. Lab. Clin. Med.* 68: 206–223, 1966.
61. LINDEMAN, R. D., J. D. TOBIN, and N. W. SHOCK. Association between blood pressure and the rate of decline in renal function with age. *Kidney Int.* 26: 861–868, 1984.
62. LINDEMAN, R. D., J. D. TOBIN, and N. W. SHOCK. Longitudinal studies on the rate of decline in renal function with age. *J. Am. Geriatr. Soc.* 33: 278–285, 1985.
63. LINDEMAN, R. D., H. C. VAN BUREN, and L. G. RAISZ. Osmolar renal concentrating ability in healthy young men and hospitalized patients without renal disease. *N. Engl. J. Med.* 262: 1306–1309, 1960.
64. LINDEMAN, R. D. Overview. Renal physiology and pathophysiology of aging. *Am. J. Kidney Dis.* 16: 275–282, 1990.
65. LJUNGVIST, A. Structure of the arteriole–glomerular units in different zones of the kidney. *Nephron* 1: 329–337, 1964.
66. LOWENSTEIN, J., D. A. FAULSTICK, M. J. YIENGST, and N. W. SHOCK. The glomerular clearance and renal transport of hemoglobin in adult males. *J. Clin. Invest.* 40: 1172–1177, 1961.
67. MAEDA, H., C. A. GLEISER, E. J. MASORO, I. MURATA, C. A. MCMAHON, and B. P. YU. Nutritional influences on aging of Fisher 344 rats. II. Pathology. *J. Gerontol.* 40: 671–688, 1985.
68. MASORO, E. J., and B. P. YU. Diet and nephropathy [Editorial]. *Lab. Invest.* 60: 165–167, 1989.
69. MCCONNELL, J. D., J. D. WILSON, F. W. GEORGE, J. GELLER, F. PAPPAS, and E. STONER. Finasteride, an inhibitor of 5α-reductase, suppresses prostatic dihydrotestosterone in men with benign prostatic hyperplasia. *J. Clin. Endocrinol. Metab.* 74: 505–508, 1992.
70. MCDONALD, R. F., D. H. SOLOMON, and N. W. SHOCK. Aging as a factor in the renal hemodynamic changes induced by a standardized pyrogen. *J. Clin. Invest.* 5: 457–462, 1951.
71. MCLACHLAN, M. S. F. The aging kidney. *Lancet* 2: 143–145, 1978.
72. MCLACHLAN, M. S. F., J. C. GUTHRIE, C. K. ANDERSON, and M. J. FULKER. Vascular and glomerular changes in the aging kidney. *J. Pathol.* 121: 65–78, 1977.
73. MEYER, T. W., S. ANDERSON, H. G. RENNKE, and B. M. BRENNER. Reversing glomerular hypertension stabilizes established glomerular injury. *Kidney Int.* 31: 751–759, 1987.
74. MILLER, I. J., M. SUTHANTHIRAN, R. R. RIGGIO, J. J. WILLIAMS, R. A. RIEHLE, E. D. VAUGHN, W. T. STUBENBORD, J. MOURADIAN, J. S. CHEIGH, and K. H. STENZEL. Impact of renal donation. Long-term clinical and biochemical follow-up of living donors in a single center. *Am. J. Med.* 79: 201–208, 1985.
75. MILLER, J. H., and N. W. SHOCK. Age difference in the renal tubular response to antidiuretic hormone. *J. Gerontol.* 8: 446–450, 1953.
76. MILLER, J. H., R. D. MCDONALD, and N. W. SHOCK. The renal extraction of p-aminohippurate in the aged individual. *J. Gerontol.* 6: 213–216, 1951.
77. MILLER, J. H., R. D. MCDONALD, and N. W. SHOCK. Age changes in the maximal rate of renal tubular reabsorption of glucose. *J. Gerontol.* 7: 196–200, 1952.
78. MILLER, M., J. E. MORLEY, L. Z. RUBENSTEIN, J. OUSLANDER, and S. STROME. Hyponatremia in a nursing home population [Abstract]. *Gerontologist* 25: 118, 1985.
79. NATH, K. A., S. M. KREN, and T. H. HOSTETTER. Dietary protein restriction in established renal injury in the rat: selective role of glomerular capillary pressure in progressive glomerular dysfunction. *J. Clin. Invest.* 78: 1199–1205, 1986.
80. NICOLLE, L. E., J. BJORNSON, G. K. M. HARDING, and J. A. MACDONELL. Bacteriuria in elderly institutionalized men. *N. Engl. J. Med.* 309: 1420–1425, 1983.
81. NORDENSTAM, G. R., C. A. BRANDBERG, A. S. ODEN, C. M. SVANBORG-EDEN, and A. SVANBORG. Bacteriuria and mortality in an elderly population. *N. Engl. J. Med.* 314: 1152–1156, 1986.
82. OHASHI, M., N. FUJIO, H. NAWATA, K. KATO, H. IBAYASHI, K. KANGAWA, and H. MATSUO. High plasma concentration of human atrial natriuretic polypeptide in aged men. *J. Clin. Endocrinol. Metab.* 64: 81–85, 1987.
83. PASCUAL, J., L. OROFINO, F. LIANO, R. MARCEN, M. T. NAYA, L. ORTE, and J. ORTUNO. Incidence and prognosis of acute renal failure in older patients. *J. Am. Geriatr. Soc.* 38: 25–30, 1990.
84. PHILLIPS, P. A., B. J. ROLLS, J. J. G. LEDINGHAM, M. L. FORSLING, J. J. MORTON, M. J. CROWE, and L. WOLLNER. Reduced

thirst after water deprivation in healthy elderly men. *N. Engl. J. Med.* 311: 753–759, 1984.
85. PHILLIPS, T. L., and G. LEONG. Kidney cell proliferation after unilateral nephrectomy as related to age. *Cancer Res.* 2: 286–292, 1967.
86. PRESTON, R. A., C. L. STEMMER, B. J. MATERSON, E. PEREZ-STABLE, and V. PARDO. Renal biopsy in patients 65 years of age or older. An analysis of the results of 334 biopsies. *J. Am. Geriatr. Soc.* 38: 669–674, 1990.
87. PROVERBIO, F., T. PROVERBIO, and R. MARIN. Ion transport and oxygen consumption in kidney cortex slices from young and old rats. *Gerontologia* 31: 166–123, 1985.
88. RESNICK, N. M. Urinary incontinence—a treatable disorder. In: *Geriatric Medicine,* edited by J. W. Rowe and R. W. Besdine. Boston: Little, Brown, 1988, p. 246–265.
89. RESNICK, N. M. Voiding dysfunction in the elderly. In: *Neurourology and Urodynamics: Principles and Practice,* edited by S. V. Yalla, E. J. McGuire, A. Elbadawi, and J. G. Blaivas. New York: Macmillan, 1988, p. 303–330.
90. RESNICK, N. M., and S. V. YALLA. Detrusor hyperactivity with impaired contractility: an unrecognized but common cause of incontinence in elderly patients. *JAMA* 257: 3076–3081, 1987.
91. RODGERS, H., J. R. STANIL, G. W. LIPKIN, and J. H. TURNEY. Acute renal failure: a study of elderly patients. *Age Aging* 19:36–42, 1990.
92. RONDEAU, E., J. DELIMA, H. CALLIENS, R. ARDAILLOU, A. VAHANIAN, and J. ACAR. High plasma antidiuretic hormone in patients with cardiac failure: influence of age. *Miner. Electrolyte Metab.* 8: 267–274, 1982.
93. ROWE, J. W., and R. L. KAHN. Human aging: usual and successful. *Science* 237: 143–149, 1987.
94. ROWE, J. W., R. ANDRES, J. D. TOBIN, A. H. NORRIS, and N. W. SHOCK. The effect of age on creatinine clearance in men: a cross sectional and longitudinal study. *J. Gerontol.* 31: 155–163, 1976.
95. ROWE, J. W., K. L. MINAKER, D. SPARROW, and G. L. ROBERTSON. Age-related failure of volume-pressure mediated vasopressin release. *J. Clin. Endocrinol. Metab.* 54: 661–664, 1982.
96. ROWE, J. W., N. W. SHOCK, and R. A. DEFRONZO. The influence of age on the renal response to water deprivation in man. *Nephron* 17: 270–278, 1976.
97. SERRA-CARDUS, A., and J. S. CAMERON. Renal vasculitis in the aged. In: *Renal Function and Disease in the Elderly,* edited by J. F. M. Nunez and J. S. Cameron. London: Butterworths, 1987, p. 321–347.
98. SHOCK, N. W., and M. J. YIENGST. Age changes in the acid-base equilibrium of the blood of males. *J. Gerontol.* 5: 1–4, 1950.
99. SMITH, M. C., M. D. GHOSE, and A. R. HENRY. The clinical spectrum of renal cholesterol embolization. *Am. J. Med.* 71: 174–180, 1981.
100. SNYDER, N. A., D. W. FEIGAL, and A. I. ARIEFF. Hyponatremia in elderly patients. A heterogenous, morbid, and iatrogenic entity. *Ann. Intern. Med.* 107: 308–319, 1987.
101. SORENSON, F. H. Quantitative studies of the renal corpuscles. *Acta Pathol. Microbiol. Scand.* 85: 356–366, 1977.
102. STONER, E., and the Finasteride Study Group. The clinical effects of a 5α-reductase inhibitor, finasteride, on benign prostatic hyperplasia. *J. Urol.* 147: 1298–1302, 1992.
103. SUNDERAM, S. G., and G. D. MANKIKER. Hyponatremia in the elderly. *Age Aging* 12: 77–80, 1983.
104. TAKAZAKURA, E., N. WASABA, A. HANDA, A. TAKADA, A. SHINODA, and J. TAKEUCHI. Intrarenal vascular changes with age and disease. *Kidney Int.* 2: 224–230, 1972.
105. TAUCHI, H., K. TSUBOI, and J. OKUTOMI. Age changes in the human kidney of different races. *Gerontologia* 17: 87–97, 1971.
106. TOLSETH, T., P. FAUCHALD, S. SKREDE, O. DJOSELAND, K. J. BERG, J. STENSTROM, A. HEILO, E. K. BRODWALL, and A. FLATMARK. Long-term blood pressure and renal function in kidney donors. *Kidney Int.* 29: 1072–1076, 1986.
107. TORRES, V. E., K. P. OFFORD, C. F. ANDERSON, J. A. VELOSA, P. P. FROHNERT, J. V. DONADIO, JR., and D. M. WILSON. Blood pressure determinants in living related allograft donors and their recipients. *Kidney Int.* 31: 1383–1390, 1987.
108. TSUNODA, K., K. ABE, T. GOTO, M. YASUJIMA, M. SATO, K. OMATA, M. SEINO, and K. YOSHINAGA. Effect of age on the renin–angiotensin–aldosterone system in normal subjects: simultaneous measurements of active and inactive renin, renin substrate, and aldosterone in plasma. *J. Clin. Endocrinol. Metab.* 62: 384–389, 1986.
109. VINCENTI, F., W. J. C. AMEND, JR., G. KAYSEN, N. FEDUSKA, J. BIRNBAUM, R. DUCA, and O. SALVATIERRA. Long-term renal function in kidney donors. Sustained compensatory hyperfiltration with no adverse effects. *Transplantation* 36: 626–629, 1983.
110. WATKIN, D. M., and N. W. SHOCK. Age-wise standard value for C_{PAH} and Tm_{PAH} in adult males. *J. Clin. Invest.* 34: 969, 1955.
111. WEIDMANN, P., S. DEMYTTENAERE-BURSZTEIN, M. H. MAXWELL, and J. DELIMA. Effect of aging on plasma renin and aldosterone in normal men. *Kidney Int.* 8: 325–333, 1975.
112. WEILAND, D., D. E. R. SUTHERLAND, B. CHAVERS, R. L. SIMMONS, H. L. ASCHER, and J. S. NAJARIAN. Information on 628 living-related kidney donors at a single institution, with long-term follow-up in 472 cases. *Transplant. Proc.* 16: 5–7, 1984.
113. WEISSMAN, P. H., L. SHENKMAN, and R. GREGERMAN. Chlorpropamide hyponatremia: drug-induced inappropriate antidiuretic hormone activity. *N. Engl. J. Med.* 284: 65–71, 1971.
114. WESSON, L. G., JR. Renal hemodynamics in physiological states. In: *Physiology of the Human Kidney,* edited by L. G. Wesson, Jr. New York: Grune and Stratton, 1969, p. 98–100.
115. WILSON, P. D., and L. M. FRANKS. Enzyme patterns in young and old mouse kidneys. *Gerontologia* 17: 16–32, 1971.
116. YAMAGUCHI, T., T. OMAF, and S. KATSUKI. Quantitative determination of renal vascular changes related to age and hypertension. *Am. Heart. J.* 10: 248–258, 1969.
117. YAMAMOTO, T., H. HARADA, J. FUKUYAMA, T. HAYASHI, and I. MORI. Impaired arginine–vasopressin secretion associated with hypoangiotensinemia in hypernatremic dehydrated elderly patients. *JAMA* 259: 1039–1042, 1988.
118. ZECH, P., S. COLON, and P. H. PONTET. The nephrotic syndrome in adults aged over 60: etiology, evaluation and treatment of 76 cases. *Clin. Nephrol.* 18: 232–236, 1982.

20. The gastrointestinal tract

PETER R. HOLT | *Division of Gastroenterology, Department of Medicine, College of Physicians & Surgeons of Columbia University, New York, New York*

CHAPTER CONTENTS

Salivary Glands
Stomach
    Gastric secretion
        Gastric acid
        Secretion of other components
Small Intestine
    Morphology
    Brush border membranes
    Enzymes
    Intestinal permeability
    Protein synthesis
    Intestinal absorption
        Methods of studying intestinal absorption
        Carbohydrate, digestion and absorption
        Protein
        Lipids
        Ion and micronutrient absorption
        Calcium
        Water-soluble vitamins
        Fat-soluble vitamins
Gut-Associated Immune System
Splanchnic Blood Flow
Gastrointestinal Motility
    Esophagus
    Stomach
    Neuromuscular functioning
    Colon and rectum
        Colonic transit
        Anorectal function
Pancreas
Liver and Biliary Tree
    Morphology
    Age-associated effects
    Consequences of aging
    Bile
Gastrointestinal Hormones
Cellular Proliferation
    Esophagus and stomach
    Small intestine
    Colon
    Effects of caloric restriction

FROM MOUTH TO ANUS, THE GASTROINTESTINAL TRACT and its accessory organs—the salivary glands, pancreas, liver, and gallbladder—present a remarkable array of differing tissues that undergo physiological changes with aging. These tissues include both long-lived postmitotic cells and cells that divide throughout the life span. As characteristic secretory and transport tissues, they are involved in the complex process of postprandial motility and also are the seat of major immunological activity and peptide hormone production. It is this array of tissues and functions that challenges the gerontological physiologist.

SALIVARY GLANDS

The salivary glands consist of clusters of acini at the extremity of the ductular system. Parotid acini contain one secretory cell type, whereas mandibular or sublingual glands usually contain two or more. The acini are supported by myoepithelial cells. The ductular system also often contains secretion granules. A parasympathetic and a sympathetic secretory motor innervation derive from the superior cervical ganglion as well as from the otic and trigeminal ganglia.

Salivary glands form a primary fluid in acini which is modified during passage through the intralobular and extralobular ductal system. The parotid, submandibular, and sublingual glands are situated around the oral cavity. Salivary secretions are controlled principally by the autonomic nervous system and stimulation of sympathetic or parasympathetic nerves elicits a salivary secretion. Neurohumoral agonists bind to acini cell-surface receptors and stimulate intracellular second messengers via two separate signal transduction systems, a cyclic AMP-dependent pathway and a pathway involving mobilization of intracellular calcium (which produces a secretion of increased fluid volume). The cyclic AMP pathway stimulates a salivary secretion rich in amylase. The fluid is modified as it passes from the salivary gland through the ductal system by absorption of sodium and hydrogen ions, resulting in an increase in sodium chloride concentrations with increasing flow rate. At modest to high secretory rates, bicarbonate concentrations may be significantly higher in saliva than in plasma.

A wide variety of proteins are secreted by the salivary glands, including amylase, mucins, lysozymes, proteases, lipases, immunoglobulins, and growth factors, such as epidermal growth factor (EGF). Immunoglobulin A (IgA) secretion provides important local mucosal immunity. In humans, there are three salivary amylase genes (compared to two that are primarily pancreatic and two that are truncated pseudogenes). Human salivary amylase hydrolyses glycogen and starch with the production of maltase, maltotriose, and oligosaccharides of 5–10 glucose units. The enzyme initiates the digestion of carbohydrates, which is nutritionally important only when serious pancreatic insufficiency is present.

Because of the accessibility of salivary gland secretions, the compactness and accessibility of the glands for study, and the potential importance of secretions in maintaining the health of the oral mucosa, age-associated effects have been extensively studied.

Morphological changes in rat salivary gland structure were described with increased age in early studies (10, 54, 55). The rate of basal salivary flow and stimulated secretion of saliva were described as falling in advanced age (297). The content of amylase in mixed saliva declined with age (77), suggesting reduction in secretory protein content. Other studies suggested that the rate of salivary gland cellular protein synthesis declined with age, as determined by reduced rates of incorporation of radioactive precursors into trichloracetic acid–precipitable and acid-soluble proteins (238, 240, 241). The salivary gland content of α amylase was found to be reduced in 24-month-old compared to 4–7-month-old Wistar rats (239). The 50% reduction in amylase activity per mg of DNA in the saliva of older rodents suggested an alteration in immunoreactive amylase, implying a change in enzyme structure. Amylase release from rat parotids in vitro is stimulated by β agonists such as the catecholamines (27, 41), a signal system which involves cyclic AMP (68) and can be blocked with the β-adrenergic blocker propranolol (27, 280). More recent studies have shown that the in vitro release of proteins from parotid lobules following secretory stimulants such as isoproterenol is not reduced in 24-month-old rats (217, 240). The volume of parotid saliva obtained following pilocarpine stimulation in old rats was about one-half that in young animals, but the saliva had similar sodium concentrations and a 40% greater protein concentration (53). A more recent study showed no changes in the density of β-adrenergic receptors in the parotid or submandibular glands in 3–24-month-old Fischer 344 rats (351).

In one large study of humans, unstimulated and 2% citrate–stimulated parotid and submandibular salivary flow rates were not altered in subjects 24–93 yr of age. Only patients with Sjogren's syndrome or radiation-induced damage had low salivary gland performance (39, 455). Other groups have confirmed this finding in normal volunteers (74) but not in patients with dementia of the Alzheimer's type (379). Baum and co-workers (40) subsequently studied a group of salivary acidic–rich proteins thought to be of particular importance in the maintenance of mucosal health. In 220 adults ranging from 20 to 80 yr of age, no difference in the ability of individuals of different ages to secrete this group of exocrine secretory proteins was detected. Furthermore, secretion of secretory IgA from parotid glands was unchanged with age, although modest elevations of lactoferrin and lysozyme were detected (135). These data are consistent with maintenance of the protective functions of parotid salivary proteins during aging.

Salivary gland dysfunction with age, whether due to physiological changes, the effects of disease, or drugs, can induce insufficient lubrication of the mouth. This causes some difficulty in initiating swallowing and impairs protection of the mucosa and of the teeth following minor injury. The repair of tooth enamel may be altered, resulting in more caries, and IgA-mediated immune defenses to external noxious agents may be lowered.

STOMACH

The stomach consists of the cardiac region, containing oxyntic mucosa; the acid-secreting body, containing principally parietal cells; and the nonacid-secreting antrum, containing pyloric glands and enterochromaffin cells. The enterochromaffin cells include G and D cells, the G cells synthesizing and secreting gastrin and the D cells synthesizing and secreting somatostatin.

For many years atrophic gastritis was believed to be a result of the aging process. Following the introduction of peroral biopsy instruments around 1955, it was shown that atrophic gastritis occurred with increasing frequency in the elderly population and was accompanied by the loss of chief and parietal cells (83). Chief and parietal cells were replaced by goblet cell metaplasia. These histological findings were paralleled by a reduction of gastric acid output and intrinsic factor secretion (12, 220). The normal responses of the human stomach as a function of age remained quite unclear, except for the presence of atrophic gastritis, which is now believed to be an acquired disease.

In 24-month-old Sprague-Dawley rats, Hollander et al. (187) demonstrated prominent thickening of the entire gastric wall, including a broadened oxyntic mucosa, an increase in connective tissue, and a loss of glands. Periodic acid-Schiff (PAS) staining of (hyaline-containing) connective tissue separated and partly replaced gastric glands. In the basal area there was evidence of glandular tissue loss accompanied by an increase in connective tissue. Gastric glands were dilated and contained cells with clear cytoplasm resembling endocrine cells. Surface epithelial cells contained mostly neutral, PAS-positive mucus. In addition, birefringent

TABLE 20.1. *Gastric Mucosal Morphometry*

	Young (n = 15)	Old (n = 15)
Total gastric wall thickness (μm)	936 ± 100	2,272 ± 640
Mucosal height (μm)	484 ± 100	1,122 ± 240
Connective tissue area (μm^2, average per microscopic field at 125×)	17,856 ± 4,000	53,228 ± 1,812

± SEM. [From (187) with permission.]

collagen fibers were seen with a polarizing microscope, and occasional focal lymphoid aggregates were found in oxyntic and antral mucosa. Morphometric data (Table 20.1) showed a twofold greater thickness of the gastric wall compared to younger animals, accompanied by an increase in mucosal height. No significant changes were seen by electronmicroscopy. One possible explanation for the increased mucosal thickness is increased proliferation. Majumdar et al. (277) studied differences in gastric morphology between 4- and 24-month-old male Fischer 344 rats and found a 32% reduction in mucosal glandular height in the older rats (745 ± 49 μm vs. 516 ± 33 μm ($P < 0.05$) and fewer parietal cells. Despite fewer parietal cells, the labeling index was 28% higher in the older animals. Majumdar's group (274, 277) agreed with the findings of Hollander's group, showing increased connective tissue around and between glands with thickening of the muscularis mucosa due to collagen deposition in the 24-month-old rats, resulting in an increase in the overall thickness of the gastric mucosa.

Gastric Secretion

The stomach secretes acid hydrogen ions (H$^+$), pepsinogen, intrinsic factor, and lipase and contains and secretes prostaglandins, gastrin, and somatostatin. Changes in the secretion of one or all of these components would be important in the elderly.

Gastric Acid. Gastric acid increases peptic hydrolysis of dietary protein, destroys microorganisms after they have been swallowed, facilitates intestinal absorption of micronutrients—including iron, food-bound vitamin B$_{12}$, folic acid, possibly calcium, and drugs—and dissociates micronutrients from their binding to dietary components such as protein and fiber.

Acid is secreted by parietal cells in oxyntic glands present in the fundus and the body of the stomach. Acid is secreted at a relatively low rate in the fasting, interdigestive period but increases abruptly following food ingestion to near maximal rates within 1.5–2 h. Postprandial gastric acid secretion is stimulated by chemical reactions of several food constituents with the gastric mucosa and by gastric distention. Following a meal, gastric hydrogen ion secretion falls to basal secretory rates in about 4–5 h. Gastric acid secretion rates are described during the fasting period as the basal acid output (BAO) and postprandially as the maximal acid (MAO) or peak acid (PAO) output.

The rates of gastric acid secretion are determined by age and as a function of body weight and body composition. Gastric acid secretion is quite low after birth but reaches adult levels by about 18 months of age. Gastric acid secretion is controlled by hormones such as gastrin, which acts directly upon parietal cells in oxyntic glands, and by cholinergic stimuli, which probably serve as accessory modulators of other primary stimulants. A variety of other peptides and mucosal prostaglandins can either increase or decrease gastric acid secretion. If acid secretion falls as a physiological function of age, any or all of these factors may play a role.

Many older studies claimed that gastric acid secretion decreased with age and that there was an increased incidence of achlorhydria in the elderly (52, 99). In the majority of these studies, single samples of gastric juice were obtained in medical clinics from patients with a variety of symptoms and disorders (428, 457). The effects of age on gastric acid secretion in patients with either duodenal ulcers or gastric ulcers have not been clarified; for instance, reduced acid secretion, no difference in acid secretion, and even increased acid secretion all have been described (130, 312).

It now is well recognized that the prevalence of atrophic gastritis increases progressively by decade with age (220) and differs markedly between different locations in the world. It is the presence of atrophic gastritis that results in hypochlorhydria or achlorhydria and, therefore, an overall increase in the percent of older individuals with reduced gastric acid secretion. The recent recognition of the frequency of the organism *Helicobacter pylori* has added another dimension to studies that aim to determine physiological changes in acid secretion with age. At the present time, such studies must exclude the presence of atrophic gastritis, either by multiple gastric biopsies or by measurement of serum pepsinogen A and B. It also is crucial to ensure the absence of *H. pylori* either by direct or indirect testing. It is clear that these criteria were not used in the many earlier studies that described age-related effects (149).

Using strict exclusion criteria, Feldman and co-workers studied elderly volunteers without current or past history of gastrointestinal disease or symptoms and specifically without atrophic gastritis or *H. pylori* infestation (150). In these studies, mean basal and gastrin-stimulated acid secretion were higher in older (mean age 57 yr) than in younger (mean age 33 yr) subjects. This was particularly evident in older men. Mean fasting serum gastrin concentration was similar in the older and younger volunteers. Higher overall acid secretion appeared to be a reflection of basal output, suggesting that the older volunteer had either a larger stomach or a larger parietal cell mass or that the cells were more sensitive to the action of gastrin. It appears likely that in this study the differences in acid secretion in elderly volunteers reflected differences in anti-secretory inhibition and not secretory stimulation. One possible explanation is that mucosal prostaglandin concentrations in the stomach are lower in older individuals than in younger ones (91). There overall results have since been confirmed (223a).

Similar conclusions were reached by Kekki and Sipponen (232), who randomly selected more than 400 subjects, aged 15 yr and over, in whom gastric disease was excluded by endoscopy and biopsy and gastric secretory studies performed. When reduced gastric acid output was found in older subjects, this correlated directly with the severity of atrophic changes. When subjects with a normal gastric mucosa were evaluated, gastric acid output did not decrease with age. Indeed, when expressed as a function of fat-free body weight, there was a significant increase in acid output with age in women. A recent study confirmed these data (173).

It also is important to point out that several studies that initially concluded that there was an age-related fall in gastric acid secretion, when re-analyzed to exclude confounding factors such as body composition or gastric mucosal morphology, concluded that data supporting an age-associated reduction in gastric acid secretion disappeared. Nevertheless, the prevalence of achlorhydria due to gastritis clearly does increase with age and may have major consequences (89, 384).

Experiments in animals have shed little light on the physiological basis of age-associated changes in gastric acid secretion. Fasting and gastrin-stimulated acid secretions have been reported to be lower in 32-month-old (very senescent) than in 3-month-old Fischer 344 rats (276). Studies of Maitra et al. (273) suggested that basal acid secretion decreased steadily between 4 and 21 months in pyloric-ligated rats and reached 50% of the level in young animals by 21 months. Pentagastrin had little effect on gastric acid secretion in the older rats, implying a loss of gastric mucosa responsiveness to this hormone in aging animals. The data of Singh et al. suggested that 24-month old Fischer rats had a marked reduction in fundal gastrin-binding sites (383), which would provide one explanation for these findings.

Secretion of Other Components. There have been relatively few studies of the secretion of enzymes by the stomach as a function of age. Basal pepsin output was found to be 40% higher in 14-month-old than in 3-month-old rats (273). There was, however, a poor response of pepsin output to gastrin in 14-month-old animals. In 21-month-old rats, there was significantly less pepsinogen than at 3 or 14 months of age. In addition, mucosal pepsinogen content was considerably reduced between 4 and 21 months. Gargouri and co-workers (144) studied the concentration of gastric lipase in biopsies obtained from human volunteers of different ages and reported a very considerable reduction in those over 60 yr of age. Unfortunately, these investigators did not report on the concentrations of other gastric enzymes nor did they exclude the possibility that biopsies were obtained from areas of atrophic gastritis.

There is little information on changes in intrinsic factor secretion as a function of age. It is likely that elderly individuals with atrophic gastritis secrete reduced amounts of intrinsic factor. However, only in those with severe gastric atrophy is intrinsic factor secretion reduced sufficiently to produce clinical pernicious anemia.

Endogenous gastroduodenal mucosal prostaglandins are thought to assist in preventing peptic ulcer disease. Furthermore, many of the elderly use drugs that reduce mucosal prostaglandin synthesis (such as aspirin and nonsteroidal antiinflammatory drugs) and thus may be at greater risk of ulcer disease. Therefore, studies of the effect of aging upon gastrointestinal tissue prostaglandin levels and mucosal synthesis are both physiologically and clinically important.

There is already some evidence that senescence may be associated with reduced prostaglandin formation. Senescent fibroblasts have been shown to respond to stimulation with reduced prostaglandin and prostanoid formation (402). Cryer et al. (91) measured gastric and duodenal mucosal prostaglandin concentrations in 35 young and 11 older (52–72 yr) volunteers. Fundal, antral, and duodenal prostaglandin F_2 (PGF_2) and E_2 (PGE_2) concentrations were found to be reduced by about 40–50% in the older subjects. Mean BAO was correlated with lower prostaglandin concentrations. Mean mucosal conversion of ^{14}C arachidonic acid to prostaglandins was not significantly lower in six older compared to six younger subjects. However, with the small number of individuals studied, a type II error could not be excluded. Inflammatory cells also contain prostaglandins, and the authors attempted to exclude an increase in inflammatory cells associated with differences in prostaglandin concentrations by studying the histology of biopsy specimens. A preliminary report from Japan confirmed some of these findings (154).

Kim and co-workers (242) reported that acid-stimulated duodenal bicarbonate secretion was reduced in aging Fischer rats. Duodenal bicarbonate secretion is mediated in part by endogenous PGE_2 release, and the authors speculated that prostaglandins might be involved, though duodenal PGE_2 production was not measured. It is possible that these rats had a reduced acid-stimulated duodenal bicarbonate secretion consequent upon reduced prostaglandin synthesis. The author is unaware of additional studies on prostaglandin concentrations or synthesis in upper gastrointestinal tissues of aging humans or rodents.

Shortly after the introduction of methods for measuring the concentrations of gastrin in the serum, mean fasting gastrin concentrations were shown to be higher in elderly than in young humans (415). This probably represents the contribution of a population of hypochlorhydric or achlorhydric individuals in whom the lack of intraluminal H^+ ions is a stimulus for antral gastrin production (443). Maitra and co-workers (273) found that serum gastrin levels were modestly lower in 21-month-old than in 4-month-old Fischer 344 rats (120 pg/ml at 4 months of age falling to 90 pg/ml at 21 months of age). These authors correlated the reduction in circulating serum gastrin with the degree of gastric mucosal atrophy. Holt and Yeh (198) found that fed 25–27-month-old male Fischer 344 rats had an insignificantly lower serum gastrin concentration than 4–5-month-old animals. Older starved rats had lower serum gastrin concentrations than younger animals and showed a poor response to refeeding. Antral gastrin concentrations, measured per gram of mucosa, were higher in the younger than in the older animals, fell appropriately after 3 days' starvation in the young, but not in the old, but then fell inappropriately during refeeding in the older rats. These studies were interpreted as demonstrating a failure of response of antral gastrin synthesis and gastrin secretion to changes in food intake in older animals.

Singh and co-workers (383) principally evaluated age-associated changes in gastrin receptors in the stomach (as well as other gastrointestinal tissues) of 4–6-month-old and 24-month-old animals. In the fundus and body of the stomach, 24-month-old rats demonstrated very low specific gastrin-binding sites per unit of crude membrane protein.

Goldschmiedt et al. (150) showed higher responses of gastrin concentration to a meal in older volunteers than in younger ones.

Thompson's group (248) has presented preliminary data on somatostatin concentrations in the antrum of aging rodents, reporting a significant age-related reduction. Somatostatin down-regulates gastrin secretion in the gastric antrum. A fall in somatostatin could be responsible for the somewhat aberrant responses of antral gastrin to meals seen in older rodents and humans.

A very important potential pathophysiological result of the age-related changes is the response to injury. There appears to be some evidence for greater injury with noxious stimuli in elderly animals. Majumdar and co-workers (278) noted greater erosions in the gastric mucosa of 24-month-old compared to 4-month-old rats, following administration of $2M$ NaCl. However, neither bleeding nor extensive ulceration was observed. Hinsull (171) also found larger erosions after administration of aspirin in 22-month-old compared to 9-wk-old rats, lesions that were abolished following administration of colloidal bismuth subnitrate in drinking water. In a preliminary report (331), cysteamine-induced gastric and duodenal ulceration were considerably greater in 16- and 24-month-old than in 3-month-old Fischer 344 rats and also resulted in more perforations. Similar data were obtained by Lee and Feldman (259) following administration of aspirin to 3-, 12-, and 21-month-old Fischer 344 rats. However, a single small study in young and elderly human volunteers found no differences in the number and extent of ulceration evaluated by endoscopy following 325 or 1,300 mg of aspirin (308).

There are several possible causes which may be responsible for the greater degree of injury and the reduced responsiveness to injury with age. In a preliminary report, Greenberg et al. (156) showed more inhibition of mucosal PGF_2 following administration of 2.5 mg per kg of aspirin in 27–28-month-old than in 3–4-month-old Fischer 344 rats. Reduced prostaglandin concentration and synthesis after aspirin was subsequently confirmed by Lee and Feldman (259). In addition, increased ulceration and reduced healing rate could reflect changes in proliferative response of the stomach to injury. This has been a focus of the studies of Majumdar's group over the last few years. They used the $2M$ NaCl hypertonic saline model of gastric injury and evaluated the response by studying the increase in mucosal DNA synthesis, ornithine decarboxylase, and tyrosine kinase–specific activity, as well as tyrosine-specific phosphorylation (278). The same group also described diminished activation of tyrosine encoded protein kinases in mucosal cells from aging animals (436). This overall impairment of the aging gastrointestinal tract to proliferate appropriately as a response to noxious stimuli is discussed in greater detail later in this chapter.

In a singular study, Kawano et al. (229) evaluated possible changes in mucosal energy metabolism with age by measuring ATP metabolism in biopsies obtained from subjects less than and more than 65 yr of age. No histological data were provided in this study, but the conclusions were that there was a significant reduction in energy charge in the older individuals as well as lower

ATP levels (6.48 ± 1.14 vs. 9.63 ± 1.92) in the antrum. These data suggest that the energy metabolism in human gastric mucosal biopsies may be impaired and might contribute to damage to the stomach from noxious agents.

SMALL INTESTINE

The small intestine, starting from the pyloric end of the stomach and ending at the ileocecal valve, is a specialized organ that digests and absorbs dietary and endogenously secreted substrates, excludes macromolecules from the body, metabolizes a variety of extraneous agents including drugs, induces specific immune responses, and moves intestinal contents through the lumen into the colon at an appropriate rate.

To achieve digestive and absorptive function, mucosal epithelial cells are specialized to provide a very large surface area to allow for enzyme digestion at the mucosal border and to permit transport through the mucosal membrane. It has been estimated that the total mucosal area of the small bowel is about the size of a doubles tennis court (257). This expanse is brought about by macroinvaginations (the valves of Kerkring) and microinvaginations (epithelial cell villi and microvilli). Any changes in intestinal epithelial cell structure that reduce the length or density of microvilli or villi as a result of disease or aging will have a very large effect on intestinal absorptive capacity.

The small intestinal epithelium may be conveniently divided into a crypt compartment, a villus compartment, and clusters of cells forming follicular domes at sites covering dense accumulation of lymphoid cells called Peyer's patches. The crypts contain undifferentiated cells, which are actively dividing, and enteroendocrine cells, Paneth cells, and goblet cells. The undifferentiated crypt cell acts as a progenitor from which each parenchymal and specialized cell originates. It recently has been established, using mouse aggregation chimeras, that during fetal development entire crypts arise from a single progenitor cell (84). Except for Paneth cells, which remain at the crypt base, other crypt cell types migrate toward the villus surface, and undifferentiated crypt cells acquire structural and functional characteristics of absorptive cells found on the villus. As absorptive cells migrate up the villus axis to the villus tip, they continue to acquire mature differentiated functions. This overall process takes approximately 3 days in the rat and probably 7 days in humans. Peyer's patches are an important part of the gut-associated lymphoid system and contain a distinctive intestinal epithelial cell, the microfold or M cell, which is able to pinocytose macromolecules from the lumen. These macromolecules then are passed to antigen-recognizing macrophages of the Peyer's patch germinal centers containing actively dividing, IgA-containing B cells. These antigen-sensitized B lymphocytes then migrate to mesenteric lymph nodes, enter the circulation, and hone in on mucosal surfaces.

An important functional component of the anatomical structure of the small intestine is the exclusion of macromolecules (except through M cells). This occurs in great part because of the presence of occluding tight junctions, where the lateral membranes of adjacent epithelial cells are closely opposed. Manipulation of the tight junction greatly alters intestinal epithelial cell permeability.

In addition to parenchymal intestinal absorbing cells, in which surface areas are greatly expanded, Paneth cells secrete mucus, endocrine cells produce a wide variety of peptides, and intramucosal and submucosal plasma cells secrete large quantities of immunoglobulins. Bacterial numbers in the lumen are controlled by a combination of the reduction of bacterial input to the small intestine from the stomach by the bacteriocidal and bacteriostatic action of gastric pH, by local antibacterial effects of lysozyme and IgA secretion, and by the normal propulsive action of intestinal motility. As described below, under Gastrointestinal Motility, the interdigestive motor function (housekeeper function, when little food is passing down the bowel) is particularly important in sweeping bacteria aborally. Small intestinal epithelial cells possess a very considerable metabolic activity, which is maintained by utilizing both fatty acids and glucose as substrates. Most of the mass of metabolizable substrates that are used for the mucosa are derived from circulating lipids and glucose and not from newly absorbed dietary components. Under conditions of starvation and mucosal substrate deprivation, newly absorbed solutes may be utilized. Relatively few studies of age-associated effects on the functional structure of the small intestine have been performed under appropriate experimental conditions.

Morphology

Since the small intestinal mucosa represents the major absorbing surface of the gastrointestinal tract, any anatomical change that might occur with age must greatly affect the efficacy of the absorptive process. As stated before, it is the functional surface area that determines the rate of absorption of most solutes.

The small bowel mucosal cell contains numerous hydrolytic enzymes that rapidly digest epithelia, so the effect of aging on human gastrointestinal tissues cannot be studied adequately postmortem. Only since the advent of peroral jejunal biopsy have the normal architecture and the changes with age and disease in the human small bowel been described. In animals, several investigators have evaluated the effect of aging on intestinal structure (Table 20.2). In one of the first published studies, Mathis (286), in 1928, described a change with age from finger-like villi present at birth to leaf-like villi in the mature and aging animal. These overall findings were confirmed by Van Lennep (425) in the long-nosed bandicoot and by Baker and colleagues (33) in the rat and were interpreted as representing the consequences of prolonged exposure to toxic intestinal contents. Andrew and Andrew (11) and Suntzeff and Angeletti (394) described an increase of connective tissue that separated and surrounded small intestinal crypts of aging rodents. This increased fibrosis was thought to interfere with proliferation. Increased numbers of goblet cells also were described (394). More complete quantitative histological studies of villi and crypts were initiated in the early 1970s by Clarke and have continued to the present day. Clarke (81, 82) evaluated changes in intestinal architecture in Wistar rats that ranged in age from less than 1 month to about 1 yr. He noted an increase in the ratio of the number of crypts to the number of villi in the oldest group, a finding that was seen at all levels of the small intestine between the pylorus and the ileocecal valve. The height of villi rose with age except in the oldest rats. Höhn et al. (175) described a fall in duodenal and jejunal villus height accompanied by the presence of irregular microvilli in rats that had reached the age of 30 months. The ileum of these animals apparently was spared. Jakab and Penzes (219) compared glucose absorption rate and villus dimensions in 6-, 12-, and 24-month-old Wistar rats, describing a very significant fall of villus height in all levels of the intestine in the oldest group. However, Penzes et al. showed only modest microvillus changes (339). In contrast, Moog (305) demonstrated an increase in villus height in older mice and Ecknauer et al. (114) some reduction in villus height but a significant increase in both villus and crypt number. No effect of aging upon gut surface area was described (296). All of these studies were performed in rodents whose clinical and nutritional status was not

TABLE 20.2. *Age-Associated Changes in Small Intestinal Epithelial Morphology*

First Author	Year	Reference	Species	Age	Findings*
Mathis	1928	286	Bat	4–8, 25–28 months	↑ Leaf- shaped villi.
Andrew	1957	11	Mouse	4–8, 25–28 months	Jejunum connective tissue ↓
Suntzeff	1961	394	Mouse	3–6, 22–27 months	Duodenum, ↓ ileum-connective tissue and goblet cells.
Van Lennep	1962	425	Long-nosed bandicoot		↑ Leaf- shaped villi.
Baker	1963	33	Rat		↑ Leaf-shaped villi.
Clarke	1972 1977	81 82	Rat Rat	1–12 months	↑ Crypt-villus ratio, ↑ villus height.
Moog	1977	305	Mouse	6–24 months	↑ Villus height at 24 months
Höhn	1978	175	Rat	4–30 months	↓ Duodenal and jejunal villus height. Irregular microvilli-ileum no change.
Jakab	1981	219	Rat	6–24 months	↓ Duodenal, jejunal, and ileal villus height.
Pénzes	1988	339	Rat	6–24 months	Modest microvillus changes in duodenum and ileum.
Meshkinpour	1981	296	Rat	3–24 months	No change in surface area.
Ecknauer	1982	114	Rat	60–75 yr	Jejunal villi shorter and broader.
Cullan	1982	93	Mouse	3–34 months	↑ Intestinal crypt.
Keelan	1985	231	Rabbit	1½–12 months	↓ Jejunal villus height.
Holt	1983 1984	202 200	Rat Rat	4–5, 27 months	No change villus height in duodenum and jejunum but ↑ in ileum crypt depth in proximal gut.
Heller	1990	169	Rat	4–5, –27 months	
Webster	1975	447	Human	60–75 yr	Jejunal villi shorter and broader.
Warren	1978	445	Human	16–20, 60–73 months	↓ Jejunum surface area.
Rowlatt	1975	360			
Corraza	1986	88	Human		Jejunal villus height unchanged.
Chin	1973	78	Mouse	15 months	Peyer's patches no involution deposition of elastin.
Kawanishi	1989	226	Mouse	24 months	Some involution of Peyer's patches with age.

* ↑ Increased, ↓ decreased.

described. Cullan and co-workers (93) investigated the intestinal morphology and the proliferation responses to gastrin and glucagon of mice aged 3–12 months and 24–30 months. Both the villus and the crypt of aging mice were described as larger and the proliferative zone was reported as increased.

When Holt and co-workers initiated a more comprehensive evaluation of the changes that occurred with advancing age in the intestine of the rat, they decided to use the National Institute on Aging (NIA) colony of Fischer 344 rats and carefully standardized their experimental conditions of food intake, absence of illness, and full recovery after transfer from the NIH animal holding facility. the light-microscopic appearance of villi in the proximal intestine of the rat from 4 to 5 months to 25 to 27 months of age did not differ (202). Villus dimensions, calculated as height or as cell number, remained constant (200). However, crypt depth initially was found to be greater in the older rats (202), a finding that was observed as early as 21 months in subsequent studies (169). These phenomena were maintained when rats were starved and was abolished by long-term food restriction to 60% of the caloric intake of the ad libitum–fed rats (231). Villus height also was found to be increased with age in the ileum.

These findings did not suggest that any physiological functional change with age was due to a paucity of absorbing cells, even if ileal hypertrophy did imply increased caloric load reaching the distal small intestine. The data also suggested that there was some alteration in proliferative activity with age.

The observations of Corrazza and co-workers (88) in human biopsies gave support to the rodent data and demonstrated no change in villus cellularity in patients up to the age of 75 yr. These data contradicted earlier studies (445, 447), which found pathological changes in biopsies taken from the small bowel of older individuals. However, these earlier studies used patients whose clinical and nutritional conditions were not defined.

Overall, the weight of the small intestine increases with the age and weight of the animal. For example, the weight of the small intestine of SWR/J strain mice that lived for 27 months was studied by Moog (305), who found an increase in weight between 5 and 24 months. In the Fischer 344 rat, Holt and co-workers (202) did not find any major changes in the weight or composition of the small intestine. Changes in Peyer's patches (78, 226) are discussed later, in the section GUT-ASSOCIATED IMMUNE SYSTEM.

Brush Border Membranes

Solute and water transport through the intestinal brush border membrane (BBM) as well as the activity of intrinsic proteins in the membrane are affected by membrane composition and fluidity. Data on changes in these components are restricted to studies in experimental animals and cell culture systems. Aging is known to be associated with numerous changes in membrane structure and function, and age-dependent changes in lipid composition of biological membranes have been observed frequently (319). Indeed, alteration in membrane composition and fluidity and associated changes in lipid peroxidation form the basis of one of the theories of cellular aging. Brasitus et al. (62) studied BBM derived from 6-wk-old, 4-month-old, and 27-month-old Fischer 344 rats. In the youngest animals, major compositional differences, such as a lower cholesterol–phospholipid ratio, were found when BBM were compared between young adult and aging rats. These compositional changes were associated with a lower membrane fluidity, indicated by a lower critical temperature of the lipid thermotropic transition, that is, 17.5°C at 6 wk compared to 22.5°–23.5°C in BBM from older rats. Compositional differences between the 4- and 27-month-old rats were minor and membrane fluidity was unaltered. In a subsequent study, Wahnon and colleagues (437) separated microvillus membranes from the upper two-thirds of the small intestine in 1-month-old, 9-month-old, and 19-month-old ad libitum–fed Charles River CD strain rats, whose body weight varied from 86 to 606 g, and reported an increase in anisotropy parameter values over a temperature range of 5°–40°C. These authors reported the highest fluidity in 1-month-old rats and the lowest in 19-month-old animals and calculated transition temperatures of 16.3°C at 1 month, 23°C at 9 months, and 28.2°C at 19 months. They did not study membrane compositional changes in parallel. The recent demonstration of the relationship between lipid peroxidation and membrane fluidity in the liver of aging animals which could be modulated by dietary restriction (462) emphasizes the importance of further studies to delineate potential membrane changes in the intestine of humans and experimental animals.

Enzymes

Changes in the intensity of BBM staining by antibodies to intestinal alkaline phosphatase using histochemical techniques have been described by several authors to demonstrate age-related changes in the gut (175, 305, 368). It is important to remember that the weight of the intestine of many rodents increases with age, particularly in those species in which body weight increases progressively, so that the total protein content and enzyme activity frequently are higher. Intestinal distribution of individual enzymes, however, may not be different.

The available quantitative data on individual enzymes involved with intestinal digestion and absorption are presented below. However, our own group has made an interesting observation that involves all of the epithelial cell enzymes that were studied. The specific activities of proximal intestinal mucosal disaccharidases (sucrase, maltase, and lactase), alkaline phosphatase, and adenosine deaminase were somewhat lower in 26–27-month-old compared to 4–5-month-old Fischer 344 rats. This reduction was not due to a lessened capability for synthesis but rather to a delay in the rate of maturation of the enzymes in epithelial cells during their migration toward the villus tip (203). Whether this "immaturity" of epithelial cells is restricted to the maturation of enzyme activity or involves other cell functions is presently unknown.

Shub et al. (380) reported an age-related difference in the type of mucosal glycoproteins synthesized by the rat small intestine. These authors initially compared the glycoprotein compositions of newborn and adult female rats and demonstrated changes in glycoprotein buoyant density, as well as biochemical differences as judged by SDS polyacrylamide gel electrophoresis and changes in the molar ratio of carbohydrate to protein and fucose and n-acetylgalactosamine content.

Intestinal Permeability

The small intestinal mucosal membrane is an important protective barrier against the absorption of potentially harmful macromolecules. The mucosa generally allows substances of less than 0.4 mm in diameter to be absorbed but prevents larger molecules from entry (123, 265). Hollander and Tarnawski (183) studied intestinal membrane function by administering solutions of polyethylene glycol (PEG 400) by gavage to Sprague-Dawley rats 34–133 wk of age. PEG absorption was evaluated from the appearance in the urine of PEG as analyzed by gas chromatography. Urinary PEG recovery was significantly higher in 124- or 133-wk-old rats than in younger animals. Urinary recovery of the higher-molecular-weight PEGs was considerably greater than the lower-molecular-weight PEG species. A study of human intestinal permeability using the uptake of cellobiose–rhamnose, which was confirmed using lactulose mannitol (50), did not find an age-associated increase in permeability (367).

Protein Synthesis

The small intestinal mucosa has a very rapid turnover rate. It makes proportionally a much larger contribution to the rate of protein synthesis than to protein mass. Thus any age-related effect on protein synthesis or turnover that occurred in older animals would be expected to induce significant biochemical effects. In early experiments, Hellthaler and co-workers (170) studied the incorporation of [^{14}C]leucine into intestinal proteins of rats aged between 3 and 14 months. Although they found a significant increase in ^{14}C incorporation between 2–3-month-old and 5–6-month-old animals when rings of upper intestine were incubated in vitro, no differences from 6 to 14–15 months of age were detected. Goldspink et al. (151), using the method of phenylalanine flooding of the precursor pool, studied protein synthesis in the small and large intestine of intact rats varying in age from 3 to 105 wk. Fractional rates of protein synthesis fell from 82% to 64% per day, associated with a reduction in total synthesis per gram of RNA protein (151). These changes were present in the small intestinal mucosal and the serosal compartments. One group of investigators studied the turnover of ribosome and soluble RNA in several tissues from 12- and 24- month-old Wistar rats obtained from the Gerontology Research Center in Baltimore and found no differences in the half-life of small intestinal mucosal ribosomes, though some changes were found in the soluble compartment (295). Turnover rate of ribosomes was calculated to be 8.1–8.3 days, somewhat longer than the turnover rate of renal and liver ribosomes (294). It seems clear that these intestinal ribosomal components must be re-utilized since the half-life of intestinal mucosa in rodents of this age is approximately 36 h. Restriction to 50% of an ad libitum diet was shown to significantly increase the intestinal mucosal protein fractional synthesis rate of 24-month-old Sprague-Dawley rats (295).

Intestinal Absorption

Since malnutrition and depletion of micronutrients are felt to be common in the elderly, understanding potential defects in intestinal absorption with age has become very important. At one time it was believed that many biological functions slowed with age, including the absorption of lipids, carbohydrates, fat-soluble and water-soluble vitamins, etc. (293). However, a reduced intake of macro- and micronutrients in the elderly compared to younger subjects is well accepted. In an early and relatively flawed study by Montgomery et al. (304), intestinal malabsorption was frequently found in healthy elderly subjects. Furthermore, in a review of over 500 healthy elderly individuals evaluated in an ambulatory geriatric care facility, 12% were found to be malnourished, and of these cases 40% were believed to involve intestinal malabsorption (289). The issue that is unsettled is whether intestinal absorption is impaired as a physiological function of age or is found only in the presence of malnutrition or intestinal disease.

The cellular physiological mechanisms that operate during intestinal absorption include (1) active absorptive processes, which involve energy-dependent, receptor-mediated uptake shown experimentally as intestinal uptake against a concentration gradient; *(2)* passive absorption, which is energy-independent, occurs experimentally down a concentration gradient, and is rate-dependent upon membrane surface area, membrane composition, and membrane fluidity; and *(3)* facilitated diffusion, which is a nonenergy-dependent process by which substrate can accumulate against a concentration gradient. Although it was initially believed that the absorption of water-soluble substances for which BBM receptors are present is completely limited by the rate of receptor-mediated uptake, it is now recognized that this is incorrect. Even glucose absorption occurs principally by diffusion, because postprandial concentrations of carbohydrates in the intestinal lumen are so very high. At low luminal glucose concentrations, receptor-mediated uptake is predominant. Furthermore, it should be remembered that the uptake of many substrates is dependent on the unstirred water layer around the intestinal microvillus BBM. Although the unstirred water layer was believed to be a very important rate-limiting barrier to intestinal solute absorption, more recent studies by Levitt and co-workers (263) have thrown doubt on this idea and have demonstrated a much smaller unstirred water layer than had been previously calculated. This is of importance because some studies of the intestine have suggested that the unstirred water layer differs markedly in aging rodents when compared to the young.

Another factor of some importance is that the denominator used to calculate intestinal absorptive rate may be inappropriate. Most animal studies have been performed in rodents. As rodents age, many species gain body weight and increase intestinal dimensions at a different rate. Although the absorptive rate of a substrate may be shown to be reduced as a function of intestinal weight in older animals, total intestinal absorption capacity may not differ from that found in young controls. The use of total animal body weight as a denominator also can be questioned because body composition changes dramatically as most animals grow old. Human studies have been limited because investigators have avoided using accurate direct perfusion techniques requiring intestinal intubation. Most of the indirect techniques that have been used to study absorption in human volunteers provide only qualitative, not quantitative, absorption data. Thus much of the available information on the effects of aging on intestinal absorption is inadequate.

Methods of Studying Intestinal Absorption. In humans, absorption may be measured by the difference between dietary intake and fecal output. This is the most accurate method for measuring absorption capacity, but it requires the collection of several days of fecal output, assumes that there is little secretion of the study substance from the body into the gut (that is, that luminal input of the substrate occurs only from the diet), and also that there is little bacterial substrate degradation to metabolites that are not detected in the feces. Human triglyceride absorption is measured by this method as the difference between calculated dietary intake and measured fecal excretion. Dietary components, such as carbohydrates or proteins, if not completely absorbed in the small intestine, will enter the colon where bacterial enzyme metabolism actively degrades these components, leaving little or none to be detected in the feces. This active bacterial metabolism is utilized as a method for estimating carbohydrate absorption in humans since bacteria rapidly metabolize all carbohydrates with the production of hydrogen (262). Hydrogen then is absorbed by the colonic mucosa, circulates to the lungs, and is excreted in the breath. The measurement of breath hydrogen following the ingestion of various carbohydrate-containing meals has been utilized as a method for estimating small intestinal carbohydrate absorption and to study differences in the absorptive capacity between young and aging humans (127). This technique is limited by the potential confounding effect of bacterial overgrowth in the small intestine and perhaps stomach (289). Intestinal absorption also can be determined by measuring the appearance and concentration curve of the substrate in the circulation. This method may be misleading, however, since peak absorption may occur at different times in young and elderly subjects and any concentration in the blood is dependent both on input (absorption rate) and on disposition rate from the circulation. For example, it was initially thought that vitamin A absorption was greater in elderly humans than in young controls (252) until it was recognized that the disappearance rate of vitamin A–containing lipoproteins from the circulation is lower in the elderly, resulting in artificially higher plasma levels (251).

Animal studies in vivo also have used the difference between oral intake and fecal excretion, but this method has the limitations described for humans above. Absorption can be measured following perfusion of intestinal loops or segments in anesthetized rodents or from loops of canine intestine. Absorption also can be studied by injecting or perfusing in vivo intestinal segments and measuring the appearance of test substrates in the serum or their disappearance from the lumen. In vitro studies can be performed using organ culture techniques; by resecting intestinal segments; by creating filled sacs, mucosal side out (everted sacs), and measuring substrate appearance in the serosal compartment; by measuring substrate uptake in intestinal slices; by measuring substrate flux in mucosal segments mounted between two chambers (Ussing chamber); or by studying uptake in isolated epithelial cells or vesicles prepared from BBM or basal lateral membranes. Many of these experimental methods provide different types of information and have been used to evaluate changes in the absorptive mechanism as a function of aging.

Carbohydrate, Digestion and Absorption. About 70% of dietary carbohydrate is consumed as polysaccharides, such as starch, and about 20% as disaccharides. On the basis of physiological information, the reserve capacity for intestinal carbohydrate absorption by the human intestine is less than that for fat (189). Only monosaccharides can be absorbed by the small intestinal mucosa; therefore, complete digestion of carbohydrate is required for effective intestinal absorption. Digestion of polysaccharides occurs principally by the action of alpha amylase, an enzyme that can hydrolyze the endo-1,4-glycosidic bonds of polysaccharides. Amylase is secreted in excess by the salivary glands and the pancreas. Subsequent hydrolysis of disaccharides and short-chain polysaccharides occurs by enzymes on the intestinal mucosal surface and depends on the functional integrity of intestinal epithelial cells. When mucosal epithelial cell function is disordered, the activity of these intestinal digestive enzymes is reduced so that the final steps of carbohydrate digestion are impaired. Hydrolysis by these enteric enzymes results in the production of glucose, fructose, and galactose, which then are absorbed by an active carrier-mediated process or by diffusion at high intraluminal concentrations. Up to 5% of carbohydrate is not absorbed by the human small intestine and passes into the colon. In the colonic lumen, bacterial hydrolytic enzymes then will hydrolyze and metabolize all carbohydrates with the production of CO_2, hydrogen, and short-chain fatty acids, among other products. The short-chain fatty acid metabolites may be very important for the health of colonic epithelial cells.

There is no evidence that amylase secretion and polysaccharide hydrolysis are affected by aging. Initially, there were some suggestions that intestinal lactase concentrations might fall as a function of age. This concept was based on data in population groups susceptible to lactase deficiency and in whom lactose intolerance occurs with greater frequency with increasing age. However, subsequent data in humans have failed to demonstrate any universal age-related alteration in disaccharidase activity (452), despite the fact that sucrase- and lactase-specific activities are significantly, though only modestly, reduced in the proximal intestine of 21- and 27-month-old Fischer 344 rats (201). Darmenton and colleagues (96) studied sucrose digestion in everted intestinal segments of jejunum and ileum from 3- and 24-month-old rats and suggested that the intestinal segments of the older animals, specifically the ileum, showed greater ability to hydrolyze sucrose and absorbed more monosaccharides than younger animals. These studies were evaluated per cm^2 of intestine and therefore did not take into account the possibility that there was a higher concentration of sucrase because of an increase in surface membrane of the older animals.

There have been extensive studies to determine whether monosaccharide absorption, such as glucose, is altered in aging animals or in humans. Since glucose absorption is so difficult to measure in vivo, for the reasons described above, early studies often used the absorption of the pentose xylose, which is not metabolized extensively by the body, as an indirect reflection of potential monosaccharidase absorption.

Our group (127) evaluated carbohydrate absorption in a small group of active, clinically healthy individuals over the age of 65 yr by administering 25–200 g of carbohydrate in a mixed meal. The absorptive capacity of the small intestine was determined on the assumption that any carbohydrate that escaped absorption and passed into the large intestine would be rapidly metabolized by colonic bacteria with the production of hydrogen, which then is detected in the breath. In our studies, young control volunteers were able to consume up to 200 g of carbohydrate in a meal without detecting any excess hydrogen in the breath. In contrast, in the over-65-yr-old group of volunteers, one-third were unable to eat a mixed meal containing 100 g of carbohydrate without an increase of breath hydrogen output, suggesting the presence of small intestinal malabsorption. Using lower concentrations of glucose and constructing a dose–response curve, we demonstrated an age-related reduction in carbohydrate absorption, which was progressive in the very old up to the age of 85 yr (127).

Using xylose as a probe molecule, reduction in absorption in the elderly was regularly emphasized in early studies that measured urinary excretion rates (233). However, since urinary xylose output is dependent on glomerular filtration rate and since this falls progressively in the elderly, these early studies were discounted. In subsequent studies, absorption was measured using both orally and I.V. administered xylose and a mathematical calculation of absorption rate from the ratio of the urinary appearance from these two routes of administration. These studies implied that there was a slight reduction in xylose absorptive capacity (287, 448), resulting in a shift of absorption to more distal intestinal sites (451).

Some of the early studies of glucose absorption were performed in rats of varying ages who were fed 600 mg of glucose per 100 g body weight and killed 3 h later. Glucose absorption was calculated as the difference between the amount of glucose administered and that remaining in the gastrointestinal tract. When glucose absorption was calculated per body surface area per h, a small but distinct reduction with weight was found (341). In 1968, Klimas (245) reported a study in CD strain rats aged 2, 5, 10, 15, 20, 26, and 32 months in which the absorption of glucose was evaluated out of an in situ loop of intestine for 1 h in anesthetized animals and calculated per 100 g of body weight. Although the 2- and 5-month-old animals were significantly smaller than their older counterparts, intestinal weight and length did not change between 10 and 32 months of age. In these experiments Klimas found minimal change in glucose absorption with age. Most studies of intestinal glucose absorption in aged animals were performed in the 1980s. It is important to point out that differing results in reported studies are often due to differences in methodology. Doubek and Armbrecht (107) evaluated changes in intestinal glucose transport over the life span of the rat using male F344 animals from the NIA colony. Using everted sacs of jejunum, they demonstrated a reduction in the intestinal absorption of 3-O-methylglucose, a nonmetabolizable glucose analog. Twelve- and 24-month-old rats transported significantly less glucose per mg of intestinal tissue than 2-month-old animals. When phloridzin (an inhibitor of the active transport process for glucose) was added, no differences in transport were detected. The data demonstrated a marked decline in carrier-mediated glucose uptake between 2 and 12 months of age. These investigators extended their studies to an evaluation of glucose uptake by BBM vesicles from 2- and 12-month-old rats (107). The study of the sodium-dependent overshoot peak showed a major difference in sodium-dependent uptake between 2- and 12-month-old rats. This difference was eliminated by replacing the sodium gradient with potassium or by adding phloridzin. The data were not due to an age-related change in sodium permeability. The conclusions of this study are complementary to those of Esposito's group (120, 267) for Wistar rats. In a parallel in vitro study (405) in intestinal segments from VC3FL male mice between 2 and 30 months of age, glucose uptake per milligram of tissue was significantly greater in the 30-month-old intestine (duodenum, jejunum, ileum) than at younger ages.

Vinardell and Bolufer (434) perfused the gut of Wistar rats with D-glucose and D-galactose at various concentrations and concluded that the jejunum of 18-month-old animals demonstrated some decrease in apparent permeability coefficient and a reduced active transport. Active transport was reduced by as much as 50% in another of their studies (433). A direct relationship between glucose absorption and villus height leading to age-dependent differences in glucose absorption has been suggested by Jakab and Penzes (219) based on their observations of a reduction in proximal intestinal villus dimensions in aging rats. These authors did not find a reduction in villus mass in the distal intestine. In one unique human study, five groups of subjects had an evaluation of passive and active carbohydrate absorption using lactulose and mannitol to reflect passive absorption and 3-O-methylglucose to measure active absorption. The data suggested that passive absorption of carbohydrate was not impaired with advanced age in healthy elderly subjects or even in long-term hospital patients. However, the percent urinary recovery of 3-O-methylglucose to that of mannitol was significantly reduced in healthy elderly subjects. These data also suggested an impairment in active sugar transport in the elderly (46). Thomson (406) also found increased glucose uptake in 12-month-old rabbits. In contrast, using the everted gut sac technique in the mouse, Chen et al. demonstrated a 55% decrease in glucose and 3-O-methylglucose uptake (75) and decreased D-glucose metabolism at 36 months of age.

Esposito and co-workers (120) used Wistar rats designated as very young (35–45 days old), young (45–60 days old), adult (2–12 months old), old (12–24 months old), and senescent (older than 24 months). In this strain, body weight increases progressively with age. Studies were performed in everted sacs in which jejunal transport of glucose increased from the very young to the young but then fell in older animals per g of intestine in parallel with changes in sodium transport and net fluid transport. In preliminary studies of membrane vesicles, these authors reported a total abolition of the sodium-dependent initial overshoot in animals greater than 24 months of age (267). In other studies, brush border vesicles of older animals did not show a complete loss of sodium-driven glucose uptake but did show some reduction (441). Rat intestinal microvillus membrane vesicles were studied in rats varying in age from 2 to 27 months by Freeman and Quamme (137), who demonstrated high-capacity, low-affinity and low-capacity, high-affinity transport processes in the small intestine. Their data suggested a greater capacity for sodium-dependent glucose transport based on milligrams of protein in younger animals.

Two studies of BBMs from human intestine have been reported. Wallis and co-workers (442) reported some reduction in brush border glucose transport, which they interpreted as reflecting changes in bacterial contamination of the small intestine. In one 76-yr-old subject, almost complete loss of the sodium-dependent active glucose transport has been reported (435).

Recently, Ferraris et al. (128) studied the absorption of D-glucose, D-fructose, L-glucose, and a series of amino acids in isolated everted sleeves of mouse small intestine using a well-validated intestinal transport method. The animals used were COBS-SFW mice purchased from the NIA breeding colonies and the older animals were aged 21–24 months. The data on these mice were compared with animals 6 months of age. It is important to emphasize that these mice were stabilized at the experimental site for 2 months prior to study. Studies were performed in everted intestine, representing the middle 60% of the gut, thus including both jejunum and proximal ileum. Uptake rates of test substances were performed at concentrations previously determined to yield V_{max} using short incubation periods. To determine glucose transporter concentration and density, [^{3}H]phlorizin–binding measurements were performed. There was a 16% decrease in food consumption between the 23.7- and 6-month-old mice so that the authors pair-fed some mice for 1 wk before the uptake experiments. D-glucose uptake per milligram of tissue fell significantly between 6 and 24 months and then further up to 27 months. There was no difference in passive permeability to glucose. Specific-binding studies of the membrane glucose transporter using phlorizin indicated a 30% fall in transporter site density per mg of intestine between the 6–7-month and the 24-month-old mice but no further fall in the 27-month-old animals. Apparent kd was similar in all rodents. Western blot analysis of the Na$^+$ D-glucose co-transporter showed a band of about 76 kd which was similar in the 23.7- and 6.7-month-old mice. It is important to point out, however, that although the aged mice had a smaller number of D-glucose transporters per milligram of jejunum, they had more jejunal tissue per cm than young animals. As a result of such mucosal hyperplasia, the total number of glucose transporters in the aging intestine may not have been less than that in young animals.

There also is indirect evidence that proximal intestinal absorption of carbohydrate substrates is somewhat reduced in aging rodents. Ileal villus mass in 21- and 27-month-old ad libitum chow-fed Fischer 344 rats was shown to be greater than in younger rats (169, 202). In these older animals, no difference could be detected in duodenal or jejunal villus mass (169). Such ileal hypertrophy could have resulted from increased luminal substrate reaching the distal intestine. Reville et al. (355) have also concluded that the ileum compensates for age-dependent loss of jejunal functions in the rat.

In any case, it seems unlikely in healthy elderly humans that reduction in overall carbohydrate absorption is sufficiently great to result in malnutrition. Most available evidence for the mechanism responsible for reduced intestinal monosaccharide absorption with age would suggest a change in intestinal receptor density or affinity for actively absorbed substrates. Future studies will need to determine whether such age-related changes in membrane receptors are limited to glucose or other monosaccharides or are a reflection of more generalized depression of intestinal BBM receptors responsible for solute absorption.

Protein. Very little information is available on the effects of aging on intestinal protein absorption. Most elderly individuals studied in a steady state are found to be in positive nitrogen balance. There are, however, major contradictions in the recommendations about the amount of protein that should be consumed to maintain the elderly in positive nitrogen balance. Some investigators have suggested that the elderly require more (56, 250), less, or no change (76) in protein intake to maintain protein balance. Albumin synthesis also may respond less well to altered dietary protein with advanced age, which suggests that the adaptive responses to changing protein needs may be diminished (147). In one early study, the concentrations of ^{131}I in blood and collected urine following ingestion of [^{131}I]-labeled albumin in water indicated no difference in digestion or absorption between young and elderly subjects (79).

Penzes' group (333–338) has performed the most comprehensive studies of the effects of age on the absorption of amino acids. They used female Wistar rats aged between 6 and 28 months that were bred and maintained in the Institute of Gerontology in Budapest and whose body weight did not differ markedly. Absorption rates were determined in anesthetized animals in which the test amino acids with tracer radioactive label were perfused through the intestinal lumen at differing concentrations. In some studies, various concentrations of amino acids were injected into closed loops of intestine in groups of animals and the contents were washed out after 20 min, absorption being measured by difference in amino acid concentration between the beginning and the end of the study. Amino acid absorption rates were calculated per 100 g body weight and intestinal affinity was determined from the K_m based on the Lineweaver–Burk equation. Initially, Penzes' group studied the absorption of radiomethionine (333), finding an increased absorption of this amino acid with age. Subsequently, they also showed greater absorption of lysine and cysteine (334) but not arginine (335), glycine, L-alanine and L-leucine (336), finding no differences in the absorption of any of these amino acids between animals aged 6, 12, and 25–28 months. In other studies, the same group found no real differences in the absorption of tryptophan (337, 338) but some reduction in the affinity of phenylalanine and proline for their intestinal receptors. More recently, Navah and Winter (320) studied the uptake of aromatic amino acids into rings of jejunum from 6-, 12-, and 24-month-old Fischer 344 rats. These authors demonstrated a progressive fall in V_{max} and increased k_m with age for phenylalanine and L-tryptophan.

It is of interest that when amino acid uptake was studied in human fibroblasts at different ages (differing doubling levels), the rate of L-phenylalanine transport declined. Although uptake was studied for several other amino acids in this experiment, only detailed evaluation of L-phenylalanine was reported (322).

Lipids. Sn triacylglycerols, the major form of dietary lipid, are insoluble in aqueous systems, such as those in the intestinal luminal contents. Triacylglycerols (TG), therefore, must first be hydrolyzed to more polar derivatives, which then are solubilized in the lumen prior to intestinal mucosal uptake. Hydrolysis is initiated by gastric lipase (1) and is completed by pancreatic lipase in association with pancreatic co-lipase to form free fatty acids and Sn 2-monoacylglycerol (MG). In the presence of conjugated bile acids and diacylphosphatidyl cholines (PC), these digestion products form both liquid crystalline and micellar phases from which mucosal uptake of the digestion products of ingested lipids can occur. PCs subsequently are hydrolyzed by phospholipase A_2 to lysophosphatidyl cholines and nonesterified fatty acids, which are absorbed by the intestinal mucosa. Although the method of entry of lipid digestion products through the cell membrane has not been fully clarified, mucosal epithelial cell uptake processes differ for long-chain and medium-chain fatty acids. Within the cell, absorbed lipids are transferred to the endoplasmic reticulum, possibly in association with the mucosal fatty acid binding protein. Subsequently, re-esterification of absorbed fatty acid and MG to TG occurs. These esterified lipids then associate with apoprotein B_{48} and are transferred to the Golgi complex, where further modification occurs to form chylomicrons and very low-density lipoprotein (VLDL) particles. The relative proportion of absorbed lipids that are transported in chylomicrons and VLDL is determined by the chemical composition of ingested TG lipid. Medium-chain, nonesterified fatty acids are principally transported directly into the portal vein bound to albumin.

The capacity for intestinal absorption of long-chain TG in humans is very large and greatly exceeds the usual dietary intake. Caloric intake tends to fall in the elderly, further reducing the need for optimal absorption of fat. These factors must be taken into account when evaluating the significance of studies of overall fat absorption performed either in elderly humans or in animals. Early studies testing fat absorption in the elderly used experimental techniques that now are not accepted and experimental volunteer subjects who were poorly defined (42, 449). Recent studies have used nutritionally stable, disease-free volunteers and have demonstrated no difference in fecal fat excretion throughout the life span in subjects consuming approximately 100 g of fat per day (22). An earlier study in eight elderly subjects suggested that more fat was excreted in the feces when 120 g than when 80 g were consumed (453), implying a reduced lipid absorption capacity. In a unique study by Simko and Michael (382), however, emulsified high fat formulas were perfused intragastrically in seriously undernourished older patients suffering from metastatic cancer, and no steatorrhea occurred in most when as much as 400 g of fat was provided. The measurement of $^{14}CO_2$ breath excretion following a standard (60 g) fat meal containing ^{14}C triolein showed lower $^{14}CO_2$ production in volunteers aged 65–85 yr (316); however, the health and nutritional status of these subjects was not described. Excretion of $^{14}CO_2$ in the breath may be delayed in the elderly because chylomicron lipid turnover is prolonged and/or fatty acid oxidation is reduced.

Perfusion studies in animals have shown contradictory results. Holt and Dominguez (193) perfused an emulsified triolein solution intraduodenally in 4–5-month-old and 19–20-month-old retired breeder Sprague-Dawley rats and reported reduced TG absorption per g wet weight of intestine in the older animals. However, intestinal weight was found to increase as total body weight increased and was much higher in the older rats than the young. Hollander's group studied the absorption of micellar oleic (177) and linoleic (185) acids out of intestinal segments using a single-pass intestinal infusion system at high rates and calculated their data per 100 cm of intestine. In contrast to other studies, their results suggested that fatty acid absorption increased with age. Hollander's group also reported greater overall cholesterol (180), vitamin A (181), vitamin D (182), and vitamin E (179) absorption in older rats per 100 cm of intestine.

The effect of age on biliary lipid composition and gallbladder contractility is described elsewhere in this chapter (see under LIVER AND BILIARY TREE). Whether these changes in bile components and output affect intraluminal bile acid and phospholipid composition is unknown since no data are available. Gastric lipase is thought to initiate dietary TG lipolysis (1) and to be of major importance if pancreatic insufficiency is present. Gargouri and co-workers have reported a fivefold reduction in gastric lipase activity in gastric biopsy specimens from human volunteers over the age of 70 yr (145). These authors unfortunately did not present data on the histological status of their biopsies or on the secretory function of the stomach in these patients, who may have had atrophic gastritis. Although these are some data suggesting that pancreatic secretion falls with age (see under PANCREAS), there is no convincing evidence that any changes are of sufficient magnitude to impair the intraluminal phase of fat absorption. Nevertheless, the intraluminal phase may be affected by increases in the concentration of bacterial flora in the small bowel lumen. Gram-positive and -negative bacteria are known to rapidly deconjugate bile acids. The resulting deconjugated bile acids can be either absorbed in the duodenum and jejunum or precipitated in the lumen, leading to lower luminal bile acid concentrations and possible secondary maldigestion and malabsorption.

The transfer of luminal digestion products from the bulk phase in the lumen to the mucosa involves two major barriers: the unstirred water layer and the cell membrane. As discussed earlier (see Intestinal Absorption), recent studies suggest that the unstirred water layer is much less of a barrier than previously thought (263). Some studies have suggested differences in the thickness of the unstirred water layer barrier between young and older animals. Thomson examined the in vitro uptake of a homologous series of saturated fatty acids and of cholesterol in jejunal disks obtained from young and older rabbits (407, 408). Fatty acid and cholesterol uptake were less in the older animals when the unstirred water layer was decreased with stirring. These data suggested that the mucosal membrane of younger animals was more permeable than that of older rabbits. The intestinal permeability of high-molecular-weight compounds in the lumen declines shortly after birth in rodents and before birth in the human fetus. In some studies, intestinal permeability of polyethylene glycol of various molecular weights (184) was found to increase with age (184). These observations were in contrast to those of Thomson (407).

Studies of the absorption of fatty acids, cholesterol, and vitamins A and D in young and aging animals have yielded very conflicting results. Overall, lymphatic transport was not evaluated in these studies. Hollander and co-workers (176) perfused in vivo intestinal segments in rats of varying ages. The experiments were performed within 2–3 h of surgical cannulation, a time when the experimental animals may not have fully recovered from surgery and anesthesia. From these data, the authors concluded that the absorption of lipids from micellar solutions was increased in advanced age. The explanation provided for these surprising findings was that there was an increase in mucosal surface area per unit length of gut in the old rats, as well as a decrease in the unstirred water layer thickness. It is important to point out that very high perfusion rates of micellar lipids (30–60 ml/h) were used in these experiments, 10–20 times greater than those used by other investigators. It is possible that these very high rates of perfusion might alter the unstirred water characteristics. It is also pertinent to mention that the findings of this group are not totally consistent, since in a study of linoleate absorption, decreased unstirred water layer resistance was reported but in another report no difference was seen.

Using low perfusion rates and emulsified lipid in rats that had been allowed to recover for 48 h after thoracic duct cannulation, Holt and Dominguez found no difference in the intraluminal lipolysis and uptake of test lipids but some reduction in transmucosal transport (193). It is of interest that essentially no studies of the intracellular phase of intestinal lipid transport nor of lymphatic transport and intestinal lipoprotein formation have been performed in aging rodents.

Overall, there appears to be little evidence for major changes in intestinal lipid transport with age. However, physiological changes in mucosal lipid transfer and lipoprotein formation have not been fully explored and will require further study (192).

Ion and Micronutrient Absorption. Age-related effects on intestinal electrolyte absorption have received little attention in the literature. Korbuly (249) studied the disappearance of sodium and potassium out of in vivo loops of cannulated jejunum in anesthetized Wistar rats aged 3–44 months. There was considerable variation in uptake rates calculated by the method used, but no age-dependent differences could be detected.

Since the elderly may be at risk for developing zinc deficiency because of marginal zinc intake (364) and since hyperzincuria may occur because of the use of diuretics (306), Mooradian and Song (307) studied zinc absorption in Fischer 344 rats aged 3, 12, and 24 months. Previous studies had suggested that zinc uptake was reduced (418). In Mooradian and Song's study (307), excised intestine was examined with Ussing type chambers and short circuit current and substrate transfer was measured. Zinc transport from mucosa to serosa in 24-month-old rats was calculated as 55 ± 3.5 nmoles/h/cm^2, significantly greater than that found in 12-month-old animals, 30.1 nmoles/h/cm^2.

In a limited study of iron and copper absorption, six healthy young men did not differ significantly (419) from elderly men (420). Decreased iron absorption previously was reported in old age (218). The weight of the evidence implies that the absorption of this mineral is not altered (190). The fact that many older subjects have increased total body iron stores (67) requires further study but militates against decreased intestinal absorption of iron.

Calcium. Calcium is a divalent cation crucial for the maintenance of cellular homeostasis and for bone stability. Since bone calcium loss is a major problem in the elderly, the absorption of calcium and of other nutrients that determine bone stability and calcium homeostasis has received much attention.

Calcium from the small intestinal lumen enters the intestinal absorptive cell by crossing the BBM via a carrier-mediated mechanism. Overall, this is thought to be a passive process since luminal calcium concentrations are much higher than intracellular calcium concentrations. Calcium entry may be facilitated by integral BBM proteins known collectively as the calcium-binding protein complex. Calcium then moves across the absorptive cell to the basolateral surface. Intracellular calcium may be sequestered by intracellular organelles or bound to cytosolic proteins. One of these cytoplasmic proteins, which may play a role in the translocation of calcium, is the vitamin D–dependent calcium-binding protein recently named "calbindin," which binds calcium with high affinity, is markedly stimulated by 1,25-dihydroxy vitamin D, and correlates well with calcium absorption. At the basolateral surface of the intestinal epithelial cell, calcium is translocated out of the cell and into the blood by either an ATP-dependent pump or an Na/Cl exchange mechanism, the former probably being the more important. It appears clear that 1,25 dihydroxy vitamin D acts at several sites to stimulate intestinal calcium absorption. It may enhance calcium entry into the epithelial cell across the BBM, perhaps by altering its lipid composition. The quantity of the calcium-binding complex and the cytosolic calcium-binding protein also are dependent on vitamin D stimulation. Furthermore, 1,25-dihydroxy D increases the capacity of basolateral membranes to actively pump calcium out of the cell. Most of these effects of vitamin D are mediated by transcription and synthesis of new protein (125). The vitamin D–dependent mechanisms play a major role in human calcium absorption at relatively low luminal calcium concentrations and are stimulated by lowering calcium intake. However, vitamin D–independent processes may function at higher calcium concentrations (378).

It is clear that calcium absorption falls with advanced age (66, 143). When isotopic calcium became available, Avioli et al. (25) initially reported reduced ^{45}Ca absorption in elderly and osteoporotic women compared with premenopausal controls. Their assessment of calcium absorption was based entirely on measurements of plasma radioactivity after an oral dose of the calcium isotope. In 1970, Bullamore and co-workers (66) studied calcium absorption in 75 men and women aged 20–95 yr from the appearance of radioactivity in plasma after oral administration of calcium isotopes. After age 60 yr, absorption of calcium appeared to fall, and over the age of 80 yr all subjects had lower calcium absorption than younger individuals. These authors initially suggested that decreased 1,25 vitamin D may be playing an important role in this process. Nordin's group (325) continued to study calcium absorption as a function of advanced age, extending their studies to more sophisticated methodology. They expanded the concept that reduced calcium absorption in the elderly might be due to aberrations of vitamin D metabolism or its effects. This group (324) as well as others (271, 311) were able to show that plasma 1,25 dihydroxy D levels were lower in elderly subjects and particularly in those who had undergone a femoral fracture. They also suggested that vitamin D "resistance" might be playing a role in this malabsorption and initially suggested that vitamin D supplementation would be an appropriate method of treating elderly patients to prevent bone loss and fractures. In the studies of Ireland and Fordtran (214), an intestinal perfusion technique using different concentrations of calcium was performed on elderly and young volunteers. They showed that calcium absorption following a diet containing high levels of calcium did not differ significantly in young and aging volunteers. However, the adaptation of the intestinal absorption of calcium by elderly subjects to a diet low in calcium for a 4–5-wk period clearly was defective (Fig. 20.1); whereas the young group increased calcium absorption by 55% on the low-calcium diet, the older subjects increased absorption only 14%. This important study implied that the responses of the intestine to lower calcium intake were altered as a function of age. Subsequent investigations used experimental animals to expand this concept and to evaluate the individual steps operating in normal calcium absorption as a function of age. Early studies suggested that calcium absorption decreased with age in the rat. Armbrecht and co-workers (20) have performed a large number of studies in this regard. Initially, they demonstrated that active calcium transport, studied in everted intestinal sacs, declined rapidly with adult age in Sprague-Dawley rats. The response of the intestine to reduction in dietary calcium also was muted (21). They studied the active basolateral pump mechanism for calcium (19), using vesicles derived from basolateral membranes isolated by differential and gradient centrifugation in rats aged 2–12 months. In vesicles isolated from 12-month-old (adult) animals, ATP-stimulated calcium uptake was only one-quarter of that seen at 2 months of age. In the absence of ATP, there were no differences in calcium uptake with age. These data suggested that aging was accompanied by a defect in the energy-dependent pump mechanism. There were no differences in the apparent affinity of the calcium transport system for calcium. However, the V_{max} at 12 months was only 20% of that seen at 2 months of age. These data suggested that the older rats had a decreased number of calcium transporters in the basolateral membranes.

Armbrecht also studied the BBM calcium transport system (17), which did not change significantly with age. However, further studies suggested that these uptake measurements probably represented mainly binding to the BBM rather than transport. Age-related changes in the cytosolic components of the calcium transport system also have been studied in the rat. A large decrease in the concentration of the vitamin D–dependent calbindin was seen between 2 and 6 months of age and a further modest decrease from 6 to 15 months of age, without much of a change thereafter

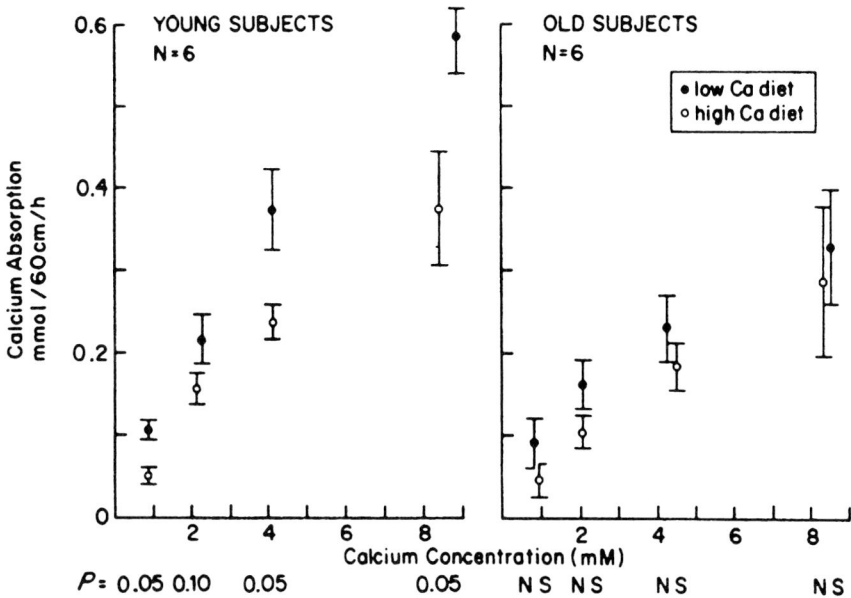

FIG. 20.1. Effect of calcium diet in young and old subjects. Each subject was studied twice, once on the low-calcium diet and once on the high-calcium diet. P values are by paired analysis. [Reprinted from Ireland and Fortran (214) with permission.]

(17). Stimulation of the calcium-binding protein by 1,25-hydroxy D was much less in adult than in very young animals. Calbindin mRNA stimulation by 1,25-dihydroxy vitamin D was unaltered by age, suggesting that defective action resulted from a translational change. Recent studies have demonstrated clearly that dietary calcium restriction results in an up-regulation of the intestinal vitamin D receptor (440). This increase in receptor binding is not associated with an increase in vitamin D receptor mRNA, suggesting that the process results primarily from a posttranslational decrease in degradation of the receptor, with an increase in receptor synthesis responsible for only a negligible portion of the accumulation. It is important to point out that other data, including those of DeLuca's group (143) suggest that defects in vitamin 1,25 dihydroxy D metabolism may be responsible for reduced calcium absorption in the elderly. Their data suggest that inadequate metabolism of vitamin 25 D to vitamin 1,25 D contributes significantly to decreased calcium absorption and adaptation to a low-calcium diet. After showing that calcium uptake into isolated duodenal cells from aging rats was impaired, Liang et al. (264) compared total and unoccupied intestinal vitamin 1,25 D receptor sites in 6- and 24-month-old rats, finding a reduction in the older animals (400). In another study, Horst and colleagues (207) have suggested that there is a reduction in calcitriol receptors in both intestine and bone as a function of age, based on a study of 1- and 15–18-month-old male rats. They studied unoccupied vitamin D receptors in the intestines of young and aging Sprague-Dawley rats and found that they were manyfold lower in the older animals (162 femtomol/mg of protein) than in the young counterparts (666 femtomol/mg of protein), with no significant difference in receptor affinity between the two groups. Similar findings were found in bone. Even the provision of vitamin 1,25 D to the elderly rats did not increase unoccupied receptor numbers anywhere close to what was found in young animals. Some of the discrepancies in data may reflect strain differences in the experimental animals.

It is pertinent to mention that the colon may play a major role in calcium absorption. A saturable calcium transport system sensitive to vitamin 1,25 D is present in the descending colon, which is inhibited by dexamethasone (223). In the ascending colon, unidirectional calcium absorption is independent of vitamin 1,25 D. Short-chain fatty acids, such as acetate and butyrate, have been shown to significantly increase calcium absorption in the distal colon but not in the proximal colon (269). Overall, studies suggest that vitamin 1,25 D can significantly increase the absorption of calcium from the colon in humans (159). The small intestinal absorption of dietary vitamin D also may be reduced in the elderly (35). In achlorhydria, when gastric acid secretion is minimal, calcium absorption from calcium carbonate is impaired in the fasting state (354). However, calcium absorption appears to be maintained normally even in achlorhydrics when calcium is provided with a meal (166). Clinical observations suggest that gastric acid plays some role in chronic calcium absorption in humans (26) on a high-fiber diet containing large amounts of wheat bran. This was found in volunteers who had normal gastric acid secretion as well as in those who had achlorhydria (246).

Milk lactose may specifically increase intestinal calcium absorption (65, 206). The substitution of lactose for other carbohydrates in the diet of laboratory animals has been shown to improve calcium absorption and to increase the retention of calcium in bone. In the studies of Schuette et al. (375), the addition of lactose but not other carbohydrates increased calcium absorption by approximately 25% in humans. Individuals with the lowest absorption in the absence of carbohydrates had the greatest increase with lactose. Calcium absorption was the same from skim milk as from lactase-treated skim milk. Since the elderly are encouraged to consume greater amounts of dairy products to enhance calcium intake, these observations are of clinical importance.

It is also important that aging is associated with reduced capacity of the human skin to produce vitamin D_3 from sunlight (270). Thus the fact that intestinal vitamin 1,25 D absorption also is reduced in the elderly becomes very important and may disturb calcium homeostasis (35).

Intestinal phosphate absorption is not as well regulated as calcium, and body phosphate stores generally are maintained by the balance between dietary intake and renal excretion. A recent review summarizes the evidence for a modest reduction in phosphate absorption with age (18). Total body magnesium stores are crucial for the maintenance of metabolic homeostasis, yet few data are available on changes in magnesium absorption as a function of age.

Water-Soluble Vitamins

Thiamine. Since thiamine deficiency has been reported in elderly subjects and the methods for measuring thiamine are well accepted and relatively simple, the absorption of this vitamin has been given much attention. In 1943, Rafsky and Neuman (350) assessed intestinal thiamine absorption based on the amount of thiamine needed to achieve a constant urinary excretion of the vitamin. These authors reported that more thiamine had to be administered in elderly than in young volunteers (350). Draper (108) showed that the absorption of an oral dose of radiolabeled thiamine decreased substantially in rats after the age of 20 months. In contrast, Kirk and Chieffi (243) measured thiamine excretion in the feces of human volunteers and found little change in the percent absorbed with increasing age at the dose levels used. Thomson (409) found no difference in the absorption of ^{35}S thiamine in young and elderly volunteers. These studies lead one to conclude that physiological doses of thiamine are well absorbed in the elderly. In another study, Jusco et al (221) concluded that the intestinal absorption of riboflavin was greater in the young than in the elderly. In contrast, when biotin uptake into brush border vesicles from 3-, 12-, and 24-month-old Fischer 344 rats was studied (363), the V_{max} of the carrier-mediated transport process was found to be higher in the 24-month-old animals than in the younger animals, whereas K_m was similar. Niacin transport also is unchanged with age (134).

Folate. Most dietary folate exists in conjugated complex forms as pteroylpolyglutamates. The absorption of such complex dietary folate requires enzymatic hydrolysis of the gammaglutamyl peptide bond of polyglutamate to form a monoglutamate by the enzyme pteroylpolyglutamate hydrolase, also known as folate conjugase. The monoglutamate derivative then is absorbed by a saturable, pH-dependent process. The hydrolysis of polyglutamyl folate to simple forms generally has not been considered to be the rate-limiting step in the process of overall absorption of dietary folate. Folate conjugase is found in the pancreas, in the contents of the intestinal lumen, and on the intestinal mucosal surface.

Intestinal folate absorption at low concentrations occurs by an active receptor-mediated process but at higher concentrations is dependent more on passive diffusion. Folate is converted to a neutral un-ionized species in the acidic microenvironment generated at the glycocalyx, where uptake can then occur by passive diffusion. If these mechanisms are disturbed as a function of aging, then folate malabsorption might result. In one of the earliest studies, Bhanthumnavin et al. (49) measured [^{3}H]folic acid absorption in everted sacs from Wistar rats obtained from the NIA colony in Baltimore and aged 1.5, 6, 12, and 24 months. No difference in absorption rate across the intestine from the luminal to the serosal side was detected in this study.

Hurdle and Picton-Williams (210) also measured the absorption of folic acid in elderly subjects and were unable to find differences from data obtained in younger individuals. Nevertheless, folate depletion can itself result in folic acid malabsorption, which then can respond to repletion with folic acid (117). Folic acid absorption also can be reduced in the presence of achlorhydria. This has been directly demonstrated by studies showing significant increase of monofolate absorption when achlorhydric elderly subjects with atrophic gastritis were given a test meal of [^{3}H]folic acid together with 0.1N HCl (362).

Alternatively it has been suggested that aging may be associated with a reduction in intestinal folate conjugase activity. Baker and co-workers (32) studied 24 elderly subjects ranging in age from 73 to 101 yr and 12 healthy young controls aged 24–42 yr. They evaluated the hydrolysis of folylpolyglutamates, which are the preponderant folates in yeast, by comparing plasma folate concentrations following administration of yeast or similar amounts of synthetic folic acid in young and elderly volunteers. They concluded that folate deficits in the elderly could be caused by impaired hydrolysis of ingested folate-containing foods. This possibility was evaluated in one study in which Wistar rats aged 2, 3, and 28–30 months were killed at varying time periods after oral administration of a single dose of 40 mg/kg body weight of either synthetic folic acid or conjugated folates (234). No differences in the absorption of folic acid were found between young and aging rats, but the older animals appeared to absorb 40% less polyglutamate. These authors suggested that there was an impaired induction of pancreatic and intestinal conjugase activity after ingestion of conjugated folate with age. In contrast, data from our laboratory (157) clearly demonstrate no significant difference in folate conjugase activity obtained from duodenum, jejunum, ileum, pancreas, and brain of 4-, 18-, and 27-month-old Fischer 344 rats. In the study by Bailey et al. (28) jejunal folate conjugase activities also were not found to differ between healthy elderly and young males. These authors used a jejunal perfusion method and found that aging did not affect intestinal absorption of either ^{3}H monoglutamate or pteroylhexaglutamate. Thus on the available information, there is no evidence that folate absorption is decreased as a function of age, except perhaps as the monoglutamate in achlorhydric individuals.

Vitamin B_{12}. Serum vitamin B_{12} levels generally are lower in advanced age than in the young (29), which has been ascribed to reduced dietary intake or to intestinal vitamin B_{12} malabsorption. Although vitamin B_{12} malabsorption was suggested by early experimental studies in older individuals (80, 148), the data of Hyams (212) clearly demonstrated that the intestinal uptake of a test dose of ^{58}Co-labeled vitamin B_{12} was not different from that in younger controls. The results of this study were based on fecal excretion of vitamin B_{12} following an oral bolus of the labeled vitamin. An important potential mechanism for vitamin B_{12} malabsorption involves reduced secretion of an intrinsic factor that may accompany atrophic gastritis in the elderly or possibly hypochlorhydria. Although crystalline vitamin B_{12} absorption may be normal, malabsorption of food-bound vitamin B_{12} may occur with hypochlorhydria because of failure of digestion of the R-binder–vitamin B_{12} complex in the upper small intestine (100) or absorption and metabolism by bacteria (395). Some investigators have claimed that this is an important cause for reduced absorption of vitamin B_{12} in the elderly (72). In the presence of intestinal bacterial overgrowth, vitamin B_{12} malabsorption may occur. The available evidence indicates that vitamin B_{12} malabsorption does not occur as a physiological function of age except when gastrointestinal disease is present.

Fat-Soluble Vitamins

Vitamin D. The changes in calcium absorption that occur with advanced age have been summarized above. It is clear that reduction in intestinal calcium absorption is related to a considerable extent to altered effects of 1,25 dihydroxy vitamin D. Human studies have suggested that vitamin D supplementation improves calcium homeostasis in the elderly. There are data showing that plasma vitamin D levels are lower in older individuals, particularly when exposure to sunlight is reduced in winter months in the Northern Hemisphere (261). It has been claimed that plasma 25 hydroxy vitamin D concentration in older patients was only marginally greater when they were provided 2,000 IU daily than 500 IU (273). Intestinal perfusion studies in the rat performed in our laboratory demonstrated impaired intestinal absorption of vitamin D (193). In one study of ^{3}H vitamin D absorption, significantly lower plasma levels of unchanged ^{3}H vitamin D and vitamin metabolites were found in elderly female volunteers than in younger volunteers, also suggesting impaired absorption of this vitamin (35).

Vitamin K. Vitamin K_1 (phylloquinone) has an essential role in blood clotting but also is involved in the binding of calcium to osteoblasts during bone formation. Thus changes in vitamin K absorption might have a crucial effect on bone mineralization. In a recent study, plasma vitamin K and its metabolites were measured in the blood of 11 apparently normal young individuals aged 20–36 yr and 17 elderly aged 56–86 yr. The circulating levels of total vitamin K_1 in the two groups did not differ. However, the levels of the important vitamin K_1 metabolite menaquinone-8 were approximately half of those found in the young (174). These data do not support a decreased absorption of the vitamin but rather altered hepatic metabolism.

Vitamin A. Normally the liver contains 90%–95% of the body's total vitamin A stores in the form of retinyl esters. Hepatic vitamin A stores in animals increase with age either because of the aging process itself or because of continued accumulation over time. Chronic ethanol ingestion depletes total liver vitamin A content considerably and increases the vitamin A levels of other tissues. Because of the large hepatic stores of vitamin A in the elderly described above, ethanol ingestion has less of an effect on hepatic vitamin A stores than in the young (302). The alternative explanation, that ethanol increases the absorption of vitamin A in the elderly, seems less likely. The study of Hollander and Morgan (181) suggested that there was a progressive increase in the intestinal uptake of vitamin A with age, data that paralleled other studies from this group and implied that all intestinal lipid absorption increases in older animals. Although initial studies by Russell's group (252) also suggested an increase in the absorption of vitamin A in elderly humans, subsequent careful re-evaluation by the same group (251) demonstrated that this was due to an altered metabolism of vitamin A–containing lipoproteins and not an increase in intestinal absorption. Hollander's group also demonstrated that 40% caloric restriction reduced vitamin A absorption in older rats (186). Although there are many assumptions about changes in drug absorption with age, the evidence indicates that there are no significant changes other than those due to gastrointestinal disease processes (73).

GUT-ASSOCIATED IMMUNE SYSTEM

Aging is characterized by an overall decline in the effectiveness of the immune system in older individuals (279). Most studies of immunity in the elderly to data have concentrated on the systemic immune system because the components are readily available for experimental observations. The gut-associated lymphoid tissue (GALT) consists of cells in isolated follicles within the intestine, aggregates of follicles found principally in the more distal small bowel (Peyer's patches), mesenteric lymph nodes, effector lymphocytes and plasma cells within the lamina propria, and intraepithelial cells of the intestine. The GALT represents about 60% of the body's immune cells but is more difficult to study in vivo. Age-associated changes may affect one or more of the components that make up the GALT.

There is some evidence that Peyer's patches change as an effect of age. Most studies suggest that the number or functional size of Peyer's patches decrease in the elderly, though according to some investigators, this change begins only in middle age in the human and mouse gut (87, 152).

Kawanishi and Kiely (226) have performed a series of studies to determine the responsiveness of various immune functions in the GALT to defined stimuli. Initially, they demonstrated a reduction in the number of Peyer's patches and mesenteric lymph node lymphoid cells in 24–27-month-old BALB/c mice compared to 3–4-month-old animals, with a remarkable decrease in the L3T4 helper/inducer T cell marker-positive subpopulations. There was, however, no reduction in the number of isolated lymphocytes from the lamina propria between mice over 24 months and those aged 14–16 months. The distribution of T cells, B cells, and their subpopulations also changed. Kawanishi and Kiely described less of a decline with age in suppressive/cytotoxic marker expressing T cells. It is possible that the decrease in thymus-derived small intestinal cells is responsible for reduced proliferative responses following stimulation with some B cell mitogens. Overall, there was only a slight reduction in the absolute number of Peyer's patch and mesenteric lymph node B cells derived from senescent mice. Using an immunohistochemical technique, reduced numbers of cytoplasmic Ig (immunoglobin) cells were observed with age both in mesenteric lymph nodes and in Peyer's patches in the CBA mouse (161, 162). In Kawanishi and Kiely's initial study (226), there was over a twofold decrease in IgA levels obtained from intestinal washings, a finding which does not agree with reports on mixed salivary secretion in elderly humans (112, 132). A recent study in volunteers aged over 70 yr demonstrated more immunoglubulin secretions and higher intraepithelial IgA plasma cell counts than younger controls aged 25–50 yr (23).

Kawanishi's subsequent studies (228) were more concerned with the effect of stimulation on GALT cell responsiveness. Peyer's patch B cells derived from 24-month-old BALB/C mice stimulated with autoreactive Peyer's patch T cell-derived, B cell stimulatory factors proliferated considerably more and contained more than tenfold the amount of total IgA as that found in mature animals, but the ratio of intracellular dimeric IgA to total IgA in the aged B cell lysates was reduced by almost one-half. Recombinant IL2 was able to partially correct aberrant humoral immune responses in the GALT from these aged mice, probably due principally to improved suppressor T cell function, suggesting that the production of this interleukin was defective (3). Peyer's patch cells from 26–28-month-old C57 black mice retained the capacity to respond to mitogens and alloantigens (119). Senescence-related alterations of the local gut mucosal immune response to enteric microbacterial antigens also were determined (227). The functional activity of specific T (CD3 + CD4) cells in the GALT was not affected much by senescence, whereas there was a qualitative defect in the suppressor T (CD3 + CD8) cell. These observations suggest that oral tolerance to exogenous stimuli is impaired, manifested as hyporeactive humoral responses to enteric microbial antigens. This presumably is due to hyporeactivity of the T-cell system.

To better understand the cellular mechanism for reduced reactivity of the GALT immunoregulatory lymphocytes, the proliferative activity of T and B cells was studied after stimulation by phorbol esters or ionomycin and a calcium ionophore. Proliferative responses of the GALT T cells of 24–28-month-old mice to concanavalin A (Con A) were considerably reduced compared to responses of 4-month-old mice, an effect which could be partially corrected by administration of IL-2. Aged GALT T cells respond to phorbol esters plus ionomycin more efficiently than to Con A. The responses to lipopolysaccharide (LPS) do not differ; thus some of the age-associated changes in the gut mucosal immune system may be related to altered second-messenger signal transduction by protein kinase C and calcium. Clearly, this depends on the specific type of exogenous signal. In contrast, B cells from the GALT of aging mice showed only minor ion responsiveness (3, 225).

It is of interest, however, that other studies (from the Host Resistance Program of McMaster University Medical Center using C57 black mice in the age range of 2–24 months) demonstrated a reduction in the heterogeneity index of IgM and IgG in splenic cells of 24-month-old animals compared to their younger counterparts, but a similar reduction in mesenteric or mediastinal cells was not seen (397). Modestly reduced heterogeneity of IgA cells from these sites in 24-month-old animals compared to younger mice was detected. These studies clearly demonstrate the contrasting changes in the GALT and in the systemic circulation. Vigorous anti-trinitnophenol (TNP) plaque-forming cell responses in mesenteric lymph nodes from mice of advanced age also were maintained (396).

Dimeric IgA also enters the intestinal lumen through the biliary system. Since there is an age-related decline of the secretion of all of the biliary components into the intestine, including dimeric IgA (374), this might reduce gastrointestinal IgA concentrations in older animals (401). Although shown in rats, the importance of this pathway in humans is less clear (106). IgA receptors and enterocytes also are unaffected in rats up to 24 months of age (95). The intestine of rodents becomes populated with organisms that are potentially pathogenic in increasing numbers as the animal ages (340, 369). Modest changes in the concentrations of gut organisms in humans with age also have been reported (153, 413). A group of Japanese investigators utilized a unique approach to study potential mechanisms for the acquisition of more pathogenic organisms in the intestine of aging rodents. These investigators fed hyperimmunized milk derived from cows immunized with antigens of various human gut microorganisms. This product was shown to be highly specific for intestinal bacteria and was fed to C57 black mice from the age of 2 months for either 6 months or 16 months. The 18-month-old mice (those fed the milk for 16 months) showed higher directed cytotoxicity of intestinal intraepithelial lymphocytes, higher proliferative response of mesenteric lymph node cells against mitogenic stimulation, and greater capacity of spleen cells to produce antisheep erythrocytic IgG antibody than control mice that did not receive hyperimmunized milk. Lower levels of circulating autoantibodies also were found in the hyperimmunized milk-fed mice. These data suggest that the senescence of the murine immune system might be delayed by consumption of milk from immunized cows (215).

SPLANCHNIC BLOOD FLOW

Older studies suggest that splanchnic blood flow declines as a fraction of cardiac output in advanced age and that changes in the enteric vasculature may underline a variety of gastrointestinal problems in the elderly (403). Cardiac output also may decrease in the elderly (see Chapter 17), which may alter splanchnic blood flow.

Varga and Csaky (430) noticed that subepithelial blood flow through distal small intestine decreased with an increase in body weight. They also reported that the blood flow to the gastrointestinal tract of Sprague-Dawley rats fell between 20 and 240 days of age. Lin and Hayton (266) evaluated subepithelial blood flow determined by studying the blood to lumen clearance of barbital in senescent and mature rats and detected no evidence for a senescence-related alteration in intestinal blood flow. The noradrenergic innervation of the superior mesenteric vessels was not altered in senescent rats (298). Vasodilator responses to a variety of drugs were studied in isolated perfused mesenteric preparations obtained from rats of different ages (444). There was an overall decrease in the response of vasodilator drugs in the older animals, and the responses to dopamine and isoprenaline were reported as negligible at the age of 24 months. Whether impaired vasoactive responses to these agents reflect differences in receptor number or in the efficacy of cellular coupling or postreceptor events is unclear. Further studies of the effect of aging on the control of intestinal, particularly mucosal, blood flow are urgently needed.

GASTROINTESTINAL MOTILITY

The flow of luminal contents along the gastrointestinal tract results from contractions of the muscular wall of the gut. The precise pattern of these contractions is affected by the intrinsic properties of the smooth muscle and by the action of the autonomic nervous system innervation. Peptides (hormones), such as secretin, cholecystokinin (CCK), motilin, vasointestinal peptide (VIP), and somatostatin, also have an influence on gastrointestinal motility.

Smooth muscle intrinsic myogenic activity involves brief initiating contractions that are themselves controlled by pacemaker electrical signals originating in the fundic muscles of the stomach and upper small intestine. These signals are generated by the muscle itself and many do not result in actual contractions. Muscle contractions are generated by slow waves, which are initiated by spike bursts that induce electrical short waves.

Autonomic nerves induce or suppress contractions. These autonomic nerves are found in intramural plexuses which are connected to autonomic centers in the central nervous system (CNS). Cholinergic nerves stimulate contractions, adrenergic nerves inhibit contractions, and noninhibiting nerves cause relaxation of sphincters. There are peptidergic nerve endings that secrete a variety of peptides that modulate gastrointestinal motor function. Recently, the importance of nitric oxide in effecting muscle responses has been recognized. Studies on the aging gut have not been performed. It is clear from this brief description that aging could interfere with one or more of these complex processes and result in disordered gastrointestinal motor function.

Esophagus

Pharyngeal and esophageal motor function determine the controlled entry of swallowed food and saliva that passes through the upper esophageal sphincter. Striated muscle is found in the upper one-third of the esophagus and smooth muscle in the lower two-thirds. The combined action of these muscles passes food down the esophagus. The extrinsic innervation of these sections differs significantly and each may be affected by the aging process. Transfer of esophageal contents into the stomach is controlled by the opening of the lower esophageal sphincter. This sphincter usually opens immediately as a pharyngeal swallow occurs and therefore before the bolus reaches the sphincter.

The upper esophageal sphincter consists of the cricopharyngeus muscle, plus contributions of the cervical esophagus and the inferior pharyngeal constrictor. It is about 1 cm in length axially and generates a pressure of 40–120 mm Hg.

The lower esophageal sphincter (LES) is a high-pressure zone of about 10–35 mm Hg, 2–3 cm in length, which is located approximately 40–45 cm from the teeth. The LES relaxes just before the arrival of esophageal contractions, which have a mean pressure of 50–150 mm Hg in the esophageal body. The sphincter closes immediately after esophageal clearing. Any defect in muscular activity of the esophagus will cause abnormal esophageal function.

The principal physiological functions of the esophagus involve rapid and sequential transport of food boluses and swallowed mouth contents into the stomach. This process usually takes no more than 2–3 s. In addition, the sphincters of the esophagus function to prevent reflux of esophageal contents through the upper esophageal sphincter into the pharynx and the lung, and also to reduce reflux of gastric contents into the esophagus. This complex of functions results in effective esophageal clearance or emptying of its contents.

Esophageal motor function is best studied by manometry, using slowly infused water-filled catheters connected to external transducers or catheters containing small intraluminal transducers. Pharyngoesophageal motor function also can be measured using either radiological or sophisticated nuclear medicine techniques to determine transit time or to detect short-lived motor dysfunction. Age-associated effects on esophageal motor function have been measured only in humans as far as this reviewer has been able to determine.

Normal swallowing, when carefully evaluated by radiographic techniques, is quite uncommon in the very old (116, 414). Dysynchrony of deglutition and respiration has been reported to occur commonly in the elderly (376). One study of 10 subjects aged 62–79 yr showed that the upper esophageal sphincter pressure was significantly (about 25%) lower and delayed relaxation compared to young controls (141). In 60–69-year-old volunteers, the LES pressure was found to be similar to younger volunteers (188). In other studies, even nonagenarian volunteers had no change in LES pressure (386). Furthermore, LES relaxation following a swallow also appears to be normal; that is, it occurs promptly after all swallows in some studies, but in subjects over 90 yr less than 50% of swallows were followed by complete relaxation of the LES. Some fall in mean resting LES pressure was recorded in another study in subjects over age 65 yr (92).

In most studies, contractions in the body of the esophagus are unchanged up to the age of 80 yr but may be less in older subjects. In the unique study of nonagenarians by Soergel et al. (386), swallows often did not result in effective propulsive contractions of the body of the esophagus.

Tertiary contractions represent simultaneous contractions of the body of the esophagus usually found by chance during routine radiography. When severe, it will be described as a "corkscrew esophagus." Tertiary contractions are frequently seen without inducing symptoms in the elderly. These changes probably result from minor degrees of neuropathy that occur increasingly with age. Distal esophageal pressures are higher and nonperistaltic contractions are more frequent in the elderly (356). Examination of autopsy material from young adults and elderly patients (aged 59–95 yr) who died of various diseases demonstrated a significant decrease in esophageal ganglion cells without a change in smooth muscle thickness (113).

A number of clinical conditions associated with altered esophageal motor activity occur much more frequently in the elderly than in the young. Thus if one evaluates the older population by esophageal manometry, many may show some motor dysfunction. Diabetes mellitus, Raynaud's phenomenon, and a number of neuromuscular disorders all may affect the normal physiology of the esophagus and/or esophageal transit. Rarely do these changes result in clinical disorders.

Esophageal transit of solid and liquid test boluses

laced with Tc.99m was evaluated in volunteers over and under the age of 50 yr. An increase in transit time for a water bolus of 5.93 ± 1.4 s to 7.5 ± 2.0 s ($P < .05$) was found (326). In a comprehensive study of 109 individuals referred for nuclear medicine evaluation of esophageal transit time, a considerable number demonstrated a delay in transit in the upper esophagus (399).

Pharyngeal (Zenker's) diverticulum is an esophageal disorder most commonly seen in the elderly and represents herniations of the posterior portion of the hypopharynx proximal to the cricopharyngeus muscle through Killian's dehiscence. As long ago as 1878, Zenker and Ziemssen (463) proposed that this herniation was due to a high hypopharyngeal pressure. Only recently has this hypothesis been confirmed, by an elegant study (86). Using a combination of a dense barium suspension viewed by high-speed videofluoroscopy and manometry with a sleeve assembly, 14 consecutive patients with Zenker's diverticulum ranging in age from 46 to 83 yr and a comparable series of control subjects were studied. Cricopharyngeal sphincter opening was reduced, resulting in an increase in intrabolus pressure in the hypopharynx without pharyngosphincteric incoordination. It seems likely that this lesion may result from an alteration in sphincter compliance. Changes in sphincter compliance might be responsible for other cases of dysphagia in the elderly, without the anatomical lesion represented by Zenker's diverticulum.

Prolonged pH monitoring of the esophagus increasingly is being used to evaluate gastroesophageal reflux in a variety of physiological, pharmacological, and disease states. A small number of investigators have reported on the results of ambulatory pH monitoring in elderly volunteers or subjects referred for evaluation of esophageal function.

Spence and co-workers (388) compared pH monitoring in 14 middle-aged subjects (age range 39–61, mean 49 yr) and a young control group (19–30 yr of age). No significant difference in reflux as defined by pH measurement < 4, < 3, or < 5 was observed between these groups. In another study, ambulatory monitoring was performed in a group of 54 volunteers over the age of 62 yr (303), 20% (11/54) of whom showed an increase in acid contact time compared to young normal subjects. Furthermore, 29 of the 54 volunteers showed abnormal alkalinity (a pH > 7 for more than 20% of the tracing). Zhu et al. (464) in a preliminary report demonstrated greater reflux and more severe degrees of esophagitis in a study group of elderly subjects.

Barrett's esophagus, a condition in which normal squamous epithelium is replaced by columnar epithelium, is associated with gastroesophageal reflux and an increased rate of development of adenocarcinoma. In reviewing over 50,000 patients undergoing upper endoscopic procedures, Cameron and Lomboy (71) evaluated 377 patients with more than 3 cm of columnar epithelium (Barrett's epithelium) and found that the prevalence of this condition increased steadily with age before reaching a plateau in the seventh decade. Whether the aging esophagus is more susceptible to cellular transformation and the development of Barrett's esophagus and subsequent cancer remains to be determined. Achalasia of the esophagus also increases progressively with age (284).

Stomach

Gastric emptying has been measured in humans by infusing fixed amounts of saline or a fluid meal (usually 500 or 750 ml) and measuring the gastric residue by aspirating gastric contents after 30–60 min, by following the passage of liquid barium or barium-impregnated particles radiographically, or by nuclear medicine detection of the passage of gastric contents out of the stomach following ingestion of a solution or meal containing ^{51}Cr- or ^{99m}Tc-labeled substrates.

Gastric emptying of solids and liquids is dependent on the contraction and relaxation of different portions of the stomach. Emptying of solid food is dependent on antral propulsive movement and the retropulsive emulsifying action of the antrum. The major factor controlling the emptying of liquids is the pressure gradient across the gastroduodenal junction, which depends mainly on the tone of the fundus.

Many of the older reviews of the effects of age on drug metabolism have stated that gastric emptying is delayed with increasing age (43, 90). These conclusions were almost entirely based on reported studies of a delay in the rate of absorption of drugs in aged subjects. More recent studies have questioned the validity of these observations.

Davies et al. (98), using a ^{51}Cr-labeled meal, found no correlation between gastric emptying and age. This result was contradicted by the studies of Evans and co-workers (121), who measured liquid emptying in 11 subjects (mean age 77 yr) and found that gastric emptying times were much prolonged. However, most of the subjects of this study had diseases that could have affected gastrointestinal motility, such as Parkinson's disease and hypothyroidism, and many probably also were taking medications that could have interfered with the results of the study.

Another group of investigators reported a delay in gastric emptying with age among 14 elderly individuals with a mean age of 79 yr, many of whom had cardiovascular disease and were hospitalized, compared with a group of young volunteers aged 24 yr (254). They used a diluted orange juice cordial with an isotopic label, raising questions about both how ill the older test subjects were and the quantitative method that was employed.

One of the earliest reported studies used fluoroscopy to measure gastric emptying of a concentrated carbohydrate meal containing barium sulphate and showed no difference in gastric emptying with age (426). However, contrast studies using such techniques have limited usefulness. In a later study, Horowitz et al. (205) used a dual isotope technique, which was able to measure both liquid and solid gastric emptying simultaneously. Although gastric emptying of both the solid and liquid phases of the test meal was slightly quicker in young volunteers than in active elderly volunteers up to age 84 yr, the differences are unlikely to be of clinical significance.

Halvorson et al. (164) studied gastric emptying of water using an intubation technique in a small number of subjects aged 22–63 yr and found no changes in emptying. Wright et al. (458) also found no correlation between solid or liquid gastric emptying rates and age in 31 control subjects, but the maximum age was only 62 yr. The study of Moore et al. (309) showed differences in liquid emptying between young and aging volunteers: at 60 min the young retained 53% of the meal compared to 64% in those over 60 yr. This suggests a reduced ability to generate gastric fundal pressures, which the authors ascribed to weakness of the oblique muscular layer.

Using a different technique, Madson (272) studied gastric emptying (as well as small and large colonic transit) using a meal containing ^{99m}Tc-labeled cellulose fiber and indium-labeled plastic particles. He compared transit in 17 healthy young subjects aged 21–27 yr and 16 healthy older subjects aged 55–74 yr. Although a difference in gastric emptying between radiolabeled cellulose fiber and plastic particles was found, no difference was detected with age. However, Wegener et al. (450) did find a significant delay in gastric emptying of technetium-labeled breakfast in all the subjects.

Two studies in aging rats have failed to find significant differences in gastric emptying rates of a meal (288, 429).

Overall, these studies led to the conclusion that by the best nuclear medicine techniques that examine passage of both solid and liquid meals, gastric emptying of food is little reduced as a function of age, though gastric emptying of the liquid part of a meal may be slightly delayed. In none of these studies, however, were patients with achlorhydria excluded. Since achlorhydria has been shown to impair gastric emptying (136), this may be a factor in some of the contradictory data obtained.

Evaluation of transit distal to the stomach is more difficult. Overall gastrointestinal transit can be measured radiographically by providing subjects radiopaque markers and following the aboral progress of the markers with multiple abdominal films on successive days (172). Eastwood (111) used this technique to evaluate younger and older constipated and nonconstipated volunteers and found that 75% of the constipated group had prolonged transit time irrespective of age. No major difference in overall transit in the older volunteers was detected. The results of this study were in accord with the observations of Connell et al. (85), who found no alteration of bowel habit in healthy ambulatory older subjects compared to younger individuals.

Another method that was used to determine overall gastrointestinal transit was that of Wegener and coworkers (450), who measured the first appearance of ^{99m}Tc-labeled coffee in the stool. He found no age-dependent differences in a study population consisting of 21 young controls (mean age of 33.5 yr) and 25 elderly subjects (mean age 81.7 yr). Radioisotope capsules also have been used to evaluate transit through the small intestine. One study by Melkersson et al. (292) did not find any age-related change in overall intestinal transit in young and aging volunteers who did not have constipation.

Small intestinal transit has been measured also by studying the progress of radiolabeled particles using nuclear medicine techniques. More commonly, orocolonic transit has been measured by determining breath hydrogen excretion following ingestion of a dose of unabsorbable carbohydrate, such as lactulose. This method has been used extensively for such studies but clearly has some limitations (104, 255). Using breath-hydrogen testing, transit in older healthy volunteers did not differ from that measured in the young (254, 342, 450). Delayed transit by 50% was reported in one preliminary communication (163) in healthy aging individuals (mean age of 81 yr). Piccione et al. (342) found unchanged transit time in 22 geriatric facility residents (mean age of 82 yr) using a similar technique.

When transit was determined from the distribution of polyethylene glycol 4,000 along the gastrointestinal tract after administration to mature (16-month-old) and senescent (31-month-old) Fischer 344 rats (266), it was significantly shorter through the proximal small intestine in the older animals but longer through the distal small intestine. Varga (429), in an earlier study, failed to find any difference in small intestinal transit in 17–20-month-old rats when compared to young animals using labeled microspheres as unabsorbable markers, a finding that was confirmed by McDougal et al. (288). This group in 1980 studied transit using unabsorbable markers in 5-, 12-, and 20-month-old Fischer 344 rats with implanted cannulas. Colon transit was reduced by 15% in the 12-month-old animals and by 45% in the senescent rats when compared to 5-month-old animals.

Madsen, in 1992 (272), administered ^{111}indium-labeled plastic particles and ^{99m}Tc-labeled cellulose fiber to 17 healthy young individuals aged 21–27 yr and 16 older subjects aged 55–74 yr. There was much intersubject variability, and no overall changes in gastric emptying or mean small intestinal transit time could be determined. By multiple regression analysis, however, there was a positive association between age and mean colonic transit time. It should be mentioned that only two of the subjects in this study were over the age of 70 yr. Thus there is almost uniform agreement that postprandial small intestinal transit times are unaffected by age.

Overall, small intestinal motor patterns are maintained in old age. Anuras and Sutherland (15) initially compared jejunal motor patterns in ten healthy elderly female subjects (mean age 72 yr) and five younger healthy females and concluded that the fasting pattern (migrating motor complex) did not differ but that the frequency of contractions and the motility index were less in the older group. Fich and co-workers (129) found no significant change in motor patterns in volunteers up to age 69 yr. These normal findings were confirmed in 15 healthy elderly volunteers (mean age 84 yr) (211), though in this study propagated clustered contractions were more frequently present in the older subjects both after a meal and during fasting. A prior preliminary communication showed some changes in interdigestive motor motility patterns in the elderly associated with elevated serum motilin concentrations and without the normal cyclical fluctuations in the concentrations of this hormone usually seen in younger subjects (58). Bartolotti's group developed the hypothesis that intestinal motilin changes were due to altered acid secretory capacity of the stomach, but they were unable to confirm this concept (57). Altered fasting motor patterns have been described in patients with intestinal bacterial overgrowth (427), a pathophysiological state encountered with considerable frequency in the elderly (167, 191).

Neuromuscular Functioning

Although much research has been directed toward a better understanding of age-dependent changes in the anatomy and physiology of the CNS, relatively little data are available in regard to the gastrointestinal tract. The available information was summarized in 1989 (398). Gabella (142) performed unique ultrastructural studies of the small intestine of 3–4-month-old and 26–30-month-old guinea pigs. Myenteric neuron number, calculated as spatial density of myenteric neurons per unit serosal area, was markedly less in aged animals, and the total number of myenteric neurons calculated to be in the small intestine, ranging from 1.1 to 1.6 million, was only about 50% of the value obtained in young adult guinea pigs. Furthermore, the microscopic appearance of neurons of the two groups of animals differed. The cytological features of muscle cells of the older animals were indistinguishable from those of the younger animals. In addition, the dendritic profiles were reduced and there appeared to be more synapses of the cell body, suggesting reorganization of the remaining neurons in the older animals.

Baker and Santer (30) studied noradrenergic nerves in Auerbach's plexus and longitudinal muscles of the proximal jejunum of Wistar rats and demonstrated a breakdown of plexus regularity and less axonal fluorescence at 18 months of age compared to 12 months. These data were interpreted as showing a decrease in the density of noradrenergic innervation with age and implied a reduction of the potential of the sympathetic nervous system to control motility. Subsequently, the same group evaluated the stimulatory response of carbachol and isoprenaline to induce motor activity of intestinal smooth muscle in rats aged 6 and 24 months (365). The concentration response curve to carbachol did not differ with age; however, the action of isoprenaline to relax longitudinal smooth muscle was significantly reduced in the older age group, due mainly to a decrease in maximal relaxation (31). In a preliminary study, Dunlap and co-workers (110) noted an increase in the average area of myenteric ganglia without a change in neuron density and an increase in the length of the small intestine in aging humans. These data were interpreted as implying that the number of neurons continues to increase in old age. Studies of Auerbach's myenteric plexus of the esophagus, stomach, and small and large intestines in 18 patients with Alzheimer's disease, eight older patients with other dementias, and nondemented older (aged 71 ± 10 yr) and young controls revealed a reduction of the functional area and fewer neurons per neural structure in the Auerbach's plexus in all areas of the gastrointestinal tract (377).

Further functional studies of the autonomic nervous system supply to smooth muscle are urgently needed. A paucity of substance P and vasoactive intestinal polypeptide and somatostatin in immunoreactive nerve elements was described in the intestine of 24- and 36-month-old female rats by Fehèr and Penzes (126). Culpepper-Morgan et al. (94) reported evidence of increased opiate receptor affinity in the ileum of aging guinea pigs.

The small and large intestines consist of layers of smooth muscle (the circular and the transverse layer) innervated by nerve plexuses (the myenteric Auerbach's plexus and, on the luminal side, Meissner's plexus). The efferent innervation is derived from parasympathetic and sympathetic fibers, and the preganglionic parasympathetic fibers originate from vagal nuclei and pass through vagal nerves and from the sacral cord by pelvic and splanchnic nerves. Postganglionic fibers may be cholinergic, adrenergic, or peptidergic. Preganglionic sympathetic fibers originate in the thoracic and lumbar spinal cord, passing through the celiac superior and inferior mesenteric ganglia. Postganglionic sympathetic fibers pass along blood vessels.

Circular, slow waves generate segmentation and peristaltic contraction. During fasting, there is an interdigestive migrating myoelectric complex every 2–2.5 h, which clears intraluminal bacteria and other debris into the colon. This interdigestive migrating myoelectric complex, which is most important to prevent bacterial overgrowth, is thought to be initiated by motilin and is interrupted by feeding. The third pattern involves frequent intermittent contractions lasting for at least 4 h after feeding. As we have seen evaluation of small intestinal patterns in older subjects has been very limited, but some authors suggest that the changes seen may be of pathogenic importance.

Colon and Rectum

Although there are many assumptions regarding changes in colonic muscular strength and structure, few reports have been published. Reduced colonic muscle mass and mucous gland number have been reported in older subjects, but the health of subjects studied was not defined. Fewer mucous cells in the colon of older individuals also were described. Some studies suggest that the colon of aging mammals shows an increase in tone and a relative inelasticity compared to the colon of younger animals (69).

Functionally, the colon can be divided into two segments: the *proximal colon,* consisting of the cecum and the ascending colon, which is responsible primarily for the absorption of fluid and electrolytes and bacterial fermentation, and the *distal colon,* which is responsible for the formation of fecal contents and evacuation.

The functional anatomy of the colon is essentially similar to that of the small bowel. Slow waves occur at 9–10 cycles per min in the proximal colon and at about 6 cycles per min in the distal colon. During fasting, bursts of spike potential occur that appear to be unrelated to slow wave activity. During feeding, more of the waves appear to be propulsive. In the transverse colon, frequent movements propel colonic contents back to the ascending colon and cecum. Haustral shuttling permits these contents to be moved, which is important for the absorption of water and electrolytes as well as for the mixing of intestinal contents. Mass contractions propel contents from the transverse colon into the sigmoid colon and the rectum.

The colon is stimulated by a gastrocolic reflex which is cholinergically mediated and increases colonic spike and contractile activity with feeding. Food is the major stimulus of colonic contraction. In addition, two classes of regulatory peptide alter colonic contractions: *(1)* the gastrin family, including gastrin and CCK, and *(2)* the secretin family, which includes secretin, glucagon, gastric inhibitory peptide (GIP), and VIP, motilin, and opioid peptides such as metenkephalin.

Neurons modulate colonic activity but do not tend to initiate it. The gastrin family are stimulants and the secretin family inhibitors of contraction. Atropine and naloxone inhibit the gastrocolic reflex so that muscarinic neurons and endogenous opioids may modulate the gastrocolic response.

The rectum functions as a reservoir for the sigmoid contents prior to defecation. The anal canal, which is continuous with the rectal ampulla, contains the internal and external sphincters that are responsible for continence and normal defecation. The internal sphincter of the rectum is a continuation of the muscularis externa. The external sphincter is continuous with the puborectalis muscle. The anus and rectum possess a basal electrical rhythm over which spike activity is superimposed.

Contraction of the sigmoid colon induces filling of the rectal ampulla, and distention of the rectal ampulla induces reflex contraction of the external sphincter and puborectalis muscle and relaxation of the internal sphincter. The sense of distention also reaches the higher cortical centers as the desire to defecate.

Continence is maintained primarily by the external sphincter. Tonic activity is due to a spinal reflex that is maintained even if the cord is transected. Phasic activity may be initiated consciously, but it cannot be maintained for more than a few minutes. Decreased anal sphincter pressure will result in incontinence, since pressures in the upper anal canal usually are about 35 mm Hg and in the lower canal about 10 mm Hg.

Defecation is the inhibition of tonic activity of the external sphincter and puborectalis, which increases the angle of defecation. The defecatory urge depends on the speed at which the ampulla is filled as well as the volume. The need to defecate usually is experienced at about 25% of maximum tolerable volume and pressure (greater than 100 ml and 18 mm Hg). At maximum tolerance, the phasic activity of the external sphincter is all that keeps the sphincter closed. Tonic activity disappears during rectal distention and straining (Valsalva).

Very few observations of changes in colonic cellular function with age have been reported. A preliminary report (61) described data on active electrolyte transport through mucosal sheets of the descending colon of 2–3-month- and 3.5–5-yr-old New Zealand white rabbits. Using the Ussing chamber–voltage clamp technique, basal and amiloride–stimulated sodium absorption did not differ when calculated as a function of the number of colonic cells. However, maximal cyclic AMP secretion induced by 5 mM theophylline was found to be significantly less in aging compared to younger colon. The authors ascribed these findings to a reduced number of goblet cells in colonic crypts.

Most studies of changes in biochemical detoxication with age have been performed with liver tissue. There has been the assumption that the changes found in the liver would be universally observed in other tissues. In 1986, one group of investigators evaluated detoxication capacity in the liver and a number of other tissues in Sprague-Dawley rats aged 2 wk to 18 months (392). Benzopyrene hydroxylation did not change with age in colon (or kidney and lung) in contrast to findings in the liver. Phenobarbital induced benzopyrene hydroxylation to a higher level in the colon of 18-month-old compared to 6-month-old rats. Napthoflavone induction of cytochrome P450 also occurred appropriately in the aging colon. Another group has studied several other biotransformation enzymes in the colon of Fischer 344 rats up to 24 months of age (290). These observations emphasize the need for more physiological studies of detoxication reactions in gastrointestinal tissues from aging animals.

Colonic Transit. Since colonic transit is the major determinant for overall gastrointestinal transit time, which is unaltered in the elderly, it is unlikely that major changes result from advanced age. Most studies in humans would agree with this conclusion. However, colonic transit is much more difficult to measure accurately in isolation than gastric emptying and small bowel transit.

Fiber is accepted as an important dietary constituent that greatly alters the biology and function of the colon and is thought to be important in maintaining optimum human colonic activity particularly in advanced age. The insoluble hydrated forms of fiber hold water in interstices and thereby increase stool water and stool frequency. Soluble fiber is susceptible to bacterial fermentation, which increases the total mass of fecal bacteria, with a subsequent quantitative increase in bacterial enzyme reactions. Dietary soluble fiber is extensively degraded to volatile short-chain fatty acids, methane, hydrogen, and carbon dioxide. Distribution of these products of bacterial metabolism and of individual short-chain fatty acids varies with diet and in differing individuals. Thus dietary fiber regulates many gastrointestinal processes, including absorption, steroid metabolism, colonic fermentation, and stool weight.

Southgate and Durnin (387) have compared apparent fiber digestibility in young and elderly subjects. In this study, the authors found that elderly men digested significantly more cellulose than the young, attributing this observation to a longer transit time in the elderly. In another study, apparent fiber digestibility was determined in nine elderly healthy subjects aged 65–85 yr and was compared to young volunteers aged 22–28 yr. The mean apparent digestibility of nondigestible fiber that supplemented the regular diet in elderly women was 62.5% compared to 70% observed in younger women, a difference that was not statistically significant in this small group of subjects (63). No differences in transit time were detected, though mean daily wet and dry fecal weights were somewhat higher in the elderly. Few comparisons have been made between the number and type of fecal bacteria in young and older animals and human volunteers. Those studies suggest minor differences (134, 363) but have never been directly compared to changes in dietary fiber degradation. Since fiber is frequently recommended to reduce transit time and prevent constipation, further studies of fiber digestibility may need to be performed. On the whole, studies in the elderly suggest that wheat bran may readily alter transit time (8).

Anorectal Function. Fecal incontinence and constipation are frequently found in the elderly, making an understanding of the normal physiology of evacuation with age most important.

The complex process of stool evacuation and the maintenance of continence have been evaluated by radiological, manometric, and electrophysiological techniques and measurement of sensory responses to rectal distention. Radioproctography evaluates appropriate relaxation responses to evacuation signals and changes in the rectal angle during defecation. Manometric studies of the rectum are performed at multiple sites above the anal verge with and without distention by a rectal balloon. The electrical activity of the external sphincter can be recorded. Subjective sensation to graded expansion of the rectal balloon is compared to the contraction and the electrical activity of the rectum. These techniques can evaluate the contractions of the internal and external sphincters, increased or decreased rectal ampulla sensation, abnormal internal sphincter contractile activity, and abnormal rectal contractions. They also evaluate the rectoanal inhibitory reflex and the inflation reflex as well as changes in rectal tone.

In 1974 Ihre (213) reported that a group of older women aged between 52 and 69 yr had higher rectal pressures as a response to a distending volume than a group of younger women aged between 19 and 44 yr. The older women were unable to tolerate as high a rectal volume as the young. Maximal basal and squeeze pressure in the anal canal were found to be significantly lower in older than in younger subjects (285, 353). Furthermore, electrophysiological studies showed that elderly individuals had evidence of a greater degree of neuropathic damage to the external anal sphincter than the young (36). In contrast to these observations, Devroede and co-workers (103) were not able to show changes in rectal compliance in healthy controls up to 77 yr of age. Changes in the rectum with age are thought to reflect loss in tissue elasticity or perhaps rectal ischemia and fibrosis (103).

Subsequently, a careful series of studies of anorectal function in 37 elderly volunteers aged 66–87 yr compared to younger subjects aged 19–55 yr was published (34). The elderly subjects had decreased anal basal and squeeze pressure compared to the younger volunteers, particularly in females. The anal response to rectal distention also differed in older subjects. No significant difference in the rectal volume required to cause initial anal relaxation was detected, but lower volumes were needed to cause sustained relaxation, a finding that might contribute to incontinence. The older volunteers responded to differing volumes of distention with higher rectal pressures than the young, though this was significantly different only in females. Maximal tolerable volumes were somewhat lower in the older subjects. Upon straining, the anorectal angle was less obtuse in elderly compared to young women. Elderly female volunteers had significantly greater degrees of perineal descent at rest and upon straining than young women or elderly men. The differences between men and women are probably explained by damage to the nerve supply of the pelvic floor sustained during childbirth. Changes in rectal pressure were associated with more sensitive rectoanal inhibitory reflexes and with increases in rectal sensitivity. The combination of higher rectal pressure upon rectal distention and lower anal pressure would contribute to the risk of incontinence in the elderly group. Incontinence, the inability to control the passage of feces and/or gas through the anus, can be associated with a variety of pathophysiological states, some of which represent the end result of injury or disease and some progressive changes with age (393).

PANCREAS

The exocrine pancreas of humans and other mammals consists of clusters of acini that form lobules separated by loose connective tissue. Individual acini are composed of 20–50 pyramidal cells arranged with the broad bases around the circumference and the apices pointed toward a central lumen. Each acinus is drained by a ductule which passes into a series of ducts of increasing caliber until the main ducts are reached. Separately distributed within the pancreas are the Islets of Langerhans, containing the cells of the endocrine pancreas. Of the endocrine hormones, glucagon, somatostatin, and pancreatic polypeptide all inhibit pancreatic exocrine secretion. Insulin may potentiate the stimulatory effect of CCK on pancreatic exocrine secretion.

The human pancreas secretes about 1 l of pancreatic fluid daily, consisting mostly of water, electrolytes, and digestive enzymes. The acinar cells secrete digestive enzymes, while the ductular cells are mainly responsible for an electrolyte secretion rich in bicarbonate. The protein mixture secreted by the pancreas includes proteolytic enzymes, such as trypsinogen, chymotrypsinogen, proelastase, procarboxypeptidases A and B, amylase, lipase, phospholipases A1 and A2, and nonspecific esterase, and nucleases, such as ribonuclease. Human pancreatic juice contains proteins in concentrations varying from less than 1% to 10%. In addition to enzymes, plasma proteins, trypsin inhibitors, and mucous proteins are found.

Postprandial pancreatic secretion occurs as a response to the action of the hormones secretin and CCK, which are synthesized in the gastrointestinal mucosa, and to vagovagal reflexes that activate cholinergic postganglionic neurons in the pancreas. Secretin stimulates fluid and bicarbonate secretion. Plasma secretin levels may be increased by acid as well as by all of the major components of a mixed meal. CCK is released from the duodenal and jejunal walls by hydrolytic products of digestion, such as amino acids and FAs. CCK release appears to be controlled by the level of active intraluminal proteinases. Proteins may bind or inhibit intraluminal endopeptidases which would otherwise inactivate CCK-releasing peptide from the duodenum. CCK is the principal stimulant of postprandial pancreatic enzyme secretion. In addition, gastrin stimulates pancreatic enzyme secretion, bombesin (gastrin-releasing peptide) stimulates a secretion containing small amounts of bicarbonate, and high concentrations of enzymes and neurotensin may stimulate pancreatic fluid and enzyme secretions. Neural mechanisms, particularly the parasympathetic nervous system, stimulate the bicarbonate secretory response. Parasympathetic fibers pass to the pancreas directly through the vagus and indirectly through the celiac ganglion and splanchnic nerves, whereas adrenergic innervation of the pancreas is mainly through the splanchnic nerves. In addition, VIP is the neurotransmitter mediating much of the bicarbonate secretory response to vagal electrical stimulation. Most hormones and neurotransmitters directly regulate acinar and duct cell response via receptors by interaction with membrane G proteins. Pancreatic acinar intracellular messengers include calcium, cyclic AMP, and phosphoinositol.

Some investigators have reported a decrease in the weight and size of the pancreas with aging (9), but this has not been uniformly described (70). Ultrasound examination also has suggested that the pancreas of individuals over the age of 65 yr is smaller than that of the young (466). Intrapancreatic and peripancreatic fat increases with aging, and this may result in increased echogenicity during ultrasound examination (310, 439).

The ductal system also may be altered. An autopsy study of pancreatic ductules in a large number of subjects older than 60 yr showed an increase of the caliber of the main pancreatic duct along its whole length and some dilatation of the interlobular and intralobular ducts with small cyst formation (370). This most probably represents a response to some reduction in parenchymal cell number, resulting in passive enlargement of the ducts. Some fibrosis, fat accumulation, and lesions of the interlobular and intralobular duct, which include proliferation and squamous metaplasia, have been described (16, 208, 253). These observations suggest modest loss of exocrine parenchymal cells with fibrosis and fat accumulation, perhaps secondary to modest vascular impairment to the organ. Major loss of pancreatic organ cell mass does not appear to be a general feature of the aging process. However, some observations suggest that pancreatic atrophy of severe degree may occur in some elderly individuals and result in pancreatic insufficiency. The studies of Ammann and Sulser (7) showed that three-fourths of patients with idiopathic pancreatic insufficiency sent to their referral center were over age 55 yr and implied that this idiopathic pancreatic exocrine deficiency in the elderly results from atherosclerosis and ischemia, though no direct evidence for this statement was provided (6). Calcified stones were present in the majority of these patients. It is of interest that Nagai and Ohtsubo (317) also have reported a high incidence of pancreatic lithiasis at autopsy in elderly patients. No pancreatic stones were found at autopsy in their Japanese patients under the age of 70 yr, but after this age there was a progressive increase in pancreatic stones, reaching 16.5% in individuals in their 90s. The chemical composition of these stones is similar to that found in younger patients with chronic calcific pancreatitis. Similar findings were reported earlier and also in a group of older women by Laugier and Sarles (258). One theory about the formation of pancreatic stones holds that the concentration of a stabilizing protein in pancreatic fluid is reduced (313). It is conceivable that this protein is defective in some aging individuals.

Since the pancreas demonstrates greater rates of protein synthesis per weight of organ mass than most other organs in the body and protein synthesis is impaired as a function of age in several tissues, Kim et al. (242) evaluated protein synthetic activity in the pancreas of rats of different ages. These authors studied the incorporation of ^{3}H leucine into the total acid-soluble fraction of the pancreas obtained from 6-, 12-, 24-, and 30-month-old rats. They described some loss of ^{3}H leucine incorporation with age per mg of pancreatic DNA between 12 and 24 months. However, light microscopic evaluation of the pancreas in parallel studies did not find much loss of parenchymal cells, though fewer granules were said to be present. Some increase in the amount of fat distributed in the periphery of the lobules in 24- and 30-month-old rats was described. Majumdar and Dubick (275) evaluated the response of the pancreas of rats aged 3, 6, 12, and 16 months to a constant gastrin infusion of 250 µg/kg/h for 14 days. Baseline data suggested very modest reduction in pancreatic protein and DNA; following gastrin infusion, pancreatic protein fell more in old than in young animals. The authors suggested that gastrin stimulates growth of the pancreas in young rats but that it inhibits the proliferative response of the glands of old rats. They supported these observations by studying steady-state mRNA for amylase and trypsinogen in these glands and described some increase in 4-month-old rats but a decrease at 16 months of age after gastrin (275). In another study, they reported that phorbol esters also inhibited pancreatic protein synthesis relative to DNA in 21-month-old Fischer rats but stimulated synthesis in 4-month-old animals (109).

In an early study, Snook (385) evaluated changes in pancreatic chemical composition in Charles River CD strain rats varying in age from 12 to 28 months. The rats continued to gain body weight between 4 and 28 months of age. Furthermore, the weight of the pancreas and the amount of DNA and RNA also increased, whereas total pancreatic contents of chymotrypsin, trypsinogen, and lipase fell. The author claimed that no amylase could be detected in the pancreas of 28-month-old animals. Greenberg and Holt (155) studied 3- and 27-month-old male Fischer 344 rats that had been well stabilized in our animal care facility and whose total pancreatic weights were almost identical. Pancreatic weight per 100 g of rat was less in the 27-month-old animals. However, protein concentration and content, DNA concentration and content, as well as protein:DNA ratios did not differ in these groups of animals. Although trypsinogen concentration per mg of protein did not differ at the two ages, amylase concentration was significantly lower and lipase concentration significantly higher in the older animals. We then studied the effect of a high-sucrose or a high-fat diet for 7 days on the response of pancreatic lipase and amylase. The high-fat diet increased lipase concentrations and the high-carbohydrate diet amylase concentration following 7 days of fat or carbohydrate feeding in young rats. However, the pancreas of aging animals did not show any significant changes in the concentrations of these enzymes. These observations suggest that the response of the aging pancreas to changes in dietary intake is impaired or delayed. In another study, Greenberg and co-workers (158) evaluated the growth response of the pancreas to the stimulus of cerulein plus secretin administered every 8 h for 7 days. In young rats, pancreatic weight increased by 211% and by 175% in aging animals when compared to their respective control groups. Protein and DNA contents also rose in both groups, indicating pancreatic hyperplasia. In addition, there was some evidence of pancreatic hypertrophy, as reflected by changes in protein:DNA ratios. This was significantly greater in young than in aging animals. The treatment also increased trypsinogen and lipase content much more in young than in aging rats. Examination of pancreatic polyamines indicated that putrescine and spermidine contents were also increased significantly more in the younger animals (158). Again, the response of the pancreas in the older rats appeared to be impaired.

A number of investigators have studied pancreatic volume protein and enzyme secretion in response to several physiological stimuli in humans and other animals. The early studies of Necheles et al. (321) and Rosenberg et al. (359) indicated that basal pancreatic secretions were somewhat less in older individuals who were evaluated for the presence of pancreatic disease. The first carefully performed physiological study in humans was that of Firky (133), who measured pancreatic secretion following secretin stimulation (1 unit per kg body weight) in a small group of subjects between 60 and 72 yr of age, finding normal lipase output but a 33% reduction in amylase and trypsin and up to a two-thirds reduction in secreted volume. CCK was not administered with secretin in this study, so total stimulated pancreatic output could not be adequately determined. Subsequently, Bartos and Groh (37) studied ten subjects (mean age 67 yr) with repeated stimulation following I.V. administration of secretin plus CCK. In this study, exocrine pancreatic function was normal after the first dose, but volume, bicarbonate, and amylase output fell after the sixth dose, which suggested decreased responsiveness due to acquired insensitivity of the pancreas to the CCK-secretin regimen. Gullo et al. (160) administered secretin and cerulein by continuous infusion to 25 elderly patients and collected duodenal secretion through a double lumen tube which had proximal and distal occluding balloons. They found no significant differences in pancreatic fluid volume, bicarbonate, trypsin, chymotrypsin, or lipase output when compared to a young control group. Subsequent reports from Vellas et al. (431) and Tiscornia et al. (412) demonstrated some minor changes in output of the human pancreas but no consistent effect of age. Even if modest reduction in pancreatic enzyme output occurs in elderly humans, this is unlikely to have clinical significance since over 90% of pancreatic enzyme output must be lost before malabsorption becomes evident (105).

Some experiments in animal systems also have evaluated the effects of aging upon pancreatic fluid and enzyme secretion. Khalil and co-workers (235) measured pancreatic exocrine secretion in 6- and 26-month-old Sprague-Dawley rats with pancreatic and duodenal fistulae. The studies were performed 24 h after surgery, pancreatic juice continuing to enter the duodenum until the studies were performed. Basal pancreatic secretion and secretion after stimulation with graded doses of CCK 8 were measured. Basal and stimulated secretion of pancreatic fluid, bicarbonate, and protein all were lower in the older animals. The doses of CCK used in this study were submaximal; since serum CCK concentrations are higher in older rats, it is possible that higher CCK doses may have induced similar maximal secretion rates in the aging rodents.

Hollander's group (178, 332) evaluated basal and secretin-stimulated pancreatic exocrine secretion in 3-, 4-, 13-, 24-, and 27-month-old Sprague-Dawley rats with drainage of pancreatic and gastric secretions. These authors described a drastic reduction of basal and stimulated pancreatic flow, as well as of bicarbonate, total protein, and amylase secretion. This study has been criticized because the pancreatic response was studied 24 h after surgery (299). Miyasaka and co-workers, in a series of papers, have reported on the effect of basal and stimulated pancreatic exocrine functions in 6–12- and 24–26-month old male (299) and female (300) Fischer 344 rats studied several days after surgery. Basal secretion was not significantly different between young and older animals. However, secretion was regularly reduced following stimulation either by biliary-pancreatic-jejunal diversion, which greatly increases pancreatic flow, or by CCK 8 or secretin administration. In the younger animals, stepwise increases in protein output were observed, whereas in older rats, the increments in response to the larger doses of CCK were considerably less than those for smaller doses. These authors concluded that, although basal secretion in the older animal was comparable, the reserve capacity for protein secretion was decreased in old compared to young animals. In another study, the pancreatic response and CCK release from the duodenum were studied after intragastric administration of a synthetic protease inhibitor (camostate) which usually elicits CCK release from the duodenum and produces pancreatic secretion and pancreatic hypertrophy (301). Following acute administration of camostate, plasma CCK concentrations increased less in aged than in young rats. Following 5 days of the camostate, pancreatic wet weight, protein, and DNA increased in both groups, but the overall response in the aging pancreas was less. These data parallel those of Greenberg and co-workers (158), suggesting that the response of the pancreas to exogenous and endogenous stimuli is impaired as a function of age.

From these data one can conclude that pancreatic function is relatively well maintained in advanced age. There is evidence for a number of physiological changes, such as reduced responsiveness of secretion to exogenous stimuli, a delay in responsiveness of pancreatic growth to proliferative signals, and an impaired or delayed response of pancreatic enzyme synthesis to changes in nutrient substrate intake. Although the mechanism for these changes has not been established, it probably reflects either changes in the concentration of circulating hormones, altered cellular receptors, or cellular signaling or response mechanisms. Elucidation of these causes may be important to further understand the physiology of cellular aging and pancreatic responsiveness. However, these age-related physiological changes do not appear to be of sufficient magnitude to result in clinical problems. Thus pancreatic insufficiency in any elderly individual results from a disease process.

LIVER AND BILIARY TREE

In addition to its many synthetic and metabolic functions, the liver acts as a gastrointestinal secretory organ, secreting into the biliary tract fluid; bicarbonate; vesicular proteins, including immunoglobulins, bile salts, and phospholipids; and sterols, including cholesterol and sterol vitamins. Furthermore, many exogenous compounds, particularly agents that are conjugated in the liver, including many drugs, pass into bile. The process of conjugation usually makes lipophilic compounds more water-soluble, permitting them to be excreted from the liver and into the gut.

Bile is diluted by the passage of water and electrolytes into bile ductules. It then passes into the gallbladder, where it is concentrated by a process in which some of its contents are absorbed. Mucins and other substances are secreted into the bile in the gallbladder. When the gallbladder contracts, as a result of stimulation by peptides released from the upper gastrointestinal tract after eating, bile is passed into the duodenum.

Bile is important in food digestion and functions also as a carrier for substances that are excreted out of the body in feces. Biliary acids and phospholipids principally aid in the digestion of dietary lipids, leading to normal absorption of triglyceride and phospholipid digestion products. Age-related changes in function, therefore, could alter crucial digestive and absorptive functions.

Morphology

The liver consists primarily of parenchymal cells (hepatocytes), which occupy 90% of its volume. Kupffer cells are part of the body's reticuloendothelial system and are present throughout the liver. Parenchymal cells are bathed in sinusoidal fluid, which is fed by hepatic arterial and portal venous blood, and are organized in sinusoids, which are arranged like the spokes of a wheel from the portal space where the hepatic arterioles and bile ducts are found to the centrilobular area, which is drained by hepatic venules. On the opposite side of parenchymal cells is found the canaliculus, into which the biliary components are secreted. The biliary canaliculae join to form ductules which enter the bile duct; bile then passes through the cystic duct into the gallbladder, where it is stored. The gallbladder acts as a reservoir until it contracts postprandially due to the action of peptides, such as CCK.

Age-Associated Effects

The size of the liver declines with age (59) and may become very small indeed in nonagenarians (209). This occurs probably because of a fall in total hepatic blood flow (432, 459) and in part because of less portal venous flow (467). In infants, the liver represents 4% of total body weight, but this drops to 2% in the elderly (314). The decrease in hepatic volume is accompanied by a modest fall in galactose elimination capacity, an index of overall hepatic function (281), but not in bromsulphalein excretion (247).

The livers of older individuals, aged between 69 and 91 yr, exhibit only minor histological changes, which may be associated with, but not specific to, the effects of aging. Thus no reliable marker of liver aging can be directly derived from histological findings. Normal and age-induced cell death occur by apoptosis in which hepatocytes disintegrate into fragments, which then are phagocytosed by macrophages without an inflammatory reaction. The life span of hepatocytes is extraordinarily long. Under normal circumstances, in the absence of cell damage, hepatocytes are thought to replicate only once or twice in a lifetime. Watanabe and Tanaka (446) carefully evaluated changes with aging from autopsy cases and described some cell enlargement relative to nucleus size, an increase in nuclear DNA, and an increased number of binucleated cells (an increase in ploidy). The studies of David and Reinke in the rat showed many nuclei with five and six lobules (97). The number of large nuclei with higher DNA levels also was found to be increased in the human liver. One study demonstrated that the number of large nuclei increased from 10.3% in the third decade of life to 22.5% in the eighth decade (38). In another study, Findor and coworkers (131) showed an increase in nucleoli in patients aged 69–91 yr. Ploidy was shown to be more frequent in aging male than female animals (329) and could be delayed by dietary restriction (118). Medvedev (291) has suggested that increased hepatic nuclear size and nuclear ploidy is a response mechanism for the liver to avoid cell replication. He believes that replicative activity in the aging organism may be accompanied by increased chromosomal aberrations. Mitochondrial number falls in individuals over age 60 yr, associated with an increase in the number of christae (366). Lysosome number also increases and peroxisome number falls (97).

Age-associated changes in the lipid composition of hepatocyte plasma membranes and intracellular organelles occur, which are associated with altered membrane microviscosity, which increases steadily with age (321). Accompanying this are changes in the activity of membrane enzymes, (323) in peroxidation (461), and perhaps in hepatocyte transport functions (328). Some studies have shown a reduction in bile flow and bile acid secretion, with changes in bile acid composition occurring between 3.5 and 24 months of age in Sprague-Dawley rats (416, 461). Dietary restriction delayed or prevented many of these changes (416, 461).

Whereas the liver shows minimal regenerative activity under normal steady-state conditions, it displays remarkable capacity to replicate following injury or hepatic resection. This has been well demonstrated both in rodents and in humans. In young rats, following a 68% resection, hepatic mass is restored within 7–10 days (4). This process is accompanied by a well-characterized sequence of cellular events involving gene activation, increase in replicative enzymes, and proliferation and is dependent on several circulating growth factors (124).

In rats 1 yr of age and older, the beginning of ^{3}H thymidine incorporation is delayed to 24 h or more, from about 18 h after hepatic resection in young control rats aged 2 months. Peak activity of incorporated ^{3}H thymidine also is less. These observations initially led to the conclusion that there is age-related decline in liver regeneration in rats (64, 327, 349). However, Beyer et al. (48) demonstrated that regeneration could be completed but over a longer period in 1-yr-old than in 6-wk-old rats, accompanied by a difference in thymidine kinase expression. Altered ornithine decarboxylase and polyamines also were found (47). A study in rats up to 24 months of age suggested that EGF would increase liver DNA synthesis following partial hepatectomy (51). It is believed, however, that these changes in hepatic regenerative capacity are not intrinsic to the liver but more likely are a reflection of alteration in circulating growth factors. Therefore, liver transplantation has become increasingly possible using livers from older donors (2, 438), and the success rate with such transplanted livers is almost as good as that with livers from younger donors (390).

Consequences of Aging

Overall, liver function tests do not change with age in humans, though hepatic blood flow falls, resulting in some reduction in the first-pass clearance of drugs. Furthermore, the storage capacity for bromsulphalein (BSP) may be reduced. There have been extensive studies of the microsomal monooxygenase system of the aging liver because these enzymes are involved in the biotransformation of many exogenous and endogenous substrates. Many rodent studies have reported a fall in monooxygenase enzyme activities and in P450 isozyme concentrations during aging. These animal data generally were used to explain a potential decline in drug-metabolizing functions that might occur in elderly humans. On the basis of this work, several mechanisms for alteration in enzyme activity were suggested, including changes in the structure of the enzymes, in microsomal membrane fluidity and structure, and in lipid peroxidation. However, these changes generally are seen only in the male rat (371). In the baboon (372) as well as in humans (456), there is no evidence for a significant fall in microsomal detoxification and hydroxylation reaction enzymes. Furthermore, the synthetic capacity of the liver is relatively well maintained and, although regenerative capacity may be delayed, the final mass of liver may be well replaced. A delay in the restoration to normal of a co-factor important in drug metabolism following acute toxic suppression may be seen. One example of this phenomenon comes from a study showing that, whereas no age-dependent differences in baseline hepatic glutathione levels were found, following acute ethanol administration, the return of hepatic glutathione content to normal following a toxic dose of ethanol was delayed in 14- and 25-month-old female Fischer 344 rats compared to animals 4 months of age. This observation is consistent with some delay in glutathione synthesis.

Bile

The prevalence of human cholesterol gallstone disease increases dramatically with advanced age, at least in the Western world. Therefore, researchers have sought to determine whether age-associated alterations in the composition of bile, changes in the hepatic secretion of biliary components, and deranged gallbladder function may be at fault. Physiological changes that accompany cholesterol gallstone formation include a reduction in the body's bile acid pool, changes in cholesterol and phospholipid secretion into bile, and the presence of nucleating proteins, all leading to supersaturation of bile with cholesterol and precipitation of cholesterol crystals.

Chilean women over age 50 yr show a very high prevalence of cholelithiasis. In one study, a group of such women were shown to have increased cholesterol saturation (423). In a large series of gallstone-free healthy Scandinavians of varying age, an increase in cholesterol saturation of bile with increasing age was detected from both sexes (115) (Fig. 20.2). The degree of bile satura-

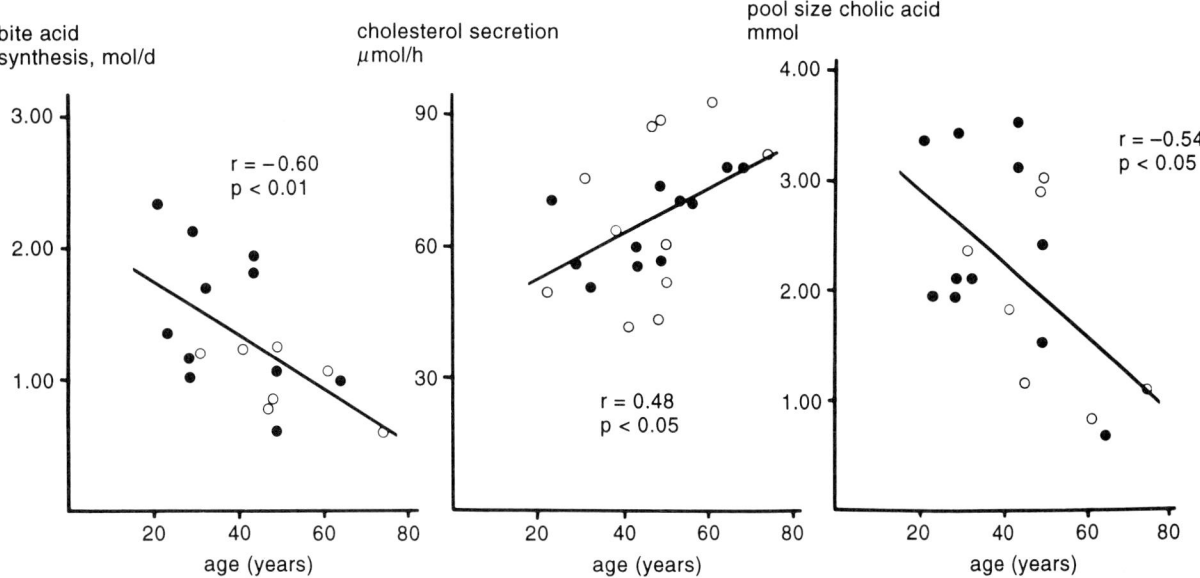

FIG. 20.2. Relation between age and hepatic secretion of cholesterol (n = 22), total bile acid synthesis (n = 18), and size of cholic acid pool (n = 18). Open circles denote women and closed circles men. To convert values for bile acids and cholesterol to milligrams, multiply by 400 and 0.39, respectively. [Reprinted from Einarsson et al. (115) with permission.]

tion was positively correlated with the secretion rate of cholesterol, a finding that also occurs in gallstone patients. In this study, bile acid production rate was seen to be less in older subjects than in the young (13). A few changes in biliary acid composition with age have been reported, including an increase in deoxycholic acid content (423). Using isotopically labeled deoxycholic and cholic acids simultaneously, van der Werf et al. (424) found a higher fractional turnover rate of cholic acid in elderly compared to younger subjects. These studies suggested that older subjects had less ileal cholic acid and greater colonic deoxycholic acid absorption. Other studies by the same group demonstrated that elderly volunteers had increased fecal secondary bile acid excretion than the young (318). One explanation for these changes in biliary acid composition with age is an increase in 7-α-dehydroxylation reactions resulting from an increase in bacterial growth in the small bowel of aging individuals.

Altogether, these data suggest that hepatic secretion of cholesterol may be greater in advanced age, that bile acid synthesis or hepatic secretion may be reduced in some individuals, and that intestinal bile acid absorption may be impaired.

Animal studies have not been very useful in this field because daily hepatic bile acid and cholesterol excretion and turnover in the rat differs greatly from that seen in humans. In older rodents, serum and hepatic cholesterol concentrations are increased. Kitani (244) has stated that there are no significant age-related changes in bile acid kinetics in the rat. In other studies, biliary cholesterol and acid excretion appear to be less in older than younger rats when calculated per 100 g of body weight (422).

Important data relating to age-related changes in gallbladder contraction have been obtained from both animal and human studies. Any reduction in the contraction of the gallbladder can result in stasis of gallbladder bile and therefore an increased opportunity for cholesterol precipitation and cholesterol crystal formation. Early studies suggested that gallbladder contraction may be reduced in older patients, but these may have reflected the clinical state of sick patients (60). When a high-fat formula was fed to fasting young and old volunteers, similar degrees of gallbladder contraction were observed, but these were accompanied by a significantly higher serum CCK level in the elderly (237). This initial clinical observation suggested that the sensitivity of the aging gallbladder to the hormone CCK was impaired. The same group of investigators then studied CCK receptor density in gallbladders from guinea pigs 24 months of age (347). The data from receptor affinity studies suggested lower CCK receptor density and reduced mobilization of cellular calcium in the 24-month-old animals than at 2 or 12 months of age (317). Subsequently, young and old guinea pigs were placed on a cholelithogenic diet with and without administration of CCK and more gallstones formed in 3-year-old guinea pigs than in rats of 1 month and 12 months of age. In the aged rats, gallstone formation was reduced by simultaneous CCK administration. Furthermore, the gallbladders of 1- and 12-month-old guinea pigs were more sensitive to exogenous CCK infusion than those of 3-year-old guinea pigs (343). From this series of studies the authors concluded that impaired gallbladder contraction may significantly contribute to increased gallstone formation in the elderly. The cellular mechanism responsible involves either altered CCK receptor density or changes in cellular responsiveness or both. Serum CCK levels have been found to be elevated, and duodenal CCK concentrations were greater both in guinea pigs (348) and in elderly patients with gallstones (224).

Any detailed description of age-related changes in hepatic function is beyond the scope of this review. Sulfobromophthalein sodium excretion capacity has been studied with varying results—probably because the test subjects had differing illnesses (138, 247, 404); however, the data suggest that overall excretion is unchanged, though reduced storage capacity may occur in advanced age. Two studies have shown a modest reduction in galactose elimination capacity (373) in elderly healthy subjects. It is likely that reduced overall functional capacity may result from a smaller liver in elderly men (352), independent of reduced body weight with age. Other indices of hepatic function are not altered in the healthy elderly (222).

GASTROINTESTINAL HORMONES

The gut is said to be the largest endocrine organ of the body. The gastrointestinal tract clearly is an organ specialized for the production of a wide variety of peptides which can alter the function of the gastrointestinal tract itself or, possibly, affect the structure and function of numerous other tissues of the body. The term "hormone" usually is restricted to peptides that are secreted from the cells of one organ to circulate and alter the properties of cells in a distant tissue. Many gastrointestinal peptides, however, do not act as classical hormones but, instead, function in a paracrine (acting upon cells close to or adjacent to the site of peptide formation) or an autocrine (acting upon cells synthesizing the peptide) fashion. These peptides are present in a wide variety of molecular forms, some or all of which may have a variety of functional activity.

It is not surprising that aging can alter the production or the effects of circulating hormones (or other active gastrointestinal peptides) in many different ways (Table 20.3). The tissue levels of the peptide in the organ where it is produced may be altered because of a change in the synthesis of the precursor, in the molecular heterogeneity of the peptide in the tissue, or in the release of the peptide from the tissue of origin. Circulating concentrations may be altered because of differences in production and secretion, in peptide catabolism, or in the levels of peptide receptors on target tissues. The response of target tissues may be altered by changes in receptor number or binding affinity, in intracellular signaling transduction mechanisms, or at the site of final intracellular action. Aging may have several differing effects either singly or in combination. The production, circulating levels, or tissue effects of peptides may differ with either greater or lesser action. Circadian rhythms of peptide actions also may be altered. There are three main families of gastrointestinal hormones plus a series of additional individual peptides. These include (1) the gastrin–CCK family; (2) the secretin–glucagon family, including GIP, VIP, and peptide–histidine–methionine; and (3) the pancreatic–polypeptide family, including pancreatic polypeptide (PP), peptide YY, and neuropeptide Y. Other hormones of importance, whose structure does not appear to permit classification into specific families, include bombesin, gastrin-releasing peptide, neurotensin, somatostatin, motilin, substance P, and chromogranin A–pancreostatin.

It must be emphasized that these peptides not only modify gut function but also modulate the proliferative activity of various gastrointestinal tissues, affect the metabolic functions of the body at a distance, and exist in large quantities in other tissues, such as the brain. The precise function of peptides in the brain is not clear, but CCK, for example, is believed to affect appetite control.

Despite the potential importance of understanding changes in peptide secretion and action in advanced age, relatively few investigators have studied elderly humans or aging animals in a comprehensive manner. It must be emphasized that some of the changes detected in the rat—the animal species most commonly studied—may not correspond to observations in humans; for example, fasting levels of pancreatic polypeptide are increased in elderly humans but are not altered with age in the rat.

TABLE 20.3. *Potential Age-Related Changes in the Effects of Gastrointestinal Hormones*

Tissue production
 Peptide synthesis
 Peptide release
 Molecular peptide processing

Circulating levels
 Peptide degradation
 Peptide excretion
 Receptor availability

Cellular effects
 Receptor number or binding
 Intracellular signaling
 End effect on intracellular organelles or gene activation

Changes in fasting and postprandial serum gastrin concentrations were described above under STOMACH. In summary, mean fasting serum gastrin concentrations in elderly human volunteers are higher than in the young, possibly because of the inclusion of subjects with hypochlorhydria, but postprandial levels also may be increased. These data contrast with those in the aging rat, in which postprandial serum levels and antral concentrations are found to be slightly lower and may not respond to fasting and refeeding but are responsive to stimulants such as bombesin. At the tissue level, crude preparations of gastric mucosal membranes from older rats show different specific gastrin-binding sites with relatively low affinity, which were not found in the young (383). The few observations of tissue somatostatin concentrations or somatostatin release also described earlier, suggest reduced production and tissue release of this peptide, an important observation that may explain the increased levels of gastrin found in older human volunteers. One report described higher plasma somatostatin concentrations in an unselected group of individuals aged 76–90 yr (357). Carbachol-stimulated release of somatostatin also was found to be impaired in one study of the isolated perfused rat stomach (248).

Experiments that have explored age-related changes in target tissue responses suggest some alteration in response mechanisms. For example, gastrin stimulation of pancreatic growth was described as being blunted (275). Several observations on age-related changes in pancreatic receptors have also been described in this chapter (see PANCREAS). One showed a decrease or delay in the trophic responses of the rat pancreas to cerulein (158), another to bombesin (345), and in another the number of CCK receptors in pancreatic lobules was shown to be less in 24- than in 3-month-old guinea pigs (346).

A major change in serum gastrointestinal peptides with aging involves a dramatic increase in the fasting and postprandial concentrations of serum PP. Up to an eightfold difference in serum PP concentrations following a meal have been demonstrated in 60–84-year-old nondiabetic volunteers (237). Although many of the physiological effects of this peptide recently have been described, neither the cause nor the consequences of this major change in serum PP concentration is known. Another gastrointestinal hormone whose concentration is higher in the elderly is serum motilin (57). The significance of this change also is unknown, though some investigators have suggested that changes in serum motilin may be a response to altered gastrointestinal motility. Neurotensin levels may be higher in older volunteers (236), an observation that has been associated with gut proliferative changes. Hyperglucanonemia also has been described (44, 282). Careful studies of the tissue production, circulation, and effects of these peptides may yield extremely valuable information about the effect of age on gastrointestinal hormones as a whole.

More data are available on the effects of age on the function of the gallbladder, particularly from the studies of Thompson's group in Galveston (237, 315, 343, 347). As described in the section LIVER AND BILIARY TREE, gallstone formation increases greatly with age in humans, and altered gallbladder motility is seen experimentally in the aging guinea pig. Daily injections of CCK in a guinea pig experimental model of gallstone disease appear to reduce the high incidence of gallstones in 3-year-old animals (315). The authors of this study believe, therefore, that the aging guinea pig gallbladder demonstrates a major impairment of motor function. Furthermore, serum CCK concentrations are higher in the aging rat (as well as in aging humans) (45), indicating altered interaction of this hormone with the gallbladder. The contraction of gallbladder muscle strips in vitro also showed age-dependent changes. Strips from 12-month-old guinea pigs achieved almost twofold greater contraction than those from 24-month-old guinea pigs and the response to CCK 8 was markedly reduced in the older animals (315). Keane et al. (230) showed an age-associated increased sensitivity of muscle strips from human gallbladder to acetylcholine in males (but not females) but no overall change in contraction with age in response to CCK 8 (230). In vivo, gallbladders from younger guinea pigs contracted more forcefully at lower concentrations of CCK 8 (317). The concentration of CCK receptors on gallbladder muscle cells was far greater in young adult guinea pigs than in aging animals. As an extension of these studies, the same group of investigators (315) measured the mobilization of intracellular calcium in muscle strips obtained from young adult and aged guinea pigs. The change in intracellular calcium concentration resulting from stimulation was similar at both ages. This result suggests that contraction response to calcium is maintained in aged animals. Whether or not there are changes in gallbladder muscle calcium channels associated with aging has not been determined. It is clear that the gallbladder represents a useful experimental model to explore age-related changes in peptide interaction with target tissues.

There are a number of examples that suggest that gastrointestinal peptides may induce different proliferative responses of the gastrointestinal tract in aging animals. These are discussed in more detail below.

CELLULAR PROLIFERATION

A basic tenet of a change that is associated with aging is that proliferative activity falls prior to the death of the tissue. This idea is based on in vitro tissue culture systems, as described in detail in Chapter 4. In vitro, experimental systems are limited to simple cells that can be propagated readily in a petri dish. The results do not apply to more complex organ systems that function in the body.

The gastrointestinal tract is a highly proliferative organ. Generally, the gastrointestinal mucosa consists of a series of cell types that demonstrate similar patterns of cell production. There is a layer of stem cells, cells distinct from stem cells but still actively dividing, and a larger zone of nondividing cells that undergo progressive differentiation to a more mature state before being extruded into the gastrointestinal lumen (454). The rate of cell turnover in the gastrointestinal tract from production to extrusion into the intestinal lumen is very rapid. In the rat, cell turnover occurs in as little as 2 days in the small and large intestine and about 2 wk in the esophagus. Although data from the human gastrointestinal tract are more limited, calculated turnover rates in the small and large intestine are only slighter greater than in rodents, ranging from about 3 to about 8 days. As a result of this rapid turnover rate, large amounts of proliferating cells are shed into the gut from the mucosa daily. Clearly, any change in proliferation that may occur as a result of aging will have profound effects on the morphology and functioning of gastrointestinal mucosal cells.

Proliferation in gastrointestinal tissues is controlled primarily by food intake. When food is removed from the gastrointestinal lumen (starvation), proliferation is reduced in the stomach, the small intestine, and the colon. The effects of starvation do not result solely from the removal of nutrients from gastrointestinal cells, because when parenteral nutrition maintains calorie balance, reduced gastrointestinal proliferation still occurs. The mechanism by which food intake stimulates gastrointestinal proliferation has not been completely established (454). Proliferative activity is stimulated to a major extent by the presence of food calories within the gastrointestinal lumen, but in addition, it is maintained by upper small intestinal secretions and even by nonnutrient, nondigestible fiber. Systemic signals, such as through various gastrointestinal peptides, also are important in the maintenance of gut proliferative activity. These peptides may act as a hormone, that is, via the action of chemical messages through the circulation, or luminally in a paracrine or autocrine fashion. Furthermore, gastrointestinal mucosal proliferation also may be affected by up-regulation of a series of early intermediate genes (194), possibly through the action of EGF. It must be emphasized that the proliferative response of all of the gastrointestinal mucosal tissues is tightly regulated to the apparent need of the organism for newly synthesized functioning epithelial cells.

It is well recognized that gastrointestinal proliferative activity varies with age. Proliferative activity in the small and large intestine of the rat is relatively low during late fetal and early postnatal life but increases abruptly during the second postnatal developmental period, between 14 and 21 days. Concurrently, maturation of epithelial cells involves an increase in mucosal sucrase activity, a rapid fall in mucosal lactase activity, and a fourfold increase in proliferation. Experiments on altered gastrointestinal proliferation generally have been performed in rodents. After the period of early development, most functional activities of the small and large intestine are maximal during the period of rapid body tissue growth, from approximately 3 wk to approximately 4 months of age, and then decrease to a relatively steady state until the rodent ages. The following section will discuss experiments that shed light on changes that occur at advanced ages. Many of these studies have been performed in only one of the gastrointestinal tissues, so each organ needs to be discussed separately.

Esophagus and Stomach

Studies of esophageal proliferation in aging animals are sparse. The original data of Thrasher (410) showed lower rates of esophageal epithelial cell proliferation in concert with data on other parts of the gastrointestinal tract from the same investigators, to be described below. A preliminary report by Simanowski et al. (381) found no change in baseline esophageal proliferation between 2–12 and 22 months of age in Fischer 344 rats. In this study, alcohol administration markedly impaired cell proliferation in all animal groups older than 2 months.

As described in the section STOMACH, the thickness of the gastric wall is increased in aging rodents, though that of the mucosal layer is decreased. Work by Majumdar and colleagues (277) has described an increase in the labeling index of gastric mucosal cells after administration of tritiated thymidine in vivo in 18-month-old Fischer 344 rats when compared to 4-month-old animals. Not only is the mucosal layer not broadened despite the increase in proliferation, but total mucosal DNA and protein content of the antrum of aging 24-month-old Fischer 344 rats also is not increased (276). In these studies, there was a marked increase in the specific activities of thymidine kinase (by 75%) and ornithine decarboxylase (by over 100%) (274). Mucosal tyrosine kinase activity also was increased in aging compared to young control animals (331), and the production of several phosphorylated tyrosine membrane proteins and myc gene expression was enhanced (274).

Gastric mucosal growth and maturation responds to several gastrointestinal peptides, including gastrin and EGF. When EGF was administered to young and aging rats, the response of the stomach in the older animals to DNA synthesis, thymidine kinase, and tyrosine kinase activities, as well as the production of phosphorylated tyrosine M55 proteins (436) was significantly less than in younger animals. Similarly, although the control baseline levels of these enzymes that reflect proliferation are greater in the stomach of older rats, following injury the response is significantly reduced (274, 331). Majumdar's group (276) has speculated that this impaired response occurs because replication is already expressed at maximum rates. The proliferative response of the antral mucosa to gastrin stimulation also is impaired in older rodents, perhaps because of reduced gastrin-binding sites in the gastric mucosa (383).

Small Intestine

The replicative activity of the small intestine is greater than other parts of the gastrointestinal tract. Furthermore, it has been known for many years that small intestinal morphology changes dramatically when food is withdrawn or animals are refed after a period of starvation. Therefore, the proliferative responses of the small bowel have been used as a model of the effect of aging on gastrointestinal proliferation.

Initially, a series of studies were performed which suggested that small intestinal proliferation was greatly reduced as a function of age. On the basis of these studies, the investigators suggested that lowered rates of proliferation were accompanied by prolongation of cell cycling and a lower transit rate of cells migrating from the proliferative zone at the crypt base to the villus tip. Although the validity of these studies has been challenged (24), it is important to describe the early studies because they have been extensively quoted.

Shortly after the development of the method of labeling proliferating epithelial cell nuclear DNA by ^{3}H thymidine (348), Fry et al. (139, 140, 260) studied intestinal proliferative changes with age. These studies were performed in male and female BALB-C mice 1 wk after transfer to the experimental site in young (3 months old), middle-aged (12 months old), and aged (30 months old) mice, whose nutritional state was not described (260). The data in the duodenum and jejunum suggested an increase in epithelial cell generation time in 30-month-old mice when compared to both younger groups (139). It must be pointed out that the investigators themselves noted more interanimal variation in old animals and speculated that this resulted from the toxic effect of ^{3}H thymidine on cellular DNA. Clearly, this interanimal variation could reflect other factors and raises some questions regarding the data. The same group failed to demonstrate any differences in replication or in epithelial transit times in the ileum of groups of animals varying from 3 to 30 months of age (140). Thrasher and Greulich (411) studied Swiss albino mice aged 10 days (infants), young rats (varying from 30 to 70 days), adult rats (about 12–13 months), and senescent mice (about 21–23 months). The body weight of these animals increased progressively with age. The authors found that the proliferative cycle lengthened with age, though the data based on DNA synthetic rate did not agree with those based on metaphase labeling. The number of labeled mitotic cells decreased in older animals. Analysis included animals of all ages, calculated by nonparametric analysis of variance. Since infant and young mice were rapidly growing, this may have obscured the overall data. Very little difference in DNA synthetic index and length of cycling could be found between adult and senescent animals.

In 1982, no decrease in jejunal and ileal proliferation was found in 25-month-old gnotobiotic Wistar rats when compared to younger animals varying from 3 to 12 months of age (114). At about the same time, observations by Cullan et al. (93) also implied that reduced proliferation did not occur with aging of the gastrointestinal tract. The studies of our own laboratory, initiated early in the 1980s, re-examined in detail the effects of aging on gastrointestinal cellular proliferation, morphology, and function, using as a model the well-defined Fischer 344 rats from the NIA. Our initial observations showed that the number of villus-absorbing cells of the upper small intestine (duodenum and jejunum) and the mucosal protein and DNA content did not differ between 4–5-month-old young mature rats and 25–27-month-old aging animals if care was taken to exclude animals that failed to recover from transport to our animal care facility and to ensure similar food intake (202). In the same studies, ileal villus cell numbers were found to be greater in old than in young animals. In addition, we noted an increase in crypt depth and the number of crypt cells in the proximal small intestine. When ^{3}H thymidine was administered, more crypt cells were labeled, suggesting greater proliferative activity. Increased proliferation was confirmed using the well-established metaphase arrest technique after the administration of vincristine. By this method, crypt cell production rates were found to be increased by one-third in the jejunum of fed aged rats compared to young controls (204).

Since starvation and refeeding induces a well-established physiological perturbation of the small intestine, this was tested in young and aging animals. Starvation was found to reduce the number of cells in both the villus and crypt in young and aging rats, and refeeding increased numbers to close to control levels at both ages. However, duodenal crypt cell production rate in young starved rats was 40% less than in fed controls but only 11% less in older starved animals (196). Refeeding resulted in a similar percent increase in proliferation rate, but the older rats still demonstrated 30% more proliferation. In addition, the distribution of proliferating cells in the small intestinal crypt of old rats was greatly altered, particularly in the refeeding model, accompanied by a dramatic expansion of the crypt cell proliferating zone. This phenomenon is similar to that seen in colonic crypts of patients at risk for colon cancer and after administration of some carcinogens (268).

The jejunal and ileal contents of several polyamines, which are associated with initiation of proliferation, were greater in aging rats (195). More ornithine decarboxylase activity was found in the ileum of older rats. Data from Thompson's group (460) similarly showed increased levels of the polyamines in 26–27-month-old Fischer 344 rats compared to 4-month-old animals. The tight control of polyamine metabolism that normally occurs as a response to starvation and refeeding also was disturbed in the aging rats. Partial small intestinal resection provides a reproducible stimulus to proliferation of the residual gut. Poston and co-workers (344) studied the adaptive response of 3- and 26-month-old Fischer 344 rats to a 60% mid-gut resection. They found that young rats completed hyperplasia of the remaining intestine within 2 wk, whereas restoration took 3 wk in the 26-month-old animals. These data indicate that there is retention of the capacity to regenerate in the older animal but some delay in the overall process. These investigators attributed altered proliferative responses to changes in the small intestinal response of aging animals to humoral stimuli. For example, the acute (216) and chronic (122) effects of neurotensin on gut hyperplasia are altered in 24-month-old Fischer 344 rats. They are beginning to investigate the molecular basis of this change in gut epithelial proliferative response to trophic hormones.

Colon

Although early studies suggested a reduction in colonic proliferation in 19-month-old compared to 3-month-old mice, Ecknauer et al. (114) described more crypts per unit serosal area in 25-month-old gnotobiotic rats. Our own laboratory extended studies of small intestine proliferation to the colon and demonstrated crypt hyperplasia, an increased rate of proliferation, and a broader proliferative zone in both proximal and distal colon of 26–28-month-old Fischer 344 rats compared to 3–4-month-old controls. As with the small intestine, the control of colonic proliferation as a response to starvation and refeeding was impaired in the older animals (197). In concert with these findings, increased thymidine kinase and ornithine decarboxylase activity has been demonstrated in the colon of 24-month-old rats (256), and phorbol ester infusion increased the activity of tyrosine kinase in the distal colon of 24-month-old far more than in 4-month-old Fischer rats. Accompanying this was an increase in membrane EGF receptor levels following administration of the phorbol ester. Rectal mucosal ornithine decarboxylase was higher in elderly than in young patients with adenomatous polyps (417).

Control of colonic proliferation in 24-month-old mice was described as much less precise than that seen in 4-month-old mice subjected to repeated irradiation (165). Data on the effect of tumorigenic agents on colon tumor formation are quite contradictory (14), but some studies do show increased susceptibility to carcinoma formation with age (421). Senescent fibroblasts also are more sensitive to the effects of phorbol esters, resulting in increased proliferation and loss of proliferative controls (101). This may be important since phorbol esters stimulate colonic protein kinase C, which is felt to increase cancer formation.

There is some evidence for an alteration in the zones of proliferation in the rectum of older human subjects. Under normal circumstances, epithelial cell DNA synthesis ceases as cells move from the proliferative zone near the crypt base in the distal colon toward the differentiating zone near the crypt mouth (268). Rectal biopsies from older human volunteers without adenomatous polyps have demonstrated a shift upward in the crypt labeling index toward the surface of the colon (102, 330, 358). This change has been defined as a phase I colon proliferative lesion, which occurs in altered proliferative states associated with colon neoplasia. Older patients with adenomatous polyps also were found to have more mucosal ornithine decarboxylase activity, which was reduced following calcium administration (417).

Effects of Caloric Restriction

Caloric restriction is well known to extend life span, to delay the development of age-associated biochemical and physiological changes in many organs (283), and to delay the appearance of naturally occurring and carcinogen-induced tumors (361). In Fischer 344 rats, when caloric intake was reduced to 60% of ad libitum food intake in the postweaning period, there was no significant effect on proximal small intestinal villus architecture or villus morphology, but caloric restriction prevented the age-associated crypt hyperplasia that was seen in ad libitum–fed animals at 20–21 months and 27 months of age. Duodenal crypt hyperplasia and ileal villus hyperplasia only became apparent in calorie-restricted animals at 33 months of age (168). Caloric restriction also delayed the loss of the specific and the total activities of disaccharidases and alkaline phosphatase that are found in ad libitum–fed aging animals (199). Caloric restriction, which reduces the incidence of carcinogen-induced colonic neoplasia, also lowers colonic epithelial cell proliferative indices in animals as early as 10 wk after initiation of the diet (391).

Since replication has been suggested as being critical for carcinogenesis (5) and one of the functions of tumor-suppressive genes is to inhibit mitogenesis (389), the findings of increased proliferation with aging might be accompanied by an increase in the risk of tumor formation. There is some evidence for this possibility as a function of aging in other tissues (465).

Because the gastrointestinal tract shows such a rapid rate of proliferation, aging effects may be an important physiological perturbation which can lead to a better understanding of the control of replicative activity in gastrointestinal epithelial cells. The data presented above allow for speculation that such information could lead to a better understanding of the cellular changes that lead to tumor formation in these gastrointestinal epithelial cells.

REFERENCES

1. ABRAMS, C. K., M. HAMOSH, S. K. DUTTA, S. VAN HUBBARD, and P. HAMOSH. Role of nonpancreatic lipolytic activity in exocrine pancreatic insufficiency. *Gastroenterology* 92: 125–129, 1987.
2. ADAM, R., I. ASTARCIOGLU, D. AZOULAY, M. MORINO, Y. M. BAO, D. CASTAING, and H. BISMUTH. Age greater than 50 years is not a contraindication for liver donation. *Transplant. Proc.* 23: 2602–2603, 1991.
3. AJITSU, S., S. MIRABELLA, and H. KAWANISHI. In vivo immunologic intervention in age-related T cell defects in murine gut-associated lymphoid tissues by IL2. *Mech. Ageing Dev.* 54: 163–183, 1990.
4. ALISON, M. R. Regulation of hepatic growth. *Physiol. Rev.* 66: 499–541, 1986.
5. AMES, B. N., and L. S. GOLD. Endogenous mutagens and the causes of aging and cancer. *Mutat. Res.* 250: 3–16, 1991.
6. AMMANN, R. Zur vaskularen Genese der chronischen pankreatitis. *Dtsch. Med. Wochenschr.* 101: 867–868, 1976.
7. AMMANN, R., and H. SULSER. Die senile chonische Pankreatitis-eine neue nosologische einheit? *Schweiz. Med. Wochenschr.* 106: 429–437, 1976.
8. ANDERSSON, H., I. BOSAEUS, T. FALKHEDEN, and M. MELKERSSON. Transit time in constipated geriatric patients during treatment with a bulk laxative and bran: a comparison. *Scand. J. Gastroenterol.* 14: 821–826, 1979.
9. ANDREW, W. Senile changes in the pancreas of Wistar Institute rats and of man with special regard to the similarity of locule and cavity formation. *Am. J. Anat.* 74: 97–127, 1944.
10. ANDREW, W. Age changes in the parotid glands of Wistar Institute rats with special reference to the occurrence of oncocytes in senility. *Am. J. Anat.* 85: 157–197, 1949.
11. ANDREW, W., and N. V. ANDREW. An age involution in the small intestine of the mouse. *J. Gerontol.* 12: 136–149, 1957.
12. ANDREWS, G. R., B. HANEMAN, J. ARNOLD, J. C. BOOTH, and K. TAYLOR. Atrophic gastritis in the aged. *Aust. Ann. Med.* 16: 230–235, 1967.
13. ANGELIN, B., and K. EINARSSON. Influence of age on biliary lipid metabolism in man. In: *Aging in Liver and Gastrointestinal Tract* edited by L. Bianchi, P. R. Holt, O. F. W. James, and R. N. Butler. Lancaster, UK: MTP Press, Falk Symposium 47, Titisee, 1987, p. 161–168.
14. ANISIMOV, V. N. *Carcinogenesis and Aging*, Boca Raton, FL: CRC Press, 1987, vols. 1, 2.
15. ANURAS, S., and J. SUTHERLAND. Small intestinal manometry in healthy elderly subjects. *J. Am. Geriatr. Soc.* 32: 581–583, 1984.
16. AOYAMA, S., S. KAWAMURA, K. NISHIO, K. HARIMA, T. AIBE, and T. TAKEMOTO. Histopathological study on aging of the pancreas from 423 autopsy cases. *Nippon Ronen Igakkai Zasshi* 6: 574–579, 1979.
17. ARMBRECHT, H. J. Changes in the components of the intestinal calcium transport system with age. In: *Aging in Liver and Gastrointestinal Tract*, edited by L. Bianchi. Lancaster, UK: MTP Press, 1988, p. 131–138.
18. ARMBRECHT, H. J. Effect of age on calcium and phosphate absorption. Role of 1,25-dihydroxyvitamin D. *Miner. Electrolyte Metab.* 16: 159–166, 1990.
19. ARMBRECHT, H. J., W. G. DOUBEK, and S. B. PORTER. Calcium transport by basal lateral membrane vesicles from rat small intestine decreases with age. *Biochim. Biophys. Acta.* 944: 367–373, 1988.
20. ARMBRECHT, H. J., T. V. ZENSER, M. E. H. BRUNS, and B. B. DAVIS. Effect of age on intestinal calcium absorption and adaptation to dietary calcium. *Am. J. Physiol.* 236 (*Endocrinol. Metab. Gastrointest. Physiol.* 5): E769–E774, 1979.
21. ARMBRECHT, H. J., T. V. ZENSER, C. J. GROSS, and B. B. DAVIS. Adaptation to dietary calcium and phosphorus restriction changes with age in the rat. *Am. J. Physiol.* 239 (*Endocrinol. Metab.* 2): E322–327, 1980.
22. ARORA, S., S. HASSARJIAN, S. D. KRASINSKI, B. CROFFEY, M. M. KAPLAN, and R. M. RUSSELL. Effect of age on tests of intestinal and hepatic function in healthy humans. *Gastroenterology* 96: 1560–1565, 1989.
23. ARRANZ, E., S. O'MAHONY, J. R. BARTON, and A. FERGUSON. Immunosenescence and mucosal immunity: significant effects of old age on secretory IgA concentrations and intraepithelial lymphocyte counts. *Gut* 33: 882–886, 1992.
24. ATILLASOY, E., and P. R. HOLT. Gastrointestinal proliferation and aging. *J. Gerontol.* 48: B43–B49, 1993.
25. AVIOLI, L. V., J. E. MCDONALD, and S. W. LEE. The influence of age on the intestinal absorption of ^{47}Ca in women and its relation to ^{47}Ca absorption in post-menopausal osteoporosis. *J. Clin. Invest.* 44: 1960–1967, 1965.
26. AXELSON, J., P. PERSON, R. GAGNERMO-PERSSON, and R. K'KANSON. Importance of the stomach in maintaining calcium homeostasis in the rat. *Gut* 32: 1298–1302, 1991.
27. BABAD, H., R. BEN-ZVI, A. BDOLAH, and M. SCHRAMM. The mechanism of enzyme secretion by the cell. 4. Effects of inducers, substrates and inhibitors on amylase secretion by rat parotid slices. *Eur. J. Biochem.* 1: 96–101, 1967.
28. BAILEY, L. B., J. J. CERDA, B. S. BLOCH, M. J. BUSHBY, L. VARGAS, C. J. CHANDLER, and C. H. HALSTEAD. Effect of age on poly- and monoglutamyl folacin absorption in human subjects. *J. Nutr.* 114: 1770–1776, 1984.
29. BAILEY, L. B., P. A. WAGNER, G. J. CHRISTAKIS, P. E. ARAUJO, H. APPLEDORF, C. G. DAVID, E. DORSEY, and J. S. DINNING. Vitamin B$_{12}$ status of elderly persons from urban low-income households. *J. Am. Geriatr. Soc.* 28: 276–278, 1980.
30. BAKER, D. M., and R. M. SANTER. A quantitative study of the effects of age on the noradrenergic innervation of Auerbach's plexus in the rat. *Mech. Ageing Dev.* 42: 147–158, 1988.
31. BAKER, D. M., S. P. WATSON, and R. M. SANTER. Evidence for a decrease in sympathetic control of intestinal function in the aged rat. *Neurobiol. Aging* 12: 363–365, 1991.
32. BAKER, H., S. P. JASLOW, and O. FRANK. Severe impairment of dietary folate utilization in the elderly. *J. Am. Geriatr. Soc.* 26: 218–221, 1978.

33. BAKER, S. J., V. I. MATHAN, and V. CHERIAN. The nature of the villi in the small intestine of the rat. *Lancet* i: 860, 1963.
34. BANNISTER, J. J., L. ABOUZEKRY, and N. W. READ. Effect of aging on anorectal function. *Gut* 28: 353–357, 1987.
35. BARRAGRY, J. M., M. W. FRANCE, D. CORLESS, S. P. GUPTA, S. SWITALA, B. J. BOUCHER, and R. D. COHEN. Intestinal cholecalciferol absorption in the elderly and in younger adults. *Clin. Sci. Mol. Med.* 55: 213–220, 1978.
36. BARTOLO, D. C. C., J. A. JARRATT, and N. W. READ. The use of conventional electromyography to assess external sphincter neuropathy in man. *J. Neurol. Neurosurg. Psychiatry* 46: 1115–1118, 1983.
37. BARTOS, V., and J. GROH. The effect of repeated stimulation of the pancreas on the pancreatic secretion in young and aged men. *Gerontol. Clin.* 11: 56–62, 1969.
38. BARZ, H., K. D. KUNZE, K. VOSS, and H. SIMON. Image processing in pathology. IV. Age dependent changes of morphometric features of liver cell nuclei in biopsies. *Exp. Pathol.* 14: 55–64, 1977.
39. BAUM, B. Evaluation of stimulated parotid saliva flow rate in different age groups. *J. Dent. Res.* 60: 1292–1296, 1981.
40. BAUM, B. J., E. E. KOUSVELARI, and F. G. OPPENHEIM. Exocrine protein secretion from human parotid glands during aging: stable release of the acidic proline-rich proteins. *J. Gerontol.* 37: 392–395, 1982.
41. BAUM, B. J., R. L. LEVINE, B. L. KUYATT, and D. B. SOGIN. Rat parotid gland amylase: evidence for alterations in an exocrine protein with increased age. *Mech. Ageing Dev.* 19: 27–35, 1982.
42. BECKER, G. H., J. MEYER, and H. NECHELES. Fat absorption in young and old age. *Gastroenterology* 14: 80–92, 1950.
43. BENDER, A. D. Effect of age on intestinal absorption: implication for drug absorption in the elderly. *J. Am. Geriatr. Soc.* 16: 1331–1339, 1968.
44. BERGER, D., R. CROWTHER, J. C. FLOYD, Jr., S. PEK, and S. S. FAJANS. Effects of age on fasting levels of pancreatic hormones in healthy subjects. *Diabetes* 26: 381a, 1977.
45. BERTHELEMY, P., M. BOUISSON, B. VELLAS, J. MOREAU, N. VAYSSE, J. L. ALBAREDE, and A. RIBET. Postprandial cholecystokinin secretion in elderly with protein-energy undernutrition. *J. Am. Geriatr. Soc.* 40: 365–369, 1992.
46. BEUMONT, D. M., I. COBDEN, W. L. SHELDON, M. F. LAKER, O. F. W. JAMES. Passive and active carbohydrate absorption by the ageing gut. *Age Ageing* 16: 294–300, 1987.
47. BEYER, H. S., M. ELLEFSON, R. SHERMAN, and L. ZIEVE. Aging alters ornithine decarboxylase and decreases polyamines in regenerating rat liver but putrescine replacement has no effect. *J. Lab. Clin. Med.* 119: 38–47, 1992.
48. BEYER, H. S., R. SHERMAN, and L. ZIEVE. Aging is associated with reduced liver regeneration and diminished thymidine kinase mRNA content and enzyme activity in the rat. *J. Lab. Clin. Med.* 118: 101–108, 1991.
49. BHANTHUMNAVIN, K., J. R. WRIGHT, and C. H. HALSTED. Intestinal transport of tritiated folic acid (^{3}H-PGA) in the everted gut sac of different aged rats. *Johns Hopkins Med. J.* 135: 152, 1974.
50. BLACK, D. A., and I. S. MENZIES. Intestinal absorption and renal clearance of sugar markers in the elderly. *Br. Geriatr. Soc.* Spring meeting, 1987.
51. BLAND, G., A. BANKS, M. NICHOLSON, and A. L. JONES. Decreased liver DNA synthesis in old rats following partial hepatectomy is restored by epidermal growth factor. In: *Liver and Aging*, edited by K. Kitani. Amsterdam: Elsevier, 1991, p. 279–290.
52. BLOOMFIELD, A. L., and C. S. KEEFER. Gastric acidity: relation to various factors such as age and physical fitness. *J. Clin. Invest.* 5: 205–227, 1928.
53. BODNER, L., and B. J. BAUM. Characteristics of stimulated parotid gland secretion in the aging rat. *Mech. Ageing Dev.* 31: 337–342, 1985.
54. BOGART, B. I. The effect of aging on the histochemistry of the rat submandibular gland. *J. Gerontol.* 22: 372–375, 1967.
55. BOGART, B. I. The effect of aging on the rat submandibular gland: an ultrastructural, cytochemical and biochemical study. *J. Morphol.* 130: 337–351, 1970.
56. BOGDONOFF, M. D., N. W. SHOCK, and M. P. NICHOLS. Calcium, phosphorus, nitrogen and potassium balance studies in the aged male. *J. Gerontol.* 8: 272–288, 1953.
57. BORTOLOTTI, M., G. FRADÀ, P. VEZZADINI, G. BONORA, G. BARBAGALLO-SANGIORGI, and G. LABÒ. Influence of gastric acid secretion on interdigestive gastric motor activity and serum motilin in the elderly. *Digestion* 38: 226–233, 1987.
58. BORTOLOTTI, M., G. J. R. FRADÀ, G. BARBAGALLO-SANGIORGI, and G. LABÒ. Interdigestive gastroduodenal motor activity in the elderly. *Gut* 25: A1320, 1984.
59. BOYD, E. Normal variability of the adult human liver and spleen. *Arch. Pathol.* 16: 350–372, 1933.
60. BOYDEN, E. A., and S. A. GRANTHAM. Evacuation of the gallbladder in old age. *Surg. Gynecol. Obstet.* 62: 34–42, 1926.
61. BRAATEN, B., and M. DONOWITZ. Stimulated active CL secretion is decreased in descending colon of aged rabbits. *Gastroenterology* 88: A1333, 1985.
62. BRASITUS, T. A., K.-Y. YEH, P. R. HOLT, and D. SCHACTER. Lipid fluidity and composition of intestinal microvillus membranes isolated from rats of different ages. *Biochim. Biophys. Acta.* 778: 341–348, 1984.
63. BRAUER, P. M., J. L. SLAVIN, and J. A. MARLETT. Apparent digestibility of neutral detergent fiber in elderly and young adults. *Am. J. Clin. Nutr.* 34: 1061–1070, 1981.
64. BUCHER, N. L. R., M. N. SWAFFIELD, and J. F. DITROIA. The influence of age upon the incorporation of thymidine-2-^{14}C into DNA of regenerating rat liver. *Cancer Res.* 24: 509–512, 1964.
65. BUCHOWSKI, M. S., and D. D. MILLER. Lactose, calcium source and age affect calcium bioavailability in rats. *J. Nutr.* 121: 1746–1754, 1991.
66. BULLAMORE, J. R., K. WILKINSON, J. C. GALLAGHER, B. E. C. NORDIN, and D. H. MARSHALL. Effect of age on calcium absorption. *Lancet* ii: 535–537, 1970.
67. BURKHARDT, R. Iron overload of bone marrow and bone. In: *Iron Metabolism and its Disorders, ICS 366*, edited by H. Kief. Amsterdam: Excerpta Medica, 1975, p. 264–272.
68. BUTCHER, F. R., J. A. GOLDMAN, and M. NEMEROVSKI. Effect of adrenergic agents on α-amylase release and adenosine 3′, 5′-monophosphate accumulation in rat parotid tissue slices. *Biochim. Biophys. Acta.* 392: 82–94, 1975.
69. BUTT, W., S. KAUFMAN, M. WANG, S. COHEN, and J. RYAN. Altered mechanical properties of the aged rat colon. *Gastroenterology* 98: A332, 1990.
70. CALLOWAY, N. O., C. F. FOLEY, and P. LANGERBLOOM. Uncertainties in geriatric data. II. Organ size. *J. Am. Geriatr. Soc.* 13: 20–28, 1965.
71. CAMERON, A. J., and C. T. LOMBOY. Barrett's esophagus: age, prevalence, and extent of columnar epithelium. *Gastroenterology* 103: 1241–1245, 1992.
72. CARMEL, R., R. M. SINOW, M. E. SIEGEL, and I. N. SAMLOFF. Food cobalamin malabsorption occurs frequently in patients with unexplained low serum cobalamin levels. *Arch. Intern. Med.* 148: 1715–1719, 1988.
73. CASTLEMEN, C. M., C. N. VOLANS, and K. RAYMOND. The

effect of ageing on drug absorption from the gut. *Age Ageing* 6: 138–143, 1977.

74. CHAUNCEY, H. H., G. A. BORKAN, A. H. WAYLER, R. P. FELLER, and K. K. KAPUR. Parotid fluid composition in healthy aging males. *Adv. Physiol. Sci.* 28: 323–328, 1981.

75. CHEN, T. S., G. J. CURRIER, and C. L. WABNER. Intestinal transport during the life span of the mouse. *J. Gerontol.* 45: B129–B133, 1990.

76. CHENG, A. H. R., A. GOMEZ, J. G. BERGAN, T. C. LEE, F. MONCKEBERG, and C. O. CHICHESTER. Comparative nitrogen balance study between young and aged adults using three levels of protein intake from a combination wheat-soy-milk mixture. *Am. J. Clin. Nutr.* 31: 12–22, 1978.

77. CHILLA, R., H. NIEMANN, C. ARGLEBE, and B. F. DOMAGK. Age-dependent changes in the α-isoamylase pattern of human and rat parotid glands. *Otorhinolaryngol. Relat. Spec.* 36: 372–382, 1974.

78. CHIN, K. N. Ultrastructure of Peyer's patches in the aged mouse. *Acta Anat.* 84: 523–533, 1973.

79. CHINN, A. B., P. S. LAVIK, and D. B. CAMERON. Measurement of protein digestion and absorption in aged persons by a test meal of I^{131}-labeled protein. *J. Gerontol.* 11: 151–153, 1956.

80. CHOW, B. F., J. P. GILBERT, K. OKUDA, and C. ROSENBLUM. The urinary excretion test for absorption of vitamin B_{12}. I. Reproducibility of results and agewise variation. *Am. J. Clin. Nutr.* 4: 142–146, 1956.

81. CLARKE, R. M. The effect of growth and of fasting on the number of villi and crypts in the small intestine of the albino rat. *J. Anat.* 112: 27–33, 1972.

82. CLARKE, R. M. The effects of age on mucosal morphology and epithelial cell production in rat small intestine. *J. Anat.* 123: 805–811, 1977.

83. COGHILL, M. F. The significance of gastritis. *Postgrad. Med. J.* 36: 433, 1960.

84. COHN, S. M., K. A. ROTH, E. H. BIRKENMEIER, and J. I. GORDON. Temporal and spatial patterns of transgene expression in aging adult mice provide insights about the origins, organization, and differentiation of the intestinal epithelium. *Proc. Natl. Acad. Sci. U.S.A.* 88: 1034–1038, 1991.

85. CONNELL, A. M., C. HILTON, G. IRVINE, J. E. LENNARD-JONES, and J. J. MISIEWICZ. Variations in bowel habits in two sample populations. *Br. Med. J.* ii: 1095–1099, 1965.

86. COOK, I. J., M. GABB, V. PANAGOPOULOS, G. G. JAMIESON, W. J. DODDS, J. DENT, and D. J. SHEARMAN. Pharyngeal (Zenkers) diverticulum is a disorder of upper esophageal sphincter opening. *Gastroenterology* 103: 1229–1235, 1992.

87. CORNES, J. S. Number, size, and distribution of Peyer's patches in the human small intestine. I. The effect of age on Peyer's patches. *Gut* 6: 230–233, 1965.

88. CORRAZA, G. R., A. STROCCHI, R. ROSSI, D. SIROLA, and G. GASBARRINI. Sorbitol malabsorption in normal volunteers and in patients with coeliac disease. *Gut* 29: 44–48, 1988.

89. CORREA, P., C. CUELLO, D. DUQUE, L. C. BURBANO, F. T. GARCIA, O. BOLANOS, C. BROWN, and W. HAENSZEL. Gastric cancer in Columbia. III. Natural history of precursor lesions. *J. Natl. Cancer Inst.* 57: 1027–1035, 1976.

90. CROOKS, J., K. O'MALLEY, and L. H. STEVENSON. Pharmacokinetics in the elderly. *Clin. Pharmacokinet.* 1: 280–296, 1976.

91. CRYER, B., J. S. REDFERN, M. GOLDSCHMIEDT, E. LEE, and M. FELDMAN. Effect of aging in gastric and duodenal mucosal prostaglandin concentrations in humans. *Gastroenterology* 102: 1118–1123, 1992.

92. CSENDES, A., E. GUIRALDES, A. BANCALARI, I. BRAGHETTO, and M. AYALA. Relation of gastroesophageal sphincter pressure and esophageal contractile waves to age in man. *Scand. J. Gastroent.* 13: 443–447, 1978.

93. CULLAN, C. E., D. A. CROUSE, and T. G. SHARP. Adaptive changes in intestinal cell proliferation studies in situ and in ectopic petal intestinal grafts in ageing mice. In: *Mechanisms of Intestinal Adaptation*, edited by J. W. L. Robinson, R. H. Dowling, and E. O. Riecken. Lancaster, UK: MTS Press, Falk Symposium 30, 1982, p. 29–46.

94. CULPEPPER-MORGAN, J. A., P. R. HOLT, and M. J. KREEK. Aging changes in colonic opiate receptors in the guinea pig. *Gerontologist* 27: 88a, 1987.

95. DANIELS, C. K., D. L. SCHMUCKER, H. BAZIN, and A. L. JONES. Immunoglobulin A receptor of rat small intestinal enterocytes in unaffected by aging. *Gastroenterology* 94: 1432–1440, 1988.

96. DARMENTON, P., F. RAUL, M. DOFFOEL, and J. Y. WESSELY. Age influence on sucrose hydrolysis and on monosaccharide absorption along the SI of rat. *Mech. Ageing Dev.* 50: 49–55, 1989.

97. DAVID, H., and P. REINKE. Liver morphology with aging. In: *Aging in Liver and Gastrointestinal Tract*, edited by L. Bianchi, P. R. Holt, O. F. W. James, and R. N. Butler. Lancaster, UK: MTP Press, Falk Symposium 47, Titisee, 1987, 1988, p. 143–159.

98. DAVIES, W. T., J. R. KIRKPATRICK, G. M. OWEN, and R. SHIELD. Gastric emptying in atrophic gastritis and carcinoma of the stomach. *Scand. J. Gastroenterol.* 6: 297–301, 1971.

99. DEDICHEN, L. Anacidity in old persons. *Acta Med. Scand.* 7: 345–350, 1924.

100. DEL CORRAL, A., and R. CARMEL. Transfer of cobalamin from the cobalamin-binding protein of egg yolk to R binder of human saliva and gastric juice. *Gastroenterology* 98: 1460–1466, 1990.

101. DERVENTZI, A., S. I. S. RATTAN, and B. F. C. CLARK. Senescent human fibroblasts are more sensitive to the effects of a phorbol ester on macromolecular synthesis and growth characteristics. *Biochem. Int.* 27: 903–911, 1992.

102. DESCHNER, E. E., and H. T. LYNCH. The influence of age and genetic risk for colonic epithelial cell proliferation. *Proc. Am. Assoc. Cancer Res.* 28: 179, 1987.

103. DEVROEDE, G., S. VOBECKY, S. MASSE, et al. Ischaemic fecal incontinence and rectal angina. *Gastroenterology* 83: 970–980, 1982.

104. DI LORENZO, D., C. P. DOOLEY, and J. E. VALENZUELA. Role of fasting gastrointestinal motility in the variability of gastrointestinal transit time assessed by hydrogen breath test. *Gut* 32: 1127–1130, 1991.

105. DI MAGNO, E. P., and W. H. J. SUMMERSKILL. Relations between pancreatic enzyme output and malabsorption in severe pancreatic insufficiency. *N. Engl. J. Med.* 288: 813–815, 1977.

106. DOOLEY, J. S., B. J. POTTER, H. C. THOMAS, et al. A comparative study of the biliary secretion of human dimeric and monomeric IgA in rat and man. *Hepatology* 2: 232–237, 1982.

107. DOUBEK, W. G., and H. J. ARMBRECHT. Changes in intestinal glucose transport over the lifespan of the rat. *Mech. Ageing Dev.* 39: 91–102, 1987.

108. DRAPER, H. H. Physiologic aspects of aging. I. Efficiency of absorption and phosphorylation of radiothiamine. *Proc. Soc. Exp. Biol. Med.* 97: 121–124, 1958.

109. DUBICK, M. A., P. R. MORRILL, and A. P. N. MAJUMDAR. Aging: effect of phorbol ester administration on pancreatic enzymes in rats. *Gastroenterology* 98: A-410, 1990.

110. DUNLAP, C. E., J. MATTOX, J. B. NELSON, and D. O. CASTELL. Morphometric analysis of enteric neurons in small intestine of the Fischer rat across age. *Gastroenterology* 94: A107, 1988.

111. EASTWOOD, H. D. H. Bowel transit studies in the elderly radio-

opaque markers in the investigation of constipation. *Gerontol. Clin.* 14: 154–159, 1972.

112. EBERSOLE, J. L., D. J. SMITH, and M. A. TAUBMAN. Secretory immune responses in aging rats. 1. Immunoglobulin levels. *Immunology* 56: 345–350, 1985.

113. ECKARDT, V. F., and P. M. LECOMPTE. Esophageal ganglia and smooth muscle in the elderly. *Dig. Dis.* 23: 443–448, 1978.

114. ECKNAUER, R., T. VADAKEL, and R. WEPLER. Intestinal morphology and cell production rate in aging rats. *J. Gerontol.* 37: 151–155, 1982.

115. EINARSSON, K., K. NILSELL, B. LEIJD, and B. ANGELIN. Influence of age on secretion of cholesterol and synthesis of bile acids by the liver. *N. Engl. J. Med.* 313: 277–282, 1985.

116. EKBERG, O., and M. J. FEINBERG. Altered swallowing function in elderly patients without dysphagia: radiologic findings in 56 cases. *Am. J. Radiol.* 156: 1181–1184, 1991.

117. ELSBORG, L. Reversible malabsorption of folic acid in the elderly with nutritional folate deficiency. *Acta Haematol.* 55: 140–147, 1976.

118. ENESCO, H. E., I. SHIMOKAWA, and B. P. YU. Effect of dietary restriction and aging on polyploidy in rat liver. *Mech. Ageing Dev.* 59: 69–78, 1991.

119. ERNST, D. N., W. O. WEIGLE, and M. L. THOMAN. Retention of T cell reactivity to mitogens and alloantigens by Peyer's patch cells of aged mice. *J. Immunol.* 138: 26–31, 1987.

120. ESPOSITO, G., A. FAELLI, M. TOSCO, M. N. ORSENIGO, and R. BATTISTESSA. Age-related changes in rat intestinal transport of D-glucose, sodium, and water. *Am. J. Physiol.* 249 (*Gastrointest. Liver Physiol.* 12): G328–G334, 1985.

121. EVANS, M. A., E. J. TRIGGS, M. CHEUNG, G. A. BROE, and H. CREASEY. Gastric emptying rate in the elderly: implications for drug therapy. *J. Am. Geriatr. Soc.* 29: 201–205, 1981.

122. EVERS, M. B., M. ISUKURA, D. H. CHUNG, D. PARDKH, K. YOSHINAGA, G. H. GREELEY, JR., T. UCHIDA, C. M. TOWNSEND, JR., and J. C. THOMPSON. Neurotensin stimulates growth of colonic mucosa in young and aged rats. *Gastroenterology* 103: 86–91, 1992.

123. EWE, K. Permeation of macromolecules. In: *Intestinal Absorption and Secretion,* edited by E. Skadhauge and Y. Heintze. Lancaster, UK: MTP Press, 1984, p. S03–S04.

124. FAUSTO, N. Protooncogenes and growth factors associated with normal and abnormal liver growth. *Dig. Dis. Sci.* 36: 653–658, 1991.

125. FAVUS, M. J., D. J. MANGELSDORF, V. TEMBE, B. J. COE, and M. R. HAUSSLER. Evidence for in vivo upregulation of the intestinal vitamin D receptor during dietary calcium restriction in the rat. *J. Clin. Invest.* 82: 218–224, 1988.

126. FEHÈR, E., and L. PENZES. Density of substance P, vasoactive intestinal polypeptide and somatostatin-containing nerve fibers in the ageing small intestine of the rats. *Gerontology* 33: 341–348, 1987.

127. FEIBUSH, J. M., and P. R. HOLT. Impaired absorptive capacity for carbohydrate in the aged. *Dig. Dis. Sci.* 27: 1095–1100, 1982.

128. FERRARIS, R. P., J. HSIAO, R. HERNANDEZ, and B. HIRAYAMA. Site density of mouse intestinal glucose transporters declines with age. *Am. J. Physiol.* 264 (*Gastrointest. Liver Physiol.* 27): G285–G293, 1993.

129. FICH, A., M. CAMILLERI, and S. F. PHILLIPS. Effect of age on human gastric and small bowel motility. *J. Clin. Gastroenterol.* 11: 416–420, 1989.

130. FIRKY, M. E. Gastric secretory functions in the aged. *Gerontol. Clin.* 7: 216–226, 1965.

131. FINDOR, J., V. PEREZ, I. E. BRUSH, M. GIOVANETTI, and N. FIARAVANTI. Structure and ultrastructure of the liver in aged persons. *Acta Hepato-gastroenterol.* 20: 200–204, 1973.

132. FINKELSTEIN, M. S., M. RANNER, and M. L. GREEDMAN. Salivary and serum IgA levels in a geriatric outpatient population. *J. Clin. Immunol.* 4: 85–91, 1984.

133. FIRKY, M. E. Exocrine pancreatic functions in the aged. *J. Am. Geriatr. Soc.* 16: 463–468, 1968.

134. FLEMING, B. B., and C. H. BARROWS. The influence of aging on intestinal absorption of vitamin B_{12} of niacin in rats. *Exp. Gerontol.* 17: 121–126, 1982.

135. FOX, P. C., M. W. HEFT, M. HERRERA, M. R. BOWERS, I. D. MANDEL, and B. J. BAUM. Secretion of antimicrobial proteins from the parotid glands of different aged healthy persons. *J. Gerontol.* 42: 466–469, 1987.

136. FRANK, E. B., R. LANGE, and R. W. McCALLUM. Abnormal gastric emptying in patients with atrophic gastritis with or without pernicious anemia. *Gastroenterology* 80: A1151, 1981.

137. FREEMAN, H. J., and G. A. QUAMME. Age-related changes in sodium-dependent glucose transport in rat small intestine. *Am. J. Physiol.* 251 (*Gastrointest. Liver Physiol.* 14): G208–G217, 1986.

138. FRESTON, J. W., and E. ENGLERT. The influence of age and excessive body weight on the distribution and metabolism of bromsulphalein. *Clin. Sci.* 33: 301–312, 1967.

139. FRY, R. J. M., S. LESHER, and H. I. KOHN. Age effect on cell-transit time in mouse jejunal epithelial cell. *Am. J. Physiol.* 201: 213–216, 1961.

140. FRY, R. J. M., S. LESHER, and H. I. KOHN. Influence of age on the transit time of cells of the mouse intestinal epithelium. *Lab. Invest.* 11: 289–293, 1962.

141. FULP, S. R., C. B. DALTON, J. A. CASTELL, and D. O. CASTELL. Aging-related alterations in human upper esophageal sphincter function. *Am. J. Gastroenterol.* 85: 1569–1572, 1990.

142. GABELLA, G. Fall in the number of myenteric neurons in aging guinea pigs. *Gastroenterology* 96: 1487–1493, 1989.

143. GALLAGHER, J. C., B. L. RIGGS, J. EISMAN, A. HAMSTRA, S. B. ARNAUD, and H. F. DELUCA. Intestinal calcium absorption and serum vitamin D metabolites in normal subjects and osteoporotic patients. *J. Clin. Invest.* 54: 729–736, 1979.

144. GARGOURI, Y., H. MOREAU, G. PIERONI, and R. VERGER. Human gastric lipase: a sulfhydryl enzyme. *J. Biol. Chem.* 263: 2159–2162, 1988.

145. GARGOURI, Y., H. MOREAU, and R. VERGER. Gastric lipases: biochemical and physiological studies. *Biochim. Biophys. Acta* 1006: 255–271, 1989.

146. GARLICK, P. J., M. A. McNURLAN, and V. R. PREEDY. A rapid and convenient technique for measuring the rate of protein synthesis by injection of [^{3}H] phenylalanine. *Biochem. J.* 192: 719–723, 1980.

147. GERSOVITZ, M., H. N. MUNRO, J. UDALL, and V. R. YOUNG. Albumin synthesis in young and elderly subjects using a new stable isotope methodology: responses to level of protein intake. *Metabolism* 29: 1075–1086, 1980.

148. GLASS, G. B. J., A. A. GOLDBLOOM, L. J. BOYD, R. LAUGHTON, S. ROSEN, and M. RICH. Intestinal absorption and hepatic uptake of radioactive vitamin B_{12} in various age groups and the effect of intrinsic factor preparations. *Am. J. Clin. Nutr.* 4: 124–133, 1956.

149. GOLDSCHMIEDT, M., and M. FELDMAN. Age-related changes in gastric acid secretion. In: *Chronic Gastritis and Hypochlorhydria in the Elderly,* edited by P. R. Holt and R. M. Russell. Boca Raton, FL: CRC Press, 1993. p. 13–30.

150. GOLDSCHMIEDT, M., C. BARNETT, B. E. SCHWARZ, W. E. KARNES, J. S. REDFERN, and M. FELDMAN. Effect of age on gastric acid secretion and serum gastrin concentrations in healthy men and women. *Gastroenterology* 101: 977–990, 1991.

151. GOLDSPINK, D. F., S. E. M. LEWIS, and F. J. KELLY. Protein

synthesis during the developmental growth of the small and large intestine of the rat. *Biochem. J.* 217: 527–534.
152. GOODMAN, S. A., and T. MAKINODAN. Effect of age on cell-mediated immunity in long-lived mice. *Clin. Exp. Immunol.* 19: 533–542, 1975.
153. GORBACH, S. L., L. NAHAS, P. I. LERNER, and L. WEINSTEIN. Studies of intestinal microflora. Effects of diet, age, and periodic sampling on numbers of fecal microorganisms in man. *Gastroenterology* 53: 845–855, 1967.
154. GOTO, H., Y. TSUKAMOTO, M. KUROIWA, A. OHARA, H. HOSHINO, and K. SEGAWA. Effects of aging on gastric mucosal prostaglandins. *Gastroenterology* 100: A74, 1991.
155. GREENBERG, R. E., and P. R. HOLT. Influence of aging upon pancreatic digestive enzymes. *Dig. Dis. Sci.* 31: 970–977, 1986.
156. GREENBERG, R. E., S. BANK, and V. KRANZ. Effect of aging on aspirin induced inhibition of gastric mucosal prostaglandins. *Gastroenterology* 96: A183, 1989.
157. GREENBERG, R. E., N. COLMAN, and P. R. HOLT. Folate conjugase pteroylpolyglutamate hydrolase activity is not impaired in the aging rat. *Gastroenterology* 90: 1438, 1985.
158. GREENBERG, R. E., P. P. MCCANN, and P. R. HOLT. Trophic responses of the pancreas differ in aging rats. *Pancreas* 3: 311–316, 1988.
159. GRINSTEAD, W. C., Y. CHARLES, C. PAK, and G. J. KREJS. Effect of 1,25-dihydroxyvitamin D_3 on calcium absorption in the colon of healthy humans. *Am. J. Physiol.* 247 (*Gastrointest. Liver Physiol.* 10): G189–G192, 1984.
160. GULLO, L., P. PRIORI, C. DANIELE, M. VENTRUCCI, G. GASBARRINI, and G. LABO. Exocrine pancreatic function in the elderly. *Gastroenterology* 29: 407–411, 1983.
161. HAAIJMAN, J. J., and W. HIJMAN. Influence of age on the immunological activity and capacity of the CBA mouse. *Mech. Ageing Dev.* 3: 375–398, 1978.
162. HAAIJMAN, J. J., H. R. E. SCHUIT, and W. HIJMANS. Immunoglobulin-containing cells in different lymphoid organs of the CBA mouse during its life-span. *Immunology* 32: 427–434, 1977.
163. HABOUBI, N. Y., P. HUDSON, Q. RAHMAN, G. S. LEE, and A. ROSS. Small-intestinal transit time in the elderly. *Lancet* i: 933, 1988.
164. HALVORSON, L., G. DOTEVALL, and A. WALAN. Gastric emptying in patients with achlorhydria or hyposecretion of hydrochloric acid. *Scand. J. Gastroenterol.* 8: 395–399, 1973.
165. HAMILTON, E. Cell proliferation and ageing in mouse colon. I. Repopulation after repeated x-ray injury in young and old mice. *Cell Tiss. Kinet.* 11: 423–431, 1978.
166. HEANEY, R. P., K. T. SMITH, R. R. RECKER, and S. M. HINDERS. Meal effects on calcium absorption. *Am. J. Clin. Nutr.* 49: 372–474, 1989.
167. HELLEMANS, J., E. JOOPSTEN, Y. GHOOS, H. N. CARCHON, G. VANTRAPPEN, W. PELEMANS, and P. RUTGEERTS. Positive 14 CO_2 bile and breath test in elderly people. *Age Ageing* 13: 138–143, 1984.
168. HELLER, T., P. R. HOLT, and A. RICHARDSON. Food restriction retards age-related histological changes in rat small intestine. *Gastroenterology* 98: 387–391, 1990.
169. HELLER, T. D., P. R. HOLT, and A. RICHARDSON. Food restriction retards age-related histologic changes in rat small intestine. *Gastroenterology* 98: 387–391, 1990.
170. HELLTHALER, VON G., H. KÖHLER, and W. ROTZSCH. Alternsabhängige veränderungen der proteinsynthese von dündarmringen. *Z. Alternsforsch.* 24: 243–247, 1971.
171. HINSULL, S. M. Effect of colloidal bismuth subcitrate on age related gastric lesions in the rat. *Gut* 32: 355–360, 1991.
172. HINTON, J. M., J. E. LENNARD-JONES, and A. C. YOUNG. A new method for studying gut transit times using radiopaque markers. *Gut* 10: 842–847, 1969.
173. HIRSCHOWITZ, B. I., and A. LANAS. Effect of aging on gastric acid and pepsin secretion-cross-sectional studies in du and nondu humans and longitudinal studies in fistula dogs. *Gastroenterology* 102: A83, 1992.
174. HODGES, S. J., M. J. PILKINGTON, M. J. SHEARER, L. BITENSKY, and J. CHAYEN. Age-related changes in the circulating levels of congeners of vitamin D_2, menaquinone-7 and menaquinone-8. *Clin. Sci.* 78: 63–66, 1990.
175. HÖHN, P., H. GABBERT, and R. WAGNER. Differentiation and aging of the rat intestinal mucosa. II. Morphological, enzyme histochemical and disc electrophoretic aspects of the aging of the small intestinal mucosa. *Mech. Ageing Dev.* 7: 217–226, 1978.
176. HOLLANDER, D., and V. D. DADUFALZA. Aging: its influence on the intestinal unstirred water layer thickness. *J. Physiol. Pharmacol.* 61: 1501–1508, 1983.
177. HOLLANDER, D., and V. D. DADUFALZA. Intestinal exsorption of oleic acid: influence of aging, bile, pH and ethanol. *J. Nutr.* 113: 511–518, 1983.
178. HOLLANDER, D., and V. D. DADUFALZA. Aging associated pancreatic exocrine insufficiency in the unanesthetized rat. *Gerontology* 30: 218–222, 1984.
179. HOLLANDER, D., and V. D. DADUFALZA. Lymphatic and portal absorption of vitamin E in aging rats. *Dig. Dis. Sci.* 34: 768–772, 1989.
180. HOLLANDER, E., and D. MORGAN. Increase in cholesterol intestinal absorption with aging in the rat. *Exp. Gerontol.* 14: 201–204, 1979.
181. HOLLANDER, E., and D. MORGAN. Aging: its influence on vitamin A intestinal absorption in vivo by rat. *Exp. Gerontol.* 14: 301–305, 1979.
182. HOLLANDER, D., and H. TARNAWSKI. Influence of aging on vitamin D absorption and unstirred water layer dimensions in the rat. *J. Lab. Clin. Med.* 103: 462–469, 1984.
183. HOLLANDER, D., and H. TARNAWSKI. Aging-associated increase in intestinal absorption of macromolecules. *Gerontology* 31: 133–137, 1985.
184. HOLLANDER, D., and H. TARNAWSKI. Age-associated increase in intestinal absorption of macromolecules. *Gerontology* 31: 133–137, 1985.
185. HOLLANDER, D., V. D. DADUFALZA, and E. G. SLETTEN. Does essential fatty acid absorption change with aging? *J. Lipid Res.* 25: 129–134, 1984.
186. HOLLANDER, D., V. DADUFALZA, R. WEINDRUCH, and R. L. WALFORD. Influence of life-prolonging dietary restriction on intestinal vitamin A absorption in mice. *Age* 9: 57–60, 1986.
187. HOLLANDER, D., A. TARNAWSKI, J. STACHURA, and H. GERGELY. Morphologic changes in gastric mucosa of aging rats. *Dig. Dis. Sci.* 34: 1692–1700, 1989.
188. HOLLIS, J. B., and D. O. CASTELL. Esophageal function in elderly men. A new look at "presbyesophagus." *Ann. Intern. Med.* 80: 371–374, 1974.
189. HOLT, P. R. The problem of fat in defined-formula diets; pros and cons. In: *Defined Formula Diets for Medical Purposes*, edited by M. Shils. Chicago: American Medical Association, 1977, p. 34–38.
190. HOLT, P. R. Effects of aging upon intestinal absorption. In: *Nutritional Approaches to Aging Research,* edited by G. B. Moment. Boca Raton, FL: CRC Press, 1982, p. 157–177.
191. HOLT, P. R. Clinical significance of bacterial overgrowth in elderly people. *Age Ageing* 21: 1–4, 1992.
192. HOLT, P. R., and J. BALINT. The effects of aging upon intestinal lipid absorption. *Am. J. Physiol.* 264 (*Gastrointest. Liver Physiol.* 27): G1–G6, 1993.

193. HOLT, P. R., and A. A. DOMINGUEZ. Intestinal absorption of triglyceride and vitamin D3 in aged and young rats. *Dig. Dis. Sci.* 26: 1109–1115, 1981.
194. HOLT, P. R., and R. N. DUBOIS. In vivo immediate early gene expression induced in intestinal and colonic mucosa by refeeding. *FEBS Lett.* 287: 102–104, 1991.
195. HOLT, P. R., and G. D. LUK. Aging intestinal polyamine metabolism in the rat. *Exp. Gerontol.* 25: 173–181, 1990.
196. HOLT, P. R., and K. Y. YEH. Small intestinal crypt cell proliferation rates are increased in senescent rats. *J. Gerontol.* 44: B9–B14, 1988.
197. HOLT, P. R., and K. Y. YEH. Colonic proliferation is increased in senescent rats. *Gastroenterology* 95: 1556–1563, 1988.
198. HOLT, P. R., and K.-Y. YEH. Aging and gastrin production: changes in serum and antral gastrin concentrations in the rat. *J. Gerontol.* 44: M62–M65, 1989.
199. HOLT, P. R., T. D. HELLER, and A. G. RICHARDSON. Food restriction retards age-related biochemical changes in rat small intestine. *J. Gerontol.* 46: B89–B94, 1991.
200. HOLT, P. R., D. P. KOTLER, and R. R. PASCAL. A simple method for determining epithelial cell turnover in small intestine—studies in young and aging rat gut. *Gastroenterology* 84: 69–74, 1983.
201. HOLT, P. R., D. P. KOTLER, and R. R. PASCAL. Delayed enzyme expression: a defect of aging rat gut. *Gastroenterology* 89: 1026–1034, 1985.
202. HOLT, P. R., R. R. PASCAL, and D. P. KOTLER. Effect of aging upon small intestinal structure in the Fisher rat. *J. Gerontol.* 39: 642–647, 1984.
203. HOLT, P. R., A. R. TIERNEY, and D. P. KOTLER. Delayed enzyme expression: a defect of aging rat gut. *Gastroenterology* 89: 1026–1034, 1985.
204. HOLT, P. R., K. Y. YEH, and D. P. KOTLER. Altered controls of proliferation in proximal small intestine of the senescent rat. *Proc. Natl. Acad. Sci. U.S.A.* 85: 2771–2775, 1988.
205. HOROWITZ, M., G. J. MADDERN, B. E. CHATTERTON, P. J. COLLINS, P. E. HARDING, and D. J. C. SHEARMAN. Changes in gastric emptying rates with age. *Clin. Sci.* 67: 213–218, 1984.
206. HOROWITZ, M., J. WISHART, L. MUNDY, and B. E. C. NORDIN. Lactose and calcium absorption in postmenopausal osteoporosis. *Arch. Intern. Med.* 147: 524–536, 1987.
207. HORST, R. L., J. P. GOFF, and T. A. REINHARDT. Advancing age results in reduction of intestinal and bone 1,25-dihydroxyvitamin D receptor. *Endocrinology* 126: 1053–1057, 1990.
208. HOUCKE, E., M. HOUCKE, and J. LEBLOIS. The pancreas of older adults: a histological study. *Presse Med.* 72: 1887–1892, 1964.
209. HOWELL, T. H. Organ weights in nonagenarians. *J. Am. Geriatr. Soc.* 26: 385–390, 1978.
210. HURDLE, A. D. F., and T. C. PICTON-WILLIAMS. Folic-acid deficiency in elderly patients admitted to hospital. *Br. Med. J.* ii: 202–205, 1966.
211. HUSEBYE, E., and K. ENGEDAL. The patterns of motility are maintained in the human small intestine throughout the process of aging. *Scand. J. Gastroenterol.* 27: 397–404, 1992.
212. HYAMS, D. E. The absorption of vitamin B_{12} in the elderly. *Gerontol. Clin.* 6: 193–206, 1964.
213. IHRE, T. Studies on anal function in continent and incontinent patients. *Scand. J. Gastroenterol.* 9(suppl. 25): 1–64, 1974.
214. IRELAND, P., and J. S. FORDTRAN. Effect of dietary calcium and age on jejunal calcium absorption in humans studied by intestinal perfusion. *J. Clin. Invest.* 52: 2673–2681, 1973.
215. ISHIDA, A., Y. YOSHIKAI, S. MUROSAKI, C. KUBO, Y. KIDAKA, and K. NOMOTO. Consumption of milk from cows immunized with intestinal bacteria influences age-related changes in immune competence in mice. *J. Nutr.* 122: 1875–1883, 1992.
216. ISUKURA, M., D. PAREKH, B. M. EVERS, K. YOSHINAGA, G. H. GREELEY, Jr., C. M. TOWNSEND, Jr., and J. C. THOMPSON. Effect of aging on neurotensin-stimulated intestinal growth in rats. *Gastroenterology* 98: A416, 1990.
217. ITO, H., B. J. BAUM, and G. S. ROTH. β- Adrenergic regulation of rat parotid gland exocrine protein secretion during aging. *Mech. Ageing Dev.* 15: 177–188, 1981.
218. JACOBS, A. M., and G. M. OWEN. The effect of age on iron absorption. *J. Gerontol.* 24: 95–96, 1969.
219. JAKAB, L., and L. PENZES. Relationship between glucose absorption and villus height in aging. *Experientia* 37: 740–742, 1981.
220. JOSKE, R. A., E. S. FINCKH, and I. J. WOOD. A study of 100 consecutive successful gastric biopsies. *Q. J. Med.* 24: 269–294, 1955.
221. JUSKO, W. L., G. LEVY, and S. J. YAFFA. Effect of age on intestinal absorption of riboflavin in humans. *J. Pharm. Sci.* 59: 487–490, 1970.
222. KAMPMANN, J. P., J. SINDING, and I. MOLLER-JORGENSEN. Effect of age on liver function. *Geriatrics* 30: 91–95, 1975.
223. KARBACH, U., and W. RUMMEL. Calcium transport across the colon ascendens and the influence of 1,25-dihydroxyvitamin D_3 and dexamethasone. *Eur. J. Clin. Invest.* 17: 368–374, 1987.
223a. KATELARIS P. H., F. SEOW, B. P. C. LIN, et al.: Effect of age, *Helicobacter pylori* infection, and gastritis with atrophy on serum gastrin and gastric acid secretion in healthy men. *Gut* 34: 1032–1037, 1993.
224. KATAOKA, S., and K.-I. SYOJI. Elevated cholecystokinin-like activity in the duodenal mucosa in patients with cholecystolithiasis. *Tohoku J. Exp. Med.* 145: 395–401, 1985.
225. KAWANISHI, H. and K. JOSEPH. Effects of phorbol myristate and ionomycin on in vitro growth of aged Peyer's patch T and B cells. *Mech. Ageing Dev.* 65: 289–300, 1992.
226. KAWANISHI, H., and J. KIELY. Immune-related alterations in aged gut-associated lymphoid tissues in mice. *Dig. Dis. Sci.* 34: 175–184, 1989.
227. KAWANISHI, H. H., S. AJITSU, and S. MIRABELLA. Impaired humoral immune responses to mycobacterial antigen in aged murine gut-associated lymphoid tissues. *Mech. Ageing Dev.* 54: 143–161, 1990.
228. KAWANISHI, H., S. SHIGERU, and A. SHIN. Aging-associated intrinsic defects in IgA production by murine Peyer's patch B cell stimulated by autoreactive Peyer's patch T cell hybridoma-derived B cell stimulatory factors (BSF). *Mech. Ageing Dev.* 49: 61–78, 1989.
229. KAWANO, S., H. TANIMURA, N. SATO, K. NAGANO, S. TSUJI, Y. TAKEI, M. TSUJII, N. HAASHI, E. MASUDA, T. KASHIWAGE, H. FUSAMOTO, and T. KAMADA. Age-related change in human gastric mucosal energy metabolism. *Scand. J. Gastroenterol.* 26: 701–706, 1991.
230. KEANE, P., D. COLWELL, H. P. BAER, A. S. CLANACHAN, and G. W. SCOTT. Effects of age, gender and female sex hormones upon contractility of the human gallbladder in vitro. *Surg. Gynecol. Obstet.* 163: 555–560, 1986.
231. KEELAN, M., K. WALKER, and A. B. R. THOMSON. Intestinal morphology, marker enzymes and lipid content of brush border membranes from rabbit jejunum and ileum: effect of aging. *Mech. Ageing Dev.* 31: 49–68, 1985.
232. KEKKI, M., and P. SIPPONEN. Age behavior of gastric acid secretion in males and females with a normal antral and body mucosa. *Scand. J. Gastroenterol.* 18: 1009–1016, 1983.
233. KENDALL, M. J. The influence of age on the xylose absorption test. *Gut* 11: 498–501, 1970.

234. KESAVAN, V., and J. M. NORONHA. Folate malabsorption in aged rats related to low levels of pancreatic folyl conjugase. *Am. J. Clin. Nutr.* 37: 262–267, 1983.
235. KHALIL, T., M. FUJIMURA, C. M. TOWSEND, G. H. GREELY, and J. C. THOMPSON. Effect of aging on pancreatic secretion in rats. *Am. J. Surg.* 149: 120–125, 1985.
236. KHALIL, T., and J. C. THOMPSON. Aging and gut peptides. In: *Gastrointestinal Endocrinology*, edited by J. C. Thompson, C. H. Greeley, Jr., P. L. Rayford, and C. M. Townsend, Jr. New York: McGraw-Hill, 1987, p. 147–157.
237. KHALIL, T., J. P. WALKER, I. WIENER, et al. Effect of aging on gallbladder contraction and release of cholecystokinin-33 in humans. *Surgery* 98: 423–429, 1985.
238. KIM, S.-K. Age-related changes in the cellular level of amylase and protein synthesis in the rat parotid gland. *J. Dent. Res.* 60: 738–747, 1981.
239. KIM, S. K., D. W. CALKINS, P. A. WEINHOLD, and S. S. HAN. Changes in the synthesis of exportable and non-exportable proteins in parotid glands during aging. *Mech. Ageing Dev.* 18: 239–250, 1982.
240. KIM, S. K., P. A. WEINHOLD, D. W. CALKINS, and V. W. HARTOG. Comparative studies of the age-related changes in protein synthesis in the rat pancreas and parotid gland. *Exp. Gerontol.* 16: 91–99, 1981.
241. KIM, S. K., P. A. WEINHOLD, S. S. HAN, and D. J. WAGNER. Age-related decline in protein synthesis in the rat parotid gland. *Exp. Gerontol.* 15: 77–85, 1980.
242. KIM, S. W., D. PAREKH, C. M. TOWNSEND, and J. C. THOMPSON. Effects of aging on duodenal bicarbonate secretion. *Ann. Surg.* 212: 332–338, 1990.
243. KIRK, J. E., and M. CHIEFFI. Effect of oral thiamine administration on thiamine content of the stool. *Proc. Soc. Exp. Biol. Med.* 77: 464–466, 1951.
244. KITANI, K. Bile acids in aging. In: *Aging in Liver and Gastrointestinal Tract*, edited by L. Bianchi, P. R. Holt, O. F. W. James, and R. N. Butler. Lancaster, UK: MTP Press, 1988, Falk Symposium 47, Titisee, 1987, p. 169–180.
245. KLIMAS, J. E. Intestinal glucose absorption during the life-span of a colony of rats. *J. Gerontol.* 23: 529–532, 1968.
246. KNOX, T. A., Z. KASSARJIAN, B. DAWSON-HUGHES, B. B. GOLNER, G. E. DALLAL, S. ARORA, and R. M. RUSSELL. Calcium absorption in elderly subjects on high- and low-fiber diets: effect of gastric acidity. *Am. J. Clin. Nutr.* 53: 1480–1486, 1991.
247. KOFF, R. S., A. J. GARVEY, S. W. BURNEY, and B. BELL. Absence of an age effect on sulphobromphthalein retention in healthy men. *Gastroenterology* 65: 300–302, 1973.
248. KOGIRE, M., D. PAREKH, J. ISHIZUKA, G. H. GREELEY, Jr., C. M. TOWNSEND, Jr., and J. C. THOMPSON. Effects of aging on gastrin and somatostatin secretion from the isolated perfused rat stomach. *Dig. Dis. Sci.* 38: 303–308, 1993.
249. KORBULY, D. Note on the influence of age on sodium- and potassium-absorption from the intestine of the rat. *Gerontologia* 12: 99–105, 1966.
250. KOUNTZ, W. B., L. HOFSTATER, and P. G. ACKERMANN. Nitrogen balance studies on elderly people. *Geriatrics* 2: 173–182, 1947.
251. KRASINSKI, S. D., J. S. COHN, E. J. SCHAEFER, and R. M. RUSSELL. Postprandial plasma retinyl ester response is greater in older subjects compared with younger subjects. *J. Clin. Invest.* 85: 883–892, 1990.
252. KRASINSKI, S. D., R. M. RUSSELL, C. L. OTRADOVE, J. A. SADOWSKI, S. C. HARTZ, R. A. JACOB, and R. B. MCGANDY. Relationship of vitamin A and vitamin E intake to fasting plasma retinol, retinol binding protein, retinyl esters, carotene, α-tocopherol and cholesterol among elderly and young adults: increased plasma retinyl esters among vitamin A supplement users. *Am. J. Clin. Nutr.* 49: 112–120, 1989.
253. KREEL, L., and B. SANDIN. Changes in pancreatic morphology associated with aging. *Gut* 14: 962–970, 1973.
254. KUPFER, R. M., M. HEPPELL, J. W., HAGGITH, and D. N. BATEMAN. Gastric emptying and small-bowel transit rate in the elderly. *J. Am. Geriatr. Soc.* 33: 340–343, 1985.
255. LA BROOY, J. S., P. J. MALE, A. K. BEAVIS, and J. J. MISIEWICZ. Assessment of the reproducibility of the lactulose H_2 breath test as a measure of mouth to caecum transit time. *Gut* 24: 893–896, 1983.
256. LANS, J., R. JASZEUSKI, F. ARLOW, J. JUREAD, J. GLARIAN, G. D. LUK, and A. MAJUMDAR. Supplemental calcium suppresses colonic mucosal odc activity in elderly pts with adenomatous polyps. *Gastroenterology* 98: A2902, 1990.
257. LASTER, L., and F. J. INGELFINGER. Intestinal absorption—aspects of structure, function and disease of the small-intestine mucosa. *N. Engl. J. Med.* 264: 1138–1148, 1961.
258. LAUGIER, R., and H. SARLES. The pancreas. In: *Clinics in Gastroenterology*, edited by O. F. W. James. London: Saunders, 1985, p. 749.
259. LEE, M., and M. FELDMAN. Age-related changes in gastric mucosal prostaglandin (PG) synthesis and aspirin-induced injury in rats. *Gastroenterology* 102: A563, 1992.
260. LESHER, S., R. J. M. FRY, and H. I. KOHN. Age and the generation time of the mouse duodenal epithelial cell. *Exp. Cell Res.* 24: 335–343, 1961.
261. LESTER, E., R. K. SKINNER, and M. R. WILLIS. Seasonal variation in serum 25-hydroxyvitamin D concentrations in the elderly in Britain. *Lancet* i: 979–980, 1977.
262. BOND, J. H. and M. D. LEVITT. Use of pulmonary hydrogen (H_2) measurements to quantitate carbohydrate absorption. *J. Clin. Invest.* 51: 1219–1225, 1972.
263. LEVITT, M. D., J. M. KNEIP, and D. G. LEVIT. Use of laminar flow and unstirred layer models to predict intestinal absorption in the rat. *J. Clin. Invest.* 81: 1365–1369, 1988.
264. LIANG, C. T., J. BARNES, S. TAKAMOTO, and B. SACKTOR. Effect of age on calcium uptake in isolated duodenum cells. Role of 1,25 dihydroxyvitamin D3. *Endocrinology* 124: 2830–2836, 1989.
265. LIN, C.-F., and L. HAYTON. Absorption of polyethylene glycol 400 administered orally to mature and senescent rats. *Age* 6: 52–56, 1981.
266. LIN, C. F., and W. L. HAYTON. GI motility and subepithelial blood flow in mature and senescent rats. *Age* 6: 46–51, 1983.
267. LINDI, C., P. MARCIANI, A. FAELLI, and G. ESPOSITO. Intestinal sugar transport during aging. *Biochim. Biophys. Acta* 816: 411–414, 1985.
268. LIPKIN, M. Phase 1 and phase 2 proliferative lesions of colonic epithelial cells in diseases leading to colonic cancer. *Cancer* 34: 878–888, 1974.
269. LUTZ, T., and E. SCHARRER. Effect of short-chain fatty acids on calcium absorption by the rat colon. *Exp. Physiol.* 76: 615–618, 1991.
270. MACLAUGHLIN, J., and M. F. HOLLOCK. Aging decreases the capacity of human skin to produce vitamin D_3. *J. Clin. Invest.* 76: 1536–1538, 1985.
271. MACLENNAN, W. J., and J. C. HAMILTON. Vitamin D supplements and 25-hydroxyvitamin D concentration in the elderly. *Br. Med. J.* ii: 859–861, 1977.
272. MADSEN, J. L. Effects of gender, age, and body mass index on gastrointestinal transit times. *Dig. Dis. Sci.* 37: 1548–1553, 1992.
273. MAITRA, R. S., E. A. EDGERTON, and A. P. NANDI MAJUMDAR. Gastric secretion during aging in pyloric-ligated rats and effects of pentagastrin. *Exp. Gerontol.* 23: 463–472, 1988.

274. MAJUMDAR, A. P. N. Regulation of gastric mucosal cell proliferation during advancing age. *Facts Res. Gerontol.* 2: 27–34, 1992.
275. MAJUMDAR, A. P. N., and M. A. DUBICK. Gastrin affects enzyme activity and gene expression in the aging rat pancreas. *Exp. Gerontol.* 26: 57–64, 1991.
276. MAJUMDAR, A. P., E. A. EDGERON, Y. DAYAL, and S. N. S. MURTHY. Gastrin levels and trophic action during advancing age. *Am. J. Physiol. (Gastrointest. Liver Physiol.* 17): G538–G542, 1988.
277. MAJUMDAR, A. P. N., S. JASTI, J. S. HATFIELD, J. TUREAUD, and S. E. G. FLIEGIEL. Morphological and biochemical changes in gastric mucosa of aging rats. *Dig. Dis. Sci.* 35: 1364–1370, 1990.
278. MAJUMDAR, A. P. N., J. A. MOSHIER, F. L. ARLOW, and G. D. LUK. Biochemical changes in the gastric mucosa after injury in young and aged rats. *Biochim. Biophys. Acta* 992: 35–40, 1989.
279. MAKINODAN, T., and M. M. B. KAY. Age influence on the immune system. *Adv. Immunol.* 29: 287–330, 1990.
280. MALAMUD, D. Amylase secretion from mouse parotid and pancreas the role of cyclic AMP and isoproterenol. *Biochim. Biophys. Acta* 279: 373–376, 1972.
281. MARCHESINI, G., V. BUA, A. BRUNORI, G. BIANCHI, P. PISI, A. FABBRI, M. ZOLI, and E. PISI. Galactose elimination capacity and liver volume in aging man. *Hepatology* 8: 1079–1083, 1988.
282. MARCO, J., J. A. HEDO, and M. L. VILLANUEVA. Hyperglucagonism in the elderly. *Diabetes* 26: 381a, 1977.
283. MASORO, E. J. Food restriction in rodents: an evaluation of its role in aging. *J. Gerontol.* 43: B59–B64, 1988.
284. MASSEY, B. T., S. SONNENBERG, and D. J. MCCANTY. Achalasia epidemiology and comorbidity in a geriatric population: an analysis of medicare data. *Gastroenterology* 98: A85, 1990.
285. MATHESON, D. M., and M. R. B. KEIGHLEY. Manometric evaluation of rectal prolapse and faecal incontinence. *Gut* 22: 126–129, 1981.
286. MATHIS, J. Beitrage zur konntris das fledermaus darmes. *Z. Mikr-anat. Forsch.* 12: 595–647, 1928.
287. MAYERSOHN, M. The xylose test to assess gastrointestinal absorption in the elderly: a pharmacokinetic evaluation of the literature. *J. Gerontol.* 37: 300–305, 1982.
288. MCDOUGAL, J. W., M. S. MILLER, and T. F. BURKS. Intestinal transit and gastric emptying in young and senescent rats. *Dig. Dis. Sci.* 25: A-15, 1980.
289. MCEVOY, A., J. DUTTON, and O. F. W. JAMEMS. Bacterial contamination of the small intestine is an important cause of occult malabsorption in the elderly. *Br. Med. J.* 287: 789–793, 1983.
290. MCMAHON, T. F., W. P. BEIERSCHMITT, and M. WEINER. Changes in phase I and phase II biotransformation with age in male Fischer 344 rat colon: relationship to colon carcinogenesis. *Cancer Lett.* 36: 273–282, 1987.
291. MEDVEDEV, Z. A. Age-related polyploidization of hepatocytes: the cause and possible role. *Exp. Gerontol.* 21: 277–282, 1986.
292. MELKERSSON, M., H. ANDERSON, I. BOSAEUS, and T. FALKHENDEN. Intestinal transit time in constipated and non-constipated geriatric patients. *Scand. J. Gastroenterol.* 18: 593–597, 1983.
293. MEL TUNE, J., D. P. MCGINTY, F. NAVAB, G. K. PATEL, and TEXTER, E. C., JR. The spectrum of mesenteric vascular insufficiency. In: *The Aging Gut, Pathophysiology, Diagnosis, and Management,* edited by E. C. Texter, Jr. New York: Masson, 1983, p. 105–115.
294. MENZIES, R. A., R. K. MISHRA, and P. H. GOLD. The turnover of ribosomes and soluble RNA in a variety of tissues of young adult and aged rats. *Mech. Ageing Dev.* 1: 117–132, 1972.
295. MERRY, B. J., E. M. SHEENA, and D. F. GOLDSPINK. The influence of age and chronic restricted feeding on protein synthesis in the small intestine of the rat. *Exp. Gerontol.* 27: 191–200, 1992.
296. MESHKINPOUR, H., M. SMITH, and D. HOLLANDER. Influence of ageing on the surface area of the small intestine in the rat. *Exp. Gerontol.* 16: 399–404, 1981.
297. MEYER, J., and H. NECHELES. Studies in old age. IV. The clinical significance of salivary, gastric and pancreatic secretion in the aged. *JAMA* 115: 2050–2055, 1940.
298. MIONE, M. C., S. L. ERDO, B. KISS, A. RICCI, and F. AMENTA. Age-related changes of noradrenergic innervation of rat splanchnic blood vessels: a histofluorescence and neurochemical study. *J. Auton. Nerv. Sys.* 25: 27–33, 1988.
299. MIYASAKA, K., and K. KITANI. Aging and pancreatic exocrine function: studies in conscious male rats. *Pancreas* 2: 523–530, 1987.
300. MIYASAKA, K., and K. KITANI. Aging and pancreatic exocrine function: studies in female conscious rats. *Dig. Dis. Sci.* 34: 841–848, 1989.
301. MIYASAKA, K., R. NAKAMURA, and K. KITANI. Effects of trypsin inhibitor (camostate) on pancreas and CCK release in young and old female rats. *J. Gerontol.* 44: M136–M140, 1989.
302. MOBARHAN, S., H. K. SEITZ, R. M. RUSSELL, R. MEHTA, J. HUPERT, H. FRIEDMAN, T. J. LAYDEN, M. MEYDANI, and P. LANGENBERG. Age-related effects of chronic ethanol intake on vitamin A status in Fisher 344 rats. *J. Nutr.* 121: 510–517, 1991.
303. MOLD, J. W., L. E. REED, A. B. DAVIS, M. P. H. MELVIN, L. ALLEN, D. L. DECKTOR, and M. ROBINSON. Prevalence of gastroesophageal reflux in elderly patients in a primary care setting. *Am. J. Gastroenterol.* 86: 965–970, 1991.
304. MONTGOMERY, R. D., M. R. HAINEY, I. N. ROSS, et al. The ageing gut: a study of intestinal absorption in relation to nutrition in the elderly. *Q. J. Med.* 47: 197–211, 1978.
305. MOOG, R. The small intestine in old mice: growth, alkaline phosphatase and disaccharidase activities, and deposition of amyloid. *Exp. Gerontol.* 12: 223–234, 1977.
306. MOORADIAN, A. D., and J. E. MORLEY. Micronutrient status in diabetes mellitus. *Am. J. Clin. Nutr.* 45: 877–895, 1987.
307. MOORADIAN, A. D., and M. K. SONG. The intestinal zinc transport in aged rats. *Mech. Ageing Dev.* 41: 189–197, 1987.
308. MOORE, J. G., D. J. BJORKMAN, M. D., MITCHELL, and A. AVOTS-AVOTINS. Age does not influence acute aspirin induced gastric mucosal damage. *Gastroenterology* 100: 1626–1629, 1991.
309. MOORE, J. G., C. TWEEDY, P. E. CHRISTIAN, and F. I. DATZ. Effect of age on gastric emptying of liquid-solid meals in man. *Dig. Dis. Sci.* 14: 340–344, 1983.
310. MORGAN, Z., and M. FELDMAN. The liver, biliary tract and pancreas in the aged: an anatomic and laboratory evaluation. *J. Am. Geriatr. Soc.* 5: 59–65, 1957.
311. MORRIS, H. A., B. E. C. NORDIN, V. FRASER, T. F. HARTLEY, A. G. NEED, and M. HOROWITZ. Calcium absorption and serum 1,25 dihydroxyvitamin D levels in normal and osteoporotic women. *Gastroenterology* 88: A1508, 1985.
312. MOZCIK, G. Y., E. VETNTER, M. SCHMELCZER, J. KUTAS, L. NAGY, and F. TARNOK. A critical analysis of the gastric secretory response of patients with duodenal ulcer in dependence of their age and duration of symptoms. *Acta Med. Hung.* 38: 117–128, 1981.
313. MULTIGNER, L., H. SARLEX, D. LOMBARDO, and A. DE CARLO. Pancreatic stone protein II. Implication in stone formation during the course of chronic calcifying pancreatitis. *Gastroenterology* 89: 387–391, 1985.

314. MUNROE, H. N., and V. R. YOUNG. Protein metabolism in the elderly. *Postgrad. Med.* 63: 143–148, 1978.
315. MURAKAMI, M., J. ISHIZUKA, K. YOSHINAGA, S. SUMI, G. A. NICHOLS, C. W. COOPER, G. H. GREELEY, and J. C. THOMPSON. Age-related changes in gallbladder contractility and cytoplasmic Ca^{++} concentration in the guinea pig. *Gastroenterology* 100: A539, 1991.
316. MYLVAGANAM, K., P. R. HUDSON, A. HERRING, and C. P. WILLIAMS. ^{14}C-triolein breath test: an assessment in the elderly. *Gut* 30: 1082–1086, 1989.
317. NAGAI, H., and K. OHTSUBO. Pancreatic lithiasis in the aged— its clinicipathology and pathogenesis. *Gastroenterology* 86: 331–338, 1983.
318. NAGENGAST, F. M., M. HECTORS, S. D. J. VAN DER WERF, and J. H. M. VAN TONGEREN. Age dependent differences in secondary bile acid concentration in human feces. *Gastroenterology* 88: A1514, 1985.
319. NAGY, ZS. The role of membrane structure and function in cellular aging: a review. *Mech. Ageing Dev.* 9: 237–246, 1979.
320. NAVAH, F., and C. G. WINTER. Effect of aging on intestinal absorption of aromatic amino acids in vitro in the rat. *Am. J. Physiol.* 254 (*Gastrointest. Liver Physiol.* 17): G630–G636, 1988.
321. NECHELES, H., F. PLOTKE, and J. MEYER. Studies on old age. V. Active pancreatic secretion in the aged. *Am. J. Dig. Dis.* 9: 157–159, 1942.
322. NEWTON, R. B., J. L. SULLIVAN, and A. G. DEBUSK. Neutral amino acid transport and in vitro aging. *Mech. Ageing Dev.* 27: 63–72, 1984.
323. NOKUBO, M. Physical-chemical and biochemical differences in liver plasma membranes in aging F-344 rats. *J. Gerontol.* 40: 409–414, 1985.
324. NORDIN, C., V. FRASER, T. F. HARTLEY, A. G. NEED, and M. HOROWITZ. Calcium absorption and serum 1,25 dihydroxyvitamin D levels in normal and osteoporotic women. *Gastroenterology* 88: A1508, 1985.
325. NORDIN, B. E. C., R. WILKINSON, D. H. MARSHALL, J. C. GALLAGHER, A. WILLIAMS, and M. PEACOCK. Calcium absorption in the elderly. *Calc. Tissue Res.* 21: 442–451, 1976.
326. O'CONNOR, M. K., D. H. KIM, C. J. Y. HUNG, and M. L. BROWN. The effects of age, sex and bolus composition on esophageal transit. *Gastroenterology* 96: A371, 1989.
327. OGAWA, K., H. MUKAI, and M. MORI. Effect of ageing on proliferative activity of normal and carcinogen-altered hepatocytes in rat liver after a two-thirds partial hepatectomy. *Jpn. J. Cancer Res.* 76: 779–784, 1985.
328. OHTA, M., and K. KITANI. Age-dependent decrease in the hepatic uptake of taurocholic acid resembles that for ouabain. *Biochem. Pharmacol.* 39: 1223–1228, 1990.
329. OHTSUBO, K., and T. A. NOMAGUCHI. A flow cytofluorometric study on age-dependent ploidy class changes in mouse hepatocyte nuclei. *Mech. Ageing Dev.* 36: 125–131, 1986.
330. PAGANELLI, G. M., R. SANTUCCI, G. BIASCO, M. MIGLIOLI, and L. BARBARA. Effect of sex and age on rectal cell renewal in humans. *Cancer Lett.* 53: 117–121, 1980.
331. PAREKH, D., K. Y. YOSHINAGA, J. ISHIZUKA, C. M. TOWNSEND, Jr., and J. C. THOMPSON. Age-related increase in the severity and outcome of experimental peptic ulceration. *Gastroenterology* 100: A541, 1991.
332. PELOT, D., J. V. LORUSSO, and D. HOLLANDER. The influence of aging on basal and secretin stimulated pancreatic exocrine secretion in the unanesthetized rat. *Age* 10: 1–4, 1987.
333. PÉNZES, L., G. SIMON, and M. WINTER. Intestinal absorption and utilization of radiomethionine in old age. *Exp. Gerontol.* 3: 257–263, 1968.

334. PÉNZES, L. Effect of concentration on the intestinal absorption of 1-lysine in ageing rats. *Exp. Gerontol.* 4: 223–230, 1969.
335. PÉNZES, L. Intestinal transfer of 1-Arg in relation to age. *Exp. Gerontol.* 5: 193–201, 1970.
336. PÉNZES, L. Intestinal absorption of glycine, L-alanine and L-leucine in the old rat. *Exp. Gerontol.* 9: 245–252, 1974.
337. PÉNZES, L., and M. BOROSS. Intestinal absorption of some heterocyclic and aromatic amino acids from the ageing gut. *Exp. Gerontol.* 9: 253–258, 1974.
338. PÉNZES, L. Further data on the age-dependent intestinal absorption of dibasic amino acids. *Exp. Gerontol.* 9: 259–262, 1974.
339. PÉNZES, L., D. KRANZ, K. KRETSCHMAR, V. ROSENTHAL, D. JANUSCHKEWITZ, M. KRÄMER, and O. REGIUS. Alterations in the intestinal microvillous surface area during the whole life span of the female rat. Ileum. *Z. Alternsforsch.* 43: 251–258, 1988.
340. PESTI, L., and J. A. GORDON. Effects of age and isolation on the intestinal flora of mice. *Gerontologia* 19: 153–161, 1973.
341. PHILLIPS, R. A., and H. GILDER. Metabolism studies in the albino rat. *Endocrinology* 27: 601–604, 1940.
342. PICCIONE, P. R., P. R. HOLT, J. A. CULPEPPER-MORGAN, et al. Intestinal dysmotility syndromes in the elderly: measurements of orocecal transit time. *Am. J. Gastroenterol.* 82: 161–164, 1990.
343. POSTON, G. J., E. J. DRAVIAM, C. Z. YAO, C. M. TOWNSEND, JR., and J. C. THOMPSON. Effect of age and sensitivity to cholecystokinin on gallstone formation in the guinea pig. *Gastroenterology* 98: 993–999, 1990.
344. POSTON, G. J., R. SAYDJARI, J. LAWRENCE, R. W. ALEXANDER, C. M. TOWNSEND, JR., and J. C. THOMPSON. The effect of age on small bowel adaptation and growth after proximal enterectomy. *J. Gerontol.* 45: B220–B225, 1990.
345. POSTON, G. J., R. SAYDJARI, J. P. LAWRENCE, C. M. TOWNSEND JR., and J. C. THOMPSON. Trophic effect of CCK, bombesin and pentagastarin on the aged rat pancreas. *Pancreas* 4: A637, 1989.
346. POSTON, G. J., P. SINGH, E. J. DRAVIAM, J. R. UPP, and J. C. THOMPSON. Development and age-related changes in pancreatic cholecystokinin receptors and duodenal cholecystokinin in guinea pigs. *Mech. Ageing Dev.* 46: 59–66, 1988.
347. POSTON, G. J., P. SINGH, and D. G. MACLELLAN, et al. Age-related changes in gallbladder contractibility and gallbladder cholecystokinin receptor population in the guinea pig. *Mech. Ageing Dev.* 46: 225–236, 1988.
348. QUASTLER, H., and F. G. SHERMAN. Cell population kinetics in intestinal epithelium in the mouse. *Exp. Cell Res.* 17: 420–438, 1959.
349. RABES, H. M. Liver cell turnover in man and animals during aging. In: *Aging in Liver and Gastrointestinal Tract*, edited by L. Bicuchi, P. R. Holt, O. F. W. James and R. N. Butler. Lancaster, UK: MTP Press, 1988, Falk Symposium 47, Titisee, 1987, p. 225–238.
350. RAFSKY, H. A., and B. NEWMAN. Vitamin B_1 excretion in the aged. *Gastroenterology* 1: 737–742, 1943.
351. RAJAKUMAR, G., M. K. MARKUS, and P. J. SCARPACE. β-Adrenergic receptors and salivary gland secretion during aging. *Growth, Dev. Aging* 56: 215–223, 1992.
352. RASMUSSEN, S. N. Liver volume determination by ultrasonic scanning. *Dan. Med. Bull.* 25: 1–45, 1978.
353. READ, N. W., W. V. HARFORD, A. C. SCHMULEN, M. G. READ, C. SANTA ANA, and J. S. FORDTRAN. A clinical study of patients with fecal incontinence and diarrhoea. *Gastroenterology* 76: 747–756, 1979.
354. RECKER, R. R. Calcium absorption and achlorhydria. *N. Engl. J. Med.* 313: 70–73, 1985.

355. REVILLE, M. F., F. GOOSE, J. KACHELHOFFER, M. DOFFOEL, and F. RAUL. Ileal compensation for age-dependent loss of jejunal function in rats. *J. Nutr.* 121: 498–503, 1991.
356. RICHTER, J. E., W. C. WU, D. N. JOHNS, J. N. BLACKWELL, J. L. NELSON, J. A. CASTELL, and D. O. CASTELL. Esophageal manometry in 95 healthy adult volunteers. Variability of pressures with age and frequency of "abnormal" contractions. *Dig. Dis. Sci.* 32: 583–592, 1987.
357. ROLANDI, E., R. FRANCESCHINI, V. MESSINA, et al. Somatostatin in the elderly: diurnal plasma profile and secretory response to meal stimulation. *J. Gerontol.* 33: 296–301, 1987.
358. RONCUCCI, L., M. PONZ DE LEON, A. SCALMATI, G. MALAGOLI, S. PRATISSOLI, M. PERINE, and N. J. CHAHIN. The influence of age on colonic epithelial cell proliferation. *Cancer* 62: 2373–2377, 1988.
359. ROSENBERG, T. I., N. FRIEDLAND, H. D. JANOWITZ, and D. A. DREILING. The effect of age and sex upon human pancreatic secretion of fluid and bicarbonate. *Gastroenterology* 50: 191–194, 1966.
360. ROWLATT, C. Cell aging in the intestinal tract. In: *Advances in Experimental Medicine and Biology. Vol. 53. Cell Impairment in Aging Development*, edited by V. Cristofalo and E. Holeckova. New York: Plenum Press, 1975, p. 215–217.
361. RUGGERI, B. The effects of caloric restriction on neoplasia and age-related degenerative processes. In: *Cancer and Nutrition*, edited by R. B. Alfin-States and D. Kritchevsky. New York: Plenum Press, 1991, p. 197–210.
362. RUSSELL, R. M., S. D. KRASINSKI, I. M. SAMLOFF, et al. Folic acid malabsorption in atrophic gastritis. *Gastroenterology* 91: 1476–1482, 1986.
363. SAID, H. M., D. HORNE, and D. MOCK. Influence of aging on intestinal biotin transport in the rat. *Gastroenterology* 96: A435, 1989.
364. SANSTEAD, H. H., L. K. HENRIKSEN, J. L. GREGER, et al. Zinc nutriture in the elderly in relation to taste acuity, immune response and wound healing. *Am. J. Clin. Nutr.* 36: 1046–1059, 1982.
365. SANTER, R. M., and D. M. BAKER. Enteric neuron numbers and sized in Auerbach's plexus in the small and large intestine of young adult and aged rats. *J. Auton. Nerv. Syst.* 25: 59–67, 1988.
366. SATO, T., and H. TAUCHI. The formation of enlarged and giant mitochondria in the aging process of human hepatic cells. *Acta Pathol. Jap.* 25: 403–412, 1975.
367. SAWEIRS, W. M., D. J. ANDREWS, and T. S. LOW-BEER. The double sugar test of intestinal permeability in the elderly. *Age Ageing* 14: 312–315, 1985.
368. SAYEED, M. Age-related changes in intestinal phosphomonoesterases. *Fed. Proc.* 26: 259, 1967.
369. SCHAEDLER, R. W., R. DUROS, and R. COSTELLO. The development of the bacterial flora in the gastrointestinal tract of mice. *J. Exp. Med.* 122: 59–66, 1965.
370. SCHMITZ-MOORMAN, P., G. W. HIMMELMANN, J. W. BRONDES, et al. Comparative radiological and morphological study of human pancreas: pancreatitis-like changes in post-mortem ductograms and their morphological pattern. *Gut* 26: 406–414, 1985.
371. SCHMUCKER, D. L., and R. K. WANG. Age-dependent alterations in rat liver microsomal NADPH-cytochrome c (P-450) reductase: a qualitative and quantitative analysis. *Mech. Ageing Dev.* 21: 137–156, 1983.
372. SCHMUCKER, D., and R. WANG. Effects of aging on the properties of rhesus monkey liver microsomal NADPH cytochrome c (P-450) reductase. *Drug Metab. Disp.* 15: 225–232, 1987.
373. SCHNEGG, M., and B. H. LAUTERBURG. Quantitative liver function in the elderly assessed by galactose elimination capacity, aminopyrine demethylation and caffeine clearance. *J. Hepatol.* 3: 164–171, 1986.
374. SCHMUCKER, D. L., R. GILBERT, A. L. JONES, G. T. HRADEK, and H. BAZIN. Effect of aging on the hepatobiliary transport of dimeric immunoglobulin A in the male Fisher rat. *Gastroenterology* 88: 436–443, 1985.
375. SCHUETTE, S. A., N. J. YASILLO, and C. M. THOMPSON. The effect of carbohydrates in milk on the absorption of calcium by postmenopausal women. *J. Am. Coll. Nutr.* 10: 132–139, 1991.
376. SHAKER, R., Q. LI, J. REN, W. F. TOWNSEND, W. J. DODDS, B. J. MARTIN, M. K. KERN, and A. RYNDERS. Coordination of deglutition and phases of respiration: effect of aging tachypnea, bolus volume, and chronic obstructive pulmonary disease. *Am. J. Physiol.* 263 (*Gastrointest. Liver Physiol.* 26): G750–755, 1992.
377. SHANKLE, W. R., B. H. LANDING, S. M. A. H. CHUI, G. VILLARREAL-ENGELHARDT, and C. ZAROW. Studies of the enteric nervous system in Alzheimer disease and other dementias of the elderly: enteric neurons in Alzheimer disease. *Mod. Pathol.* 6: 10–14, 1993.
378. SHEIKH, M. S., A. RAMIREZ, M. EMMETT, C. SANTA ANA, L. R. SCHILLER, and J. S. FORDTRAN. Role of vitamin D-dependent and vitamin D-independent mechanisms in absorption of food calcium. *J. Clin. Invest.* 81: 126–132, 1988.
379. SHIP, J. A., C. DECARLI, R. P. FRIEDLNAND, and B. J. BAUM. Diminished submandibular salivary flow in dementia of the Alzheimer type. *J. Gerontol.* 45: M61–M66, 1990.
380. SHUB, M. D., K. Y. PANG, D. A. SWANN, and W. A. WALKER. Age-related changes in chemical composition and physical properties of mucus glycoproteins from rat small intestine. *Biochem. J.* 215: 405–411, 1983.
381. SIMANOWSKI, U. A., P. SUTER, F. STICKEL, H. MAIER, R. WALDHERR, R. M. RUSSELL, and H. K. SEITZ. Esophageal epithelial hyperregeneration following chronic ethanol consumption: effect of age and saliva. *Gastroenterology* 102: A398, 1992.
382. SIMKO, V., and S. MICHAEL. Absorptive capacity for dietary fat in elderly patients with debilitating disorders. *Arch. Intern. Med.* 149: 557–560, 1989.
383. SINGH, P., B. RAE-VENTER, C. M. TOWNSEND, JR., T. KHALIL, and J. C. THOMPSON. Gastrin receptors in normal and malignant gastrointestinal mucosa: age-associated changes. *Am. J. Physiol.* 249 (*Gastrointest. Liver Physiol.* 12): G761–G769, 1985.
384. SIURALA, M., M. ISOKOSKI, K. VARIS, and M. KEKKI. Prevalence of gastritis in a rural population. *Scand. J. Gastroenterol.* 3: 211–223, 1968.
385. SNOOK, J. T. Effect of age and long-term diet on exocrine pancreas of the rat. *Am. J. Physiol.* 228: 262–268, 1975.
386. SOERGEL, K. H., F. F. ZBORALSKE, and J. R. AMBERG. Presbyesophagus: esophagus motility in nonagenarians. *J. Clin. Invest.* 48: 1472–1478, 1964.
387. SOUTHGATE, D. A. T., and J. V. G. A. DURNIN. An experimental reassessment of the factors used in the calculation of the energy value of human diets. *Br. J. Nutr.* 24: 517–535, 1970.
388. SPENCE, R. A. J., B. J. COLLINS, T. G. PARKS, and A. H. G. LOVE. Does age influence normal gastro-oesophageal reflux? *Gut* 26: 799–801, 1985.
389. STANBRIDGE, E. S. Human tumor suppressor genes. *Annu. Rev. Genet.* 24: 615–657, 1990.
390. STARZL, T. E., R. GORDON, A. TZAKIS, W. MARSH, and D. VAN THIEL. Liver transplantation in older patients. *N. Engl. J. Med.* 316: 484–485, 1987.
391. STEINBACH, G., S. P. KUMAR, B. S. REDDY, M. LIPKIN, and P. R. HOLT. Divergent effects of dietary calories and fat on rat colonic cell proliferation. *Cancer Res.* 33: 2745–2749, 1993.

392. Sun, J., and H. W. Strobel. Aging affects the drug metabolism systems of rat liver, kidney, colon and lung in a differential fashion. *Exp. Gerontol.* 21: 523–534, 1986.
393. Sun, W. M., T. C. Donnelly, and N. W. Read. Utility of a combined test of anorectal manometry, electromyography, and sensation in determining the mechanism of "idiopathic" faecal incontinence. *Gut* 33: 807–813, 1992.
394. Suntzeff, V., and P. Angeletti. Histological and histochemical changes in intestines of mice with aging. *J. Gerontol.* 16: 225–229, 1951.
395. Suter, P. M., B. B. Golner, B. R. Goldin, F. D. Morrow, and R. M. Russell. Reversal of protein-bound vitamin B_{12} malabsorption with antibiotics in atrophic gastritis. *Gastroenterology* 101: 1039–1045, 1991.
396. Szewczuk, J. R., and R. J. Campbell. Differential effect of aging on the heterogeneity of the immune response to a T-dependent antigen in systemic and mucosal-associated lymphoid tissues. *J. Immunol.* 126: 472–477, 1981.
397. Szewczuk, M. R., R. J. Campbell, and L. K. Jung. Lack of age-associated immune dysfunction in mucosal-associated lymph nodes. *J. Immunol.* 128: 2200–2204, 1981.
398. Szurszewski, J. H., P. R. Holt, and M. Schuster. Proceedings of a workshop entitled "Neuromuscular function and dysfunction of the gastrointestinal tract in aging." *Dig. Dis. Sci.* 34: 1135–1146, 1989.
399. Taillefer, R., M. Jadiawalla, E. Pellerin, E. Lafontaine, and A. Duranceau. Radionuclide esophageal transit study in detection of esophageal motor dysfunction: comparison with motility studies (manometry). *J. Nucl. Med.* 31: 1921–1926, 1990.
400. Takamoto, S., Y. Seino, B. Sackor, and C. T. Liang. Effect of age on duodenal 1,25-dihydroxyvitamin D-3 receptors in Wistar rats. *Biochim. Biophys. Acta* 1034: 22–28, 1990.
401. Taylor, L. D., C. K. Daniels, and D. L. Schmucker. Does aging impair gastrointestinal mucosal immunity. *Aging* 2: 205–209, 1990.
402. Taylor, L., E. Schneider, J. Smith, and P. Polgar. Prostaglandin production and cellular aging. *Mech. Ageing Dev.* 16: 311–317, 1981.
403. Texter, E. C., and H. J. Jordan. The effect of vascular factors on nutrient absorption. In: *Handbook of Nutrition and Food*, edited by M. Rechcigl. Boca Raton, FL: CRC Press, 13–20, 1983.
404. Thompson, E. N., and R. Williams. Effect of age on liver function with particular reference to bromsulphalein excretion. *Gut* 6: 266–269, 1965.
405. Thompson, J. S., D. A. Crouse, S. I. Mann, S. K. Saxena, and J. G. Sharp. Intestinal glucose uptake is increased in aged mice. *Mech. Ageing Dev.* 46: 135–143, 1988.
406. Thomson, A. B. R. Unstirred water layer and age dependent changes in rabbit jejunal D glucose transport. *Am. J. Physiol.* 236 (*Endocrinol. Metab. Gastrointest. Physiol.* 5): E685–691, 1979.
407. Thomson, A. B. R. Effect of age on uptake of homologous series of saturated fatty acids into rabbit jejunum. *Am. J. Physiol.* 239 (*Gastrointest. Liver Physiol.* 2): G363–371, 1980.
408. Thomson, A. B. R. Aging and cholesterol uptake in the rabbit jejunum. Role of the bile salt micelle and the unstirred water layer. *Dig. Dis. Sci.* 26: 890–896, 1981.
409. Thomson, A. D. Thiamine absorption in old age. *Gerontol. Clin.* 8: 354–361, 1966.
410. Thrasher, J. D. Age and the cell cycle of the mouse esophageal epithelium. *Exp. Gerontol.* 6: 19–24, 1971.
411. Thrasher, J. D., and R. C. Greulich. The duodenal progenitor population. I. Age related increase in the duration of the cryptal progenitor cycle. *J. Exp. Zool.* 159: 39–46, 1965.
412. Tiscornia, O., M. A. Cresta, E. S. de Lehmann, D. Celener, and D. A. Dreiling. Effects of sex and age on pancreatic secretion. *Int. J. Pancreatol.* 1: 95–118, 1986.
413. Tomotari, M. Intestinal flora and aging. *Nutr. Rev.* 50: 438–446, 1992.
414. Tracy, J. F., J. A. Logemann, P. J. Kahrilas, P. Jacob, M. Kobara, and C. Krugler. Preliminary observations on the effects of age on oropharyngeal deglutition. *Dysphagia* 4: 90–94, 1989.
415. Trudeau, W. L., and J. E. McGuigan. Serum gastrin levels in patients with peptic ulcer disease. *Scand. J. Gastroenterol.* 6: 9–46, 1970.
416. Tuchweber, B., A. Perea, G. Ferland, and I. M. Yousef. Dietary restriction influences bile formation in aging rats. *Life Sci.* 41: 2091–2099, 1987.
417. Turead, J., and A. P. N. Majumdar. Phorbol ester induced changes in colonic mucosal tyrosine kinase and epidermal growth factor receptor during aging. *Gastroenterology* 98: A434, 1990.
418. Turnland, J. R., N. Durkin, F. Costa, and S. Margen. Stable isotope studies of zinc absorption and retention in young and elderly men. *J. Nutr.* 116: 1239–1247, 1986.
419. Turnlund, J. R., M. C. Michel, W. R. Keyes, Y. Schutz, and S. Margen. Copper absorption in elderly men determined by using ^{65}Cu. *Am. J. Clin. Nutr.* 36: 587–591, 1982.
420. Turnlund, J. R., D. Reager, B. S. Reager, and F. Costa. Iron and copper absorption in young and elderly men. *Nutr. Res.* 8: 333–343, 1988.
421. Turusov, V. S., N. S. Lanko, and Y. D. Parfenov. Effect of age on induction of intestinal tumors in mice by 1,2-dimethylhydrazine. *Oncology* 1681–1683, 1982.
422. Uchida, K., Y. Nomura, M. Kadowaki, H. Takase, K. Takano, and N. Takeuchi. Age-related changes in cholesterol and bile acid metabolism in rats. *J. Lipid Res.* 19: 544–552, 1978.
423. Valdivieso, V., R. Palma, R. Wunkhaus, C. Antezana, C. Severin, and A. Contreras. Effect of aging on biliary lipid composition and bile acid metabolism in normal Chilean women. *Gastroenterology* 74: 871–874, 1978.
424. van der Werf, S. D. J., A. W. M. Huijbregts, H. L. M. Lamers, G. P. van Berge Henegouwen, and J. H. M. van Tongeren. Age dependent differences in human bile acid metabolism and 7-alpha-dehydroxylation. *Eur. J. Clin. Invest.* 11: 425–431, 1981.
425. Van Lennep, E. W. The histology of the mucosa of the small intestine of the long-nosed bandicoot with special reference to the intestinal secretion. *Acta Anat.* 50: 73–89, 1962.
426. Van Liere, E. J., and D. W. Northup. The emptying time of the stomach of old people. *Am. J. Physiol.* 134: 719–722, 1941.
427. Vantrappen, G., J. Janssens, J. Hellemans, and Y. Ghoos. The interdigestive motor complex of normal subjects and patients with bacterial overgrowth of the small intestine. *J. Clin. Invest.* 59: 1158–1166, 1977.
428. Vanzant, F. R., W. C. Alverez, G. B. Essterman, H. L. Dunn, and J. Berkson. The normal range of gastric acidity from youth to old age. *Arch. Intern. Med.* 49: 345–359, 1932.
429. Varga, F. Transit time changes with age in the gastrointestinal tract of the rat. *Digestion* 14: 319–324, 1976.
430. Varga, F., and T. Z. Csaky. Changes in the blood supply of the gastrointestinal tract in rats with age. *Pflugers Arch.* 364: 129–133, 1976.
431. Vellas, B., D. Balas, J. Moreau, M. Bouisson, F. Senegas-Balas, M. Guidet, and A. Ribet. Exocrine pancreatic secretion in the elderly. *Int. J. Pancreatol.* 3: 497–502, 1988.
432. Vestal, R. E., A. J. J. Wood, R. J. Branch, et al. Studies of drug disposition in the elderly using model compounds. In:

Liver and Aging, edited by K. Kitani. Amsterdam: Elsevier, 1978, p. 343–355.

433. VINARDELL, M. P., and J. BOLUFER. Age dependent changes in jejunal sugar absorption by rat in vivo. *Exp. Gerontol.* 19: 73–78, 1984.

434. VINARDELL, M. P., and J. BOLUFER. Active/diffusion ratio of sugars intestinal absorption at different ages in rats. *Nutr. Rep. Int.* 33: 199–209, 1986.

435. VINCENZINI, M. T., T. IANTOMASI, M. STIO, F. FAVILLI, P. VANNI, F. TONELLI, and C. TREVES. Glucose transport during ageing by human intestinal brush-border membrane vesicles. *Mech. Ageing Dev.* 48: 33–41, 1989.

436. WAHBY, M. A., and P. N. MAJUMDAR. Diminished activation of tyrosine kinases by gastrin in isolated gastric mucosal cells from aged rats. *Proc. Soc. Exp. Biol. Med.* 202: 365–370, 1993.

437. WAHNON, R., S. MAKADY, and U. COGAN. Age and membrane fluidity. *Mech. Ageing Dev.* 50: 249–255, 1989.

438. WALL, W. J., R. MIMEAULT, D. R. GRANT, and M. BLOCK. The use of older donor livers for hepatic transplantation. *Transplantation* 49: 377–381, 1990.

439. WALLACE, S., and C. ASHWORTH. Early degenerative lesions of the pancreas. *Tex. State J. Med.* 37: 584–587, 1942.

440. WALLING, M. W., and S. S. ROTHMAN. Apparent increase in carrier affinity for intestinal calcium transport following dietary calcium restriction. *J. Biol. Chem.* 245: 5007–5011, 1970.

441. WALLIS, J. L., and B. H. HIRST. Glucose uptake by aged mouse jejunal brushborder membrane vesicles. *Proc. Int. Union Physiol. Sci.* XCII: 52, 1989.

442. WALLIS, J. L., P. S. LIPSKI, J. C. MATHERS, O. F. W. JAMES, and B. H. HIRST. Duodenal brush-border mucosal glucose transport and enzyme activities in ageing man and the effect of bacterial contamination of the small intestine. *Dig. Dis. Sci.* 38: 403–409, 1993.

443. WALSH, J., C. RICHARDSON, and J. FORTRAN. pH dependence of acid secretion and gastrin release in normal and ulcer patients. *J. Clin. Invest.* 55: 462–469, 1972.

444. WANSTALL, J. C., and S. R. O'DONNELL. Vasodilator responses to dopamine in rat perfused mesentery are age-dependent. *Br. J. Pharmacol.* 98: 302–308, 1989.

445. WARREN, P. M., M. A. PEPPERMAN, and R. D. MONTGOMERY. Age changes in small intestinal mucosa. *Lancet* ii: 849, 1978.

446. WATANABE, T., and Y. TANAKA. Age-related alternations in the size of human hepatocytes. A study of mononuclear and binucleate cells. *Virchows Arch. (B) Cell Pathol. Incl. Mol. Pathol.* 39: 9–20, 1982.

447. WEBSTER, S. G. P., and J. T. LEEMING. The appearance of the small bowel mucosa in old age. *Age Ageing* 4: 168–174, 1975.

448. WEBSTER, S. G. P., and J. T. LEEMING. Assessment of small bowel function in the elderly using s modified xylose tolerance test. *Gut* 16: 109–113, 1975.

449. WEBSTER, S. G. P., E. M. WILKINSON, and E. GOWLAND. A comparison of fat absorption in young and old subjects. *Age Ageing* 6: 113–117, 1977.

450. WEGENER, M. G., J. SCHARFFSTEIN, J. LÜTH, R. RICKELS, and D. RICKEN. Effect of ageing on the gastro-intestinal transit of a lactulose supplemental solid-liquid meal in humans. *Digestion* 39: 40–46, 1988.

451. WEINER, P. G., F. DIETZE, and R. LAUE. Age-dependent alterations of intestinal absorption. II. A clinical study using a modified D-xylose absorption test. *Arch. Gerontol. Geriatr.* 3: 97–108, 1984.

452. WELSH, J. D., J. R. POLEY, M. BHATIA, and D. E. STEVENSON. Intestinal disaccharidase activities in relation to age, race and mucosal damage. *Gastroenterology* 75: 847–855, 1978.

453. WERMER, I., and L. HAMBRAEUS. The digestive capacity of elderly people. In: *Nutrition in Old Age,* edited by L. A. Carlson. Uppsala, Sweden: Almquist and Wicksell, 1972, p. 55–60.

454. WILLIAMSON, R. C. N. Intestinal adaptation: structural, functional, and cytokinetic changes. *N. Engl. J. Med.* 298: 1393–1401, 1978.

455. WOLFF, A., P. C. FOX, J. A. SHIP, J. C. ATKINSON, A. A. MACYNSKI, and B. J. BAUM. Oral mucosal status and major salivary gland function. *Oral Surg. Oral Med. Oral Pathol.* 70: 49–54, 1990.

456. WOODHOUSE, K. W., F. WILLIAMS, E. MUTCH, H. WYNNE, M. RAWLINS, and O. F. W. JAMES. Phase 1 drug metabolism in aging. In: *Aging in Liver and Gastrointestinal Tract,* edited by L. Bianchi, P. R. Holt, O. F. W. James, and R. N. Butler. Lancaster, UK: MTP Press, 1988, Falk Symposium 47, Titisee, 1987, p. 255–265.

457. WORMSLEY, K. G., and M. I. GROSSMAN. Maximal histalog test in control subjects and patients with peptic ulcer. *Gut* 6: 427–435, 1965.

458. WRIGHT, R. A., S. KRINSKY, L. FLEEMAN, J. TRUJILLO, and E. TEAGUE. Gastric emptying and obesity. *Gastroenterology* 84: 747–751, 1983.

459. WYNNE, H. A., L. H. COPE, E. MUTCH, M. D. RAWLINS, K. W. WOODHOUSE, and O. F. W. JAMES. The effect of age upon liver volume and apparent liver blood flow in healthy men. *Hepatology* 9: 297–301, 1989.

460. YOSHINAGA, K., J. ISHIZUKA, R. SAYDJARI, C. M. TOWNSEND, Jr., and J. C. THOMPSON. Effect of aging on polyamine pathway of small intestine in the rat. *Dig. Dis. Sci.* 38: 410–416, 1993.

461. YU, B. P., E. A. SUESCUN, and S. Y. YANG. Effect of age-related lipid peroxidation on membrane fluidity and phospholipase A_2 modulation by dietary restriction. *Mech. Ageing Dev.* 65: 17–33, 1992.

462. YU, B. P., E. A. SUESCUN, and S. Y. YANG. Effect of age-related lipid peroxidation on membrane fluidity and phospholipase A_2: modulation by dietary restriction. *Mech. Ageing Dev.* 65: 17–33, 1992.

463. ZENKER, F. A., and H. VON ZIEMSSEN. Dilatations of the esophagus. In: *Cyclopaedia of the Practice of Medicine.* London: Low, Marston, Searle and Rivington, 1878, p. 46–68.

464. ZHU, H., F. PACE, O. SANGALETTI, and B. PORRO. Features of symptomatic gastroesophageal reflux in elderly patients. *Scand. J. Gastroenterol.* 28: 235–238, 1993.

465. ZIMMERMAN, J. A., and T. H. CARTER. Altered cellular responses to chemical carcinogens in aged animals. *J. Gerontol.* 44: B19–B24, 1989.

466. ZIMMERMAN, V. W., N. FRANK, C. WEIB-SIMON, et al. Das normals pankreas-darstellung in sonogramm in abhangigkeit zum lebensalter. *Fortschr. Med.* 99: 1178–1182, 1981.

467. ZOLI, M., T. IERVESE, S. ABBATI, G. P. BIANCHI, G. MARCHESINI, and E. PISI. Portal blood velocity and flow in aging man. *Gerontology* 35: 61–65, 1989.

21. Immune system

RICHARD A. MILLER

Department of Pathology, University of Michigan School of Medicine; Institute of Gerontology, University of Michigan; GRECC, Ann Arbor Veterans Affairs Medical Center, Ann Arbor, Michigan

CHAPTER CONTENTS

T Lymphocyte Subsets
    Helper (CD4) and cytotoxic (CD8) T cell subsets
    Naive and memory T cell subsets
    Other T cell subsets
T Lymphocyte Function
    IL-2 production
    Response to IL-2
    Production of other lymphokines
    T cell activation
        Activation of protein kinases
        Calcium signal generation
        Inositol phosphate metabolism
        Calcium influx and efflux
        Control of membrane potential
        Gene expression
    Clonal diversity: a "mosaic" model for T cell senescence
T Cell Development
    Thymic involution
    Prothymocytes
B Lymphocytes
    B cell number and subsets
    Proliferation and antibody production
    Antibodies: levels, repertoire, and autoreactivity
B Cell Development
Accessory Cells and Their Cytokines
    Dendritic cells and Langerhans cells
    Cytokine production
Natural Cytotoxicity
Restoration of Immune Function
Immunity, Disease, and Longevity
Summary: Immune Models for Aging Research

THE UNIQUE VALUE OF THE IMMUNE SYSTEM as a model for age-dependent change in cell physiology comes from its nonsessile character: unlike other complex, multicomponent cellular systems in mammals, the immune system is made up principally of cells that recirculate through the blood and lymphoid vasculature. As a consequence, immunocytes can be prepared in single-cell suspensions, treated, separated, reassorted, and then recombined in culture or in adoptive hosts under circumstances that permit (nearly) full restoration of functional properties. Fortunately, gerontologists are not alone in their esteem for immunological models and are thus able to benefit from the industry of the larger cadre of basic immunologists whose insights and reagents have provided the needed infrastructure for progress in immunogerontology. The potential therapeutic implications of work on immunosenescence lend this subdiscipline additional urgency and earn it additional support from medically oriented funding agencies. This review summarizes current knowledge of how aging alters immune function, with particular emphasis on areas of investigation that have been especially fruitful or that have useful implications for other areas of gerontological cell biology or medical research.

Over the years immunologists have developed a technical vocabulary and an armament of acronyms that are often confusing to the uninitiated. This chapter uses specialized terms sparingly, but where they are indispensible they are defined at their first use. Table 21.1 presents these definitions for convenient reference, together with abbreviations of other terms used in the chapter.

Specific protective immune responses to foreign antigens depend on three varieties of cells: T lymphocytes, B lymphocytes, and a set of accessory cells (AC) that includes macrophages, dendritic cells, and under certain circumstances B lymphocytes. Immune responses to foreign proteins typically begin when the protein molecule is ingested, and then digested to smaller peptides, by a macrophage. Some of these peptide fragments are then bound noncovalently to proteins encoded by the major histocompatibility complex (Ia molecules). The Ia/peptide complexes relocate to the extracellular face of the plasma membrane, where they are subject to recognition by those T cells that express receptors (TCR) specifically complementary to the peptide-containing complex. Recognition of the immunogenic complex initiates a series of biochemical changes within the T cell, leading to proliferation, clonal expansion, and differentiation into several distinct kinds of effector T cell. In parallel to this T cell activation, B lymphocytes are also able to bind to the foreign protein via their own antigen-specific surface receptors—the immunoglobulin (Ig) proteins—digest the antigen, and generate their own Ia/peptide complexes for surface presentation. Once the activated T cells come in contact with B cells displaying the appropriate cognate Ia/peptide complex, they can deliver signals to the B cells ("T cell help") allowing them to

TABLE 21.1. *Some Useful Abbreviations and Definitions*

AC	Accessory cell: processes antigen and presents it to T cells and produces cytokines	IL-2R	IL-2 receptor
CD25	A component of the IL-2 receptor, thus a marker for activated T cells	IL-3	A helper T cell product with effects on several stages of hematopoiesis
CD3	Present on all T cells: the signal-transducing component of the T cell receptor	IL-4	A helper T cell product that acts on T cells, B cells, macrophages, etc.
CD4	Present on class II restricted helper T cells	IL-5	A helper T cell product with effects on B cell maturation
CD44	A marker for memory T cells, formerly known as PGP-1	IL-6	A cytokine produced by macrophages and many other cell types, with multiple effects on diverse cell types
CD45RA	A marker for naive T cells (human)	LAK	Lymphokine-activated killer: a cell, related to the NK cell, that develops in culture in the presence of IL-2 and can lyse some tumor targets
CD45RB	A marker for naive T cells (mouse)		
CD45RO	A marker for memory T cells (human)		
CD8	Present on class-I restricted cytotoxic T cells	LN	Lymph node
Con A	Concanavalin A, a plant lectin that stimulates T cell proliferation	MW	Molecular weight
		NK	Natural killer cell: present in unprimed animals and humans, can lyse some tumor cells and some virus-infected cell types
CTL	Cytotoxic T lymphocyte ("killer" cell)		
DTH	Delayed-type hyersensitivity: A T cell–mediated response often used to assess human immune function as a "skin test"	PBL	Peripheral blood lymphocytes
		PC	Phosphorylcholine: a principal antigen of pneumococcal cell walls
FDC	Follicular dendritic cell: an accessory cell found in lymphoid follicles in spleen and lymph nodes	PG	Prostaglandin
		P-Gp	P-glycoprotein: a 170 kDa plasma membrane pump that mediates multiple drug resistance in some tumor cells
GH	Growth hormone		
Ia	Immune-response-associated antigen; a class II histocompatibility protein present on accessory cells that can activate helper T cells	PHA	Phytohemagglutinin: a plant lectin that is mitogenic for T cells
		PK	Protein kinase
IFNγ	Interferon-γ: a product of T cells that has antiviral and macrophage-activating effects	PKC	Protein kinase C
		PPN	Phosphoprotein
Ig	Immunoglobulin (antibody): can be a surface protein (on B cells) or a secreted molecule	PMA	Phorbol myristate acetate (also known as TPA): a potent stimulator of PKC
IL	Interleukin	SEB	Staphylococcal enterotoxin B: A superantigen that stimulates T cells through the β chain of the T cell receptor
IL-1	A cytokine produced by macrophages (and many other cell types) with effects on helper T cells (and many other cell types)		
IL-2	A lymphokine produced by helper T cells: a T cell growth factor with effects on B cells, NK cells, and other cell types	TCR	T-cell receptor: most T cells express an αβ heterodimer, while a minority instead use a γδ heterodimer as receptor

undergo their own process of activation, proliferation, and eventual differentiation into antibody-secreting plasma cells. Several stages in B cell growth and maturation are dependent on and channeled by additional, soluble T cell products called "lymphokines," including interleukin-2 (IL-2), IL-4, and interferon-γ (IFNγ).

Responses to antigens produced intracellularly, including viral and neoplastic determinants, are more often mediated by the T cells alone. Peptide fragments of these moieties are presented by many cell types, including endothelial and parenchymal cells of most organs, in conjunction with class I histocompatibility molecules. T cell recognition of the presented peptides leads to proliferation and differentiation into effector cells, including cytotoxic T lymphocytes (CTL) that can lyse the infected or neoplastic target cells. Lymphokines produced by these activated T cells can also attract and activate cells of the macrophage series to generate delayed-type hypersensitivity (DTH) reactions.

In principle, then, immune senescence could reflect alterations in the functions of T cells, B cells, or AC. We will consider each of these possibilities in turn and then more global issues of immune restoration, the relation of immunosenescence to disease, and the interaction of the immune with other age-sensitive systems.

T LYMPHOCYTE SUBSETS

Helper (CD4) and Cytotoxic (CD8) T Cell Subsets

The realization that the T lymphocyte population actually consists of many different subpopulations with distinct expressions of surface marker molecules and differing functional capabilities led quickly to the hypothesis that aging might alter the relative proportions of cells within the T subsets. Initial work focused on the CD4 and CD8 markers. Among functionally mature, peripheral T cells, CD4 is present on cells of the "helper" subpopulation, which recognize foreign antigens in combination with Ia molecules and secrete lymphokines, including IL-2 and IL-4, to support the activities of B cells, other T cells, and nonlymphoid effectors. CD8, in contrast, is present on cells of the cytotoxic T cell subset, which recognizes foreign antigens in the context of the class I histocompatibility molecules and can differentiate into CTL effectors that can lyse tumor- or virus-infected targets. As a rule, mature T cells express either CD4 or CD8 but not both.

Many laboratories have now studied the proportions of CD4 and CD8 T cells in aging humans or rodents. Their reports are listed in Table 21.2. There is clearly a good deal of disagreement among the various groups: some report relative increases in CD4, others find relative increases in the CD8 subset, and still others observe no effect of age. Some of the variation may reflect differences in health status among populations. Hallgren et al. (115), for example, have noted differences in the proportions of cells expressing CD4 and CD8 antigens between young adults and apparently healthy elderly adults that were not observed in a subset of elderly adults selected for especially good health. In other cases, discrepancies may reflect variation among laboratories in the criteria used to distinguish marker-positive from marker-negative cells. Grossmann et al. (108), for example, have noted an increase with age in the fraction of human T cells that express low but detectable levels of CD8 but no change in the total number of CD8 cells; a laboratory that classified these $CD8^{dim}$ cells as $CD8^-$ might have drawn different conclusions from the same data. In still other cases, differences in the age composition of the young and old groups may account for some of the discrepancies: Armanini et al. (12), for example, found no overall difference between young and old humans in CD4 and CD8 proportions but did note a significant age-associated decline in the proportions of the CD4 cells within the elderly population (aged 62–97 yr). It should be noted, moreover, that the extent of the age effect on CD4 and CD8 cell numbers seems quite small even in cases where the change is statistically significant, and a consensus has emerged that changes in the proportions of CD4 and CD8 cells cannot in themselves account for much of the functional decline in protective immunity with age.

There is also some disagreement as to whether aging leads to any change in the density of marker molecules in those cells that express detectable levels of the markers. This question is of considerable importance, since CD3 (and its associated TCR), CD4, and CD8 all play important roles in T cell activation, and a change in molecular density might affect signalling efficacy. Most authors who have reported data on the fractions of marker-positive cells in aged individuals have not commented specifically on marker density, and the few reports of age-dependent shifts in marker density have not always been consistent. Thus CD3 density has been reported to be unchanged in human peripheral blood T cells (108, 292) and mouse spleen and lymph nodes (LN) (109) but to increase in both CD4 and CD8 subsets of mouse peripheral blood (109). Another group finds a decrease in CD3 density in very old mice, particularly in those mice that proliferate least well in response to anti-CD3 antibody (127), and a further report has suggested a decline in CD3 density in older humans (295). Similarly, while two groups (294, 295) find no change in CD4 or CD8 density in peripheral blood cells from healthy human donors, Grossmann et al. (108) report a shift toward cells with lower CD8 levels in humans, and Komuro et al. (165) also note a decline in CD8 density in a study of spleen cells from old mice. All of these studies have relied on flow cytometric methods that are not ideally suited for quantitative analyses, in that the level of fluorescence intensity per cell may not provide a linear index of marker antigen concentration per mm^2 of plasma membrane, let alone of the capacity of the marker itself to participate in target recognition and signal transduction.

Naive and Memory T Cell Subsets

Although these studies using CD4 and CD8 determinants have not provided especially helpful insights into functional immunosenescence, it has more recently become clear that aging does lead to a dramatic shift in the proportions of naive and memory T cells within the

TABLE 21.2. *Changes with Age in CD4 and CD8 T-Cell Subpopulations*

Result	Cell Type	Reference
No change	Human PBL	(108)
		(177)
		(184)
		(241)
		(12)
		(141)
No change	Mouse spleen	(266)
		(97)
		(127)
		(158)
No change	Rat spleen	(91)
		(60)
Increased CD4/CD8	Human PBL	(289)
		(204)
		(24)
		(295)
Increased CD4/CD8	Mouse spleen	(165)
Decreased CD4/C8	Human PBL	(39)
		(182)
		(285)
		(292)
Decreased CD4/CD8	Mouse spleen, LN, blood	(109)
	Mouse LN	(158)
	Mouse blood	(30)

CD4 and the CD8 pools. T lymphocytes that leave the thymus and reach the peripheral immune system are referred to as "naive" or "virgin" cells to indicate that they have not yet encountered the stimulating cognate antigen in an immunogenic form. Once such a cell is triggered by the antigen (in a complex with histocompatibility protein), it undergoes one or more rounds of clonal proliferation. Some of the progeny cells thus produced return to the resting state and are termed "memory" T cells. These memory cells help to insure a rapid and vigorous secondary immune response should the original antigen be encountered again in later life. It has become clear over the last 10 yr that naive and memory T cells differ not only in their history but also in their requirements for activation and in their functional abilities (3, 249), in particular their ability to secrete high levels of certain lymphokines, including IL-4, IL-5, and IFNγ.

Naive and memory T cells can be discriminated using antibodies to surface markers, and several groups have used immunofluorescence to show an age-related increase in the relative proportion of memory cells. Five reports have shown in humans a decline in the proportions of peripheral blood CD4 T cells that express the CD45RA marker characteristic of naive cells (59, 236, 263, 289, 295). Memory cells, quantitated by expression of the CD45RO or CD29 markers, have been reported to increase in parallel to the decline in naive cell number (236, 289). In a study of B6D2F$_1$ mice, Lerner et al. (173) observed an age-dependent increase in the proportion of T cells that express the CD44 marker characteristic of memory T cells and found that the increase affected both CD4 and CD8 cells within the blood, spleen, and LNs. Similar results using the CD44 marker have been reported by Grossmann et al. (109) for CD4 and CD8 cells in blood, spleen, and LN of WBB6F$_1$ mice; by Flurkey et al. (75) for splenic CD4 cells in (B6 × CBA)F$_1$ mice; and by Ernst et al. (67) for splenic CD4 cells in C57BL/6 mice. An age-dependent decrease in the proportion of mouse splenic CD4 cells expressing the CD45RB^{hi} phenotype of naive cells has also been reported (67, 75). CD4 T cells from older mice also express lower levels (67, 123) of another marker, 3G11, which, like CD45RB, is expressed preferentially by naive T cells within the CD4 subset (124).

Thus a large body of evidence now supports the idea that aged mice and humans accumulate T cells with the surface markers of memory T cells and have lower numbers of naive T cells. The extent of the shift is impressive, representing an increase of approximately 2.5-fold in the number and percentage of naive or memory T cells over the life span of the mouse (174). Further, such a shift is also developmentally plausible, since the maintenance of high levels of naive T cells has been shown to require the presence of the thymus (34), which undergoes morphological and functional involution with normal aging (97, 130, 214, 259). There is some controversy as to whether the conversion of cells with the naive phenotype to the memory phenotype is irreversible (19, 188), and some immunologists maintain that the CD45RO^{hi} and CD45RB^{lo} or CD45RA^{lo} cells should be considered to be in an activated (or transient) condition rather than in a permanently altered memory state. In this context it is worth noting that the proportion of T cells expressing Ia or CD25 (IL-2 receptor p55 chain) molecules, both of which are good markers of recent activation, does not seem to change with age in humans (154, 289). The extent to which the functional changes seen with aging can be attributed to the shift from naive to memory T cells and the topic of age-dependent change in function within the naive and memory populations will be considered below under T LYMPHOCYTE FUNCTION.

Other T Cell Subsets

One of the earliest observations (241) of an age-dependent change in T cell subset composition was of a threefold increase in the proportion of human peripheral blood T cells bearing the 3G5 glycoprotein; the functional implications of this change are unclear. CD4 T cells that express an antigen called "6C10," which apparently distinguishes cells specialized for IL-4 rather than IL-2 production (124), are said to increase somewhat during the first year of life (123), but the antibody has proven technically inconvenient for routine use and does not seem to have been further exploited for gerontological work.

Although the antigen-binding receptor of most T cells consists of a heterodimer encoded by the TCR α and β genes, a small proportion of peripheral T cells express instead a receptor encoded by the closely related γ and δ TCR genes (which are easily confused with, but distinct from, the γ and δ chains that make up part of the CD3 complex). The function, specificity, and activation requirements of the $\gamma\delta$ T cell subset are currently matters of controversy and investigation. The two initial reports on $\gamma\delta$ T cells in aging are in conflict and so not entirely satisfying. One group (222) examined human peripheral blood T cells, using an antibody to the $\alpha\beta$-heterodimer to infer the proportions of the reciprocal $\gamma\delta$ set; they found a decrease in $\gamma\delta$ T cells in a subset of elderly humans who sought medical attention. In contrast, a second study (185) inferred an increase in the proportion of $\gamma\delta$ T cells in mice (aged 8–40 wk) from an increase in the corresponding mRNA and in cells with the CD3$^+$/CD4$^-$/CD8$^-$ phenotype characteristic of $\gamma\delta$ cells. Thus neither of these reports measured $\gamma\delta$ T cells directly, and further descriptive work is clearly needed.

A recent study (307) has reported an increase with age in the proportion of mouse splenic CD4 and CD8

T cells that express high-level activity of the 170 kDa P-glycoprotein (P-Gp), the plasma membrane pump responsible for the multidrug-resistant phenotype of human and murine cancer cells. Interestingly, T cells with high levels of P-Gp function (not to be confused with the CD44 marker discussed above, which was originally referred to as "PGP-1") were found to make up an increasing proportion of both the naive and the memory T cell subsets with increasing age. Cells with high and low P-Gp activity can be separated by flow cytometry using dyes (such as rhodamine 123) that are removed from the cell by this plasma membrane pump, and thus differential expression of P-Gp may provide a way to subdivide the naive and memory populations into new subsets, transitions among which might prove to contribute to functional immunosenescence. Although the function of the P-Gp pump in normal (that is, nontransformed) cells is still uncertain, the observation (45) that P-Gp gene expression is regulated by *ras* and p53, both of which play critical roles in growth control and cell-cycle progression, is consistent with the idea that an age-dependent increase in P-Gp function could reflect underlying changes in T cell activation.

T LYMPHOCYTE FUNCTION

IL-2 Production

Work as early as the 1970s established that most in vivo and in vitro assays of T cell functional competence suffered an age-dependent decline in both rodents and humans. These classical reports included measures of proliferation induced by plant mitogens, such as concanavalin A (Con A) and phytohemagglutinin (PHA) (18, 140, 152, 215, 296) or antibodies to components of the TCR (215, 256); generation of cytotoxic effector cells (15); rejection of transplanted tumors (72, 98); DTH responses to protein antigens (209, 244); and ability to provide help for B lymphocytes (37). Lymphocyte proliferative responses to alloantigens (165, 294), to protein antigens (85), and to syngeneic stimuli (264) also seem to decline with age. T cell responses to superantigens, which stimulate the $\alpha\beta$ antigen-binding T cell receptor (TCR) through invariant determinants on the β chain and thus provide a model for activation directly through the TCR, have been variously reported to decline (75) or not to decline (97) with age in mice. This largely descriptive literature has been more extensively reviewed elsewhere (102, 122, 179, 283) and has led to the general consensus that the age-associated loss of T cell proliferative capacity in vitro may provide a useful model for the parallel decline in T cell function in intact animals.

The first critical mechanistic insight into age-related T cell proliferative failure came with the understanding that T cell division required the synthesis of both IL-2 and its receptor, both of which were made by activated, but not by resting, T cells. A large body of evidence has now shown that IL-2 production by human and mouse T cells clearly declines with age under most experimental culture conditions (55, 68, 90, 127, 141, 199, 211, 213, 279, 294). The data on rats are more equivocal: two groups have reported no effect of age on rat IL-2 production (104, 137), while three others have found evidence for an age-related decline analogous to that seen in mice and humans (54, 221, 310). One of these positive reports, however, did note that IL-2 synthesis was relatively well preserved in aged female rats, in comparison to aged male rats (54). In addition, one group documented an age-dependent loss of IL-2 production by rat splenocytes in allogeneic mixed lymphocyte cultures but saw no age effect in mitogen-stimulated cultures (91). It thus seems plausible that differences in colony health, sex, and estrous cycle status, as well as details of culture methodology, might in some cases be masking an age effect on IL-2 production in rats. IL-2 mRNA production by activated T cells has been reported to decline with age in humans (211) and mice (76), while two studies in rats have produced conflicting results, with one (310) but not the other (137) observing an age-dependent loss. In situ hybridization analysis showed that the decline in IL-2 mRNA levels in Con A–stimulated T cells from old mice represented a three-fold decline in the proportion of cells that could synthesize IL-2 mRNA, rather than a decline in the amount of mRNA produced by each productive cell (76). The evidence for a decline in IL-2 mRNA production suggests that the age-dependent decline in accumulation of IL-2 in culture supernatants is unlikely to represent differential absorption of IL-2 by the activated cells, a suggestion rendered even more implausible by the results of IL-2 receptor studies described below under response to IL-2. Hobbs et al. (135) have noted that immobilized anti-CD3 antibody, which in contrast to soluble anti-CD3 is a very potent and AC-independent stimulus for mouse CD4 cells, stimulates roughly equal levels of both IL-2 and IL-2 mRNA in cultures of splenic CD4 cells from old and young mice. This demonstration suggests that the age-related decline in IL-2 production observed under most conditions may be overcome by unusually strong stimuli that bypass the need for AC-linked co-stimuli.

Response to IL-2

The demonstration that aging diminished IL-2 production led to the idea that restoration of IL-2, for example, by addition of exogenous IL-2 to cultures or to the site of in vivo immune responses, might repair the age-dependent loss in protective immunity. Indeed, several reports have shown that addition of high doses of IL-2 to cultures (18, 93, 280) or injection of IL-2 during the course of an immune response in vivo (281) can overcome age-associated immune defects. In most cases, however, exogenous IL-2 restores only part, if any, of the diminished responsiveness of T cells from old donors (68, 90, 91, 103, 127, 192, 226, 294).

The failure of added IL-2 to overcome functional impairments in old T cells seems to represent a loss with age in the ability to generate functional IL-2 receptors (IL-2R). The IL-2R that transduces the IL-2 growth signal into activated T cells contains at least two components: a 55 kDa chain (termed IL-2Rα, TAC, or CD25) and a 70 kDA chain (IL-2Rβ). Although the β chain is present on the surface of many resting T cells and has itself a moderate affinity for IL-2, its affinity is not high enough to permit signal transduction at physiological IL-2 concentrations. The CD25 IL-2Rα chain, which can associate with the IL-2Rβ chain to produce the physiologically relevant high-affinity receptor, is not present on resting T cells but is synthesized over the first 6–48 h after stimulation to render the T cells IL-2-responsive. In the physiological immune response to antigens, the restriction of the functional IL-2R to T cells that have been stimulated by cognate antigen helps to prevent the inappropriate activation of bystander T cells.

The initial report of an age-related decline in IL-2 production by human T cells (90) also showed a decline with age in the ability of activated T cells to absorb IL-2, consistent with a diminution of IL-2R. Subsequent studies using antibodies to the IL-2Rα chain have documented an age-dependent decline in the proportion of mouse and human T cells that can express this component of the IL-2R after activation (68, 84, 217, 226, 293). The proportion of activated T cells that can respond to added IL-2 by proliferation and differentiation also declines with age (220, 227, 239). IL-2 binding experiments have been used to estimate the number of high-affinity receptors on activated T cells and have consistently shown a decline in this index of IL-2R expression (83, 212, 217, 239, 257); the change represents a decrease in the proportion of cells that can express the high-affinity receptor rather than in the number of high-affinity receptors per positive cell or the binding affinity of the receptor for its ligand (212, 257). Direct measurement of the 55 kDa and the 70 kDa subunits of the IL-2R has shown an age-dependent decline in both components (117), although this point is somewhat controversial (257). Thus the large majority of evidence suggests that aging leads to a decline not merely in IL-2 production but also in the production of T cells that can express the IL-2R needed for response to this growth factor. In this context the ability of IL-2 to restore immunocompetence in some assay systems seems most likely to represent a pharmacological effect, overcoming the defects in both IL-2 production and reactivity, rather than a physiological restoration of the single, rate-limiting factor missing from the aged immune system.

There is also some evidence that the response of even IL-2R$^+$ T cells to IL-2 may be impaired by aging. Three groups (212, 217, 278) have shown that IL-2R$^+$ lymphoblasts from older donors, freshly purified from nonresponding cells after activation in culture, proliferate less strongly in the presence of added IL-2 than cells prepared from parallel cultures from young donors. Whether the molecular defects that lead to diminished expression of IL-2 and IL-2R also contribute to the poor responsiveness of IL-2R$^+$ cells remains to be determined.

A recent report (141) has noted an unanticipated but suggestive relationship between IL-2 production and vaccination responses with a subset (31%) of elderly humans (mean age 86 yr) who had high levels of serum IL-2 compared to both young controls and other elderly subjects. Individuals with high serum IL-2 were found to generate low levels of IL-2 in vitro in cultures stimulated with PHA and phorbol myristate acetate (PMA). Furthermore, it was noted that the combination of high serum IL-2 and poor in vitro production of IL-2 tended to predict poor generation of antiinfluenza antibodies in response to influenza vaccination. Since vaccination (of intact subjects) was found to cause a transient depression in the levels of IL-2 produced in vitro after 15 (but not 30) days, these authors hypothesized that the poor responses of unvaccinated elderly subjects might be caused by an undiagnosed infection or other immunologically relevant event in the weeks just prior to in vitro assessment. The suggestion that depressed immune responsiveness may represent a common but transient state in the elderly is supported by a study (31) that showed especially poor test–retest correlations in PHA-induced proliferation using T cells from elderly donors, though this report did not attempt to relate changes in responsiveness to concurrent infections or other potential immunomodulatory events.

It seems very likely that these defects in IL-2 production and response account for much of the age-dependent loss in the T cell proliferative response in culture assays. To the extent—probably quite considerable—that T cell proliferation is critical to effective humoral and cell-mediated immune responses to microbes and (perhaps) tumors, age-associated defects in IL-2 production and effect may well explain a good part of the medically relevant immunodeficiency in the aged.

Production of Other Lymphokines

The question of whether aging also impairs the production by T cells of other lymphokines is of considerable practical and theoretical importance. On the one hand, one might predict that whatever factors interfere with the activation of resting T cells to produce IL-2 and IL-R would also inhibit the production of other lymphokines by activated T cells. On the other hand, the transition in the elderly from naive T cells to memory T cells might be predicted to lead to enhanced—or at least maintained—production of those lymphokines, including IL-4 and IFNγ, thought to be generated principally by memory T cells in young donors.

Furthermore, studies of cloned mouse CD4 T cell lines have shown that most such long-term cultures eventually develop one of two patterns of lymphokine production (206). So-called "T_{H1}" cells are said to produce predominantly IL-2 and IFNγ but only low levels of IL-4 and IL-5, while T_{H2} cells generate the opposite pattern. Although additional work, especially using human T cell clones, has shown that this initial dichotomizing classification was greatly oversimplified, there remains a good deal of evidence to suggest that circumstances (strains, cell lines, immunogens, stimuli) that promote IL-4 production often also increase secretion of a second T cell lymphokine, IL-5, that, like IL-4, has potent effects on B lymphocyte maturation. To complicate matters, memory T cells are thought to be particularly good producers of both IFNγ (a T_{H1} product) and IL-4 and IL-5 (T_{H2}) products. Thus observations of age-related changes in the production of IL-4, IL-5, and IFNγ—in addition to the work on IL-2 just reviewed—could help to test a number of models for cellular changes in immune aging. Evidence for increased production of IL-4, IL-5, and IFNγ, for example, would suggest that aged subjects might have high function in memory cells of both the T_{H1} and T_{H2} varieties, while alterations in the ratio of IL-4 and IL-5 to IFNγ might suggest a tilt toward the T_{H1} or T_{H2} pattern of differentiation. IL-4 and IFNγ play vital roles in regulating cell-mediated and humoral immune responses, and alterations of the balance between IL-4 mediated and IFNγ-mediated responses could thus have profound implications for antimicrobial and antineoplastic defenses in the elderly.

Studies of IL-4 production are most abundant and most pertinent to this problem but are not yet entirely consistent or convincing. Five groups (48, 55, 67, 169, 213) have shown an increase with age in IL-4 production by activated murine T cells. Studies of IL-4 mRNA production (135, 136) have also provided evidence for increased IL-4 production in short-term cultures of activated murine T cells. These researchers have inferred from their data that the increase with age in memory T cells (discussed above, see Naive and Memory T Cell Subsets) may lead to an increase in the products, including IL-4, of the memory T cell population. Three other studies, however, sound a note of caution. One recent report has documented a twofold decline in IL-4 production by T cells from older human donors (7), consistent with the age-dependent decline in IgE production and allergic symptomatology. One study (106), using immunofluorescent detection of mouse IL-4 in single cells after primary and secondary stimulation with PHA, showed a dramatic decline with age in production of IL-4 positive cells from both spleen and LN; the number of mice tested, however, was too small (2–5/point) to allow a powerful test of the statistical significance of the finding, and the authors concluded (perhaps too hastily) that there was no evidence for an alteration of IL-4 production with age. Lastly, Li and Miller (175a) have carried out a direct test of the hypothesis that memory cell accumulation leads to increased IL-4 production and have shown that purified CD4 memory T cells from old mice are significantly less able to secrete this lymphokine than memory T cells from younger donors. Unseparated CD4 T cells from old mice were also found to produce less IL-4 than CD4 cells from young mice in this study. The discrepancy between the earlier reports (48, 55, 67, 169, 213) and the data of Li and Miller may reflect differences in kinetics and availability of IL-2: the latter experiments employed a relatively long culture interval in which the impaired ability of the IL-4-producing cells from aged donors to proliferate in response to IL-2 could have been decisive. Since AC are known to differ in their ability to promote IL-2 vs. IL-4 secretion (124), it may well prove that the ability of T cells to generate IL-4 depends critically on the amount and variety of AC and other co-stimuli during the activation period. A good deal more work needs to be done before we can produce a coherent account of how aging alters the many factors that influence the level of IL-4 production.

Although the evidence is so far limited, two reports have shown an increase with age in production of IL-5 protein and mRNA (55, 136) by activated mouse T cells. Neither report can be considered definitive: one (55) used a very short culture period in serum-free medium, and the other (136) used immobilized anti-CD3 antigen in an AC-free culture. Additional studies using a variety of AC preparations and co-stimuli will be needed to clarify the effects of age on IL-5 production by T cells under other circumstances. Nonetheless, most of the evidence on IL-4 and IL-5 production to date is consistent with the suggestion that aging may increase the tendency of T cells to generate IL-4 and IL-5 rather than IL-2. Whether this change reflects an underlying alteration in cell type (for example, the shift from naive to memory T cells) or instead alterations in the stimulatory environment [as suggested by studies on dehydroepiandrosterone under effects to be discussed below under RESTORATION OF IMMUNE FUNCTION; see (55)], also needs further clarification.

Many laboratories have studied the effects of age on

IFNγ production, but the published studies are somewhat inconsistent. Table 21.3 summarizes much of the published work. Five groups listed in the table have found evidence for increased production of IFNγ (or in one case both IFNγ and its mRNA) by mouse splenic T cells in response to either Con A or anti-CD3 antibody. A sixth paper, however, observed a decline in IFNγ secretion in 24-h Con A cultures (48). A seventh report (106) used PHA to stimulate mouse cells and employed a "spot" enzyme-linked immunosorbent assay (ELISA) to count the number of IFNγ-producing T cells; the data suggested an increase with age in IFNγ-producing spleen or LN cells between 4 and 20 months but then a fivefold decline between 20 and 30 months of age. Although this study used only small numbers of animals (as few as three per age group) and thus did not produce statistically significant differences between groups, the large difference between 20- and 30-month-old animals suggests that studies of other stimulating agents might be informative. The studies of human peripheral blood cells shown in Table 21.3 are not consistent among themselves or with the mouse data. Con A, used for most of the murine studies, was in most reports found to induce less IFNγ in T cells from older humans (7). Of the three studies that used PHA, two reported an age-related decline in IFNγ and one reported no change with donor age. Three groups used PMA and a calcium ionophore to bypass receptor-dependent events and to stimulate intracellular pathways directly: of these three studies, one reported an increase, one a decrease, and one no change with age in production of IFNγ (or its mRNA). It is possible that the discrepancies between murine and human studies could reflect either species differences or differences attributable to the use of blood cells in human work and spleen (or LN) cells in murine work, but this suggestion clearly cannot account for the lack of agreement among the studies of human T cells. It seems safe to conclude that further insight into this theoretically and practically important question will require studies that pay careful attention to the effects of AC environment and to differences among stimuli, including stimuli that mimic natural antigens more closely than do mitogenic plant lectins.

Studies on production of IL-3, a T cell lymphokine with wide-ranging effects on the development of several hematopoietic cell lineages, have also generated inconsistent findings. An initial study (144) reported an age-related increase in murine IL-3 secretion and has been supported by a second study using PMA and calcium ionophore as stimuli (169). Three other groups, however, have reported an age-associated decline in IL-3 production (43, 55, 175). A sixth group (166) has reported a statistically significant but very small (10%) decline in IL-3 production in Con A–stimulated supernatants. Studies of IL-3 mRNA have included one report of an increase (136) in responses to immobilized anti-CD3 and one of a decrease (175) in responses to Con A. Limiting dilution studies have also been used to estimate the number of T cells that are able to produce IL-3 after stimulation. The first of these (169) argued that aging induced an increase in the frequency of IL-3-producing T cells (from 1/20,000 to 1/5,700 cells) in responses stimulated by PMA and a calcium ionophore. The second, in contrast, reported a fourfold decline in the proportion of IL-3-producing T cells (from 1/6 in young mice to 1/25 in old mice) in response to Con A (75); responses to the superantigen SEB were found to decline with age to a similar extent. It is clear from the reported frequencies that the methods used in the initial report (169) were able to detect only a very small fraction of the potential IL-3-secreting T cell population. There is even controversy over the class of T cell principally responsible for IL-3: analysis in high-density cultures suggests that the $CD44^{hi}$ memory cell is largely responsible for IL-3 production in response to anti-CD3, while limiting dilution cultures have shown a higher frequency of IL-3-producing cells within the $CD44^{lo}$, $CD45RB^{hi}$ naive subset (75). It is clear that the data so far confound consensus and that detailed analysis of stimulatory conditions, cell source, strain, and subset interactions may be required to clarify the situation.

Finally, two papers have examined the effects of aging on production of another T cell factor, granulocyte-macrophage colony-stimulating factor (GM-CSF), which helps to promote production of new myeloid cells. GM-CSF secretion to stimulated mouse T cells appears to decline with age in cultures activated by anti-CD3 (55) or Con A plus PMA (36).

TABLE 21.3. *Changes with Age in Secretion of IFNγ*

Species	Stimulus	Effect	Citation
Mouse	Con A	Increase	(126)
Mouse	Con A	Increase	(253)
Mouse	Con A	Increase	(158)
Mouse	Anti-CD3	Increase	(55)
Mouse	Anti-CD3	Increase*	(136)
Mouse	Con A	Decrease	(48)
Mouse	PHA	See Text	(106)
Human	PMA/ionophore	No change	(4)
Human	PHA	No change	(248)
Human	PMA/ionophore	Increase*	(47)
Human	Con A	Decrease	(4)
Human	PHA or virus	Decrease	(1)
Human	PHA, anti-CD3, PMA/ionophore	Decrease†	(87)

*Both IFNγ and its mRNA were measured. †Only mRNA measured.

In summary, the bulk of evidence to date suggests that aging of the immune system may increase the ability of T cells to produce IFNγ and IL-4 (both products of memory T cells, though of the T_{H1} and T_{H2} types, respectively) while decreasing IL-2 production. However, studies that compare responses in the presence of different stimuli and AC types show that this simple model is unlikely to account for all of the data, and more detailed analysis of how lymphokine secretion patterns are regulated in old and young T cells will be informative.

T Cell Activation

The studies reviewed above provide good evidence for an age-dependent decline in the production of IL-2 and in the expression of the high-affinity IL-2R needed for T cell clonal growth, though the issue of activation of T cells specialized for production of other lymphokines cannot yet be summarized as confidently. IL-2 and IL-2R production, however, are undetectable until approximately 6 h after the encounter of the T cell with an activator. Several research groups have wrestled with the question of whether diminution of IL-2 and IL-2R gene expression can be attributed to age-related alterations at earlier stages of the activation cascade.

Although the process by which resting lymphocytes respond to activators is far from fully understood, work over the last decade has emphasized several critical biochemical events that take place within the first few minutes of activation. These include (1) activation of protein kinases, including kinases that phosphorylate on serine or threonine residues and those that phosphorylate on tyrosine residues; (2) activation of phospholipase C, which in turn cleaves the membrane phospholipid phosphoinositol bisphosphate (PIP2) to generate diacylglycerol and inositol trisphosphate (IP_3); and (3) increases in intracellular free calcium ion levels ($[Ca]_i$) through a combination of IP_3-mediated release from intracellular stores and a change in the balance of Ca^{2+} exchange between the cytoplasm and the extracellular space. Activation of new gene expression begins within about 15 min and eventually involves alterations in the expression of at least 100 genes (51). Although T cell activation is, under normal circumstances, initiated by contact with an antigenic fragment on an antigen-presenting AC, it is also possible to stimulate T cell proliferation by a combination of two factors that act at intracellular sites: phorbol esters, such as PMA, which mimic diacylglycerol to activate protein kinase C, and a calcium ionophore that increases $[Ca]_i$ and thereby activates calcium-dependent processes, presumed to include calcium-dependent protein kinases (183). Many of the steps in T cell activation are thought to be induced or regulated by members of the *src* family of tyrosine-specific protein kinases, of which several *(lck, fyn)* are known to be tightly coupled to the T cell receptor/CD3 complex.

Activation of Protein Kinases. Protein kinases—enzymes that add phosphate groups to other proteins and in so doing often alter their function—fall into two broad classes. Approximately 99% of protein–phosphate groups are added on serine and threonine residues by one of a large number of kinases, among which protein kinase C (PKC) has been particularly well scrutinized. The tyrosine-specific protein kinases, although quantitatively less important in protein–phosphate balance, include several families of enzymes that play critical roles in cell, including T cell, activation.

Shi and Miller (265) have examined the ability of anti-CD3 antibody to alter the patterns of tyrosine-specific protein phosphorylation in T cells of aging mice, using antibody specific for phosphotyrosine groups. They found three proteins—molecular weight 40, 80, and 120 kd—to be rapidly phosphorylated on tyrosine within 0.5–2 min of addition of anti-CD3 antibody to T cells. Each of these three activation-sensitive substrates was found to be more vigorously phosphorylated in T cells from young than from old mice. The responses of all three proteins to Con A and to anti-TCR antibody were also shown to decline with age (except that the 40 kd substrate did not respond to anti-TCR antibody in mice of any age). Although the data showed a statistically significant effect of age, the effect was only about twofold, and it is not clear which (if any) of these three substrates might play a role in the activation process. Further work (Shi and Miller, 265a) has shown that both CD4 and CD8 cells are affected, though to different extents for different substrates, and that the age-related decline in the responses of CD4 cells can be attributed to the relatively poor response of CD4 memory cells (which accumulate with age) compared to cells in the CD4 naive subset. Additional progress will depend on the identification and analysis of specific substrates, tyrosine protein kinases and phosphatases known to be involved in T cell activation.

The activities of serine- and threonine-specific protein kinases have also been examined in T cells from young and old mice (228), using two-dimensional electrophoretic separation of labeled phosphoproteins (PPNs) present in T cell lysates before or after addition of a variety of activating stimuli. Of 16 PPNs that responded vigorously (at least fivefold increase in phosphorylation level within 10 min) to anti-CD3 antibody in T cells from 2-4- month-old mice, all 16 were found to be essentially unresponsive in T cells from mice 22–24- months old. A decline in responsiveness could be measured in each of the 16 PPN substrates in mice as young as 10–12 months, which progressively worsened over the second year of life. These changes could not be attributed simply to a disruption in signal transduction through the CD3 complex, since anti-CD3 induced the phosphorylation of a new set of three PPNs in T cells from old mice, PPNs that did not respond in T cells from young donors.

This report (228) also described experiments using PMA and ionomycin to stimulate intracellular targets thought to be involved in T cell activation, thus bypassing the TCR/CD3 complex. All ten of the PPNs phosphorylated in young T cells after exposure to ionomycin were found to be essentially unreactive in old T cells, demonstrating a defect in the ability to respond to increases in $[Ca]_i$. Of 12 PPNs that respond in young T cells to the PKC activator PMA, ten were found to be unresponsive in old T cells but two others were fully reactive, as were the three new PPNs that responded to anti-CD3 in old, but not in young, mice. These PMA data suggest that aged T cells may well have important alterations in PKC-dependent pathways but are not consistent with models that propose a simple decline in PKC level or functional responsiveness. Interestingly, the PPN defect could not be explained simply by the age-dependent accumulation of memory cells, since defects were noted in PPNs whose activation was apparently subset-specific. It is not clear, unfortunately, whether any of the substrates detected by the autoradiographic method play an important role in T cell activation, nor whether the changes seen contribute to age-associated defects in calcium signal generation or gene expression (see below under Calcium Signal Generation), and additional studies of specific kinases and substrates will be needed to flesh out this idea. The data of Proust et al. (238) on IP_3-mediated PKC translocation are also relevant to these issues and are discussed in the following section.

Calcium Signal Generation. Resting T cells have a $[Ca]_i$ of approximately 100 nM, that is, approximately 10^4-fold lower than the $[Ca^{2+}]$ of the extracellular space (1 mM). This difference is maintained through the function of an ATP-requiring membrane transporter with high affinity for intracellular Ca^{2+}, the "calcium pump" (38). Stimulation of T cells by receptor-dependent agonists, such as Con A, PHA, or antibody to the TCR/CD3 complex, leads within a few minutes to a two- to tenfold increase in $[Ca]_i$ and then a fall in $[Ca]_i$ to a plateau level, stable for hours, that is still somewhat above the baseline value seen in resting T cells. The initial surge of $[Ca]_i$ is thought to depend in part on IP_3-mediated Ca release from intracellular depots and in part on alterations in the balance of Ca^{2+} influx and efflux across the plasma membrane. The IP_3-dependent contribution to $[Ca]_i$ changes in normal T cells (as opposed to lymphoma cells) is typically less than 50% even at early stages and dwindles further after the first few minutes of activation (88). The factors that regulate Ca^{2+} influx are not well understood, though some data have hinted at the existence of calcium channels activated by a combination of IP_3 and its metabolite IP_4 (174) or by IP_3 alone (170). Thus in principle, $[Ca]_i$ level is subject to complex regulation by a combination of regulated Ca^{2+} influx, pump-mediated Ca^{2+} efflux, and interchange with intracellular stores.

The availability of dyes that permit the measurement of $[Ca]_i$ in living cells under nearly physiological conditions (111) has allowed assays for age-related changes in calcium signal generation. Three groups have reported a decline with age in the ability of T cells to increase $[Ca]_i$ after stimulation with either Con A (202, 238) or anti-CD3 (109) antibody. There is some discrepancy, however, in the nature of the proposed alteration one group finding a change in baseline Ca^{2+} levels but not in induced peak levels (238) and two others (109, 202) reporting alterations in peak levels that cannot be attributed to the small or absent changes in baseline Ca^{2+} levels. It seems possible that the reports of high baseline Ca^{2+} levels in T cells from old donors may relate to the use of an ionic lysis step in the T cell preparation method employed by one of these groups (238). The defect in calcium signal production affects both CD4 and CD8 cells, responding to Con A or to anti-CD3 antibody, in at least four strains of mouse (109, 110, 233). LN T cells seem to be somewhat more resistant to this age-associated defect than T cells from blood or spleen (109). In most circumstances, the decline in the average level of calcium signal generation seems to reflect a decline in the proportion of T cells that can generate a signal significantly above baseline levels (109, 233). Calcium responses of mouse T cells to some signals (PHA and anti-Ly6 antibody) seem to be unimpaired by aging (234).

Do defects in calcium signal generation contribute significantly to age-related declines in lymphokine production, lymphokine response, and cell proliferation? This question was tested by Philosophe and Miller (232), who used electronic cell sorting to prepare T cell subsets that differed in their ability to produce a change in $[Ca]_i$ after short-term activation by Con A, anti-CD3, or the calcium ionophore ionomycin. In all three cases, the pool of T cells whose $[Ca]_i$ levels changed most dramatically upon activation was found, by limit dilution analysis, to contain high levels of cells able to produce IL-2 and to respond to IL-2 by proliferation and differentiation into CTL effectors. Conversely, T cells that were unable to alter $[Ca]_i$ after stimulation did not produce or respond to IL-2. Furthermore, the calcium-resistant T-cell subset was shown to consist predominantly of memory T cells (233), though differences between naive and memory T cells in Con A-induced and anti-CD3-induced calcium signal generation were statistically significant for CD4 cells but not for CD8 cells. Since memory cells had been previously found to be hyporesponsive to Con A–mediated induction of IL-2 production, proliferation, and CTL production (173), the data suggested that these functional declines could be accounted for by the increased resistance of memory T cells, from mice of any age, to changes in [Ca]$_i$. An independent method that separated T cells based on differences in the ability to increase [Ca]$_i$ after ionomycin challenge also revealed functional defects in those T cells that were most resistant to increases in [Ca]$_i$ and showed that these calcium-resistant cells were predominantly of the memory phenotype (201). These results suggest that the accumulation of memory T cells, and more particularly resistance of memory T cells to calcium signal development, might underlie several important functional defects in aged T cell pools. However, a second group (110) has noted that the improved proliferative responses due to caloric restriction in aging mice cannot be attributed to alterations in calcium signals, which decline in aged mice regardless of dietary regimen, and studies of calcium signal development in human T cells do not provide support for the idea that alterations in calcium flux contribute greatly to immunosenescence in that species.

The bulk of the evidence reviewed above suggests that aging mice exhibit a decline in their ability to generate calcium signals and that this change contributes to some extent to the decline in T cell proliferative responses. Studies of human T cells, however, have not shown the same degree of consistency. Six groups have reported on mitogen-induced [Ca]$_i$ in human T cells. Two of these found no difference between old and young T cells in calcium signals after stimulation by PHA (177) or anti-CD3 antibody (215). Three other groups, however, have reported an age-dependent decline in the ability of human T cells to generate Ca^{2+} signals after stimulation by PHA or anti-CD3 or both (7, 113, 303), similar to the bulk of the data in mice. A sixth group (108) observed small, statistically significant declines in PHA- and anti-CD3-induced Ca^{2+} signals but noted that these affected primarily CD4 cells and thus could not account for proliferative defects, which affected primarily CD8 cells. These changes in calcium response do not seem to reflect any increase in [Ca]$_i$ levels in resting T cells from old mice in that baseline levels have been reported either to remain unaltered (108, 215, 303) or to decrease (113) in T cells from older donors. Experiments to assess the implications of calcium signal defects in aging humans have not yet been reported, although studies of T cells from young adults (254) have suggested that CD8 memory cells exhibit poor mitogen-induced proliferation despite excellent Ca^{2+} signals.

Inositol Phosphate Metabolism. Two studies of IP generation in T cells from old mice have produced conflicting results. Proust et al. (238) have reported a decline with age in Con A–stimulated IP$_3$ generation by mouse T cells; in this instance the alteration seemed to reflect a change in the amount of IP$_3$ synthesis in resting T cells rather than in the levels of synthesis after activation. IP$_3$ is produced by the action of phospholipase C on PIP2, and the other product of this cleavage, diacylglycerol, is thought to be the principal stimulus for PKC translocation from cytoplasm to membrane. This group (238) also noted an age-associated decline in Con A–induced PKC translocation, which suggests a decline in IP$_3$ production and is thus not entirely consistent with the observed absence of an age effect on peak IP$_3$ levels after stimulation. In contrast to the Proust report, Lerner et al. (172) found no effect of age on production of IP$_2$, IP$_3$, or IP$_4$ in mouse T cell responses to Con A. The one study (303) of IP$_3$ production by human T cells found no change with donor age in either baseline or stimulated IP$_3$ levels. The data (228) on PPN phosphorylation in response to PMA, summarized above, also suggest that the effects of aging on PKC activation by IP$_3$ and other regulators may be more complicated than a simple increase or decrease in enzyme function. None of the studies has yet addressed the question of age-related changes in response to internally generated IP$_3$ or IP$_4$, in particular their ability to alter calcium transport across the plasma membrane that seems to account for most of the calcium signal produced.

Calcium Influx and Efflux. The principal source of Ca^{2+} for T cell signal development is the extracellular space (88, 176). Calcium influx can be measured by exposing T cells to ^{45}Ca as a radiotracer and then measuring cell-associated calcium at various intervals after activation. Similar studies in other cell types have proven technically challenging, in particular because of rapid saturation of the very small internal pool of free calcium (6). An early study of calcium uptake by aging T cells (262) was rendered less useful in that it failed to include studies of peripheral T cells, adult animals, or time points earlier than 10 min after agonist addition. A more recent study (172) examined Ca^{2+} uptake into splenic T cells in the first 60 s after Con A addition. Ca^{2+} uptake was found to be linear between 20 and 60 s after ^{45}Ca addition, and thus the rate of change in cell-associated calcium over this interval was taken as an index of calcium influx rate. The "leak rate" of Ca^{2+} into unstimulated T cells was found to be slightly (about 50%) but consistently higher in older mice (172, 201), which might reflect alterations in either membrane permeability or baseline activity of a calcium channel. Con A led to a 4.5-fold increase in Ca^{2+} influx into young T cells but a much smaller increase in old T cells, and the final rate of influx into old T cells was only 55% that of the rate in T cells from young animals. These data suggest that the ability of Con A to induce Ca^{2+} influx is substantially diminished in T cells from older mice. Additional insight into the mechanism of this change will depend on new ideas about the role of protein kinases and inositol metabolites in the control of calcium influx channels. It seems unlikely, however, that changes in Ca^{2+} influx rate can account for much of the age effect on calcium concentrations, since earlier work (82) has shown that the mitogen-induced change in influx rates is very transient and that influx has returned to baseline levels at times (5 min after agonist addition) when $[Ca]_i$ levels are still well above baseline.

The activity of the high-affinity calcium pump responsible for calcium efflux is not easily measured in intact cells: the simple approach of following ^{45}Ca release from labeled cells provides data not about calcium efflux per se but about the ability of intracellular pools (protein, mitochondrial, and endoplasmic) to replenish the free cytoplasmic pool. An indirect method of estimating calcium pump activity, however, is based on the ability of the cell to maintain its $[Ca]_i$ in the face of ionomycin-facilitated Ca^{2+} influx (203). The steady-state $[Ca]_i$ level attained in the presence of very low ionomycin doses was found to be regulated by agents (PKC agonists and calmodulin antagonists) known to control calcium pump function. In experiments using this indirect ionomycin challenge method, T cells from old mice were found (203) to be more resistant than T cells from young animals to ionomycin-induced changes in $[Ca]_i$, consistent with the hypothesis that aging leads to an increase in pump activity or sensitivity to changes in $[Ca]_i$. Flow cytometric work later showed that these ionomycin-resistant T cells were predominantly in the memory subset of both CD4 and CD8 cells (233) and that isolated ionomycin-resistant T cells from old or young mice were relatively depleted of functional helper, cytotoxic, and proliferative cells (232). A second group has reported that ionomycin induces a greater change in $[Ca]_i$ in T cells from young than from old mice (216), though two other reports have found no such age effect in studies of rats (79) and humans (303).

The use of calcium ionophores (usually ionomycin or A23187) in combination with phorbol esters to stimulate T cell proliferation or gene expression provides an independent, if somewhat indirect, approach to the question of whether alterations in the generation of internal signals (calcium increases, PKC activation) are critical to T cell immunodeficiency. Several groups (193, 213, 216, 282) have found that mixtures of PMA and ionomycin or A23187 can usually induce levels of proliferation, IL-2 production, or IL-2R expression substantially above those induced by receptor-dependent ligands like Con A or anti-CD3 antibody in mice. The difference between young and old T cells is often less in response to PMA plus ionophore than to receptor-dependent stimuli, suggesting that the components of the activation process that lie downstream from the generation of calcium and diacylglycerol may be relatively unimpaired by aging. Studies of human T cells using PMA and ionomycin to stimulate proliferation or IL-2 production have also suggested that aged T cells are often less responsive to these agonists, but the difference between old and young donors has ranged from twofold (47) to tenfold (215). The latter of these papers also reported that the PMA-associated reduction in induced calcium signals was more severe in young than in old donors, suggesting that PKC-mediated signals are relatively diminished in old T cells. It should be understood, however, that the internal signals induced by ionophores and phorbol esters are likely to be far stronger and longer-lasting than those generated under physiological conditions by antigen or in vitro by receptor-dependent ligands. Experiments with PMA and ionophores are thus hard to interpret with much confidence, because these agents might be expected either to induce feedback effects not seen in more natural responses or to overcome (and therefore obscure) downstream defects that actually do affect T cells from older donors. It is worth noting that two groups (193, 216) have found that the maximal stimulatory effects of ionomycin on proliferation require higher ionophore concentrations in old than in young mice, consistent with the idea that T cells from older donors may be resistant to ionomycin-induced changes in calcium concentrations. Similarly, early work has shown that PHA-induced human T cell proliferation from old donors is especially susceptible to inhibition by calcium chelators and channel blockers (155).

In most species calcium ionophores do not by themselves induce strong T cell proliferation, which requires co-stimulation by a PKC activator. In rats, however, A23187 or ionomycin do seem to induce T cell proliferation, provided that the growth medium contains a reducing agent (for example, reduced glutathione or 2-mercaptoethanol). Curiously, this proliferation does not seem to involve synthesis of either IL-2 or IL-4 and is substantially higher in old than in young rats (79). In this species there does not appear to be a difference between old and young animals in the level of ionomycin-induced changes in $[Ca]_i$ (79). The biochemical bases for these unusual phenomena and their possible relationship to differences in IL-2 production between mice and rats await further study.

Control of Membrane Potential. T-cell activation also involves alterations in cellular control of pH, size, and K^+ ion concentrations through a complex set of interacting pumps and channels. Resting T cells have a membrane potential (inside negative) whose magnitude is controlled largely by the factors that regulate K^+ ion transport, including the ATP-dependent Na^+/K^+-pump that maintains the high K^+/Na^+- ratio in the intracellular space. Using vital dyes whose distribution is sensitive to membrane potential, Witkowski and Micklem (305) noted that the T cells of old mice had a relatively lower (that is, less negative) membrane potential than T cells from younger animals and argued that this could result from the diminished activity of the Na^+/K^+-pump, previously demonstrated in T cells from older humans (308). In other laboratories, the resting potential in T cells from older human donors has, however, variously been reported to decrease (113), increase (292), or remain unchanged (53). The response of potential to activating agents has also been reported to be affected by aging. In young mice, for example, Con A induces an initial depolarization, which returns to baseline within 5 min, while in old mice, Con A leads to a paradoxical hyperpolarization (306); a similar age effect has also been noted in human T cells (113). Calcium ionophores induce a hyperpolarization in mouse T cells, but this change seems to be slower in T cells of old mice (306) and humans (292). These observations are consistent with an age-related loss in Ca^{2+}-dependent K^+ channels but might also reflect an increased activity of the calcium pump, as discussed above. The significance of these differences in resting potential and in changes in potential after activation is still obscure and will require new insights into the role of membrane potential in the regulation of T cell activation.

Gene Expression. The signals generated by changes in $[Ca]_i$, protein kinase function, and (perhaps) membrane potential lead, by still poorly understood pathways, to the transcription and translation of genes whose products are critical for the activation, proliferation, and functional differentiation of the resting T cell. Studies of production of mRNA for lymphokines and lymphokine receptors have been reviewed above, see under Production of Other Lymphokines, and have in general supported the sensible notion that diminished gene expression may account for diminished production of the key proteins these genes encode during the first day or two after activation. It seems likely, however, that the genes for lymphokine and receptor production are themselves controlled by transcriptional factors, including the products of the protooncogenes c-*fos* and c-*myc*, among others, whose synthesis is itself regulated by early intracellular transitions. There is some evidence that aging leads to alterations in expression of these early, activation-sensitive genes, although there is still considerable disagreement about the details. Mouse T cells activated by Con A (33) and human T cells activated by PHA (86) have been reported to generate peak levels of c-*myc* mRNA and protein (235) that are lower in cells from older donors. Expression of the c-myb protein, which is produced later than c-myc and seems to be regulated at a later stage of the activation cascade, is also reported to decline with age in PHA-treated human T cells (235). One of these studies (86) noted, using in situ hybridization, that the amount of c-*myc* mRNA per positive cell did not seem to decline with age, suggesting that the change reflected a decline in the proportion of reactive cells, in good agreement with the data on c-myc and c-myb protein (235), as well as with studies of IL-2, IL-2R, and calcium signal generation. The two studies that have included measures of gene transcription (as opposed to mRNA accumulation) reached opposite conclusions, with one (86) finding evidence for an age-dependent change in primary transcript production and the other (33) suggesting instead an alteration in the rate of conversion of primary transcripts to mature mRNA molecules. A great deal of additional work will be needed to extend these initial observations to a comprehensive analysis of the early activation genes and to connect changes to defects in both earlier and later steps of the activation process. In this context it is worth noting that PMA and ionomycin seem to induce equal levels of c-*myc* mRNA in human T cells, although these conditions seem to induce a more rapid rate of mRNA turnover in young than in old T cells (57).

Clonal Diversity: A "Mosaic" Model for T Cell Senescence

Many of the reports cited above have included evidence that the age-related decline in T cell responsiveness does not take the form of a progressive change that affects each cell in parallel but instead involves a change—usually a decline—in the proportion of T cells that can generate a functional effect. In many, though not all, cases there is little or no effect of age on the strength of the response among those (few) cells that can respond. This general point has been illustrated by limiting dilution analyses of helper, cytotoxic, and proliferative functions in response to alloantigens, lectins, and superantigens (75, 192, 220, 294); by in situ hybridization analysis of IL-2 production (76) and expression of the c-*myc* protooncogene (86); by flow cytometric studies of IL-2R and other early activation antigens (68, 84, 293); and by studies of calcium signal generation at the single cell level (109, 202, 233). These data led to the suggestion that the immune system might be seen as a "mosaic" of responsive and hyporesponsive cells, with the latter becoming more frequent at advanced ages. Some of this transition seems to reflect the age-related accumulation of memory T cells and the corresponding depletion of naive T cells, with their greater propensity for IL-2 production and calcium signal development (194). The suggestion that the memory cells which accumulate in old mice may remain highly competent for some purposes, including IL-4 production, has led to the idea that the aging immune system ought to be viewed as different rather than simply defective, thus prompting a reassessment of the original mosaic model. In my view, the notion that some aspects of immune function may be preferentially retained or even exaggerated in the aging immune system deserves enthusiastic exploration but should not cause investigators to lose sight of the need to find an explanation for the well-documented loss of protective immunity to infections and perhaps tumors discussed in more detail later in this chapter. The old immune system is defective, and the evidence that shifts in the relative proportion of its component cell types contribute to the loss of protective function seems strong though not yet irrefutable. The idea that a shift among component cell types might contribute to age-related declines in the functions of other organs and tissues also seems worthy of further exploration.

T CELL DEVELOPMENT

The development of mature T cells from their progenitors is a complex process regulated at multiple stages. Pluripotent bone marrow stem cells give rise to prothymocytes, which can migrate to the thymus gland and therein undergo a process of proliferation, differentiation, functional maturation, and cell selection that results in the apoptotic death of the 95%–99% of cells whose stochastically chosen TCR sequence is either too autoreactive or insufficiently able to recognize antigenic complexes on antigen-presenting cells. The few cells with acceptable TCRs then migrate to the peripheral immune organs (spleen, LN, blood, and marrow), where their survival, life span, and clonal expansion are further regulated by poorly understood mechanisms (245, 272). Of the three major stages in the production of mature T cells, most attention has been paid to the intrathymic stage, some to the prethymic stage, and all too little to the postthymic aspects.

Thymic Involution

The dramatic age-dependent involution of the thymus gland, marked by declines in organ weight, organ cellularity, and ratio of parenchyma to fat and connective tissue is certainly the most striking morphological change in the aging immune system, and it has long seemed reasonable that this shrinkage might contribute to functional immunosenescence (122). In normal young adults, about 3% of thymocytes have the double negative (that is, $CD4^-$, $CD8^-$) phenotype characteristic of the earliest cells in the developmental sequence. Most thymocytes are double positive (that is, $CD4^+$, $CD8^+$), and it is during this stage that T cell gene rearrangements and selection take place. About 10%–15% of the cells in a young adult thymus are single positive (that is, they express either CD4 or CD8 but not both); these cells lie primarily in the inner medullary area of the gland and are in most respects functionally mature. Recent work has emphasized changes in the relative proportions of thymocytes whose position along this developmental lineage can be assessed by expression of CD4 and CD8 markers. Thus aging in mice leads to a relative decline in the proportions of thymocytes with the intermediate, double positive phenotype and a relative increase in the proportions of both the least mature (double negative) and the most mature (single positive) cells (65, 97). An analysis of human thymic specimens obtained at cardiac surgery from individuals 0–40 yr of age has noted a decline with age in the size of the cortical area (mostly double positives) compared to the medullary area (214) and is thus consistent with the mouse data.

The functional implications of thymic involution have been assessed in several ways, all of them informative but none of them entirely satisfactory. Thus direct fluorescence labeling of thymus cells has shown that the number of cells that reach the periphery drops about 20-fold within the first quarter of the mouse life span (259). The export rate in mature animals, however, is far too low to account for the known turnover of cells within the periphery, and it seems likely that regulation of peripheral self-renewal also contributes to immunosenescence to a great extent. The functional capacities of thymus glands from donors of different ages have also been tested directly by transplantation studies: transplanted thymuses from newborn and very young (< 3 months) mice were found to be able to support the differentiation of bone marrow cells in a young host into immunocompetent cells, while thymuses of donors as young as 3 months of age were severely impaired in this regard, with a further decline evident at 12 and 24 months of age (129). More recent experiments, involving thymic transplants into athymic (nude) host mice, have suggested that the capacity to produce T cells declines by about 50% within the first 4 wk of life but does not decline further thereafter (290); this seems quite surprising in view of the earlier results (129, 259). Two groups have suggested that the aged thymus may show a greater defect in production of CD8 cells than of CD4 cells (97, 290), although (as reviewed above under Lymphocyte Subsets) the ratio of CD8 to CD4 cells does not show a consistent or dramatic change in aging mice or humans. All in all, the hypothesis that thymic involution is the fundamental cause of T cell immunosenescence, though still plausible, may be considered far from certain, particularly in view of the relatively mild effects of thymectomy in adult life (148, 191, 267) and the evidence that thymus-independent peripheral self-renewal plays a major role in maintenance of the peripheral T cell pool (200, 245). Analysis of peripheral immunity in strains of rat (133) and mouse (M. Kronenberg, personal communication) that show a retardation of morphological thymic involution may throw additional light on this debate.

These studies have dealt largely with quantitative changes in thymic function rather than alteration in the ability of the thymus to mold the T cell recognition repertoire through positive and negative selection of cells based on their TCR antigen-binding receptors, which are heterodimers of α and β chains. A comprehensive analysis (97) of Vβ gene utilization has shown that there is no major change in the relative abundance of the different Vβ chains in mouse thymus or in splenic CD4 or CD8 subsets. No comparable survey of Vα expression has yet been carried out. The force of negative selection, in which the thymus weeds out T cells expressing specific Vβ chains that bind too well to autologous molecules, was also reported not to become any less efficient with age (97). There is very little evidence, moreover, on the details of TCR gene expression at finer levels of resolution than mere β chain selection, and it is possible that subtle shifts in gene recombination or selection are yet to be discovered. There is some indirect evidence (258), for example, for age-related alterations in T cell specificities, although this report is based largely upon analysis of T cell clones whose properties may not accurately reflect those of the initial starting population, particularly in that only a minority of the clones studied expressed the $\alpha\beta$ TCR found on most mature peripheral T cells. Similarly, a study of CTL responses to fibrosarcoma tumors (72) provided suggestive but indirect evidence for an alteration in the fine specificity of CD8 effectors but relied upon arcane methodology not easily extended to other systems.

Prothymocytes

The loss of thymic function in older individuals could reflect a decline in the ability of the bone marrow to supply functional prothymocytes to the thymic stroma. Although aging seems to dramatically diminish the number of prothymocytes in the spleen (17, 147), marrow prothymocyte numbers seem to remain unaltered (17). Nonetheless, when competitive repopulation assays are used to detect subtler effects of age on prothymocyte function, marrow from older mice is less able to initiate thymocyte maturation after inoculation into thymic organ rudiments in an in vitro organ culture system (66), and limit dilution analysis of this system suggests a loss with age in functional prothymocyte numbers within the marrow. When marrow is tested for its ability to regenerate peripheral immune function in an intact host mouse, the results appear to vary depending in part on the length of time that elapses between the time of marrow transplantation and the time of assessment of its functional progeny. Thus assays of peripheral function carried out within a few months after bone marrow transplantation into irradiated recipients usually reveal no difference between marrow from old and from young donors (105, 120). Experiments that examine immune function at extended posttransplant intervals, however, often (14, 105, 131), though not invariably (120), reveal an age-dependent loss of immune function in recipients of marrow from older donors. Old marrow also appears to function less well than young marrow when tested in old recipients, even when thymic function is provided by a grafted infant thymus (13). Recent work of Harrison's group (121) has suggested that the most primitive hematopoietic stem cells, that is, those capable of sustained reconstitution of myeloid, erythroid, and lymphoid lineages, do not decrease in frequency with age, though aging may lead to an increase in a subset of stem cells whose capacity for very long-term reconstitution is somewhat lower than that of the most primitive stem cells.

In summary, there is not as yet any definitive developmental explanation for the dramatic functional and phenotypic changes seen in the T cell component of the peripheral immune system of aging rodents and humans. Although thymic involution seems likely to play a critical role, we still know essentially nothing about the mechanism of the involutionary process or the relative significance of postthymic maturation events.

B LYMPHOCYTES

B Cell Number and Subsets

Most surveys find little evidence for a dramatic effect of age on the number of B lymphocytes in either human blood (289) or mouse spleen (152, 229, 275), although exceptions have been noted in some strains of mouse (74). There are, however, reports of alterations in subsets of B cells whose functional capabilities are still somewhat uncertain. Thus Subbarao et al. (275) distinguished three B cell subsets based on alterations in the ratio of surface IgM to IgD and noted that, although there were no major changes with age in the relative proportions of these subsets, individual old mice were much more likely than younger mice to have an unusually high or low proportion of one or more B cell subtypes. Similarly, the proportion of B cells that express surface Ia antigens was found to not alter, on average, with age, but the proportion of individual mice with unusually high or low levels of Ia$^+$ B cells did increase in older mice. The absence of an age effect on the average levels of Ia expression has also been noted by a second group (264), while a third group (266) observed an increase in Ia expression in murine spleen cells but did not determine if this reflected changes in B cells or in the nonlymphoid AC population. B cells that express high levels of both surface Ig and the Ly5 marker antigen, which are thought to represent a late stage in B cell maturation, are said to increase with age in mouse bone marrow (242), although data for spleen, LN, and blood were not reported. There is a report (301) of a twofold increase with age in the fraction of peritoneal B cells expressing the CD5 antigen characteristically present on a subset of autoantibody-producing, leukemia-prone B cells, but it is unclear whether this change represents a normal senescent change or a prodrome of a form of B cell malignancy common at advanced ages in the mouse strain used.

Proliferation and Antibody Production

The principal challenge for those who wish to test the effects of aging on B lymphocyte function is to design experiments in such a way as to avoid the objection that any differences actually reflect the effects of T cells that may be present in the B cell preparation under examination. Several early attempts relied on so-called T-independent antigens, which are known to be able to stimulate B cells even in the absence of T cells, but these reports failed to account for the possibility that T cells, even if not necessary for the response, could nonetheless alter its characteristics by help or suppression. Two other approaches have proven more useful, one relying on tests of rigorously T-depleted B cell preparations and the other providing the B cells from old or young donors with equal amounts of T cell help, in the form of either purified T cells or T cell clones. Table 21.4 lists the results of these classical studies. About half of the studies report evidence for an age-dependent decline in intrinsic B cell function; the others find no evidence for any effect of age, and none reports an increase in older mice or humans. The mouse data show some evidence for strain-specific effects. Thus IgM responses to a pneumococcal vaccine are said to decrease with age in C57BL/6 mice but to increase with age in BALB/c mice (218); possible reasons for the unusual response to this antigen will be considered below. In one instance (275) aging was found to lead to an increase in the proportion of mice whose B cells were relatively unresponsive to either anti-IgM antibody or anti-Lyb2 antibody; unre-

TABLE 21.4. *Tests for Intrinsic B-Lymphocyte Function*

Species	Stimulus	Assay	Result	Citation
Mouse	LPS	Proliferation	Decline	(2)
Mouse	LPS	Proliferation	No change	(269)
Mouse	Anti-Ig	Proliferation	Decline	(261)
Mouse	Fc fragments + T	Proliferation	Decline	(205)
Human	Anti-Ig	Proliferation	No change	(300)
Human	Staphylococcus	Proliferation	Decline	(116)
Rat	Anti-Ig	Proliferation	No change	(91)
Mouse	LPS	Antibody	No change	(269)
Mouse	Fc fragments + T	Antibody	Decline	(205)
Mouse	Protein Ag + T	Antibody	Decline	(37)
Mouse	Protein Ag + T-cell clone	Antibody	No change	(269)
Human	Various mitogens	Ig secretion	Decline	(309)
Human	Pokeweed mitogen	Ig secretion	Decline	(39)
Human	Pokeweed mitogen	Ig secretion	No change	(159)
Human	Tetanus toxoid	Ig secretion	Decline	(160)

sponsive mice were more frequent among those with unusually low levels of a specific B cell subset with a high IgD/IgM ratio.

Several groups have explored the question of whether altered B cell responsiveness to specific lymphokines can account for any of the functional defects. An initial study (284) of the effect of IL-4 in mice documented an age-related decline in three aspects of B cell response: Ia expression, proliferation, and IgE production. T cell proliferation in response to PMA and IL-4 was, however, unimpaired. In contrast, a study of the responses of IgE-secreting human B cells to IL-4 found no age effect (7). Neither purified IL-2 nor IL-4 was found to be able to restore the age-associated decline in human B cell-proliferative responses to a variety of mitogens (304), although a poorly characterized mixture of B cell growth factors was able to restore responsiveness to one of the activators (anti-IgM coupled to insoluble beads). Ig production by these human B cells in response to anti-IgM beads produced unexpected results: IL-4 appeared to induce higher levels of IgM production by old B cells, in contrast to mouse results (284), while IL-2 tended to decrease production of IgG only in B cells from old donors (304). It is clear that a good deal of additional work, using purified B cells at various stages of activation in combinations of T cells and purified lymphokines, will be needed to generate a coherent picture of the effects of age on lymphokine reactivity.

Many studies of T cells (reviewed above) have supported a mosaic model for immunosenescence in which the proportion of cells able to generate some specific functional response declines more dramatically with age than the amount of response per responding cell. Studies of B cell proliferation by limit dilution have been fewer and less consistent. An initial study (8) demonstrated a 95% decline in the proportion of mouse B cells that could respond to lipopolysaccharide (LPS) by proliferation. A second group, however, found no such age effect in tests of the original and three other mouse strains (139). There is at present no obvious explanation for this discrepancy. Another in vitro clonal assay system, which uses filter paper disks in an LPS-stimulated B cell colony assay, has shown a modest (50%–70%) decline in the proportion of mouse splenic B cells that can form colonies, as well as a twofold reduction in average colony size (255). In a third approach, Zharhary and Klinman (313) have used a "splenic focus" method for counting the proportion of B cells that can react to a specific antigen, given saturating amounts of T cell help, after injection into a recipient mouse; their data show that the frequency of these responsive B cells declines approximately twofold in older mice for a range of arbitrarily chosen synthetic haptens. The frequency of responders for influenza antigens, however, was found to not change with age (314), and the response to a pneumococcal antigen, phosphorylcholine, was found to increase with age (315) for reasons that will be discussed further below. Thus it is not yet clear whether a decline in responsive B cell frequency makes an important contribution to the immunodeficiency of aging nor is there currently any insight into the developmental or phenotypic differences between responsive and nonresponsive B cells in the older subject.

Knowledge about the biochemistry of B cell activation has lagged several years behind the T cell story, and there is so far only a single report of age-related changes in the early phases of the B cell response. Whisler et al. (302) have reported a loss with age in the ability of human B cells to generate calcium signals after stimulation by anti-IgM or staphylococcal protein A; the changes reflected alterations in the peak and plateau levels after stimulation but not in the baseline levels of resting cells. This group also found a combination of anti-IgM and a phorbol ester–induced phosphorylation of PPNs at 35–37 kd and 43 kd, the latter of which was phosphorylated at least partially on tyrosine residues. Phosphorylation of both substrates was reduced approximately 50% in B cells from older donors in response to anti-IgM plus phorbol ester. Some, but not all, older subjects also exhibited a defect in the ability to translocate PKC from cytosol in response to anti-IgM, but neither total nor membrane PKC levels was measured. Additional work along these lines may help to define a molecular basis for age-related changes in B cell activation, though it must be noted that physiological B cell responses usually involve the delivery of signals by T cells in direct contact with the B cell surface and that so far little is known about the nature and consequences of these contact-mediated signals even in cells from young donors.

Antibodies: Levels, Repertoire, and Autoreactivity

The result of B cell activation, proliferation, and differentiation is antibody secretion by the plasma cells that emerge at the end of the B cell maturation pathway. An early, comprehensive analysis (178) showed little obvious change with age in human serum antibody concentrations: no change in IgM levels, less than a 10% change in IgG levels over the life span, and a slow upward trend in IgA levels that amounted to about a 25% increase between ages 20 and the 80 yr. In contrast, a study of several mouse strains produced evidence (94) for much larger age-associated increases in IgM and all four subclasses of IgG; similar increases have been reported for C3H mice in another colony as well (56). Another study of mouse Ig isotypes (5), however, found no major age effect on Ig levels, except for an increase in IgG2a and a decrease in IgG1 in aged C3H mice and a decrease in IgG3 levels in aged C57BL/6 mice; this report did not, however, provide enough information to evaluate the replicability of the results. It may be, then, that aging leads to an increase in Ig levels in some mouse strains, but more work is needed to determine if this suggestion can be confirmed and, if so, whether the unexpectedly large age effect is related to underlying alterations in B cell biology and immune reactivity.

Just as work with probes specific for TCR variable genes has shown no systematic effect of age on V gene usage (97), analogous studies in B cells have, in general, yielded null results in individual mouse strains on the average expression of heavy- and light-chain variable region genes in LPS-responsive clones of splenic B cells (255); the sole exception was a 2.4-fold increase in the use of the V_HS107 gene by aging BALB/c mice.

Despite these negative results, it is possible that aging could result in alterations of antibody gene assembly and selection that are not obvious at the level of V gene family expression. Analysis of the response of BALB/c mice to phosphorylcholine (PC), a major immunogen present on pneumococci, has been particularly provocative. In young mice, the overwhelming majority of the anti-PC antibodies produced after immunization utilize a single combination of heavy- and light-chain variable region genes; this unusually restricted response results in the production of antibodies that can themselves be detected immunochemically, using antiidiotypic antibodies. Thus nearly all of the anti-PC antibody molecules produced by young BALB/c mice react with the T15 antiidiotype antibody, and these anti-PC antibodies are thus said to be T15-positive. We have noted the atypical increase with age in the frequency of anti-PC-reactive B cells (315). Further analysis of this system (243) at the level of V_H gene utilization noted both an increase with age in the proportion of B cells that express the particular V_H gene (V_HS107) used in the restricted anti-PC response of young mice (see also ref. 255). More remarkably, this group also noted that the anti-PC antibodies of old mice frequently utilized V_H gene segments that were essentially absent from the anti-PC response of young and middle-aged animals. This set of experiments tested V gene usage in a population of bone marrow B cell progenitors at a stage of B cell development at which surface antibody is not yet expressed; the unusual preponderance of non-V_HS107 gene segments must therefore reflect a still obscure selective process that works at an antigen-independent step in the B cell maturation process. A later study (219) established that the shift in V gene usage in the anti-PC response affected mature B cells (as tested by analysis of B cell hybrids) in mice of three strains (BALB/c, C57BL/6, and D1.LP) and involved increasing diversity of the light chain used in anti-PC responses (V_κ22 in young mice). The anti-PC system clearly deserves a good deal of further exploration, in the hope that its analysis will throw light on the details of V gene selection and how these genes are affected by aging, even though it is far from clear whether the age-dependent changes apply to more typical antigens or affect protective immune defenses in the elderly.

The generation of B cell antibody diversity does not depend on selection of combinations of variable region genes alone but employs a range of other mechanisms, including splicing in of other small protein-coding regions encoded by the D- and J-gene segments; splice-site ambiguities that can alter amino acid sequences by frame-shifting; variation in the length of the D and J regions present in the finished sequences; nontemplated interposition of additional nucleotides at the junctions between V, D, and J segments; and somatic hypermutation in the portions of the antibody sequence responsible for contact with antigen. Analysis of these mechanisms at the molecular level has so far generated only a single, but a very provocative, report (16). Polymerase chain reaction was used to amplify and then sequence a specific high-variability region of a large set of V_H antibody genes of one 15-month-old mouse and one 8-week-old mouse of the BALB/c strain. Comparison of the set of sequences suggested many aging effects: *(1)* major changes in the use of specific D gene segments, *(2)* some shift in the pattern of J-segment utilization, *(3)* a great increase in the proportion of sequences that were recovered more than once in the set of sequenced antibody genes, and *(4)* a major increase in the length of the D-encoded DNA left in the finished antibody sequence. This sort of high-resolution detail is obviously costly to obtain, and analysis of other sections of the antibody molecule, in a diversity of B cells from different ages and at several stages of the immune response, will be needed to produce a coherent model, but even the very limited data now available suggest that aging may well lead to major changes in the molecular processes by which antibody genes are assembled and then selected.

Numerous reports have suggested that aging leads to an increase in serum titers of autoreactive antibodies with specificities for a broad range of proteins, cells, and organelles in mice and humans (71, 100, 125, 161, 180, 207, 246, 251). Studies of B cell hybridomas (187) and single B cells (162) have suggested that individual cells from older mice are increasingly likely to produce antibodies with broad cross-reactive specificity for foreign and autologous antigens. The significance of these changes is at best uncertain: in most cases the autoantibodies seem to be broadly reactive, of low affinity, and without apparent pathological sequelae. Many of the classical autoimmune syndromes exhibit a peak incidence in midlife, and the contribution of autoreactivity to the degenerative and neoplastic diseases of aging is still no more than speculation. Experimental models of induced autoimmunity have produced a confusing mix of results. One group (27) has found an increase with age in the severity of autoimmune encephalomyelitis after inoculation with myelin basic protein. Another group (286), however, has reported an age-dependent decline in the severity of a lupus-like syndrome induced by injection of immunogenic anti-DNA antibodies. A third report (247), using a mouse model for autoimmune thyroiditis, demonstrated a decline in humoral and cell-mediated anti-thyroglobulin responses in old mice but saw no age-dependent decline in the severity of autoimmune pathology. On balance, current evidence suggests that production in older mice and humans of cross-reactive autoreactive antibodies does not have significant effects on health, but investigation of the cellular and molecular mechanisms that underlie the shift may yet provide important insights into developmental immunology in the last half of the life span.

B CELL DEVELOPMENT

Immunocompetent B lymphocytes emerge from a developmental process, largely localized in the bone marrow of adults, that involves a number of well-defined stages, distinguished in part by the progress of immunoglobulin gene splicing and expression. The earliest pro-B cells are first identifiable by the initiation of gene rearrangements at the Ig loci. Several varieties of pre-B cells synthesize and then express complete Ig (μ) heavy chains and give rise to B cells whose surface IgM contains both heavy- and light-chain components. These early B cells are relatively easy to render tolerant but eventually give rise to more mature B cells that express both IgM and IgD, which when appropriately triggered can generate clones of proliferating B cells, antibody-producing plasma cells, and memory B cells.

Several investigators have examined the effects of aging on this developmental progression. Zharhary (312), for example, used antibodies specific for B cell progenitors to demonstrate a decline in the numbers of pro- and pre-B cells in the marrow of older mice. Bone marrow of older mice was also found to be defective in several in vitro tests for functional B cell precursors. Riley et al. (242) have examined the numbers and functional competence of two sorts of murine pre-B cell: small ones that give rise to B cells and larger ones from which the former arise. They observed a decline with age in both progenitor types, noting also that the smaller (more mature) form seemed to decline at earlier ages and to a greater extent than the larger (less mature) cell type. No changes were seen, however, in the mitotic fraction and cytokine responsiveness of the larger pre-B cells. Adoptive transfer studies (78) have suggested that B cell maturation from bone marrow precursors may also be impaired in vivo after transplantation into depleted hosts. Although all of these papers suggest that the marrow of older mice may be relatively impaired in B cell generation, it is not yet clear if these changes actually lead to qualitative or quantitative changes in the mature B cell population, either under normal circumstances or in situations of immunological stress.

In addition to these intrinsic changes in B cell development, there is a good deal of evidence that T cell abnormalities in the older animal may lead to secondary alterations in the later stages of B cell differentiation. The twofold age-related decline in the responder cell frequencies of mature B cells, for example, is not seen in studies of the Ig$^-$ pre-B cell populations (313), suggesting that some alterations in B cells affect only the later Ig$^+$ stages. Further work (311) showed directly that these response defects occurred only in B cells allowed to develop in the presence of T cells from old mice. Molding by T cells of B cell maturation may be mediated in part by the T cell-dependent production of antiidiotypic antibodies that are thought to regulate B cell function at several levels. Several investigators (95, 187, 277) have argued that these regulatory antibodies play an important role in diminishing the production by old mice of high-affinity IgG antibodies, and follow-up studies have suggested (157, 288) that T cells from old mice are required for the development of B cells able to generate such an antiidiotypic response. Some of the strongest evidence that these idiotype-specific interactions can alter B-cell responsiveness comes from studies (163) showing that T cells from aged mice are able to inhibit B cells, after co-transplantation to an adoptive host, only if the T cells and B cells come from mice that share genetic alleles at the immunoglobulin loci. These results suggest that T cells from aged mice may be able to recognize specific determinants on the B cell's own receptor immunoglobulins and consequently alter B cell responsiveness. These idiotype-specific interactions, however, are difficult to study even in genetically malleable mice and thus do little more than raise the possibility that some portion of B cell hyporesponsiveness in aged animals may reflect perturbation by aged T cells of some aspect of B cell development.

ACCESSORY CELLS AND THEIR CYTOKINES

Accessory cells (AC), also sometimes referred to as "antigen-presenting cells" (APC), play a vital role in initiating antigen-specific immune responses to presenting antigenic fragments to helper T cells. Some AC, particularly dendritic cells, also serve as depots for antigen in the form of antigen–antibody complexes that adhere tightly to receptors on the dendritic cell surface that are specific for the F_c carboxy terminal sequences on antibodies; dendritic cell antigen depots can persist for many months, even years, after an initial encounter with antigen and are thought to play a role in the maintenance of T cell memory by constant low-level presentation of antigens to memory T cells. Macrophages have specialized functions that allow them to ingest particulate antigens (bacteria, fungi, etc.) into digestive organelles that generate peptide fragments for presentation. B cells can serve as especially potent AC for those antigens which the individual B cell recognizes through its surface Ig; antigen-specific B cells can be 10^4-fold more potent than macrophages for presentation of recognized antigens. A good deal of work has been done in the last 5 yr to elucidate the various steps of the antigen-processing pathway in different AC types.

Unfortunately, most of the work done to date to assess the role of AC function in the aging immune system has relied on methods that do not take full account of current models for AC diversity and function. The majority of published work has used in vitro cultures in which mixed AC populations, usually including macrophages, dendritic cells, and often B cells from donors of different ages, are added to old and young T cells to see if the age of the macrophage donor influenced the resulting response to some poorly characterized antigen or mitogenic stimulus. Table 21.5 lists eight studies of this kind. Most of the reports provide no support for an important effect of age on AC cell function at this crude level of analysis. Of the two studies that did report an aging effect, one (62) is flawed by the presence of T cells (from young or old donors) in the preparation used for antigen presentation. Since in most cases the responses of old T cells are not repaired by addition of young AC, nor are the responses of young T cells impaired by AC from older donors, most authorities

TABLE 21.5. *In Vitro Assays of Accessory Cell Function*

Species	Stimulus	Result*	Citation
Human	Lectins	No change	(9)
Mouse	Con A	No change (IL-2)	(107)
Mouse	Lectins	No change	(32)
Mouse	Con A	Decline (IL-2)	(41)
Mouse	F_c fragments	No change	(205)
Mouse	Protein	No change	(231)
Mouse	Alloantigens	No change	(103)
Mouse	Influenza	Decline (LD)	(62)

*Endpoint was proliferation except as indicated: IL-2 = measurement of IL-2 production; and LD = limit dilution analysis of cytotoxic T cell production.

have concluded that poor AC function is not responsible for altered T cell reactivity in aging.

A number of other studies, however, have begun to paint a more complicated picture. There is some evidence that T cells from aged humans may be more sensitive than T cells from young controls in their response to the inhibitory effects of prostaglandins (PG) produced by macrophages (58). In accord with this idea, PG synthesis inhibitors were found (99) to overcome much of the age-dependent decline in mitogen-stimulated proliferation of human T cells. Aged mice whose diet has been supplemented with vitamin E, which lowers PG production in cultured macrophages, also show improved T cell responses in vitro (190). However, proliferation of T cells from old donors is clearly impaired under conditions in which AC function has been replaced by saturating amounts of anti-CD28 antibodies (108), and some laboratories are unable to find any effect of PG inhibition on the responses of aged T cells (270). It also seems possible that some aspects of T cell/macrophage interaction may be particularly sensitive to the effect of PG: inhibition of PG synthesis has been found to reverse the age-dependent loss of mitogen-induced transferrin receptor expression, but not IL-2R expression, by T cells from old humans (10).

A recent study (18) of PHA-mediated human T cell proliferation has pointed to alterations in IFNγ production as a potential complicating factor. AC preparations from young donors were found to be superior to those from old donors in their ability to support proliferation of old T cells in nine of ten cases, although old AC were able to support the proliferation of T cells from young donors. Overnight treatment of the old AC with IFNγ was found to restore the ability of these cells to provide accessory function to old T cells, perhaps through IFNγ-mediated inhibition of PGE$_2$ production.

It also seems likely that a more complete understanding of the functional implications of diversity within the macrophage/monocyte lineage may shed further light on questions of aging. Smith et al. (268), for example, have studied an unusual macrophage subset that expresses the Thy-1 surface marker and is restricted to germinal centers, a key location for T cell/B cell interaction. These tingible body macrophages are easily identified by their staining properties in LN of young mice but are essentially absent from LN in older animals. Their absence may contribute to the small size and number of germinal centers in old mice and thus to declines in the secondary antibody response.

Little work has so far been done on senescent changes in the critical interactions between T cells and AC-presented cognate antigens, which are now known to involve a complex set of interactions between antigen-nonspecific co-stimulatory molecules on the surface of both cell types, among which interactions between B7 and CD28 and between LFA-1 and ICAM-1 are thought to be particularly influential. A glimpse of the progress likely to emerge from this line of investigation comes from a study (123) of heterogeneity within the murine CD4 population in which aging was shown to lead to an increase in a subset of T cells, for which mature B cells rather than macrophages were required for optimal stimulation. Systems for analysis of T cell co-stimulation by combinations of ligands have been developed (291) but not yet exploited for studies of aging.

Dendritic Cells and Langerhans Cells

Special attention has been given to a population of AC cells called "Langerhans" cells, dendritic cells in the skin that are critical for processing cutaneous antigen sources. Several groups (22, 46, 89, 271), though not all (164), have noted a mild (20%–50%) decline with age in the number of Langerhans cells per unit area of skin. In vitro tests of the stimulatory capacity of epidermal cells suggest that the decline in Langerhans cell numbers may have functional consequences (271), though other data suggest that the changes are not severe enough to account for the decline with age in contact sensitivity (22).

Tew's laboratory has published a very interesting series of studies concerning the ability of dendritic cells in the LNs to process protein antigens in aging mice. During the course of an immune response, antigen is transported by skin and other sites to the LN, where it is trapped and retained by these follicular dendritic cells (FDC); FDC-presented antigen is thought to be required for germinal center formation, strong antibody responses, and production of memory B cells. An early paper from this group (138) noted that, although LN from old mice retained the ability to trap and retain antigens, the trapped antigens remained in the subcapsular region of the LN rather than migrating into the germinal centers as they do in young mice. Since the germinal centers are the principal site of T cell/B cell interaction, a defect in migration of antigen-bearing FDC might well lead to diminished humoral responses. A later morphological analysis (276) of the LN of old mice showed atrophic areas and pycnotic cells in older mice only. More impressively, these workers found that FDC from young, but not old, mice could produce small, immune complex–coated vesicles ("iccosomes"), which had previously been shown to be crucial for conveying antigen/antibody complexes to secondary B cells in an immunogenic form. An elegant adoptive transfer study (35), in which T and memory B cells from young mice were transplanted into young or old host mice, showed that antigen associated with FDC from old mice was far less immunogenic than antigen on young FDC; sonicating the old, antigen-loaded FDC generated immunogenic vesicles that resembled the iccosomes produced naturally by FDC from younger mice. These papers taken together suggest that poor secondary antibody responses in old mice may relate, at least in part, to defects in the processing of antigen by a key AC.

Cytokine Production

In addition to their role in antigen presentation and processing, many AC promote T and B cell activation by secreting antigen-nonspecific cytokines with potent effects on immune reactivity. Original models of AC/T cell interaction focused on the role of IL-1 produced by macrophages as a co-factor for T cell activation. More recent work has complicated all aspects of this simple picture in that it is now clear *(1)* that IL-1, IL-6, TNF, and perhaps a dozen less well characterized cytokines can all affect T cell activation through a complex network of interacting signals; *(2)* that these cytokines are produced by a diversity of cell types in addition to cells in the macrophage/monocyte lineage; and *(3)* that cytokines can act at a wide range of sites within and outside of the immune system and thus serve to connect the immune system to other organ systems that play a role in perturbed homeostasis. So far, however, very little is known conclusively about how these complex interactions are altered by aging.

The earliest investigations of cytokine production and response focused on IL-1. Two of these reported an age-dependent decline in IL-1 production (32, 142), while two others found no effect of age (146, 149). Each of these reports used bioassays that are now known to not discriminate well between IL-1 and IL-6 or between the two IL-1 isoforms, IL-1α and IL-1β. A more recent report, using an ELISA method specific for IL-1β, observed no effect of age on human IL-1β production with or without addition of Con A (96). Another report using ELISA IL-1 measurements also found no difference between young and old humans in serum IL-1 or monocyte release of IL-1 into conditioned medium (240). IL-1 mRNA analyses have shown an apparent decrease in mouse skin (250). Unfortunately, many of these studies were based on macrophage preparations that had been elicited by inflammatory stimuli (to obtain high numbers of cells) and then tested IL-1 production after exposure to stimuli (LPS, PMA, Con A, etc.) that are likely to induce stronger and more prolonged activation than is typical in physiological immune responses; it is therefore difficult to judge the relevance of the findings to immunosenescence. IL-1 fails to correct defects in T cell responsiveness in vitro (32, 217), suggesting that altered IL-1 production does not by itself account for some forms of age-dependent immunodeficiency, although injection of IL-1β (along with an immunogen) into 12–15-month-old mice has been shown (81) to improve their helper T cell response to levels equal to those of young controls, though not to those of young mice whose response had been improved by IL-1 treatment. Thus, on balance, there is little reason at present to think that altered IL-1 production plays a major role in immunosenescence.

More recently, some attention has been directed to IL-6, another product of macrophages (and other cell types) with profound effects within and outside the immune system proper. Plasma IL-6 concentrations have been reported to increase with age in humans (56, 298) and in mice (56), and cultured spleen or mesenteric LN cells from aged mice are reported to produce high levels of IL-6 spontaneously (56). LPS injection led to slightly elevated levels of IL-6 in 12–15-month-old rats (compared to 3–5-month-old animals) but substantially (17-fold) elevated levels in 24–27-month-old rats (77). There is also one report of an age-related decline in IL-6 production by mouse macrophages (63). An analysis of IL-6 mRNA production by stimulated CD4 T cells (136) found no effect of age, although analogous data on non-T cells would have been more informative. TNFα, another inflammatory cytokine that can be produced by both T cells and macrophages, has been reported to increase dramatically with age in the LPS-injected rat model (77) but to decline in macrophage culture supernatants from aged mice (63), while no effect of age was noted on accumulation of TNFα (or TNFβ) mRNA in stimulated mouse CD4 cells (136). It is clear that these pioneering experiments will need to be supplemented by more systematic studies using carefully defined mixtures of T cells and AC, subjected to graded stimuli chosen for physiological relevance. Work using antibodies to cytokines thought to affect T cell and B cell responses will also permit a more critical evaluation of the possible contribution of altered cytokine production (and response) to the immunodeficiency of aging.

NATURAL CYTOTOXICITY

T cell and B cell-mediated immune responses can be primed in the sense that an initial encounter with a foreign antigen will alter the state of the immune system in such a way that responses to second and subsequent encounters are stronger and speedier. In contrast, a third variety of lymphocyte mediates a form of immune reaction that does not require (or benefit from) prior antigenic sensitization and is therefore termed "natural"-cell-mediated cytotoxicity. The natural killer (NK) cells make up a small fraction (5%–15%) of the lymphoid population in blood and internal organs, express their own set of surface marker antigens, and seem specialized for recognition and lysis of certain varieties of cancer cell and virally infected cell. These cells do not express the clonally restricted TCR or Ig receptors characteristic of the antigen-specific B and T cells, and the way in which they distinguish normal from neoplastic or infected targets is still not well understood. Since they do not require activation by prior contact with antigen, they are thought to constitute a first line of defense, and it has been postulated that declines in NK function might contribute to the increased vulnerability of elderly people to infections and neoplasias.

Table 21.6 lists reports that have examined the effect of age on NK cell function in humans and mice. Nearly all of the mouse data show an age-dependent decline in NK function, while five of the seven human studies show no age effect or a small increase with age. It is likely that much of this discrepancy reflects a technical difference: all of the human work was done with cells from peripheral blood, while nearly all of the mouse data reflect assays of spleen or LN cells. The one study of mouse blood (171) found no effect of age on NK function, in good agreement with the bulk of the reports on human blood cells. It thus seems reasonable to hypothesize that NK function may also decline in human internal lymphoid organs, despite an absence of any data putting this idea to a direct test. Most NK cells show a limited preference for leukemia and lymphoma cell targets; a related form of natural cytotoxic cell with preference for sarcoma cell targets does not seem to change with age in mice (274).

There have been a number of investigations of NK regulation and control that provide some useful insights. For one thing, NK function in human blood is known to be very sensitive to variables (emotional state, recent exercise) that are usually not controlled in routine laboratory investigations, and it is thus possible that some of the discrepancies among different reports are due to subtle variations in subject status that were not thought to be relevant and thus not controlled. Details of the assay procedure can also have an important effect. One group, for example, has found that an age-dependent decline in NK function in human peripheral blood mononuclear cells disappeared when purified lymphocytes were studied (210), suggesting that blood monocytes were able to diminish the NK activity of lymphocytes from older donors. Adherent cell-mediated inhibition has also been suggested to account for age-related declines in NK function in a mouse system (143). Recent work has also suggested that NK function may be mediated by cells of several types that can be distinguished by their surface markers and further that age-dependent increases in human NK function may be attributable to an increase in an NK subset bearing both the Leu-7 and Leu-11 markers (168). This group has also reported that increased NK function in elderly women may reflect diminished responsiveness to the inhibitory effects of exogenous purines (167). The relevance of the subset and purine-receptor data seems, however, somewhat questionable in view of the reports from most other workers that show NK function remaining constant or decreasing in aged humans (see Table 21.6). The number of human peripheral blood cells that express the CD56 marker thought to be characteristic for NK cells has been shown to remain constant between the ages of 20 and 60 yr, to increase slightly between 60 and 80 yr, and then to fall in the very old (289). NK numbers also increase somewhat in old rats (92).

NK function can be increased by several lymphokines, including IL-2 and IFNγ, and several groups have examined whether or not low NK responses can be

TABLE 21.6. *Age-Associated Changes in NK Cell Function*

Species	Result	Citation
Human	No change	(23)
Human	No change	(208)
Human	No change	(237)
Human	No change	(285)
Human	Increase	(168)
Human	Decline	(210)
Human	Decline	(287)
Mouse	Decline	(134)
Mouse	Decline	(4)
Mouse	Decline	(29)
Mouse	Decline	(150)
Mouse	Decline	(252)
Mouse	Decline	(299)
Mouse (blood)	No change	(171)

improved by these modulators. IFN injections into old mice can indeed restore NK function (29, 299), and it thus seems plausible that a decline in NK function in old mice might reflect lower endogenous IFNγ levels, although newer data (see Table 21.3) suggest that IFNγ production may increase with age, at least in T cells stimulated in vitro. Cells cultured in vitro with high doses of IL-2 give rise to lymphokine-activated killer (LAK) cells thought to resemble NK cells in many of their properties. LAK production by cells from mouse spleen has been reported both to decrease (252) and to remain unaffected (134, 150) by aging, suggesting that IL-2 treatments might in principle be able to restore age-related losses in NK function. A single report of the effects of IFNγ on generation of LAK cells produced paradoxical findings, in which IFNγ addition increased LAK production in cultures from young donors while decreasing LAK generation in cultures from older mice (151).

RESTORATION OF IMMUNE FUNCTION

Investigations of compounds or procedures that can improve immune function in old subjects are prompted by two major motives: the hope that such studies will provide insights into the physiological basis for the age-related decline in function and the possibility that such experiments will suggest clinically useful protocols for protecting the elderly from disease. Interpreting the physiological significance of these interventive studies is fraught with difficulties, in particular the possibility that a restorative agent is improving an immunological function through a pathway other than that which is damaged by the normal aging process. Controls in which young subjects are also exposed to the intervention are clearly a necessary (but not sufficient) part of the argument but have all too often been omitted.

Caloric restriction is the most thoroughly studied and assiduously replicated method for prevention of immunosenescence in rodents, and its effects on immunity have recently been reviewed (195). These effects are presumed to be linked to the still mysterious mechanism by which it retards age-related changes in most, though not all, other age-sensitive indices (182). Newer work suggests that not all age-related immune changes are equally preserved in restricted mice: the loss of calcium signal generation, for example, seems to proceed equally in restricted and control mice (110), despite convincing effects on T cell function (64, 110, 198) and subset distribution (195). Caloric restriction per se is not useful for human interventions, but additional insights into the mechanism by which this protocol retards aging may eventually lead to useful therapeutic or preventive maneuvers.

The classical method of restoring high-level immune function to old rodents involves transplantation of young bone marrow, together with an infant thymus gland, into irradiated old host animals; early studies along these lines have been thoughtfully reviewed by Harrison (118). Repeating this procedure on individual mice as they age can maintain immune function at relatively high levels throughout the life span of the recipient (132). Multiply-transplanted mice do not have increased longevity, although it is possible that the positive effects of lifelong immune function may have been counterbalanced by the negative effects of repeated exposure to pretransplant irradiation. The age-dependent loss of the ability of the thymus to support T lineage development (130) has suggested that transplantation of live thymic epithelial cells could perhaps restore T-cell immunity without a need for marrow co-transplantation, and indeed some limited but promising data have been obtained along these lines (114). Mature, immunocompetent T and B cells from young mice can function well when transplanted into irradiated old hosts (37), except perhaps in situations that require AC functions not provided by the aged environment (35). Although the morbidity incurred by irradiation clearly limits the usefulness of this technique, there is some indication that the resistance of unirradiated animals to engraftment of mature lymphocytes may itself be diminished in old age (224), and attempts to transfer protective immunity to old individuals in the form of live mature T and B cells may be worth further investigation.

A recent report (55) that treatment with dehydroepiandrosterone (DHEA) can correct a number of immunological deficits in aged mice has elicited a good deal of excited speculation. Chronic oral administration of DHEA sulfate, which is metabolized internally to DHEA at sites of action, was said to increase the ability of mouse T cells to generate IL-2, IL-3, and GM-CSF in in vitro cultures stimulated by anti-CD3 and at the same time to diminish production of IL-4 and IL-5, thus producing a pattern of lymphokine secretion similar to that seen in younger (untreated) mice. Surprisingly, similar effects were seen in old mice given a single injection of DHEA sulfate a mere 24 h before sacrifice. The acute effect was local in that the response of cells from LN draining a site of topical DHEA application was altered, whereas the response of cells on the contralateral site was unaffected. Even more impressively, DHEA treatment was found to restore the ability to make strong primary antibody responses to a protein immunogen and to improve the ability of immunized mice to generate memory B cells primed for a later, secondary response. These results, if eventually confirmed by other groups and extended to other antigens, may at least provide new avenues for improving the specific immune reactivity of elderly humans to vaccines. It is worth noting, however, that the in vitro results make use of an unusual culture system that provides information only about the very earliest (24 h) phases of immune responses and that an earlier paper from this group (11) included data to suggest that the DHEA effect on IL-4 production was dependent on co-administration of dihydrotestosterone. DHEA treatment of old mice is also said to diminish plasma IL-6 levels and production of IL-6 by cultured splenocytes, as well as serum levels of autoantibodies and acute phase reactants arguably dependent on IL-6 production in the intact animal (56).

Is the DHEA effect, assuming that it can be confirmed, an instance of repair of a physiological defect, or is it a pharmacological alteration of the normal hormonal milieu? DHEA levels do fall progressively with age in humans, and it thus seems plausible that age-related changes in lymphokine profiles and immune responses could reflect the decline in DHEA levels in older subjects. However, the published reports do not yet include much data about possible immunostimulatory effects of DHEA on young mice, and it would be premature to exclude the hypothesis of an adjuvant-like effect. Chronic treatment with DHEA sulfate does not seem to prevent or reverse the accumulation of cells with the surface markers of memory T cells (Daynes, personal communication), suggesting that the hormone may alter either the lymphokine response patterns of individual T cells or the relative responsiveness of subsets of cells already predisposed to the production of specific immunoregulators. Detailed characterization of cell subsets and their responsiveness in mice treated briefly or over an extended interval with DHEA is likely to prove rewarding.

The idea that an altered hormonal environment might contribute to thymic involution and/or immunodeficiencies in the elderly has prompted a number of experimental approaches at hormonal therapy. In an early attempt, a pituitary tumor cell line that secreted growth hormone (GH) among other bioactive materials was transplanted into old rats and found to induce increases in thymic weight but only modest improvements in peripheral T cell function (153). In another study, 24-month-old mice were given implants of ovine GH (186); thymic size and histology were restored to an apparently youthful condition, but there was no significant change in proliferation, IL-2 production, or CTL generation by splenocytes. Six of the seven implanted mice were found on autopsy to have developed hepatomas, which were not seen in any of the placebo-treated mice, and it is possible that alterations in liver function may have contributed to the disappointing functional results. In a third study (156), BALB/c mice were given twice-weekly injections of GH for 13 wk beginning at age 17 months. This protocol led to statistically significant increases in splenocyte production of IL-2 and mitogenic response to pokeweed mitogen (a stimulus for both T cell and B cell proliferation) but no change in Con A–induced proliferation. GH-treated mice were found to have higher levels of IL-1 and TNF than either young or old controls. Interestingly, GH-treated mice lived longer than placebo-treated controls: over the initial 13-wk period, 16 of the 26 control mice died, compared to only two of the 26 GH-treated mice. The very low survival of the control group (nearly all dead by 21 months of age) suggests that death in this colony may well reflect infectious causes, and it is thus unclear whether survival was influenced by GH-induced improvements in immune function or whether the poor immune function in control mice reflected ongoing illness.

A related study (52) focused on immune responses in aged mice that had received implants of pituitary gland under the kidney capsule; such preparations have been shown to have prompt immunostimulatory effects in young recipients. Older recipients, however, showed no evidence of functional or morphological improvement at the 10-day interval and by 28 days showed statistically significant increases in IgG and IgM that were still substantially (90%) lower than the responses of young controls. Thus, on balance, the evidence that the immunodeficiencies of aging can be corrected by administration of pituitary-derived hormones is not strong. Indeed, two groups (119, 260) have reported that surgical removal of the pituitary can lead to improvements of immune function in aged rodents. There are several varieties of mutant mice that are genetically deficient in one or more hormones, and data on their immune functions in middle and old age could prove informative; preliminary results along these lines have already been published (73).

Another line of investigation has involved the idea that thymic involution might impair immune function by lowering levels of thymic hormones with extrathymic sites of action. It should be said at the outset that most immunologists consider the evidence that the thymus does indeed produce endocrine factors with effects on extrathymic T cell maturation to be unconvincing, and early reports of age-dependent changes in serum thymic hormone levels were undermined by demonstrations that the hormone preparations used were in fact mixtures of substances, some of them produced by many different tissues (273). Systematic surveys of the ability of various proposed thymic hormones to alter immune function in aging rodents have not, in general, produced encouraging results (128). Nonetheless, a number of reports have now appeared to suggest that injection of synthetic oligopeptide analogs of thymic proteins can improve immune function in aged mice and humans (48, 80, 101, 189). In one of the most dramatic of these reports (101), a single injection of 160 pg/

mouse of an octapeptide derivative of THFγ2 was found to increase by sixfold the production of IL-2 by 12-month-old mice and to lead to a fourfold increase in carrier-specific T helper function in an in vitro assay system. The effect of this octapeptide was found to be dose-dependent and to increase the fraction of spleen cells that could proliferate or produce helper factors in limit dilution assays. Two other thymic hormones were also found to work in this system but at molar doses 50-fold (TP5) or 400-fold (thymosin α1) higher than those needed for THFγ2.

The effects of thymopentin (TP) on immune responses of aged mice have also been examined in the context of *Leishmania major* infection (48). BALB/c mice of 8, 16, and 30 months of age were found to be more susceptible to *L. major* infection than were 2.5-month-old controls and to produce more IL-4, less IL-2, and less IFNγ in 24-h Con A splenocyte cultures. Treatment of the mice with TP five times per week starting from the day of infection was found to retard disease progression in old and middle-aged mice and to prevent the lethality seen in the oldest cohort. Both uninfected and infected aged mice were found to respond to TP treatment by increases in IL-2 and IFNγ production and decreased IL-4 production. Since progression of *L. major* infection in young mice has been shown to depend critically on IL-4 and IFNγ production, with IL-4 favoring and IFNγ opposing disease (44), it seems entirely plausible that the changes in lymphokine profile could account for the change in disease severity. In summary, despite the absence of a compelling theoretical justification for use of thymic proteins as immunological rejuvenators, empirical data have begun to suggest that this area deserves further investigation by appropriately skeptical laboratories.

A variety of other pharmacological approaches have also been judged to be mildly promising in isolated reports. Injection of the opioid pentapeptide Met-enkephalin for 1 day before and 4 days after immunization with sheep erythrocytes was found to increase the hemagglutinin response of old rats to levels seen in untreated young rats, though not to levels seen in treated young controls (145); Arthus and DTH responses were also improved. In another study 3 months of treatment with phosphatidylserine (in drinking water) was found to reverse the age-related decline in the ability of rats to produce antialbumin IgG antibodies after priming and boosting (112); incorporation of phosphatidylserine into culture medium was also found in this report to increase the ability of human T cells to express the IL-2 receptor after stimulation by anti-CD3 and PMA. In vitro assays have also suggested the ability of isoprinosine to improve several age-sensitive indices of human T cell, NK cell, and neutrophil responses (287). While each of these reports suggests areas for further work, none seems to provide either useful insights into the mechanism of immune senescence or a compelling empirical basis for clinical trials.

Reports of interaction between the sympathetic nervous system and the immune system represent an area for potential therapeutic intervention that has yet to be exploited. The work of Felten and colleagues (20, 21, 70) has shown an unexpectedly high level of sympathetic innervation of the peripheral immune system in the rat and further that aging leads to a loss of innervation parallel with immune decline. The observation that drug-induced sympathetic denervation can itself induce immunodeficiency suggests that the natural loss of innervation in aged animals could contribute to immunosenescent failure. This provocative set of studies clearly suggests new ideas for both developmental immunogerontologists and therapeutic strategies.

Interestingly, one of the most intriguing of the recent therapeutic reports involves one of the most old-fashioned approaches. Chandra (40) hypothesized that mild micronutrient deficiencies might contribute to immunological deficits in some apparently healthy elderly humans and to test this administered a 12-month course of vitamin and mineral supplements at levels similar to or only slightly above the minimum recommended daily doses for young adults. The proportion of the elderly population that had abnormally low blood levels of one or more micronutrients was found to decline after treatment, as expected. Immunological assays showed that the treated subjects, in comparison to placebo controls, exhibited improvements in mitogen response, IL-2 production, antibody response, and NK function. Even more impressively, the treated group was significantly less likely to suffer from infectious illness over the 12-month treatment course (23 vs. 48 days/yr, $P < 0.002$). Although vitamin-treated young controls were not tested, this report clearly suggests that some of the immune deficits in the elderly population might reflect a mild, remediable deficiency of one or more micronutrients.

IMMUNITY, DISEASE, AND LONGEVITY

It seems plausible that age-related declines in immune function might contribute to the vulnerability of the elderly to infectious and perhaps neoplastic disease and thus increase the risk of mortality. Nearly all of the evidence on this attractive hypothesis, however, is lamentably indirect, usually taking the form of a demonstration that an immune mechanism (IL-2 production, for example, or generation of CTL effectors) thought to protect against some illness does indeed decline at advanced ages. A more powerful approach, involving longitudinal analyses of morbidity and mortality in individuals shown to differ in immune indices thought to influence disease susceptibility, has seldom been attempted and even less frequently been successful. Such studies are very expensive to perform in humans and require many years to generate definitive results, while studies in rodents have often been stymied by a need to develop nonlethal microassays suitable for analysis of function in these smaller animals.

One approach has been to test elderly humans for immune competence and then to assess the rate at which members of the tested population succumb to illness. None of the three published reports has been entirely satisfactory. The earliest (244) reported a significant negative correlation between immune anergy as measured by skin DTH testing and subsequent 2 yr survival in a population of nursing home residents aged 80 yr or more, each of whom was said to be "ambulant, cooperative, and well-nourished" at the beginning of the study but who were no longer able to live alone, and an unspecified number of whom also suffered from one or more major degenerative illnesses. The central weakness of this study is the absence of any test of the idea that preexisting illness might have contributed to both the immune anergy and the risk of mortality. None of the 34 deaths recorded in the 2 yr follow-up period was attributable to neoplasia, making this population a poor one for testing some aspects of the relation between immune senescence and disease. A second study (209) reported a positive correlation between poor in vitro responsiveness to the T cell mitogen PHA and subsequent mortality but like the earlier work failed to adjust for potential confounding effects of latent illness or even for the effects of subject age. A third study (297) also noted a correlation between skin test anergy and subsequent all-cause mortality in its elderly test population, but after adjustment for age the relationship was found to be statistically insignificant, though provocative (relative risk of 1.89). Perhaps the strongest evidence that immune status might predict mortality risk comes from an analysis (26) of the survival statistics of the Baltimore Longitudinal Study on Aging, in which healthy men found to have lower peripheral blood lymphocyte counts were found to be at greater risk of mortality at any age. The study design used very thorough laboratory and physical examinations to rule out detectable preexisting illness as a confounding variable but did not, unfortunately, include a more detailed analysis of immunological status, so it is difficult to know if the alterations in blood lymphocyte count represented a loss in one particular T cell or B cell subset or were accompanied by evidence of a functional deficit.

Thus none of the human studies to date has produced convincing correlative evidence that aged individuals with lowered immune function are indeed more vulnerable to illness and mortality in part because the very long human life span makes it difficult to carry out longitudinal studies in which proposed prognostic indices are measured at ages at which most subjects are free of diseases that could themselves alter immune function. Nonetheless, each of the published human studies has provided some support for the hypothesis that immunosenescence may contribute to mortality risk. Further indirect support has come from two animal models. In one, the proportion of $CD8^-$ T cells in the peripheral blood at any age was found to predict remaining life expectancy (30) in CBA mice. The same relationship was also seen in young and old, though not in middle-aged, C57BL/6 mice. In this study, however, there seemed to be an age-related decline in the proportion of $CD8^-$ T cells in the blood which has not been noted in most other laboratories, and it is therefore unclear to what extent the conclusions are likely to prove generalizable. In a second approach, immune function and longevity were measured in groups of genetically heterogeneous mice that had been selected over many generations for differences in early-life humoral immune responsiveness (50). Lines bred for high immune response were found to have higher longevity and lower age-adjusted incidence of both neoplastic and nonneoplastic mortality compared to lines selectively bred for low early-life immunity. Genetic experiments using F1 hybrids and backcrosses between the high-immune and low-immune groups showed a good correlation between immune measures and life expectancy both between groups and within those groups that had substantial genetic variability. Calculations suggested that the interline differences in immune responses and life span were controlled by allelic variance at as few as three to seven genetic loci. Although this study provides fairly strong evidence in support of the idea that interindividual differences in immunity may protect from or predispose to lethal illness, the relatively short life span of even the longest-lived groups of mice suggests that the effects might not be reproducible in specific-pathogen-free colonies. Furthermore, the absence of an unselected group leaves some uncertainty as to whether the direction of selection was for higher or lower immunity (or was perhaps bidirectional). Despite these ambiguities, this provocative study suggests that detailed analysis of immune function and inheritance patterns in similarly selected animals could provide useful insights into both the cellular basis of immunosenescence and the relation between immunity and longevity.

Immune reconstitution experiments have provided some additional support for the idea that T cell deficiency in the aged may predispose to infection. Thus the vulnerability of old mice to polio virus (28), tuberculosis (223), and Listeria (230) has been shown to be diminished by administration of T cells from younger hosts. Detailed analysis of a murine model for recrudescence of latent pulmonary tuberculosis (TB) (225) has shown that the development of lethal TB in old mice that had been infected when young was preceded by a loss in protective antibacterial T cell function assessed by adoptive transfer protocols. Additional analysis of this promising system may provide insights into the waning of protective immunity within the memory T cell pool, with direct relevance to an important disease of elderly humans. Evidence on the relation between immunity and infection in humans is limited and indirect, but in vitro cell mixing experiments have shown that in some circumstances addition of helper T cells from responsive donors could correct the poor responses of aged individuals who were unresponsive to hepatitis vaccination (49). In an analysis of human responses to influenza vaccination, one group (141) has noted that those elderly subjects who exhibited both low serum IL-2 levels and good production of IL-2 in an in vitro test were as likely to respond well to vaccination as were young controls, while poor vaccination responses were typical of elderly subjects with high serum IL-2 and low in vitro IL-2 production. Murine models of influenza infection have also begun to yield some insights into the cellular basis for age-related increases in susceptibility to viral disease (25, 61). It seems likely that further work along these lines, in humans or mice, might lead to the development and validation of prognostic assays that separate the elderly population into subsets with differential vulnerability to infectious agents.

The question of whether age-related alterations in immune function predispose to cancer is controversial, and the arguments have recently been reviewed at great length (69, 196, 197). It seems very likely, based on species differences in aging and cancer incidence rates, on the parallel effect of food restriction on cancer and longevity, and on the low cancer incidence of long-lived mice selected for high immune function (50), that the rate of cancer development is tightly coupled to the underlying aging process, but whether the altered immunity seen in old age is among the coupling mechanisms cannot yet be answered with any confidence. It is clear that fairly small (two- to fourfold) changes in the strength of in vitro indices of antitumor immunity can lead to very large (400-fold) increases in cancer susceptibility (98), but whether they actually do so remains uncertain. Longitudinal studies in which early- and mid-life immune status variables are tested for their ability to predict later cancer incidence in rodents may eventually provide better evidence, particularly if carried out in genetically heterogeneous populations in which large variations in both immunity and cancer susceptibility can be expected.

SUMMARY: IMMUNE MODELS FOR AGING RESEARCH

The potential of the immune system for exploring the basic cellular and physiological bases of aging is still largely untapped. Each of the key problems—cellular heterogeneity, signal transduction, intercellular communication within the immune system and between immune cells and other cell types, developmental processes and their modulation—has so far attracted the attention of only a small number of dedicated investigators, and there is thus no lack of uncharted and unclaimed territory for the intrepid prospector. A detailed mechanistic understanding of immune senescence in developmental and molecular terms will have broad implications not just for clinical researchers who wish to protect the elderly by repairing damaged defenses but also for basic scientists in search of the fundamental principles that time the parallel disintegration of neural, endocrine, connective, musculoskeletal, and sundry other systems in synchrony with immunological decline.

Preparation of this review was supported by grants from the National Institutes of Health (AG03978, AG09801, and AG08808).

REFERENCES

1. ABB, J., H. ABB, and F. DEINHARDT. Age-related decline of human interferon alpha and interferon gamma production. *Blut* 48: 285–289, 1984.
2. ABRAHAM, C., Y. TAL, and H. GERSHON. Reduced in vitro response to concanavalin A and lipopolysaccharide in senescent mice: a function of reduced number of responding cells. *Eur. J. Immunol.* 7: 301–304, 1977.
3. AKBAR, A. N., M. SALMON, and G. JANOSSY. The synergy between naive and memory T cells during activation. *Immunol. Today* 12: 184–188, 1991.
4. ALBRIGHT, J. W., and J. F. ALBRIGHT. Age-associated impairment of murine natural killer activity. *Proc. Natl. Acad. Sci. U.S.A.* 80: 6371–6375, 1983.
5. ALBRIGHT, J. W., K. L. HOLMES, and J. F. ALBRIGHT. Fluctuations in subsets of splenocytes and isotypes of Ig in young adult and aged mice resulting from *Trypanosoma musculi* infections. *J. Immunol.* 144: 3970–3979, 1990.
6. ALKON, D. L., and H. RASMUSSEN. A spatial–temporal model of cell activation. *Science* 239: 998–1005, 1988.
7. AL-RAYES, H., W. PACHAS, N. MIRZA, D. J. AHERN, R. S. GEHA, and D. VERCELLI. IgE regulation and lymphokine patterns in aging humans. *J. Allergy Clin. Immunol.* 90: 630–636, 1992.
8. ANDERSSON, J., A. COUTINHO, and F. MELCHERS. Frequencies of mitogen-reactive B cells in the mouse. I. Distribution in different lymphoid organs from different inbred strains of mice at different ages. *J. Exp. Med.* 145: 1511–1530, 1977.
9. ANTEL, J. P., J. F. D. E. OGER, D. P. RICHMAN, H. H. HUO, and B. G. W. ARNASON. Reduced T-lymphocyte cell reactivity as a function of human aging. *Cell. Immunol.* 54: 184–192, 1980.

10. ANTONACI, S., C. TORTORELLA, A. POLIGNANO, A. OTTOLENGHI, E. JIRILLO, and L. BONOMO. Modulating effects on CD25 and CD71 antigen expression by lectin-stimulated T lymphocytes in the elderly. *Immunopharmacol. Immunotoxicol.* 13: 87–100, 1991.
11. ARANEO, B. A., T. DOWELL, M. DIEGEL, and R. A. DAYNES. Dihydrotestosterone exerts a depressive influence on the production of interleukin-4 (IL-4), IL-5, and γ-interferon, but not IL-2 by activated murine T cells. *Blood* 78: 688–699, 1991.
12. ARMANINI, D., I. KARBOWIAK, M. SCALI, E. ORLANDINI, V. ZAMPOLLO, and G. VITTADELLO. Corticosteroid receptors and lymphocyte subsets in mononuclear leukocytes in aging. *Am. J. Physiol.* 262(*Endocrinol. Metab.* 25): E464–E466, 1992.
13. ASTLE, C. M., and D. E. HARRISON. Effects of marrow donor and recipient age on immune responses. *J. Immunol.* 132: 673–677, 1984.
14. AVERILL, L. E., and N. S. WOLF. The decline in murine splenic PHA and LPS responsiveness with age is primarily due to an intrinsic mechanism. *J. Immunol.* 134: 3859–3863, 1985.
15. BACH, M. A. Lymphocyte-mediated cytotoxicity: effects of ageing, adult thymectomy and thymic factor. *J. Immunol.* 119: 641–647, 1977.
16. BANGS, L. A., I. E. SANZ, and J. M. TEALE. Comparison of D, J_H, and junctional diversity in the fetal, adult, and aged B cell repertoires. *J. Immunol.* 146: 1996–2004, 1991.
17. BASCH, R. S. Thymic repopulation after irradiation in aged mice. *Aging: Immunol. Infect. Dis.* 2: 229–235, 1990.
18. BECKMAN, I., K. DIMOPOULOS, X. N. XU, J. BRADLEY, P. HENSCHKE, and M. AHERN. T cell activation in the elderly: evidence for specific deficiencies in T cell/accessory cell interactions. *Mech. Ageing Dev.* 51: 265–276, 1990.
19. BELL, E. B., and S. M. SPARSHOTT. Interconversion of CD45R subsets of CD4 T cells in vivo. *Nature* 348: 163–166, 1990.
20. BELLINGER, D. L., S. Y. FELTEN, T. J. COLLIER, and D. L. FELTEN. Noradrenergic sympathetic innervation of the spleen: IV. Morphometric analysis in adult and aged F344 rats. *J. Neurosci. Res.* 18: 55–63, 126–129, 1987.
21. BELLINGER, D. L., D. LORTON, S. Y. FELTEN, and D. L. FELTEN. Innervation of lymphoid organs and implications in development, aging, and autoimmunity. *Int. J. Immunopharmacol.* 14: 329–344, 1992.
22. BELSITO, D. V., R. M. DERARKISSIAN, G. J. THORBECKE, and R. L. BAER. Reversal by lymphokines of the age-related hyporesponsiveness to contact sensitization and reduced Ia expression on langerhans cells. *Arch. Dermatol. Res.* 279: S76–S80, 1987.
23. BENDER, B. S., F. J. CHREST, and W. H. ADLER. Phenotypic expression of natural killer cell associated membrane antigens and cytolytic function of peripheral blood cells from different aged humans. *J. Clin. Lab. Immunol.* 21: 31–36, 1986.
24. BENDER, B. S., F. J. CHREST, J. A. NAGEL, W. H. ADLER, D. M. BENTLEY, and R. E. MORRIS. Peripheral blood CD8+ subsets in young and elderly adults: enumeration by two-color immunofluorescence and flow cytometry T cell subsets required for protection against age-dependent polioencephalomyelitis of C58 mice. *J. Immunol.* 128: 530–534, 1982.
25. BENDER, B. S., M. P. JOHNSON, and P. A. SMALL. Influenza in senescent mice: impaired cytotoxic T-lymphocyte activity is correlated with prolonged infection. *Immunology* 72: 514–519, 1991.
26. BENDER, B. S., J. E. NAGEL, W. H. ADLER, and R. ANDRES. Absolute peripheral blood lymphocyte count and subsequent mortality of elderly men. The Baltimore Longitudinal Study of Aging. *J. Am. Geriatr. Soc.* 34: 649–654, 1986.
27. BEN-NUN, A., Y. RON, and I. R. COHEN. Spontaneous remission of autoimmune encephalomyelitis is inhibited by splenectomy, thymectomy or ageing. *Nature* 288: 389–390, 1980.
28. BENTLEY, D. M., and R. E. MORRIS. T cell subsets required for protection against age-dependent polioencephalomyelitis of C58 mice. *J. Immunol.* 128: 530–534, 1982.
29. BLAIR, P. B., M. O. STASKAWICZ, and J. S. SAM. Suppression of natural killer cell activity in young and old mice. *Mech. Ageing Dev.* 40: 57–70, 1987.
30. BOERSMA, W. J. A., F. A. STEINMEIER, and J. J. HAAIJMAN. Age-related changes in the relative numbers of Thy-1 and Lyt-2-bearing peripheral blood lymphocytes in mice: a longitudinal approach. *Cell. Immunol.* 93: 417–430, 1985.
31. BRILL, S., T. KUKULANSKY, E. TAL, L. ABEL, Y. POLGIN, C. DASSA, and A. GLOBERSON. Individual changes in T lymphocyte parameters of old human subjects. *Mech. Ageing Dev.* 40: 71–79, 1987.
32. BRULEY-ROSSET, M. and I. VERGNON. Interleukin-1 synthesis and activity in aged mice. *Mech. Ageing Dev.* 24: 247–264, 1984.
33. BUCKLER, A., H. VIE, G. SONENSHEIN, and R. A. MILLER. Defective T lymphocytes in old mice: diminished production of mature c-*myc* mRNA after mitogen exposure not attributable to alterations in transcription or RNA stability. *J. Immunol.* 140: 2442–2446, 1988.
34. BUDD, R. C., J. C. CEROTTINI, C. HORVATH, C. BRON, T. PEDRAZZINI, R. C. HOWE, and H. R. MACDONALD. Distinction of virgin and memory T lymphocytes. Stable acquisition of the Pgp-1 glycoprotein concomitant with antigenic stimulation. *J. Immunol.* 138: 3120–3129, 1987.
35. BURTON, G. F., M. H. KOSCO, A. K. SZAKAL, and J. G. TEW. Iccosomes and the secondary antibody response. *Immunology* 73: 271–276, 1991.
36. CAI, N. S., D. D. LI, H. T. CHEUNG, and A. RICHARDSON. The expression of granulocyte/macrophage colony-stimulating factor in activated mouse lymphocytes declines with age. *Cell Immunol.* 130: 311–319, 1990.
37. CALLARD, R. E., and A. BASTEN. Immune function in aged mice. IV. Loss of T cell and B cell function in thymus-dependent antibody responses. *Eur. J. Immunol.* 8: 552–558, 1978.
38. CARAFOLI, E. Intracellular calcium homeostasis. *Annu. Rev. Biochem.* 56: 395–433, 1987.
39. CEUPPENS, J. L., and J. S. GOODWIN. Regulation of immunoglobulin production in pokeweed mitogen-stimulated cultures of lymphocytes from young and old adults. *J. Immunol.* 128: 2429–2434, 1982.
40. CHANDRA, R. K. Effect of vitamin and trace-element supplementation on immune responses and infection in elderly subjects. *Lancet* 340: 1124–1127, 1992.
41. CHANG, M., T. MAKINODAN, W. J. PETERSON, and B. L. STREHLER. Role of T cells and adherent cells in age-related decline in murine interleukin 2 production. *J. Immunol.* 129: 2426–2430, 1982.
42. CHANG, M. P., D. C. NORMAN, and T. MAKINODAN. Immunotoxicity of alcohol in young and old mice. I. In vitro suppressive effects of ethanol on the activities of T and B immune cells of aging mice. *Alcohol Clin. Exp. Res.* 14: 210–215, 1990.
43. CHANG, M. P., M. UTSUYAMA, K. HIROKAWA, and T. MAKINODAN. Decline in the production of interleukin-3 with age in mice. *Cell Immunol.* 115: 1–12, 1988.
44. CHATELAIN, R., K. VARKILA, and R. L. COFFMAN. IL-4 induces a Th2 response in Leishmania major-infected mice. *J. Immunol.* 148: 1182–1187, 1992.
45. CHIN, K. V., K. UEDA, I. PASTAN, and M. M. GOTTESMAN. Modulation of activity of the promoter of the human MDR1 gene by Ras and p53. *Science* 255: 459–462, 1992.
46. CHOI, K. L., and D. N. SAUDER. Epidermal Langerhans cell

density and contact sensitivity in young and aged BALB/c mice. *Mech. Ageing Dev.* 39: 69–79, 1987.
47. CHOPRA, R. K., N. J. HOLBROOK, D. C. POWERS, M. T. MCCOY, W. H. ADLER, and J. E. NAGEL. Interleukin 2, interleukin 2 receptor, and interferon-gamma synthesis and mRNA expression in phorbol myristate acetate and calcium ionophore A23187-stimulated T cells from elderly humans. *Clin. Immunol. Immunopathol.* 53: 297–308, 1989.
48. CILLARI, E., S. MILANO, M. DIELI, F. ARCOLEO, R. PEREGO, F. LEONI, G. GROMO, A. SEVERN, and F. Y. LIEW. Thymopentin reduces the susceptibility of aged mice to cutaneous leishmaniasis by modulating CD4 T cell subsets. *Immunology* 76: 362–366, 1992.
49. COOK, J. M., N. GUALDE, L. HESSEL, M. MOUNIER, J. P. MICHEL, F. DENIS, and M. H. RATINAUD. Alterations in the human immune response to the hepatitis B vaccine among the elderly. *Cell. Immunol.* 109: 89–96, 1987.
50. COVELLI, V., D. MOUTON, V. DI MAJO, Y. BOUTHILLIER, C. BANGRAZI, J. C. MEVEL, S. REBESSI, G. DORIA, and G. BIOZZI. Inheritance of immune responsiveness, life span, and disease incidence in interline crosses of mice selected for high or low multispecific antibody production. *J. Immunol.* 142: 1224–1234, 1989.
51. CRABTREE, G. R. Contigent genetic regulatory events in T lymphocyte activation. *Science* 243: 355–361, 1989.
52. CROSS, R. J., J. L. CAMPBELL, W. R. MARKESBERY, and T. L. ROSZMAN. Transplantation of pituitary grafts fail to restore immune function and to reconstitute the thymus glands of aged mice. *Mech. Ageing Dev.* 56: 11–22, 1990.
53. DAMJANOVICH, S., and C. PIERI. Electroimmunology: membrane potential, ion-channel activities, and stimulatory signal transduction in human T lymphocytes from young and elderly. *Ann. N. Y. Acad. Sci.* 621: 29–39, 1991.
54. DAVILA, D. R., and K. W. KELLEY. Sex differences in lectin-induced interleukin-2 synthesis in aging rats. *Mech. Ageing Dev.* 44: 231–240, 1988.
55. DAYNES, R. A., and B. A. ARANEO. Prevention and reversal of some age-associated changes in immunologic responses by supplemental dehydroepiandrosterone sulfate therapy. *Aging: Immunol. Infect. Dis.* 3: 135–154, 1992.
56. DAYNES, R. A., B. A. ARANEO, W. B. ERSHLER, C. MALONEY, G.-Z. LI, and S.-Y. RYU. Altered regulation of interleukin-6 production with normal aging: possible linkage to the age-associated decline in dehydroepiandrosterone (DHEA) and its sulfated derivative. *J. Immunol.* (in press), 1993.
57. DEGUCHI, Y., S. NEGORO, H. HARA, S. NISHIO, and S. KISHIMOTO. Age-related changes of proliferative response, kinetics of expression of protooncogenes after the mitogenic stimulation and methylation level of the protooncogene in purified human lymphocyte subsets. *Mech. Ageing Dev.* 44: 153–168, 1988.
58. DELFRAISSY, J. F., P. GALANAUD, C. WALLON, J. F. BALAVOINE, and J. DORMONT. Abolished in vitro antibody response in elderly: exclusive involvement of prostaglandin-induced T suppressor cells. *Clin. Immunol. Immunopathol.* 24: 377–385, 1982.
59. DE PAOLI, P., S. BATTISTIN, and G. F. SANTINI. Age-related changes in human lymphocyte subsets: progressive reduction of the CD4 CD45R (suppressor inducer) population. *Clin. Immunol. Immunopathol.* 48: 290–296, 1988.
60. EBERSOLE, J. L., M. J. STEFFEN, and J. PAPPO. Secretory immune responses in ageing rats. II. Phenotype distribution of lymphocytes in secretory and lymphoid tissues. *Immunology* 64: 289–294, 1988.
61. EFFROS, R. B., and R. L. WALFORD. The immune response of aged mice to influenza: diminished T-cell proliferation, interleukin 2 production and cytotoxicity. *Cell. Immunol.* 81: 298–305, 1983.
62. EFFROS, R. B., and R. L. WALFORD. The effect of age on the antigen-presenting mechanism in limiting dilution precursor cell frequency analysis. *Cell. Immunol.* 88: 531–539, 1984.
63. EFFROS, R. B., K. SVOBODA, and R. L. WALFORD. Influence of age and caloric restriction on macrophage IL-6 and TNF production. *Lymphokine Cytokine Res.* 10: 347–351, 1991.
64. EFFROS, R. B., R. L. WALFORD, R. WEINDRUCH, and C. MITCHELTREE. Influences of dietary restriction on immunity to influenza in aged mice. *J. Gerontol. Biol. Sci.* 46: B142–B147, 1991.
65. EL DEMELLAWY, M., and R. EL RIDI. Age-associated decrease in proportion and antigen expression of $CD8^+/CD4^+$ thymocytes in BALB/c mice. *Mech. Ageing Dev.* 62: 307–318, 1992.
66. EREN, R., D. ZHARHARY, L. ABEL, and A. GLOBERSON. Age-related changes in the capacity of bone marrow cells to differentiate in thymic organ cultures. *Cell. Immunol.* 112: 449–455, 1988.
67. ERNST, D. N., M. V. HOBBS, B. E. TORBETT, A. L. GLASEBROOK, M. A. REHSE, K. BOTTOMLY, K. HAYAKAWA, R. R. HARDY, and W. O. WEIGLE. Differences in the expression profiles of CD45RB, Pgp-1, and 3G11 membrane antigens and in the patterns of lymphokine secretion by splenic $CD4^+$ T cells from young and aged mice. *J. Immunol.* 145: 1295–1302, 1990.
68. ERNST, D. N., W. O. WEIGLE, D. N. MCQUITTY, A. L. ROTHERMEL, and M. H. HOBBS. Stimulation of murine T cell subsets with anti-CD3 antibody. Age-related defects in the expression of early activation molecules. *J. Immunol.* 142: 1413–1421, 1989.
69. ERSHLER, W. B. The influence of an aging immune system on cancer incidence and progression. *J. Gerontol. Biol. Sci.* 48: B3–B7, 1993.
70. FELTEN, S. Y., D. L. BELLINGER, T. J. COLLIER, P. D. COLEMAN, and D. L. FELTEN. Decreased sympathetic innervation of spleen in aged Fischer 344 rats. *Neurobiol. Aging* 8: 159–165, 1987.
71. FIELDS, R. A., H. TOUBBEH, R. P. SEARLES, and A. D. BANKHURST. The prevalence of anticardiolipin antibodies in a healthy elderly population and its association with antinuclear antibodies. *J. Rheumatol.* 16: 623–625, 1989.
72. FLOOD, P. M., J. L. URBAN, M. L. KRIPKE, and H. SCHREIBER. Loss of tumor-specific and idiotype-specific immunity with age. *J. Exp. Med.* 154: 275–290, 1981.
73. FLURKEY, K. and D. E. HARRISON. Use of genetic models to investigate the hypophyseal regulation of senescence. In: *Genetic Effects on Aging II*, edited by D. E. Harrison. Caldwell, NJ: Telford Press, p. 437.
74. FLURKEY, K., R. A. MILLER, and D. E. HARRISON. Cellular determinants of age-related decrements in the T-cell mitogen response of B6CBAF1 mice. *J. Gerontol.* 47: B115–B120, 1992.
75. FLURKEY, K., M. STADECKER, and R. A. MILLER. Memory T lymphocyte hyporesponsiveness to non-cognate stimuli: a key factor in age-related immunodeficiency. *Eur. J. Immunol.* 22: 931–935, 1992.
76. FONG, T. C., and T. MAKINODAN. In situ hybridization analysis of the age-associated decline in IL-2 mRNA expressing murine T cells. *Cell. Immunol.* 118: 199–207, 1989.
77. FOSTER, K. D., C. A. CONN, and M. J. KLUGER. Fever, tumor necrosis factor, and interleukin-6 in young, mature, and aged Fischer 344 rats. *Am. J. Physiol.* 262: R211–R215, 1992.
78. FRANCUS, T., Y. W. CHEN, L. STAIANO-COICO, and J. M. HEFTON. Effect of age on the capacity of the bone marrow and the

spleen cells to generate B lymphocytes. *J. Immunol.* 137: 2411–2417, 1986.
79. FRANKLIN, R. A., S. ARKINS, and K. W. KELLEY. The proliferative response of rat T cells to calcium ionophores increases with age. *Cell Immunol.* 130: 416–428, 1990.
80. FRASCA, D., L. ADORINI, and G. DORIA. Enhanced frequency of mitogen-responsive T cell precursors in old mice injected with thymosin alpha-1. *Eur. J. Immunol.* 17: 727–730, 1987.
81. FRASCA, D., D. BORASCHI, S. BASCHIERI, P. BOSSU, A. TAGLIABUE, L. ADORINI, and G. DORIA. In vivo restoration of T cell functions by human IL-1 beta or its 163–171 nonapeptide in immunodepressed mice. *J. Immunol.* 141: 2651–2655, 1988.
82. FREEDMAN, M. H., M. C. RAFF, and B. GOMPERTS. Induction of increased calcium uptake in mouse T lymphocytes by concanavalin A and its modulation by cyclic nucleotides. *Nature* 255: 378–382, 1975.
83. FROELICH, C. J., J. S. BURKETT, S. GUIFFAUT, R. KINGSLAND, and D. BRAUNER. Phytohemagglutinin induced proliferation by aged lymphocytes: reduced expression of high affinity interleukin-2 receptors and interleukin-2 secretion. *Life Sci.* 43: 1583–1590, 1988.
84. FULOP, T., JR., M. UTSUYAMA, and K. HIROKAWA. Determination of interleukin 2 receptor number of con A stimulated human lymphocytes with aging. *J. Clin. Lab. Immunol.* 34: 31–36, 1991.
85. GAHRING, L. C., and W. O. WEIGLE. The effect of aging on the induction of humoral and cellular immunity and tolerance in two long-lived mouse strains. *Cell Immunol.* 128: 142–151, 1990.
86. GAMBLE, D. A., R. SCHWAB, M. E. WEKSLER, and P. SZABO. Decreased steady state c-myc mRNA in activated T cell cultures from old humans is caused by a smaller proportion of T cells that transcribe the c-myc gene. *J. Immunol.* 144: 3569–3573, 1990.
87. GAUCHAT, J. F., A. L. DEWECK, and B. M. STADLER. Decreased cytokine mRNA levels in the elderly. *Aging: Immunol. Infect. Dis.* 1: 191–204, 1988.
88. GELFAND, E. W., R. T. CHEUNG, G. B. MILLS, and S. GRINSTEIN. Uptake of extracellular Ca^{2+} and not recruitment from internal stores is essential for T lymphocyte proliferation. *Eur. J. Immunol.* 18: 917–922, 1988.
89. GILCHREST, B. A., G. F. MURPHY, and N. A. SOTER. Effect of chronologic aging and ultraviolet irradiation on Langerhans cells in human epidermis. *J. Invest. Dermatol.* 79: 85–88, 1982.
90. GILLIS, S., R. KOZAK, M. DURANTE, and M. E. WEKSLER. Immunological studies of aging. Decreased production of and response to T cell growth factor by lymphocytes from aged humans. *J. Clin. Invest.* 67: 937–942, 1981.
91. GILMAN, S. C., J. S. ROSENBERG, and J. D. FELDMAN. T lymphocytes of young and aged rats. II. Functional defects and the role of interleukin-2. *J. Immunol.* 128: 644–650, 1982.
92. GILMAN-SACHS, A., Y. B. KIM, M. POLLARD, and D. L. SNYDER. Influence of aging, environmental antigens, and dietary restriction on expression of lymphocyte subsets in germ-free and conventional Lobund-Wistar rats. *J. Gerontol.* 46: B101–B106, 1991.
93. GOIDL, E. A., J. B. INNES, and M. E. WEKSLER. Immunological studies of aging. II. Loss of IgG and high avidity plaque-forming cells and increased suppressor cell activity in aging mice. *J. Exp. Med.* 144: 1037–1048, 1976.
94. GOIDL, E. A., P. W. STASHAK, S. J. M. MCEVOY, and J. R. HIERNAUX. Age-related changes in serum immunoglobulin isotypes and isotype sub-class levels among standard long-lived and autoimmune and immunodeficient strains of mice. *Aging: Immunol. Infect. Dis.* 1: 227–236, 1988.
95. GOIDL, E. A., G. J. THORBECKE, M. E. WEKSLER, and G. W. SISKIND. Production of auto-anti-idiotypic antibody during the normal immune response: changes in the auto-anti-idiotypic antibody response and the idiotype repertoire associated with aging. *Proc. Natl. Acad. Sci. U.S.A.* 77: 6788–6792, 1980.
96. GOLDBERG, T. H., D. G. BAKER, and H. R. SCHUMACHER. Interleukin-1 and the immunobiology of aging. *Aging: Immunol. Infect. Dis.* 3: 81–89, 1991.
97. GONZALEZ-QUINTIAL, R., and A. N. THEOFILOPOULOS. V beta gene repertoires in aging mice. *J. Immunol.* 149: 230–236, 1992.
98. GOODMAN, S. A., and T. MAKINODAN. Effect of age on cell-mediated immunity in long-lived mice. *Clin. Exp. Immunol.* 19: 533–542, 1972.
99. GOODWIN, J. S., and R. P. MESSNER. Sensitivity of lymphocytes to prostaglandin E2 increases in subjects over age 70. *J. Clin. Invest.* 64: 434–439, 1979.
100. GOODWIN, J. S., R. P. SEARLES, and K. S. K. TUNG. Immunological responses of a healthy elderly population. *Clin. Exp. Immunol.* 48: 403–410, 1982.
101. GOSO, C., D. FRASCA, and G. DORIA. Effect of synthetic thymic humoral factor (THF-γ2) on T cell activities in immunodeficient ageing mice. *Clin. Exp. Immunol.* 87: 346–351, 1992.
102. GOTTESMAN, S. R. S. Changes in T-cell-mediated immunity with age: an update. *Rev. Biol. Res. Aging* 3: 79–111, 1987.
103. GOTTESMAN, S. R. S., R. L. WALFORD, and G. J. THORBECKE. Proliferative and cytotoxic immune functions in aging mice. III. Exogenous interleukin-2 rich supernatant only partially restores alloreactivity in vitro. *Mech. Ageing Dev.* 31: 103–113, 1985.
104. GOYA, R. G., K. BROOKS, and J. MEITES. A comparison between hormone levels and T lymphocyte function in young and old rats. *Mech. Ageing Dev.* 61: 275–285, 1991.
105. GOZES, Y., T. UMIEL, and N. TRAININ. Selective decline in differentiating capacity of immunohemopoietic stem cells with aging. *Mech. Ageing Dev.* 18: 251–259, 1982.
106. GREEN-JOHNSON, J. M., J. A. HAQ, and M. R. SZEWCZUK. Effects of aging on the production of cytoplasmic interleukin-4 and 5, and interferon-γ by mucosal and systemic lymphocytes after activation with phytohemagglutinin. *Aging: Immunol. Infect. Dis.* 3: 43–57, 1991.
107. GRINBLAT, J., K. SCHAUENSTEIN, E. SALTZ, N. TRAININ, and A. GLOBERSON. Regulatory effects of thymus humoral factor on T cell growth factor in aging mice. *Mech. Ageing Dev.* 22: 209–218, 1983.
108. GROSSMANN, A., J. A. LEDBETTER, and P. S. RABINOVITCH. Reduced proliferation in T lymphocytes in aged humans is predominantly in the $CD8^+$ subset, and is unrelated to defects in transmembrane signaling which are predominantly in the $CD4^+$ subset. *Exp. Cell Res.* 180: 367–382, 1989.
109. GROSSMANN, A., L. MAGGIO-PRICE, J. C. JINNEMAN, and P. S. RABINOVITCH. Influence of aging on intracellular free calcium and proliferation of mouse T-cell subsets from various lymphoid organs. *Cell. Immunol.* 135: 118–131, 1991.
110. GROSSMANN, A., L. MAGGIO-PRICE, J. C. JINNEMAN, N. S. WOLF, and P. S. RABINOVITCH. The effect of long-term caloric restriction on function of T-cell subsets in old mice. *Cell Immunol.* 131: 191–204, 1990.
111. GRYNKIEWICZ, G., M. POENIE, and R. Y. TSIEN. A new generation of Ca^{2+} indicators with greatly improved fluorescence properties. *J. Biol. Chem.* 260: 3440–3448, 1985.
112. GUARCELLO, V., G. TRIOLO, M. CIONI, M. C. MORALE, Z. FARINELLA, U. SCAPAGNINI, and B. MARCHETTI. Phosphatidylserine counteracts physiological and pharmacological suppression of humoral immune response. *Immunopharmacology* 19: 185–195, 1990.
113. GUPTA, S. Membrane signal transduction in T cells in aging humans. *Ann. N. Y. Acad. Sci.* 568: 277–282, 1989.

114. HAAR, J. L., J. K. TAUBENBERGER, L. DOANE, and N. KENYON. Enhanced in vitro bone marrow cell migration and T-lymphocyte responses in aged mice given subcutaneous thymic epithelial cell grafts. *Mech. Ageing Dev.* 47: 207–219, 1989.

115. HALLGREN, H. M., N. BERGH, K. J. RODYSILL, and J. J. O'LEARY. Lymphocyte proliferative response to PHA and anti-CD3/Ti monoclonal antibodies, T cell surface marker expression, and serum IL-2 receptor levels as biomarkers of age and health. *Mech. Ageing Dev.* 43: 175–185, 1988.

116. HARA, H., S. NEGORO, S. MIYATA, O. SAIKI, K. YOSHIZAKI, T. TANAKA, T. IGARASHI, and S. KISHIMOTO. Age-associated changes in proliferative and differentiative response of human B cells and production of T cell-derived factors regulating B cell function. *Mech. Ageing Dev.* 38: 245–258, 1987.

117. HARA, H., T. TANAKA, S. NEGORO, Y. DEGUCHI, S. NISHIO, O. SAIKI, and S. KISHIMOTO. Age-related changes of expression of IL-2 receptor subunits and kinetics of IL-2 internalization in T cells after mitogenic stimulation. *Mech. Ageing Dev.* 45: 167–175, 1988.

118. HARRISON, D. E. Cell and tissue transplantation: a means of studying the aging process. In: *Handbook of the Biology of Aging* (2nd ed.), edited by C. E. Finch and E. L. Schneider. New York: Van Nostrand Reinhold, 1985, p. 322–356.

119. HARRISON, D. E., J. R. ARCHER, and C. M. ASTLE. The effect of hypophysectomy on thymic aging in mice. *J. Immunol.* 129: 2673–2677, 1982.

120. HARRISON, D. E., C. M. ASTLE, and J. A. DELAITTRE. Loss of proliferative capacity in immunohemopoietic stem cells caused by serial transplantation rather than aging. *J. Exp. Med.* 147: 1526–1531, 1978.

121. HARRISON, D. E., C. M. ASTLE, and M. STONE. Numbers and functions of transplantable primitive immunohematopoietic stem cells. Effects of age. *J. Immunol.* 142: 3833–3840, 1989.

122. HAUSMAN, P. B., and M. E. WEKSLER. Changes in the immune response with age. In: *Handbook of the Biology of Aging* (2nd ed.), edited by C. E. Finch and E. L. Schneider. New York: Van Nostrand Reinhold, 1985, p. 414–432.

123. HAYAKAWA, K., and R. R. HARDY. Murine CD4+ T cells subsets defined. *J. Exp. Med.* 168: 1825–1838, 1988.

124. HAYAKAWA, K., and R. R. HARDY. Phenotypic and functional alteration of CD4+ T cells after antigenic stimulation. Resolution of two populations of memory T cells that both secrete interleukin 4. *J. Exp. Med.* 169: 2245–2250, 1989.

125. HAYASHI, Y., M. UTSUYAMA, C. KURASHIMA, and K. HIROKAWA. Spontaneous development of organ-specific autoimmune lesions in aged C57BL/6 mice. *Clin. Exp. Immunol.* 78: 120–126, 1989.

126. HEINE, J. W., and W. H. ADLER. The quantitative production of interferon by mitogen-stimulated mouse lymphocytes as a function of age and its effect on the lymphocytes proliferative response. *J. Immunol.* 118: 1366–1369, 1977.

127. HERTOGH-HUIJBREGTS, A., C. VISSINGA, J. ROZING, and L. NAGELKERKEN. Impairment of CD3-dependent and CD3-independent activation pathways in CD4+ and in CD8+ T cells from old CBA/RIJ mice. *Mech. Ageing Dev.* 53: 141–155, 1990.

128. HIRAMOTO, R. N., V. K. GHANTA, and S. J. SOONG. Effect of thymic hormones on immunity and lifespan. In: *Aging and the Immune. Response,* edited by E. Goidl, New York: Marcel Dekker, 1986, p. 177–198.

129. HIROKAWA, K., and T. MAKINODAN. Thymic involution: effect on T cell differentiation. *J. Immunol.* 114: 1659–1664, 1975.

130. HIROKAWA, K., J. W. ALBRIGHT, and T. MAKINODAN. Restoration of impaired immune functions in aging animals. I. Effect of syngeneic thymus and bone marrow grafts. *Clin. Immunol. Immunopathol.* 5: 371–376, 1976.

131. HIROKAWA, K., S. KUBO, M. UTSUYAMA, C. KURASHIMA, and T. SADO. Age-related change in the potential of bone marrow cells to repopulate the thymus and splenic T cells in mice. *Cell. Immunol.* 100: 443–451, 1986.

132. HIROKAWA, K., K. SATO, and T. MAKINODAN. Restoration of impaired immune functions in aging animals. V. Long-term immunopotentiating effects of combined young bone marrow and newborn thymus grafts. *Clin. Immunol. Immunopathol.* 22: 297–304, 1982.

133. HIROKAWA, K., M. UTSUYAMA, M. KASAI, A. KONNO, C. KURASHIMA, and E. MORIIZUMI. Age-related hyperplasia of the thymus and T-cell system in the Buffalo rat. *Virchows Arch. B. Cell Pathol. Incl. Mol. Pathol.* 59: 38–47, 1990.

134. HO, S. P., K. E. KRAMER, and W. B. ERSHLER. Effect of host age upon interleukin-2-mediated anti-tumor responses in a murine fibrosarcoma model. *Cancer Immunol. Immunother.* 31: 146–150, 1990.

135. HOBBS, M. V., D. N. ERNST, B. E. TORBETT, A. L. GLASEBROOK, M. A. REHSE, D. N. MCQUITTY, M. L. THOMAN, K. BOTTOMLY, A. L. ROTHERMEL, and D. J. NOONAN. Cell proliferation and cytokine production by CD4+ cells from old mice. *J. Cell. Biochem.* 46: 312–320, 1991.

136. HOBBS, M. V., W. O. WEIGLE, D. J. NOONAN, B. E. TORBETT, R. J. MCEVILLY, R. J. KOCH, G. J. CARDENAS, and D. N. ERNST. Patterns of cytokine gene expression by CD4+ T cells from young and old mice. *J. Immunol.* 150: 3602–3614, 1993.

137. HOLBROOK, N. J., R. K. CHOPRA, M. T. MCCOY, J. E. NAGEL, D. C. POWERS, W. H. ADLER, and E. L. SCHNEIDER. Expression of interleukin 2 and the interleukin 2 receptor in aging rats. *Cell Immunol.* 120: 1–9, 1989.

138. HOLMES, K. L., C. T. SCHNIZLEIN, E. H. PERKINS, and J. G. TEW. The effect of age on antigen retention in lymphoid follicles and in collagenous tissue of mice. *Mech. Ageing Dev.* 25: 243–255, 1984.

139. HOOIJKAAS, H., A. A. PREESMAN, A. VAN OUDENAREN, R. BENNER, and J. J. HAAIJMAN. Frequency analysis of functional immunoglobulin C and V gene expression in murine B cells at various ages. *J. Immunol.* 131: 1629–1633, 1983.

140. HORI, Y., E. H. PERKINS, and M. K. HALSALL. Decline in phytohemagglutinin responsiveness of spleen cells from aging mice. *Proc. Soc. Exp. Biol. Med.* 144: 48–53, 1973.

141. HUANG, Y. P., J. C. PECHERE, M. MICHEL, L. GAUTHEY, M. LORETO, J. A. CURRAN, and J. P. MICHEL. In vivo T cell activation, in vitro defective IL-2 secretion, and response to influenza vaccination in elderly women. *J. Immunol.* 148: 715–722, 1992.

142. INAMIZU, T., M. P. CHANG, and T. MAKINODAN. Influence of age on the production and regulation of interleukin-1 mice. *Immunology* 55: 447–455, 1985.

143. IRIMAJIRI, N., E. T. BLOOM, and T. MAKINODAN. Suppression of murine natural killer cell activity by adherent cells from aging mice. *Mech. Ageing Dev.* 31: 155–162, 1985.

144. IWASHIMA, M., T. NAKAYAMA, M. KUBO, Y. ASANO, and T. TADA. Alterations in the proliferative response of T cells from aged and chimeric mice. *Int. Arch. Allergy Appl. Immunol.* 83: 129–137, 1987.

145. JANKOVIC, B. D., and D. MARIC. Enkephalin-induced stimulation of humoral and cellular immune reactions in aged rats. *Ann. N. Y. Acad. Sci.* 621: 135–147, 1991.

146. JONES, P. G., C. A. KAUFFMAN, A. G. BERGMAN, C. M. HAYES, M. J. KLUGER, and J. G. CANNON. Fever in the elderly. Production of leukocytic pyrogen by monocytes from elderly persons. *Gerontology* 30: 182–187, 1984.

147. KADISH, J. L., and R. S. BASCH. Hematopoietic thymocyte precursors. I. Assay and kinetics of the appearance of progeny. *J. Exp. Med.* 143: 1082–1099, 1976.

148. KAPPLER, J. W., P. C. HUNTER, D. JACOBS, and E. LORD. Functional heterogeneity among the T-derived lymphocytes of the mouse. I. Analysis by adult thymectomy. *J. Immunol.* 113: 27–38, 1974.
149. KAUFFMAN, C. A. Endogenous pyrogen/interleukin-1 production in aged rats. *Exp. Gerontol.* 21: 75–78, 1986.
150. KAWAKAMI, K., and E. T. BLOOM. Lymphokine-activated killer cells and aging in mice: significance for defining the precursor cell. *Mech. Ageing Dev.* 41: 229–240, 1987.
151. KAWAKAMI, K., and E. T. BLOOM. Lymphokine-activated killer cells derived from murine bone marrow: age-associated difference in precursor cell populations demonstrated by response to interferon. *Cell Immunol.* 116: 163–171, 1988.
152. KAY, M. M. B., J. MENDOZA, J. DIVEN, T. DENTON, N. UNION, and M. LAJINESS. Age-related changes in the immune system of mice of eight medium and long-lived strains and hybrids. I. Organ, cellular and activity changes. *Mech. Ageing Dev.* 11: 295–346, 1979.
153. KELLEY, K. W., S. BRIEF, H. J. WESTLY, J. NOVAKOFSKI, P. J. BECHTEL, J. SIMON, and E. B. WALKER. GH3 pituitary adenoma cells can reverse thymic aging in rats. *Proc. Natl. Acad. Sci. U.S.A.* 83: 5663–5667, 1986.
154. KENDIG, N. E., F. J. CHREST, J. E. NAGEL, R. E. CHAISSON, A. J. SAAH, and W. H. ADLER. Age-related changes in the immune function of HIV-1 seropositive adults. *Aging: Immunol. Infect. Dis.* 3: 67–80, 1991.
155. KENNES, B., C. L. HUBERT, D. BROHEE, and P. NEVE. Early biochemical events associated with lymphocyte activation in ageing. I. Evidence that Ca^{2+} dependent processes induced by PHA are impaired. *Immunology* 42: 119–126, 1981.
156. KHANSARI, D. N., and T. GUSTAD. Effects of long-term, low-dose growth hormone therapy on immune function and life expectancy of mice. *Mech. Ageing Dev.* 57: 87–100, 1991.
157. KIM, Y. T., E. A. GOIDL, C. SAMARUT, M. E. WEKSLER, G. J. THORBECKE, and G. W. SISKIND. Bone marrow function. I. Peripheral T cells are responsible for the increased auto-anti-idiotype response of older mice. *J. Exp. Med.* 161: 1237–1242, 1985.
158. KIRSCHMANN, D. A., and D. M. MURASKO. Splenic and inguinal lymph node T cells of aged mice respond differently to polyclonal and antigen-specific stimuli. *Cell Immunol.* 139: 426–437, 1992.
159. KISHIMOTO, S., S. TOMINO, K. INOMATA, S. KOTEGAWA, T. SAITO, M. KUROKI, H. MITSUYA, and S. HISAMITSU. Age-related changes in the subsets and functions of human T lymphocytes. *J. Immunol.* 121: 1773–1780, 1978.
160. KISHIMOTO, S., S. TOMINO, H. MITSUYA, and H. NISHIMURA. Age-related decrease in frequencies of B-cell precursors and specific helper T cells involved in the IgG anti-tetanus toxoid antibody production in humans. *Clin. Immunol. Immunopathol.* 25: 1–10, 1982.
161. KLINMAN, D. M. Cross-reactivity of IgM-secreting B cells from normal BALB/c mice. *J. Immunol.* 149: 3569–3573, 1992a.
162. KLINMAN, D. M. Similarities in B cell repertoire development between autoimmune and aging normal mice. *J. Immunol.* 148: 1353–1358, 1992b.
163. KLINMAN, N. R. Antibody-specific immunoregulation and the immunodeficiency of aging. *J. Exp. Med.* 154: 547–551, 1981.
164. KOMATSUBARA, S., B. CINADER, and S. MURAMATSU. Functional competence of dendritic cells of ageing C57BL/6 mice. *Scand. J. Immunol.* 24: 517–525, 1986.
165. KOMURO, T., K. SANO, Y. ASANO, and T. TADA. Analysis of age-related degeneracy of T-cell repertoire: localized functional failure in $CD8^+$ T cells. *Scand. J. Immunol.* 32: 545–553, 1990.
166. KOYAMA, K., T. HOSOKAWA, and A. AOIKE. Aging effect on the immune functions of murine gut-associated lymphoid tissues. *Dev. Comp. Immunol.* 14: 465–473, 1990.
167. KRISHNARAJ, R. Negative modulation of human NK cell activity by purinoceptors. 2. Age-associated, gender-specific partial loss of sensitivity to ATP. *Cell Immunol.* 144: 11–21, 1992.
168. KRISHNARAJ, R., and G. BLANDFORD. Age-associated alterations in human natural killer cells. 2. Increased frequency of selective NK subsets. *Cell Immunol.* 114: 137–148, 1988.
169. KUBO, M., and B. CINADER. Polymorphism of age-related changes in interleukin (IL) production: differential changes of T helper subpopulations, synthesizing IL 2, IL 3 and IL 4. *Eur. J. Immunol.* 20: 1289–1296, 1990.
170. KUNO, M., and P. GARDNER. Ion channels activated by inositol 1,4,5-trisphosphate in plasma membrane of human T-lymphocytes. *Nature* 326: 301–304, 1987.
171. LANZA, E., and J. Y. DJEU. Age-independent natural killer cell activity in murine peripheral blood. In: *NK Cells and Other Natural Effector Cells,* edited by R. B. Herberman, New York: Academic, 1982, p. 335–340.
172. LERNER, A., B. PHILOSOPHE, and R. A. MILLER. Defective calcium influx and preserved inositol phosphate generation in T cells from old mice. *Aging: Immunol. Infect. Dis.* 1: 149–157, 1988.
173. LERNER, A., T. YAMADA, and R. A. MILLER. PGP- 1^{hi} T lymphocytes accumulate with age in mice and respond poorly to concanavalin A. *Eur. J. Immunol.* 19: 977–982, 1989.
174. LEVINE, R. F. Inositol phosphates and Ca^{2+} entry: toward a proliferation or a simplification? *FASEB J.* 6: 3085–3091, 1992.
175. LI, D. D., Y. K. CHIEN, M. Z. GU, A. RICHARDSON, and H. T. CHEUNG. The age-related decline in interleukin-3 expression in mice. *Life Sci.* 43: 1215–1222, 1988.
175a. LI, S. P., and R. A. MILLER. Age-associated decline in IL-4 production by murine T lymphocytes in extended culture. *Cell. Immunol.* 151: 187–195, 1993.
176. LICHTMAN, A. H., G. B. SEGAL, and M. A. LICHTMAN. The role of calcium in lymphocyte proliferation (an interpretive review). *Blood* 61: 413–422, 1983.
177. LUSTYIK, G., and J. J. O'LEARY. Aging and intracellular free calcium response in human T cells after stimulation by phytohemagglutinin. *J. Gerontol.* 44: B30–B36, 1989.
178. LYNGBYE, J., and J. KROLL. Quantitative immunoelectrophoresis of proteins in serum from a normal population: season-, age-, and sex-related variations. *Clin. Chem.* 17: 495–500, 1971.
179. MAKINODAN, T., and M. M. B. KAY. Age influence on the immune system. *Adv. Immunol.* 29: 287–330, 1980.
180. MANOUSSAKIS, M. N., A. G. TZIOUFAS, M. P. SILIS, P. J. E. PANGE, J. GOUDEVENOS, and H. M. MOUTSOPOULOS. High prevalence of anti-cardiolipin and other autoantibodies in a healthy elderly population. *Clin. Exp. Immunol.* 69: 557–565, 1987.
181. MASCART-LEMONE, F., G. DELESPESSE, G. SERVAIS, and M. KUNSTLER. Characterization of immunoregulatory T lymphocytes during ageing by monoclonal antibodies. *Clin. Exp. Immunol.* 48: 148–154, 1982.
182. MASORO, E. J. Food restriction in rodents: an evaluation of its role in the study of aging. *J. Gerontol.* 43: B59–B64, 1988.
183. MASTRO, A. M., and M. C. SMITH. Calcium-dependent activation of lymphocytes by ionophore, A23187, and a phorbol ester tumor promoter. *J. Cell. Physiol.* 116: 51–56, 1983.
184. MATOUR, D., M. MELNICOFF, D. KAYE, and D. M. MURASKO. The role of T cell phenotypes in decreased lymphoproliferation of the elderly. *Clin. Immunol. Immunopathol.* 50: 82–99, 1989.
185. MATSUZAKI, G., Y. YOSHIKAI, K. KISHIHARA, K. NOMOTO, and

T. YOKOKURA. Age-associated increase in the expression of T cell antigen receptor gamma chain genes in mice. *Eur. J. Immunol.* 18: 1779–1784, 1988.
186. MCCORMICK, K. R., J. L. HARR, J. K. TAUBENBERGER, and R. J. KRIEG. A murine model for regeneration of the senescent thymus using growth hormone therapy. *Aging: Immunol. Infect. Dis.* 3: 19–26, 1991.
187. MCELVOY, S. J. M., AND E. A. GOIDL. Studies on immunological maturation. II. The absence of high-affinity antibody producing cells early in the immune response is only apparent. *Aging: Immunol. Infect. Dis.* 1: 47–54, 1988.
188. MERKENSCHLAGER, M. Confusion over CD45 isoform. *Nature* 352: 28, 1991.
189. MERONI, P. L., W. BARCELLINI, D. FRASCA, C. SGUOTTI, M. O. BORGHI, G. DE BARTOLO, G. DORIA, and C. ZANUSSI. In vivo immunopotentiating activity of thymopentin in aging humans: increase of IL-2 production. *Clin. Immunol. Immunopathol.* 42: 151–159, 1987.
190. MEYDANI, S. N., M. MEYDANI, C. P. VERDON, A. A. SHAPIRO, J. B. BLUMBERG, and K. C. HAYES. Vitamin E supplementation suppresses prostaglandin E2 synthesis and enhances the immune response of aged mice. *Mech. Ageing Dev.* 34: 191–201, 1986.
191. MILLER, J. F. A. P. Effect of thymectomy in adult mice on immunological responsiveness. *Nature* 208: 1337–1338, 1965.
192. MILLER, R. A. Age-associated decline in precursor frequency for different T cell-mediated reactions, with preservation of helper or cytotoxic effect per precursor cell. *J. Immunol.* 132: 63–68, 1984.
193. MILLER, R. A. Immunodeficiency of aging: restorative effects of phorbol ester combined with calcium ionophore. *J. Immunol.* 137: 805–808, 1986.
194. MILLER, R. A. Accumulation of hyporesponsive, calcium extruding memory T cells as a key feature of age-dependent immune dysfunction. *Clin. Immunol. Immunopathol.* 58: 305–317, 1991a.
195. MILLER, R. A. Caloric restriction and immune function: developmental mechanisms. *Aging: Clin. Exp. Res.* 3: 395–398, 1991b.
196. MILLER, R. A. Gerontology as oncology: research on aging as the key to the understanding of cancer. *Cancer* 68: 2947–2951, 1991c.
197. MILLER, R. A. Aging and cancer—another perspective. *J. Gerontol. Biol. Sci.* 48: B8–B9, 1993.
198. MILLER, R. A. and D. E. HARRISON. Delayed reduction in T cell precursor frequencies accompanies diet-induced lifespan extension. *J. Immunol.* 136: 977–983, 1984.
199. MILLER, R. A., and O. STUTMAN. Decline, in aging mice, of the anti-TNP cytotoxic T cell response attributable to loss of Lyt-2⁻, IL-2 producing helper cell function. *Eur. J. Immunol.* 11: 751–756, 1981.
200. MILLER, R. A., and O. STUTMAN. T cell repopulation from functionally restricted splenic precursors: 10,000 fold expansion documented by using limiting dilution analyses. *J. Immunol.* 133: 2925–2932, 1984.
201. MILLER, R. A., K. FLURKEY, M. MOLLOY, T. LUBY, and M. J. STADECKER. Differential sensitivity of virgin and memory T lymphocytes to calcium ionophores suggests a buoyant density separation method and a model for memory cell hyporesponsiveness to con A. *J. Immunol.* 147: 3080–3086, 1991.
202. MILLER, R. A., B. JACOBSON, G. WEIL, and E. R. SIMONS. Diminished calcium influx in lectin-stimulated T cells from old mice. *J. Cell. Physiol.* 132: 337–342, 1987.
203. MILLER, R. A., B. PHILOSOPHE, I. GINIS, G. WEIL, and B. JACOBSON. Defective control of cytoplasmic calcium concentration in T lymphocytes from old mice. *J. Cell. Physiol.* 138: 175–182, 1989.
204. MOODY, C. E., J. B. INNES, L. STAIANO-COICO, G. S. INCEFY, H. T. THALER, and M. E. WEKSLER. Lymphocyte transformation induced by autologous cells. XI. The effect of age on the autologous mixed lymphocyte reaction. *Immunology* 44: 431–438, 1981.
205. MORGAN, E. L., M. L. THOMAN, and W. O. WEIGLE. The immune response in aged C57BL/6 mice. I. Assessment of lesions in the B-cell and T-cell compartments of aged mice utilizing the Fc fragment-mediated polyclonal antibody response. *Cell. Immunol.* 63: 16–27, 1981.
206. MOSMANN, T. R., and R. L. COFFMAN. TH1 and TH2 cells: different patterns of lymphokine secretion lead to different functional properties. *Ann. Rev. Immunol.* 7: 145–173, 1989.
207. MOULIAS, R., J. PROUST, A. WANG, F. CONGY, M. R. MARESCOT, A. DEVILLE CHABROLLE, A. PARIS HAMELIN, and B. LESOURD. Age-related increase in autoantibodies [Letter]. *Lancet* 1: 1128–1129, 1984.
208. MURASKO, D. M., B. J. NELSON, R. SILVER, and D. MATOUR. Immunologic response in an elderly population with a mean age of 85. *Am. J. Med.* 81: 612–618, 1986.
209. MURASKO, D. M., P. WEINER, and D. KAYE. Association of lack of mitogen-induced lymphocyte proliferation with increased mortality in the elderly. *Aging: Immunol. Infect. Dis.* 1: 1–6, 1988.
210. MYSLIWSKA, J., A. MYSLIWSKI, P. ROMANOWSKI, J. BIGDA, D. SOSNOWSKA, and J. FOERSTER. Monocytes are responsible for depressed natural killer (NK) activity in both young and elderly low NK responders. *Gerontology* 38: 41–49, 1992.
211. NAGEL, J. E., R. K. CHOPRA, F. J. CHREST, M. T. MCCOY, E. L. SCHNEIDER, N. J. HOLBROOK, and W. H. ADLER. Decreased proliferation, interleukin 2 synthesis, and interleukin 2 receptor expression are accompanied by decreased mRNA expression in phytohemagglutinin-stimulated cells from elderly donors. *J. Clin. Invest.* 81: 1096–1102, 1988.
212. NAGEL, J. E., R. K. CHOPRA, D. C. POWERS, and W. H. ADLER. Effect of age on the human high affinity interleukin 2 receptor of phytohaemagglutinin stimulated peripheral blood lymphocytes. *Clin. Exp. Immunol.* 75: 286–291, 1989.
213. NAGELKERKEN, L., A. HERTOGH-HUIJBREGTS, R. DOBBER, and A. DRAGER. Age-related changes in lymphokine production related to a decreased number of CD45RB^{hi} CD4$^+$ T cells. *Eur. J. Immunol.* 21: 273–281, 1991.
214. NAKAHAMA, M., N. MOHRI, S. MORI, G. SHINDO, Y. YOKOI, and R. MACHINAMI. Immunohistochemical and histometrical studies of the human thymus with special emphasis on age-related changes in medullary epithelial and dendritic cells. *Virchows Arch. B. Cell Pathol. Incl. Mol. Pathol.* 58: 245–251, 1990.
215. NAYLOR, J. R., S. R. JAMES, and L. K. TREJDOSIEWICZ. Intracellular free Ca^{2+} fluxes and responses to phorbol ester in T lymphocytes from healthy elderly subjects. *Clin. Exp. Immunol.* 89: 158–163, 1992.
216. NEGORO, S., and H. HARA. The effect of taurine on the age-related decline of the immune response in mice: the restorative effect on the T cell proliferative response to costimulation with ionomycin and phorbol myristate acetate. *Adv. Exp. Med. Biol.* 315: 229–239, 1992.
217. NEGORO, S., H. HARA, S. MIYATA, O. SAIKI, T. TANAKA, K. YOSHIZAKI, T. IGARASHI, and S. KISHIMOTO. Mechanisms of age-related decline in antigen-specific T cell proliferative response: IL-2 receptor expression and recombinant IL-2 induced proliferative response of purified TAC-positive T cells. *Mech. Ageing Dev.* 36: 223–241, 1986.
218. NICOLETTI, C., and J. CERNY. The repertoire diversity and

magnitude of antibody responses to bacterial antigens in aged mice: I. Age-associated changes in antibody responses differ according to the mouse strain. *Cell Immunol.* 133: 72–83, 1991.

219. NICOLETTI, C., C. BORGHESI-NICOLETTI, X. YANG, D. H. SCHULZE, and J. CERNY. Repertoire diversity of antibody response to bacterial antigens in aged mice. II. Phosphorylcholine-antibody in young and aged mice differ in both V_H/V_L gene repertoire and in specificity. *J. Immunol.* 147: 2750–2755, 1991.

220. NORDIN, A. A., and G. D. COLLINS. Limiting dilution analysis of alloreactive cytotoxic precursor cells in aging mice. *J. Immunol.* 131: 2215–2218, 1983.

221. ODIO, M., A. BRODISH, and M. J. RICARDO, JR. Effects on immune responses by chronic stress are modulated by aging. *Brain Behav. Immun.* 1: 204–215, 1987.

222. O'LEARY, J. J., R. FOX, N. BERGH, K. J. RODYSILL, and H. M. HALLGREN. Expression of the human T cell antigen receptor complex in advanced age. *Mech. Ageing Dev.* 45: 239–252, 1988.

223. ORME, I. M. Aging and immunity to tuberculosis: increased susceptibility of old mice reflects a decreased capacity to generate mediator T lymphocytes. *J. Immunol.* 138: 4414–4418, 1987.

224. ORME, I. M. An age-related loss of the isogeneic barrier to the successful passive cell transfer of antimicrobial immunity in mice. *Mech. Ageing Dev.* 46: 29–32, 1988a.

225. ORME, I. M. A mouse model of the recrudescence of latent tuberculosis in the elderly. *Am. Rev. Respir. Dis.* 137: 716–718, 1988b.

226. ORSON, F. M., C. K. SAADEH, D. E. LEWIS, and D. L. NELSON. Interleukin 2 receptor expression by T cells in human aging. *Cell. Immunol.* 124: 278–291, 1989.

227. OWEN, J. A., M. ALLOUCHE, and P. C. DOHERTY. Limiting dilution analysis of the specificity of influenza-immune cytotoxic T cells. *Cell. Immunol.* 67: 49–59, 1982.

228. PATEL, H. R., and R. A. MILLER. Age-associated changes in mitogen-induced protein phosphorylation in murine T lymphocytes. *Eur. J. Immunol.* 22: 253–260, 1992.

229. PATEL, P. J. Aging and cellular defense mechanisms: age-related changes in resistance of mice to Listeria monocytogenes. *Infect. Immun.* 32: 557–562, 1981a.

230. PATEL, P. J. Aging and antimicrobial immunity. Impaired production of mediator T cells as a basis for the decreased resistance of senescent mice to Listeriosis. *J. Exp. Med.* 154: 821–831, 1981b.

231. PERKINS, E. H., J. M. MASSUCCI, and P. L. GLOVER. Antigen presentation by peritoneal macrophages from young adult and old mice. *Cell. Immunol.* 70: 1–10, 1982.

232. PHILOSOPHE, B., and R. A. MILLER. T lymphocyte heterogeneity in old and young mice: functional defects in T cells selected for poor calcium signal generation. *Eur. J. Immunol.* 19: 695–699, 1989.

233. PHILOSOPHE, B., and R. A. MILLER. Diminished calcium signal generation in subsets of T lymphocytes that predominate in old mice. *J. Gerontol. Biol. Sci.* 45: B87–B93, 1990.

234. PHILOSOPHE, B., and R. A. MILLER. Calcium signals in murine T lymphocytes: preservation of responses to PHA and to an anti-Ly-6 antibody. *Aging: Immunol. Infect. Dis.* 2: 11–18, 1991.

235. PIERI, C., R. RECCHIONI, F. MORONI, F. MARCHESELLI, and G. LIPPONI. Phytohemagglutinin induced changes of membrane lipid packing, c-myc and c-myb encoded protein expression in human lymphocytes during aging. *Mech. Ageing Dev.* 64: 177–187, 1992.

236. PILARSKI, L. M., B. R. YACYSHYN, G. S. JENSEN, E. PRUSKI, and H. F. PABST. β1 integrin (CD29) expression on human postnatal T cell subsets defined by selective CD45 isoform expression. *J. Immunol.* 147: 830–837, 1991.

237. PROSS, H. F., and M. G. BAINES. Studies of human natural killer cells. I. In vivo parameters affecting normal cytotoxic function. *Int. J. Cancer* 29: 383–390, 1982.

238. PROUST, J. J., C. R. FILBURN, S. A. HARRISON, M. A. BUCHHOLZ, and A. A. NORDIN. Age-related defect in signal transduction during lectin activation of murine T lymphocytes. *J. Immunol.* 139: 1472–1478, 1987.

239. PROUST, J. J., D. S. KITTUR, M. A. BUCHHOLZ, and A. A. NORDIN. Restricted expression of mitogen-induced high affinity IL-2 receptors in aging mice. *J. Immunol.* 141: 4209–4216, 1988.

240. PUTNAM, A. D., and T. C. PETERSON. Effect of aging and other factors on monocyte aryl hydrocarbon hydroxylase activity. *Mech. Ageing Dev.* 60: 61–74, 1991.

241. RABINOWE, S. L., R. C. NAYAK, K. KRISCH, K. L. GEORGE, and G. S. EISENBARTH. Aging in man. Linear increase of a novel T cell subset defined by antiganglioside monoclonal antibody 3G5. *J. Exp. Med.* 165: 1436–1441, 1987.

242. RILEY, R. L., M. G. KRUGER, and J. ELIA. B cell precursors are decreased in senescent BALB/c mice, but retain normal mitotic activity in vivo and in vitro. *Clin. Immunol. Immunopathol.* 59: 301–313, 1991.

243. RILEY, S. C., B. G. FROSCHER, P. J. LINTON, D. ZHARHARY, K. MARCU, and N. R. KLINMAN. Altered V_h gene segment utilization in the response to phosphorylcholine of aged mice. *J. Immunol.* 143: 3798–3805, 1989.

244. ROBERTS-THOMSON, I. C., S. WHITTINGHAM, U. YOUNGCHAIYUD, and I. R. MACKAY. Ageing, immune response, and mortality. *Lancet* 2: 368–370, 1974.

245. ROCHA, B. B. Population kinetics of precursors of IL 2-producing peripheral T lymphocytes: evidence for short life expectancy, continuous renewal, and post-thymic expansion. *J. Immunol.* 139: 365–372, 1987.

246. RODRIGUEZ, M. A., J. L. CEUPPENS, and J. S. GOODWIN. Regulation of IgM rheumatoid factor production in lymphocyte cultures from young and old subjects. *J. Immunol.* 128: 2422–2428, 1982.

247. ROMBALL, C. G., and W. O. WEIGLE. The effect of aging on the induction of experimental autoimmune thyroiditis. *J. Immunol.* 139: 1490–1495, 1987.

248. RYTEL, M. W., K. S. LARRATT, P. A. TURNER, and J. H. KALBFLEISCH. Interferon response to mitogens and viral antigens in elderly and young adult subjects. *J. Infect. Dis.* 153: 984–987, 1986.

249. SANDERS, M. E., M. W. MAKGOBA, and S. SHAW. Human naive and memory T cells: reinterpretation of helper-inducer and suppressor-inducer subsets. *Immunol. Today* 9: 195–199, 1988.

250. SAUDER, D. N., U. PONNAPPAN, and B. CINADER. Effect of age on cutaneous interleukin 1 expression. *Immunol. Lett.* 20: 111–114, 1989.

251. SAWIN, C. T., S. T. BIGOS, S. LAND, and P. BACHARACH. The aging thyroid. Relationship between elevated serum thyrotropin level and thyroid antibodies in elderly patients. *Am. J. Med.* 79: 591–595, 1985.

252. SAXENA, R. K., Q. B. SAXENA, and W. H. ADLER. Interleukin-2-induced activation of natural killer activity in spleen cells from old and young mice. *Immunology* 51: 719–726, 1984.

253. SAXENA, R. K., Q. B. SAXENA, and W. H. ADLER. Lectin-induced cytotoxic activity in spleen cells from young and old mice. Age-related changes in types of effector cells, lymphokine production and response. *Immunology* 64: 457–461, 1988.

254. SCHLUNCK, T., W. SCHRAUT, G. RIETHMULLER, and H. W. ZIEGLER-HEITBROCK. Inverse relationship of Ca^{2+} mobilization

and cell proliferation in CD8$^+$ memory and virgin T cells. *Eur. J. Immunol.* 20: 1957–1963, 1990.
255. SCHULZE, D. H., P. MANCILLAS, A. KAUSHIK, C. BONA, and G. KELSOE. Mitogen-induced V$_H$ and V$_K$ expression is similar in young adult and aged mice. *Aging: Immunol. Infect. Dis.* 3: 127–134, 1992.
256. SCHWAB, R., P. B. HAUSMAN, E. RINNOOY-KAN, and M. E. WEKSLER. Immunological studies of ageing. X. Impaired T lymphocytes and normal monocyte response from elderly humans to the mitogenic antibodies OKT3 and Leu 4. *Immunology* 55: 677–684, 1985.
257. SCHWAB, R., L. M. PFEFFER, P. SZABO, D. GAMBLE, C. M. SCHNURR, and M. E. WEKSLER. Defective expression of high affinity IL-2 receptors on activated T cells from aged humans. *Int. Immunol.* 2: 239–246, 1990.
258. SCHWAB, R., C. RUSSO, and M. E. WEKSLER. Altered major histocompatibility complex-restricted antigen recognition by T cells from elderly humans. *Eur. J. Immunol.* 22: 2989–2993, 1992.
259. SCOLLAY, R. G., E. C. BUTCHER, and I. L. WEISSMAN. Thymus cell migration. Quantitative aspects of cellular traffic from the thymus to the periphery in mice. *Eur. J. Immunol.* 10: 210–218, 1980.
260. SCOTT, M., R. BOLLA, and W. D. DENCKLA. Age-related changes in immune function of rats and the effect of long-term hypophysectomy. *Mech. Ageing Dev.* 11: 127–136, 1979.
261. SCRIBNER, D. J., H. L. WEINER, and J. W. MOORHEAD. Anti-immunoglobulin stimulation of murine lymphocytes. V. Age-related decline in Fc receptor-mediated immunoregulation. *J. Immunol.* 121: 377–382, 1978.
262. SEGAL, J. Studies on the age-related decline in the response of lymphoid cells to mitogens: measurements of concanavalin A binding and stimulation of calcium and sugar uptake in thymocytes from rats of varying ages. *Mech. Ageing Dev.* 33: 295–303, 1986.
263. SERRA, H. M., J. F. KROWKA, J. A. LEDBETTER, and L. M. PILARSKI. Loss of CD45R (Lp220) represents a post-thymic T cell differentiation event. *J. Immunol.* 140: 1435–1441, 1988.
264. SETH, A., M. NAGARKATTI, P. S. NAGARKATTI, B. SUBBARAO, and V. UDHAYAKUMAR. Macrophages but not B cells from aged mice are defective in stimulating autoreactive T cells in vitro. *Mech. Ageing Dev.* 52: 107–124, 1990.
265. SHI, J., and R. A. MILLER. Tyrosine-specific protein phosphorylation in response to anti-CD3 antibody is diminished in old mice. *J. Gerontol. Biol. Sci.* 47: B147–B153, 1992.
265a. SHI, J., and R. A. MILLER. Differential tyrosine-specific protein phosphorylation in mouse T lymphocyte subsets. Effect of age. *J. Immunol.* 151: 730–739, 1993.
266. SIDMAN, C. L., E. A. LUTHER, J. D. MARSHALL, K. A. NGUYEN, D. C. ROOPENIAN, and S. M. WORTHEN. Increased expression of major histocompatibility complex antigens on lymphocytes from aged mice. *Proc. Natl. Acad. Sci. U.S.A.* 84: 7624–7628, 1987.
267. SIMPSON, E., and H. CANTOR. Regulation of the immune response by subclasses of T lymphocytes. II. The effect of adult thymectomy upon humoral and cellular responses in mice. *Eur. J. Immunol.* 5: 337–343, 1975.
268. SMITH, J. P., A. M. LISTER, J. G. TEW, and A. K. SZAKAL. Kinetics of the tingible body macrophage response in mouse germinal center development and its depression with age. *Anat. Rec.* 229: 511–520, 1991.
269. SNOW, E. C. An evaluation of antigen-driven expansion and differentiation of hapten-specific B lymphocytes purified from aged mice. *J. Immunol.* 139: 1758–1762, 1987.
270. SOHNLE, P. G., S. E. LARSON, C. COLLINS-LECH, and A. R. GUANSING. Failure of lymphokine-producing lymphocytes from aged humans to undergo activation by recall antigens. *J. Immunol.* 124: 2169–2174, 1980.
271. SPRECHER, E., Y. BECKER, G. KRAAL, E. HALL, D. HARRISON, and L. D. SCHULTZ. Effect of aging on epidermal dendritic cell populations in C57BL/6J mice. *J. Invest. Dermatol.* 94: 247–253, 1990.
272. STUTMAN, O. Two main features of T-cell development: thymus traffic and postthymic maturation. *Contemp. Top. Immunobiol.* 7: 1–46, 1977.
273. STUTMAN, O. Role of thymic hormones in T cell differentiation. *Clin. Immunol. Allergy* 3: 9–81, 1983.
274. STUTMAN, O., C. J. PAIGE, and E. F. FIGARELLA. Natural cytotoxic cells against solid tumors in mice. I. Strain and age distribution and target cell susceptibility. *J. Immunol.* 121: 1819–1826, 1978.
275. SUBBARAO, B., J. MORRIS, and R. J. KRYSCIO. Phenotypic and functional properties of B lymphocytes from aged mice. *Mech. Ageing Dev.* 51: 223–241, 1990.
276. SZAKAL, A. K., J. K. TAYLOR, J. P. SMITH, M. H. KOSCO, G. F. BURTON, and J. G. TEW. Morphometry and kinetics of antigen transport and developing antigen retaining reticulum of follicular dendritic cells in lymph nodes of aging mice. *Aging: Immunol. Infect. Dis.* 1: 7–22, 1988.
277. SZEWCZUK, M. R., and R. J. CAMPBELL. Lack of age-associated auto-anti-idiotypic antibody regulation in mucosal-associated lymph nodes. *Eur. J. Immunol.* 11: 650–656, 1981.
278. THOMAN, M. L. Impaired responsiveness of IL-2 receptor-expressing T lymphocytes from aged mice. *Cell Immunol.* 135: 410–417, 1991.
279. THOMAN, M. L., and W. O. WEIGLE. Lymphokines and aging: interleukin-2 production and activity in aged animals. *J. Immunol.* 127: 2101–2106, 1981.
280. THOMAN, M. L., and W. O. WEIGLE. Cell-mediated immunity in aged mice: an underlying lesion in IL 2 synthesis. *J. Immunol.* 128: 2358–2361, 1982.
281. THOMAN, M. L., and W. O. WEIGLE. Reconstitution of in vivo cell-mediated lympholysis responses in aged mice with interleukin 2. *J. Immunol.* 134: 949–952, 1985.
282. THOMAN, M. L., and W. O. WEIGLE. Partial restoration of con A-induced proliferation, IL-2 receptor expression, and IL-2 synthesis in aged murine lymphocytes by phorbol myristate acetate and ionomycin. *Cell. Immunol.* 114: 1–11, 1988.
283. THOMAN, M. L., and W. O. WEIGLE. The cellular and subcellular bases of immunosenescence. *Adv. Immunol.* 46: 221–261, 1989.
284. THOMAN, M. L., E. A. KEOGH, and W. O. WEIGLE. Response of aged T and B lymphocytes to IL-4. *Aging: Immunol. Infect. Dis.* 1: 245–253, 1988.
285. THOMPSON, J. S., D. R. WEKSTEIN, J. L. RHOADES, C. KIRKPATRICK, S. A. BROWN, T. ROSZMAN, R. STRAUS, and N. TIETZ. The immune status of healthy centenarians. *J. Am. Geriatr. Soc.* 32: 274–281, 1984.
286. TOMER, Y., S. MENDLOVIC, T. KUKULANSKY, E. MOZES, Y. SHOENFELD, and A. GLOBERSON. Effects of aging on the induction of experimental systemic lupus erythematosus (SLE) in mice. *Mech. Ageing Dev.* 58: 233–244, 1991.
287. TSANG, K. Y., J. F. PAN, D. L. SWANGER, and H. H. FUDENBERG. In vitro restoration of immune responses in aging humans by isoprinosine. *Immunopharmacology* 7: 199–206, 1985.
288. TSUDA, T., Y. T. KIM, G. W. SISKIND, and M. E. WEKSLER. Old mice recover the ability to produce IgG and high-avidity antibody following irradiation with partial bone marrow shielding. *Proc. Natl. Acad. Sci. U.S.A.* 85: 1169–1173, 1988.
289. UTSUYAMA, M., K. HIROKAWA, C. KURASHIMA, M. FUKAYAMA, T. INAMATSU, K. SUZUKI, W. HASHIMOTO, and K. SATO.

Differential age-change in the numbers of CD4⁺CD45RA⁺ and CD4⁺CD29⁺ T cell subsets in human peripheral blood. *Mech. Ageing Dev.* 63: 57–68, 1992.

290. UTSUYAMA, M., M. KASAI, C. KURASHIMA, and K. HIROKAWA. Age influence on the thymic capacity to promote differentiation of T cells: induction of different composition of T cell subsets by aging thymus. *Mech. Ageing Dev.* 58: 267–277, 1991.

291. VAN SEVENTER, G. A., W. NEWMAN, Y. SHIMIZU, T. B. NUTMAN, Y. TANAKA, K. J. HORGAN, T. V. GOPAL, E. ENNIS, D. O'SULLIVAN, H. GREY, and S. SHAW. Analysis of T cell stimulation by superantigen plus major histocompatibility complex class II molecules or by CD3 monoclonal antibody: costimulation by purified adhesion ligands VCAM-1, ICAM-1, but not ELAM-1. *J. Exp. Med.* 174: 901–913, 1991.

292. VARGA, Z., N. BRESSANI, A. M. ZAIA, L. BENE, T. FULOP, A. LEOVEY, N. FABRIS, S. DAMJANOVICH, and A. M. ZAID. Cell surface markers, inositol phosphate levels and membrane potential of lymphocytes from young and old human patients. *Immunol. Lett.* 23: 275–280, 1990. [Erratum appears in *Immunol Lett* 26: 111, 1990.]

293. VIE, H., and R. A. MILLER. Decline, with age, in the proportion of mouse T cells that express IL-2 receptors after mitogen stimulation. *Mech. Ageing Dev.* 33: 313–322, 1986.

294. VISSINGA, C., A. HERTOGH-HUIJBREGTS, J. ROZING, and L. NAGELKERKEN. Analysis of the age-related decline in alloreactivity of CD4⁺ and CD8⁺ T cells in CBA/RIJ mice. *Mech. Ageing Dev.* 51: 179–194, 1990.

295. WALKER, D., J. F. GAUCHAT, A. L. DE WECK, and B. M. STADLER. Analysis of leukocyte markers in elderly individuals. *Aging: Immunol. Infect. Dis.* 2: 31–43, 1990.

296. WALTERS, C. S., and H. N. CLAMAN. Age-related changes in cell-mediated immunity in BALB/c mice. *J. Immunol.* 115: 1438–1443, 1975.

297. WAYNE, S. J., R. L. RHYNE, P. J. GARRY, and J. S. GOODWIN. Cell-mediated immunity as a predictor of morbidity and mortality in subjects over 60. *J. Gerontol. Med. Sci.* 45: M45–M48, 1990.

298. WEI, J., H. XU, J. L. DAVIES, and G. P. HEMMINGS. Increase of plasma IL-6 concentration with age in healthy subjects. *Life Sci.* 51: 1953–1956, 1992.

299. WEINDRUCH, R., B. H. DEVENS, H. V. RAFF, and R. L. WALFORD. Influence of dietary restriction and aging on natural killer cell activity in mice. *J. Immunol.* 130: 993–996, 1983.

300. WEINER, H. L., D. J. SCRIBNER, A. L. SCHOCKET, and J. W. MOORHEAD. Increased proliferative response of human peripheral blood lymphocytes to anti-immunoglobulin antibodies in elderly people. *Clin. Exp. Immunol.* 9: 356–362, 1978.

301. WEKSLER, M. E., R. SCHWAB, F. HUETZ, Y. T. KIM, and A. COUTINHO. Cellular basis for the age-associated increase in autoimmune reactions. *Int. Immunol.* 2: 329–335, 1990.

302. WHISLER, R. L., L. BEIQING, Y. G. NEWHOUSE, J. D. WALTERS, M. B. BRECKENRIDGE, and I. S. GRANTS. Signal transduction in human B cells during aging: alterations in stimulus-induced phosphorylations of tyrosine and serine-threonine substrates and in cytosolic calcium responsiveness. *Lymphokine Cytokine Res.* 10: 463–473, 1991.

303. WHISLER, R. L., Y. G. NEWHOUSE, R. L. DONNERBERG, and C. M. TOBIN. Characterization of intracellular ionized calcium responsiveness and inositol phosphate production among resting and stimulated peripheral blood T cells from elderly humans. *Aging: Immunol. Infect. Dis.* 3: 27–36, 1991.

304. WHISLER, R. L., J. W. WILLIAMS, JR., and Y. G. NEWHOUSE. Human B cell proliferative responses during aging. Reduced RNA synthesis and DNA replication after signal transduction by surface immunoglobulins compared to B cell antigenic determinants CD20 and CD40. *Mech. Ageing Dev.* 61: 209–222, 1991.

305. WITKOWSKI, J., and H. S. MICKLEM. Decreased membrane potential of T lymphocytes in ageing mice: flow cytometric studies with a carbocyanine dye. *Immunology* 56: 307–313, 1985.

306. WITKOWSKI, J. M., and H. S. MICKLEM. Transmembrane electrical potential of lymphocytes in ageing mice. Flow cytometric analysis of mitogen-stimulated cells. *Mech. Ageing Dev.* 62: 167–179, 1992.

307. WITKOWSKI, J. M., and R. A. MILLER. Increased functions of P-glycoprotein in T lymphocytes of aging mice. *J. Immunol.* 150: 1296–1306, 1993.

308. WITKOWSKI, J. M., A. MYSLIWSKI, and J. MYSLIWSKA. Decrease of lymphocyte (Na⁺,K⁺)ATP-ase activity in aged people. *Mech. Ageing Dev.* 33: 11–17, 1985.

309. WRABATZ, L. G., J. P. ANTEL, J. J. F. OGER, B. G. W. ARNASON, J. M. GOUST, and J. E. HOPPER. Age-related changes in vivo immunoglobulin secretion: comparison of responses to T-dependent and T-independent polyclonal activators. *Cell. Immunol.* 74: 398–403, 1982.

310. WU, W. T., M. PAHLAVANI, H. T. CHEUNG, and A. RICHARDSON. The effect of aging on the expression of interleukin 2 messenger ribonucleic acid. *Cell. Immunol.* 100: 224–231, 1986.

311. ZHARHARY, D. T cell involvement in the decrease of antigen-responsive B cells in aged mice. *Eur. J. Immunol.* 16: 1175–1178, 1986.

312. ZHARHARY, D. Age-related changes in the capability of the bone marrow to generate B cells. *J. Immunol.* 141: 1863–1869, 1988.

313. ZHARHARY, D., and N. R. KLINMAN. Antigen responsiveness of the mature and generative B cell populations of aged mice. *J. Exp. Med.* 157: 1300–1308, 1983.

314. ZHARHARY, D., and N. R. KLINMAN. B cell repertoire diversity to PR8 influenza virus does not decrease with age. *J. Immunol.* 133: 2285–2287, 1984.

315. ZHARHARY, D., and N. R. KLINMAN. A selective increase in the generation of phosphorylcholine-specific B cells associated with aging. *J. Immunol.* 136: 368–370, 1986.

22. Loss of integration and resiliency with age: a dissipative destruction

F. EUGENE YATES
LAUREL A. BENTON | *Department of Medicine, University of California, Los Angeles, California*

CHAPTER CONTENTS

Senescence
    Models in science
    Senescence is not the same as aging
    What senesces?
        Evolution and senescence
        Mitosis, senescence, and multicellularity
    System death or component death
        Death is a poor indicator
        Weighing counterexamples
Regular Phenomena
    Increases in regularity with senescence
    Regularity of a variable's time history
        Programmatic phenomena
        Execution-driven phenomena
Physical Background of Senescence
    Complexity
    Order
    Vertical integration (hierarchy)
    Horizontal integration (heterarchy)
    Causality
    Stability
        Marginal dynamic stability: resiliency
    Energy vs. entropy in self-organization
General Principle of Homeodynamic Senescence
    Homeodynamics instead of homeostasis
    Irreversibility and constraints
        Fractal time, "1/f noise," and near-periodicity of homeodynamic systems
    Biological markers of age
Homeodynamics and Predictability
    Specifying the homeodynamic construct
    Fluctuations and chance
Counterintuitive Effects of Clamping a Homeodynamic System
    Environmental potentials
    Clamping
Redefinition of Senescence
    Escape from senescence-induced fatal failures by re-initialization
    Summary of characteristics of senescence as homeodynamic instability
Aspects of Senescence
    Aspect theories
    Generalizations from aspect theories
Wear-and-Tear Revisited
    Reliability theory for machines
        Three mathematical models
        Manifestations of unreliability
Human Senescence as Dissipative Destruction
    Component failure—cell culture senescence
    Dissipative destruction as basis of Gompertz mortality kinetics
        Model of reliability theory
        Use it and lose it or use it or lose it?
        Model of data
Summary

SENESCENCE

THE EMERGENCE OF A COMPREHENSIVE AND COHERENT THEORY OF BIOLOGICAL AGING might easily be expected, given the intense interest in human mortality and the successful application of methods of molecular and cellular biology to the study of senescence, as well as the maturation of reliability theories pertaining to technological devices and machines. Unfortunately, the reality is otherwise: we have only "aspect" viewpoints, each partial and incomplete, in which investigators with different disciplinary backgrounds perceive many diverse starting points for the development of theories about aging (80). It has even been claimed that senescence is not a fact at all because the idea has no basis from which nontrivial predictions can be made that are not merely tautologous rearrangements of the facts out of which they were constructed in the first place (54). The literature on senescence has been described as a "froth of uninterpretable data, based on a substratum of speculations" (75), but in biology one always has great difficulty making or justifying anything resembling a general statement (11). In this chapter we seek a new model for senescence.

Models in Science

In a mature physical science two kinds of models are found: *(1)* models *on* theory (specified by auxiliary equations or statements of boundary conditions and constraints) and *(2)* models *of* data fitted by a deterministic or statistical formalism. Complete scientific explanation in a particular case requires joining the two types of model to show that they are identical or that the data model is a special instance of the more general theory model (89). In the study of biological aging, we have only models of data and the high probability that the data themselves are incomplete, inaccurate, or obtained under unnatural conditions.

In this chapter we offer a physical, thermodynamic perspective on senescence as a prototheory—*homeodynamics*—to encourage the maturation of gerontological theorizing and the convergence of physics and biology (104). We begin by distinguishing senescence from aging.

Senescence Is Not the Same as Aging

We define "aging" as any changes in a system of interest that occur seemingly in association with the directional flow of external time. Those changes may be judged as good, bad, or indifferent, as in the aging of wine or cheese (43, 51); however, the term "aging" is neutral. We shall use the term "senescence" to describe damage, harm, loss, fragility, or failure associated with the aging of living systems. It is senescence, not aging, that is the prelude to death from "old age." Senescence is usually defined with respect to a *population* as an increase in morbidity and in mortality rates with time, implying a progressive deterioration in age-specific fitness. *Mortality rate* is the number dying per population unit (typically for humans 100,000) per time unit (typically 1 yr). It is often normalized for humans by reference to the age structure of the U.S. population in some given year. (Botanists sometimes make a restricted use of the term "senescence" to denote a narrow class of phenomena, including seasonal loss of leaves in deciduous trees. This idiosyncratic usage is irrelevant to the gerontological phenomena we analyze here.)

Stable atoms do not age, but an aggregate of radioactive isotopes does; its chemical composition changes with time. Simple molecules (for example, H_2) do not age, but complex molecules, such as biologically synthesized proteins, age by spontaneous racemization of the L-isomers of their amino acids; they lose their broken symmetries (for example, dentin). Inanimate, suspended life or crypto- or frozen life can age. Dehydrated tardigrades, spores, seed embryos, and some frozen organisms are examples of pure, dead organic structures without biological processes. If they show any change with time, such as spontaneous oxidation of lipids when they are exposed to air, it is only aging, but, carried too far, that aging may prevent the regaining of the living state under later, favorable conditions of hydration or thermalization that usually revivify.

A zygote exposed to environmental conditions under which it will grow, develop, and differentiate is changing with time (that is, aging; in this case favorably with respect to survival, so we can regard it as developing or *maturing*, the opposite of senescing).

What Senesces?

Inanimate matter does not senesce. Viruses are inanimate and do not senesce. To be animate, matter must be so organized that the three processes of autonomous morphogenesis, teleonomic (goal-directed) behavior, and (nearly) invariant reproduction can be observed (53). Among living states of matter, a subset of organisms senesces. The problem is to define that subset and extract some generalization from it. If an organism itself cannot be clearly defined—as in the case of the slime mold with its separate stages of a population of free-swimming amoebae and the multicellular, aggregated, differentiated stage with fruiting bodies, spores, stalks, etc.,—it falls outside of the domain of the prototheory of senescence we shall propose. Rose (71) has attempted a comparative (evolutionary) analysis of senescence, which exposes the substantial difficulty in extracting generalizations from biodiversity.

Below we sketch some evolutionary pathways and try to locate senescence phenomena in them. In doing so we take an organismal, not a populational, view of senescence. The former focuses on deleterious effects of aging on individuals and, in the case of human beings, serves as the foundation for geriatric medicine. The latter is the evolutionary view and depends on population genetic hypotheses. Both are valid approaches but differ in emphasis. For example, the evolutionary perspective puts great weight on the fact that as time passes for a population, the age-specific distributions of probability of dying in the next time interval and of reproductive capability both change, mortality increasing and fecundity decreasing (in most cases). Our interest here, however, is to examine and explain the viability trajectory of an individual organism from the beginning to the end of its life.

To anticipate the evidence, we point out that certain organisms do not seem to senesce. These include all prokaryotes and some coelenterates. Some plants have vegetative reproduction and may not senesce. Semelparous reproducers die dramatically after reproduction, but it is debatable whether or not that death is from senescence. Porifera (sponges) are double-walled cell colonies permanently attached as adults, but the organisms themselves are ambiguous, being either single-celled or multicellular (as is the slime mold already mentioned). Pieces of sponge can regenerate a whole sponge. Diatoms are unicellular or colonial algae and present similar ambiguities. Most algae are more clearly multicellular and senesce. Some have the capability for

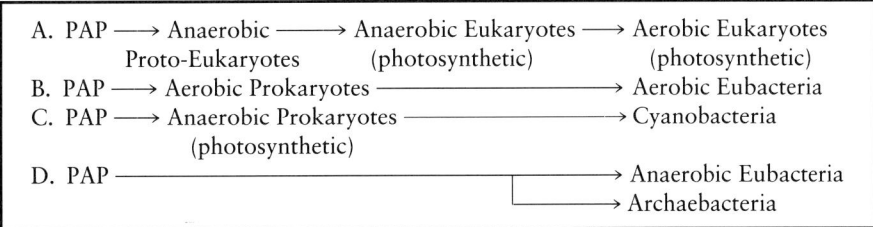

Scheme I

secondary growth, and older cells of stipes become nonfunctional while new trumpet cells appear.

We conclude that senescence is most evident in multicellular forms with highly differentiated subsystems that require compromises in overall design, such that the performance of every function cannot be simultaneously optimized. Senescence appears when some threshold of evolutionary complexity has been exceeded. We do not know the exact distribution of senescence phenomena among existing taxa or in the history of the biosphere. Finch (26) has provided a splendid account of the problem.

Evolution and Senescence. Here we summarize interpretatively a large body of observations (see refs. 71, 26, 32, and chapter 1 in this volume). Impressive as such compendia are, they pale in the face of the estimated 8–10 million contemporary living species, including roughly 9,000 kinds of bird, 4,500 kinds of mammal, 20,000 species of butterfly, and 250,000 plant species. Sixty-nine thousand kinds of fungus have been named, but it is estimated that 20 times that number are so far unnamed (69). Furthermore, this impressive biodiversity, now waning, is thought to be much less than it was 500,000 yr ago. Recognizing the small size of the available sample of organisms carefully studied under defined and understood conditions, we shall base our prototheory on the least doubtful instances of senescence leading to death. Our own species is the cynosure, and we adopt the working hypothesis that only a subset of multicellular organisms senesces.

The evolutionary lines of single cells from primordial anaerobic prokaryotes (PAP), and, perhaps, a precursor RNA system (24a), to the contemporary diversity of the biosphere are conjectured to have followed four pathways before multicellular forms appeared (Scheme I).

Scheme I does not show the postulated symbioses between anaerobic, photosynthetic pro- and eukaryotes leading to chloroplasts as organelles. A similar symbiosis may have occurred between aerobic prokaryotes and photosynthetic eukaryotes. The notion that mitochondria are the result of another symbiosis is weakened by the fact that mitochondrial DNA has reiterated sequences more like eukaryotes than bacteria.

Nowhere in Scheme I do we find organisms that clearly senesce. We assume, on the present limited evidence, that they all die by accumulated mutations, accident, or predation or that they achieve immortality through reproduction. [The question of whether or not some unicellular organisms must occasionally reproduce sexually to avoid senescence has been discussed by Rose (71). Sexual reproduction is not an absolute requirement for immortality of single-celled organisms, and in the case of some multicellular organisms it may actually be a contributing cause of senescence.]

Senescence appears unambiguously only in the further evolution (A′, Scheme II) that continued pathway A (Scheme I) to multicellular forms. In the continuation shown in Scheme II, protozoa are single-celled; slime molds are ambiguous, as noted above; and algae, fungi, animals, and plants are multicellular. The multicellular forms may senesce.

Mitosis, Senescence, and Multicellularity. Among animals we find some species in which adults are composed almost entirely of postmitotic cells (for example, many

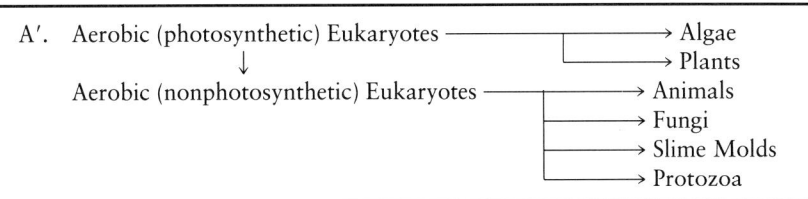

Scheme II

insects). These organisms senesce, but others that can reproduce asexually, in whom most or all cells can continue proliferation indefinitely, have life spans of individual organisms that are also indefinite (26, p. 61). Plants have somatic adult cells that can become totipotent and immortal under certain laboratory conditions, as discussed later under Escape from Senescence-Induced Fatal Failures by Re-Initialization.

All postmitotic cells of a multicellular organism, though not organisms themselves, will manifest senescence and die if not accidentally killed or experimentally dedifferentiated. However, senescence is not always to be found in cell lines that can continuously grow and divide (for example, transformed cells), even if highly differentiated (for example, some cells of the gastrointestinal tract). Senescence may appear among facultative dividers (for example, fibroblasts) and certain cells that regularly divide in the normal life of the multicellular organism (for example, skin cells). Wei et al. (95) found a strictly linear decrease of 0.61% per year using a quantitative measure of DNA repair capability of small samples of normal human skin from men and women ranging in age from 20 to 60 yr. This constant rate was alleged to imply a uniform senescence process for normal skin, accelerated in persons with a history of repeated sunburn or in women (untreated) after menopause. Therefore, over the 40-yr period in this cross-sectional study, 23% of the initial repair capacity was normally lost. Note, however, that 77% was left. The authors supposed that skin cancer rates increase with age because of the decreasing DNA repair capacity and that the phenomenon might be generalizable to explain age-dependence of many cancer types. However, it has not been shown how much DNA repair capacity is needed to protect cells from becoming transformed. It is important to note that cellular senescence, where present in a multicellular organism, is not synonymous with organismal senescence (see the following section for the distinction between component and system failure).

System Death or Component Death

If it avoids fatal accidents, a multicellular organism can die either a *system death* or a *component failure death*. Component failure death requires that some particular, local structural change causes a process to lose the dynamic range required for organismal stability. For component failure death we have the multiple "aspect theories" of aging (discussed later under Aspect Theories), each addressing failure of one or more of the basic maintenance processes—for example, those that sustain human life (36), including *(1)* healing, *(2)* protecting DNA, *(3)* guaranteeing fidelity in the replication of DNA, *(4)* degrading defective protein molecules, *(5)* eliminating reactive free radicals that are generated continually by respiration or other cellular processes, *(6)* detoxifying, *(7)* immunologically protecting against threats, *(8)* inducing protective mechanisms against environmental shock (such as the heat shock response), *(9)* maintaining activity of specialized genes in differentiated cells and repressing activity of other specialized genes to be expressed only in other cell types, *(10)* sustaining chromosomal integrity, *(11)* defending the milieu interieur.

System death occurs when a network of interrelated parts and processes experiences a shrinkage of dynamic range, chiefly through loss of connectivity, beyond some critical minimum for stability in a fluctuational environment. Understanding system death requires a global view, such as seeing senescence as a continuation past maturity of those metabolic processes supporting growth and development in the first place, leading to both an overdifferentiation and a destruction of connections and constraints (107). The result is a loss of cooperativity, integration, and adaptability, as will be explained. A complex system can fail and die in ways unique to its level of global organization and not seen in the local failure modes of its components (72, 73). A loss of connectedness among components is a powerful example, which can lead to counterintuitive increases in the regularity of component behaviors, as discussed later under Increases in Regularity with Senescence.

Death Is a Poor Indicator. An organism can die from many causes: accident, predation, or (in the case of organisms showing senescence) dynamic instability induced by component or system failure through senscence. There are many models of data showing nonlinear dependence of the probability of death on the age of the organism (32). These models provide a framework for theorizing about senescence, but they are limited by the constraint that the death of an organism can be observed only once per individual and that the not fully developed statistics of extreme values are required for analysis of life span distribution. When we try to escape that limitation by studying groups of organisms supposedly genetically identical, we encounter the difficulty that their environments and experiences, even though very similar, cannot be made exactly identical. Finally, the death that is inevitably consequent to senescence may not have any obvious immediate cause if it occurs through system failure. In contrast, death by component failure usually has a conspicuous immediate cause (for example, ventricular tachycardia progressing to ventricular fibrillation and death in a human being who happens to be wearing a Holter monitor at the time of death). About the only good thing that can be said about death as an endpoint datum for proving a scientific theory is that it is an unambiguous and decisive event, a dynamic singularity.

Weighing Counterexamples. In physics a single confirmed counterexample to an established theory can send shock waves through the scientific community and force revisions of thought. Physics features many simple objects lacking intraspecies diversity (all electrons in the universe are exactly alike, although in different contexts, as in making, breaking, or exchanging chemical bonds they may show varied behaviors). In contrast, biology is about complex objects, most of which are unique or nearly so. Consequently, in biology a single counterexample, or even a few, to a hypothesis or an intuition carries less weight. Observations could be wrong or wrongly interpreted. Perhaps too little is known about the organism involved. Under such nonideal circumstances, counterexamples must be taken only as cautions that a theoretical view may be mistaken or limited in generality, but they need not slaughter the theory. Rather, they encourage its further development or critical examination.

REGULAR PHENOMENA

Increases in Regularity with Senescence

The stable motions of physiological variables show some degree of regularity, reflecting the underlying recurrent thermodynamic processes guaranteeing the persistence of the system (115, 99). Regularity can be represented in phase space (an abstract space whose coordinates describe the possible states of the system) as a point (constancy—this is rare), a cycle (near-periodicity), a strange attractor of chaotic dynamics, or as some other, undefined, nonrandom, bounded behavior (for example, asymptotic orbital stability). Empirically we see that near-periodicity superimposed on a $1/f^\beta$ noisy background (discussed below under Regularity of a Variable's Time History) is a common spectral view of the behavior of a single physiological variable (99, 100, 109).

Intuitively one might suppose that the degradations of senescence would always lead to a loss of regularity, but the reverse is often observed. Many of the constraints in a living system determine the strength of couplings among processes. It is well known that networks of coupled, nonlinear oscillators, mutually entrained or interacting, as is typical of organisms, are highly likely to exhibit complex behaviors, including chaos (77, 88). As constraints weaken, couplings loosen, and the simpler dynamics of separate subsystems begin to emerge (62). These may impose a more regular, near-periodic motion on their variables. Thus we have the paradox that complex dynamics often appear irregular and that as the dynamics are altered by the senescent weakening or breaking of coupling constraints, with subsystems becoming increasingly isolated, complexity is lost and regularity increases. Lipsitz and Goldberger (48) have expressed a similar idea. It should not be a surprise that for human beings some behavioral correlates increase with age and may go still higher in some forms of dementia (21, 45). Increasing regularity is a senescent manifestation of the loss of complexity through the weakening of coupling constraints (simplification by a loss of internal inputs).

Regularity of a Variable's Time History

The admixture of near-periodicity and $1/f^\beta$ background power (variance) in a stochastic–deterministic time series requires a new kind of analysis to describe the motion (f is frequency; β is a small constant, usually 1 or 2). Classical spectral analysis is too limited and too focused on exact periodicities. Pincus et al. (63–65) have provided a needed analysis through the new statistic *approximate entropy* (ApEn). ApEn provides a model-free estimate of the regularity of time series data. An equilibrium point is regular. A strictly periodic process is regular. Chaotic dynamics are less regular, though fully deterministic. Random behavior is even more irregular by this same measure. Applications of ApEn have shown that physiological variables normally may move in their stable modes with a regularity less than that of a periodic process but greater than that of a random process, and that senescence often leads to increases in component or nodal regularity.

Programmatic Phenomena. Regular phenomena, as a class, have a particular set of antecedents which generally lead to a particular set of consequences with a high probability. Stent (87) has distinguished between programmatic phenomena as a subset and the full class of regular phenomena:

> Of the large class of regular phenomena, programmatic phenomena form only a small subset, almost all the members of which are associated with human activity. For membership of a phenomenon in the subset of programmatic phenomena, it is a necessary condition that, in addition to the phenomenon itself, there exists a "program," whose structure is isomorphic with, i.e., can be brought into one-to-one correspondence with, the phenomenon.... The operation of a digital computer has programmatic aspects, insofar as there exists a program, or set of instructions separate from the hardware, whose structure is isomorphic with the sequence of operations performed by the machine. However, in the example of computer programs the demand for isomorphism has to allow for the possibility that the structure of the program is actually more elaborate than that of the phenomenon. Here the program often calls for one of two or more alternative operations at various stages of the process, depending on the result of earlier computations (and hence on the initial

state). In such cases the phenomenon is evidently isomorphic with only part of the program.

One of the very few regular phenomena independent of human activity that can be said to have a programmatic component is the formation of proteins. Here the assembly of amino acids into a polypeptide chain of a particular primary structure is programmatic, because there exists a stretch of DNA polynucleotide chain—the gene—whose nucleotide base sequence is isomorphic with the sequence of events that unfold at the ribosomal assembly site. *However, the subsequent folding of the completed polypeptide chain into its specific tertiary structure lacks programmatic character, since the three-dimensional conformation of the molecule is the automatic consequence of its contextual situation and has no isomorphic correspondent in the DNA.* (emphasis added)

Stent goes on to remark that the fact that gene mutations lead to altered phenotypes, for example in the nervous system, shows only that genes are part of the causal antecedents of the adult organism but does not in any way indicate that the mutant gene is part of a program for the development of the nervous system. Neuronal circuitry is not prespecified in detail (20).

Execution-Driven Phenomena. Execution-driven phenomena are a larger subset of regular phenomena than are programmatic phenomena (105). Development of biological systems might be better connected to physics if biologists took a more execution-driven view in which some genes serve as modifiable constraints on cooperative kinetic processes that generate new structures as new constraints at the next stage. In an execution-driven process, the execution of one stage of processing leads to a change in the master program itself (if there is a program) or in the hardware available for subsequent stages. In programmatic phenomena everything must be on hand and ready in advance, contrary to the conditions of truly execution-driven processes, which are self-organizing. Execution-driven processes in biology include activation and inhibition, cooperation and competition, symmetry-breaking (3), and chemical complementarities as major kinds of activity (105, 106). Thom (91) showed that four morphologies of flow (birth, stopping, confluence, and ramification) express many dynamic features needed to describe embryonic morphogenesis in metazoa: canalization of dynamics, coupling to a potential to obtain a direct flow, entrainment, nonlinear catastrophic escapements, dissipation of free energy, and periodic behavior. In our opinion, the development of a theoretical biology is impeded by a continuing failure to distinguish, among regular phenomena, between programmatic and execution-driven processes. The unfortunate consequence is that too many biologists and journalists invest DNA with intentionality (as in the sophistry, "DNA directs development," whereas in reality a gene can do nothing by itself).

The morphogenesis of a multicellular individual from a single-celled zygote stands out as the most amazing execution-driven process in the universe of which we are aware. It involves three cellular processes: *(1)* determination or commitment, *(2)* differentiation, and *(3)* pattern formation. All three require a succession of proteins as gene products. The driving forces are cell division, cell motion, and cell death (apoptosis [96a]), guided by adhesion processes (24). At maturity these processes have nearly exhausted their constructive possibilities under the physical and genetic constraints then present.

PHYSICAL BACKGROUND OF SENESCENCE

Senescence occurs only in certain, viable, animate, self-organizing, living systems, all of which are complex by any measure. Senescence is observable as the terminal phase of a life-span trajectory that begins with growth, development, and differentiation, all of which are anabolic, "negentropic," constructive processes that initially mask the ongoing senescence. In that sense it is a counterpart to development (12). Senescence may actually start at the initiation of an individual multicellular organism's life but does not become dominant or manifest until the maturation phase of development is completed. To give these claims a physical basis and explanation, we next comment on complexity, order, integration, causality, stability—all essential concepts for a theory of senescence. We then turn to our proposal for a physical theory of senescence that is progressive, *homeodynamic instability*.

Complexity

A complex system manifests a property of nonreducibility (3); it cannot be described fully by a superposition of models of simple subsystems or of parts and their interactions (73, 112). The more ways we can interact with a system of interest, the more complex it seems to us. It will always have the potential to reveal behavior that some observers will regard as counterintuitive. Complex systems are nonlinear, with high bulk/shear viscosity ratios, so that there can be long, internal processing delays between inputs and outputs (40, 99, 112). Their behavioral modes are dominated by action (energy × time) rather than by momentum, and their motions are governed by nonholonomic constraints so that the relation of states and rates must be specified independently at every level (73, 111, 112). They are causal systems, but their causality arises from multiple entailments and is not expressed adequately by mechanistic schemes that generate only next state from present state under given parameters and forces (74). They do not have a Lagrangian or Hamiltonian.

Order

The concept of order appears separately in mathematics, physics, and biology. Physical order is a regularity in simple structures or events that can be measured. Order parameters determine the enslavement of short-lasting quantities by long-lasting quantities. Mathematical order originally concerned number and geometry but now extends to include invariance, symmetry, and probability. Biological order is a *functional* order that serves to correlate biochemical and physiological events (19), whereas *physical* order has invariance explicit in it; it is difficult to formulate the condition of invariance met by biological systems that keep the characters of one species constant during all of the transformations of biochemical or physiological events, including development, metabolism, and senescence. The functional order of living systems may be achieved largely through biomembranes as event correlators (19).

Vertical Integration (Hierarchy)

The conventional view of the hierarchical organization and experience of a complex biological organism, such as a human being, lists atoms, simple molecules, macromolecules, organelles, cells, tissues, organs, organ systems, organism, tribe or clone, society, and biosphere in ascending order of complexity of level. These levels are not disjoint sets, and some boundaries are arbitrary. Each level in the hierarchy is constrained from above (by the next higher level in which it is embedded) and from below (by the next lower level of which it is composed). Thus a complex organization is a vertical series of "sandwiches," mutually interdependent. Each sandwich level has its own constraints, degrees of freedom, rules of change, and emergent properties.

Horizontal Integration (Heterarchy)

At any hierarchical level (for example, organs) there are many components interacting directly or through intermediates. Those interacting, same-level components constitute a *heterarchy*. Any particular organ locus is capable of receiving and contributing only partial information concerning the overall status of the organism. Thus to model the resulting integration we are forced to use awkward constructs such as team decision theory, which invokes partial differential equations and suboptimizations as ill-defined objective functions. Even the modern versions of control theory do not handle such problems well (86). The overall dynamics of a complex system are profoundly affected by changes in constraints and strength of couplings (interactions) within or between levels. Changes in these coupling strengths are the motor of senescence, as we shall explain.

Causality

Causality within a complex system arises globally from many entailments. In contrast, classically causal Newtonian dynamical laws (equations of motion) in physics and engineering express only locally how next state arises from present state under a given set of parameter values and under the influence of a given force. As Rosen (74) remarks, "There is not much causality manifested in such a system; only next state from present state. Almost everything in such a system is uncaused within the system; the forces themselves, the parameter values. The initial states need to be posited, and only then can we invoke what little causality is allowed within the system. But organisms have too much causality for that; almost everything about them is entailed by something else about them." In Newtonian physics, the classical Aristotelian material, formal and efficient causes appear separately, but not equivalently, in the initial conditions, equations of motion, and trajectories. In contrast, in biological dynamics multiple causes overlap (72, 76).

Stability

Health, vigor, vitality, hardiness, robustness, resiliency, and well-being are familiar, informal terms that we regard as synonyms for the more technical concept of stability. Health equals stability; poor health is instability. The ultimate instability is the collapse of dynamics of each process to the singular point equilibrium of death. Stability, like order, appears variously in physics, mathematics, computation, and biology but in essence always expresses the two ideas that (*1*) the system of interest can recover from a (limited) range of perturbations without losing its identity or characteristic function; and (*2*) in the long run, after a disturbance, or from a set of initial conditions, behavior will settle down into a bounded, finite domain (of phase space) and remain there (2).

Marginal Dynamic Stability: Resiliency. The stability of living organisms must not be so strict that they fail to grow and adapt within their lifetimes. (We do not here address the possibility of a population to evolve.) In other words, life must exhibit a *marginal stability* that is supple and flexible, allowing some change. It is a global, nonlinear, dynamic stability and not a structural stability in the topological sense. It does not require local stability. Parallel-processing Boolean networks poised between order and chaos show flexible adaptations that may serve as analogies for such marginal dynamic stability (42, 42a). This peculiar kind of stability that has high fault tolerance we designate as *resilience*.

Energy vs. Entropy in Self-Organization

An essential feature of self-organization is a competition between energy and entropy, between broken symmetry and symmetry. Life is a broken symmetry. Energy is associated with asymmetry, manifested, for example, through potential gradients, whereas entropy favors symmetry. For a system to construct itself, there must be a throughput of matter and energy under an execution-driven succession of constraints. The consequence of this thermodynamic openness is at first locally negentropic in the net: new structures appear against an entropic background of internal processes. Total entropy of the system and its environment shows a net increase, as required by the second law of thermodynamics. Later, after maturation of the self-constructing system is achieved, the exchanges of matter and energy between system and environment become both locally and globally entropic in the net. This scenario reflects the fundamental physical aspects of self-organizing systems (see ref. 102 for a variety of perspectives) and the inevitability of senescence in any system that must operate continuously but lacks the capacity for re-initialization (as we explain later) under Redefinition of Senescence. A different view of the role of the second law in evolving life has been presented by Schneider and Kay (82a).

GENERAL PRINCIPLE OF HOMEODYNAMIC SENESCENCE

Homeodynamics Instead of Homeostasis

Homeostasis (18) is a stability theory for an organism, but because the stability of a living system is motional and not still (stillness being the equilibrium of death), the term "homeodynamics" seems more suitable. Elsewhere, following Iberall and Soodak (39–41, 85), we have described some physical principles of stability and offered homeodynamics as a new, generalized mechanics for biology (99, 111, 112). Those principles, consisting of 14 conjectures that extend standard physics heuristically to encompass complex systems, will not be repeated here. (Physics normally addresses simple systems and objects.) Homeodynamics allows for an interaction of deterministic and stochastic processes and leads to a new stability regime we call "asymptotic orbital stability" that is not one of the classical topological attractors of fully deterministic, nonlinear systems (78). It proposes that all complex, open systems that are persistent and whose operations are sustained over very long periods of time, compared to the characteristic process and interactional times within, must have recurrent thermodynamic engine cycles (*clocks*) imposed by the second law, which assure the dissipative aspects of the dynamics. The persistence or survival of the clocks is dependent on the performance of some kind of nonlinear, escapement-like coupling by which a potential is tapped (typically once per cycle) to sustain the repetitive motion in spite of dissipative loss of free energy.

Three questions of physics arise repeatedly in discussions of aging and senescence: (*1*) How can the historical, evolutionary arrow of time that predicts increasing order in certain locations in open systems be reconciled with the irreversible and inevitable degradation of order imposed by the second law of thermodynamics operating in isolated systems? (The answer to this seems to lie in the distinction between open and isolated systems, but the actuality is more subtle because the second law operates also in open systems.) (*2*) In an open system, why can repair and maintenance processes not keep pace with degradations to achieve an immortal steady-state? (*3*) Do biological systems operate too far from equilibrium for the classical laws of thermodynamics to apply? We have argued elsewhere that, contrary to conventional wisdom, organisms have low duty cycles—ΔG is not large—and they do not "knock." They work sufficiently close to equilibrium for thermodynamic constructs to account for most of their energetic and entropic phenomena (103).

Irreversibility and Constraints

Senescence is irreversible. In an open system two different kinds of irreversible process occur: kinetic or thermodynamic. *Kinetic irreversibility* can be constructive and stabilizing. In an execution-driven system the appearance of new structures and functions during self-construction leads to behavioral restrictions we can conceptualize topologically as dynamic basins of attraction with separatrices (2). In our model abstractions, certain allowable regions of phase space become inaccessible because the energy cost of reaching them from the present region is higher than the system can provide. More generally, the appearance of new structures and functions during self-organization freezes out degrees of freedom on configurations and/or motions. That loss of degrees of freedom is *differentiation*. A differentiated system, therefore, can be created and stabilized kinetically. Paradoxically, such a constrained, differentiated system can have richer behavior than a less constrained system (52).

Any constraint that eliminates a configurational variable causes a loss of two degrees of freedom: one on the structure of the system and one on the motion that the configurational variable could have had, were it not eliminated or pinned down. Such constraints are called *holonomic constraints*. (Rigidity is an example.) Much more common in living systems are *nonholonomic constraints* that place a restriction on velocities rather than on configurational coordinates (44). Wherever a many-to-few mapping occurs, as from genes to proteins, a nonholonomic constraint is also operating. A powerful consequence of the prevalence of nonholonomic constraints in living systems is that states do not imply rates across levels, contrary to ordinary technological engineering designs. In living systems, states (configurations and velocities) and rates (accelerations) have to be independently specified for each level (111).

Thermodynamic irreversibility is inevitable for some processes even within open systems. Entropy is always produced internally by the operation of the system. The question then is: Can the entropy be "exported" from the system by inputs of energy? (Entropy cannot itself be exported; it is a field characteristic arising from distributions of matter and energy, both of which can be transported.) In these terms, the question reduces to: Why can negentropic effects of the importation of free energy from the environment not offset the degradative effects of thermodynamically irreversible processes occurring within an open system? The key to answering the question lies in the recognition that all self-organizing systems are execution-driven and that an inevitable consequence is that energy throughput and transformation initially is constructive until the maximum number of degrees of freedom that can be frozen out at that scale of time and space has been reached, starting from the given initial conditions. After that, energy throughput and transformation no longer can drive a net gain in constructive processes. The ongoing, previously background, thermodynamic, irreversible processes now dominate the transformations. We hypothesize that senescence begins to manifest itself the moment maturity is reached. Of course, some irreversible processes occur even during the start-up stage and leave permanent effects, such as the stiffening of the lens of the human eye. Senescence runs concurrent with growth, development, and differentiation in a self-organizing system; but until the constructive phase is completed, senescence is masked and not easily detected. At maturity it becomes dominant and manifests through the decay of constraints and connections.

If any constraint is particularly vulnerable to the consequences of matter or energy throughputs or challenges, a component failure becomes likely. More interesting are the manifestations of impending system death, which arise from alterations in multiple constraints so that global homeodynamic stability decreases, and environmental fluctuations previously well-tolerated become potentially lethal. This idea is captured in Figures 3.8 and 8.1 from Fries and Crapo (28), and we have expanded the notion (106).

Fractal Time, "1/f Noise," and Near-Periodicity of Homeodynamic Systems. The basic dynamic structure of a complex, open, persistent, resilient system is that of a collection of loosely coupled, limit cycle–like oscillators. As a consequence of that coupling, the mean levels of most of the state variables are closely determined, but the variances around them can be large and will have temporal organization. The mean level is kept bounded by dynamic regulation. Feedback control may add to the stability of the mean operating point.

When seen through spectral analysis, the repetitive thermodynamic processes generate a power spectrum that is peaked, although the peaks may be broad and nonharmonically related. As noted above (under Regularity of a Variable's Time History), there is also likely to be a fractal background of "1/f" noise or, simply and more accurately, decreasing power with increasing frequency. Fractal time, like fractal space, has the features of heterogeneity, self-similarity, and the absence of a characteristic scale (109). The basis for the ubiquitousness of the appearance of a $1/f^\beta$ spectral background has been explained variously by Bak et al. (5), Shlesinger (83), Bassingthwaighte et al. (10), and Pincus (62). A technique for decomposing spectra into periodicities, $1/f^\beta$ power, and white noise residues has been introduced by Yamamoto and Hughson (98). Thomson (93) has provided a critical review of time series analyses and emphasizes the "multiple-data-window technique" as the surest approach. Although the theory of 1/f spectra is not complete, the characteristic that power, variance, or amplitude decreases with increasing frequency is ubiquitous in physical and biological domains. With respect to biological signals, we suggest that the 1/f component reflects the effects of internal inputs, or connectivity, in networks.

Because homeodynamics asserts that complex systems will have many near-periodic, regular action modes (99, 112), we expect to find peaks in the spectra of many physiological variables, as is indeed the case. The possible functional importance of such modes can be seen in a series of papers carefully applying mathematical modeling to problems of signal transmission in biological systems. Goldbeter and colleagues have demonstrated that pulsatile, periodic, or near-periodic variations in the thermodynamic activity of a chemical signal provide greater sensitivity and more efficient communication than do random or chaotic signals (23, 33, 34, 46, 47). Earlier, Rapp et al. (68) had made a similar suggestion.

Biological Markers of Age

Given the inadequacy of attempts to read genomic tea leaves to predict life trajectories, and the inherent unpredictability of internal nonlinear dynamics and of environmental contingencies, we are left to seek some kind of marker of biological, as opposed to chronological, age (114). This is, of course, an old problem. No one has yet succeeded at finding a reasonably small set of biochemical, physiological, and psychological assessments that can adequately define human biological age. However, in mammals, generally, a strong case can be made for choosing changes in the immune system as one index of senescence (84). Because biological and chronological time will be partially correlated through entrainment of circadian clocks by geophysical rhythms, chronological age will always be a relevant indicator of risk of morbidity and mortality. The true independent variable, however, is not external time; it is constrained energy throughput and internal transformation, and the metric of internal time so generated is nonlinearly related to external time (70).

HOMEODYNAMICS AND PREDICTABILITY

A theory of everything is a theory of nothing. In biology, theories of great scope usually lack precision, and theories of great precision usually lack scope. Homeodynamics is intended to have great scope and to apply to all self-organizing systems (99, 112, 113). As such, it serves more as a heuristic construct than as a scientific theory. To confront it with experimental tests requires that it be specified for an individual or for a prepared experimental set-up. However, such specification is extremely difficult.

Specifying the Homeodynamic Construct

Some of the specification of homeodynamic principles for human beings arises through the genome plus the maternal, mitochondrial DNA, which serve as initial conditions and constraints for dynamics, but the aleatory aspects of development, which depend in part on internal and external fluctuations, by definition cannot be specified in advance; and to the extent that physiology comprises deterministic, chaotic dynamics, it is inherently unpredictable in the long run (78). Experimental set-ups can attempt to minimize chance effects, but these effects cannot be eliminated entirely in a contingent universe. The environment always has an epigenetic influence. Both deterministic, chaotic dynamics and stochastic fluctuations severely limit our ability to predict long-term outcomes.

Fluctuations and Chance

Random fluctuations or noise contribute to development, senescence, morbidity, and mortality. As some control parameter is extended in nonlinear systems capable of dynamic bifurcations, critical values may emerge at which sensitivity to fluctuations becomes intense. Thom (92, translated by Barham (7) has pointed out: "A careful study allows us to predict in advance the possible outcomes of the bifurcation, which already exist prior to the triggering fluctuation. The role of the latter is, on the one hand, to get the process under way, and also to determine by an apparently arbitrary choice the actual course of subsequent evolution out of all the possible outcomes. But the fluctuation does not create the outcome." Stochastic fluctuations are necessary for the emergence of order and complexity, but they are not sufficient. They express themselves uniquely only under a given set of initial conditions and execution-driven processes, creating a succession of constraints as regular phenomena.

Under controlled laboratory conditions, external fluctuations can be minimized. Internal fluctuations are not necessarily minimized at the same time and may even be enhanced. For example, restraint is a powerful stressor, leading to huge internal neuroendocrine perturbations. Clamping any variable can have unexpected effects, as discussed in the following section.

COUNTERINTUITIVE EFFECTS OF CLAMPING A HOMEODYNAMIC SYSTEM

Environmental Potentials

Resilient open systems sustain their required cyclic, thermodynamic, dissipative processes by repetitively tapping some environmental potentials to offset partially the inevitable degradations of energy or materials. Seven available physical–chemical potentials at terrestrial scales are listed in Table 22.1 (1a–g). (If one

TABLE 22.1. *Potentials That Support Terrestrial Life*

1. Physical–chemical (environmental)
  a. Radiation flux (e.g., for photosynthesis)
  b. Temperature
  c. Mechanical pressure
  d. Chemical potential for required material species (e.g., CHNOPS)
  e. Chemical potential for free energy (e.g., caloric value of food)
  f. Gravitational potential
  g. Electromagnetic potential

2. Genetic (internal)
Information content of genome (including maternal, mitochondrial DNA where present)

3. Cultural (for human beings and, perhaps, some few other primates)
Value potential of culture, society, or tribe

includes play and the making of artifacts, human beings draw upon all seven potentials at least occasionally.)

Because living systems uniquely combine information and symbol systems with dynamics (6, 39, 57–60, 73, 76, 82, 94, 101, 108, 110), they may be thought of as also having an internal informational potential that is drawn upon for growth, development, reproduction, repair, and maintenance. Finally, because human behavior in the aggregate affects much or all of the earth's surface and because economic drives, political disputes, and religious fervor profoundly shape behavior and entrain resources, we must acknowledge the authority of some kind of cultural value potential for our species. This potential is both environmental (social, economic, political) and internal (memories, beliefs, plans, goals).

In examining senescence, particularly if we focus on its apparent rate, we must make some assumptions about the typical environment in which the subject or population lives. That environment will present a typical mean value and a fluctuational spectrum for each of the physical–chemical potentials (1a–g in Table 22.1.) The resilient organism is adapted to those typical levels and vicissitudes to which it has been long exposed.

Clamping

If we now introduce a *clamping* on any variable in the system, either within the organism or on one of its environmental potentials, thereby resetting its operating point and/or reducing its fluctuations, surprising results can be obtained as a consequence of properties of nonlinear dynamical systems. Yates and Poston (113) have presented a formal demonstration of the counterintuitive effects of such clamping of endogenous variables, including clamping a variable that already seems to be showing a steady value. If there could be another value, then clamping becomes a new constraint, and the dynamics change, sometimes dramatically. New attractors can form, as well as new action modes.

We call attention to the remarkable effects of clamping because they are underappreciated and their influence is usually ignored in the choice of experimental controls. We do not hesitate to regulate temperature, lighting, etc., in an effort to reduce variability in our data. These controls, however, are clamps, and they may have large effects on dynamics. When an environmental potential such as food supply is clamped, as in caloric restriction experimental designs, we should expect the dynamics to change. In this case, the fascinating result is that even though the specific metabolism of the animal does not change, its life-span potential increases. The clamping constraint on food intake profoundly alters the homeodynamic stability of the animal under the influence of additional environmental constraints affecting lighting, temperature, protection from predators, etc.

It is the proper business of reductionistic analysis to seek the mechanism by which caloric clamping seems to cause the byproducts of metabolism to be less harmful. Unfortunately, we cannot yet appeal to any theory (not even to the broad construct of homeodynamics) to predict life extension as an outcome of limited caloric restriction. Nevertheless, homeodynamic theory would predict some change in the dynamics as caloric supply is varied. As a reductio ad absurdum, if caloric supply is reduced to zero, the animal dies. Less obviously, if an animal is forcibly fed beyond its adapted intake, we observe fatty livers, renal failure, atherosclerosis, or other morbidities, depending on the species. The curiosity is that in the controlled, clamped laboratory setting the maximum life-span potential is reached at a caloric intake less than that freely chosen by the animal adapted to the study environment. This surprising result, we propose, is partly a consequence of the act of clamping (or clipping) the potential for free energy supply in the presence of other environmental clamps (such as protection from predation).

REDEFINITION OF SENESCENCE

Senescence of a living, multicellular, self-organized, open, complex system (such as a human being) is a steady, unremitting degradation of structure and function. It inevitably shows when energy throughputs and transformations have frozen out the maximal number of degrees of freedom in configurations and motions during differentiation of the system from its initial conditions. The freezing-out occurs as a result of the execution-driven creation of structures as constraints, both holonomic and nonholonomic. Further energy throughput and transformations under the final, mature set of constraints then finds few or no new net constructive outlets and so serves only the irreversible, dissipative processes that continue to drive reproduction, maintenance, catch-up repair, synthesis, turnover, transports, and movement. These metabolic processes, both anabolic and catabolic, are thermodynamically dissipative in the net under the constraints of differentiated maturity. Energy transformations cannot keep pace to eliminate the entropic consequences, because the energy transformations themselves are irreversible. (An infinite regress would result.)

A differentiated, complex, self-organized system scales itself with respect to its energy transformations. The specific metabolism of an animal is an example (calories/unit of metabolically active body weight/day). For each species there is a robust, typical mean operating level and range at maturity that is dynamically regulated. The energy throughput at that scale of continuous operation is dissipative in the net, as required by the second law in open systems lacking a deus ex machina, and the dissipations consist of destruction of constraints and connections, leading to component degradation and isolation and thus system disintegration. Beyond a certain degree of disintegration, the system must fail in a fluctuational environment. Senescence is progressing homeodynamic instability, finally fatal. (Even calorically restricted laboratory animals showing increased longevity, compared to those eating ad libitum, ultimately die.)

Escape from Senescence-Induced Fatal Failures by Re-Initialization

There is an escape from the fatal outcome of senescence, viz., *re-initialization*. Re-initialization refers to resetting a system to its set of initial conditions. When that is done, all memory or trace effects of previous operations or experiences are lost and cease to have any historical influence. Because the biosphere is so rich in diversity, we might expect that some living systems have evolved one of at least several methods of re-initializing, thus gaining immortality.

Single-celled organisms can re-initialize by copying in toto their relatively simple, single-chromosomal genome, packaging it with a small set of enzymes and energy sources, and launching it to proceed on its own (budding, binary fission). Some multicellular organisms can reactivate their total genome from any or most of their cells under conditions of separation of a cell from the organism.

More complex multicellular forms of life have overdifferentiated with respect to this escape path and have sharply separated a germ line and a soma. Under these conditions the organism as a whole cannot re-initialize itself or any somatic cell and can only offer a gamete to a gene pool to which other organisms must also contribute to perpetuate the species. (Gynogenetic, all-female species that reproduce clonally, are a fascinating, ambiguous case.) Most organisms undergo homeodynamic instability, as must any open thermodynamic, complex system that cannot re-initialize. To call this circumstance a theory of "throw-away soma" or "antagonistic pleiotropy" seems gratuitous and adds nothing fundamental to our understanding of the general principles involved.

Plants, all multicellular, can regenerate under experimental conditions a complete new organism from perhaps any of their individual differentiated cells, thus revealing a potential for immortality not ordinarily realized under natural environments. The phenomenon of totipotency of each cell observed under certain laboratory conditions of tissue culture has either of two outcomes: *(1)* undifferentiated callus formation or (if appropriate growth factors are added) *(2)* further differentiation of callus into a new entire plant (30). These well-substantiated abilities of plant cells to re-initialize by dedifferentiation and regeneration of whole multicellular organisms suggest that adult human somatic cells might have a similar potential under certain conditions not yet discovered (human embryos have already been cloned). Even if the cloning of an adult human being (now merely science-fiction) should be achieved, it would not help answer the question we address here: Why do we senesce and die?

Summary of Characteristics of Senescence as Homeodynamic Instability

From the general principles of homeodynamics we can form some broad impressions.

1. There is no unique senescence process.
2. Ultimate system failure is latent in the beings and becomings of self-organizing systems and is an inevitable consequence of energy throughput at all levels.
3. The only escape from fatal failure is re-initialization (available only to single-celled organisms or some multicellular forms that have not strongly differentiated a separation of germ line and somatic cells).
4. Progressing senescence tears down the constraints and connections that originally differentiated the living system and defined its mature status.
5. For some individuals, as a consequence of their particular differentiated state, the senescence process may reveal itself by attack on a "weak link" constraint, and the organism will ultimately die a component death, such as renal failure.
6. In other individuals the senescence process may attack many constraints rather evenly. These organisms die from old age—a system death consisting of dynamic instability in a fluctuational environment—while individual components studied in isolation seem to be still in a viable range of performance. Global resiliency requires connectivity as well as component competence.
7. A system without energy throughput will not show senescence, although it may age. Frozen or dehydrated, inactive life forms, when rethermalized or rehydrated, can resume where they left off, as if their time had stopped. They may deteriorate while inactive if mechanically stressed or noncatalytically oxidized by air; lipids go rancid.
8. Human senescence and the inevitability of death are less mysterious than the multifarious aspect theories below (see Aspect Theories) seem to indicate. Confusions abound because of the failure to distinguish between program-driven and execution-driven systems.

Confusions also result from the inadequacy of our knowledge about how the second law of thermodynamics operates in self-organized open systems. Classically, it was defined only in the case of isolated systems.

ASPECTS OF SENESCENCE

We do not expect that any single, overarching, predictive theory of senescence will ever be found for our species, because aging human beings undergo changes in all domains of life: genetic, biochemical/metabolic, physiological, psychological, social, and, for some, even spiritual. Although age-related decrements in function have been described in nearly every system examined, there is no common program of functional decline with age in the absence of recognizable disease. In view of individual variability, these decrements cannot be considered as biomarkers of either aging or mortality, if such markers require that aging and mortality have exactly the same specific bases in all humans. Almost all bodily functions in every person are found to decline with increasing chronological age, even in the absence of clinical disease, but the apparent rate of decline, which partly determines life span, differs even between closely related species, individuals, or processes. Cutler (22) notes that persons who are unusually long-lived and live past 100 yr do so apparently not because they age more slowly but instead because they age more uniformly; that is, they appear to not suffer from any particular weak link in their body functions, such as from heart disease or diabetes, but to die instead from what we call a "system death."

Aspect Theories

Recent discussions of the different aspects of senescence (25–27, 29, 32, 61, 61a, 71, 79, 117) demonstrate that very little stays the same over time and that changes are likely to be found anywhere one looks. The problem is to assign significance and causality to the observations, and there are many competing and overlapping partial theories. The diversity of aspect theories does not express incompatibility as much as the fact that senescence is a multifaceted problem.

Every aspect theory of senescence has one or more conspicuous defects. Masoro (see Chapter 1) addresses the weaknesses of many of these theories. For example, consider the "brain size" and the "rate of living" theories. Austad and Fischer (4) examined these theories using a database consisting of body mass and maximum recorded longevity for 580 mammalian species gleaned from standard sources. They came to the following conclusion:

The linear logarithmic relationship between mammalian body mass and maximum longevity, deleting bats and marsupials, is used as a standard against which to measure lifespans of particular mammal groups. Bats have maximum lifespans a minimum of three times those of non-flying eutherians—a trend resulting from neither low basal metabolic rate, the ability to enter torpor, nor large relative brain size. Marsupials live about 80% as long as non-flying eutherians despite averaging lower basal metabolic rates; similarly, there is no effect of heterothermy or relative brain size. These results directly conflict with predictions of both "rate of living" and brain-size mediated theories of aging.

Generalizations from Aspect Theories

From the jumble of current views, certain modest generalizations can be made about human senescence:

1. There are no obvious reasons human beings should age and die.

2. Human senescence takes place concurrently at different levels of a hierarchy (molecules, organelles, cells, tissues, organs, organisms, populations, societies), a fact accounted for more plausibly by stochastic and dynamic processes than by genetic mechanism.

3. In view of the stochastic character of senescence, the relationship between genotype and phenotype is unpredictable. Regardless of the degree of genetic homogeneity of a population, individuals die across an enormous range of ages. Even in inbred animal strains, with greater than 99% genetic homogeneity, we observe about the same coefficient of variation in age of death as in (mongrel) human beings (81). These facts imply that, although stochastic processes have effects that depend (within limits) on genotype, the course of stochastic damage is so sensitive to small perturbations that the genotype of an individual within a species is not a useful indicator of life-span potential.

4. Ecological factors (such as predators, crowding, microbes, and toxins) have a strong bearing on life expectancy for individuals (although the exact strengths of these influences are partially dependent on the phenotype, which in turn is partially dependent on the genotype). Traumatic life experiences can strongly affect the appearance of age-associated, detrimental changes (38), and there may be permanent, cumulative trace effects of stress responses long after the stressors are gone.

5. There is a monotonically increasing human mortality with chronological age, expressible from ages (approximately) 25–85 yr, according to the Gompertz exponential model. (See Chapter 1 for evidence that the mortality vs. time relationship is not monotonic all the way to the maximum life span. Furthermore, not all of the elderly are decrepit.)

6. There are regular changes in the chemical composition of the body with age.

7. There is a broad spectrum of progressive deteriorative changes seen as declines in physiological, immunological, and biochemical functions.

8. There is reduced ability of older individuals to respond adaptively to environmental change.

9. There is increased vulnerability to certain diseases with age (increased morbidity).

10. There is a slowing down of many processes, even before there is detectable mean operating point degradation.

11. Some aspects of brain function ("wisdom") may improve with age until late in life.

We must emphasize that Masoro (Chapter 1) and Yu (116) have shown that specific metabolic rate (oxygen utilization per unit of lean body mass) cannot be the measure or determinant of senescence rate. This is an important fact that any rate of living theory must include. Furthermore, Boxenbaum (17) called attention to the paradox of "longevity hormesis" in which the Gompertzian hazard function can be reduced in some cases by low-dose exposure to agents usually considered toxic. A powerful gerontological theory should explain not only the above facts but more generally the longevity, senescence, and death of individuals and the population kinetics of morbidity and mortality; answer "why do we live so long?" (rather than only "why do we die?"); and show why biomarkers of senescence do not serve well as biomarkers of mortality. Manton and colleagues have developed a detailed mathematical account of the problem (49, 50, 97).

One might hope that a general gerontological theory under stated conditions would be able to explain the changes of senescence in a given individual of a given cohort of a particular species at a given period. In other words, we need not only a general theory but knowledge about how to specify it for particular applications. Out of those changes it will be necessary to show how the observed disintegration, death of individuals, and population mortality data arise. Under what conditions, if any, would the theory allow for human life-span prolongation (life extension) in the form of an increase in the maximum life-span potential for our species (which is not a specifically determined number of years)? Under what conditions could that extension be associated with a delay in morbidity? We have no such theory today. Birren and Bengtson have presented a collection of emerging theories (13).

WEAR-AND-TEAR REVISITED

Of the many aspect theories of senescence, including brain and body size effects, wear-and-tear, hysteretic disinhibition, biological life events, throw-away soma, antagonistic pleiotropy, error catastrophe, defective proteins, glycation, aberrant immune function, clonal senescence, somatic mutations, free radicals, failure of DNA repair, rate of living, dis-differentiation, membrane stiffening, gerontogenes, programmed aging, diffusion limitation, desynchronosis, storage disease, etc., only wear-and-tear provides an inherently physical–chemical perspective, and for that reason alone it is worth close reexamination. From this perspective, the life span of a system is a result of its activity and not a predetermined parameter, and there is no fixed, maximum life-span potential. There is, however, a median time to failure for a population. Almost alone among gerontologists, Gavrilov and Gavrilova (32) have chosen the wear-and-tear perspective, through reliability theory, as the methodological foundation for research into the mechanisms which determine life span. This is a position we strongly endorse as the basis for gerontological theory-building, recognizing that in its superficial forms, to date, it has proved inadequate.

An obvious starting point for examination of wear-and-tear phenomena is a study of the failure modes and failure rates of machines of all kinds—mechanical, electro-mechanical, electronic—that can do work or process information. These technological devices are biological objects created through the human mind. They are not natural. Unfortunately, there is an awkwardness inherent in starting with the reliability of machines to find clues to the senescence of organisms, because organisms differ profoundly from machines (73–75).

Reliability Theory for Machines

Because human beings are continuously operating during their lifetimes, with activity superimposed on a basal metabolic rate that never goes to zero until death, for comparison we should address machines that also operate continuously. Many computers and their hard-disk drives are left running continuously; many electrical generators similarly are always going; and airline companies, noting that their aircraft make no profits while on the ground, strive for the highest possible ratio of flying time to down time compatible with scheduling of flights and maintenance crews. If a continuously running machine has a maintenance program that requires occasional shutting down and human intervention, it can provide relevant data on wear but not on life span, because the human intervention may re-initialize components by part replacement, an eventuality not analagous to anything that autonomous living systems experience. (Genetic engineering and organ transplants are changing that situation.)

Machines reveal a significant start-up mortality rate analogous to infant mortality in human beings. The "burn-in" testing of new electronic equipment is an attempt to reveal it. To expose the failure rate, the equipment may be initially tested at a temperature near the upper extreme of its designed operating range. The temperature coefficient of failure modes of electronic devices often resembles that of a simple physical–chemical diffusion process.

Because infant mortality and early childhood deaths are not ordinarily considered in the kinetics of mortality for human beings, we consider here only the reliability of machines that have survived their start-up "burn-in" and begun their mature performance under continuous operation.

Three Mathematical Models. Barlow and Proschan (8, 9) have illuminated the mathematical theory of reliability for machines. The theoretical models include the Weibull power distribution, which in generalized form (31, 32) is given as:

$$\mu(x) = A + Bx^c \qquad (1)$$

where μ is some force of mortality (the fraction of survivors dying in the next designated time interval) and x is age. A, B, and c are parameters. Other models include a generalized binomial mortality law:

$$\mu(x) = A + (B + Cx)^n \qquad (2)$$

where A, B, C, and n are parameters (time-invariant), and the Gompertz–Makeham law:

$$\mu(x) = A + B\exp(Cx) \qquad (3)$$

where A is age-independent failure rate, B is initial failure rate [in the case of human beings, Finch (26) suggests that the initial mortality rate be chosen at puberty], and C is a parameter not sensitive to environments.

The range of applicability of the Gompertz–Makeham rule for human mortality is approximately ages 25–85 yr. At either extreme, infancy and childhood or very old age, the rule does not provide a satisfactory description of data. We find a striking similarity in the distribution of life spans of machines and biological systems in that at extremely high ages there seems to be a stage of saturation of failure, leading to an approximately constant failure rate instead of a continuing exponential. This period might depend on the high mortality rate at extreme age, such that defective elements are eliminated at a rate close to that at which they accumulate. If so, the result would be a stationary distribution of organisms according to the number of defects, and the force of mortality would become constant rather than exponential.

Manifestations of Unreliability. When machines become less reliable as a function of age, the effects of aging show up in at least four different ways: *(1)* a decrease in stability, both static and dynamic; *(2)* a decrease in accuracy in carrying out operations; *(3)* a decrease in speed of operations; and *(4)* a change in loading characteristic (the response of the system to an ordinary demand or stimulus). These empirical observations about machines seem remarkably parallel to what we observe in aging human beings, but with this caveat: the kinetics of mortality of populations of living systems do not usually follow Equation 1, as many machines do, but seem closer to Equation 3. However, Gavrilov and Gavrilova (32, p. 46) note that Equation 2 is rather flexible: under certain parameter values it can imitate the Weibull rule of Equation 1, and under other parameter values the Gompertz–Makeham formula of Equation 3. It may be the best model, but it requires a fourth parameter, thereby weakening its specificity in fitting data.

HUMAN SENESCENCE AS DISSIPATIVE DESTRUCTION

The prototheory of homeodynamics (99, 112) cited above, addressing the competition between energetic and entropic processes in self-organizing systems, rests on a combination of statistical thermodynamics and nonlinear mechanics. One of its antecedants is dissipative structure theory (66, 67). It belongs to the wear-and-tear category of theories of senescence, but it does not predict any particular kinetic model for rates of failure or probability of dying. Some special justification for the commonly observed Gompertz–Makeham kinetics of human mortality is required.

Component Failure—Cell Culture Senescence

We emphasize again that a complex, highly connected system has failure modes stemming from a loss of connectivity, even when the components, separated, are still reliable. Thus the justification of the Gompertz–Makeham kinetics should include both component death and system death. Abernethy (1) compared the exponential increase in mortality rate with age to the wearing out of biological components.

Swim (90) observed that serial cultivation of strains of fibroblasts from many different sources indicated that "in most instances where growth occurs, the cells eventually undergo nonspecific degeneration" (p. 145). This now well-known phenomenon was confirmed and popularized by a series of studies and articles by Hayflick's group, beginning in 1961 (35). Weismann, in his two classic books of 1882 and 1884 (96), had already suggested that the life span of multicellular organisms was determined by some restriction on the capacity of their somatic cells for division. However, today we recognize that, even in the case of cells taken from very old individuals, the residual capacity for division can be substantial. Therefore, it is not compelling that the limitation on the number of times cells in a confluent monolayer culture can double is pertinent to senescence of a whole multicellular organism. It has even been doubted that the cessation of doubling, which does not occur at any fixed number and which can be affected by the addition of certain growth factors, represents cell senescence. It could be a form of differentiation of the cells into something that is postmitotic. Fibroblasts can differentiate into osteoblasts or fat cells, etc. Their various functions include production of cytokines, procollagen, proelastin, matrix glycosaminoglycans, as well as proliferation and migration. Fibroblasts are versatile.

There is no doubt that after repeated divisions in culture, even when the fibroblasts can still make DNA, the cell-cycle stage arrests and mitosis stops. (For details see Chapter 4.) It is as if there is some dominant failure of signal transduction. A fusion of old and young cells acts old. The addition of certain modulators can get mitosis going again for awhile. In this arrested stage of cell cycle, for which there is no name, some genes are overexpressed and some are underexpressed, with respect to earlier, younger stages. As the gene expression profile changes with time, there is a loss of cellular, integrative functioning; many processes appear to become uncoupled, as suggested by our prototheory of senescence as progressive, homeodynamic, dissipative destruction. As suggested in Chapter 4, the first or early events in the aging of these cells may be deterministic, but as disintegration progresses, stochastic events dominate. Diminished reliability of DNA polymerase (37) may be a consequence.

Dissipative Destruction as Basis of Gompertz Mortality Kinetics

To rationalize the Gompertz–Makeham model as a descriptor of human mortality, we draw upon the homeodynamic principle that in the postmaturational stage, beginning roughly at age 25–30 yr for human beings, entropic processes will dominate over negentropic processes; and connections, constraints, and components will be lost as an inevitable byproduct of dissipative energetic transactions of chemical reactions, such as uncatalyzed glycation, of free-radical production during synthesis of dopamine in substantia nigra, or during oxidative metabolism. It is not necessary to seek or postulate a unique cause; the dissipative energetic overhead of continuing persistence will inevitably tear the system down by one means or another. The common morphological effect is a loss of connectivity and redundancy; the common functional effect is loss of control. An absolute requirement for senescence to appear in a living organism is that the system initially be highly connected both in series and in parallel and that it contain multiple negative feedback regulations.

Model of Reliability Theory. Gavrilov and Gavrilova (32, p. 254–276) develop in detail mathematical models of the population mortality kinetics for systems that are nonideal initially, having numerous defects, leading to a heterogeneous population. In that case the force of mortality of an organism grows exponentially with age, following the Gompertz law. We believe that their approach is fundamentally correct but would qualify it by adding the notion of progressive dissipative destruction, which relieves the requirement that the organism be saturated with defects initially. Defects will appear spontaneously and inevitably through the operation of the system. We believe that this view is close to the idea that senescence is caused by a cascade of dependent and independent failures, leading to an avalanche-like mechanism of breakdown. This is not the error catastrophe theory of Orgel (55, 56) resuscitated. That theory, now rejected, focused on defects in information handling, whereas we emphasize the inevitable consequences of dynamics for which informational structures act only as one class of constraints.

Use It and Lose It or Use It or Lose It? Any theory of senescence belonging even remotely to the wear-and-tear class must face the hard fact that desuetude is also destructive. Disuse atrophy and the cardiovascular deconditioning that results from prolonged immobilization or bed rest give vivid testimony in favor of what we call "use it or lose it." Elsewhere we have suggested a thermodynamic justification for this maxim (106). Bortz has clearly and colorfully made a strong case for the invigorating power of exercise (14–16), and mental activity seems similarly powerful. What are we to make of this if, over time, entropy is gaining on us because of the energetic wear-and-tear cost of being?

We suggest that the anabolic enterprises of growth, maintenance, and repair are nonlinearly—roughly parabolically—coupled to catabolic metabolism, such that the gap between the destructive costs of being and becoming and the benefits of activity is minimal at an energy throughput that lies between basal metabolic rate at the low end and exhausting activity at the high end. The dissipative destruction rate of senescence is least at that minimum. Nevertheless, the net effect of any integral of physical action (energy × time) over any time interval is inevitably entropic both internally and externally.. "Use it or lose it" (activity should exceed basal rates of metabolism) and "use it and lose it" (ultimate death from the entropic costs of being) are both correct maxims, and they are not contradictory.

Model of Data. There is no unique set of assumptions that forces the choice of Equations 1, 2, or 3, nor do we have any continuous, constant parameter model that purports to fit the data describing human mortality from birth to extreme old age. Some options are to do piecewise modeling separately for infancy, childhood, youth, maturity, and old age or to invoke time-varying parameters. Noting that the Gompertz model is inconsistent with studies showing mortality tending to high constant values at late ages, Manton et al. (50) argue that a model of mortality should (1) be multidimensional, (2) reflect stochasticity in physiological change, (3) reduce under special conditions to simpler models, (4) use multiple time-varying covariants, and (5) describe the effects of observed age-related factors. They offer a model with these properties and arrive at the important conclusion that the concept of a fixed determined life span should be replaced by a dynamic one where physiological heterogeneity significant at late ages probabilistically determines life span.

As we noted, models are not theories. They may specify a theory or fit data. In either case, they serve as tools, not goals, in a scientific program. The model of Gavrilov and Gavrilova (32) attempts to specify a theory of reliability; the equally admirable model of Manton et al. (50) attempts to fit data from the Framingham study. These models are too detailed mathematically to present here, but we close with the thought that formal reconciliation of the two models would represent an advance in the maturation of gerontological theory. Both models are compatible with the broad principles of homeodynamics, but the heuristic character of homeodynamics in its present stage of development (99, 112) is not sufficiently formal to support derivation of these models. Nevertheless, we expect that a comprehensive gerontological theory, if ever completed, will draw upon elements present in these three concepts. All three are level-independent and can be brought to bear at any level in a biological organization that involves transformation of energy and the making, breaking, or exchanging of bonds. Meanwhile, specialists investigating senescence at any organizational level of interest will continue to have rich possibilities for specific new discoveries, some of which, no doubt, will have medical applicability. However, for a general principle of senescence, we believe the homeodynamic construct will be needed, rationalizing a ubiquitous, dissipative destruction for living, multicellular, self-organizing systems.

SUMMARY

Many of the seemingly disparate and even counterintuitive features of increases with time of human morbidity and probability of dying can be comprehended, if not understood exactly, from the standpoint of a global theory of stability for complex, persistent, open, nonlinear systems. We have introduced homeodynamics as such a theoretical construct to extend the more limited and more linear concept of homeostasis. The application of homeodynamics to senescence we designate as dissipative destruction theory. The theory expresses a set of contrasts between (1) the first and second laws of thermodyanmics (energy vs. entropy), (2) broken symmetry and symmetry, (3) information and dynamics, (4) constructive and destructive processes, and (5) program-driven and execution-driven regular phenomena.

Homeodynamics is a scheme of functional organization of open systems with a marginally stable hierarchy and heterarchy of loosely coupled, nonlinear, dissipative, wobbly oscillators, each expressing a thermodynamic process cycle. Such a constellation of highly entailed and constrained processes generates near-periodicity and $1/f^\beta$ background noise reflecting internal inputs, seen in the spectral analysis of the behavior of many physiological variables. Stochastic fluctuations, both internal and external, further shape the behaviors. Global homeodynamic stability arises from constraints and couplings. Energy throughput, after maturity, weakens or destroys these constraints once the available degrees of freedom for construction have been frozen out by execution-driven energy transformations.

Senescence is here regarded as an inevitable, post-maturational consequence of persistence in an energetic, open, self-organized, complex, living system. As energy transfers and transformations degrade constraints, many of the behaviors lose their irregularity (complexity) and simplify. Some correlations can then increase. Resiliency is progressively lost.

Clamping environmental potentials, such as food intake, or some internal variables has the capability of profoundly affecting the dynamics of nonlinear systems. Most of the changes are likely to be detrimental or destabilizing, but a few may increase stability. Life-span extension by caloric restriction may be an example of the latter case.

Constraints differentiate living organisms and give them both their species and individual identities. Even though senescence is a broad, nonspecific attack on constraints, it will be manifested rather particularly in each person, according to his or her set of constraints at maturity. To the extent that we share some constraints with other individuals and species, we also share some manifestations of senescence, but there always will be a unique residue of changes peculiar to each individual and a personal rate of deterioration for each constrained process.

Health is homeodynamic resiliency. It represents a compromise between two independent, competing truths: (1) use it or lose it; and (2) use it and lose it.

Reliability theories for machines lead to three mathematical models of life spans: Weibull, binomial, and Gompertz–Makeham rules. Although living systems differ profoundly from machines, they share the same senescence kinetics models. These models for inanimate machines (not self-constructing) reflect wear-and-tear; for self-organizing living systems with repair capabilities they reflect instead the dissipative destruction required by homeodynamics.

Conventional or traditional aspect theories of senescence that try to stretch one process or loss to cover all the phenomena that lead to Gompertz-Makeham population mortality kinetics suffer from too many counterexamples or lack of fundamental basis in either biology or physics. Meanwhile, evolutionary biology suffers still from its ancient and abiding curse of the tautological "what survives, survives"; its inability to define fitness independently; and its limitation to retrodiction without prediction, as must be the case with all purely historical theories in an aleatory, contingent universe. Evolutionary games, running as computer simulations, have revealed many useful strategies for different situations, but none can be proved optimal for all instances of unknowable futures, where "winning" means only that for some population of players the game goes on.

REFERENCES

1. ABERNETHY, J. D. The exponential increase in mortality rate with age attributed to wearing-out of biological components. *J. Theor. Biol.* 80: 333–354, 1979.
2. ABRAHAM, R. H., and C. D. SHAW. Dynamics: a visual introduction. In: *Self-Organizing Systems: The Emergence of Order*, edited by F. E. Yates. New York: Plenum Press, 1987, p. 543–598.
3. ANDERSON, P. W. More is different. *Science* 177: 393–396, 1972.
4. AUSTAD, S. N., and K. E. FISCHER. Mammalian aging, metabolism, and ecology: evidence from bats and marsupials. *J. Gerontol. (Biol. Sci.)* 46: B47–B53, 1991.
5. BAK, P., C. TANG, and K. WIESENFELD. Self-organized criticality: an explanation of 1/f noise. *Phys. Rev. Lett.* 59: 381–384, 1987.
6. BARHAM, J. A Poincaréan approach to evolutionary epistemology. *J. Soc. Biol. Struct.* 13: 193–258, 1990.
7. BARHAM, J. From enzymes to $E = mc^2$: A reply to critics. *J. Soc. Evol. Sys.* 15: 249–306, 1992.
8. BARLOW, R. E., and F. PROSCHAN. *Mathematical Theory of Reliability*. New York: Wiley, 1965.
9. BARLOW, R. E., and F. PROSCHAN. *Statistical Theory of Reliability and Life Testing Probability Models*. New York: Holt, Rinehart and Winston, 1975.
10. BASSINGTHWAIGHTE, J. B., R. B. KING, J. E. SAMBROOK, and B. VAN STEENWYK. Fractal analysis of blood-tissue exchange kinetics. *Adv. Exp. Med. Biol.* 222: 15–23, 1988.
11. BEATTY, J. What's wrong with the received view of evolutionary theory? In: *Philosophy of Science Association*, edited by P. D. Asquith and A. M. Giere, 1981, Greenwich, CT; JAI Press, vol. 2, p. 397–426.
12. BIRREN, J. E. A contribution to the theory of the psychology of aging: as a counterpart of development. In: *Emergent Theories of Aging*, edited by J. E. Birren and V. L. Bengtson. New York: Springer, 1988, p. 153–176.
13. BIRREN, J. E., and V. L. BENGTSON (Eds). *Emergent Theories of Aging*. New York: Springer, 1988.
14. BORTZ, II, W. M. Aging as entropy. *Exp. Gerontol.* 21: 321–328, 1986.
15. BORTZ, II, W. M. *We Live Too Short and Die Too Long*. New York: Bantam, 1991.
16. BORTZ, II, W. M. The physics of frailty. *J. Am. Geriatr. Soc.* 41: 1004–1008, 1993.
17. BOXENBAUM, H. Gompertz mortality analysis: aging, longevity hormesis and toxicity. *Arch. Gerontol. Geriatr.* 13: 125–138, 1991.
18. CANNON, W. B. Organization for physiological homeostasis. *Physiol. Rev.* 9: 399–431, 1929.
19. CARERI, G. *Order and Disorder in Matter*, translated by K. Jarratt. Menlo Park, CA: Benjamin/Cummings, 1984.
20. CEPKO, C. What do progenitor cells tell their daughters during development of the cerebral cortex? *J. N.I.H. Res.* 4: 60–62, 1992.
21. CUNNINGHAM, W. R., and J. E. BIRREN. Age changes in the factor structure of intellectual abilities in adulthood and old age. *Educ. Psychol. Measurement* 40: 271–290, 1980.
22. CUTLER, R. G. Human longevity and aging: possible role of reactive oxygen species. In: *Physiological Senescence and Its Postponement*, edited by W. Pierpaoli and N. Fabris. New York: New York Academy of Sciences, 1991, vol. 621, p. 1–28.
23. DECROLY, O., and A. GOLDBETER. Birhythmicity, chaos, and other patterns of temporal self-organization in a multiply regulated biochemical system. *Proc. Natl. Acad. Sci. U.S.A.* 79: 6917–6921, 1982.
24. EDELMAN, G. M. *Topobiology: An Introduction to Molecular Embryology*. New York: Basic Books, 1988.
24a. EIGEN, M. *Steps Towards Life*. New York: Oxford University Press, 1992.
25. FABRIS, N., D. HARMAN, D. L. KNOOK, E. STEINHAGEN-THIESSEN, and I. ZS-NAGY (Eds). *Physiopathological Processes of Aging: Towards a Multi-Causal Interpretation*. New York: New York Academy of Sciences, 1992, vol. 673.
26. FINCH, C. E. *Longevity, Senescence, and the Genome*. Chicago: University of Chicago Press, 1990.
27. FRANCESCHI, C., G. CREPALDI, V. J. CRISTOFALO, and J. VIJG (Eds). *Aging and Cellular Mechanisms*. New York: New York Academy of Sciences, 1992, vol. 663.
28. FRIES, J. F., and L. M. CRAPO. *Vitality and Aging*. San Francisco: Freeman, 1981.
29. FROLKIS, V. V., and K. K. MURADIAN. *Life Span Prolongation*. Boca Raton, FL: CRC Press, 1991.
30. GALSTON, A. W. *Life Processes of Plants*. New York: Scientific American Library, 1994.
31. GAVRILOV, L. A. Investigation of life span genetics using kinetic analysis. Ph.D. diss., Moscow State University, Moscow (in Russian), 1980.
32. GAVRILOV, L. A., and N. S. GAVRILOVA. *The Biology of Life Span: A Quantitative Approach*. English edition translated by J. Payne and L. Payne. New York: Harwood, 1991. (Originally in Russian, edited by V. P. Skulachev, Moscow: Nauka, 1986.)
33. GOLDBETER, A. Periodic signaling as an optimal mode of intercellular communication. *News in Physiological Science* 3: 103–105, 1988.
34. GOLDBETER, A., and G. DUPONT. Allosteric regulation, cooperativity, and biochemical oscillations. *Biophys. Chem.* 37: 341–353, 1990.
35. HAYFLICK, L., and P. S. MOORHEAD. The serial cultivation of human diploid cell strains. *Exp. Cell Res.* 25: 585–621, 1961.
36. HOLLIDAY, R. The ancient origins and causes of ageing. *NIPS* 7: 38–40, 1992.
37. HOLLIDAY, R., and T. C. L. KIRKWOOD. Predictions of the somatic mutation and mortalization theories of cellular ageing are contrary to experimental observations. *J. Theor. Biol.* 93: 627–642, 1981.
38. HOUX, P. J., F. W. VREELING, and J. JOLLES. Age-associated

cognitive decline is related to biological life events. In: *Alzheimer's Disease: Basic Mechanisms, Diagnosis and Therapeutic Strategies,* edited by K. Iqbal, D. R. C. McLachlin, B. Winblad, and H. M. Wisniewski. Chichester, UK: Wiley, 1991, p. 353–358.

39. IBERALL, A. S. What is "language" that can facilitate the flow of information? A contribution to a fundamental theory of language and communication. *J. Theor. Biol.* 102: 347–359, 1983.
40. IBERALL, A. S., and H. SOODAK. Physical basis for complex systems—some propositions relating levels of organizations. *Collect. Phenom.* 3: 9–24, 1978.
41. IBERALL, A. S., and H. SOODAK. A physics for complex systems. In: *Self-Organizing Systems: The Emergence of Order,* edited by F. E. Yates. New York: Plenum Press, 1987, p. 499–520.
42. KAUFFMAN, S. A. Antichaos and adaptation. *Sci. Am.* 265: 78–84, 1991.
42a. KAUFFMAN, S. A. *The Origins of Order.* New York: Oxford University Press, 1993.
43. KENYON, G. M., J. E. BIRREN, and J. J. F. SCHROOTS (Eds). *Metaphors of Aging in Science and the Humanities.* New York: Springer, 1991.
44. LANCZOS, C. *The Variational Principles of Mechanics* (3rd ed.), Toronto: University of Toronto Press, 1966.
45. LEUCHTER, A. F., J. E. SPAR, D. O. WALTER, and H. WEINER. Electroencephalographic spectra and coherence in the diagnosis of Alzheimer's-type and multi-infarct dementia. *Arch. Gen. Psychiatry* 44: 993–998, 1987.
46. LI, Y.-X., and A. GOLDBETER. Frequency specificity in intercellular communication: influence of patterns of periodic signaling on target cell responsiveness. *Biophys. J.* 55: 125–145, 1989.
47. LI, Y.-X., and A. GOLDBETER. Pulsatile signaling in intercellular communication: periodic stimuli are more efficient than random or chaotic signals in a model based on receptor desensitization. *Biophys. J.* 61: 161–171, 1992.
48. LIPSITZ, L. A., and A. L. GOLDBERGER. Loss of "complexity" and aging. *JAMA* 267: 1806–1809, 1992.
49. MANTON, K. G., and M. A. WOODBURY. A mathematical model of the physiological dynamics of aging and correlated mortality selection. II: Application to the Duke Longitudinal Study. *J. Gerontol.* 38: 406–413, 1983.
50. MANTON, K. G., E. STALLARD, M. A. WOODBURY, and J. E. DOWD. Time-varying covariates in models of human mortality and aging: multidimensional generalizations of the Gompertz. *J. Gerontol. (Biol. Sci.)* 49: B169–B190, 1994.
51. MEDAWAR, P. B. *An Unsolved Problem of Biology.* London: Lewis, 1952.
52. MEDAWAR, P. A geometric model of reduction and emergence. In: *Studies in the Philosophy of Biology,* edited by F. J. Ayala and C. H. Waddington. Berkeley: University of California Press, 1975, p. 57–64.
53. MONOD, J. *Chance and Necessity.* New York: Knopf, 1971.
54. MURPHY, E. A. Muddling, meddling, and modeling. In: *Genetic Basis of Epilepsy,* edited by V. E. Anderson, W. A. Hauser, J. K. Penry, and C. F. Sing. New York: Raven Press, 1982, p. 333–348.
55. ORGEL, L. E. The maintenance of the accuracy of protein synthesis and its relevance to ageing. *Proc. Natl. Acad. Sci. U.S.A.* 49: 517–521, 1963.
56. ORGEL, L. E. The maintenance of the accuracy of protein synthesis and its relevance to ageing: a correction. *Proc. Natl. Acad. Sci. U.S.A.* 67: 1476, 1970.
57. PATTEE, H. H. Dynamic and linguistic modes of complex systems. *Int. J. Gen. Sys.* 3: 259–266, 1977.
58. PATTEE, H. H. Instabilities and information in biological self-organization. In: *Self-Organizing Systems: The Emergence of Order,* edited by F. E. Yates. New York: Plenum Press, 1987, p. 325–338.
59. PATTEE, H. H. Simulations, realizations, and theories of life. In: *Artificial Life,* edited by C. G. Langton. Menlo Park, CA: Addison-Wesley, 1989, p. 63–77.
60. PATTEE, H. H. The limitations of formal models of measurement, control, and cognition. *Appl. Math. Comput.* (in press), 1994.
61. PIERPAOLI, W., and N. FABRIS (Eds). *Physiological Senescence and Its Postponement: Theoretical Approaches and Rational Interventions.* New York: New York Academy of Sciences, 1991, vol. 621.
61a. PIERPAOLI, W., W. REGELSON, and N. FABRIS (Eds). *The Aging Clock.* New York: New York Academy of Science 719, 1994.
62. PINCUS, S. M. Greater signal regularity often indicates increased system isolation. *Math. Biosci.* (in press), 1994.
63. PINCUS, S. M. How and when to look for evolution from order to randomness in practical time-series analysis. *Meth. Enzymol.* (in press), 1994.
64. PINCUS, S. M., and A. L. GOLDBERGER. Physiological time-series analysis: what does regularity quantify? *Am. J. Physiol.* 266 (Heart Circ. Physiol. 35): H1643–H1646, 1994.
65. PINCUS, S. M., I. M. GLADSTONE, and R. A. EHRENKRANZ. A regularity statistic for medical data analysis. *J. Clin. Monitor.* 7: 335–345, 1991.
66. PRIGOGINE, I. Time, structure and fluctuations. *Science* 201: 777–784, 1978.
67. PRIGOGINE, I. *From Being to Becoming: Time and Complexity in the Physical Sciences.* San Francisco: Freeman, 1980.
68. RAPP, P. E., A. I. MEES, and C. T. SPARROW. Frequency encoded biochemical regulation is more accurate than amplitude-dependent control. *J. Theor. Biol.* 90: 531–544.
69. RAVEN, P. H. Defining biodiversity. *Nature Conservancy* 44: 11–15, 1994.
70. RICHARDSON, I. W., and R. ROSEN. Aging and the metrices of time. *J. Theor. Biol.* 79: 415–423, 1979.
71. ROSE, M. R. *Evolutionary Biology of Aging.* New York: Oxford University Press, 1991.
72. ROSEN, R. Feedforward and global system failure: a general mechanism for senescence. *J. Theor. Biol.* 74: 579–590, 1978.
73. ROSEN, R. *Life Itself: A Comprehensive Inquiry into the Nature, Origin, and Fabrication of Life.* New York: Columbia University Press, 1991a.
74. ROSEN, R. Beyond dynamical systems. *J. Soc. Biol. Struct.* 14: 217–220, 1991b.
75. ROSEN, R. Cells and senescence. In: *Fundamentals of Medical Cell Biology, Vol. 7: Developmental Biology.* Greenwich, CT: JAI Press, 1992, pp. 191–203.
76. ROSEN, R. The Schrödinger question: what is life 50 years later? (preprint available from author, Dept. of Physiology and Biophysics, Dalhausie University, Halifax, Nova Scotia, Canada B3H 4H7, 1993.)
77. RÖSSLER, O. E. Chaos in coupled optimizers. In: *Perspectives in Biological Dynamics and Theoretical Medicine,* edited by S. H. Koslow, A. J. Mandell, and M. F. Shlesinger. New York: New York Academy of Sciences, 1987, vol. 504, p. 229–240.
78. RUELLE, D. *Chance and Chaos.* Princeton: Princeton University Press, 1991.
79. RUSTING, R. L. Why do we age? *Sci. Am.* 267: 130–141, 1992.
80. SACHER, G. A. Theory in gerontology, part I. *Ann. Rev. Gerontol. Geriatr.* 1: 3–25, 1980.
81. SACHER, G., and P. H. DUFFY. Genetic relation of lifespan to metabolic rate for inbred mouse strains and their hybrids. *Fed. Proc.* 38: 184–189, 1979.
82. SEARLS, D. B. The linguistics of DNA. *Am. Sci.* 80: 579–591, 1992.

82a. SCHNEIDER, E. D., and J. J. KAY. Life as a manifestation of the Second Law of Thermodynamics. *Math. Comput. Modelling.* 19: 25–48, 1994.
83. SHLESINGER, M. F. Fractal time and 1/f noise in complex systems. In: *Perspectives in Biological Dynamics and Theoretical Medicine,* edited by S. H. Koslow, A. J. Mandell, and M. F. Shlesinger. New York: New York Academy of Science, 1987, vol. 504, p. 214–228.
84. SOLOMON, G. F., M. A. FIATARONE, D. BENTON, J. E. MORLEY, E. BLOOM, and T. MAKINODAN. Psychoimmunologic and endorphin function in the aged. *Ann. N. Y. Acad. Sci.* 521: 43–57, 1988.
85. SOODAK, H., and A. S. IBERALL. Homeokinetics: a physical science for complex systems. *Science* 201: 579–582, 1978.
86. STEAR, E. B. Control paradigms and self-organization in living systems. In: *Self-Organizing Systems: The Emergence of Order,* edited by F. E. Yates. New York: Plenum Press, 1987, p. 351–397.
87. STENT, G. S. Programmatic phenomena, hermeneutics and neural biology. In: *Self-Organizing Systems: The Emergence of Order,* edited by F. E. Yates. New York: Plenum Press, 1987, p. 339–345.
88. STROGATZ, S. H., and I. STEWART. Coupled oscillators and biological synchronization. *Sci. Am.* 269: 102–109, 1993.
89. SUPPES, P. *Studies in the Methodology and Foundations of Science.* New York: Humanities Press, 1969, p. 18.
90. SWIM, H. E. Microbiological aspects of tissue culture. *Ann. Rev. Microbiol.* 15: 141–176, 1959.
91. THOM, R. *Mathematical Models of Morphogenesis.* New York: Halstead Press, 1983.
92. THOM, R. Halte au hasard, silence au bruit. In: *La Querelle du Déterminisme: Philosophie de la Science d'Aujourd'hui,* edited by K. Pomian. Paris: Le Débat/Gallimard, 1990, p. 61–78.
93. THOMSON, D. J. Time series analysis of Holocene climate data. *Phil. Trans. R. Soc. Lond. A* 330: 601–616, 1990.
94. WEBER, B. H., D. J. DEPEW, C. DYKE, S. N. SALTHE, E. D. SCHNEIDER, R. E. ULANOWICZ, and J. S. WICKEN. Evolution in thermodynamic perspective: an ecological approach. *Biol. Philos.* 4: 373–405, 1989.
95. WEI, Q., G. M. MATANOSKI, E. R. FARMER, M. A. HEDAYATI, and L. GROSSMAN. DNA repair and aging in basal cell carcinoma: a molecular epidemiology study. *Proc. Natl. Acad. Sci. U.S.A.* 90: 1614–1618, 1993.
96. WEISMANN, A. *Essays Upon Heredity and Kindred Biological Problems.* Oxford: Clarendon Press, 1889.
96a. WHITE, K., M. E. GRETHER, J. M. ABRAMS, L. YOUNG, K. FARRELL, and H. STELLER. Genetic control of programmed cell death in *Drosophila. Science* 264: 677–683, 1994.
97. WOODBURY, M. A., and K. G. MANTON. A mathematical model of the physiological dynamics of aging and correlated mortality selection. I: Theoretical development and critiques. *J. Gerontol.* 38: 398–405, 1983.
98. YAMAMOTO, Y., and R. L. HUGHSON. Course-graining spectral analysis: new method for studying heart rate variability. *J. Appl. Physiol.* 71: 1143–1150, 1991.
99. YATES, F. E. Outline of a physical theory of physiological systems. *Can. J. Physiol. Pharmacol.* 60: 217–248, 1982a.
100. YATES, F. E. Systems analysis of hormone action: principles and strategies. In: *Biological Regulation and Development, Vol. 3A: Hormone Action,* edited by R. F. Goldberger and K. R. Yamamoto. New York: Plenum Press, 1982b, p. 25–97.
101. YATES, F. E. Semiotics as a bridge between information (biology) and dynamics (physics.) *Rech. Semiot./Semiot. Inqui.* 5: 347–360, 1985.
102. YATES, F. E. (Ed). *Self-Organizing Systems: The Emergence of Order.* New York: Plenum Press, 1987a.
103. YATES, F. E. Physics of self-organization. In: *Self-Organizing Systems: The Emergence of Order,* edited by F. E. Yates. New York: Plenum Press, pp. 409–416, 1987b.
104. YATES, F. E. Quantumstuff and biostuff: a view of patterns of convergence in contemporary science. *Self-Organizing Systems: The Emergence of Order,* edited by F. E. Yates. New York: Plenum Press, 1987c, p. 617–644.
105. YATES, F. E. Evolutionary computing by dynamics in living organisms. In: *Advances in Cognitive Science: Steps Toward Convergence,* edited by M. Kochen and H. M. Hastings. AAAS Selected Symposia Series. Boulder, CO: Westview Press, 1988a, p. 26–49.
106. YATES, F. E. The dynamics of aging and time: how physical action implies social action. In: *Emergent Theories of Aging,* edited by J. E. Birren and V. L. Bengtson. New York: Springer, 1988b, p. 90–117.
107. YATES, F. E. Aging as prolonged morphogenesis: a sorcerer's apprentice. In: *Metaphors of Aging in Science and the Humanities,* edited by J. E. Birren and G. Kenyon. New York: Springer-Verlag, 1991a, p. 199–218.
108. YATES, F. E. Pharmacosemiotics: where is the message in the drug? In: *Semiotic Perspectives on Clinical Theory and Practice—Medicine, Neuropsychiatry and Psychoanalysis,* edited by R. E. Litowitz and P. S. Epstein. New York: Mouton de Gruyter, 1991b, p. 65–79.
109. YATES, F. E. Fractal applications in biology: scaling time in biochemical networks. In: *Methods in Enzymology: Numerical Computer Methods,* edited by L. Brand and M. L. Johnson. New York: Academic Press, 1992a, vol. 210, p. 636–675.
110. YATES, F. E. On the emergence of chemical languages. In: *Biosemiotics: The Semiotic Web 1991,* edited by T. A. Sebeok and J. Umiker-Sebeok. New York: Mouton de Gruyter, 1992b, p. 471–486.
111. YATES, F. E. Self-organizing systems. In: *The Logic of Life,* edited by D. Noble. Oxford: Oxford University Press, 1993, p. 189–217.
112. YATES, F. E. Order and complexity in dynamical systems: homeodynamics as a generalized mechanics for biology. *Mathl. Comput. Modelling,* 19: 49–74, 1994.
113. YATES, F. E., and T. POSTON. Rate-controlled delivery of endocrine agents: some paradoxical consequences of controlling the inputs. In: *Principles and Applications of Rate-Controlled Drug Administration and Action,* edited by H. A. J. Struyker-Boudier. Boca Raton, FL: CRC Press, 1986, p. 247–272.
114. YATES, F. E., L. A. BENTON, and J. C. BECK. Risk assessment and early detection of functional decline. In: *Health, Aging, and Competence: The Next Generation of Longitudinal Studies,* edited by J. J. F. Schroots. Amsterdam: Elsevier, 1993, p. 87–107.
115. YATES, F. E., D. J. MARSH, and A. S. IBERALL. Integration of the whole organism—a foundation for a theoretical biology. In: *Challenging Biological Problems: Directions Toward Their Solution,* edited by J. A. Behnke. New York: Oxford University Press, 1972, p. 110–122.
116. YU, B. P. Food restriction research: past and present status. *Rev. Biol. Res. Aging* 4: 349–371, 1990.
117. ZS.-NAGY, I., D. HARMAN, and K. KITANI. (Eds). *Pharmcology of Aging Processes.* New York: New York Academy of Science vol. 717, 1994.

V PROPOSED MODIFIERS OF AGING PROCESSES OR AGING PHENOTYPE

23. Putative interventions

BYUNG P. YU | Department of Physiology, University of Texas Health Science Center, San Antonio, Texas

CHAPTER CONTENTS

Criteria for Claiming Retardation of Aging Processes
    Life span extension
    Modulation of functional, structural, and morphological changes as evidence for aging retardation
    Modulation of pathology
Dietary Restriction, a Robust Antiaging Intervention
    Historical notes
    Dietary restriction, an aging intervention
    Population mortality characteristics
    Age-related disease processes
    Physiological characteristics
        Bone metabolism
        Immune function
        Protein metabolism
        Other metabolic and endocrine characteristics
    Cellular actions
        Membrane structure
        Other cellular constituents
        Protection against senescent cellular deterioration
Modulation of the Aging Process by Other Interventions
    Antioxidant feeding
    Deprenyl
    Melatonin
    Hypophysectomy
    Dehydroepiandrosterone
Concluding Remarks

CRITERIA FOR CLAIMING RETARDATION OF AGING PROCESSES

AGING PROCESSES APPEAR TO DIFFER among different cells, organs, and organ systems within the same organism (166). Among gerontologists, there is no consensus concerning a biomarker or a panel of biomarkers to provide a quantitative measure of the aging processes (167), nor is it likely that such a marker will be found in the near future (4, 167). Historically, gerontologists have looked to such mortality characteristics of populations as life span or age-specific mortality rate as primary tools in assessing the effectiveness of an intervention on aging (30, 79). However, secondary attention has been focused on age-associated diseases and on age changes in the function and structure of organisms (110).

Life Span Extension

Life span is the most widely used quantitative assessment of interventions of aging processes (16, 157) and indeed provides a simple, clear endpoint (196). However, the term "life span" is used in two different ways: as the mean (or median) or as the maximum length of life of a population. The mean length of life is influenced by many factors unrelated to aging processes. Therefore, the use of this measurement as an index of a putative antiaging intervention is questionable (16).

Maximum life span, which refers to the age of the last survivors of a population cohort, is widely used as an index of aging. It is generally agreed that if an intervention increases the maximum life span, it is an antiaging intervention. Yet Finch et al. (49) caution that the rate of aging is not the only biological factor influencing maximum life span. Moreover, population size can influence maximum life span (see Chapter 1). The latter problem can be partially circumvented by using the age of the tenth-percentile survivors as an index of maximum life span (123). Therefore, although widely used in assessing the influence of an intervention on aging, maximum life span cannot be considered an unambiguous measure.

Although not as widely used, Gompertzian and related analyses probably provide a more rigorous assessment of putative antiaging interventions (49). Mortality rate doubling time is a convenient expression of this kind of analysis and inversely relates to the rate of aging (see Chapter 1).

Modulation of Functional, Structural, and Morphological Changes as Evidence for Aging Retardation

Functional deterioration and structural damage have been examined for reliability as indices of the rate of aging, but at this time no biological marker or panel of biomarkers of aging has been validated (4). Nevertheless, several functional and structural measures have given evidence of the extent of aging. Examples are collagen cross-linkage, nonenzymatic glycosylation, lipofuscin deposition, and many other physiological and biochemical parameters, such as immune competence and endocrine functions (167).

Modulation of Pathology

A hallmark of aging is an increased incidence of age-associated disease processes (112). A delay in onset and a slowing of progression of these disease processes have been viewed as evidence that an intervention modifies the aging process (107, 208). For example, retardation of age-associated leukemia and nephropathy by dietary means has been considered evidence of the retardation of aging processes by nutritional interventions (70, 165, 166).

DIETARY RESTRICTION, A ROBUST ANTIAGING INTERVENTION

Historical Notes

The concept of intervention into the aging process is not a novel idea or a product of modern scientific advancements. For centuries, people have dreamed of attaining a long life and have proposed a variety of interventions for extending the life span. Of the many methods, nutritional interventions involving modifications of dietary composition, including dietary supplements, and alterations in food intake have been the most frequent.

An old notion purports that the life span can be extended through growth retardation during the developmental phase; that is, a slower growth means a longer life. In 1832, Edmonds (38) stressed the relationship between retardation of maturity and extension of the adult life span and hypothesized that life span can be predicted from growth rate. This concept probably arose from the common observation that life spans of various species appeared related to growth patterns (120).

In 1917, Osborne et al. (135) experimentally explored this relationship between growth rate and longevity in rodents using diet to modulate growth rate and obtained evidence generally supportive of the concept. However, shortly thereafter, Robertson and Ray (152) evaluated the complete life span of colony mice from birth to death, testing the hypothesis that growth retardation lengthens life span, and found just the opposite. Conflicting results possibly occurred in these early studies because experimental conditions did not prevent infection and malnutrition, and consequently premature death.

McCay et al. (119) evaluated these conflicting results and concluded that "the relationship between growth rate and life span cannot be determined upon a heterogeneous group of animals permitted to grow at the maximum rate of which they are capable." Using a low-protein diet to retard the growth rate of trout, McCay and his colleagues found that fish with slower growth outlived those allowed to grow normally (120). They confirmed this finding in studies with rats in which reducing food intake *(caloric restriction)* resulted in a reduction in growth rate and an increase in longevity. The key to their success was the use of diets containing all known nutrients essential to the maintenance of a healthy colony of experimental rodents. These seminal findings demonstrated that both the median and the maximum life spans of rodents can be extended. Since this discovery, significant advances have been made in the evaluation of caloric restriction on aging processes. This nutritional intervention is considered to be the most effective, if not the only, known means of slowing the aging process in mammalian species.

Dietary Restriction, an Aging Intervention

The observation that dietary restriction extends both maximum and median life spans is strong evidence that it slows the aging process in rodents. The magnitude and reproducibility of its effect is shown by the survival curves in Figure 23.1 (207) from studies on male Fischer 344 rats fed ad libitum or restricted to 40% of ad libitum intake. In addition, a large body of information demonstrates that much age-related functional deterioration is modified by dietary restriction (111, 115, 190). An extensive literature (70, 107, 202, 208) details the effects of dietary restriction on population mortality characteristics, age-associated disease processes, and physiological characteristics. Each warrants in-depth discussion.

Population Mortality Characteristics

Mathematical evaluation of life span and age-specific mortality rate of populations originated in 1825 with Gompertz (56). His analysis revealed that the age-specific mortality rate of a human population increases exponentially during much of the postmaturational period of life. When this is plotted on a logarithmic scale as function of age, the slope of the straight-line exponential increase component of the relationship is expressed algebraically as follows:

$$G_t = G_o + \alpha_t$$

where G_t is the "force of mortality," α is a rate constant (the proposed measure of the rate of actuarial aging), and G_o (often called the "vulnerability factor") is the y intercept (that is, age = 0).

The Gompertzian analysis is widely used to determine the influence of an intervention on the rate of aging. Mortality rate doubling time (MRDT), which relates

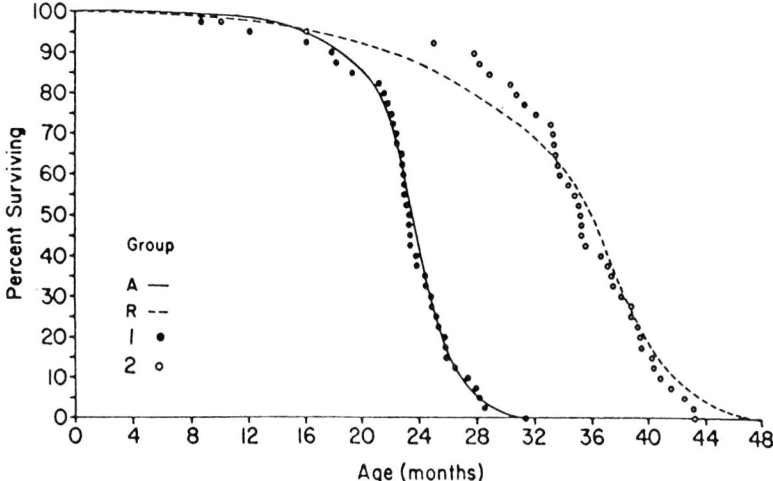

FIG. 23.1. Survival curves from two separate studies of male F344 rats. The *lined curves* (*solid*, ad libitum–fed; *broken*, diet-restricted) indicate the study of Yu et al. (208) with 115 rats in each group. The *circled curves* (*closed*, ad libitum–fed; open, diet-restricted) indicate the study of Yu et al. (207) with 40 rats in each group. [Reproduced with permission.]

inversely to α, is often used because of its obvious relation to other longevity measures (49, 197).

Sacher (157) effectively utilized the Gompertzian analysis to assess the life-prolonging characteristics of dietary restriction. He found that dietary restriction decreases the mortality rate constant (α), that is, that it increases the MRDT. Neafsey (130) recently used this approach to assess the effects of food restriction initiated at different ages and/or applied for varying periods of time, demonstrating that dietary restriction, regardless of age of implementation and length of restriction, retarded the rate of aging (decreased α) but did not invariably alter G_o. Thus Gompertzian analysis strongly points to dietary restriction as an effective antiaging intervention, confirming what had already been concluded based on extension of maximum life span. Although dietary restriction has been shown to retard aging processes in several nonmammalian species (190), it has not been sufficiently studied in mammals, other than rodents.

Age-Related Disease Processes

Suppression of disease by dietary restriction was an early observation by McCay et al. (119). Since then, dietary restriction has been found to retard a wide variety of age-associated disease processes (20, 70, 107, 139, 181).

The ability of dietary restriction to retard chronic nephropathy, a major age-associated disease of rats, is well documented (8, 161, 208). Maeda et al. (107) questioned whether the pathogenesis of nephropathy can be influenced through dietary restriction initiated at different ages. Restriction was begun at 6 wk or 6 months of age and either maintained throughout life or limited to only a short period of early life (4–5 months), then discontinued. Dietary restriction initiated at 6 months of age was as effective as restriction initiated at 6 wk of age in retarding the progression of chronic nephropathy. In contrast, rats in which dietary restriction was limited to 4–5 months of early life exhibited at advanced ages an incidence and severity of nephrotic lesions similar to those of ad libitum–fed rats. Restricting protein intake in the absence of caloric restriction (107) and using soy protein as the dietary protein source (70) also delayed the onset of nephropathy but much less effectively than simple caloric restriction. It was questioned whether dietary restriction influenced nephropathy because of restricted energy intake or restricted protein intake. Masoro et al. (112) clarified this area by showing that the age-related progression of nephropathy in male Fischer 344 rats is markedly slowed by restricting dietary energy intake by 40% while maintaining protein intake. Thus it is clear that the reduction in protein intake cannot be the major reason caloric restriction retards age-associated nephropathy (70). Caloric restriction is the obvious overriding factor in the beneficial effects of dietary restriction on age-related nephropathy and life-span extension (115).

Caloric restriction also markedly decreases the incidence of neoplastic diseases, which, along with nephropathy, are the major lesions associated with aging in rats (166). Ross and Bras (153) demonstrated a direct correlation between caloric intake and the incidence of neoplastic lesions. Also, dietary restriction exhibits some selectivity in its reduction of tumorigenesis since it does not suppress all tumors. In male Fischer 344 rats, it effectively suppresses leukemia (165) and tumors of the pituitary (166) but is less effective in suppressing thyroid or soft-tissue tumors (107).

As with chronic nephropathy, the question arises as to whether or not energy intake, rather than any specific dietary constituent, influences the incidence of carcinogenesis (7). Tannenbaum (179) documented the suppressive action of underfeeding on the initiation and growth of tumors. Later, Lavik and Baumann (101) showed that mice fed a diet low in calories but high in fat exhibited a much lower incidence of skin tumors than mice fed a diet low in fat but high in calories. Kritchevsky (94) concluded that, although an individual dietary constituent, for example, fat, can play a role in experimental tumorigenesis, reduced energy intake is the overriding factor modulating tumorigenesis.

Much thought and research have been aimed at identifying mechanisms by which caloric restriction delays the onset of neoplastic lesions. An important clue was obtained by Pashko and Schwartz (136), who examined the initiation phase of tumorigenesis. These authors investigated binding of the highly mutagenic polycyclic hydrocarbon carcinogen dimethylbenzene (a)anthracene (DMBA) to DNA from mouse skin. Dietary restriction for 5, 7, and 10 wk significantly reduced DMBA binding to DNA, which suggests a possible mechanism by which dietary restriction suppresses the initiation of tumorigenesis. Pollard et al. (140) reported in rats treated with methylazoxymethanol (MAM) that 25% restriction of food intake started 10 days after a single subcutaneous injection of MAM reduced the number of intestinal tumors.

Physiological Characteristics

Dietary restriction alters physiological characteristics, including the course of age-related deterioration of physiological systems (190). Recent reviews have highlighted the remarkable breadth of these actions (110, 116, 202). Examples of some of the major physiological effects are presented below.

Bone Metabolism. Bone loss is a commonly observed aging phenomenon. Since almost all body calcium (>99%) is associated with bone, the status of bone metabolism must be assessed in relation to whole-body calcium homeostasis (76). Studies of the rat skeleton demonstrate that substantial age-related changes in bone metabolism occur during senescence (that is, after 24 months of age), reflected in loss in bone weight, calcium content, lipid content, and strength. However, this terminal bone loss in rats may be related to and/or exacerbated by chronic nephropathy, which occurs in rats with age, rather than to the aging process per se (76).

McCay et al. (119) produced the earliest report on the influence of dietary restriction on bone. They noted that the femurs of diet-restricted rats became fragile when compared to those of ad libitum–fed animals. This adverse effect was unexpected, given the overall beneficial effect of dietary restriction. In retrospect, it is clear that this fragility was due to severe food restriction, which resulted in calcium malnutrition.

The effect of dietary restriction on bone metabolism also has been examined in the absence of calcium malnutrition. Kalu and his colleagues (74, 75) found that when calcium intake was sufficient, dietary restriction delayed bone growth and maturation but also prevented senile bone loss up to 30 months of age. Three major calcium-regulating hormones, calcitonin, parathyroid hormone, and 1,25-dihydroxy vitamin D, were measured. The plasma concentration of calcitonin, a potent plasma calcium-lowering hormone, progressively increased with age in ad libitum–fed animals. However, serum Ca^{2+} concentrations still were unaltered, which suggests that sensitivity to this hormone is blunted with age. Dietary restriction prevents age-related increases in calcitonin. Also, the plasma concentration of parathyroid hormone, the major hormone responsible for bone resorption and Ca^{2+} mobilization, increases with age in ad libitum–fed rats, and this increase is prevented by dietary restriction. Finally, the plasma concentration of 1,25 dihydroxy vitamin D, which plays a role in Ca^{2+} metabolism by regulating intestinal absorption of calcium, declines with age in ad libitum–fed rats but not in food-restricted rats (73).

Mishimoto et al. (125), measuring age-related changes in bone matrix mineral content in rats, reported that both magnesium and calcium contents of the tibia significantly declined between 6 and 18 months, which agrees with the earlier study of McDonald et al. (121). Age-related changes in matrix mineral content were unaffected by dietary restriction. It seems, then, that the effects of dietary restriction on the age changes in bone are selective, some parameters being modulated and others uninfluenced.

Immune Function. Senescence and the deterioration of immune function are proven to be closely associated (78, 191), and dietary restriction retards this deterioration (46, 71). Dietary restriction influences many different components of the immune system. For example, it delays thymus involution (65), thereby enhancing T cell or B cell functions, and it alters spleen cell responses to mitogens such as phytohemagglutinin (PHA) and concanavalin A (Con A) by enhancing lymphocyte proliferation (148) and IL-2 induction (68). Fernandes et al. (47) proposed that dietary restriction enhances both T- and B-cell functions in the production of antibodies to thymus-dependent antigens and the response to alloantigens, probably by increased IL-2 production. In diet-restricted rats, an increased IL-2

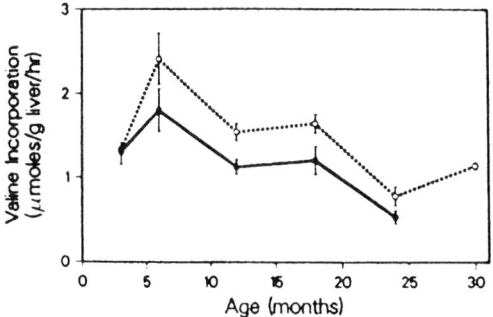
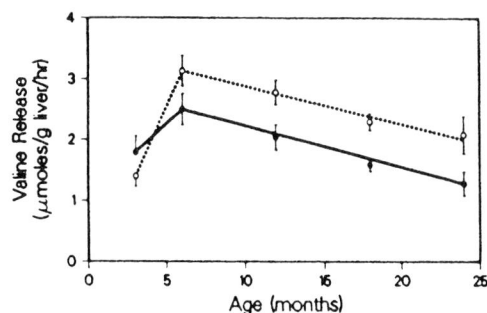

FIG. 23.2. Effects of age and dietary restriction on protein synthesis (*left*) and protein degradation (*right*). *Solid line, dotted line* refer to ad libitum–fed and diet-restricted rats, respectively. [Reproduced from Ward (187, 188) with permission.]

receptor expression was correlated with increased IL-2 production (21). Also, an age-related decline in T cell responses to mitogens or antibodies has been linked to alterations in intracellular Ca^{2+} regulation (124). Dietary restriction seems to act by maintaining proper functioning of the Ca^{2+} in the signal transduction system of T lymphocytes. For example, the Ca^{2+} response to Con A in splenocytes is much enhanced by dietary restriction compared to the responses of ad libitum–fed rats of the same age (47). Deterioration in membrane fluidity associated with lipid peroxidation has also been implicated in age-related Ca^{2+} malfunction in the signal transduction system of lymphocytes (47, 184). Although it is clear there is a loss of T cell function with age, the precise mechanism by which dietary restriction retards this loss is not known.

Protein Metabolism. Interest in protein metabolism in aging was stimulated by Orgel's "Error Catastrophe" hypothesis (133, 134) in which abnormal protein synthesis was causally linked to the aging process. Although this theory of aging has been discarded by most, strong evidence has emerged that during senescence protein biosynthetic activity declines. This decline has been observed in both in vivo and in vitro systems (see Chapter 9 for a detailed discussion). Many of the studies were carried out with liver preparations (189). Although intensively studied, the biochemical basis for this decline in protein biosynthesis is not clear.

In the renewal or turnover of cellular proteins, degradative processes are as important as synthetic ones. Comparatively little work has been done in regard to aging and protein degradation, and the findings have not been consistent, which may be due to the technical difficulties encountered in measuring protein degradation. Whole-body protein turnover was studied by Goldspink and Kelley (54, 55), who showed that in rats between the ages of 3 and 105 wk, protein breakdown declined by 50%. Reduction in this rate of protein degradation may causally relate to the accumulation of altered proteins with age (176). For instance, Dice (35) showed that the degradation rate of modified RNase was much delayed in human senescent fibroblasts.

Dietary restriction modulates age-related changes in protein metabolism. Using hepatocytes isolated from Fischer 344 rats, Birchenall-Sparks et al. (11) showed that protein biosynthesis decreased 55% between 2.5 and 19 months of age in ad libitum–fed rats but only slightly in diet-restricted rats. Indeed, the protein synthetic activity of hepatocytes from 19-month-old diet-restricted rats was similar to that of 7-month-old ad libitum–fed rats. Ward (187) confirmed these findings using perfused livers. Protein synthesis observed in livers from diet-restricted rats was maintained throughout life at a rate about 35% higher than that of ad libitum–fed rats. This study involved valine incorporation into protein, which peaked at 6 months of age and progressively declined to 24 months of age. As shown in Figure 23.2, age-related changes in protein synthesis of the diet-restricted group paralleled those of the ad libitum–fed rats, peaking at 6 months and progressively declining thereafter.

Several investigators (108, 188) have attempted to determine the mechanisms through which dietary restriction prevents age-related decline in protein synthesis. Altered ribosomal aggregation appears to play a role in reducing the number of ribosomes bound to mRNA with advancing age (109). Coniglio et al. (31) investigated the effect of age on elongation factor and found that the elongation time required for the synthesis of an average half-length of a peptide was significantly prolonged with advancing age, reducing protein synthesis significantly. Of the two elongation factors EF-1 and EF-2, only EF-1, which facilitates binding of the tRNA to ribosomal mRNA, appears affected by age (32, 52). However, Rattan et al. (144) reported that levels of protein elongation factors in rat liver were not modulated by dietary restriction. Breese et al. (15) proposed that a reduction in the plasma levels of insulin-like growth factor I (IGF-I) with age may contribute to the decline in protein synthesis and demonstrated that dietary restriction can prevent the reduction in IGF-I and the decline in protein synthesis. However, the mechanisms by which dietary restriction modifies protein biosynthesis remain to be defined.

Less is known about the effects of aging on protein degradation. A decline with age has been assumed since no apparent change in the amount of body protein occurs despite a decreased protein biosynthetic rate. In a recent study (188) using perfused liver, protein degradative capacity decreased by about 50% between 6 and 24 months of age (Fig. 23.2). Protein degradation was also found to be modulated by dietary restriction. Ishigami and Goto (69) recently reported that hepatocytes from diet-restricted mice have a higher capacity to degrade proteins than cells from ad libitum–fed mice. Caloric restriction, started at 23 months of age and lasting 70 days, reduced the half-lives of two proteins injected into the hepatocytes by 40% to a level comparable to the half-lives of these same proteins in cells from young ad libitum–fed mice. These studies revealed two important points about caloric restriction and protein degradation: first, caloric restriction is effective even when started as late as 23 months of age, and second, this effect required about 70 days of dietary restriction. Both points could be important for a further understanding of the cellular mechanisms involved during dietary restriction.

To maintain homeostasis, cells must maintain lower levels of aberrant or modified proteins. Dietary restriction enables cells to meet this challenge by maintaining a high turnover rate of proteins, even in late life.

Other Metabolic and Endocrine Characteristics. The metabolic rate theory is one of the most frequently invoked of hypotheses proposed to explain the action of dietary restriction (see Chapter 6 for discussion of this theory). Caloric restriction, or underfeeding, is generally assumed to reduce metabolic rate. Studies (114, 117, 118) have tested this assumption; the findings show that for most of the life span, diet-restricted and ad libitum–fed rats have similar metabolic rates per unit of metabolic mass. Thus it does not appear that dietary restriction retards aging processes by decreasing metabolic rate.

Although metabolic rate is not altered by dietary restriction, ad libitum–fed and diet-restricted rats exhibit different metabolic and endocrine characteristics (37, 48). These include plasma hormone levels (131, 171), responsiveness of tissues to hormones (162, 204), functioning of adipose tissue (9), and other functions related to metabolic characteristics (64). Some of these may play a role in the antiaging action of dietary restriction (111). Since these characteristics have been cataloged (190, 202), only those particularly important will be discussed here.

Dietary restriction blunts the age-related increase in adipose tissue mass (106). The lipolytic response of adipocytes to catecholamines and glucagon decreases with age, and dietary restriction prevents this (10). Moreover, the age-associated loss of adipocyte responsiveness can be reversed by dietary restriction (9).

Koizumi et al. (91) found that dietary restriction lowered fasting blood sugar levels in mice. Masoro et al. (113, 114) carried out a detailed study of plasma glucose and insulin levels in ad libitum–fed and diet-restricted rats. Diurnal patterns of plasma glucose levels showed that diet-restricted rats maintained lower concentrations through most of the day and had mean 24 h plasma glucose levels about 15 mg/dl below those of ad libitum–fed rats through the life span. Also, plasma insulin levels of these diet-restricted rats were markedly lower than those of ad libitum–fed rats. In spite of the lower levels of plasma glucose and insulin, diet-restricted rats used glucose as fuel per gram lean body mass at the same rate as ad libitum–fed rats.

Balage et al. (5) examined the insulin binding characteristics of liver and skeletal muscle for clues to the molecular events occurring during dietary restriction. This also reinforced earlier findings that caloric restriction reduced plasma glucose and postprandial insulin concentrations. Insulin binding to membranes from liver was higher in diet-restricted rats than in control rats, but insulin binding to the skeletal muscle membranes was similar for both groups. Spindler et al. (175) reported that dietary restriction increased hepatic insulin receptor mRNA levels by 15%–25% over those of mice fed ad libitum. However, dietary restriction exerts no effect on the level of mRNA for transcription factors such as Sp1, c-*jun*, or RNA polymerase II elongation factor S-II RNA (127).

Although aging is not associated with a decrease in the mRNA levels of the glucose-regulated proteins GRP78 and GRP94, these levels are down-regulated by dietary restriction for GRP78 mRNA and GRP94 mRNA by approximately 50% and 40%, respectively (174). These findings contrast with those obtained with cultured cells in which these GRPs are transcriptionally up-regulated by glucose deprivation.

Glucocorticoids, a class of metabolic hormones, are involved in the regulation of lipolysis, gluconeogenesis, and fat oxidation. The research of Landfield et al. (99) and Sapolsky et al. (159) underlies the "Glucocorticoid Cascade Hypothesis of Aging," which proposes that periodic exposure of hippocampal neurons to high levels of glucocorticoids causes the death of these neurons. Their loss is postulated to lead to impairment in the feedback inhibition of glucocorticoid secretion and consequently to a further elevation of glucocorticoid levels, which act to promote aging processes. Results from two recent studies independently challenge this theory. Sabatino et al. (156), utilizing a longitudinal design, measured the diurnal pattern of plasma corticosterone concentration of ad libitum–fed and diet-restricted male Fischer 344 rats throughout the life span. The afternoon peak levels of corticosterone were markedly higher in diet-restricted than in ad libitum–fed rats. These findings not only contradict the glucocorticoid cascade hypothesis but also raise the possibility that daily periods of moderate hyperadrenocorticism may retard the aging process. Similar elevations in plasma corticosterone levels by dietary restriction were reported in $B6C3F_1$ mice by Holson et al. (66).

Cellular Actions

The actions of dietary restriction are remarkably broad, occurring not only at the organ and organ system levels but also at the cellular, subcellular, and molecular levels (Table 23.1). This suggests that dietary restriction influences basic cellular processes, thereby maintaining cellular homeostasis (102). As discussed in the following sections, dietary restriction prevents or greatly minimizes age-related deterioration in cellular and subcellular function and structure.

Membrane Structure. Age-related deterioration in cellular and subcellular structure is evident in mitochondrial and microsomal membranes of most cell types (129, 201, 203), a fact which has promoted various membrane-related aging hypotheses (163, 185, 211). Before discussing these age-related changes and their modulation by dietary restriction, a brief description of oxidative reactions of lipids is presented, because both aging and dietary restriction substantially influence membrane lipids and their peroxidation.

Many membrane alterations are due to the oxidative damage of membrane lipids because of their vulnerability to prooxidant molecules. Initiation sites for these reactions are the reactive pi- and diene-conjugated double bonds of lipid structures. This oxidation leads to the formation of hydroperoxides, followed by molecular fragmentation through a scission process. Free radicals are then most often generated by a propagation process which continues until it is terminated or neutralized by free radical scavengers or reductants. Therefore, it is essential for cells to possess effective defense systems to protect cellular integrity against the continuous oxidative threat that occurs even under normal physiological conditions. Unfortunately, the defense components themselves, which are also targets of oxidative insult, deteriorate with age.

TABLE 23.1. *Effect of Age and Dietary Restriction on Genomic Activities*

Parameters	System	Strain	Age	Dietary Restriction	Reference
PolyA RNA/rRNA	Hepatocytes	Fischer 344 rats	NC*	NC	126
PolyA tail length	Brain, kidney, liver, hypothalamus, oviduct, hepatocytes	Fischer 344 rats	NC	NC	93
mRNA androgen receptor	α2μ-globulin	Fischer 344 rats (male)	Decrease	Attenuate	173
mRNA insulin receptor	Liver	$C3B10RF_1$ mice	Increase	Further increase	175
Gene expression Mn superoxide dismutase	Liver	$C3B10RF_1$ mice	Decrease	Attenuate	126
Gene expression catalase	Liver	Fischer 344 rats	Decrease	Attenuate	143
Gene expression Cu/Zn superoxide dismutase	Brain, heart, liver, hepatocytes, kidney, intestinal mucosa	Fischer 344 rats	Decrease	Attenuate	143, 199
HSP70 induction heat shock proteins	Hepatocytes	Fischer 344 rats	Decrease	Attenuate	199
RNA-encoding CYP1A	Cytochrome P-450	$C3B10RF_1$ mice	Decrease	Attenuate	127
Induction of P-450 isozymes	Cytochrome P-450	Fischer 344 rats	Decrease	Attenuate	67
Glucose-regulating proteins	Liver	$C3B10RF_1$ mice	NC	Decrease	174
c-*myc* mRNA	Liver	Fischer 344 rats	Increase	No effect	186
Apo-A1	Plasma	Fischer 344 rats	Increase	Attenuate	186
Apo-B	Plasma	Fischer 344 rats	Increase	No effect	186
Gene expression IGF1	Plasma	BN-F334 rats	Decrease	Attenuate	15
Senescence marker protein	Liver	Fischer 344 rats	Increase	Decrease	19

* NC = no change.

Although age-related alterations in membrane composition and structure were well documented more than 10 yr ago by Hegner (62), very little research has explored possible interventions. Our laboratory recently provided substantial evidence (96, 98, 205) that dietary restriction retards much of the age-related membrane damage. Dietary restriction maintains homeostatic protective mechanisms in the face of age-related oxidative stress (141, 206). Aging in rats has been linked to changes in fatty acid composition in both mitochondrial and microsomal membranes (95). Highly peroxidizable long-chain fatty acids such as 20:4, 22:5, and 22:6 increase with age, while the amounts of 18:2 and 18:3 concurrently decrease. In diet-restricted rats, however, membrane profiles exhibit a decrease in polyunsaturated fatty acids and an increase in 18:2 and 18:3 fatty acids, rendering the membrane lipids less peroxidizable. Remarkably, all these changes take place in the face of a constant ratio of unsaturated/saturated fatty acids, the major determinant of membrane fluidity. Thus dietary restriction maintains membrane fluidity while suppressing the peroxidizability of membrane lipids (209).

Dietary restriction also lessens age-related physical and biochemical changes in membranes. It prevents age-related decreases in cytochrome P-450 content in hepatic microsomal membranes (104) and maintains membrane fluidity and transition temperature of both mitochondria and microsomes (104, 209).

Based on its membrane-stabilizing effect, dietary restriction should improve stability of receptor–ligand interactions at the cell membrane surface. Indeed, most deterioration with age in ligand–receptor interactions can be ameliorated by dietary restriction. Roth and co-workers (154) showed that the age-related deterioration of dopaminergic receptors is effectively blunted by dietary restriction. Similarly, Scarpace and Yu (162) recently demonstrated that the adenylate cyclase membrane β-adrenergic receptors of rat lung are protected during aging by dietary restriction.

The remarkable power of dietary restriction extends to other membrane-associated events, particularly those related to free-radical generation. The two major producers of free radicals are mitochondria and endoplasmic reticulum. As reported recently (104), dietary restriction enhances the cell's cytosolic antioxidant defense systems. Production of superoxide anion, hydroxyl radicals, and hydrogen peroxide by membranes isolated from ad libitum–fed rats is consistently higher than that by membranes from diet-restricted rats.

Other Cellular Constituents. It has been suggested that the cytosolic defense systems against free-radical damage deteriorate with age, resulting in an impaired capacity to resist the increased oxidative stress with aging and that dietary restriction blunts this age change. Laganiere and Yu (97) provided supportive evidence by showing that the activities at similar ages of key scavenger enzymes (catalase, glutathione reductase, and glutathione transferase) are enhanced in diet-restricted compared to ad libitum–fed rats. Also, levels of reduced glutathione, a major physiological reducing agent, were maintained with age in diet-restricted rats (97), indicating that dietary restriction preserves defense mechanisms against oxidative attack.

Lee and Yu (104, 105) assessed the effect of caloric restriction on the overall defense capacity in vitro. Cytosolic preparations were isolated from both diet-restricted and ad libitum–fed rats at different ages, and their ability to protect against the destruction of cytochrome P-450 was assessed. Protection was consistently greater with cytosolic preparations from diet-restricted rats than those from ad libitum–fed rats. Although the factors responsible for this protective action against oxidative damage have not been identified, these results strongly indicate that dietary restriction enhances the cytosolic protective system.

DNA repair appears to be enhanced by dietary restriction. Richardson and Cheung (148) reported that the capacity to repair irradiated DNA damage declined with age and that caloric restriction prevented such loss. Old diet-restricted rats maintained DNA repair capacity at the level of young ad libitum–fed rats (193). Chung et al. (24) found that mitochondrial DNA is substantially more damaged than nuclear DNA and that dietary restriction protects both. The findings on the difference between mitochondrial and nuclear DNA agree with the earlier work of Richter et al. (149), and this difference may relate to the high levels of oxygen-derived reactive species produced by mitochondrial respiration. Dietary restriction may protect by influencing gene expression of antioxidant scavenger enzymes (126).

Protection against Senescent Cellular Deterioration. No established and defined mechanism explains all the antiaging actions of dietary restriction. As suggested above, dietary restriction may slow the aging process by protecting against oxygen free radicals and other reactive oxygen-containing molecules (58). Of the various theories proposed to explain possible cellular mechanisms responsible for senescence, the free-radical theory is particularly attractive (60, 144). Senescence and free-radical reactions share the characteristics of being intrinsic, progressive, cumulative, and deleterious. Free radicals are generated through respiration and other intrinsic processes. Free-radical reactions progress through chain reactions. The damage inflicted by free-radical reactions can be cumulative and is deleterious. Thus the antiaging and life-prolonging actions of dietary restriction could well result from its ability to partially prevent free-radical damage.

To appreciate the possible involvement of free radicals in cellular homeostatic failure, a discussion of how free radicals may perturb various cellular structures and functions, thereby upsetting homeostatic control, is in order. The membrane structure is the preferential target of free-radical attack for two reasons: *(1)* most cellular and subcellular membranes, including plasma, mitochondrial, and microsomal, are major sites of production of free radicals and other reactive molecular species, and *(2)* membrane lipids are highly vulnerable to attack and consequent peroxidation. Another major cellular component which undergoes oxidative modification is DNA. DNA repair processes appear to become inadequate with age, and the resulting accumulation of damaged DNA could have serious consequences. Oxidative damage of proteins also occurs (53).

Oxidative damage is not limited to structural constituents. Free-radical reactions can also damage metabolic substrates like glucose. Recently, Wolff and colleagues (198) showed that glucose autoxidation probably occurs even under normal physiological conditions. Moreover, glucose oxidative reactions in turn lead to increased free-radical formation, as shown by Hunt et al. (68) and Mullarkey et al. (128), who demonstrated that nonenzymatic glycosylation usually generates superoxide radicals. The possible roles of free-radical reactions in senescence have been reviewed (92, 176).

Cellular homeostatic capacity is best evaluated when the cell is challenged by some defined perturbation. Two examples illustrate this point: *(1)* in vitro challenge with UV irradiation and *(2)* in vivo challenge with aflatoxin B_1 (AFB_1). In the first example, the DNA repair process of hepatocytes damaged by UV irradiation was examined. Weraarchakul et al. (193) clearly showed that the DNA repair process was well maintained in hepatocytes from diet-restricted rats. Thus food restriction preserves the ability of hepatocytes to coordinate the complex repair process when exposed to UV irradiation, which is known to cause nondiscriminatory cellular injury. In the second example, Chou et al. (23) challenged rats with the potent carcinogen aflatoxin. In animals that consumed the carcinogen, hepatic nuclear AFB_1–DNA binding, DNA strand breaks, and thymidine incorporation into liver DNA were measured. Caloric restriction suppressed all three parameters, demonstrating again its ability to fend off such insults. These results strongly support dietary restriction as a potent protector of cellular homeostasis, a concept formally proposed by Yu et al. (206).

MODULATION OF THE AGING PROCESS BY OTHER INTERVENTIONS

Experimental interventions for the retardation of the aging process have not been limited to dietary restriction. Claims have been made for many interventions in regard to antiaging actions, and several are discussed in this section.

Antioxidant Feeding

Antioxidants have been administered as dietary supplements or by other means to test their ability to extend the life span (Table 23.2). They have been administered to a variety of species, including nematodes, rotifers, fruit flies, mice, and rats. The free-radical theory of aging was the rationale for this approach. However, the results have been disappointing. Unlike dietary restriction, the effects were not reproducible or robust, particularly in mammalian species. Even in cases where life-span extension was observed, the increase was usually confined to mean, not maximum, life span. Thus antioxidants may modulate predisposed disease processes without influencing the aging process.

Deprenyl

Deprenyl is one of the most effective therapeutic drugs in the treatment of Parkinson's disease (83, 86, 89, 183). L-deprenyl (selegiline hydrochloride), a synthetic, proparglamine derivative (Fig. 23.3), is a specific monoamine oxidase (MAO) B inhibitor known to counteract the neurotoxicity of 6-hydroxydopamine (6-OHDA) (82) and 1-methyl 4-phenyl-1,2,5,6-tetrahydropyridine (MPTP) (22, 28). The specificity of (−)deprenyl is superior to other known MAO inhibitors (87). Recently, deprenyl has been shown to have life span–extending effects in rats (84, 123), which implies an antiaging action. Thoughts on this antiaging action have been considered along with concepts on its action as a treatment for Parkinson's disease.

While the etiology of Parkinson's disease remains unknown, the basis for age-related deterioration has been traced to alterations in nigrostriatal dopaminergic neurons. Neurotoxic metabolites from endogenous dopamine are thought to be responsible for this neuronal deterioration (14, 15, 85). The decline in dopamine content of the caudate nucleus in humans has been estimated at 13% per decade over the age of 45 yr (151). If dopamine content decreases below 30% of the young adult level, symptoms of the disease appear. Changes with age in the dopamine concentration of the human striatum are presented in Table 23.3.

The biochemical basis for the action of deprenyl on dopamine metabolism seems related to its effect on MAO, a key enzyme in dopamine metabolism. MAO, located in the mitochondria, catalyzes the oxidative deamination of dopamine, thus controlling the levels of this neurotransmitter substance in the brain and protecting the liver and intestine against excessive levels of biogenic amines. MAO has two forms, A and B, which exhibit different substrate specificities. MAO-A cata-

TABLE 23.2. *Antioxidant-Supplemented Studies in Aging*

Species	Antioxidants	Concentration	Life-Span Extension Mean	Maximum	Reference
Rotifer	Vitamin E	1×10^{-4} M	Increase*	NC	39
	Vitamin C	25 μM	NC	NC	12
	TCA	400 μM	Increase*	NC	12
		800 μM			
	BHT	25 μM	NC	NC	12
	Vitamin E	25 μM	Increase*	ND	160
Fruit fly	Tocopherol-p-chlorophenoxy acetate	0.1% W	Increase (13%)	Increase (13%)	122
	NDGA	0.1% W	Increase (20%)	Increase (20%)	122
	Mg-TCA	0.1% W	Increase (20%)	Increase (20%)	122
House fly	Ascorbate	0.5% W	Decrease*	ND	172
	β-carotene	2% W	NC		
	Tocopherol	2% W	NC		
Nematode	Vitamin E	400 μM	Increase (30%)	Increase (30%)	40
Guinea pig	Cysteine	21 s.c. injection (30 mg/kg body wt) on alternate days	Marginal increase	ND	132
Mouse	Santoquin	0.5% W	Increase (18%)	ND	29
	BHT	0.75% W	Increase (30%)	NC	25
	Mixture of varying amounts of antioxidants: tocopherol, butylated hydroxy toluene, ascorbate, methionine, selenite		NC	ND	180
	Cysteine	1%	Increase (25%)	ND	132
	MEA	1% W	NC	NC	90
	BHT	0.2% W	NC	NC	90
	MEA	1.0% W	Increase (12%)	ND	59
	MEA	0.25% W	Increase (13%)	Increase (12%)	63
	Ethoxyquin/MEA	0.25% W	NC	NC	61
		0.6% W			
	α-tocopherol acetate	4.4 mg/g chow	NC	NC	103
Rat	Cysteine	21 s.c. injection (30 mg/kg body wt) on alternate days	NC	ND	132
	Folcystein	21 s.c. injection on alternate days	NC	ND	123
	Vitamin E	Oral (100 mg/wk)	NC	ND	7
	Vitamin E	200 mg/100 mg chow	Increase*	NC	142

ND, not determined; NC, no change; s.c., subcutaneous injection; folcystein, injected with thiazolidincarboxylic acid (30 mg + folic acid 0.75 mg); TCA, thiozolidine-4-carboxylic acid; BHT, butylated hydroxytoluene; MEA, 2-mercaptoethylamine hydrochloride; NDGA, nordihydroguaiaretic acid.   *Statistically significant.

lyzes the breakdown of adrenaline, noradrenaline, and serotonin. The substrates for MAO-B are benzylamine, phenylethylamine, and MPTP. Both forms are capable of metabolizing tyramine and dopamine (50). In humans, most brain dopamine is metabolized by MAO-

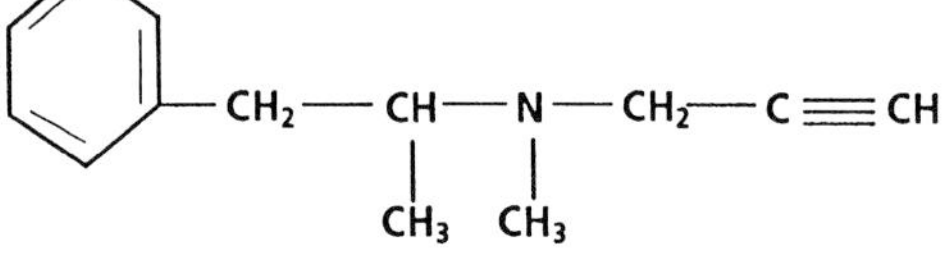

FIG. 23.3. Structure of deprenyl.

TABLE 23.3. *Age-Related Changes in Dopamine Content of Caudate Nucleus*

Age (yr)	Striatal Function (%)
45	100
55	87
65	74
75	61
85	48
95	35

Functional changes (%) were estimated by the average loss of dopamine content in caudate nucleus. [Adapted from Knoll (88) with permission.]

B, while in rats, MAO-A is prevalent (17). Differences also exist in the regional localization of these two enzymes. MAO-A is concentrated in the cortex, while MAO-B is mostly found in the subcortical nuclei and brain stem (36).

The activity of MAO-B increases markedly with age in the cortex, the hypothalamus, the hippocampus, and the nigrostriatal system (1, 150, 194), and age-related changes in MAO-B activity are closely correlated to the decline in dopamine content in the nigrostriatal system. Increased MAO-B activity is due to the increased mitochondrial content of the enzyme (51). Based on this correlation, MAO-B inhibitors such as deprenyl are being used in the treatment of Parkinsonism (13).

While deprenyl acts primarily to inhibit MAO-B when given at low doses, it also blocks dopamine uptake by presynaptic membranes (3). Therefore, deprenyl not only inhibits the age-related increase in MAO-B activity but also prolongs the length of time in which dopamine can act.

In 1988, Knoll (84) reported that deprenyl increases longevity. Rats were treated from the end of the second year of life with 0.25 mg deprenyl per kg, three times per week until death. The treated group exhibited a significant life span extension. The maximum and mean life spans of control rats (164 and 147 wk, respectively) were significantly shorter than those of the deprenyl-treated group (226 and 192 wk, respectively). Estimated life span extension was 38% for the maximum life span and 30% for the mean life span. Other investigators have also confirmed the life-prolonging action of deprenyl. Milgram et al. (123) treated 66 male Fischer 344 rats with injections of 0.25 mg deprenyl/kg every other day, starting at 23–25 months of age, and found the mean and maximum life spans to increase (Table 23.4). Food intake was not monitored, but the body weights of the deprenyl-treated rats were similar to controls, leading the authors to conclude that food intake was not suppressed by deprenyl treatment. Carrillo et al. (18) later showed that food intake is not altered by deprenyl. Kitani et al. (80) reported that male Fischer 344 rats treated three times per week with injections of 0.25 mg deprenyl/kg started at 18 months of age had a 15% increase in mean life span, and when started at 24 months of age, there was a 34% increase. Knoll (84) reported that male rats treated with deprenyl had a restored sexual activity and an improvement in learning ability, as measured by shuttle box tests.

Mechanisms underlying these actions of deprenyl are being considered. One possibility is that deprenyl functions as an antioxidant, stemming from the hypothesis introduced by Langston (100) that oxidative damage plays a causal role in the neuronal degeneration in Parkinson's disease (57). Knoll (85) has suggested that deprenyl protects nigrostriatal dopaminergic neurons from the toxic free-radical reactions associated with 6-hydroxy-dopamine. Carrillo et al. (18) reported that deprenyl induces superoxide dismutase (SOD) activity in the striatum of rats after subcutaneous daily injections for 21 days. The increase was dose-dependent, and the greatest effect was a tenfold increase in the activity in male rats treated with 2 mg/kg/day.

Deprenyl also potentiates other free-radical scavenging enzymes in the striatum, including superoxide dismutase (26), catalase, and glutathione peroxidase (84). Cohen and Spina (27) reported that deprenyl (2.5 mg/kg) suppressed the rise of oxidized glutathione (GSSG) by 71% in mice treated with the prooxidant haloperidol (1 mg/kg), which in control mice raised the concentration of GSSG in the striatum threefold. They concluded that deprenyl probably acts as an antioxidant and suppresses oxidative stress associated with increased dopamine turnover.

The usefulness of deprenyl as part of an antioxidant strategy in the treatment of Parkinsonism was confirmed by Shoulson (170) in a double-blind clinical trial of the chronic administration of deprenyl and tocopherol carried out in four treatment groups: deprenyl (10 mg/day) and tocopherol placebo, deprenyl placebo and tocopherol (2,000 IU/day), deprenyl (10 mg/day) and tocopherol (2,000 IU/day), or deprenyl placebo and tocopherol placebo. Another study suggests that deprenyl might work as an antioxidant. Fahn (45) reported beneficial effects when high dosages of tocopherol and ascorbate were administered to patients with early Parkinson's disease. The endpoint of the trial was the need to treat patients with levodopa. In the group treated with antioxidants, the time when levodopa became necessary was extended by 2.5 yr. Fahn concluded that the progression of Parkinson's disease may be retarded by the administration of antioxidants.

Not all studies are in accord with this conclusion. Bar-

TABLE 23.4. *Effect of L-Deprenyl Treatment on Longevity in Fischer 344 Rats*

Group	Mean Life Span (wk)	% Increase	Age of Tenth-Percentile Survivors (wk)	% Increase	Maximum Life Span (wk)	% Increase
Control	114 ± 7.7	—	212 ± 8.9	—	251	—
Deprenyl-treated	133 ± 8.3	11.5	248 ± 11.7	16.7	315	25.5

[Adapted from Milgram et al. (123) with permission.]

onti et al. (6) could not detect any enhancement by deprenyl in the activities of circulating glutathione peroxidase, glutathione reductase, glutathione transferase, SOD, and catalase in blood. Deprenyl also failed to enhance cerebrospinal fluid levels of total glutathione and the activities of glutathione peroxidase and SOD. Of course, these are measurements in blood and cerebrospinal fluid and not the striatum.

The current state of knowledge can thus be summarized: deprenyl slows the aging process in rats and is effective in treating Parkinson's disease. Its role as an antioxidant may underlie both actions.

Melatonin

Melatonin, a hormone of the pineal gland, is secreted into the blood in a circadian manner. Its production is age-dependent, robust in the young and progressively declining with age (147). Melatonin functions as both a neurohormone and a neurotransmitter, acting on the hypothalamo–pituitary axis and on peripheral tissues to influence metabolism and immune surveillance (147). Because of its broad range of action and decreased secretion with age, it was proposed that the aging process might be secondary to the failure of the pineal gland (2, 155, 158). This hypothesis was refined by Kloeden et al. (81), who proposed that the pineal gland provides a highly regulated melatonin circadian rhythm coupled to various age-related physiological functions.

Studies have been carried out on the effects of melatonin on longevity, reproductive function, and immune competence. Terentrini et al. (182) found that the onset of the postreproductive estrous–anovulatory state is delayed by administering 0.4 µ/ml of melatonin in the drinking water of 14–24-month-old female rats. Melatonin treatment also blunted the loss of luteinizing hormone (LH) response to naloxone in 16- and 20-month-old rats.

Although the effects of melatonin on age changes in immune function have not been studied, Pierpaoli and Maestroni (138) proposed that the ability of melatonin to antagonize the immunosuppressive effects of acute anxiety stress in mice implies an antiaging action; they found that melatonin administration increased the mean life span of mice by 20%. They postulated that the effect of melatonin is not directly exerted on immune cells but is mediated through the endogenous opioid system upon antigen activation of T cells. Reiter (146) proposes that this action on the immune system may also suppress tumor growth and in this way contribute to life-span extension. In this regard, a recent report of Pierpaoli and Regelson provides additional interesting insights into the antiaging action of melatonin: melatonin administration in drinking water to 15-month-old female mice was found to extend both median and maximum life spans in the absence of any difference in body weights. Most interesting was the finding that pineal transplantation of thymus of young mice to aged mice showed well-preserved thymic cellularity and T cell function. The authors concluded that pineal melatonin plays an important role in regulating the physical aging process (138a).

Hypophysectomy

Everitt and colleagues (41–43) showed that hypophysectomy of rats delays aging parameters such as the aging of tail tendon collagen fibers, the occurrence of kidney disease, cardiac enlargement, and endocrine and nonendocrine-related tumorigenesis. A major concern was whether or not the antiaging action of hypophysectomy was mediated by reduction in food intake. To address this important issue, Everitt et al. utilized hypophysectomized rats, subjected to hypothalamic lesions, which increased the food intake from 7 to 15 g/day (44). These hypophysectomized obese rats also exhibited retardation of the aging parameters, although they did show an increased incidence of abnormal glomeruli compared to nonobese hypophysectomized rats. Comparing the effects of hypophysectomy with those of dietary restriction, Everitt's group (168, 169) recently reported that ablation of the pituitary in rats 60 days of age resulted in cessation of the growth of type 1 fibers in gastrocnemius muscle and a reduction of the size of type 2 muscle fibers in 120-day-old rats. These findings suggest that dietary restriction is not as effective in suppressing muscle fiber growth as hypophysectomy, which appears to be more effective in preserving the smaller muscle fiber size seen in young rats. Also, Wyndham et al. (200) reported that age-related thickening of the glomerular basement membrane was suppressed more by hypophysectomy than by dietary restriction in rats consuming the same amount of food. That hypophysectomy influences many age changes in rats points to a possible involvement of pituitary hormones in aging.

Dehydroepiandrosterone

Dehydroepiandrosterone (DHEA) is the adrenal steroid hormone in highest concentration in human plasma. It is best known for its anticancer action. Administered to rodents, it protects against obesity, diabetes, autoimmunity, and tumorigenesis (164).

Schwartz (164) showed that DHEA administration suppressed the incidence of spontaneous breast tumors in mice, and Pashko and Schwartz (136) reported that feeding A/J mice a diet with 6% DHEA for 10 wk significantly reduced the binding to skin DNA of topically applied carcinogenic DMBA. Long-term administration of DHEA to NZB mice also delayed the onset of autoimmune disease (178).

Although it is claimed that DHEA exerts an antiaging action, there are concerns about the validity of this view (72). The mouse strains used in these studies are those which are genetically predisposed to tumorigenesis or autoimmune disease. Also, whether reduced food intake accompanies DHEA administration has been a matter of debate. Weindruch et al. (192) noted the insufficient data on food intake in the DHEA studies.

Recent attention has refocused on the enhancement of function by DHEA (177, 195). Daynes et al. (34) have proposed that DHEA is a physiological regulator of IL-2 biosynthesis. They showed that lymphocytes from DHEA or DHEA-sulfate-treated mice consistently produced much greater amounts of IL-2 than untreated controls. Concentration of DHEA as low as 10^{-10} M produces IL-2 secretion by lymphocytes. Both in vivo and in vitro DHEA treatments can overcome glucocorticoid suppression of IL-2 synthesis by T cells. Based on these findings, Daynes et al. have suggested that DHEA might act through receptor-mediated mechanisms similar to other types of steroid hormone and may be an important immunoregulator of IL-2 function in pathological conditions.

The mechanisms of the diversified cellular actions of DHEA and its analogs are not known (137, 145). However, it seems reasonable to assume that the enhancement of immune competence may play a role in its putative antiaging action.

CONCLUDING REMARKS

Aging processes can be characterized as time-dependent, progressive, physiological deteriorations which appear irrevocable. Numerous attempts have been made to reverse the course of these processes or to retard their deleterious effects. Modern scientific inquiry into biological aging, particularly during the last two decades, has enhanced our understanding of both the intrinsic and the extrinsic processes of aging. Recent explorations of life extension by caloric restriction, first reported by McCay and colleagues 50 yr ago, have provided insights on the aging process and possible interventions and have encouraged gerontologists to tackle the difficult task of examining the effects of this dietary intervention in nonhuman primates (33, 77).

The broad and reproducible effects of dietary restriction are remarkable and unique. It has been found to influence most systems examined, usually in a way which counteracts the progression of events which occur with aging. For this reason, it provides a powerful tool for studying the aging process. Because its effects are so robust and widespread, one is tempted to seek a unifying mechanism to explain its antiaging actions. Unfortunately, the determination of the mechanisms for its action has so far been as difficult as elucidating the aging processes themselves.

During the past two decades, early views about the nature of aging processes and mechanisms of action of dietary restriction have been eliminated. The following concepts on the mechanism of action of caloric restriction are no longer tenable: *(1)* slowing of the aging process by reduction of the metabolic rate, *(2)* increasing longevity by slowing growth rate, and *(3)* increasing longevity by reduction of adiposity. As advances in molecular techniques are applied to the dietary restriction paradigm, understanding of the mechanisms underlying this nutritional intervention on the modulation of oxidative stress and antioxidant defense systems (210) should emerge.

The author gratefully acknowledges the critical evaluation and editorial work on this manuscript by Dr. Jeremiah Herlihy and Dr. Edward Masoro. The author's work has been supported in part by the National Institute on Aging grant AGO1188.

REFERENCES

1. ARAI, J., and H. KINEMUCHI. Differences between monoamine oxidase concentrations in striatum and forebrain of aged and young rats. *J. Neural. Transm.* 72: 99–105, 1988.
2. ARMSTRONG, S. M. Melatonin: a chronobiotic with anti-aging properties? *Med. Hypotheses* 34: 300–309, 1991.
3. AZZARO, A. J., and K. T. DEMAREST. Inhibitory effect on type A and type B monoamine oxidase inhibitors on synaptosomal accumulation of [^{3}H] dopamine: a reflection of antidepressant potency. *Biochem. Pharmacol.* 31: 2195–2197, 1982.
4. BAKER, G. T., and R. L. SPROTT. Biomarker of aging. *Exp. Gerontol.* 23: 223–240, 1988.
5. BALAGE, M., J. GRIZARD, and M. MANIN. Effect of calorie restriction on skeletal muscle and liver insulin binding in growing rat. *Horm. Metab. Res.* 22: 207–214, 1990.
6. BARONTI, F., T. L. DAVIS, R. C. BOLDRY, M. M. MOURADIAN, and T. N. CHASE. Deprenyl effects on levodopa pharmacodynamics, mood and free radical scavenging. *Neurology* 42: 541–544, 1992.
7. BERG, B. N. Study of vitamin E supplements in relation to muscular dystrophy and other diseases in aging rats. *J. Gerontol.* 14: 174–180, 1959.
8. BERG, B. N., and H. S. SIMMS. Nutrition and longevity in the rat. II. Longevity and onset of disease with different levels of food intake. *J. Nutr.* 71: 255–263, 1960.
9. BERTRAND, H. A., W. R. ANDERSON, E. J. MASORO, and B. P. YU. Action of food restriction on age-related changes in adipocyte lipolysis. *J. Gerontol.* 42: 666–673, 1987.
10. BERTRAND, H. A., E. J. MASORO, and B. P. YU. Maintenance of glucagon-promoted lipolysis in adipocytes by food restriction. *Endocrinology* 107: 591–595, 1981.
11. BIRCHENALL-SPARKS, M. C., M. S. ROBERTS, J. L. STAECKER, and A. RICHARDSON. Effect of dietary restriction on liver protein synthesis in rats. *J. Nutr.* 115: 944–950, 1985.
12. BOZAVIC, V., and H. E. ENESCO. Effect of antioxidants on rotifer lifespan and activity. *Age* 9: 41–45, 1986.

13. BRANDEIS, R., M. SAPIR, Y. KAPON, G. BORELLI, S. CADEL, and B. VALSECCHI. Improvement of cognitive function by MAO-B inhibitor L-deprenyl in aged rats. *Pharmacol. Biochem. Behav.* 39: 297–304, 1991.
14. BRAVI, D., J. J. ANDERSON, F. DAGANI, T. L. DAVIS, R. FERRARI, M. GILLESPIE, and T. N. CASE. Effect of aging and dopaminomimetic therapy on mitochondrial respiratory function in Parkinson's disease. *Move. Disord.* 7: 228–231, 1992.
15. BREESE, C. R., R. L. INGRAM, and W. E. SONNTAG. Influence of age and long-term dietary restriction on plasma insulin-like growth factor-1 (IGF-1), IGF-1 gene expression, and IGF-1 binding proteins. *J. Gerontol.* 46: B180–B187, 1991.
16. BRODY, J. A., and D. B. BROCK. Epidemiologic and statistical characteristics of the United States elderly population. In: *Handbook of the Biology of Aging,* edited by C. E. Finch, and E. L. Schneider. New York: Van Nostrand Reinhold, 1989, p. 3–26.
17. BURCHINSKY, S. G., and S. M. KUZNETSOVA. Brain monoamine oxidase and aging: a review. *Arch. Gerontol. Geriatr.* 14: 1–15, 1992.
18. CARRILLO, M. C., S. KANAI, M. NOBUBO, and K. KITANI. (−) Deprenyl induces activities of both superoxide dismutase and catalase but not of glutathione peroxidase in the striatum of young male rats. *Life Sci.* 48: 517–521, 1991.
19. CHATTERJEE, B., G. FERNANDES, B. P. YU, C. SONG, J. M. KIM, W. DEMYAN, and A. K. ROY. Calorie restriction delays age-dependent loss in androgen responsiveness of the rat liver. *FASEB J.* 3: 169–173, 1989.
20. CHENEY, K. E., R. K. LIU, G. S. SMITH, R. E. LEUNG, M. R. MICKEY, and R. L. WALFORD. Survival and disease patterns in C57BL/6J mice subjected to undernutrition. *Exp. Gerontol.* 15: 237–258, 1980.
21. CHEUNG, H. T., W. T. WU, M. PAHLAVANI, and A. RICHARDSON. The effect of age on the interleukin 2 messenger RNA level. *Federation Proc.* 44: 573, 1985.
22. CHIUEH, C. C., S. J. HUANG, and D. L. MURPHY. Enhanced hydroxyl radical generation by 2′-methyl analog of MPTP: suppression by clorgyline and deprenyl. *Synapse* 11: 346–348, 1992.
23. CHOU, M. W., R. A. PEGRAM, P. GAO, and W. T. ALLABEN. Effect of calorie restriction on aflatoxin B1 metabolism and DNA modification in Fischer 344 rats. In: *Biological Effects of Dietary Restriction,* edited by L. Fishbein. New York: Springer-Verlag, 1991, p. 42–54.
24. CHUNG, M. H., H. KASAI, S. NISHIMURA, and B. P. YU. Protection of DNA damage by dietary restriction. *Free Rad. Biol. Med.* 12: 523–525, 1992.
25. CLAPP, N. K., L. C. SATTERFIELD, and N. D. BOWLES. Effects of the antioxidant butylated hydroxytoluene (BHT) on mortality in BALB/c mice. *J. Gerontol.* 34: 497–501, 1979.
26. CLOW, A., T. HUSSAIN, V. GLOVER, M. SANDLER, D. T. DEXTER, and M. WALKER. (−) Deprenyl can induce soluble superoxide dismutase in rat striata. *J. Neural Transm. Gen. Sect.* 86: 77–80, 1991.
27. COHEN, G., and M. B. SPINA. Deprenyl suppresses the oxidant stress associated with increased dopamine turnover. *Ann. Neurol.* 26: 689–690, 1989.
28. COHEN, G., P. PASIK, B. COHEN, A. LEIST, C. MYTILINEOU, and M. D. YAHT. Parglyne and deprenyl prevent the neurotoxicity of 1-methyl-4-phenyl-1,2,3,6-tetrahydropyridine (MPTP) in monkeys. *Eur. J. Pharmacol.* 106: 209–210, 1984.
29. COMFORT, A. Effect of ethoxyquin on the longevity of C3H mice. *Nature* 229: 254–255, 1971.
30. COMFORT, A. *The Biology of Senescence.* New York: Elsevier, 1979.
31. CONIGLIO, J. J., D. S. H. LIU, and A. RICHARDSON. A comparison of protein synthesis by liver parenchymal cells isolated from Fischer 344 rats of various ages. *Mech. Ageing Dev.* 11: 77–90, 1979.
32. COOK, J. R., and D. E. BUETOW. Decreased protein synthesis by polysome tRNA and aminoacyl-tRNA synthetases isolated from senescent rat liver. *Mech. Ageing Dev.* 17: 41–52, 1981.
33. CUTLER, R. G., B. J. DAVIS, D. K. INGRAM, and G. S. ROTH. Plasma concentrations of glucose, insulin and percent glycosylated hemoglobin are unaltered by food restriction in Rhesus and squirrel monkeys. *J. Gerontol.* 47: B9–B12, 1992.
34. DAYNES, R. A., D. J. DUDLEY, and B. A. ARANEO. Regulation of murine lymphokine production in vivo. II. Dehydroepiandrosterone is a natural enhancer of interleukin 2 synthesis by helper T cells. *Eur. J. Immunol.* 20: 793–802, 1990.
35. DICE, J. F. Altered degradation of proteins microinjected into senescent human fibroblasts. *J. Biol. Chem.* 257: 14624–14627, 1982.
36. DOSTERT, P. L., M. STROLIN-BENEDITTI, and K. F. TIPTON. Interaction of monoamine oxidase with substrates and inhibitors. *Med. Res. Rev.* 9: 45–89, 1989.
37. DUFFY, P. H., R. J. FEUERS, J. A. LEAKEY, A. TURTURRO, and R. W. HART. Effect of chronic calorie restriction on physiological variables related to energy metabolism in the male Fischer 344 rat. *Mech. Ageing Dev.* 48: 117–133, 1989.
38. EDMONDS, T. R. *Life Tables Founded upon the Discovery of a Numerical Law Regulating the Existence of Every Human Being Illustrated by a New Theory of the Cause Producing Health and Longevity.* London: J. Duncan, 1832.
39. ENESCO, H. E., and C. VERDONE-SMITH. α-Tocopherol increases lifespan in the rotifer PHILOVINA. *Exp. Gerontol.* 15: 335–338, 1980.
40. EPSTEIN, J., and D. GERSHON. Studies on aging in nematodes. IV. The effect of antioxidant on cellular damage and lifespan. *Mech. Ageing Dev.* 1: 257–265, 1972.
41. EVERITT, A. V., and L. M. CAVANAGH. The ageing process in the hypophysectomised rat. *Gerontologia* 11: 198–207, 1965.
42. EVERITT, A. V., G. G. OLSEN, and G. R. BURROWS. The effect of hypophysectomy on the aging of collagen fibers in the tail tendon of the rat. *J. Gerontol.* 23: 333–336, 1968.
43. EVERITT, A. V., N. J. SEEDSMAN, and F. JONES. The effects of hypophysectomy and continuous food restriction, begun at ages 70 and 400 days, on collagen aging, proteinuria, incidence of pathology and longevity in the male rat. *Mech. Ageing Dev.* 12: 161–172, 1980.
44. EVERITT, A. V., J. R. WYNDHAM, and D. L. BARNARD. The anti-aging action of hypophysectomy in hypothalamic obese rats: effects on collagen aging, age-associated proteinuria development and renal histopathology. *Mech. Ageing Dev.* 22: 233–251, 1983.
45. FAHN, S. An open trial of high dosage antioxidants in early Parkinson's disease. *Am. J. Clin. Nutr.* 53: 380S–382S, 1991.
46. FERNANDES, G. Nutritional factors: modulating effects on immune function aging. *Pharmacol. Rev.* 36: 1235–1295, 1984.
47. FERNANDES, G., J. T. VENKATRAMAN, E. FLESCHER, S. LAGANIERE, H. IWAI, and P. GRAY. Prevention in the decline of membrane-associated functions in immune cells during aging by dietary restriction. In: *Biological Effects of Dietary Restriction,* edited by L. Fishbein. New York: Springer-Verlag, 1991, p. 172–182.
48. FEUERS, R. J., D. A. CASCIANO, J. G. SHADDOCK, J. E. A. LEAKEY, P. H. DUFFY, R. W. HART, J. D. HUNTER, and L. E. SCHERING. Modification in regulation of intermediary metabolism by caloric restriction in rodents. In: *Biological Effects of Dietary Restriction,* edited by L. Fishbein. New York: Springer-Verlag, 1991, p. 198–206.

49. FINCH, C. E., M. C. PIKE, and M. WITTEN. Slow mortality rate accelerations during aging in some animals approximate that of humans. *Science* 249: 902–905, 1990.
50. FOWLER, C. J., and S. B. ROSS. Selective inhibitors of monoamine oxidase A and B: biochemical, pharmacological and clinical properties. *Med. Res. Rev.* 4: 323–358, 1984.
51. FOWLER, C. J., A. WIBERG, L. ORELAND, J. MARKUSSON, and B. WINBLAD. The effect of age on the activity and molecular properties of human brain monoamine oxidase. *J. Neural. Transm.* 49: 1–20, 1980.
52. GABIUS, H., R. ENGLEHARDT, F. DEERBURG, and F. CRAMER. Age-related changes in different steps of protein synthesis of liver and kidney of rats. *FEBS Lett.* 160: 115–118, 1983.
53. GAFNI, A. Altered protein metabolism in aging. *Ann. Rev. Gerontol. Geriatr.* 10: 117–131, 1990.
54. GOLDSPINK, D. F., and F. J. KELLY. Protein turnover and growth in the whole body, liver and kidney of the rat from the foetus to senility. *Biochem. J.* 217: 507–516, 1984.
55. GOLDSPINK, D. F., and F. J. KELLY. Pre- and post-natal growth and protein turnover in smooth muscle, heart and slow- and fast-twitch skeletal muscles of the rat. *Biochem. J.* 217: 517–526, 1984.
56. GOMPERTZ, B. On the nature of the function expressive of the low of human mortality and on a new mode of determining life contingencies. *Phil. Trans. R. Soc. (Lond.)* 115: 513–585, 1825.
57. GRIMES, J. D., M. N. HASSAN, and J. THAKER. Antioxidant therapy in Parkinson's disease. *Can. J. Neural Sci.* 14: 483–487, 1987.
58. HABIB, M. P., F. DICKERSON, and A. D. MOORADIAN. Ethane production rate in vivo is reduced with dietary restriction. *J. Appl. Physiol.* 68: 2588–2590, 1990.
59. HARMAN, D. Free radical theory of aging: effect of free radical reaction inhibitors on the mortality rate of male LAF1 mice. *J. Gerontol.* 23: 476–482, 1968.
60. HARMAN, D. Free radical theory of aging: nutritional implications. *Age* 1: 145–150, 1978.
61. HARRIS, S. B., R. WEINDRUCH, G. S. SMITH, M. R. MICKEY, and R. L. WALFORD. Dietary restriction alone and in combination with oral ethoxyquin/2-mercaptoethylamine in mice. *J. Gerontol.* 45: B141–B147, 1990.
62. HEGNER, D. Age-dependence of molecular and functional changes in biological membrane properties. *Mech. Ageing Dev.* 14: 101–118, 1980.
63. HEIDRICK, M. L., L. C. HENDRICKS, and D. E. COOK. Effect of dietary 2-mercaptoethanol on the lifespan, immune system, tumor incidence and lipid peroxidation damage in spleen lymphocytes of aging BC3F1 mice. *Mech. Ageing Dev.* 27: 341–358, 1984.
64. HERLIHY, J. T., and J. N. THOMAS. The aging of the cardiovascular system: modulation by dietary restriction. *Age Nutr.* 3: 185–191, 1992.
65. HOLEHAN, A. M., and B. J. MERRY. The experimental manipulation of ageing by diet. *Biol. Rev.* 61: 329–368, 1986.
66. HOLSON, R. R., P. H. DUFFY, S. F. ALI, and F. M. SCALZO. Aging, dietary restriction, and glucocorticoids: a critical review of the glucocorticoid hypothesis. In: *Biological Effects of Dietary Restriction*, edited by L. Fishbein. New York: Springer-Verlag, 1991, p. 123–139.
67. HORBACH, G. J. M. J., J. T. VENKATRAMAN, and G. FERNANDES. Food restriction prevents the loss of isosafrole inducible cytochrome P-450 mRNA and enzyme levels in aging rats. *Biochem. Int.* 20: 725–730, 1990.
68. HUNT, J. V., C. C. T. SMITH, and S. P. WOLFF. Autoxidative glycosylation and possible involvement of peroxides and free radicals in LDL modification by glucose. *Diabetes* 39: 1420–1424, 1990.
69. ISHIGAMI, A., and S. GOTO. Effect of dietary restriction on the degradation of proteins in senescent mouse parenchymal cell culture. *Arch. Biochem. Biophys.* 238: 362–366, 1990.
70. IWASAKI, K., C. A. GLEISER, E. J. MASORO, C. A. MCMAHAN, E. J. SEO, and B. P. YU. The influence of dietary protein source on longevity and age-related disease processes of Fischer rats. *J. Gerontol.* 43: B5–B12, 1988.
71. JUNG, L. K. L., M. A. PALLADINO, S. CALVANO, D. A. MARK, R. A. GOOD, and G. FERNANDES. Effect of calorie restriction on the production and responsiveness to interleukin 2 in (NZBXBZW)F1 mice. *Clin. Immunol. Immunopathol.* 25: 295–301, 1982.
72. KALU, D. N. Comparison of the effects of DHEA and food restriction on serum calcitonin. *Exp. Ageing Res.* 10: 3–5, 1984.
73. KALU, D. N. Bone and the calcium regulating hormones: modulation by aging and food restriction. *Age Nutr.* 3: 179–184, 1992.
74. KALU, D. N., R. R. HARDIN, R. COCKERHAM, and B. P. YU. Aging and dietary modulation of rat skeleton and parathyroid hormone. *Endocrinology* 115: 1239–1247, 1984.
75. KALU, D. N., R. R. HARDIN, R. COCKERHAM, B. P. YU, B. K. NORLING, and J. W. EGAN. Lifelong food restriction prevents senile osteopenia and hyperparathyroidism in F344 rats. *Mech. Ageing Dev.* 26: 103–112, 1984.
76. KALU, D. K., D. C. HERBERT, R. R. HARDIN, B. P. YU, G. KAPLAN, and J. W. JACOB. Mechanism of dietary modulation of calcitonin levels in Fischer rats. *J. Gerontol.* 3: B125–B131, 1988.
77. KEMNITZ, J. W., R. WEINDRUCH, E. B. BOECKER, K. CRAWFORD, P. L. KAUFMAN, and W. B. ERSHLER. Dietary restriction of adult male Rhesus monkeys: design, methodology and preliminary findings from the first years of study. *J. Gerontol.* 48: B17–B26, 1993.
78. KHANSARI, D. N., and T. GUSTAD. Effects of long-term, low-dose growth hormone therapy on immune function and life expectancy of mice. *Mech. Ageing Dev.* 57: 87–100, 1991.
79. KIRKWOOD, T. B. L. Comparative and evolutionary aspects of longevity. In: *Handbook of the Biology of Aging* (2nd ed.), edited by C. E. Finch and E. L. Schneider. New York: Van Nostrand Reinhold, 1985, p. 27–44.
80. KITANI, K., S. KANAI, Y. SATO, M. OHTA, G. O. IVY, and M. C. CARRILLO. Chronic treatment of (−) deprenyl prolongs the life span of male Fischer 344 rats. Further evidence. *Life Sci.* 52: 281–288, 1993.
81. KLOEDEN, P. E., R. ROSSLER, and O. E. ROSSLER. Does a centralized clock for ageing exist? *Gerontology* 36: 314–322, 1990.
82. KNOLL, J. The possible mechanism of action of (−) deprenyl in Parkinson's disease. *J. Neural Transm.* 43: 177–198, 1978.
83. KNOLL, J. The facilitation of dopaminergic activity in the aged brain by (−) deprenyl. A proposal for a strategy to improve the quality of life in senescence. *Mech. Ageing Dev.* 30: 109–122, 1985.
84. KNOLL, J. The striatal dopamine dependency of lifespan in male rats. Longevity study with (−) deprenyl. *Mech. Ageing Dev.* 46: 237–262, 1988.
85. KNOLL, J. (−) Deprenyl (selegiline, movergan) facilitates the activity of nigrostriatal dopaminergic neuron. *J. Neural Transm. Suppl.* 25: 45–66, 1988.
86. KNOLL, J. Extension of lifespan of rats by long-term (−) deprenyl treatment. *Mt. Sinai J. Med.* 55: 67–74, 1988.
87. KNOLL, J. The pharmacology of selegiline ((−) deprenyl). New aspects. *Acta Neurol. Scand.* 126: 83–91, 1989.

88. KNOLL, J. Nigrostriatal dopaminergic activity, deprenyl treatment, and longevity. In: *Parkinson's Disease: Anatomy, Pathology, and Therapy, Adv. Neurol.*, edited by M. B. Streifler, A. D. Korczyn, E. Mclaned, and M. B. H. Youdin. New York: Raven Press, 1990, vol. 53, p. 425–429.
89. KNOLL, J. (−) Deprenyl-medication: a strategy to modulate the age-related decline of the striatal dopaminergic system. *J. Am. Geriatr. Soc.* 40: 839–847, 1992.
90. KOHN, R. R. Effect of antioxidants on lifespan of C57BL/6J mice. *J. Gerontol.* 26: 378–380, 1971.
91. KOIZUMI, A., Y. WADA, M. TSUKADA, J. HASEGAWA, and R. L. WALFORD. Low blood glucose levels and small islets of Langerhans in the pancreas of calorie-restricted mice. *Age* 12: 93–96, 1989.
92. KRISTAL, B. S., and B. P. YU. An emerging hypothesis: synergistic induction of aging by free radicals and Maillard reactions. *J. Gerontol.* 47: B107–B114, 1992.
93. KRISTAL, B. S., C. C. CONRAD, A. RICHARDSON, and B. P. YU. Is poly(A) tail length altered by aging or dietary restriction? *Gerontology* 39: 152–162, 1993.
94. KRITCHEVSKY, D. Fat, calories and cancer. In: *Frontiers of Gastrointestinal Research*, edited by P. Rozen. Basel: Karger, 1988, vol. 14, p. 188–198.
95. LAGANIERE, S., and B. P. YU. Anti-lipoperoxidation action of food restriction. *Biochem. Biophys. Res. Commun.* 145: 1185–1191, 1987.
96. LAGANIERE, S., and B. P. YU. Effect of chronic food restriction in aging rats. I. Liver subcellular membranes. *Mech. Ageing Dev.* 48: 207–219, 1989.
97. LAGANIERE, S., and B. P. YU. Effect of chronic food restriction in aging rats. II. Liver cytosolic anti-oxidants and related enzymes. *Mech. Ageing Dev.* 48: 221–230, 1989.
98. LAGANIERE, S., and B. P. YU. Modulation of membrane phospholipid fatty acid composition by age and food restriction. *Gerontology* 39: 7–18, 1993.
99. LANDFIELD, P. W., J. C. WAYMIRE, and G. LYNCH. Hippocampal aging and adrenocorticoids: quantitative correlations. *Science* 202: 1098–1102, 1978.
100. LANGSTON, J. W. Selegiline as neuroprotective therapy in Parkinson's disease. *Neurology* 40: 61–61, 1990.
101. LAVIK, P. S., and C. A. BAUMANN. Further studies on tumor promoting action of fat. *Cancer Res.* 3: 749–756, 1943.
102. LEAKEY, J. F. A., J. J. BAZARE, J. R. HARMON, R. J. FEUERS, P. H. DUFFY, and R. W. HART. Effect of long-term calorie restriction on hepatic drug-metabolizing enzyme activities in the Fischer 344 rat. In: *Biological Effects of Dietary Restriction*, edited by L. Fishbein. New York: Springer-Verlag, 1991, p. 207–216.
103. LEDVINA, M., and M. HODANOVA. The effect of simultaneous administration of tocopherol and sunflower oil on the lifespan of female mice. *Exp. Gerontol.* 15: 67–71, 1980.
104. LEE, D. W., and B. P. YU. Modulation of free radicals and superoxide dismutases by age and dietary restriction. *Aging* 2: 357–362, 1990.
105. LEE, D. W., and B. P. YU. The age-related alterations in liver microsomal membranes: the effects of lipid peroxidation and dietary restriction. In: *Liver and Aging*, edited by K. Kitani. Amsterdam: Elsevier, 1991, p. 17–26.
106. LIEPA, G. U., E. J. MASORO, H. A. BERTRAND, and B. P. YU. Food restriction as modulator of age-related changes in serum lipids. *Am. J. Physiol.* 238 (*Endocrinol. Metab.* 1): E253–E257, 1980.
107. MAEDA, H., C. A. GLEISER, E. J. MASORO, I. MURATA, C. A. MCMAHAN, and B. P. YU. Nutritional influences on aging of Fischer 344 rats. II. Pathology. *J. Gerontol.* 40: 671–688, 1985.
108. MAKRIDES, S. Protein synthesis and degradation during aging and senescence. *Biol. Rev.* 58: 343–422, 1983.
109. MAKRIDES, S. C., and J. GOLDTHWAITE. The content and size distribution of membrane-bound and free polyribosomes in mouse liver during aging. *Mech. Ageing Dev.* 27: 111–134, 1984.
110. MASORO, E. Food restriction in rodents: an evaluation of its role in the study of aging. *J. Gerontol.* 43: B59–B64, 1988.
111. MASORO, E. Overview of the effect of food restriction. In: *Dietary Restriction and Aging*, edited by D. L. Snyder. New York: Alan R. Liss, 1989, p. 27–35.
112. MASORO, E. J., K. IWASAKI, C. A. GLEISER, C. A. MCMAHAN, E. J. SEO, and B. P. YU. Dietary modulation of the progression of nephropathy in aging rats. An evaluation of the importance of protein. *Am. J. Clin. Nutr.* 49: 1217–1227, 1989.
113. MASORO, E. J., M. S. KATZ, and A. MCMAHAN. Evidence for the glycation hypothesis of aging from the food-restricted rodent model. *J. Gerontol.* 44: B20–B22, 1989.
114. MASORO, E. J., R. J. M. MCCARTER, M. S. KATZ, and C. A. MCMAHAN. Dietary restriction alters characteristics of glucose fuel use. *J. Gerontol.* 47: B202–B208, 1992.
115. MASORO, E. J., I. SHIMOKAWA, and B. P. YU. Retardation of the aging processes in rats by food restriction. In: *Physiological Senescence and Its Postponement*, edited by W. Pierpaoli and N. Fabris. New York: New York Academy of Sciences, 1991, vol. 621, p. 337–352.
116. MASORO, E. J., B. P. YU, and H. A. BERTRAND. Action of food restriction in delaying the aging process. *Proc. Natl. Acad. Sci. U.S.A.* 79: 4239–4241, 1982.
117. MCCARTER, R., E. J. MASORO, and B. P. YU. Does food restriction retard aging by reducing the metabolic rate? *Am. J. Physiol.* 248 (*Endocrinol. Metab.* 11): E488–E490, 1985.
118. MCCARTER, R. J., and J. PALMER. Energy metabolism and aging: a lifelong study of Fischer 344 rats. *Am. J. Physiol.* 263: (*Endocrinol. Metab.* 26): E448–E452, 1992.
119. MCCAY, C., M. CROWELL, and L. MAYNARD. The effect of retarded growth upon the length of lifespan and upon the ultimate body size. *J. Nutr.* 10: 63–79, 1935.
120. MCCAY, C. M., W. E. DILLEY, and M. F. CROWELL. Growth rates of brook trout reared upon purified rations upon dry skim milk diets and upon feed combinations of cereal grains. *J. Nutr.* 1: 233–246, 1929.
121. MCDONALD, R., J. HEGENAUER, and P. SALTMAN. Age-related differences in the bone mineralization pattern of rat following exercise. *J. Gerontol.* 41: 445–452, 1986.
122. MIGUEL, J., and J. E. JOHNSON. Effects of various antioxidants and radiation protectants on the lifespan and lipofuscin of drosophila and C57BL/6J mice. *Gerontologist* 15: 25, 1975.
123. MILGRAM, N. W., R. J. RACINE, P. NELLIS, A. MENDONCA, and G. O. IVY. Maintenance on L-deprenyl prolongs life in aged male rats. *Life Sci.* 47: 415–420, 1990.
124. MILLER, R. A., B. PHILOSOPHE, I. TINIS, O. WEIL, and B. JACOBSON. Defective control of cytoplasmic calcium concentration in T-lymphocytes from old mice. *J. Cell. Physiol.* 138: 175–182, 1989.
125. MISHIMOTO, S. K., S. M. PADILLA, and D. L. SNYDER. The effect of food restriction and germ-free environment on age-related changes in bone matrix. *J. Gerontol.* 34: B164–B168, 1990.
126. MOTE, P. L., J. M. GRIZZLE, R. L. WALFORD, and S. R. SPINDLER. Influence of age and caloric restriction on expression of hepatic genes for xenobiotic and oxygen metabolizing enzymes in the mouse. *J. Gerontol.* 46: B95–B100, 1991a.
127. MOTE, P. L., J. M. GRIZZLE, R. L. WALFORD, and S. R. SPINDLER. Aging alters hepatic expression of insulin receptor and c-jun mRNA in the mouse. *Mutat. Res.* 256: 7–12, 1991b.
128. MULLARKEY, C. J., D. EDELSTEIN, and M. BROWNLEE. Free

radical generation by early glycation products: a mechanism for accelerated atherogenesis in diabetes. *Biochem. Biophys. Res. Commun.* 173: 932–939, 1990.
129. NAEIM, F., and R. L. WALFORD. Aging and cell membrane complex: the lipid bilayer integral proteins, and cytoskeleton. In: *Handbook of the Biology of Aging*, edited by C. E. Finch and E. L. Schneider. New York: Van Nostrand Reinhold, 1985, p. 272–289.
130. NEAFSEY, P. A. Longevity hormesis, a review. *Mech. Ageing Dev.* 51: 1–31, 1990.
131. NELSON, J. F. The potential role of endocrine systems in the retardation of aging by calorie restriction. *Age Nutr.* 3: 171–178, 1992.
132. OERIU, S., and E. VOCHITU. The effect of the administration of compounds which contain sulfhydryl groups on the survival rates of mice, rats and guinea pigs. *J. Gerontol.* 20: 417–419, 1965.
133. ORGEL, L. E. The maintenance of the accuracy of protein synthesis and its relevance to aging. *Proc. Natl. Acad. Sci. U.S.A.* 49: 517–521, 1963.
134. ORGEL, L. E. The maintenance of the accuracy of protein synthesis and its relevance to aging: a correction. *Proc. Natl. Acad. Sci. U.S.A.* 67: 1476, 1970.
135. OSBORNE, T. B., L. B. MENDEL, and E. L. FERRY. The effect of retardation of growth upon the breeding period and during life in rats. *Science* 40: 294–295, 1917.
136. PASHKO, L. L., and A. G. SCHWARTZ. Effects of food restriction, dehydroepiandrosterone, or obesity on the binding of 3H-7,12-dimethylbenzene(a)anthracene to mouse skin DNA. *J. Gerontol.* 38: 8–12, 1983.
137. PASHKO, L. L., D. K. FAIRMAN, and A. G. SCHWARTZ. Inhibition of proteinuria development in aging Sprague-Dawley rats and C57BL/6J mice by long-term treatment with dehydroepiandrosterone. *J. Gerontol.* 41: 433–438, 1986.
138. PIERPAOLI, W., and G. J. MAESTRONI. Melatonin: a principal neuroimmunoregulatory and anti-stress hormone: its antiaging effects. *Immunol. Lett.* 16: 355–361, 1987.
138a. PIERPAOLI, W., and W. REGELSON. Pineal control of aging: effect of melatonin and pineal grafting on aging mice. *Proc. Natl. Acad. Sci. USA* 91: 787–791, 1994.
139. POLLARD, M., and P. H. LUCKERT. Spontaneous diseases in aging Lobund-Wistar rats. In: *Dietary Restriction and Aging*, edited by D. L. Snyder. New York: Alan R. Liss, 1989, p. 51–60.
140. POLLARD, M., P. H. LUCKERT, and G. Y. PAN. Inhibition of intestinal tumorigenesis in methylazoxymethanol treated rats by dietary restriction. *Cancer Treat. Rep.* 68: 405–408, 1984.
141. PORTA, E. A. Role of oxidative damage in the aging process. In: *Cellular Antioxidant Defense Mechanisms*, edited by C. K. Chow. Boca Raton FL: CRC Press, 1988, vol. III, p. 2–52.
142. PORTA, E. A., N. S. JOUN, and R. T. NITTA. Effects of the type of dietary fat at two levels of vitamin E in Wistar male rats during development and aging. *Mech. Ageing Dev.* 13: 1–39, 1980.
143. RAO, G., E. XIA, and A. RICHARDSON. Effect of age on the expression of antioxidant enzymes in male Fischer 344 rats. *Mech. Ageing Dev.* 53: 49–60, 1990.
144. RATTAN, S. I. S., W. F. WARD, M. GLEUTING, L. SVENDSEN, B. RIIS, and B. F. C. CLARK. Dietary calorie restriction does not affect the levels of protein elongation factors in rat livers during aging. *Mech. Ageing Dev.* 58: 85–91, 1991.
145. REGELSON, W., R. LORIA, and M. KALIMI. Hormonal intervention: "buffer hormone" or "state dependency." The role of dehydroepiandrosterone (DHEA), thyroid hormone, estrogen and hypophysectomy in aging. *Ann. N. Y. Acad. Sci.* 521: 260–273, 1988.
146. REITER, R. J. The ageing pineal gland and physiological consequences. *Bioessays* 14: 169–175, 1992.
147. REITER, R. J., and B. A. RICHARDSON. Some perturbations that disturb the circadian melatonin rhythm. *Chronobiol. Int.* 9: 314–321, 1992.
148. RICHARDSON, A., and H. T. CHEUNG. The relationship between age-related changes in gene expression, protein turnover, and the responsiveness of an organism to stimuli. *Life Sci.* 31: 605–613, 1982.
149. RICHTER, C., J. W. PARK, and B. N. AMES. Normal oxidative damage to mitochondrial and nuclear DNA is extensive. *Proc. Natl. Acad. Sci. U.S.A.* 85: 6465–6467, 1988.
150. RIEDERER, P., and K. JELLINGER. Morphological and biochemical changes in the aging brain: pathophysiological and possible therapeutic consequences. In: *The Aging Brain*, edited by S. Hoyer. Berlin: Springer, 1982, p. 158–166.
151. RIEDERER, P., and S. WUKETICH. Time course of nigrostriatal degeneration in Parkinson's disease. *J. Biol. Med.* 247: 3170–3175, 1979.
152. ROBERTSON, T. B., and L. A. RAY. On the growth of relatively long-lived compared with that of relatively short-lived animals. *J. Biol. Chem.* 42: 71–107, 1920.
153. ROSS, M. H., and G. BRAS. Tumor incidence patterns and nutrition in the rat. *J. Nutr.* 87: 245–260, 1965.
154. ROTH, G. S., D. K. INGRAM, and J. A. JOSEPH. Delayed loss of striatal dopamine receptors during aging of dietarily restricted rats. *Brain Res.* 300: 27–32, 1984.
155. ROZENCWAIG, R., B. R. GRAD, and J. OCHOA. The role of melatonin and serotonin in aging. *Med. Hypotheses* 23: 337–352, 1987.
156. SABATINO, F., E. J. MASORO, A. MCMAHAN, and R. W. KUHN. Assessment of the role of the glucocorticoid system in aging processes and in the action of food restriction. *J. Gerontol.* 46: B171–B179, 1991.
157. SACHER, G. A. Life table modification and life prolongation. In: *Handbook of the Biology of Aging*, edited by C. E. Finch and L. Hayflick, New York: Van Nostrand Reinhold, 1977, p. 582–638.
158. SANDYK, R. Possible role of pineal melatonin in the mechanisms of aging. *Int. J. Neurosci.* 52: 85–92, 1990.
159. SAPOLSKY, R. M., L. C. KREY, and B. S. MCEWEN. The neuroendocrinology of stress and aging: the glucocorticoid cascade hypothesis. *Endocrinol. Rev.* 7: 284–301, 1986.
160. SAWADA, M., and H. E. ENESCO. Vitamin E extends lifespan in the short-lived rotifer Asplanchna brightwella. *Exp. Gerontol.* 19: 179–183, 1984.
161. SAXTON, J. A., JR., and G. C. KIMBALL. Relation to nephrosis and other diseases of albino rat to age and to modifications of diet. *Arch. Pathol.* 32: 951–965, 1941.
162. SCARPACE, P. J., and B. P. YU. Diet restriction retards the age-related loss of beta-adrenergic receptors and adenylate cyclase activity in rat lung. *J. Gerontol.* 42: 442–446, 1987.
163. SCHROEDER, F. Role of membrane lipid asymmetry in aging. *Neurobiol. Aging* 5: 323–333, 1984.
164. SCHWARTZ, A. G. Inhibition of spontaneous breast cancer formation in female C3H(Avy/a) mice by long-term treatment with dehydroepiandrosterone. *Cancer Res.* 39: 1129–1132, 1979.
165. SHIMOKAWA, I., B. P. YU, Y. HIGAMI, T. IKEDA, and E. J. MASORO. Dietary restriction retards onset but not progression of leukemia in male F344 rats. *J. Gerontol.* 48: B68–B73, 1993.
166. SHIMOKAWA, I., B. P. YU, and E. J. MASORO. Influence on diet on fatal neoplastic disease in male Fischer 344 rats. *J. Gerontol.* 46: B228–B232, 1991.
167. SHOCK, N. W. Physiological and chronological age. In: *Aging—Its Chemistry*. Washington: Am. Assoc. Clin. Chem., 1979, p. 3–24.

168. SHOREY, C. D., L. A. MANNING, and A. V. EVERITT. Morphometrical analysis of skeletal muscle fiber aging and the effect of hypophysectomy and food restriction in the rat. *Gerontology* 34: 97–109, 1988.
169. SHOREY, C. D., L. A. MANNING, A. L. GRANT, and A. V. EVERITT. Morphometrical analysis of the short-term effects of hypophysectomy and food restriction on skeletal muscle fibers in relation to growth and aging changes in the rat. *Growth Dev. Aging* 56: 85–93, 1992.
170. SHOULSON, I. Antioxidative therapeutic strategies for Parkinson's disease. *Ann. N.Y. Acad. Sci.* 648: 37–41, 1992.
171. SNYDER, D. L., B. S. WOSTMANN, and M. POLLARD. Serum hormones in diet-restricted gnotobiotic and conventional Lobund-Wistar rats. *J. Gerontol.* 43: B168–B173, 1988.
172. SOHAL, R. S., R. G. ALLEN, K. J. FARMER, R. K. NEWTON, and P. L. TOY. Effect of exogenous antioxidants on the levels of endogenous antioxidants, lipid-soluble fluorescent material and life span in the housefly, *Musca domestica*. Mech. Ageing Dev. 31: 329–336, 1985.
173. SONG, C. S., T. R. RAO, W. F. DEMYAN, M. A. MANCINI, B. CHATTERJEE, and A. K. ROY. Androgen receptor messenger ribonucleic acid (mRNA) in the rat liver: changes in mRNA levels during maturation, aging, and calorie restriction. *Endocrinology* 128: 349–356, 1991.
174. SPINDLER, S. R., M. D. CREW, P. L. MOTE, J. M. GRIZZLE, and R. L. WALFORD. Dietary energy restriction in mice reduces hepatic expression of glucose-regulated protein 78(BiP) and 94 mRNA. *J. Nutr.* 120: 1412–1417, 1990.
175. SPINDLER, S. R., J. M. GRIZZLE, R. L. WALFORD, and P. L. MOTE. Aging and restriction of dietary calories increases insulin receptor mRNA, and aging increases glucocorticoid receptor mRNA in the liver of female C3B10RF1 mice. *J. Gerontol.* 46: B233–B237, 1991.
176. STADTMAN, E. R. Protein oxidation and aging. *Science* 257: 1220–1224, 1992.
177. SUZUKI, T., N. SUZUKI, R. A. DAYNES, and E. G. ENGLEMAN. Dehydroepiandrosterone enhances IL2 production and cytotoxic effector function of human T cells. *Clin. Immunol. Immunopathol.* 61: 202–211, 1991.
178. TANNEN, R. H., and A. G. SCHWARTZ. Reduced weight gain and delay of Coombs' positive hemolytic anemia in NZB mice treated with dehydroepiandrosterone (DHEA). *Fed. Proc.* 41: 463, 1982.
179. TANNENBAUM, A. The initiation and growth of tumors. I. Effects of underfeeding. *Am. J. Cancer* 38: 335–350, 1940.
180. TAPPEL, A. L., B. FLETCHER, and D. DEAMER. Effect of antioxidants and nutrients on lipid peroxidation fluorescent products and aging parameters in the mouse. *J. Gerontol.* 28: 415–424, 1973.
181. TAYLOR, A., A. M. ZULINNI, R. E. HOPKINS, G. E. DALLAL, P. TREGLIA, J. F. R. KUCK, and K. KUCK. Moderate calorie restriction delays cataract formation in the Emory mouse. *FASEB J.* 3: 1741–1746, 1989.
182. TERENTRINI, G. P., A. R. GENAZZANI, M. CRISCUOLO, F. PETRAGLIA. C. DE GAETANI, G. FICARRA, B. BIDZINSKA, M. MIGALDI, and A. D. GENAZZANI. Melatonin treatment delays reproductive aging of female rat via the opiatergic system. *Neuroendocrinology* 56: 364–370, 1992.
183. TETRUD, J. W., and J. W. LANGSTON. The effect of deprenyl (selegiline) on the natural history of Parkinson's disease. *Science* 245: 519–522, 1989.
184. VENKATRAMAN, J., and G. FERNANDES. Modulation of age-related alterations in membrane composition and receptor-associated immune functions by food restriction in Fischer 344 rats. *Mech. Ageing Dev.* 63: 27–44, 1992.
185. VON ZGLINIKI, T. A mitochondrial membrane hypothesis of aging. *J. Theor. Biol.* 127: 4127–4132, 1987.
186. WAGGONER, S., M. Z. GU, W. H. CHIANG, and A. RICHARDSON. The effect of dietary restriction on the expression of a variety of genes. In: *Genetic Effects on Aging*, edited by D. Harrison. Caldwell, NJ: Telford Press, 1990, vol. II, p. 255–274.
187. WARD, W. Enhancement of food restriction of liver protein synthesis in aging Fischer 344 rat. *J. Gerontol.* 43: B50–B53, 1988a.
188. WARD, W. Food restriction enhances the proteolytic capacity of aging rat liver. *J. Gerontol.* 43: B121–B124, 1988b.
189. WARD, W., and A. RICHARDSON. Effect of age on liver protein synthesis and degradation. *Hepatology* 14: 935–948, 1991.
190. WEINDRUCH, R., and R. WALFORD. *The Retardation of Aging and Disease by Dietary Restriction*. Springfield, IL: Thomas, 1988.
191. WEINDRUCH, R., S. R. S. GOTTESMAN, and R. L. WALFORD. Modification of age-related immune decline in mice dietarily restricted from or after mid-adulthood. *Proc. Natl. Acad. Sci. U.S.A.* 79: 898–902, 1982.
192. WEINDRUCH, R., G. MCFEETERS, and R. WALFORD. Food intake reduction and immunologic alterations in mice fed dehydroepiandrosterone. *Exp. Gerontol.* 19: 297–304, 1984.
193. WERAARCHAKUL, N., R. STRONG, W. G. WOOD, and A. RICHARDSON. Effect of age and dietary restriction on DNA repair. *Exp. Cell. Res.* 181: 197–204, 1989.
194. WIENER, H. L., A. HASHIM, A. LAJTHA, and H. SERSHEN. Age and strain differences in monoamine oxidase B in mouse brain. *Res. Commun. Psychol. Psychiatr. Behav.* 13: 305–308, 1988.
195. WISNIEWSKI, T. L., C. W. HILTON, E. V. MORSE, and F. SVEC. The relationship of serum DHEA-S and cortisol levels to measures of immune function in human immunodeficiency virus-related illness. *Am. J. Med. Sci.* 305: 79–83, 1993.
196. WITTEN, M. Reliability theoretic methods and aging: critical elements, hierarchies and longevity-interpreting survival curves. In: *Molecular Biology of Aging*, edited by A. D. Woodhead, A. D. Blackett, and A. Hollaender. New York: Plenum Press, 1985, p. 345–360.
197. WITTEN, M. A return to time, cells, systems and ageing. V. Further thoughts on Gompertzian survival dynamics—the geriatric years. *Mech. Ageing Dev.* 46: 175–200, 1988.
198. WOLFF, S. P., M. J. C. CRABBE, and P. J. THORNALLY. The autoxidation of glyceraldehyde and other simple monosaccharides. *Experientia* 40: 244–246, 1984.
199. WU, B., A. R. HEYDARI, C. C. CONRAD, and A. RICHARDSON. The age-related decline in the induction of a heat shock protein is reversed by life-long dietary restriction. In: *Liver and Aging*, edited by K. Kitani, Elsevier, 1991.
200. WYNDHAM, J. R., A. V. EVERITT, A. EYLAND, and J. MAJOR. Inhibitory effect of hypophysectomy and food restriction on glomerular basement membrane thickening, proteinuria and renal enlargement in aging male Wistar rats. *Arch. Gerontol. Geriatr.* 6: 323–337, 1987.
201. YANG, S. Y., and B. P. YU. Age-related membrane alterations: modulation by dietary restriction. In: *Handbook of Nutrition in the Aged*, edited by R. R. Watson. Boca Raton, FL: CRC Press, 1994, p. 113–131.
202. YU, B. P. Food restriction research: past and present status. In: *Review of Biological Research in Aging*, edited by M. Rothstein. New York: Wiley-Liss, 1990, vol. 4, p. 349–371.
203. YU, B. P. Free radicals and lipid peroxidation of membranes in aging. In: *Free Radicals in Aging*, edited by B. P. Yu. Boca Raton, FL, CRC Press, 1993, p. 57–88.
204. YU, B. P., H. A. BERTRAND, and E. J. MASORO. Nutritional-aging influence of catecholamine-promoted lipolysis. *Metabolism* 29: 438–444, 1980.

205. YU, B. P., S. LAGANIERE, and J. W. KIM. Influence of life-prolonging food restriction on membrane lipoperoxidation and antioxidant status. In: *Oxygen Radicals in Biology and Medicine,* edited by G. M. Simic, K. A. Taylor, J. F. Ward, and C. von Sonntag. New York: Plenum Press, 1989, p. 1067–1073.
206. YU, B. P., B. W. LEE, C. G. MARLER, and J. H. CHOI. Mechanism of food restriction: protection of cellular homeostasis. *Proc. Soc. Exp. Biol. Med.* 193: 13–15, 1990.
207. YU, B. P., E. J. MASORO, and C. A. MCMAHAN. Nutritional influences on aging of Fischer 344 rats. I. Physical, metabolic and longevity characteristics. *J. Gerontol.* 40: 657–670, 1985.
208. YU, B. P., E. J. MASORO, I. MURATA, H. A. BERTRAND, and F. T. LYND. Life span study of SPF Fischer 344 male rats fed ad libitum or restricted diets: longevity, growth, lean body mass and disease. *J. Gerontol.* 37: 130–141, 1982.
209. YU, B. P., E. A. SUESCUN, and S. Y. YANG. Effect of age-related lipid peroxidation on membrane fluidity and phospholipase A2: modulation by dietary restriction. *Mech. Ageing Dev.* 65: 17–23, 1992.
210. YU, B. P. Cellular defenses against damage from reactive oxygen species. *Physiol. Rev.* 74: 139–162, 1994.
211. ZS-NAGY, I. The role of membrane structure and function in cellular aging: a review. *Mech. Ageing Dev.* 9: 237–246, 1979.

24. Exercise

JOHN O. HOLLOSZY
WENDY M. KOHRT

Department of Medicine, Washington University School of Medicine, St. Louis, Missouri

CHAPTER CONTENTS

Exercise and Longevity
    Insights regarding the extension of longevity by food restriction
    Re-evaluation of the rate-of-living concept
Decline in Maximal Oxygen Uptake Capacity with Aging
    Decline in $\dot{V}O_{2max}$ in people who exercise regularly
    Effect of exercise training on $\dot{V}O_{2max}$ in previously sedentary elderly men and women
    Effects of aging and physical inactivity on cardiovascular function: role in the decline in aerobic exercise capacity
        Studies of cardiovascular function in untrained people
        Studies of trained people
    Effect of exercise training on cardiovascular function in elderly people and rats
    Role of skeletal muscle in the decline in aerobic exercise capacity
        Role of skeletal muscle in the decline in $\dot{V}O_{2max}$ in sedentary people
        Adaptations of skeletal muscle to endurance exercise
        Role of skeletal muscle in the decline in $\dot{V}O_{2max}$ in people who exercise regularly
Decline in Muscle Mass and Strength with Aging
    Studies on humans
    Studies on rats
    Effects of strength training on muscle mass and strength in old age
Changes in Body Composition with Aging
    Age-related changes in weight and height
        Studies in untrained people
        Studies in people who exercise regularly
    Age-related changes in fat and fat-free mass
        Multicompartment models of body composition
        Studies in untrained people
        Studies in people who exercise regularly
    Age-related changes in total body water
    Age-related changes in bone mineral content
        Studies in untrained people
        Studies in people who exercise regularly
    Age-related changes in fat distribution pattern
        Studies in untrained people
        Studies in people who exercise regularly
Exercise, Aging, and Carbohydrate Metabolism
    Exercise and carbohydrate metabolism
    Aging and carbohydrate metabolism in rats
        Exercise and carbohydrate metabolism in aging rats
    Aging and carbohydrate metabolism in humans
    Effects of exercise on insulin resistance and glucose tolerance in older people
    Effects of exercise in non-insulin-dependent diabetes
    Effects of exercise in nondiabetic older people who are moderately insulin-resistant
Concluding Remarks

THROUGHOUT MAMMALIAN EVOLUTION, survival has depended on the ability to perform vigorous exercise to obtain food and to escape from predators and other dangers. As a consequence, mammals are genetically adapted for a physically active life, and a chronic lack of exercise is abnormal from a physiological perspective. A remarkable decrease in habitual level of physical activity has occurred in the wealthy nations, made possible by the technological advances of the past century. Perhaps even more remarkable is that, within a few generations, it has become common to think of a sedentary life as normal and of exercise as an intervention. As a consequence, various of the anatomical and physiological changes that occur in sedentary people and laboratory animals as the result of an exercise deficiency are commonly attributed to primary aging processes.

A major purpose of this chapter is to distinguish between the effects of primary aging and those of exercise deficiency, with particular emphasis on those components of the deterioration in structure and function that are preventable and reversible consequences of physical inactivity. We will focus on: *(1)* the effects of exercise deficiency and of exercise training on longevity, cardiovascular and skeletal muscle function as they relate to aerobic exercise capacity, skeletal muscle mass and strength, body composition, insulin resistance, and glucose tolerance and *(2)* the changes in cardiovascular and skeletal muscle structure and function caused by aging that are responsible for the declines in aerobic exercise capacity and strength. While information about some of these topics is still quite sparse, we think that enough is known to provide at least a tentative picture. Other important topics are not addressed either because of a paucity of information or because the authors lack the expertise to critically evaluate the research findings.

EXERCISE AND LONGEVITY

The rationale for the earliest studies of the effect of exercise on longevity was provided by the "rate-of-living" concept, according to which the metabolic rate determines life span (243, 275). It was reasoned that if, as postulated by the rate-of-living hypothesis, life span is inversely related to energy expenditure, interventions such as exercise or cold exposure should accelerate aging and decrease longevity. The results of studies on rats by Slonaker (290) and Benedict and Sherman (13) appeared to support the rate-of-living concept: in both of these studies exercised rats died earlier than those kept sedentary. However, in contrast to the observations of Slonaker (290) and Benedict and Sherman (13) that exercise decreases longevity, subsequent studies have consistently shown that exercised rats live longer than freely eating, sedentary controls. The early studies in which exercise decreased longevity involved small numbers of animals and were performed before the availability of pathogen-free rats. At that time, laboratory rats generally had a variety of chronic infections. When we first studied the effects of exercise on rats in the 1960s, we also used rats that were not pathogen-free and found that as the exercise stress, in the form of swimming or treadmill running, was increased, the rats would frequently lose weight, and if the exercise was continued, they would die of pneumonia or lung abscesses. As soon as we switched to working with pathogen-free rats, the problem with infections stopped, and the rats remained healthy and were able to adapt to prolonged, strenuous exercise training (144, 235, 237). In this context, it seems possible that exercise may have shortened the lives of Slonaker's (290) and Benedict and Sherman's (13) rats by activating or worsening chronic infectious processes.

Although their studies also did not involve pathogen-free rats, Retzlaff et al. (258) found that daily walking for 10 min at 11.5 m/min significantly extended average survival and maximal life span in Sprague-Dawley rats. Sedentary control rats in this study were abnormally short-lived, with an average age at death of only 474 days; the treadmill walkers were also unusually short-lived, with an average age at death of 605 days. Other abnormal findings were that the exercised male rats were heavier than the sedentary ad libitum–fed rats, which attained a peak body weight of only 401 g. Healthy sedentary male Sprague-Dawley rats usually live about 2 yr and attain a body weight of ~700 g. In another study, Edington et al. (80) reported that 20 min of daily treadmill walking at 10 m/min resulted in improved survival of young rats but reduced the survival time of older rats. However, there was a remarkable difference in the survival times of the sedentary control groups for the young and older exercisers. In the case of the controls for the young exercisers, which began exercise at age 120 days, 56% of the sedentary animals were dead before 650 days of age, while only 20% of the controls for the old exercisers were dead by 960 days of age. Thus what was interpreted as a decrease in survival of the older exercisers was actually a remarkable and unexplained increase in the longevity of their sedentary controls. In view of these problems, the studies of Retzlaff et al. (258) and Edington et al. (80) are impossible to interpret with regard to the effect of exercise on aging and longevity. Furthermore, the exercise programs used in these studies (10–20 min of slow walking) represent a negligible exercise stimulus for a rat and would not be expected to induce measurable physiological adaptations (92, 144).

Goodrick (114) followed up these studies with an investigation of the effect of voluntary wheel-running on longevity of male and female Wistar rats. At age 6 wk, rats were housed either in cages with running wheels attached to them or in conventional cages and fed ad libitum. Male rats that had access to running wheels lived an average of 4 months longer than sedentary controls, while female runners lived 3 months longer than their sedentary controls. Furthermore, the exercise appeared to also result in an increase in maximal longevity of about 3 months. Goodrick (114) hypothesized on the basis of these findings that exercise, like food restriction, slows aging. It had been hypothesized (217) that food restriction increases longevity by slowing growth, and Goodrick (114) suggested that exercise might act by the same mechanism. In a subsequent study, Goodrick et al. (116) examined the effect of housing rats in activity wheel cages beginning at either 10.5 or 18 months of age. Neither of these groups given access to running wheels showed an increase in survival time compared to the rats housed in standard cages. Goodrick et al. (116) interpreted this finding to indicate that there is an early threshold for the beneficial effect of exercise on longevity and that exercise started after this threshold age does not increase longevity. As is usually the case in older rats fed ad libitum, the rats in this study performed a minimal amount of voluntary running. Therefore, an alternative explanation is that an exercise threshold exists below which exercise does not improve the survival of rats.

Two studies on specific-pathogen-free, male Long-Evans rats have confirmed the finding of Goodrick (114) that rats given access to activity wheels, beginning at an age at which they do a considerable amount of voluntary running, have an increased average length of life compared to sedentary, freely eating or pair-fed controls (148, 152). However, in contrast to the study by Goodrick (114), the voluntary wheel-runners did not have an increase in maximal life span (148, 152). In the first of these studies, 6-month-old rats were assigned to a voluntary exercise group, a sedentary, freely eating control group, or a paired-weight group that was food-restricted to keep their weights in the same range as those of the wheel-runners (152). After becoming accustomed to the wheels, the runners were initially running

~7 km/24 h (range 3–11 km). Male rats are unusual in that they do not increase their food intake to compensate for the increase in energy expenditure due to exercise, and the runners' body weights stabilized at ~400 g on ad libitum food intake. The paired-weight, sedentary rats, whose food intake was restricted to keep their body weights the same as the runners', ate ~70% as much food as the runners. The freely eating, sedentary rats' average body weight increased to ~600 g.

After a few months the runners began to markedly reduce their distances. This decrease in running was reversed by reducing the runners' food intake to 92% of their ad libitum consumption. This slight food restriction, presumably by stimulating food-searching behavior, reversed the abrupt decrease in running but did not prevent a gradual decline in the average distance run from ~6.4 km/24 h at age 9 months to ~1.6 km/24 h at age 30 months. The 8% reduction in the runners' food intake was controlled for by converting a group of paired-weight controls to pair-fed controls that were fed the same average amount of food as was eaten by the runners. The 8% reduction in food intake required to keep the animals running did not have a significant effect on their body weights, probably because of the gradual decline in running activity.

The paired-weight, sedentary rats that were food-restricted to keep their body weights in the same range as those of the runners, that is, ~30% less food than the freely eating, sedentary rats, had significant increases in average and maximal longevity. The average age at death of the sedentary, freely eating group was 923 ± 160 days, while the paired-weight (food-restricted), sedentary rats' average age at death was 1,113 ± 150 days. As in the many previous studies of the effect of food restriction (see Chapter 23), the improved survival of the paired-weight animals was due to a later onset of mortality and an increase in maximal life span. Runners had a significantly better average survival than freely-eating, sedentary rats (1,012 ± 138 days vs. 923 ± 160 days). However, runners had no increase in maximal longevity compared to sedentary, freely eating animals; furthermore, runners' average age at death was significantly lower than that of the paired-weight, sedentary group. The pair-fed, sedentary rats that, like the runners, were food-restricted by 8% had average and maximal life spans similar to those of the freely eating, sedentary group, showing that this minimal food restriction does not improve survival. Necropsy with histopathological examination showed no significant differences in the cause of death between the wheel-runners and the sedentary, freely-eating or the sedentary, pair-fed animals. This is in contrast to the food-restricted, paired-weight controls, which had a markedly reduced incidence of neoplasms, a finding that is in keeping with the results of numerous previous studies of food restriction (see Chapter 23).

Among the hypotheses that have been suggested to explain the life-extending effect of food restriction are retardation of growth with maintenance of growth potential (217), prevention of excess body fat accumulation (15), and decreased availability of energy for cell proliferation with a shift in the physiological state to maintenance and repair pathways (314, 317). Male rats do not increase their food intake to compensate for the increase in energy expenditure that results from exercise. As a consequence, voluntary wheel-runners had a decreased availability of energy for cell proliferation, resulting in growth retardation (152). However, unlike the food-restricted, paired-weight, sedentary animals, which had the same decrease in the amount of energy available for growth and cell proliferation, runners had no extension of maximal life span.

This finding suggests that decreased availability of energy for cell proliferation and growth is not the mechanism responsible for slowing the aging process and that food restriction extends maximal life span by some other mechanism. Alternatively, exercise could have a deleterious effect that nullifies a mechanism by which decreased availability of energy prolongs life. If the second possibility were correct, exercise should counteract the prolongation of maximal longevity induced by food restriction. A second study was therefore performed to examine the combined effects of exercise and food restriction on longevity of male rats (148). Voluntary wheel-runners were again compared to sedentary, freely eating animals and paired-weight, sedentary rats that were food-restricted to keep their body weights the same as those of the runners. A second group of runners that was pair-fed with the paired-weight, sedentary controls was included in this study. Both groups of runners were given access to the running wheels at age 3 months. From 6 to 30 months of age the food intake of the food-restricted, paired-weight, sedentary rats and the food-restricted runners averaged ~30% below ad libitum intake.

As in the previous study (152), wheel-running improved average length of survival without increasing maximal longevity. Food-restricted runners, which were restricted to ~70% of ad libitum energy intake, showed an improvement in maximal life span similar to that seen in the food-restricted, paired-weight, sedentary rats with which they were pair-fed. Thus exercise did not prevent the life-extending effect of food restriction. This study was complicated by the finding that, although the food-restricted runners showed a prolongation of maximal life span, they had an increased mortality rate over the first 50% of their mortality curve (148). This finding, which was interpreted as indicating that exercise

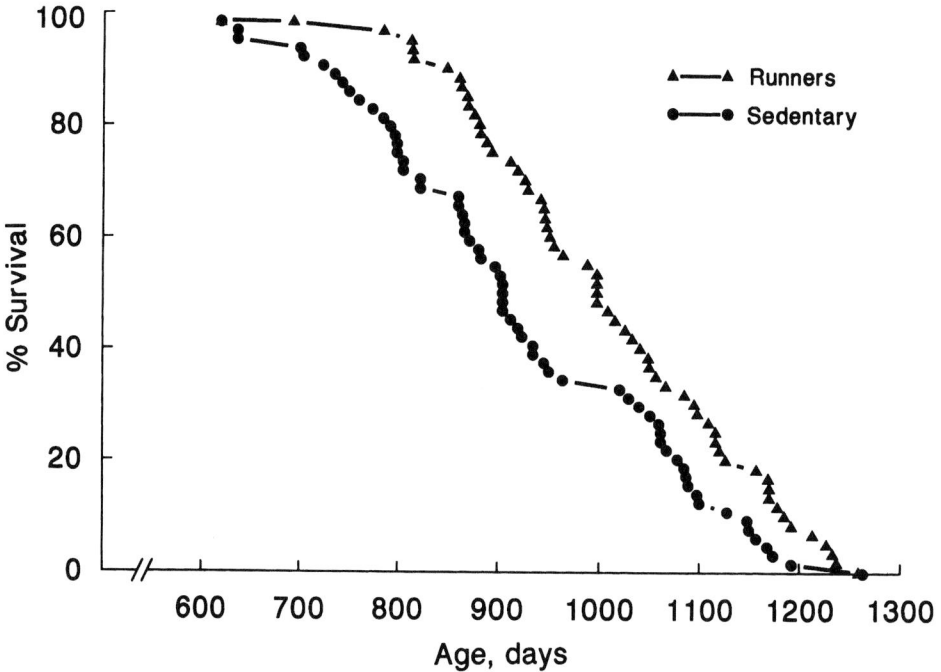

FIG. 24.1. Survival curves of female Long-Evans rats that either had free access to voluntary running wheels starting at the age of 4 months (runners) or were housed in individual cages (sedentary) (145).

has a deleterious effect on food-restricted rats, appeared to be in keeping with the findings of Goodrick et al. (115, 117) that rats fed every other day and given access to voluntary running wheels had a 14 wk shorter survival than sedentary rats that were fed every other day.

However, in contrast to these studies, McCarter and Palmer (214; personal communication, 1993) found that food restriction increased the longevity of voluntary wheel-running rats without increasing early mortality. Furthermore, in a study currently in progress (J. O. Holloszy, unpublished data), a group of male voluntary wheel-running rats that were food-restricted to 70% of ad libitum intake did not have an increased mortality. The age range over which mortality was increased in food-restricted wheel-runners in the previous study was 20–30 months (148). The reason for this difference in response to the same treatment in pathogen-free male rats of the same strain is unexplained, because, due to a funding cut-back, it was not possible to perform necropsies on the rats in the study in which the food-restricted runners had an increased early mortality. All that can be concluded at this time is that *(1)* exercise does not interfere with the slowing of aging, that is, extension of maximal life span, induced by food restriction and *(2)* for unknown reasons, exercise can sometimes result in an increased early mortality rate in food-restricted rats.

Because voluntary wheel-running does not result in an increase in food intake in male rats (148, 152), the runners in the longevity studies had a relative caloric deficiency that resulted in growth retardation, with attainment of a peak body weight about 30% lower than that of freely eating, sedentary controls. It was, therefore, not clear whether the improvement in average length of life of the wheel-runners was due to the exercise per se or to decreased availability of energy for cell proliferation and growth (317). Female rats usually increase their food intake sufficiently in response to exercise to compensate for the increased energy expenditure (236, 237, 268). This made it possible to examine the effects of exercise on longevity without the complication of decreased availability of energy for cell proliferation and growth (145).

Female pathogen-free Long-Evans rats were assigned to either a wheel-running or a sedentary group at age 4 months. Both groups were fed ad libitum. The female runners' food intake was ~37% greater than that of the sedentary animals up to age 10 months and ~20% greater thereafter. Female runners gained weight more rapidly than sedentary controls, but the two groups attained similar peak body weights. Voluntary wheel-running resulted in a rectangularization of the survival curve, with a significant (9%) prolongation of average life span, due to a later onset of mortality, but without an increase in maximal life span (Fig. 24.1). This increase in average length of life is similar to that seen in response to voluntary wheel-running in male rats of the same strain (148, 152). This finding shows that the increase in average longevity in voluntary wheel-running rats compared to freely eating or pair-fed controls is not mediated by decreased availability of energy for cell proliferation and growth. It also provides evidence that a large increase in food intake is not harmful when it is balanced by an increase in energy expenditure that prevents obesity.

Insights Regarding the Extension of Longevity by Food Restriction

Studies on the effect of exercise on longevity provide an approach to evaluating a number of the hypotheses proposed to explain how food restriction slows aging and increases maximal life span. The first of these hypotheses, suggested by McCay et al. (217) who discovered this phenomenon, is that the increased longevity of food-restricted rats is mediated by growth retardation, with retention of growth potential until late in life. Other hypotheses are that food restriction acts by *(1)* increasing spontaneous physical activity (77, 161), *(2)* preventing the development of obesity (15), and *(3)* decreasing energy availability for cell proliferation, with a shift in physiological state to maintenance and repair pathways (314, 317).

Male rats, unlike most other mammals, do not increase their food intake to compensate for the increased energy expenditure caused by exercise. As a result, male voluntary wheel-runners are similar to food-restricted rats in that they have a reduced availability of energy for cell proliferation, with growth retardation (148, 152) and reduced fat cell size and number (53). They are, of course, also much more physically active than rats housed in standard cages. Therefore, if any of the above hypotheses were correct, one would expect exercise, like food restriction, to slow aging and increase maximal longevity. However, exercise in the form of voluntary wheel-running did not increase maximal life span in male rats despite a reduced availability of energy for growth, cell proliferation, and other biological processes. In contrast, sedentary rats that were food-restricted to keep their body weights the same as the runners', and therefore had a similar decrease in energy availability, showed the expected increase in maximal life span.

These findings provide direct evidence against the hypotheses that food restriction slows aging by means of growth retardation (217), by increasing physical activity (77, 161), by protecting against development of obesity (15), or by decreasing energy availability for cell proliferation (314, 317). The alternative possibility, that decreased availability of energy does slow aging and that this beneficial effect is countered by a deleterious effect of exercise, seems unlikely in view of the finding that exercise does not prevent the increase in maximal longevity induced by food restriction. Thus the finding that exercise causes a decreased availability of energy for cell proliferation and growth in male rats but does not increase maximal life span favors the interpretation that the slowing of aging by food restriction is mediated by some aspect of decreased intake or metabolism of food, not by decreased availability of energy. Possible mechanisms include decreased formation of toxins and carcinogens and/or decreased accumulation of waste products.

Re-evaluation of the Rate-of-Living Concept

It has been hypothesized that metabolic rate is a major factor in determining longevity. Rubner (275) postulated that longevity is related to energy turnover, based on comparative studies on a variety of mammals that showed an inverse relationship between metabolic rate and life span. Rubner estimated that total energy expenditure during an animal's lifetime is approximately 200 kcal/g body weight and hypothesized that each gram of tissue can perform only a fixed amount of "work" in a lifetime. While it is true that small species with a high metabolic rate are usually shorter-lived than large species with a lower metabolic rate, there are a number of exceptions. For example, the figure of 200 kcal/g body weight/lifetime is off by a factor of more than 3 for humans. Also, this relationship does not hold within a species; for example, some small breeds of dog are longer-lived than other breeds that are tenfold larger.

Following Rubner, the rate-of-living concept was popularized by Pearl (243), who proposed that longevity is inversely proportional to metabolic rate per unit of body mass and that an organism is born with a certain amount of "vital principle," which is irreplaceable and is depleted at a rate proportional to the rate of energy expenditure, resulting in aging and death. In this, its most primitive form, the rate-of-living concept represents a survival of the philosophy of vitalism into the twentieth century and makes no sense in the context of modern biological knowledge. However, the rate-of-living concept has been restated in modern form as the "free-radical theory of aging" by Harman (131, 132). According to this hypothesis, the greater the rate of oxygen consumption the greater the rate of formation of free radicals of oxygen which cause tissue damage and thus aging.

There is considerable theoretical and some experimental support for the free-radical theory of aging (67, 99). Oxygen is toxic not only to obligate anaerobes but also to aerobic organisms. Although molecular O_2 is rather unreactive, it gives rise to dangerously reactive free radicals and derivatives in the univalent pathway of oxygen reduction, including the superoxide radical hydrogen peroxide and the hydroxy radical (67, 99).

The major defense against oxygen toxicity in aerobic organisms is avoidance of the univalent pathway of oxygen reduction by the reaction catalyzed by cytochrome oxidase. In this reaction electrons are transferred to oxygen in an apparent four-electron reduction to H_2O, during which no intermediates of oxygen reduction are released from the enzyme. However, there appears to be a "leak current" or a "univalent leak" in electron flow along the mitochondrial electron transport chain, leading to formation of some free radicals. A variety of enzymatic reactions and the spontaneous oxidation of hemoglobin, myoglobin, epinephrine, and other compounds also lead to production of superoxide radical and H_2O_2. Superoxide dismutases, catalases, and peroxidases protect against free radicals and H_2O_2 (67, 99). However, no defense is perfect, and it appears that reactive oxygen radicals cause a continual low level of damage to cells of aerobic organisms. Furthermore, the available defense mechanisms may not be able to keep pace with the rate of free-radical formation when O_2 consumption is markedly increased. In this context, the hypothesis that intermittent large increases in energy expenditure could be harmful and result in decreased longevity seems reasonable and requires evaluation. The studies of Benedict and Sherman (13) and Slonaker (290) on the effects of exercise on longevity of rats have been cited as evidence in support of the rate-of-living theory. However, as discussed earlier, subsequent studies have shown that this interpretation is incorrect and that exercise increases the average longevity of rats. Exercising male rats are not a good model for evaluating the effects of increased O_2 utilization on longevity. Male rats do have intermittent increases in energy utilization as a result of exercise, and, because of their smaller size, they have a higher average energy expenditure per gram body weight than sedentary rats eating the same amount of food. However, total daily energy intake and, after attainment of steady-state body weight, total daily caloric expenditure are usually similar in voluntary wheel-running and sedentary male rats.

Female rats are a better model because, like most mammals, they increase their food intake to compensate for the increased energy expenditure caused by exercise. The finding, reviewed above, that female voluntary wheel-runners lived longer on average than sedentary controls despite a 20%–30% higher energy intake provides evidence that the increase in the rate of living caused by exercise does not have an adverse effect on longevity. However, the possibility must be considered that the increase in the rate of energy utilization caused by exercise is harmful but that this harmful effect is counterbalanced by the beneficial effects of exercise. Another approach that has, therefore, been used to evaluate the effect of an increased rate of living on longevity is to raise the metabolic rate of rats by means of cold exposure. The effects of cold exposure are of interest in the present context because, unlike exercise, cold exposure is not known to have beneficial effects that might counter an acceleration of aging by increased energy expenditure.

A number of studies in which rats were continuously kept at 6°C (138) or 9°C (162, 169, 170) have been cited as evidence in support of the rate-of-living theory. The cold-exposed rats in these studies had a chronic increase in metabolic rate and a marked shortening of life span. Two problems complicate interpretation of these studies. One is that the rats in these studies were not specific-pathogen-free, which raises the possibility that the chronic cold stress may have aggravated the effects of chronic infections (162). The other is that most stresses, including the stimuli that raise the metabolic rate, such as cold exposure, are normally intermittent and separated by recovery periods during which reversal of the acute effects of the stress can occur. Continuous cold exposure of rats represents an unremitting stress, and chronic stress can have harmful effects on health and longevity regardless of whether or not it results in increased energy expenditure (84, 240, 286).

The effects on longevity of increasing the metabolic rate by means of cold exposure were therefore reinvestigated in a study designed to avoid these problems (149). To avoid the complicating effects of chronic infections, specific-pathogen-free rats were studied. To minimize the nonspecific effects of chronic stress, intermittent instead of continuous cold exposure was used. Six-month-old male Long-Evans rats were assigned to control and cold-exposure groups. Cold exposure consisted of immersion of rats to the upper border of the scapulae in water kept at 23°C. Cold exposure was gradually increased from 10 min/day to 4 h/day, 5 days/wk over a 3-month period, and was maintained at this level until age 32 months, at which time it was discontinued. The cold-exposed animals ate significantly more food than the freely eating controls; the increase in food intake averaged 44%. Despite this increase, the cold-exposed rats' body weights were significantly lower than those of controls between the ages of 11 and 32 months. After age 32 months the two groups' weights became similar as a result of weight gain by the cold-exposure group after cold exposure was discontinued and of aging-associated weight loss by the control group. The average age at death was 968 days for the cold-exposed group and 923 days for the controls. These values are not significantly different, and there were no major differences in the shapes of the mortality curves of the two groups.

The results of the studies on voluntary wheel-running female rats and intermittently cold-exposed male rats show that the large increases in the rate of living induced by these stimuli do not have a deleterious effect on longevity in rats that do not have chronic infections. These findings do not negate the concept that tissue damage caused by free radicals of oxygen plays a role in aging. They do, however, provide evidence that the free-radical hypothesis of aging is not relevant to the effects of exercise on longevity. It is actually well documented that exercise, particularly strenuous activity to which the muscles are unaccustomed, can cause severe muscle damage (5, 87), and it appears that this damage is mediated, at least in part, by free radicals (62, 159). Regularly performed exercise, (training) results in adaptations that protect against exercise-induced muscle damage, although some muscle damage may occur even in highly trained athletes if the exercise is sufficiently strenuous and prolonged. However, skeletal muscle has considerable capacity for repair and regeneration (320), and there is no good evidence that individuals who exercise regularly develop persistent impairment of muscle function as a result of exercise-induced damage (48, 121, 135). More importantly, skeletal muscle and brown adipocytes, the tissues in which O_2 utilization is increased by exercise and cold, are not vital organs, so even if exercise or cold were to result in some persistent free-radical-induced damage, this should not affect longevity.

DECLINE IN MAXIMAL OXYGEN UPTAKE CAPACITY WITH AGING

Maximal oxygen uptake capacity ($\dot{V}O_{2max}$) is the highest rate of oxygen consumption that one can attain while performing an exercise test of progressively increasing intensity that requires a large proportion of the total skeletal muscle mass. Uphill treadmill running is the form of exercise most generally used for determining $\dot{V}O_{2max}$ There is a progressive decline in $\dot{V}O_{2max}$ and in the capacity for aerobic exercise with aging. In humans, this decline generally begins between ages 25 and 30 yr. $\dot{V}O_{2max}$ is determined by the capacity of the cardiovascular system to deliver oxygen to the working muscles and the capacity of the muscles to extract oxygen from the blood and to utilize it to generate ATP via oxidative metabolism. $\dot{V}O_{2max}$ is therefore a function of both maximal cardiac output and maximal arteriovenous oxygen difference (7).

Evaluation of the effect of aging on $\dot{V}O_{2max}$ is complicated by a number of factors. $\dot{V}O_{2max}$ decreases with physical inactivity and increases in response to aerobic exercise training (52, 276). As a result, an individual's $\dot{V}O_{2max}$ can vary as much as twofold depending on physical activity level. Another major factor that affects $\dot{V}O_{2max}$ is the development of disease, particularly atherosclerotic heart disease. An additional complication in studies in which $\dot{V}O_{2max}$ is expressed as ml O_2/min/kg body weight is the gain in body weight (that is, fat) that occurs in a high proportion of sedentary people in our society. In such studies, a significant portion of the large decline in $\dot{V}O_{2max}$ in sedentary individuals is due to weight gain. One alternative is to express $\dot{V}O_{2max}$ in absolute terms, as liters/min, which is particularly appropriate in longitudinal studies. The other alternative is to express $\dot{V}O_{2max}$ in terms of lean body mass, (ml $O_2 \cdot$ kg lean body mass$^{-1} \cdot$ min^{-1}, when body composition data are available. Although it corrects for changes in body fat content, this method has the disadvantage of masking a portion of the decrease in total $\dot{V}O_{2max}$ because there is a loss of lean tissue with advancing age.

The studies of the decline in $\dot{V}O_{2max}$ with advancing age performed prior to 1985 have been reviewed by Buskirk and Hodgson (36) and Hagberg (127). Although most of the available data come from cross-sectional studies, there is also some information from longitudinal studies in which subjects were usually retested after a relatively short time period. Taken together, the findings provide evidence that $\dot{V}O_{2max}$ declines approximately 10% per decade in healthy sedentary men and women when those studies in which the findings were clearly affected by large changes in factors not attributable to aging are eliminated (Fig. 24.2). The latter include follow-up studies of trained individuals who stopped training.

Decline in $\dot{V}O_{2max}$ in People Who Exercise Regularly

Studies comparing well-trained endurance athletes with untrained individuals have shown that at all ages $\dot{V}O_{2max}$ expressed as ml $O_2 \cdot$ kg$^{-1} \cdot$ min^{-1} is about 60%–70% higher in the trained subjects (120, 135, 251, 252, 270). This difference falls to about 40%–50% when the results are expressed as liters/min or per kg fat-free mass. While some of this difference is genetically determined, the major factor is regularly performed, vigorous exercise. This is dramatically illustrated by the finding that when champion athletes with very high $\dot{V}O_{2max}$ values were retested after not training for 20 or more yr, their $\dot{V}O_{2max}$ was similar to that of lean, untrained men of the same age (72, 135, 265).

Because of the major role that habitual level of exercise plays in determining $\dot{V}O_{2max}$, it seems likely that some of the decline in $\dot{V}O_{2max}$ with advancing age is due to a decline in physical activity, that is, aging plus detraining. It also seems possible that chronic physical inactivity could accelerate the rate of decline in $\dot{V}O_{2max}$ with aging as a result of "disuse atrophy," such as is seen in an accelerated form with bed rest or space flight. These possibilities are of more than theoretical interest, as a low $\dot{V}O_{2max}$ can limit even ordinary activities of daily living in an otherwise healthy old individual.

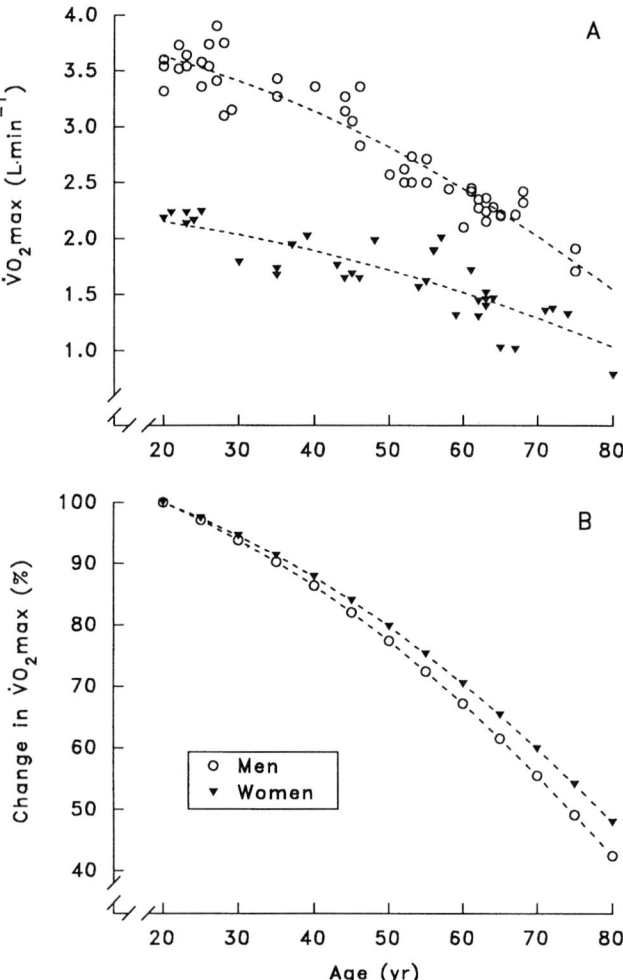

FIG. 24.2. Absolute *(A)* and relative *(B)* declines in $\dot{V}O_{2max}$ expressed as liters/min in healthy, sedentary men (○) and women (▼). Each symbol in *A* is an average $\dot{V}O_{2max}$ for groups of men or women of different ages from studies in the literature (14, 42, 45, 54, 56, 59, 66, 88, 98, 128, 135, 153, 155, 157, 173, 176, 186, 212, 223, 226, 228, 231, 234, 242, 247, 248, 250, 253, 254, 264, 265, 270, 272, 281–283, 303, 313, 322). Curves were fitted to the data points using general quadratic equations (Sigma Plot 4.1; Jandel Scientific, Corte Madera, CA). *B* is the percent decline in $\dot{V}O_{2max}$ with aging relative to the average values for young healthy, sedentary men and women. Data points were calculated using the quadratic equations generated to fit the data in *A*.

To evaluate the contribution of physical inactivity to the decline in $\dot{V}O_{2max}$, young and old active endurance (master) athletes have been compared to physically inactive subjects in a number of studies. In two cross-sectional studies in which the training stimulus was not controlled for (120, 252), the $\dot{V}O_{2max}$ values for the master athletes fall on a line well above, but parallel to, that for the decline in $\dot{V}O_{2max}$ for untrained men (cf. ref. 135). This finding could mean either that $\dot{V}O_{2max}$ declines at the same relative rate in trained and sedentary individuals or that the athletes decreased their training with advancing age. To control for the latter possibility, a study was performed in which sixteen highly trained master endurance athletes aged 59 ± 6 yr (range 50–72 yr) were compared with sixteen young athletes with whom they were closely matched in terms of training program and, when possible, best performance time in the same event (1- or 2-mile races) at approximately the same age (135). The results of this comparison suggest that the rate of decline in $\dot{V}O_{2max}$ in these master athletes averaged ~5% per decade. However, cross-sectional studies can only provide suggestive evidence on which to base a hypothesis that must then be tested in longitudinal studies.

Longitudinal studies are difficult to perform, and in the case of $\dot{V}O_{2max}$ the difficulty is increased by the need to study healthy individuals who maintain the same relative level of exercise training over many years. This is essential, because a decrease in the training stimulus will exaggerate (265), while a gradual increase in the relative intensity of the training stimulus will mask (166), the decline in $\dot{V}O_{2max}$. One approach to minimizing this problem has been to study competitive master athletes, who presumably train as hard as they can in order to do well in competition. Pollock et al. (251) studied 24 master athletes over 10 yr and found that $\dot{V}O_{2max}$ declined by an average of 9% in the total group. The data were also analyzed by comparing the athletes who continued to compete and train intensely with the athletes who had stopped competing and reduced their training intensity. $\dot{V}O_{2max}$ was unchanged in the athletes who continued to train intensely and decreased 14% in those who had reduced their training. In a second study, Rogers et al. (270) re-evaluated 15 well-trained master middle- and long-distance runners and cyclists and 14 sedentary controls after an average follow-up period of ~8 yr, when their average age was 62 yr. The athletes' initial and follow-up tests were done during their competitive season, when they judged themselves to be in top condition. There was no significant change in body weight or composition in either group. The master athletes' $\dot{V}O_{2max}$ decreased an average of 2.2 ml·kg^{-1}·min^{-1}, (from 54 ± 1.7 to 51.8 ± 1.8 ml·kg^{-1}·min^{-1} equivalent to a 5.5% decline per decade, while the sedentary subjects' $\dot{V}O_{2max}$ declined by an average of 3.3 ml·kg^{-1}·min^{-1} (from 33.9 ± to 30.6 ± 1.6 ml·kg^{-1}·min^{-1}) equivalent to 12% per decade.

These findings provide very preliminary evidence suggesting that the age-related decrease in $\dot{V}O_{2max}$ may be accelerated approximately twofold by physical inactivity. There are a number of reasons for caution in interpreting the results of the studies suggesting that the decline in $\dot{V}O_{2max}$ is speeded by lack of exercise. One is that the follow-up periods are too short to eliminate the

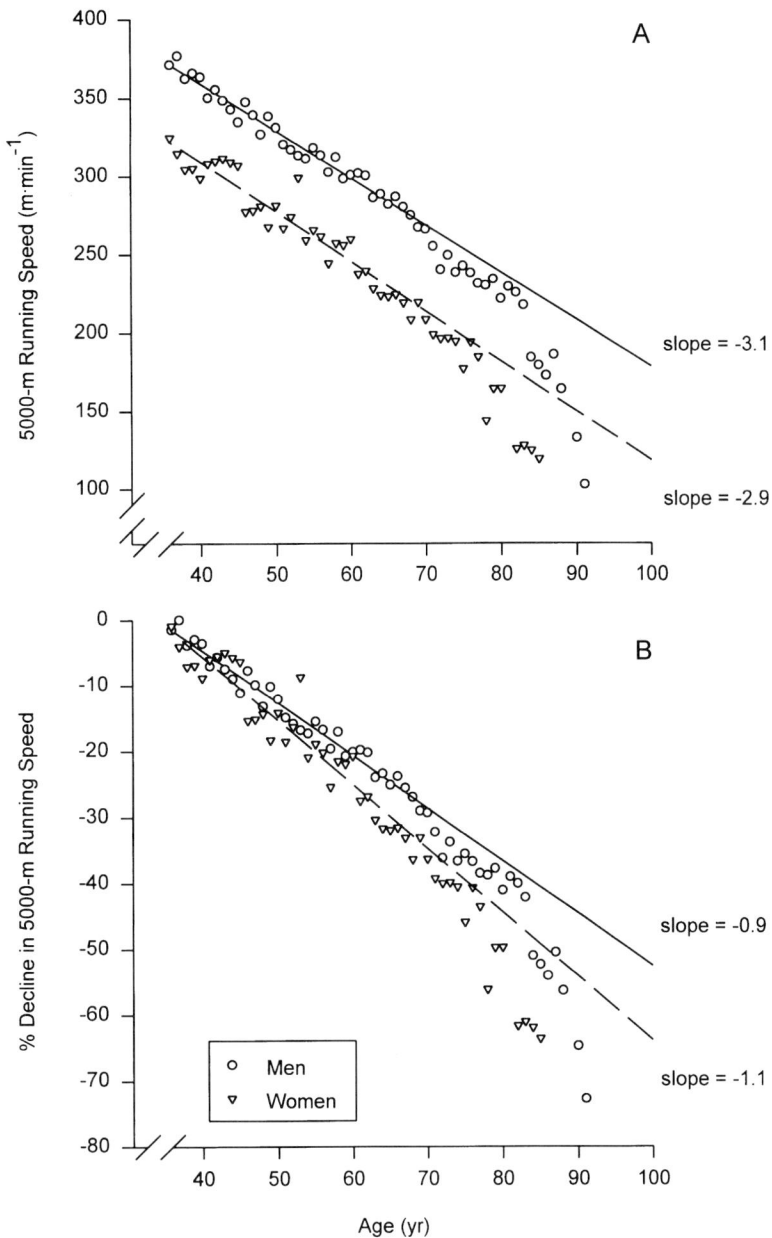

FIG. 24.3. Running speed of age group competition record holders in the 5,000 m race (3A; ○ men, ▽ women) and percent decline in world record 5,000-m running speed with aging (B) (From Masters Age Records 1991; Venice, CA).

possibility that the athletes increased their training sufficiently to temporarily compensate for the deterioration due to aging; that is, that the investigators' attempt to avoid this complication was not successful. A second reason for caution is that the results of a large-scale natural experiment, the well-documented world records for running events, ranging from 1 mile to 10,000 meters, show a steady 1% per yr deterioration in performance between the ages of 35 and ~65 yr and a more rapid decline thereafter in both men and women (Fig. 24.3).

Of course, factors other than a decline in $\dot{V}O_{2max}$, such as deterioration of muscle function, connective tissue changes, arthritic deterioration, etc. may also contribute to the decline in running speed. Furthermore, there may not be a direct one-to-one relationship between $\dot{V}O_{2max}$ and running speed in these events such that a 1% change in one results in, or reflects, a 1% change in the other. In view of these uncertainties, longer-term follow-up periods on larger numbers of athletes and sedentary subjects are needed to answer this question.

Effect of Exercise Training on $\dot{V}O_{2max}$ in Previously Sedentary Elderly Men and Women

Men and women in their 60s and 70s can adapt to endurance exercise training with an increase in $\dot{V}O_{2max}$ (23, 56, 129, 185, 284). If the training stimulus is sufficiently intense, frequent, and prolonged, the magnitude of the increase in $\dot{V}O_{2max}$ in previously sedentary older people is similar in relative magnitude (~20%–30%) to that in young people. As in young men and women, the increase in $\dot{V}O_{2max}$ in elderly men is mediated by increases in both maximal cardiac output, that is, oxygen delivery, and arteriovenous O_2 difference, that is, oxygen extraction (81, 210, 295). From a study on 16 women in their 60s, it appears that, in contrast to young women and to men, older women do not undergo adaptive increases in stroke volume and maximal cardiac output in response to a training program that elicits these adaptations in men of the same age (295, 296). In these older women who did not show the usual cardiac adaptations to exercise, the increase in $\dot{V}O_{2max}$ was entirely due to increased oxygen extraction by the working muscles, reflected in a greater arteriovenous O_2 difference. Further research is needed to confirm this finding and, if it is reproducible, to determine why the usual cardiac adaptation to endurance exercise training does not occur in elderly women.

Effects of Aging and Physical Inactivity on Cardiovascular Function: Role in the Decline in Aerobic Exercise Capacity

$\dot{V}O_{2max}$ is a function of maximal cardiac output and arteriovenous O_2 difference. It is of interest, therefore, to consider the role that cardiovascular system aging plays in the decline in aerobic exercise capacity. The differences in the cardiovascular response to exercise in young and older men have been reviewed in detail by Gerstenblith et al. (109). Maximal cardiac output is the product of maximal heart rate and the stroke volume attained during exercise at $\dot{V}O_{2max}$. A decline in maximal heart rate is a well-documented aging-related phenomenon (190).

Studies of Cardiovascular Function in Untrained People.

As is the case with $\dot{V}O_{2max}$, it is difficult to distinguish between the effects of aging and the effects of physical inactivity on stroke volume and cardiac output in sedentary people, because stroke volume and cardiac output also normally increase in response to aerobic exercise training and decrease with physical inactivity (82, 276). There is surprisingly little information on stroke volume and cardiac output in comparable healthy young and older people performing maximal exercise.

In two early studies on untrained men in which the cardiac catheterization–dye dilution technique was used, the older subjects had a lower maximal cardiac output as a result of both a lower stroke volume and a lower maximal heart rate (119, 163). More recently, Makrides et al. (210) compared young men with a reasonably well-matched group of 60–70-yr-old (average age 65 yr) men when they were sedentary and again after 12 wk of cycle ergometer exercise training. Before training, maximal stroke volume, measured with the CO_2 rebreathing method, was 16% lower in the older men, while after training it was 7% lower. Ogawa et al. (231) compared sedentary older men and women with sedentary young men and women. The average age of the older subjects was 64 yr. Cardiac output was measured with the acetylene rebreathing method during exercise that elicited $\dot{V}O_{2max}$. Stroke volume was ~12% lower in the older men and 8% lower in the older women than in their younger counterparts. The difference in maximal cardiac output between the young and older groups was considerably greater than the difference in stroke volume, averaging ~22% in both men and women, because of the lower maximal heart rates in the older people.

The results of a study by Rodeheffer et al (267) appear to be in disagreement with the studies reviewed above. Sixty-one men and women ranging in age from 25 to 79 yr were evaluated using radionuclide ventriculography during upright cycle ergometer exercise. No age-related decline in cardiac output, measured during exhausting exercise, was evident, because a higher stroke volume in the older subjects compensated for the decrease in maximal heart rate. Rodeheffer et al. (267) concluded that aging does not limit maximal cardiac output and hypothesized that the difference between their findings and those of earlier studies was due to their careful screening out of people with heart disease. It is obviously essential to differentiate between the effects of aging and disease. However, examination of their cardiac output data suggests a different explanation for the lack of a decline in maximal cardiac output with aging. The population studied by Rodeheffer et al. (267) was quite heterogeneous, with a variation in maximal cardiac output over a more than twofold range in both the younger and older groups. A number of the young men and women had exceptionally low cardiac outputs, while some of the old men, including one in his 70s, had maximal cardiac outputs in the range normally found in elite young endurance athletes and much higher than those generally found in highly trained master athletes in their 60s. These findings illustrate the important point that, because of genetic endowment, level of physical training, etc., it is not unusual for some people in their 60s to be superior to others in their 20s in a variety of physiological measures, including $\dot{V}O_{2max}$

and strength. Therefore, if a cross-sectional comparison of people of different ages is to provide any information regarding aging, it is essential that the young and old subjects be carefully matched.

The results of the studies reviewed above, with the exception of that by Rodeheffer et al. (267), provide evidence that maximal cardiac output declines with aging and that the decrease in maximal heart rate plays a major role in explaining this decline. The sparse information available suggests the possibility that the Frank-Starling mechanism may be able to compensate for the deterioration in myocardial contractile function sufficiently long to prevent maximal stroke volume from declining until early old age in some people.

Studies of Trained People. In two cross-sectional studies comparing matched young athletes and master athletes, the oxygen pulse during exercise that elicited $\dot{V}O_{2max}$ (O_2 pulse max = $\dot{V}O_{2max}$ ÷ heart rate at $\dot{V}O_{2max}$) was the same in the young and older athletes (128, 135). Thus it appears that in these master athletes the decrease in $\dot{V}O_{2max}$ with age was due solely to the decrease in maximal heart rate. This interpretation is supported by the finding in one of these studies that maximal stroke volume, measured by the CO_2 rebreathing method, was similar in the young and the master athletes (128). However, in two other studies comparing master athletes and young athletes, stroke volume during exercise that elicited $\dot{V}O_{2max}$ was approximately 15% lower in the older athletes (231, 263). One possible explanation for the difference between the study by Hagberg et al. (128) and the findings of Ogawa et al. (231) and Rivera et al. (263) relates to a difference in the ages of master athletes. In the study of Hagberg et al. (128) the average age of the master athletes was 56 yr compared to 66 yr in the study of Rivera et al. (263) and 63 yr in the study of Ogawa et al. (231). It seems possible that in healthy people who regularly perform vigorous exercise, the decline in $\dot{V}O_{2max}$ is due primarily to the decrease in maximal heart rate until late middle age or early old age and that, at some point in the aging process, the deterioration in cardiac contractile function can no longer be completely compensated for by the Frank-Starling mechanism, resulting in a decrease in maximal stroke volume. Longitudinal studies on physically active individuals who maintain a constant relative training stimulus are needed to provide a definitive answer regarding the role of a decrease in stroke volume in the decline in maximal cardiac output with aging.

Effect of Exercise Training on Cardiovascular Function in Elderly People and Rats

As reviewed above, a major component of the decline in $\dot{V}O_{2max}$ with advancing age is mediated by a reduction in maximal cardiac output. Comparisons of young untrained individuals with sedentary elderly people, along with studies on young and old laboratory animals have provided information regarding the physiological changes in cardiovascular function that are responsible for the decline in maximal cardiac output. The changes seen in the elderly include *(1)* decreased responsiveness of myocardial contractility to β-adrenergic stimulation; *(2)* increased arterial stiffness, vascular impedance, and total peripheral resistance, resulting in increased systolic pressure; *(3)* moderate compensatory hypertrophy of the pressure overload type in response to the increase in afterload; *(4)* prolongation of contraction, which appears to be mediated by increased duration of myofilament activation by Ca^{2+} and is probably also a compensatory adaptation to the increase in systolic pressure; and *(5)* lower maximal heart rate (see Chapter 17 for details and references). One of the manifestations of these changes is an impairment of early left ventricular diastolic filling (34, 75, 193, 222). Another is a smaller decrease in end systolic volume and a smaller increase in ejection fraction in response to exercise, reflecting a reduction in maximal myocardial contractile function (81, 141, 267).

While the aging process is responsible for much of this deterioration in cardiovascular function, it appears that a significant component is due to exercise deficiency and that the magnitude of the impairment in left ventricular function is considerably exaggerated in chronically sedentary individuals. Comparisons of master athletes with young athletes and young and older sedentary subjects have shown that older athletes have a "younger" pattern of left ventricular filling, with enhanced early diastolic filling more like that of untrained young adults than that of sedentary older individuals (74, 97).

Systolic function also improves with training. In a study on ten previously sedentary men with an average age of 64 yr, who were screened and found to have no evidence of ischemic heart disease, left ventricular systolic function was evaluated by radionuclide ventriculography before and after a moderately intense 12-month-long endurance exercise program that induced a ~23% increase in $\dot{V}O_{2max}$ (81). Before training, the increase in left ventricular ejection fraction from rest to peak exercise averaged 4.3% in older men, compared to 10% in young healthy, untrained men. After training the increase in ejection fraction from rest to peak exercise in the 64-yr-old men was significantly greater, averaging 10.7%, a value similar to that of the young men. Despite a similar increase in systolic pressure in response to the exercise before and after training, end systolic volume decreased significantly from rest to peak exercise after, but not before, training, with a shift to the left in the end systolic volume–systolic blood pressure relationship. This finding provides evidence for an enhanced inotropic state. Training also induced a moderate degree of the physiological, volume overload type of hypertrophy that occurs in sedentary individuals when they adapt to endurance exercise.

As mentioned earlier, there is some evidence that elderly women do not undergo an adaptive increase in maximal cardiac output in response to training (295). In a study in which cardiac function was assessed by radionuclide ventriculography it was found that older women who adapted to 9–12-months of endurance exercise training with a 21% increase in $\dot{V}O_{2max}$ did not develop left ventricular hypertrophy and showed no adaptive increase in peak exercise ejection fraction or stroke volume (296). The difference in the cardiac adaptive response to endurance training of older women as compared to men of the same age and young men and women raises the possibility that the anabolic effect of the sex steroids may be necessary for the normal cardiovascular adaptation to exercise.

Much additional research is needed on the effects of aging, exercise deficiency, and training on cardiovascular function in elderly men and women. However, considerable information that is probably relevant to humans is already available from studies on rats (194). Starnes et al. (299) evaluated the effects of a 16-wk-long program of treadmill running on cardiac function of old rats. Isolated perfused working hearts of 25-month-old male exercise-trained rats were compared with hearts of 9- and 25-month-old sedentary rats. Under high workload conditions, cardiac output and peak systolic pressure were higher in the hearts of the 25-month-old trained rats and the 9-month-old sedentary rats than in those of the 25-month-old sedentary animals. At a systolic pressure of 150 mm Hg, coronary flow in the hearts of the trained 25-month-old rats was higher than in the 25-month-old sedentary group but not as high as in the 9-month-old sedentary group. Spurgeon et al. (297) have provided insights regarding the physiological basis for the improvement in myocardial function induced by exercise training. They compared the contractile properties of trabeculae carnae muscles from the left ventricle of 24-month-old exercise-trained male rats with those of 24- and 9-month old sedentary rats. The cardiac muscle of the sedentary old rats showed a significant prolongation of contraction and relaxation times and increased dynamic stiffness. In contrast, the old runners' trabeculae carnae muscles were similar to those of the young adult rats in terms of contraction duration and dynamic stiffness coefficient.

Subsequent studies on ventricular papillary muscles have confirmed these findings (206) and provided evidence suggesting that the shorter contraction and relaxation times in heart muscle of exercise-trained compared to sedentary old rats are mediated by increased calcium transport by the sarcoplasmic reticulum (305), resulting in a shorter intracellular calcium transient (125). The results of a study by Thomas et al. (308) suggest that less collagen cross-linking in the left ventricular myocardium may play a major role in explaining why stiffness is less and contraction and relaxation are more rapid in heart muscle of exercise-trained compared to sedentary old rats.

Taken together, the information reviewed above provides evidence that much of the decline in cardiovascular function with advancing age in sedentary individuals is due to the effects of exercise deficiency rather than to aging per se. It appears that the component of the decline in cardiac function that is due to exercise deficiency is largely reversible, even in old age.

Role of Skeletal Muscle in the Decline in Aerobic Exercise Capacity

$\dot{V}O_{2max}$ is determined by both cardiac output and arteriovenous O_2 difference. The magnitude of the arteriovenous O_2 difference attained during exercise that elicits $\dot{V}O_{2max}$ reflects the ability of the working skeletal muscles to extract O_2 from the blood and utilize it to generate ATP via oxidative phosphorylation. It is, therefore, of interest to consider the role that skeletal muscle aging plays in the decline in aerobic exercise capacity. Skeletal muscle undergoes major adaptations in response to changes in the habitual level of physical activity, and it is therefore necessary to control for this variable in studies on the effects of aging.

Role of Skeletal Muscle in the Decline in $\dot{V}O_{2max}$ in Sedentary People. Comparisons of untrained young and older people have shown that the arteriovenous O_2 difference attained during exercise at $\dot{V}O_{2max}$ is lower in the elderly, accounting for ~30% of the difference in $\dot{V}O_{2max}$ (163, 210, 231). This finding fits well with the results of histochemical and biochemical studies on quadriceps and gastrocnemius muscles, showing that mitochondrial enzyme levels and capillary density are ~20%–40% lower in skeletal muscles of sedentary men and women in their 60s than in young untrained people (47, 218, 241).

Aging results in a decline in muscle mass. Fleg and Lakatta (94) used urinary creatinine excretion as an indicator of muscle mass to normalize for this decline and expressed $\dot{V}O_{2max}$ as ml $O_2 \cdot$ mg creatinine$^{-1} \cdot$ min^{-1}. Because creatinine excretion decreases with age, expressing $\dot{V}O_{2max}$ per milligram creatinine, that is, dividing by a smaller number, resulted in a less steep decline in $\dot{V}O_{2max}$. This study raises a question regarding the role of skeletal muscle mass in the decline in $\dot{V}O_{2max}$ with aging. To attain true $\dot{V}O_{2max}$ requires recruitment of as large a mass of muscle as the cardiovascular system is capable of supplying with O_2. Most individuals are unable to attain $\dot{V}O_{2max}$ during cycle ergometer exercise or upper body exercise, because the muscle mass involved is too small to attain a sufficiently high work rate. Exceptions are athletes in sports that utilize and result in hypertrophy of the muscles involved in the exercise test. Cyclists and skaters, for example, can generally attain $\dot{V}O_{2max}$ during cycle ergometer exercise. Uphill treadmill walking or running is generally the preferred exercise testing procedure for determination of $\dot{V}O_{2max}$ as it involves a large muscle mass in a familiar activity.

It seems probable that in some sedentary old people advanced muscle disuse atrophy may limit exercise capacity. However, it is unlikely that decreasing muscle mass plays a significant role in the linear decrease in $\dot{V}O_{2max}$ that begins at ~30 yr of age, because the treadmill exercise protocols used for measurement of $\dot{V}O_{2max}$ routinely result in attainment of exercise intensities higher than that required to elicit $\dot{V}O_{2max}$. In situations in which there is a question of whether or not the muscle mass involved in the exercise is limiting an individual's $\dot{V}O_{2max}$, some mild to moderate upper body exercise, such as "ski-poleing," can be combined with uphill treadmill walking. Direct evidence against the possibility that muscle mass limits $\dot{V}O_{2max}$ in normal elderly people is provided by the finding that moderate endurance exercise training can result in a 20%–30% increase in $\dot{V}O_{2max}$ in men and women in their 60s and 70s in the absence of an increase in lean body mass (129, 185, 282). Also of interest is the finding that middle-aged weight lifters have a $\dot{V}O_{2max}$, in liters/min, similar to that of sedentary men whose lean body mass is ~10 kg smaller (156).

Adaptations of Skeletal Muscle to Endurance Exercise. The capacity of an individual's skeletal muscles for aerobic exercise can vary over a wide range depending on the habitual level of physical activity. Regularly performed endurance exercise, such as prolonged running, results in an increase in the capacity of muscle for aerobic metabolism that is mediated by an increase in mitochondria, with increases in the levels of mitochondrial respiratory and citrate cycle enzymes and the enzymes involved in the oxidation of fatty acids and ketones (144, 146). There is also conversion of type IIb muscle fibers to type IIa fibers in humans (146) and an increase in capillary density with an increase in the number of capillaries per muscle fiber (2, 68). These adaptations are thought to be responsible for the greater ability of the muscles to extract oxygen from the blood during maximal exercise and for the smaller production of lactate during submaximal exercise in the trained compared to the untrained state (146). Skeletal muscles of elderly humans (46, 48, 218, 293) and rats (17, 39, 325) retain the ability to adapt to endurance exercise with an increase in the capacity for aerobic metabolism.

Role of Skeletal Muscle in the Decline in $\dot{V}O_{2max}$ in People Who Exercise Regularly. The habitual level of physical activity typically declines with advancing age (55). Studies in which this variable was controlled for suggest that the lower arteriovenous O_2 difference during exercise that elicits $\dot{V}O_{2max}$ found in older, sedentary people compared to young, untrained subjects, is a result of physical inactivity rather than aging. This interpretation is based on the finding in two studies that there is little or no difference in the maximal arteriovenous O_2 differences attained by young and older endurance athletes (128, 231). In keeping with this finding, Coggan et al. (48) have shown that mitochondrial enzyme levels and capillary density in gastrocnemius muscles of competitive master runners in their 60s are as high as or higher than those of young athletes with whom the master athletes were matched in terms of training program. It is interesting that, although endurance exercise training does not usually cause significant skeletal muscle hypertrophy, these competitive master runners did not show the usual decrease in type II muscle fiber area, that is, atrophy, that occurs in sedentary people with advancing age (48).

DECLINE IN MUSCLE MASS AND STRENGTH WITH AGING

Studies on Humans

Isometric and dynamic skeletal muscle strength generally begin to decline after age 30 yr (101, 165, 196, 298, 311). The magnitude of the decrease in strength is usually in the range of 30%–40% between the ages of 30 and 80 yr. Most of this decline occurs after age 50 yr, the reduction in strength being generally small up to this age and accelerating thereafter. The major factor underlying the decrease in strength appears to be a decrease in muscle mass caused primarily by a loss of muscle fibers (202–204), which is thought to be due to the death of motor neurons, resulting in a decrease in the number of motor units (37). With the exception of two studies by Larsson and co-workers (196, 197), who reported a selective loss of type II fibers, no difference has been observed between young and older people in the proportions of type I and type II fibers in skeletal muscle (4, 47, 86, 203, 204, 232, 298). A second contributor to the decrease in muscle mass is a reduction in the size of the type II fibers (4, 47, 197, 203), and there is evidence that the fractional rate of muscle protein synthesis is reduced in the elderly (323). Thus it seems clear that the major factor in the decrease in strength with advancing age is the loss of muscle mass (25, 101, 204, 260, 310).

In both men and women, muscle mass estimated from measurements of creatinine excretion is ~33% less in 80-year-olds than in young people (310). This finding agrees well with that of Lexell et al. (204), who examined the vastus lateralis muscle in cadavers and found an average reduction in muscle area of 40% and in the total number of muscle fibers of 39% between the ages of 20 and 80 yr. These changes in muscle mass are similar in magnitude to the decrease in strength (30%–40%) over the same age range. However, a number of investigators have reported that, in addition to the reduction in muscle mass, there is a decrease in the maximal force developed per unit of muscle cross-sectional area (33, 61, 244, 311, 324). The decreases in strength expressed in terms of muscle cross-sectional area that have been reported in some of these studies are impossibly large. For example, Davies et al. (61) reported that strength of the triceps surae muscles, corrected for cross-sectional area, was ~40% lower in 70 yr olds than in subjects in their 20s.

In view of the fact that muscle mass is decreased by 30%–40% in 70–80-year-old people (204, 310), an additional decrease in strength of 20%–40% per unit of cross-sectional area should result in a total decrease in muscle strength of some 60%–80% by age 80 yr, while the actual decrease in strength is similar in magnitude to the decrease in muscle mass. This discrepancy is explained by the overestimation of muscle cross-sectional area by the anthropometric and other indirect measures used by investigators who have reported large decreases in strength per unit muscle cross-sectional area. Studies using computed tomography (CT) have shown that the muscle mass that is lost in the elderly is largely replaced by adipose and other nonmuscle tissue (25, 238, 259). In a study in which muscle cross-sectional area was accurately measured with CT, Overend et al. (238) found that 70-year-old men had significantly smaller muscles and were 22%–32% weaker in knee flexion and extension than men in their 20s. However, isometric strength expressed per muscle cross-sectional area was not significantly different in the young and old men for either the flexor or the extensor muscles. Interestingly, dynamic, "high-speed strength" measured during isokinetic–concentric contractions at 120°/s, was significantly lower in elderly than in young men (~10% for knee extension) even when expressed in terms of cross-sectional area. A possible explanation suggested by the authors relates to the preferential atrophy of the fast contracting type II muscle fibers in the elderly.

Studies on Rats

The literature on the effects of aging on rat skeletal muscle structure and function published prior to 1980 has been reviewed in detail by Fitts (91). Studies on rats have shown that, as in humans, skeletal muscle mass decreases with aging (10, 108, 124, 150, 326). In earlier studies much of the decline in muscle mass was attributed to loss of muscle fibers (124). However, in more recent studies there was no decrease in the total number of muscle fibers in soleus and extensor digitorum longus muscles of Wistar (31) or Fischer 344 rats (79) up to the age of 30 months. Also, in a study on Long-Evans rats, the 30% decrease in plantaris muscle weight between 10 and 30 months of age could be accounted for by a 30% lower cross-sectional area of the muscle fibers in the older animals (150). From these studies, it appears that if muscle fiber loss occurs in healthy, specific-pathogen-free rats with senescence, it must occur at a very late stage of the aging process. While the majority of skeletal muscles atrophy with age in rats, some do not. Atrophy occurs in the weight-bearing muscles and is most severe in those with a high proportion of type IIb fibers (150). The muscles that have been found to not atrophy have all been non-weight-bearing and include the lateral omohyoideus (216), the flexor digitorum longus (300), the epitrochlearis (325), and the adductor longus (150).

At least up to the age of 28 months, aging has no effect on isometric peak tetanic tension, expressed per cm^2 of cross-sectional area, developed by soleus, extensor digitorum longus, or the superficial portion of the vastus lateralis muscles in Long-Evans rats (93). This finding agrees well with the results of Overend et al. (238) on elderly men. In Fisher 344 rats, there were no significant changes in the contractile properties or composition of the soleus or lateral omohyoideus muscles up to age 27 months (215).

Effects of Strength Training on Muscle Mass and Strength in Old Age

A number of recent studies have demonstrated that weight-lifting programs can induce significant skeletal muscle hypertrophy and major increases in strength in men and women ranging in age from 60 to 96 yr (30, 89, 102, 103, 129). In the studies by Frontera et al. (102, 103), 60–72-yr-old men performed three sets of eight repetitions of the extensor and flexor muscles of the knees at 80% of the one-repetition maximum (1 RM) three times per week for 12 wk. This training program resulted in ~10% increases in total thigh and quadriceps muscle areas estimated from CT, while vastus lateralis muscle biopsies showed an increase in muscle fiber area of ~30%. The ability to lift weight, as reflected in 1 RM for the exercises used in the training program, increased ~100% for the knee extensors and ~200% for the knee flexors. Isokinetic peak torque of the knee extensors and flexors measured on a Cybex II dynamometer increased ~15%. Frontera et al. attributed the large difference in the magnitudes of the improvement in 1 RM and isokinetic peak torque to neural adaptations specific to the type of training. The results of this study and of a similar study by Brown et al. (30) provide evidence that men in their 60s adapt to weight training, with increases in muscle mass and strength that are similar in relative terms to those that occur in young men in response to a comparable training regimen.

In the study by Fiatarone et al. (89), ten frail institutionalized subjects, six women and four men, aged 86–96 yr performed an 8 wk program of high-intensity weight-lifting exercise involving the quadriceps muscles. The training consisted of three sets of eight repetitions performed three times per week. Mid-thigh muscle area increased ~10%, while muscle strength, as reflected in 1 RM, increased ~175%.

In a study on male Wistar rats, Klitgaard et al. (181) evaluated the effects of weight-lifting training begun at age 20 months, on muscle weight and strength. At both 24 and 29 months of age, weight lifters had significantly larger and stronger muscles than untrained rats.

It seems clear from the studies reviewed in this section that aging skeletal muscle retains the ability to adapt to heavy resistance exercise training with hypertrophy and an increase in strength. The finding by Fiatarone et al. (89) that this adaptive response occurs even in frail people over the age of 90 yr has major practical importance relative to the maintenance of function and independence in old age. Perhaps the most important unanswered questions relating to the decrease in strength with advancing age relate to the loss of skeletal muscle fibers. What are the factors responsible for the loss of muscle fibers with advancing age? Why have recent studies not confirmed the results of earlier studies which showed a decreased number of fibers in muscles of old rats? Can muscle fiber loss be slowed or prevented in humans by interventions such as regularly performed exercise or anabolic steroids?

CHANGES IN BODY COMPOSITION WITH AGING

The true effects of aging on body composition are difficult to discern because of the confounding influence of physical activity level, the paucity of longitudinal data, and other problems inherent in assessment of body composition in humans.

Age-Related Changes in Weight and Height

Studies in Untrained People. In the United States and other industrialized countries, body weight typically increases through the seventh decade (Fig. 24.4). The open symbols in Fig. 24.4 represent mean data from cross-sectional studies that reported body weights (Fig.

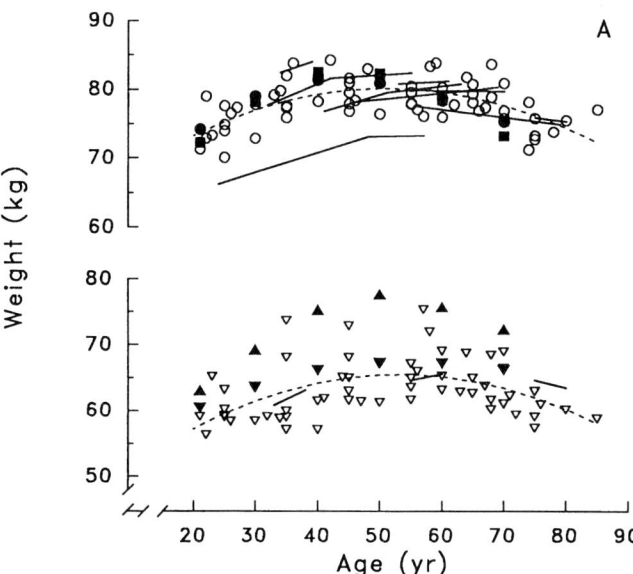

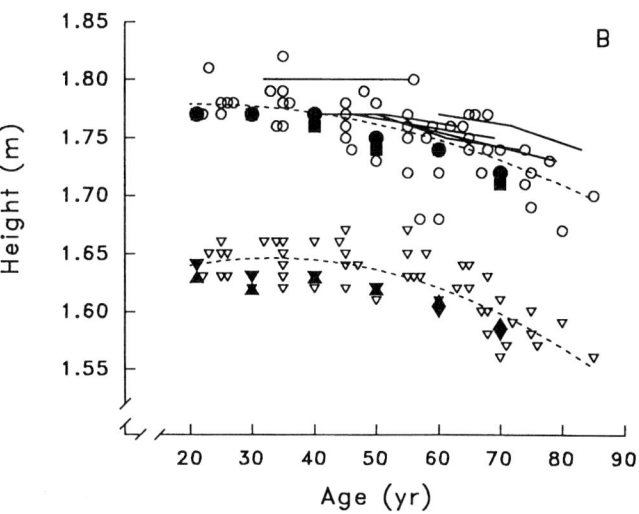

FIG. 24.4. Change in body weight *(A)* and height *(B)* with aging. The open symbols (○ men, ▽ women) are mean data from cross-sectional studies of relatively large numbers of healthy, predominantly Caucasian subjects grouped approximately by decade of life (9, 11, 21, 44, 71, 78, 95, 104, 142, 153, 179, 186, 229, 245, 248, 288, 291, 312, 321). Curves (----) were fitted to data points using general quadratic equations (Sigma Plot 4.1). *Closed symbols* (■ African-American men; ● Caucasian men; ▲ African-American women; ▼ Caucasian women) are mean data from the second National Health and Nutrition Examination Survey (224). *Open symbols:* ○ men, ▽ women; *solid lines* (——) represent changes in weight and height from longitudinal studies (38, 130, 209, 265, 288).

24.4a) and heights (Fig. 24b) for relatively large numbers of men and women grouped approximately by decade of life. The 5,353 subjects (2,851 men, 2,502 women), predominantly Caucasian, in these studies were generally reported to be healthy. The solid lines in the figure represent changes in body weight and height from longitudinal studies that followed subjects for 5–33 yr.

Although the cross-sectional data in Figure 24.4 suggest that body weight increases up to ~55 yr of age, after which it decreases, longitudinal data indicate that weight probably continues to increase or is maintained until ~70 yr of age. It is likely that true age-related changes in body weight are obscured when extrapolated from cross-sectional data, due to birth-cohort effects on body size, sampling bias, and/or survival. Whereas cross-sectional data suggest that men and women gain an average of 8–9 kg between the ages of 18 and 55 yr, longitudinal data imply that there is an additional gain of 1–2 kg over the next decade, after which body weight declines (38, 288). For example, in a 23-yr follow-up of participants in the Western Collaborative Group Study (38), body weight increased by an average of 2.2 kg in those subjects who were 42–50 yr old at the initial time of measurement and 65–73 yr old at follow-up but decreased an average of 1.6 kg in those who were 51–60 yr old at the initial test period and 74–83 yr old at follow-up. The estimated rate of loss of body weight in 65–80 year-olds is 1–2 kg per decade in both men and women based on these longitudinal and cross-sectional data. It is likely that the rate of decline accelerates with advancing age.

Height appears to be maintained up to 40–50 yr of age (Fig. 24.4b). Based on cross-sectional data, there appears to be a slow decline in height between the ages of 40 and 60 yr, averaging about 1 and 1.5 cm per decade in men and women, respectively, and a more rapid decline after age 60 yr, averaging 2 and 3.5 cm per decade in men and women, respectively. However, Borkan and colleagues (26) reported that as a consequence of birth-cohort effects, cross-sectional studies result in an overestimation of the true decline in height. They suggested that, of the 7.3 cm decline in height between the ages of 22 and 82 yr estimated from cross-sectional studies (Fig. 24.4b), 4.3 cm is due to a biological effect and 3.0 cm is due to a birth-cohort effect. Longitudinal data in men also suggest that the actual decline in height may progress more slowly, averaging ~0.8 cm per decade between 40 and 60 yr of age and ~1.2 cm per decade after age 60 yr (38, 130).

To evaluate racial differences in age-related changes in body weight and height, included in Figure 24.4 (solid symbols), are the normative data for 5,797 men (649 African-American, 5,148 Caucasian) and 6,468 women (782 African-American, 5,686 Caucasian) from the second National Health and Nutrition Examination Survey (NHANES II) conducted in the United States from 1976 through 1980 (224). It should be noted that the population for this survey included people who were not necessarily healthy and that age-related changes are therefore potentially confounded by the effects of disease and/or disability in addition to those confounds associated with cross-sectional comparisons mentioned above. The results of the NHANES II indicated that there were no differences between African-Americans and Caucasians in height in either men or women. However, the median weight of Caucasian men was ~2 kg greater than that of African-American men, and the median weight of African-American women was nearly 6 kg greater than that of Caucasian women.

Studies in People Who Exercise Regularly. It is likely that an increase in body weight between the ages of 20 and 70 yr occurs primarily in response to a sedentary lifestyle rather than to aging and/or increased food intake (28, 130). In support of this interpretation, the body weights of male and female master endurance athletes tend to be similar to or less than those of young trained people. Based on a number of cross-sectional comparisons of young and older athletes (48, 128, 135, 186, 219, 251, 252, 263, 283), the averages for weight and height of male athletes between the ages of 52 and 72 yr were 67.8 kg and 1.75 m compared to 68.1 kg and 1.77 m in 22–32-year-old trained men. The older male athletes weighed an average of 10–12 kg less than older sedentary men, despite being similar in height.

Although fewer data are available on women, cross-sectional comparisons of young and older female athletes also suggest that weight gain is prevented by regular exercise (176, 186, 226). In these studies, weight and height of the 57–62-year-old female athletes averaged 56.6 kg and 1.63 m compared to 57.5 kg and 1.67 m in young athletes. The trained older women weighed approximately 10–12 kg less than age-matched sedentary women of the same height.

Longitudinal data support the inference from cross-sectional studies that habitual exercise prevents an age-related increase in body weight (6, 251, 271). Followup studies of master athletes showed that body weight was either maintained (271) or decreased slightly (251) over 8–10 yr in men whose ages averaged 62 and 64 yr at follow-up. That the prevention of weight gain is dependent on continued physical activity rather than on a genetic predisposition toward maintenance of a low body weight is supported by the study of Robinson and colleagues (265), who found that the magnitude of weight gain in former athletes was similar to that of nonathletes. In that study, 13 men who had been American champion middle-distance runners gained an average of 7.1 kg over ~22 yr after they stopped training (Fig. 24.4a).

Age-Related Changes in Fat and Fat-Free Mass

The most common methods of estimating body composition in humans rely on the assessment of body density, total body water, or total body potassium. The estimation of fat-free mass (FFM) from each of these measures is based on assumptions that may not hold true across age groups. For example, the estimation of FFM from total body water or total body potassium assumes that these constituents remain a constant proportion of the FFM during aging. Similarly, the estimation of FFM from body density assumes that the fractional composition of the FFM (% water, % mineral, % protein, % carbohydrate) remains constant with aging. Recent technological advances have made it possible to do multicompartment modeling of body composition in humans (139).

Multicompartment Models of Body Composition. The six basic constituents of the body are fat, water, protein, osseous mineral, extraosseous mineral, and carbohydrate. In the classical two-compartment model of body composition, all nonfat constituents are grouped into a single compartment. Assuming, then, that the densities of the fat and the fat-free compartments are constant, this model provides an accurate assessment of body composition from total body density. It has been theorized, however, that the density of the fat-free compartment changes with age. For example, an age-related loss of bone mineral, which has a high density relative to other constituents of the fat-free compartment, could potentially reduce the density of the fat-free compartment and lead to an overestimation of body fat content, particularly in older women who lose larger amounts of bone mineral than men.

Recent technological improvements in neutron activation analysis and dual-energy x-ray radiography now make it possible to do six-compartment modeling of body composition in humans (139). While multicompartment models indicate that the density of the fat-free compartment does indeed vary markedly among individuals (11, 140), they also indicate that there does not appear to be a significant change in the density of the fat-free compartment with aging or differences between men and women. For example, in a study of 98 subjects 65–94 yr of age, relative body fat content estimated from body density using the equation of Brozek et al. (32) was 24.4% and 31.7% in men and women, respectively, compared to 23.3% and 31.5% by the more extensive modeling techniques. Snead et al. (291) estimated that the age-related loss of bone mineral might result in an error of ~1% when relative fat content is determined by hydrodensitometry. These studies indicate that hydrodensitometric measures provide a reasonable estimate of changes in body composition.

Studies in Untrained People. Figure 24.5 was compiled from studies that measured body density by hydrostatic weighing in relatively large numbers of men and women grouped approximately by decade of age. Because of small differences between the results obtained using the

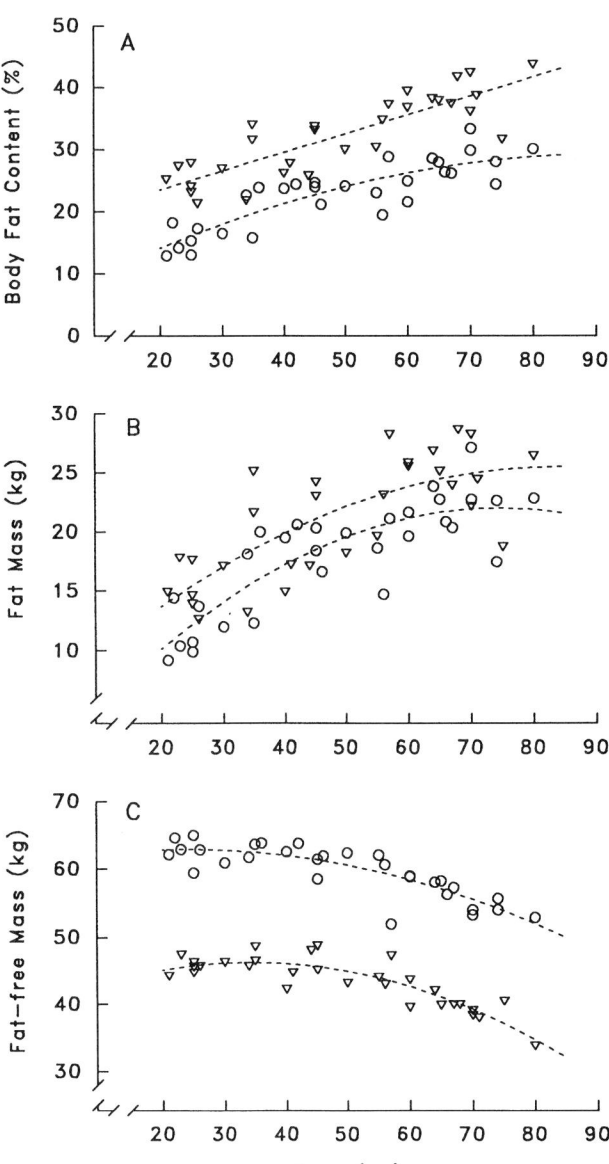

FIG. 24.5. Changes in percent body fat *(A)*, fat mass *(B)*, and FFM *(C)* with aging determined by hydrostatic weighing. *Symbols* (○ men, ▽ women) are mean values for data from cross-sectional studies of relatively large numbers of healthy, predominantly Caucasian subjects grouped approximately by decade of life (9, 11, 44, 71, 78, 142, 186, 291, 311, 321). *Curves* (----) were fitted to the data points using general quadratic equations (Sigma Plot 4.1).

equations of Siri (289) and Brozek et al. (32) to estimate body composition from body density, the mean values from these studies were standardized using the equation of Brozek et al. (32). The 2,303 subjects (958 men, 1,345 women) in these studies were generally reported to be healthy and the population was predominantly Caucasian.

These cross-sectional studies suggest that body fat content continues to increase with age (Fig. 24.5*A,B*).

In women, the change in percent body fat appears to be linear through the eighth decade, increasing from ~25% in 25-year-olds to ~41% in 75-year-olds. Cross-sectional data on men show a rate of change in percent body fat similar to that of women between the ages of 20 and 50 yr, after which the rate of increase slows. The average relative body fat content in 25-year-old men is ~16% compared to ~28% in 75-year-olds.

In absolute terms, the fat content of the body appears to increase with age similarly in men and in women (Fig. 24.5B). Between the ages of 20 and 50 yr, there is a fairly linear increase in fat mass, after which the rate of accumulation diminishes. The averages for fat mass in 25-year-old men and women are 12.2 kg and 15.5 kg, respectively, compared to 22.0 kg and 25.3 kg in 75-year-old men and women. A net increase of 10 kg of fat over 50 yr represents a caloric excess of only ~5 kcal/day.

Cross-sectional data further suggest that FFM remains relatively stable in both men and women through ~40 yr of age, after which it decreases, with the rate of decline accelerating with advancing age (Fig. 24.5C). The averages for FFM are 62.9 kg and 45.8 kg in 25-year-old men and women, respectively. Based on the curves generated to fit to these cross-sectional data, FFM appears to decrease between the ages of 40 and 60 yr by ~3.5 kg in both men (~3% per decade) and women (~4% per decade). Between the ages of 60 and 80 yr, the estimated decreases are 6.5 kg in men (~6% per decade) and 7.9 kg in women (10% per decade). These rates of decline are comparable to those calculated by Forbes (96), who reviewed cross-sectional data on the age-related decline in FFM estimated by total body potassium. However, the true rate of decline in FFM with aging is probably overestimated by cross-sectional data because of birth-cohort effects.

Regardless of whether or not the data in Figure 24.5C represent the "true" change in FFM with aging, it is interesting to note that the variance in FFM at any age is far less than the variance in fat mass. This observation suggests that most of the variability in body weight among people of a given age and height can be attributed to differences in fat mass.

Studies in People Who Exercise Regularly.
In some of the studies of master athletes, body fatness was estimated from skin-fold measurements (128, 135, 252, 271, 283), and it was concluded that body fat content was not different from that of young athletes. However, unless appropriate age-corrected algorithms are used to extrapolate total adiposity from skin-fold thicknesses, it is likely that measures of subcutaneous fat underestimate changes in total adiposity with age due to an accumulation of intraabdominal fat.

Studies in which body composition was assessed by hydrodensitometry have shown that percent body fat in middle-aged and older male and female athletes is higher than in young athletes, though markedly less than in age-matched sedentary controls (48, 176, 186, 219, 251). Pollock et al. (251) found that body fat content increased by ~2% over 10 yr even in those athletes who remained highly competitive, suggesting that exercise attenuates, but does not prevent, an age-related increase in adiposity. In general, percent body fat levels of older athletes are comparable to those of young, lean, untrained subjects. These studies further suggest that endurance exercise training does not prevent the age-related decline in FFM, as FFM of older endurance-trained athletes is significantly less than that of young endurance athletes. Furthermore, the difference in FFM between young and older athletes is at least as great as that between young and older sedentary people.

Age-Related Changes in Total Body Water

Watson et al. (316) and Schoeller (280) have reviewed studies of the age-related changes in total body water (TBW). Briefly, both cross-sectional and longitudinal data indicate a decline in TBW with aging, apparently commensurate with the decline in the nonaqueous constituents of FFM. In support of this, cross-sectional studies using independent measures of TBW and FFM generally find no significant age-related differences in the water content of FFM (11, 49, 140, 201). However, it remains uncertain whether the reduction in TBW with aging reflects changes in the intracellular and/or the extracellular water compartments. Whereas cross-sectional data imply that the decline in TBW reflects a change in the intracellular water compartment, the few longitudinal data available (302) indicate that the decline in TBW between the ages of 70 and 81 yr reflects a reduction in extracellular water.

Age-Related Changes in Bone Mineral Content

Studies in Untrained People.
A recent cross-sectional study showed that the bone mineral fraction of FFM was similar among young (21–39 yr; 4.7% ± 0.4%, mean ± SD), middle-aged (40–59 yr; 4.5% ± 0.5%), and older (≥60 yr; 4.6% ± 0.5%) men (291). The bone mineral fraction of FFM was also similar in young (5.2% ± 0.4%) and middle-aged (5.2% ± 0.4%) but significantly lower in older (4.5% ± 0.5%) women. These data suggest that the loss of osseous mineral in men with aging is proportional to the decline in FFM. Women, however, have a disproportionate loss of bone mineral after menopause. Estrogen replacement has been shown to be effective in attenuating this accelerated loss of osseous mineral in postmenopausal women (207).

Figure 24.6 depicts the relationship between total body bone mineral content and age in Caucasian men (n = 70) and women (n = 113) (W. M. Kohrt, D. B. Snead, and S. J. Birge, unpublished data). Based on the curves generated to fit these data, bone mineral content is 10% and 15% lower in 65-year-old men and women, respectively, than in 25-year-olds. Similar differences have been noted in other cross-sectional studies of men (118, 261) and women (106, 208).

Studies in People Who Exercise Regularly. There are a number of recent reviews of the effects of exercise on bone mineral status (58, 186, 292). While some cross-sectional studies provide evidence that bone mineral density is higher in athletes than in nonathletes (22, 50, 233, 262) and higher in people who are physically active than in those who are sedentary (8, 41, 304), other studies fail to find such differences (136, 176, 226, 233). Similarly, prospective studies have shown that exercise training both does (59, 191, 211, 228) and does not (110, 266) have beneficial effects on bone mass. The few longitudinal data available indicate that the rate of mineral loss in people over the age of 50 yr who exercise regularly is not different from that in age-matched sedentary people (195, 220) but that bone density is higher in the active subjects.

The importance of physical activity in preventing excess bone mineral loss is perhaps best exemplified in studies utilizing conditions where loading forces on the skeleton are minimized, such as bedrest (199), immobilization (213), or space flight (3). In general, these studies demonstrate not only a rapid loss of bone mineral when loading forces are reduced but also a very slow recovery of mineral when normal loading conditions are restored. For example, young healthy men had a 1.4% deficit in total body bone mineral density after 4 months of bedrest, or a rate of mineral loss approximately 20-fold greater than expected, with no net recovery of mineral after 6 months of reambulation (199).

Since the skeleton appears to be sensitive to reductions in loading forces, it seems likely that part of the age-related decline in bone mineral content may be a consequence of the reduction in physical activity that often accompanies aging. It should be noted, however, that in addition to the age-related decline, women experience a menopause-related loss of bone mineral that can be largely prevented with estrogen replacement therapy. At this time, there is no evidence that habitual exercise may compensate for the mineral loss associated with hormone deficiency.

Age-Related Changes in Fat Distribution Pattern

Studies in Untrained People. The increase in adiposity with aging in people who are not physically active occurs primarily in central, as opposed to peripheral, regions of the body. For example, Shimokata et al. (288) compared anthropometric measures of fat distribution in 771 men and 408 women grouped by age (17–39-year-olds, 40–54-year-olds, 55–69-year-olds, and 70–96-year-olds). They found that several ratios of central-to-peripheral adiposity (that is, waist-to-hip, arm-to-thigh, waist-to-thigh, and waist-to-arm circumference ratios and subscapular-to-triceps skin-fold ratio) increased with age in both men and women. However, whereas men appeared to have a progressive increase in measures of central adiposity with increasing age, the trend was apparent in women only after age ~54 yr, suggesting a menopause-related change in fat distribution.

Cross-sectional studies utilizing CT, magnetic resonance imaging (MRI), or dual-energy x-ray absorptiometry (DXA) to assess fat distribution confirm the findings from anthropometric studies that the increase in central or abdominal adiposity occurs at an earlier age in men than in women (24, 85, 205, 285). These studies further indicate that the increase in abdominal fat occurs primarily in visceral rather than subcutaneous regions. For example, Enzi et al. (85) found that in non-

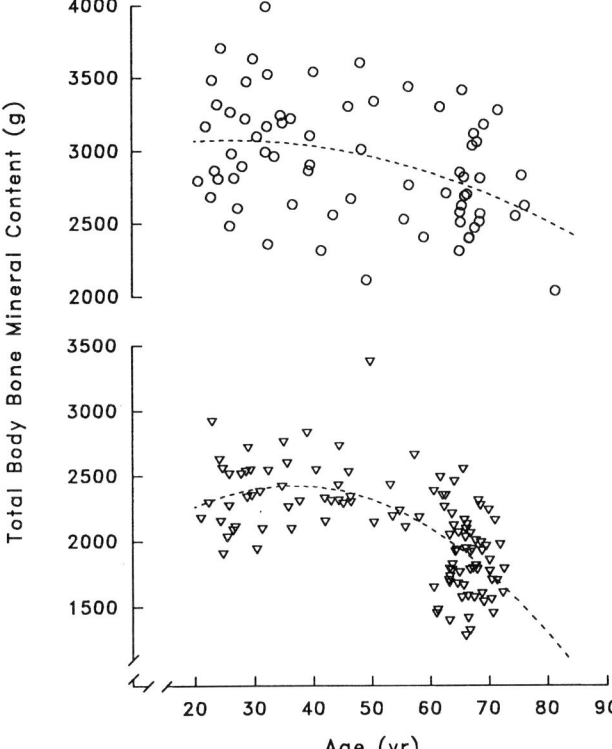

FIG. 24.6. Changes in total body bone mineral content with aging in healthy, normally active Caucasian men (○) and women (▽) (unpublished results).

obese men intraabdominal fat areas were 56.1 cm² in 20–39-year-olds, 74.0 cm² in 40–59-year-olds, and 93.7 cm² in older men. In similar age groups of nonobese women, intraabdominal fat areas were 37.2, 38.9, and 56.9 cm², respectively. There is preliminary evidence that the postmenopausal accumulation of abdominal fat may be attenuated by hormone replacement therapy (126, 133).

Studies in People Who Exercise Regularly. As mentioned above, habitual exercise appears to attenuate, but not prevent, an increase in fat accumulation with aging. There is preliminary evidence that exercise may prevent the disproportionate increase in central adiposity that typically occurs. Kohrt et al. (186) found that the mean differences in skin-fold thickness between young and older male athletes at triceps, thigh, and suprailiac sites (≤2 mm) were approximately the same as the differences between young and older untrained men (≤3 mm). At central body sites (umbilicus, subscapula, pectoralis), the differences in the athletes were of similar magnitude as those at peripheral sites (≤4 mm) but were much larger in nonathletes (7–14 mm). Similar differences were apparent in women. Furthermore, there appears to be a preferential loss of fat in central regions of the body when older, previously sedentary men and women participate in vigorous endurance exercise training (187, 281). However, it is not known whether habitual exercise specifically prevents or reverses an accumulation of intraabdominal fat.

EXERCISE, AGING, AND CARBOHYDRATE METABOLISM

Exercise and Carbohydrate Metabolism

The ability to perform prolonged, vigorous exercise depends on the availability of glucose. Endurance is, therefore, limited by the size of the glycogen stores in the skeletal muscles and liver and by the rates at which they are utilized. Depletion of muscle glycogen stores results in muscle fatigue and the inability to perform work that requires more than ~50% of $\dot{V}O_{2max}$ (154), while development of hypoglycemia results in central nervous system symptoms that prevent continued exercise (43). Repeated performance of vigorous exercise was necessary for survival throughout mammalian evolution, and acute and long-term adaptive responses to exercise evolved that make possible rapid repletion of glycogen stores when carbohydrate-containing meals are eaten in the rest intervals between exercise bouts.

Exercise has an acute, insulin-like effect on glucose transport across the plasma membrane (sarcolemma) of muscle cells (147, 315). Facilitated glucose transport into cells is mediated by a family of glucose transport proteins that differ in their tissue distribution (12). The major glucose transporter isoform in skeletal muscle is the GLUT4 protein (180), which undergoes translocation from intracellular sites into the sarcolemma in response to insulin and muscle contractions (73, 143, 180). This translocation process is the primary mechanism by which insulin and exercise increase glucose transport activity. An additional mechanism may involve an increase in the intrinsic activity of the glucose transporters (175).

The increase in glucose transport induced by exercise reverses rapidly after exercise is stopped (122). As this direct, insulin-independent effect of exercise wears off, it is replaced by a marked increase in the sensitivity of muscle glucose transport and glycogen synthesis to insulin (40, 107). If sufficient carbohydrate is eaten, the increase in insulin sensitivity results in a rapid increase in muscle glycogen concentration to a much higher level than that in the carbohydrate-fed, nonexercised state (16, 307). This phenomenon has been termed "glycogen supercompensation." The increase in muscle insulin sensitivity following exercise appears to persist until glycogen supercompensation has occurred (40).

In addition to these responses to a single exercise bout, repeated vigorous and prolonged exercise (training) induces an adaptive increase in GLUT4 protein in skeletal muscle (100, 246, 268, 269). As a consequence, the same insulin stimulus results in a larger increase in glucose transport activity in the trained state (268).

Individuals who exercise vigorously on a regular basis have a reduced plasma insulin response to glucose and other stimuli because of an adaptive decrease in insulin secretory capacity (20, 105, 164, 173, 189, 200). This adaptation, which is rapidly lost after training is stopped, serves to counterbalance the increase in insulin sensitivity and to protect against development of hypoglycemia. As a consequence of the interaction between these adaptations to exercise and to exercise training, exercise-trained individuals have unchanged or improved glucose tolerance despite their lower plasma insulin concentrations (20, 200, 283, 284). The enhanced insulin action in the trained state has been quantified in a number of studies utilizing the euglycemic clamp procedure (171, 172, 221, 278). In young athletes, the increase in insulin action is rapidly lost (within a few days) after cessation of exercise (35, 134, 171, 200).

Probably the most important effect of exercise relative to carbohydrate metabolism in older people is on body composition. In contrast to the majority of sedentary people who gain weight despite a decrease in lean body mass as they get older, individuals who regularly perform vigorous, prolonged exercise generally do not gain weight. Perhaps even more importantly they accumulate much less abdominal fat with advancing age than sedentary people (see the previous discussion of exercise and body composition).

Aging and Carbohydrate Metabolism in Rats

The most widely used animal model in studies of aging is the rat. It is frequently stated that aging is associated with the development of insulin resistance in rats. This is a misconception that has resulted from comparison of juvenile rats in the 4–10-wk age range to young adult animals aged 4–12 months (188, 225, 227, 255) and to older rats aged 20 months (188, 227). Studies in which a wide range of ages were compared have shown that insulin action decreases during growth and development, that is, between ~8 and ~26 wk, with no further decline attributable to aging (112, 113, 123, 158, 227).

For example, in studies on the perfused rat hindlimb preparation Goodman et al. (113) found that resistance of hindlimb muscles to insulin increased markedly between 3 and 24 wk of age, with no further significant change between 24 and 96 wk, while Ivy et al. (158) found that insulin-stimulated glucose uptake by hindlimb muscles was the same in 9-, 18-, and 24-month-old rats. Similarly, Gulve et al. (123) found in isolated muscles studied in vitro that insulin-stimulated glucose transport activity decreased between 1 and 4 months of age, with no further decline attributable to aging up to 25 months. There was also no decrease in the concentration of the GLUT4 glucose transporter protein in skeletal muscles between 10 and 25 months of age (123). Nishimura et al. (227) used the euglycemic clamp technique to evaluate insulin resistance and found that most of the decline in insulin action occurred between 2 and 4 months of age and that there was no decline in the rate of insulin-mediated glucose disposal due to aging from 10 to 20 months. Fat cells also become more insulin-resistant during growth and development; the primary factor that appears to influence the adipocytes' susceptibility to the action of insulin is fat cell size, with no major independent effect of aging (53, 198).

There is evidence suggesting that glucose tolerance deteriorates with advancing age in some rats (27, 111, 158). This deterioration appears to be due to decreased insulin secretion in response to a glucose stimulus (111, 158). The effect of aging on insulin secretion by the pancreatic β-cells is currently the subject of controversy. A number of investigators have provided evidence that the insulin secretory response of isolated islets to glucose and other stimuli is considerably reduced in 12-, 18-, and 24-month-old rats compared to 2-month-old rats (57, 76, 256, 277). These studies shed no light on the effect of aging, as the decrease in insulin secretion could have occurred during growth and development, that is, between 2 and 6 months of age. However, Elahi et al. (83) showed that isolated, perfused pancreas preparations from 23-month-old Wistar rats secreted less insulin than those of 12-month-old rats when perfused with 8mM glucose. While this finding is compatible with an aging effect, no such decrease in insulin secretory response was found by Starnes et al. (301), who also used the perfused pancreas preparation and studied 10-, 18-, 24-, and 30-month-old rats. This apparent discrepancy is still unexplained; however, one possibility relates to the use of Fischer 344 rats by Starnes et al. (301). Most strains of rat, including the Wistar, become grossly obese when kept sedentary and fed ad libitum; the Fischer 344 rat is an exception, and although its percent body fat does increase, it does not become grossly obese.

Exercise and Carbohydrate Metabolism in Aging Rats. In a study on male Long-Evans by Ivy et al. (158), freely eating, sedentary animals were compared to rats that were exercised by swimming 3 h/day, 5 days/wk, and to sedentary, food-restricted rats to keep their body weights in the same range as those of the swimmers. The rats' body weights plateaued by ~9 months of age, and the swimmers and paired-weight, sedentary rats weighed ~75% as much as the freely eating, sedentary animals. The rate of glucose uptake by hindlimb muscles perfused with medium containing a submaximal insulin concentration (50 μU/ml) and 8 mM glucose was the same within each treatment group at ages 9–10 months, 18 months, and 24 months. However, the swimmers had a significantly greater rate of glucose uptake by their perfused muscles than did the sedentary, freely eating animals. This beneficial effect of exercise appeared to be mediated by protection against the development of obesity rather than by short-term effects of the exercise, as the sedentary, food-restricted rats' rates of muscle glucose uptake were similar to those of the swimmers. In this study, the swimmers were not exercised for ~48 h before hindlimb perfusion to permit short-term effects of exercise on insulin sensitivity to wear off. There was essentially no difference in the plasma glucose response to an I.V. glucose tolerance test (IVGTT) between the young and old swimmers. In the freely eating, sedentary rats the average plasma glucose levels were ~20% higher in the 24-month-old than in the 9–10 month-old animals during IVGTT, but the differences did not attain statistical significance.

The effects of aging, regularly performed exercise, and food restriction on epididymal fat cell size and resistance to insulin were studied in Long-Evans rats by Craig et al. (53). The exercise group had free access to voluntary running wheels, and the rats were studied at ages 12 months and 28 months. The freely eating, sedentary rats were obese, and their large fat cells were highly insulin-resistant. The runners' adipocytes were small and were approximately ninefold more responsive to insulin, in terms of stimulation of 2-deoxyglucose uptake, than those of the freely eating, sedentary rats. The sedentary rats that were food-restricted to keep their body weights the same as those of the runners had fat cells that were intermediate in size and insulin responsiveness relative to the runners and the freely eating, sedentary animals. There was a close correlation between fat cell size and insulin sensitivity and responsiveness. Fat cell size and insulin sensitivity and responsiveness were not significantly different in the 12- and 28-month-old rats within each treatment group. Thus there appeared to be no effect of aging per se, and exercise was effective in protecting against fat cell hypertrophy and insulin resistance by preventing development of obesity.

Aging and Carbohydrate Metabolism in Humans

It is commonly stated that aging results in development of insulin resistance and glucose intolerance, independent of development of obesity, physical inactivity, or other factors (60, 63, 90, 274, 287). This belief appears to be widely accepted, and the evidence in support of it is well summarized by Jackson (160). However, while it is true that older people are, on average, more insulin-resistant and glucose-intolerant than young people in our largely sedentary and obese society, a sizeable proportion of older people are similar to young people in terms of glucose tolerance and insulin sensitivity. For example, Broughton et al. (29) and Pacini et al. (239) found that the insulin sensitivity of some lean older men was similar to that of young men.

The glucose and insulin response curves to an oral glucose tolerance test (OGTT) on such insulin-sensitive older individuals, with an average age of 65 yr, are compared to those of young lean individuals in Figure 24.7. In a study comparing such insulin-sensitive older subjects to more insulin-resistant individuals of the same age, the major difference that appeared to account for the insulin resistance was a greater accumulation of abdominal fat (184). Waist girth alone accounted for more than 40% of the variance in insulin action, whereas age explained only 10%–20% of the total variance and less than 2% of the variance when the effect of waist circumference was statistically controlled (184).

Because aging is universal, an effect due to the aging process should be present in all old people. The fact that many older people are insulin-sensitive and glucose-tolerant therefore argues against the concept that "age related glucose intolerance is the result of defects specific to the aging process" (160). An alternative possibility is that insulin resistance may, like male pattern baldness, be an age-related phenomenon that manifests itself in

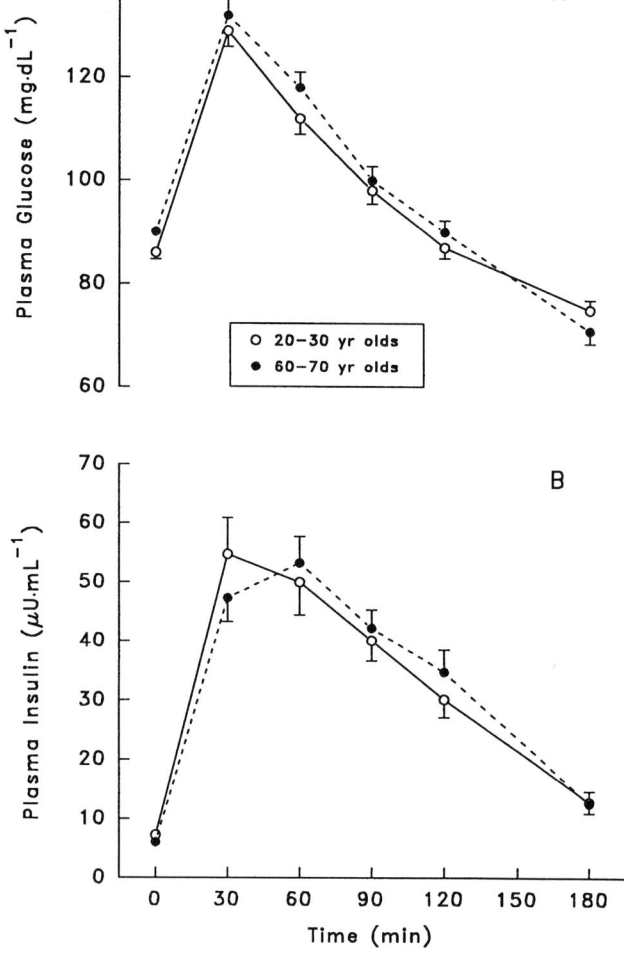

FIG. 24.7. Plasma glucose (A) and insulin (B) responses (mean ± SE) to a 75 g OGTT in 46 young (24 ± 1 yr) men and women and in 44 older (65 ± 1 yr) men and women who have no evidence of age-related deterioration in glucose tolerance (unpublished results).

genetically susceptible individuals who develop the physiological milieu necessary for its expression. While it is known that the genotype for male pattern baldness is not phenotypically expressed unless the level of dihydrotestosterone increases to a sufficiently high level, the factor(s) responsible for development of insulin resistance are still obscure. However, available evidence does suggest that accumulation of abdominal fat plays an important, and possibly primary, role.

Zavaroni et al. (327) have reported that an effect of aging on glucose tolerance was essentially eliminated after correcting for the effects of obesity and physical inactivity. However, other studies have provided evidence that total adiposity does not explain the age-related increase in insulin resistance (64, 90, 274, 287). It has, therefore, been argued that obesity is not responsible, because in most of the studies of age-related insulin resistance the subjects were not obese and the magnitude of their hyperinsulinemia was not commensurate with that found in obesity (160). The explanation for this apparent discrepancy appears to be that upper body, and particularly intraabdominal, fat accumulation rather than total body adiposity is responsible for development of insulin resistance (18, 19, 65, 69, 178, 294). Sedentary people of "normal" body weight in our society commonly increase their body fat content by 40%–80% with advancing age, often without becoming obese by the generally used criteria, and much of this fat is deposited in the abdominal area (25, 85, 294).

The abdominal obesity syndrome, which consists of "central" obesity with deposition of a large amount of intraabdominal fat, insulin resistance, hyperglycemia, hyperlipidemia, and sometimes hypertension (65), is the full-blown manifestation of the interaction between the genotype(s) for insulin resistance and a prolonged, positive energy balance. There is wide interindividual variability in the expression and severity of the various components of this syndrome. With regard to insulin resistance, those individuals who have developed full-blown diabetes are at one end of the severity spectrum. The other, least severe, end of the abdominal obesity spectrum has not been defined. However, it seems a reasonable possibility that it includes older people who are not grossly obese but who, as the result of an increase in abdominal fat, have mild insulin resistance and glucose intolerance (294).

Because of the high level of physical activity required to obtain food and avoid predators, animals living in the wild remain lean throughout life. Similarly, the abdominal obesity syndrome phenotype is not seen in hunter-gatherers or subsistence farmers, who are uniformly lean, even though the genotype underlying this syndrome occurs with high frequency in such populations (174, 182, 230, 319) and may confer a survival advantage (318). As reviewed below, endurance athletes are our society's equivalent of the hunter-gatherer in terms of energy expenditure and metabolic state. The abnormal conditions, in an evolutionary context, of a sedentary life combined with ready availability of food of high caloric density, permits the phenotypic expression of the abdominal obesity syndrome.

It seems likely that those individuals who do not become insulin-resistant or glucose-intolerant with advancing age despite a sedentary life are those who either do not have a genetic predisposition for insulin resistance or do not accumulate a sufficiently large amount of abdominal fat because of a low energy intake. From the modest amount of information available it does appear that those sedentary older people who remain insulin-sensitive have usually avoided accumulation of much abdominal fat (29, 51, 184).

Effects of Exercise on Insulin Resistance and Glucose Tolerance in Older People

Effects of Exercise in Non-Insulin-Dependent Diabetes.
It is not possible to generalize regarding the roles of exercise in the prevention and treatment of non-insulin-dependent diabetes mellitus (NIDDM) because of the genotypic and phenotypic diversity of patients classified as having NIDDM. In those patients with NIDDM in whom insulin deficiency is a major problem, insulin sensitivity generally improves in response to exercise, but this is countered by a further decrease in insulin secretion. As a consequence, exercise is usually not an effective therapeutic measure in patients with NIDDM who are insulin-deficient. In contrast, NIDDM that is due to the abdominal obesity–insulin resistance syndrome can be thought of as an exercise deficiency disease. The alternative view, that it is caused by a high energy intake, is generally not correct. With the exception of the severely obese who have eating disorders, the majority of middle-aged and elderly people with abdominal obesity have gained ~20 kg of fat gradually over 25–30+ yr as the result of underexercising, not overeating. A weight gain of 20 kg between the ages of 25 and 50 yr represents an excess energy intake of only ~20 kcal/day. Diet surveys have found no correlation between obesity and food intake. Caloric intake was either the same or lower in obese people as compared to lean people; there was, however, a strong inverse relationship between physical activity and body fatness (1, 28, 167, 192).

Physically active people are protected against development of abdominal obesity with NIDDM (137, 306), and exercise results in preferential loss of fat from the central regions of the body (70, 187, 281). People with jobs that require hard physical labor stay lean despite very high energy intakes (168). The role of occupational physical activity is illustrated by a study on the inhabitants of the Micronesian nation of Kiribati, who have over the past generation developed a high prevalence of diabetes (174). A comparison of rural and urban populations showed that prevalence of NIDDM was threefold greater in the urban population. The rural population had a moderate level of physical activity compared to the urban group, whose activity was light to moderate. The rural population had a higher total energy intake than the urban yet were leaner and, in contrast to the urban group, did not show an increase in body mass index with advancing age. Occupations requiring heavy physical exercise have become rare in the technologically advanced nations, and leisure time exercise has assumed primary importance in the prevention of obesity and NIDDM.

The results of studies of the effects of exercise in patients with NIDDM have been quite variable. While some early studies found no improvement, more recent studies have shown that exercise training can bring about an improvement in insulin resistance (151, 164, 257, 273, 279, 309). As reviewed earlier, exercise has two separate effects applicable to the treatment of NIDDM associated with the abdominal obesity–insulin resistance syndrome. One is the short-term decrease in insulin resistance, the other is the long-term effect on body fat content and distribution. Another short-term effect is the decreased insulin response of the pancreatic β-cells to glucose and other stimuli. Most of the studies of the effects of exercise in NIDDM referred to above were too short in duration and/or did not involve sufficiently prolonged and intense exercise to result in significant weight loss. The improvement in insulin resistance was therefore solely, or largely, due to the short-term improvement in insulin action. While insulin resistance generally improved in the more recent studies, the response of glucose tolerance to exercise training varied considerably, showing no improvement in some studies and large improvement in others.

The short duration of the effect of exercise on insulin action is illustrated by the study of Schneider et al. (279), who found that most of the improvement in oral glucose tolerance seen 18 h after the last exercise session was lost after 72 h. The short duration of this phenomenon is probably responsible for the lack of improvement in OGTT in response to a brief period of training in studies in which the investigators waited for 3–7 days after the last exercise bout before measuring glucose tolerance. Two additional reasons for the lack of improvement in glucose tolerance observed by some investigators are the patient population studied and insufficiently vigorous, prolonged, and frequent exercise. A number of studies have involved patients with moderate to severe insulin deficiency; as discussed earlier exercise increases insulin sensitivity but decreases insulin secretion and is, therefore, generally not effective as the sole treatment of NIDDM in patients who have a moderate to marked insulin deficiency. In a study that avoided these problems, Reitman et al. (257) found a marked improvement in glucose tolerance and insulin action in six obese Pima Indians with recent onset NIDDM who exercised vigorously 5 or 6 days per wk for an average of 8 wk.

Although regularly performed exercise is effective in preventing development of the abdominal obesity syndrome with NIDDM, it is less effective in reversing obesity. The reason for this is that obese middle-aged and elderly people are usually unwilling or unable to exercise for sufficiently long periods at a high enough intensity to result in a reasonably rapid weight loss. Therefore, once abdominal obesity with NIDDM has developed, the best practical approach is to initially combine caloric restriction with mild to moderate exercise to induce rapid weight loss and then increase food intake to a maintenance level while increasing the habitual level of exercise to maintain, or cause further, weight loss.

Effects of Exercise in Nondiabetic Older People Who Are Moderately Insulin-Resistant.

Glucose tolerance frequently deteriorates with advancing age due primarily to the development of insulin resistance (60, 63). This decline in glucose tolerance is generally associated with the development of hyperinsulinemia. There is also an increase in abdominal fat with advancing age, and abdominal fat accumulation results in the development of insulin resistance in genetically susceptible individuals (18, 19, 65, 69, 178, 294). The effects of exercise on insulin resistance, hyperinsulinemia, and abdominal fat are the reverse of those seen with advancing age in our society. The effects of exercise training on glucose tolerance, plasma insulin response, and insulin action have, therefore, been evaluated in a number of studies on nondiabetic older people. In three studies on the effects of 6–12 months of endurance exercise training in previously sedentary older individuals, the insulin response to I.V. and/or oral glucose administration was significantly reduced, while glucose tolerance was unchanged (164, 177, 283). These results provide evidence for a decrease in insulin resistance that is counterbalanced by the exercise-induced decrease in insulin secretion. As a consequence, the insulin response of these older people after training was similar to that of young people, but their age-associated deterioration in glucose tolerance was not reversed. Thus the exercise improved their insulin resistance but not to the "young" level.

The exercise in these three studies was not sufficiently vigorous, frequent, and/or prolonged to result in the loss of a large amount of fat, with the decrease in body fat content ranging from ~1–2 kg. In the study by Kirwan et al. (177), which is the only one in which circumference measurements were reported, there was no significant decrease in waist girth in response to exercise training. However, in some insulin-resistant elderly individuals who do sufficiently vigorous exercise for a long enough period of time to lose a considerable amount of abdominal fat, the decrease in insulin resistance is sufficiently great to result in an improvement in glucose tolerance despite the marked blunting of the insulin response (Fig. 24.8).

Endurance-trained master athletes who exercise vigorously on a regular basis are largely protected against the increase in abdominal fat with advancing age. While fatter, on average, than highly trained young athletes, they are as lean or leaner than young, untrained people of normal weight (48, 128, 136, 186, 249, 251, 270, 271, 282).

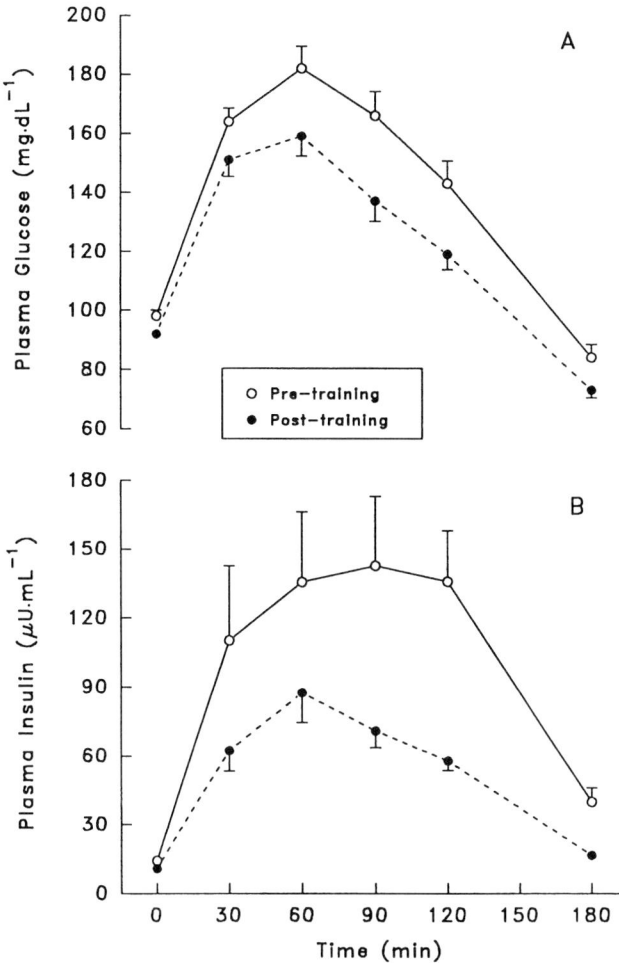

FIG. 24.8. Pre- and posttraining plasma glucose (A) and insulin (B) responses (mean ± SE) to a 75 g OGTT in 30 men and women aged 60–70 yr. Subjects' body weights decreased 5.1 ± 0.6 kg, body fat contents decreased 3.4% ± 4%, and waist circumferences decreased 5.2 ± 0.4 cm in response to 9 months of endurance exercise training (unpublished results).

In a study on 14 endurance-trained master athletes aged 60 ± 2 yr who were running ~90 km/wk, plasma glucose responses to an OGTT were similar to those of young athletes and young sedentary men, despite a low plasma insulin response (282). The area above fasting under the glucose curve during the OGTT was roughly 50% as great for the master athletes and young groups as for healthy untrained men in their 60s who had good glucose tolerance for their age group. The area above baseline under the insulin curve during the OGTT was 50% lower in both the old and the young athletes than in the young untrained men. The most remarkable findings of this study were that glucose tolerance and insulin action were as good in the 60-year-old master athletes as in the young athletes and that the master athletes cleared a 100 g glucose load as rapidly as young untrained subjects despite ~50% lower insulin levels.

To determine whether exercise training prevents the age-related changes responsible for the development of insulin resistance and deterioration in glucose tolerance or whether the changes occur despite regularly performed exercise and are countered by short-term effects of daily exercise, Rogers et al. (271) evaluated the effects of 10 days of physical inactivity on plasma glucose and insulin responses to an OGTT in master athletes who had been exercising regularly. The master athletes, aged 62 ± 2 yr, were running 60 ± 14 km/wk. There were two different patterns of response to the 10 days of physical inactivity. Ten of the master athletes responded to inactivity in the same way as young athletes, with a large increase in insulin response to an OGTT, reflected in a 67% greater area under the insulin curve, and no change in glucose tolerance. Thus in these individuals the regular performance of exercise prevented development of the changes responsible for increased insulin resistance and reduced glucose tolerance with advancing age. The other four master athletes showed a significant deterioration in glucose tolerance with 10 days of inactivity despite as great an increase in insulin response to the OGTT as that seen in the ten runners who showed no deterioration. It seems probable that the four master athletes who underwent a deterioration in glucose tolerance with 10 days of inactivity had a genetic predisposition for NIDDM and that their predisposition to develop insulin resistance was being countered both by their leanness and by the short-term effects of regularly performed exercise on insulin sensitivity.

CONCLUDING REMARKS

Mammals are genetically adapted for a physically active life. Chronic physical inactivity is physiologically abnormal and results in disuse atrophies and metabolic abnormalities that decrease physical performance capacity and increase susceptibility to injury. A sedentary life in combination with ready availability and unrestricted consumption of food leads to a progressive increase in adiposity which, in genetically susceptible individuals, results in metabolic abnormalities that greatly increase the risk of developing atherosclerosis, NIDDM, and hypertension. Exercise deficiency, therefore, is a major cause of secondary aging.

Since the physically active, that is, exercise-trained, condition is the normal state for mammals, it is unreasonable to expect exercise to favorably affect the aging process. The deterioration in structure and function that occurs in healthy, physically active individuals is, by definition, normal aging. Thus exercise training does not slow or partially reverse the decline in aerobic exercise capacity or the decrease in muscle mass and strength caused by the aging process. What regularly performed vigorous exercise can do is prevent or reverse the abnormalities that result from being sedentary. In addition, specific forms of exercise training can induce adaptations that compensate for some of the deterioration caused by aging. This is made possible by the fact that even physically active people who have avoided disuse atrophies and obesity are generally well below their attainable upper limits in terms of their physical performance capacities, that is, strength, VO_{2max}, agility, flexibility, etc. This makes it possible by specific and intense training to induce adaptive increases in various functional capacities, such as strength or VO_{2max}, that can for a time (theoretically until the full capacity to adapt has been utilized) compensate for the decline in these functions caused by aging.

Some of the effects of exercise deficiency, such as the disuse atrophies, are additive to those of primary aging, while others, such as the increase in central adiposity with the development of insulin resistance, can play a major role in secondary aging. It therefore seems essential in studies of primary aging to utilize as subjects normal, physically active people and laboratory animals to avoid confusing the effects of exercise deficiency with those of aging.

The authors are most grateful to Janet Seavitte for her help in the preparation of this chapter. The authors research is supported by NIH grants AG-05562, AG-00425, AG-00078, DK-18986, and AR-40705.

REFERENCES

1. ALBANES, D. Potential for confounding of physical risk assessment by body weight and fatness. *Am. J. Epidemiol.* 125: 745–746, 1987.
2. ANDERSEN, P., and J. HENRIKSSON. Capillary supply of the quadriceps femoris muscle of man: adaptive response to exercise. *J. Physiol. (Lond.).* 270: 677–690, 1977.
3. ANDERSON, S. A., and S. H. COHN. Bone demineralization during space flight. *Physiologist* 28: 212–217, 1985.
4. ANIANSSON, A., G. GRIMBY, M. HEDBERG, and M. KROTKIEWSKI. Muscle morphology, enzyme activity and muscle strength in elderly men and women. *Clin. Physiol.* 1: 73–86, 1981.
5. ARMSTRONG, R. B., G. L. WARREN, and J. A. WARREN. Mechanisms of exercise-induced muscle fibre injury. *Sports Med.* 12: 184–207, 1991.
6. ÅSTRAND, I., P.-O. ÅSTRAND, I. HALLBACK, and A. KILBOM. Reduction in maximal O_2 uptake with age. *J. Appl. Physiol.* 35: 649–654, 1973.
7. ÅSTRAND, P.-O., and K. RODAHL. *Textbook of Work Physiology: Physiological Bases of Exercise,* (3rd ed.) New York: McGraw-Hill, 1986, p. 330–341.
8. BALLARD, J. E., B. C. MCKEOWN, H. M. GRAHAM, and S. A. ZINKGRAF. The effect of high level physical activity (8.5 METs or greater) and estrogen replacement therapy upon bone mass in postmenopausal females, aged 50–68 years. *Int. J. Sports Med.* 11: 208–214, 1990.
9. BARLETT, H. L., S. M. PUHL, J. L. HODGSON, and E. R. BUSKIRK. Fat-free mass in relation to stature: ratios of fat-free mass to height in children, adults, and elderly subjects. *Am. J. Clin. Nutr.* 53: 1112–1116, 1991.
10. BASS, A., E. GUTMANN, and V. HANZLIKOVA. Biochemical and histochemical changes in energy supply-enzyme pattern of muscles of the rat during old age. *Gerontologia* 21: 31–45, 1975.
11. BAUMGARTNER, R. N., S. B. HEYMSFIELD, S. LICHTMAN, J. WANG, and R. N. PIERSON, JR. Body composition in elderly people: effect of criterion estimates on predictive equations. *Am. J. Clin. Nutr.* 53: 1345–1353, 1991.
12. BELL, G. I., T. KAYANO, J. B. BUSE, C. F. BURANT, J. TAKEDA, D. LIN, H. FUKUMOTO, and S. SEINO. Molecular biology of mammalian glucose transporters. *Diabetes Care* 13: 198–208, 1990.
13. BENEDICT, G., and H. C. SHERMAN. Basal metabolism of rats in relation to old age and exercise during old age. *J. Nutr.* 14: 179–198, 1937.
14. BENESTAD, A. M. Trainability of old men. *Acta Med. Scand.* 178: 321–327, 1965.
15. BERG, B. N., and H. S. SIMMS. Nutrition in the rat. II. Longevity and onset of disease with different levels of food intake. *J. Nutr.* 71: 255–263, 1960.
16. BERGSTRÖM J., and E. HULTMAN. Muscle glycogen synthesis after exercise: an enhancing factor localized to the muscle cells in man. *Nature* 210: 309–310, 1966.
17. BEYER, R. E., J. W. STARNES, D. W. EDINGTON, R. J. LIPTON, R. T. COMPTON, III, and M. A. KWASMAN. Exercise-induced reversal of age-related declines of oxidative reactions, mitochondrial yield, and flavins in skeletal muscle of the rat. *Mech. Ageing Dev.* 24: 309–323, 1984.
18. BJÖRNTORP, P. "Portal" adipose tissue as a generator of risk factors for cardiovascular disease and diabetes. *Arteriosclerosis* 10: 493–496, 1990.
19. BJÖRNTORP, P. Metabolic implications of body fat distribution. *Diabetes Care* 14: 1132–1143, 1991.
20. BJÖRNTORP, P., K. deJOUNGE, L. SJOSTROM, and L. SULLIVAN. The effect of physical training on insulin production in obesity. *Metabolism* 19: 631–637, 1970.
21. BLANCHARD, J., K. A. CONRAD, and G. G. HARRISON. Comparison of methods for estimating body composition in young and elderly women. *J. Gerontol.* 45: B119–B124, 1990.
22. BLOCK, J. E., A. L. FRIEDLANDER, G. A. BROOKS, P. STEIGER, H. A. STUBBS, and H. K. GENANT. Determinants of bone density among athletes engaged in weight-bearing and non-weight-bearing activity. *J. Appl. Physiol.* 67: 1100–1105, 1989.
23. BLUMENTHAL, J. A., C. F. EMERY, D. J. MADDEN, L. K. GEORGE, R. E. COLEMAN, M. W. RIDDLE, D. C. MCKEE, J. REASONER, and R. S. WILLIAMS. Cardiovascular and behavioral effects of aerobic exercise training in healthy older men and women. *J. Gerontol.* 44: M147–M157, 1989.
24. BORKAN, G. A., D. E. HULTS, S. G. GERZOF, and A. H. ROBBINS. Comparison of body composition in middle-aged and elderly males using computed tomography. *Am. J. Phys. Anthropol.* 66: 289–295, 1985.
25. BORKAN, G. A., D. E. HULTS, S. G. GERZOF, A. H. ROBBINS, and C. K. SILBERT. Age changes in body composition revealed by computed tomography. *J. Gerontol.* 38: 673–677, 1983.
26. BORKAN, G. A., D. E. HULTS, and R. J. GLYNN. Role of longitudinal change and secular trend in age differences in male body dimensions. *Hum. Biol.* 55: 629–641, 1983.
27. BRACHO-ROMERO, E., and G. M. REAVEN. Effect of age and weight on plasma glucose and insulin responses in the rat. *J. Am. Geriatr. Soc.* 25: 299–302, 1977.
28. BRAITMAN, L. E., E. V. ADLIN, and J. L. STANTON. Obesity and caloric intake: the national health and nutrition examination

survey of 1971–1975 (Hanes, I.). *J. Chronic Dis.* 38: 727–732, 1985.
29. BROUGHTON, D. L., O. W. F. JAMES, K. G. M. M. ALBERTI, and R. TAYLOR. Peripheral and hepatic insulin sensitivity in healthy elderly human subjects. *Eur. J. Clin. Invest.* 21: 13–21, 1991.
30. BROWN, A. B., N. MCCARTNEY, and D. G. SALE. Positive adaptations to weight-lifting training in the elderly. *J. Appl. Physiol.* 69: 1725–1733, 1990.
31. BROWN, M. Change in fibre size, not number, in ageing skeletal muscle. *Age Ageing* 16: 244–248, 1987.
32. BROZEK, J., F. GRANDE, J. T. ANDERSON, and A. KEYS. Densitometric analysis of body composition: revision of some quantitative assumptions. *Ann. N. Y. Acad. Sci.* 110: 113–140, 1963.
33. BRUCE, S. A., D. NEWTON, and R. C. WOLEDGE. Effects of age on voluntary force and cross-sectional area of human adductor pollicis muscle. *Q. J. Exp. Physiol.* 74: 359–362, 1989.
34. BRYG, R. J., G. A. WILLIAMS, and A. J. LABOVITZ. Effect of aging on left ventricular diastolic filling in normal subjects. *Am. J. Cardiol.* 59: 971–974, 1987.
35. BURSTEIN, R., C. POLYCHRONAKOS, C. J. TOEWS, J. D. MACDOUGALL, H. J. HUYDA, and B. I. POSNER. Acute reversal of the enhanced insulin action in trained athletes. Association with insulin receptor changes. *Diabetes* 34: 756–760, 1985.
36. BUSKIRK, E. R., and J. L. HODGSON. Age and aerobic power: the rate of change in men and women. *Federation Proc.* 46: 1824–1829, 1987.
37. CAMPBELL, M. J., A. J. MCCOMAS, and F. PETITO. Physiological changes in ageing muscles. *J. Neurol. Neurosurg. Psychiatry* 36: 174–182, 1973.
38. CARMELLI, D., M. R. MCELROY, and R. H. ROSENMAN. Longitudinal changes in fat distribution in the Western Collaborative Group Study: a 23-year follow-up. *Int. J. Obes.* 15: 67–74, 1991.
39. CARTEE, G. D., and R. P. FARRAR. Muscle respiratory capacity and VO_{2max} in identically trained young and old rats. *J. Appl. Physiol.* 63: 257–261, 1987.
40. CARTEE, G. D., D. A. YOUNG, M. D. SLEEPER, J. ZIERATH, H. WALLBERG-HENRIKSSON, and J. O. HOLLOSZY. Prolonged increase in insulin-stimulated glucose transport in muscle after exercise. *Am. J. Physiol.* 256 (*Endocrinol. Metab.* 19): E494–E499, 1989.
41. CHENG, S., H. SUOMINEN, T. RANTANEN, T. PARKATTI, and E. HEIKKINEN. Bone mineral density and physical activity in 50–60-year-old women. *Bone Min.* 12: 123–132, 1991.
42. CHOW, R., J. E. HARRISON, and C. NOTARIUS. Effect of two randomised exercise programmes on bone mass of healthy postmenopausal women. *Br. Med. J.* 295: 1441–1444, 1987.
43. CHRISTENSEN, E. H., and O. HANSEN. Hypoglykame, arbeitsfahigkeit und ermudung. *Skand. Arch. Physiol.* 81: 172–179, 1939.
44. CHUMLEA, W. C., A. F. ROCHE, and P. WEBB. Body size, subcutaneous fatness and total body fat in older adults. *Int. J. Obes.* 8: 311–317, 1984.
45. CLAYTOR, R. P., R. H. COX, E. T. HOWLEY, K. A. LAWLER, and J. E. LAWLER. Aerobic power and cardiovascular response to stress. *J. Appl. Physiol.* 65: 1416–1423, 1988.
46. COGGAN, A. R., R. J. SPINA, D. S. KING, M. A. ROGERS, M. BROWN, P. M. NEMETH, and J. O. HOLLOSZY. Skeletal muscle adaptations to endurance training in 60- to 70-year-old men and women. *J. Appl. Physiol.* 72: 1780–1786, 1992.
47. COGGAN, A. R., R. J. SPINA, D. S. KING, M. A. ROGERS, M. BROWN, P. M. NEMETH, and J. O. HOLLOSZY. Histochemical and enzymatic comparison of the gastrocnemius muscle of young and elderly men and women. *J. Gerontol.* 47: B71–B76, 1992.
48. COGGAN, A. R., R. J. SPINA, M. A. ROGERS, D. S. KING, M. BROWN, P. M. NEMETH, and J. O. HOLLOSZY. Histochemical and enzymatic characteristics of skeletal muscle in master athletes. *J. Appl. Physiol.* 68: 1896–1901, 1990.
49. COHN, S. H., D. VARTSKY, S. YASUMURU, A. SAWITSKY, I. ZANZI, A. VASWANI, and K. J. ELLIS. Compartmental body composition based on total body nitrogen, potassium and calcium. *Am. J. Physiol.* 239(*Endocrinol. Metab.* 2): E524–E530, 1980.
50. COLLETTI, L. A., J. EDWARDS, L. GORDON, J. SHARY, and N. H. BELL. The effects of muscle-building exercise on bone mineral density of the radius, spine, and hip in young men. *Calcif. Tissue Int.* 45: 12–14, 1989.
51. COON, P. J., E. R. BLEECKER, D. T. DRINKWATER, D. A. MEYERS, and A. P. GOLDBERG. Effects of body composition and exercise capacity on glucose tolerance, insulin, and lipoprotein lipids in healthy older men: a cross-sectional and longitudinal study. *Metabolism* 38: 1201–1209, 1989.
52. COYLE, E. F., W. H. MARTIN, D. R. SINACORE, M. J. JOYNER, J. M. HAGBERG, and J. O. HOLLOSZY. Time course of loss of adaptations after stopping prolonged intense endurance training. *J. Appl. Physiol.* 57: 1857–1864, 1984.
53. CRAIG, B. W., S. M. GARTHWAITE, and J. O. HOLLOSZY. Adipocyte insulin resistance: effects of aging, obesity, exercise and food restriction. *J. Appl. Physiol.* 62: 95–100, 1987.
54. CRESS, M. E., D. P. THOMAS, J. JOHNSON, F. W. KASCH, R. G. CASSENS, E. L. SMITH, and J. C. AGRE. Effect of training on VO_{2max}, thigh strength, and muscle morphology in septuagenarian women. *Med. Sci. Sports Exerc.* 23: 752–758, 1991.
55. CUNNINGHAM, D., H. MONTOYE, H. METZNER, and J. KELLER. Active leisure time activities as related to age among males in a total population. *J. Gerontol.* 23: 551–559, 1968.
56. CUNNINGHAM, D. A., P. A. RECHNITZER, J. H. HOWARD, and A. P. DONNER. Exercise training of men at retirement: a clinical trial. *J. Gerontol.* 42: 17–23, 1987.
57. CURRY, D. L., G. REAVEN, and E. REAVEN. Glucose-induced insulin secretion by perfused pancreas of 2- and 12-month-old Fischer 344 rats. *Am. J. Physiol.* 248(*Endocrinol. Metab.* 11): E375–E380, 1985.
58. DALSKY, G. P. Effect of exercise on bone: permissive influence of estrogen and calcium. *Med. Sci. Sports Exerc.* 22: 281–285, 1990.
59. DALSKY, G. P., K. R. STOCKE, A. A. EHSANI, E. SLATOPOLSKY, W. C. LEE, and S. J. BIRGE. Weight-bearing exercise training and lumbar bone mineral content in postmenopausal women. *Ann. Intern. Med.* 108: 824–828, 1988.
60. DAVIDSON, M. B. The effect of aging on carbohydrate metabolism: a review of the English literature and a practical approach to the diagnosis of diabetes mellitus in the elderly. *Metabolism* 28: 686–705, 1979.
61. DAVIES, C. T. M., D. O. THOMAS, and M. J. WHITE. Mechanical properties of young and elderly human muscle. *Acta Med. Scand. Suppl.* 711: 219–226, 1986.
62. DAVIES, K. J. A., A. T. QUINTANILHA, G. A. BROOKS, and L. PACKER. Free radicals and tissue damage produced by exercise. *Biochem. Biophys. Res. Commun.* 107: 1198–1205, 1982.
63. DEFRONZO, R. A. Glucose intolerance and aging. Evidence for tissue insensitivity to insulin. *Diabetes* 28: 1095–1101, 1979.
64. DEFRONZO, R. A. Glucose intolerance and aging. *Diabetes Care* 4: 493–501, 1981.
65. DEFRONZO, R. A., and E. FERRANNINI. Insulin resistance. A multifaceted syndrome responsible for NIDDM, obesity, hypertension, dyslipidemia and atherosclerotic cardiovascular disease. *Diabetes Care* 14: 173–194, 1991.
66. DEHN, M. M., and R. A. BRUCE. Longitudinal variations in maximal oxygen intake with age and activity. *J. Appl. Physiol.* 33: 805–807, 1972.

67. DEL MAESTRO, R. F. An approach to free radicals in medicine and biology. *Acta Physiol. Scand.* 492: 153–168, 1980.
68. DENIS, C., J.-C. CHATARD, D. DORMOIS, M.-T. LINOSSIER, A. GEYSSANT, and J.-P. LACOUR. Effects of endurance training on capillary supply of human skeletal muscle in two age groups (20 and 60 years). *J. Physiol. Paris* 81: 379–383, 1986.
69. DESPRÉS, J.-P., A. NADEAU, A. TREMBLAY, M. FERLAND, S. MOORJANI, P. J. LUPIEN, G. THÉRIAULT, S. PINAULT, and C. BOUCHARD. Role of deep abdominal fat in the association between regional adipose tissue distribution and glucose tolerance in obese women. *Diabetes* 38: 304–309, 1989.
70. DESPRÉS, J.-P., A. NADEAU, and C. BOUCHARD. Physical training and changes in regional adipose tissue distribution. *Acta Med. Scand.* 723(suppl.): 205–212, 1988.
71. DEURENBERG, P., K. VAN DER KOOIJ, P. EVERS, and T. HULSHOF. Assessment of body composition by electrical impedance in a population aged > 60 y. *Am. J. Clin. Nutr.* 51: 3–6, 1990.
72. DILL, D. B., S. ROBINSON, and J. C. ROSS. A longitudinal study of 16 champion runners. *J. Sports Med. Phys. Fitness* 7: 4–27, 1967.
73. DOUEN, A. G., T. RAMLAL, S. RASTOGI, P. J. BILAN, G. D. CARTEE, M. VRANIC, J. O. HOLLOSZY, and A. KLIP. Exercise induces recruitment of the "insulin-responsive glucose transporter." *J. Biol. Chem.* 265: 13427–13430, 1990.
74. DOUGLAS, P. S., and M. O'TOOLE. Aging and physical activity determine cardiac structure and function in the older athlete. *J. Appl. Physiol.* 72: 1969–1973, 1992.
75. DOWNES, T. R., A. M. NOMEIR, K. M. SMITH, K. P. STEWART, and W. C. LITTLE. Mechanism of altered pattern of left ventricular filling with aging in subjects without cardiac disease. *Am. J. Cardiol.* 64: 523–527, 1989.
76. DRAZNIN, B., J. P. STEINBERG, J. W. LEITNER, and K. E. SUSSMAN. The nature of insulin secretory defect in aging rats. *Diabetes* 34: 1168–1173, 1985.
77. DRORI, D., and Y. FOLMAN. Environmental effects on longevity in the male rat: exercise, mating, castration and restricted feeding. *Exp. Gerontol.* 11: 25–32, 1976.
78. DURNIN, J. V. G. A., and J. WOMERSLEY. Body fat assessed from total body density and its estimation from skinfold thickness: measurements on 481 men and women from 16 to 72 years. *Br. J. Nutr.* 32: 77–97, 1974.
79. EDDINGER, T. J., R. L. MOSS, and R. G. CASSENS. Fiber number and type composition in extensor digitorum longus, soleus, and diaphragm muscles with ageing in Fischer 344 rats. *J. Histochem. Cytochem.* 33: 1033–1041, 1985.
80. EDINGTON, D. W., A. C. COSMAS, and W. B. MCCAFFERTY. Exercise and longevity: evidence for a threshold age. *J. Gerontol.* 27: 341–343, 1972.
81. EHSANI, A. A., T. OGAWA, T. R. MILLER, R. J. SPINA, and S. M. JILKA. Exercise training improves left ventricular systolic function in older men. *Circulation* 83: 96–103, 1991.
82. EKBLOM, B., P.-O. ÅSTRAND, B. SALTIN, J. STENBERG, and B. WALLSTROM. Effect of training on circulatory response to exercie. *J. Appl. Physiol.* 24: 518–528, 1968.
83. ELAHI, D., D. C. MULLER, D. K. ANDERSON, J. D. TOBIN, and R. ANDRES. The effect of age and glucose concentration on insulin secretion by the isolated perfused rat pancreas. *Endocrinology* 116: 11–16, 1985.
84. ELIOT, R. S., F. C. CLAYTON, G. M. PIEPER, and G. L. TODD. Influence of environmental stress on pathogenesis of sudden cardiac death. *Federation Proc.* 36: 1719–1724, 1977.
85. ENZI, G., M. GASPARO, P. R. BIONDETTI, D. FIORE, M. SEMISA, and F. ZURLO. Subcutaneous and visceral fat distribution according to sex, age, and overweight, evaluated by computed tomography. *Am. J. Clin. Nutr.* 44: 739–746, 1986.
86. ESSÉN-GUSTAVSSON, B., and O. BÖRGES. Histochemical and metabolic characteristics of human skeletal muscle in relation to age. *Acta Physiol. Scand.* 126: 107–114, 1986.
87. EVANS, W. J., and J. G. CANNON. The metabolic effects of exercise-induced muscle damage. *Exerc. Sport Sci. Rev.* 19: 99–125, 1991.
88. FAGARD, R., E. BIELEN, and A. AMERY. Heritability of aerobic power and anaerobic energy generation during exercise. *J. Appl. Physiol.* 70: 357–362, 1991.
89. FIATARONE, M. A., E. C. MARKS, N. D. RYAN, C. N. MEREDITH, L. A. LIPSITZ, and W. J. EVANS. High intensity strength training in nonagenarians. *JAMA* 263: 3029–3034, 1990.
90. FINK, R. I., O. G. KOLTERMAN, J. GRIFFIN, and J. M. OLEFSKY. Mechanisms of insulin resistance in aging. *J. Clin. Invest.* 71: 1523–1535, 1983.
91. FITTS, R. H. Aging and skeletal muscle. In: *Exercise and Aging: The Scientific Basis*, edited by E. L. SMITH and R. C. Serfass. Hillside, NJ: Enslow, 1981, p. 31–44.
92. FITTS, R. H., F. W. BOOTH, W. W. WINDER, and J. O. HOLLOSZY. Skeletal muscle respiratory capacity, endurance and glycogen utilization. *Am. J. Physiol.* 228: 1029–1033, 1975.
93. FITTS, R. H., J. P. TROUP, F. A. WITZMAN, and J. O. HOLLOSZY. The effects of aging and exercise on skeletal muscle function. *Mech. Ageing Dev.* 27: 161–172, 1984.
94. FLEG, J. L., and E. G. LAKATTA. Role of muscle loss in the age-associated reduction in VO_{2max}. *J. Appl. Physiol.* 65: 1147–1151, 1988.
95. FLYNN, M. A., G. B. NOLPH, A. S. BAKER, W. M. MARTIN, and G. KRAUSE. Total body potassium in aging humans: a longitudinal study. *Am. J. Clin. Nutr.* 50: 713–717, 1989.
96. FORBES, G. B. *Human Body Composition: Growth, Aging, Nutrition, and Activity.* New York: Springer-Verlag, 1987, p. 169–195.
97. FORMAN, D. E., W. J. MANNING, R. HAUSER, E. V. GERVINO, W. J. EVANS, and J. Y. WEI. Enhanced left ventricular diastolic filling associated with long-term endurance training. *J. Gerontol.* 47: M56–M58, 1992.
98. FOSTER, V. L., G. J. HUME, A. L. DICKINSON, S. J. CHATFIELD, and W. C. BYRNES. The reproducibility of VO_{2max}, ventilatory, and lactate thresholds in elderly women. *Med. Sci. Sports Exerc.* 18: 425–430, 1986.
99. FRIDOVICH, I. Superoxide and evolution. In: *Horizons in Biochemistry and Biophysics,* edited by E. Quagliariello, F. Palmieri, and T. P. Singer. Menlo Park, CA: Addison-Wesley, 1974, p. 1–37.
100. FRIEDMAN, J. E., W. M. SHERMAN, M. J. REED, C. W. ELTON, and G. L. DOHM. Exercise training increases glucose transporter protein GLUT4 in skeletal muscle of obese Zucker (fa/fa) rats. *FEBS Lett.* 268: 13–16, 1990.
101. FRONTERA, W. R., V. A. HUGHES, K. J. LUTZ, and W. J. EVANS. A cross-sectional study of muscle strength and mass in 45- to 78-yr-old men and women. *J. Appl. Physiol.* 71: 644–650, 1991.
102. FRONTERA, W. R., C. N. MEREDITH, K. P. O'REILLY, and W. J. EVANS. Strength training and determinants of VO_{2max} in older men. *J. Appl. Physiol.* 68: 329–333, 1990.
103. FRONTERA, W. R., C. N. MEREDITH, K. P. O'REILLY, H. G. KNUTTGEN, and W. J. EVANS. Strength conditioning in older men: skeletal muscle hypertrophy and improved function. *J. Appl. Physiol.* 64: 1038–1044, 1988.
104. FUKAGAWA, N. K., L. G. BANDINI, and J. B. YOUNG. Effect of age on body composition and resting metabolic rate. *Am. J. Physiol.* 259 (*Endocrinol. Metab.* 22): E233–E238, 1990.
105. GALBO, H., C. J. HEDESKOV, K. CAPITO, and J. VINTEN. The effect of physical training on insulin secretion of rat pancreatic islets. *Acta Physiol. Scand.* 11: 75–79, 1981.
106. GALLAGHER, J. C., D. GOLDGAR, and A. MOY. Total body cal-

cium in normal women: effect of age and menopause status. *J. Bone Min. Res.* 2: 491–496, 1987.
107. GARETTO, L. P., E. A. RICHTER, M. N. GOODMAN, and N. B. RUDERMAN. Enhanced muscle glucose metabolism after exercise in the rat: the two phases. *Am. J. Physiol.* 246 (*Endocrinol. Metab.* 9): E471–E475, 1984.
108. GARTHWAITE, S. M., H. CHENG, J. E. BRYAN, B. W. CRAIG, and J. O. HOLLOSZY. Ageing, exercise and food restriction: effects on body composition. *Mech. Ageing Dev.* 36: 187–196, 1986.
109. GERSTENBLITH, G., D. S. RENLUND, and E. G. LAKATTA. Cardiovascular response to exercise in younger and older men. *Federation Proc.* 46: 1834–1839, 1987.
110. GLEESON, P. B., E. J. PROTAS, A. D. LEBLANC, V. S. SCHNEIDER, and H. J. EVANS. Effects of weight lifting on bone mineral density in premenopausal women. *J. Bone Min. Res.* 5: 153–158, 1990.
111. GOLD, G., K. KAROLY, C. FREEMAN, and R. C. ADELMAN. A possible role for insulin in the altered capability for hepatic enzyme adaptation during aging. *Biochem. Biophys. Res. Commun.* 73: 1003–1010, 1976.
112. GOMMERS, A., M. DEHEZ-DELHAYE, and M. JEANJEAN. The effect of age on the in vitro response to insulin in the rat. 1. Glucose metabolism in the diaphragm. *Gerontology* 23: 127–141, 1977.
113. GOODMAN, M. N., S. M. DLUZ, A. MCELANY, E. BELUR, and N. B. RUDERMAN. Glucose uptake and insulin sensitivity in rat muscle: changes during 3–96 weeks of age. *Am. J. Physiol.* 244 (*Endocrinol. Metab.* 7): E93–E100, 1983.
114. GOODRICK, C. L. Effects of long-term voluntary wheel exercise on male and female Wistar rats 1. Longevity, body weight and metabolic rate. *Gerontology* 26: 22–23, 1980.
115. GOODRICK, C. L., D. K. INGRAM, M. A. REYNOLDS, J. R. FREEMAN, and N. L. CIDER. Effects of intermittent feeding upon growth and life span in rats. *Gerontology* 28: 233–241, 1982.
116. GOODRICK, C. L., D. K. INGRAM, M. A. REYNOLDS, J. R. FREEMAN, and N. L. CIDER. Differential effects of intermittent feeding and voluntary exercise on body weight and lifespan in adult rats. *J. Gerontol.* 38: 36–45, 1983a.
117. GOODRICK, C. L., D. K. INGRAM, M. A. REYNOLDS, J. R. FREEMAN, and N. L. CIDER. Effects of intermittent feeding upon growth, activity, and lifespan in rats allowed voluntary exercise. *Exp. Aging Res.* 9: 203–209, 1983b.
118. GOTFREDSON, A., A. HARBERG, L. NILAS, and C. CHRISTIANSEN. Total body bone mineral in healthy adults. *J. Lab. Clin. Med.* 110: 362–368, 1987.
119. GRANATH, A., B. JONSSON, and T. STRANDELL. Circulation in healthy old men, studied by right heart catheterization at rest and during exercise in supine and sitting position. *Acta Med. Scand.* 176: 425–446, 1964.
120. GRIMBY, G., and B. SALTIN. Physiological analysis of physically well trained middle-aged and old athletes. *Acta Med. Scand.* 179: 513–526, 1966.
121. GRIMBY, G., and B. SALTIN. The ageing muscle. *Clin. Physiol.* 3: 209–218, 1983.
122. GULVE, E. A., G. D. CARTEE, J. R. ZIERATH, V. M. CORPUS, and J. O. HOLLOSZY. Reversal of enhanced muscle glucose transport after exercise: roles of insulin and glucose. *Am. J. Physiol.* 259 (*Endocrinol. Metab.* 22): E685–E691, 1990.
123. GULVE, E. A., E. J. HENRIKSEN, K. J. RODNICK, J. H. YOUN, and J. O. HOLLOSZY. Glucose transporters and glucose transport in skeletal muscles of 1- to 25-mo-old rats. *Am. J. Physiol.* 264 (*Endocrinol. Metab.* 27): E319–E327, 1993.
124. GUTMAN, E., and V. HANZLIKOVA. Motor unit in old age. *Nature* 209: 921–922, 1966.
125. GWATHMEY, J. K., M. T. SLAWSKY, C. L. PERREAULT, G. M. BRIGGS, J. P. MORGAN, and J. Y. WEI. Effect of exercise conditioning on excitation–contraction coupling in aged rats. *J. Appl. Physiol.* 69: 1366–1371, 1990.
126. HAARBO, J., U. MARSLEW, A. GOTFREDSEN, and C. CHRISTIANSEN. Postmenopausal hormone replacement therapy prevents central distribution of body fat after menopause. *Metabolism* 40: 1323–1326, 1991.
127. HAGBERG, J. M. Effect of training on the decline of VO_{2max} with aging. *Federation Proc.* 46: 1830–1833, 1987.
128. HAGBERG, J. M., W. K. ALLEN, D. R. SEALS, B. F. HURLEY, A. A. EHSANI, and J. O. HOLLOSZY. A hemodynamic comparison of young and older endurance athletes during exercise. *J. Appl. Physiol.* 58: 2041–2046, 1985.
129. HAGBERG, J. M., J. E. GRAVES, M. LIMACHER, D. R. WOODS, S. H. LEGGETT, C. CONONIE, J. J. GRUBER, and M. L. POLLOCK. Cardiovascular responses of 70- to 79-yr-old men and women to exercise training. *J. Appl. Physiol.* 66: 2589–2594, 1989.
130. HALLFRISCH, J., D. MULLER, D. DRINKWATER, J. TOBIN, and R. ANDRES. Continuing diet trends in men: the Baltimore Longitudinal Study of Aging (1961–1987). *J. Gerontol.* 45: M186–M191, 1990.
131. HARMAN, D. Role of free radicals in mutation, cancer, aging, and maintenance of life. *Radiat. Res.* 16: 752–763, 1962.
132. HARMAN, D. Free radical theory of aging: effect of free radical reaction inhibitors on the mortality rate of male LAF mice. *J. Gerontol.* 23: 476–482, 1968.
133. HASSAGER, C., and C. CHRISTIANSEN. Estrogen/gestagen therapy changes soft tissue body composition in postmenopausal women. *Metabolism* 38: 662–665, 1989.
134. HEATH, G. W., J. R. GAVIN, III, J. M. HINDERLITER, J. M. HAGBERG, S. A. BLOOMFIELD, and J. O. HOLLOSZY. Effects of exercise and lack of exercise on glucose tolerance and insulin sensitivity. *J. Appl. Physiol.* 55: 512–517, 1983.
135. HEATH, G. W., J. M. HAGBERG, A. A. EHSANI, and J. O. HOLLOSZY. A physiological comparison of young and older endurance athletes. *J. Appl. Physiol.* 51: 634–640, 1981.
136. HEINRICH, C. H., S. B. GOING, R. W. PAMENTER, C. D. PERRY, T. W. BOYDEN, and T. G. LOHMAN. Bone mineral content of cyclically menstruating female resistance and endurance trained athletes. *Med. Sci. Sports Exerc.* 22: 558–563, 1990.
137. HELMRICH, S. P., D. R. RAGLAND, R. W. LEUNG, and R. S. PAFFENBARGER. Physical activity and reduced occurrence of non-insulin-dependent diabetes mellitus. *N. Engl. J. Med.* 325: 147–152, 1991.
138. HEROUX, O., and J. S. CAMPBELL. A study of the pathology and life span of 6°C- and 30°C-acclimated rats. *Lab. Invest.* 9: 305–315, 1960.
139. HEYMSFIELD, S. B., and M. WAKI. Body composition in humans: advances in the development of multicompartment chemical models. *Nutr. Rev.* 49: 97–108, 1991.
140. HEYMSFIELD, S. B., J. WANG, J. J. KEHAYIAS, S. HESHKA, S. LICHTMAN, and R. N. PIERSON, JR. Chemical determination of human body density in vivo: relevance to hydrodensitometry. *Am. J. Clin. Nutr.* 50: 1282–1289, 1989.
141. HIGGINBOTHAM, M. B., K. G. MORRIS, R. S. WILLIAMS, E. COLEMAN, and F. R. COBB. Physiologic basis for the age-related decline in aerobic work capacity. *Am. J. Physiol.* 57: 1374–1379, 1986.
142. HIMES, J. H., A. F. ROCHE, and P. WEBB. Fat areas as estimates of total body fat. *Am. J. Clin. Nutr.* 33: 2093–2100, 1980.
143. HIRSHMAN, M. F., L. J. GOODYEAR, L. J. WARDZALA, E. D. HORTON, and E. S. HORTON. Identification of an intracellular pool of glucose transporters from basal and insulin-stimulated rat skeletal muscle. *J. Biol. Chem.* 265: 987–991, 1990.
144. HOLLOSZY, J. O. Biochemical adaptations in muscle. Effects of exercise on mitochondrial O_2 uptake and respiratory enzyme

activity in skeletal muscle. *J. Biol. Chem.* 242: 2278–2282, 1967.
145. HOLLOSZY, J. O. Exercise increases average longevity of female rats despite increased food intake and no growth retardation. *J. Gerontol.* 48: B97 100, 1993.
146. HOLLOSZY, J. O., and E. F. COYLE. Adaptations of skeletal muscle to endurance exercise and their metabolic consequences. *J. Appl. Physiol.* 56: 831–839, 1984.
147. HOLLOSZY, J. O., and H. T. NARAHARA. Studies of tissue permeability. X. Changes in permeability to 3-methylglucose associated with contraction of isolated frog muscles. *J. Biol. Chem.* 240: 3492–3500, 1965.
148. HOLLOSZY, J. O., and K. B. SCHECHTMAN. Interactions between exercise and food restriction: effects on longevity of male rats. *J. Appl. Physiol.* 70: 1529–1535, 1991.
149. HOLLOSZY, J. O., and E. K. SMITH. Longevity of cold exposed rats: a reevaluation of the "rate-of-living theory." *J. Appl. Physiol.* 61: 1656–1660, 1986.
150. HOLLOSZY, J. O., M. CHEN, G. D. CARTEE, and J. C. YOUNG. Skeletal muscle atrophy in old rats: differential changes in the three fiber types. *Mech. Ageing Dev.* 60: 199–213, 1991.
151. HOLLOSZY, J. O., J. SCHULTZ, J. KUSNIERKIEWICZ, J. M. HAGBERG, and A. A. EHSANI. Effects of exercise on glucose tolerance and insulin resistance. *Acta Med. Scand. Suppl.* 711: 55–65, 1986.
152. HOLLOSZY, J. O., and E. K. SMITH, M. VINING, and S. ADAMS. Effect of voluntary exercise on longevity of rats. *J. Appl. Physiol.* 59: 826–831, 1985.
153. HOSSACK, K. F., and R. A. BRUCE. Maximal cardiac function in sedentary normal men and women: comparison of age-related changes. *J. Appl. Physiol.* 53: 799–804, 1982.
154. HULTMAN, E. Physiological role of muscle glycogen in man, with special reference to exercise. *Circ. Res.* 20: 99–114, 1967.
155. HURLEY, B. F., J. M. HAGBERG, A. P. GOLDBERG, D. R. SEALS, A. A. EHSANI, R. E. BRENNAN, and J. O. HOLLOSZY. Resistive training can reduce coronary risk factors without altering VO_{2max} or percent body fat. *Med. Sci. Sports Exerc.* 20: 150–154, 1988.
156. HURLEY, B. F., J. M. HAGBERG, D. R. SEALS, A. A. EHSANI, A. P. GOLDBERG, and J. O. HOLLOSZY. Glucose tolerance and lipid-lipoprotein levels in middleaged powerlifters. *Clin. Physiol.* 7: 11–19, 1987.
157. HURLEY, B. F., P. M. NEMETH, W. H. MARTIN, III, J. M. HAGBERG, G. P. DALSKY, and J. O. HOLLOSZY. Muscle triglyceride utilization during exercise: effect of training. *J. Appl. Physiol.* 60: 562–567, 1986.
158. IVY, J. L., J. C. YOUNG, B. W. CRAIG, W. M. KOHRT, and J. O. HOLLOSZY. Ageing, exercise and food restriction: effects on skeletal muscle glucose uptake. *Mech. Ageing Dev.* 61: 123–133, 1991.
159. JACKSON, M. J., R. H. T. EDWARDS, and M. C. R. SYMONS. Electron spin resonance studies of intact skeletal muscle. *Biochim. Biophys. Acta* 847: 185–190, 1985.
160. JACKSON, R. A. Mechanisms of age-related glucose intolerance. *Diabetes Care* 13(suppl.2): 9–19, 1990.
161. JAKUBCZAK, L. F. Behavioral aspects of nutrition and longevity in animals. In: *Nutrition, Longevity, and Aging,* edited by M. Rockstein and M. L. Sussman. New York: Academic Press, 1976, p. 103–122.
162. JOHNSON, H. D., L. D. KINTNER, and H. H. KIBLER. Effects of 48°F (8.9°C) and 83°F (28.4°C) on longevity and pathology of male rats. *J. Gerontol.* 18: 29–36, 1963.
163. JULIUS, S., A. AMERY, L. S. WHITLOCK, and J. CONWAY. Influence of age on the hemodynamic response to exercise. *Circulation* 36: 222–230, 1967.
164. KAHN, S. E., V. G. LARSON, J. C. BEARD, K. C. CAIN, G. W. FELLINGHAM, R. S. SCHWARTZ, R. C. VEITH, J. R. STRATTON, M. D. CERQUEIRA, and I. B. ABRASS. Effect of exercise on insulin action, glucose tolerance, and insulin secretion in aging. *Am. J. Physiol.* 258 (*Endocrinol. Metab.* 21): E397–E943, 1990.
165. KALLMAN, D. A., C. C. PLATO, and J. D. TOBIN. The role of muscle loss in the age-related decline of grip strength: cross-sectional and longitudinal perspectives. *J. Gerontol.* 45: M82–M88, 1990.
166. KASCH, F. W., J. P. WALLACE, and S. P. VAN CAMP. Effects of 18 years of endurance exercise on the physical work capacity of older men. *J. Cardiac. Rehabil.* 5: 308–312, 1985.
167. KEEN, H., B. J. THOMAS, R. J. JARRETT, and J. H. FULLER. Nutrient intake, adiposity and diabetes. *Br. Med. J.* 1: 655–658, 1979.
168. KEYS, A. *Seven Countries. A Multivariate Analysis of Death and Coronary Disease,* Cambridge, MA: Harvard University Press, 1980.
169. KIBLER, H. H., and H. D. JOHNSON. Metabolic rate and aging in rats during exposure to cold. *J. Gerontol.* 16: 13–16, 1961.
170. KIBLER, H. H., H. D. SILSBY, and H. D. JOHNSON. Metabolic trends and life span of rats living at 9°C and 28°C. *J. Gerontol.* 18: 235–239, 1963.
171. KING, D. S., G. P. DALSKY, W. E. CLUTTER, D. A. YOUNG, M. A. STATEN, P. E. CRYER, and J. O. HOLLOSZY. Effects of exercise and lack of exercise on insulin sensitivity and responsiveness. *J. Appl. Physiol.* 64: 1942–1946, 1988.
172. KING, D. S., G. P. DALSKY, M. A. STATEN, W. E. CLUTTER, D. R. VAN HOUTEN, and J. O. HOLLOSZY. Insulin action and secretion in endurance-trained and untrained humans. *J. Appl. Physiol.* 63: 2247–2252, 1987.
173. KING, D. S., M. A. STATEN, W. M. KOHRT, G. P. DALSKY, D. ELAHI, and J. O. HOLLOSY. Insulin secretory capacity in endurance-trained and untrained young men. *Am. J. Physiol.* 259(*Endocrinol. Metab.* 22): E155–E181, 1990.
174. KING, H., R. TAYLOR, P. ZIMMET, K. PARGETER, L. R. RAPER, T. BERIKI, and J. TEKANENE. Non-insulin-dependent diabetes (NIDDM) in a newly independent pacific nation: The Republic of Kiribati. *Diabetes Care* 7: 409–414, 1984.
175. KING, P. A., M. F. HIRSHMAN, E. D. HORTON, and E. S. HORTON. Glucose transport in skeletal muscle membrane vesicles from control and exercised rats. *Am. J. Physiol.* 257 (*Cell Physiol.* 26): C1128–C1134, 1989.
176. KIRK, S., C. F. SHARP, N. ELBAUM, D. B. ENDRES, S. M. SIMONS, J. G. MOHLER, and R. K. RUDE. Effect of long-distance running on bone mass in women. *J. Bone Min. Res.* 4: 515–522, 1989.
177. KIRWAN, J. P., W. M. KOHRT, D. M. WOJTA, R. E. BOUREY, and J. O. HOLLOSZY. Endurance exercise training reduces glucose-stimulated insulin levels in 60- to 70-yr-old men and women. *J. Gerontol.* 48: M84–M90, 1993.
178. KISSEBAH, A. H. Insulin resistance in visceral obesity. *Int. J. Obes.* 15: 109–115, 1991.
179. KLINE, G. M., J. P. PORCARI, R. HINTERMEISITER, P. S. FREEDSON, A. WARD, R. F. MCCARRON, J. ROSS, and J. M. RIPPE. Estimation of VO_{2max} from a one-mile track walk, gender, age, and body weight. *Med. Sci. Sports Exerc.* 19: 253–259, 1987.
180. KLIP, A., and M. R. PAQUET. Glucose transport and glucose transporters in muscle and their metabolic regulation. *Diabetes Care* 13: 228–243, 1990.
181. KLITGAARD, H., R. MARC, A. BRUNET, H. VANDEWALLE, and H. MONOD. Contractile properties of old rat muscles: effect of increased use. *J. Appl. Physiol.* 67: 1401–1408, 1989.
182. KNOWLER, W. C., P. H. BENNET, R. F. HAMMAN, and M. MILLER. Diabetes incidence and prevalence in Pima Indians: a 19-fold greater incidence than in Rochester, Minnesota. *Am. J. Epidemiol.* 108: 497–505, 1978.
183. KOHRT, W. M., and D. B. SNEAD. Effect of exercise on bone mass in the elderly. In: *Aging, Musculoskeletal Disorders and*

Care of the Frail Elderly, edited by H. M. Perry, III, J. E. Morley, and R. M. Coe. New York: Springer, 1993, p. 214–227.

184. KOHRT, W. M., J. P. KIRWAN, M. A. STATEN, R. E. BOUREY, D. S. KING, and J. O. HOLLOSZY. Insulin resistance in aging is related to abdominal obesity. *Diabetes* 42: 273–281, 1993.

185. KOHRT, W. M., M. T. MALLEY, A. R. COGGAN, R. J. SPINA, T. OGAWA, A. A. EHSANI, R. E. BOUREY, W. H. MARTIN, III, and J. O. HOLLOSZY. Effects of gender, age, and fitness level on response of VO_{2max} to training in 60 to 71 yr-olds. *J. Appl. Physiol.* 71: 2004–2011, 1991.

186. KOHRT, W. M., M. T. MALLEY, G. P. DALSKY, and J. O. HOLLOSZY. Body composition of healthy sedentary and trained, young and older men and women. *Med. Sci. Sports Exerc.* 24: 832–837, 1992.

187. KOHRT, W. M., K. A. OBERT, and J. O. HOLLOSZY. Exercise training improves fat distribution patterns in 60- to 70-year-old men and women. *J. Gerontol.* 47: M99–M105, 1992.

188. KONO, S., H. KUZUYA, M. OKAMOTO, H. NISHIMURA, A. KOSAKI, T. KAKEHI, G. INOUE, I. MAEDA, and H. IMURA. Changes in insulin receptor kinase with aging in rat skeletal muscle and liver. *Am. J. Physiol.* 259 (*Endocrinol. Metab.* 22): E27–E35, 1990.

189. KORANYI, L. I., R. E. BOUREY, C. A. SLENTZ, J. O. HOLLOSZY, and M. A. PERMUTT. Coordinate reduction of rat pancreatic islet glucokinase and proinsulin by exercise training. *Diabetes* 40: 401–404, 1991.

190. KOSTIS, J. B., A. E. MOREYRA, M. T. AMENDO, J. DIPIETRO, N. COSGROVE, and P. T. KUO. The effect of age on heart rate in subjects free of heart disease. *Circulation* 65: 141–145, 1982.

191. KROLNER, B., B. TOFT, S. P. NIELSEN, and E. TONDEVOLD. Physical exercise as prophylaxis against involutional vertebral bone loss: a controlled trial. *Clin. Sci.* 64: 541–546, 1983.

192. KROMHOUT, D. Energy and macronutrient intake in lean and obese middle-aged men (the Zutphen Study). *Am. J. Clin. Nutr.* 37: 295–299, 1983.

193. LAKATTA, E. G. Cardiac muscle changes in senescence. *Ann. Rev. Physiol.* 49: 519–531, 1987.

194. LAKATTA, E. G., and H. A. SPURGEON. Effect of exercise on cardiac muscle performance in aged rats. *Federation Proc.* 46: 1844–1849, 1987.

195. LANE, J. E., D. A. BLOCH, H. B. HUBERT, H. JONES, U. SIMPSON, and J. F. FRIES. Running, osteoarthritis, and bone density: initial 2-year longitudinal study. *Am. J. Med.* 88: 452–459, 1990.

196. LARSSON, L., G. GRIMBY, and J. KARLSSON. Muscle strength and speed of movement in relation to age and muscle morphology. *J. Appl. Physiol.* 46: 451–456, 1979.

197. LARSSON, L., B. SJÖODIN, and J. KARLSSON. Histochemical and biochemical changes in human skeletal muscle with age in sedentary males, age 22–65 years. *Acta Physiol. Scand.* 103: 31–39, 1978.

198. LAWRENCE, J. C., J. COLVIN, G. D. CARTEE, and J. O. HOLLOSZY. Effects of aging and exercise on insulin action in rat adipocytes are correlated with changes in fat cell volume. *J. Gerontol.* 44: B88–B92, 1989.

199. LEBLANC, A. D., V. S. SCHNEIDER, H. J. EVANS, D. A. ENGELBRETSON, and J. M. KREBS. Bone mineral loss and recovery after 17 weeks of bed rest. *J. Bone Min. Res.* 5: 843–850, 1990.

200. LEBLANC, J., A. NADEAU, D. RICHARD, and A. TREMBLAY. Studies on the sparing effect of exercise on insulin requirements in human subjects. *Metabolism* 30: 1119–1124, 1981.

201. LESSER, G. T., and J. MARKOFSY. Body water compartments with human aging using fat free mass as the reference standard. *Am. J. Physiol.* 236 (*Regulatory Integrative Comp. Physiol.* 7): R215–R220, 1979.

202. LEXELL, J., D. DOWNHAM, and M. SJOSTROM. Distribution of different fibre types in human skeletal muscles. Fibre type arrangement in m. vastus lateralis from three groups of healthy men between 15 and 83 years. *J. Neurol. Sci.* 72: 211–222, 1986.

203. LEXELL, J., K. HENRIKSSON-LARSÉN, B. WINBLAD, and M. SJÖSTRÖM. Distribution of different fiber types in human skeletal muscle: effects of aging studied in whole muscle cross sections. *Muscle Nerve* 6: 588–594, 1983.

204. LEXELL, J., C. C. TAYLOR, and M. SJOSTROM. What is the cause of the ageing atrophy? Total number, size and proportion of different fiber types studied in whole vastus lateralis muscles from 15 to 83 year-old men. *J. Neurol. Sci.* 84: 275–294, 1988.

205. LEY, C. J., B. LEES, and J. C. STEVENSON. Sex- and menopause-associated changes in body-fat distribution. *Am. J. Clin. Nutr.* 55: 950–954, 1992.

206. LI, Y., T. LINCOLN, D. MENDELOWITZ, W. GROSSMAN, and J. W. WEI. Age-related differences in effect of exercise training on cardiac muscle function in rats. *Am. J. Physiol.* 251 (*Heart Circ. Physiol.* 22): H12–H18, 1986.

207. LINDSAY, R. The menopause: sex steroids and osteoporosis. *Clin. Obstet. Gynecol.* 30: 847–859, 1987.

208. LINDSAY, R., F. COSMAN, B. S. HERRINGTON, and S. HIMMELSTEIN. Bone mass and body composition in normal women. *J. Bone Min. Res.* 7: 55–63, 1992.

209. LISSNER, L., R. ANDRES, D. C. MULLER, and H. SHIMOKATA. Body weight variability in men: metabolic rate, health and longevity. *Int. J. Obes.* 14: 373–383, 1990.

210. MAKRIDES, L., G. J. F. HEIGENHAUSER, and N. L. JONES. High-intensity endurance training in 20- to 30- and 60- to 70-yr-old healthy men. *J. Appl. Physiol.* 69: 1792–1798, 1990.

211. MARGULIES, J. Y., A. SIMKIN, and I. LEICHTER. Effect of intense physical exercise on the bone-mineral content in the lower limbs of young adults. *J. Bone Joint Surg.* 68A: 1090–1093, 1986.

212. MARTI, B., M. KNOBLOCH, W. F. RIESEN, and H. HOWALD. Fifteen-year changes in exercise, aerobic power, abdominal fat, and serum lipids in runners and controls. *Med. Sci. Sports Exerc.* 23: 115–122, 1991.

213. MAZESS, R. B., and G. D. WHEDON. Immobilization and bone. *Calcif. Tissue Int.* 35: 265–267, 1983.

214. MCCARTER, R., and J. PALMER. Physical activity and metabolic rate: are they important factors in the action of food restriction on aging [Abstract]? *Gerontologist* 31: 172A, 1991.

215. MCCARTER, R. J. M., and J. MCGEE. Influence of nutrition and ageing on the composition and function of rat skeletal muscle. *J. Gerontol.* 42: 432–441, 1987.

216. MCCARTER, R. J. M., E. J. MASORO, and B. P. YU. Rat muscle structure and metabolism in relation to age and food intake. *Am. J. Physiol.* 242 (*Regulatory Integrative Comp. Physiol.* 11): R89–R93, 1982.

217. MCCAY, C. M., M. F. CROWELL, and L. A. MAYNARD. The effect of retarded growth upon length of life span and upon ultimate body size. *J. Nutr.* 10: 63–79, 1935.

218. MEREDITH, C. N., W. R. FRONTERA, E. C. FISHER, V. A. HUGHES, J. C. HERLAND, J. EDWARDS, and W. J. EVANS. Peripheral effects of endurance training in young and old subjects. *J. Appl. Physiol.* 66: 2844–2849, 1989.

219. MEREDITH, C. N., M. J. ZACKIN, W. R. FRONTERA, and W. J. EVANS. Body composition and aerobic capacity in young and middle-aged endurance-trained men. *Med. Sci. Sports Exerc.* 19: 557–563, 1987.

220. MICHEL, B. A., N. E. LANE, D. A. BLOCH, H. H. JONES, and J. F. FRIES. Effect of changes in weight-bearing exercise on lumbar bone mass after age fifty. *Ann. Med.* 23: 397–401, 1991.

221. MIKINES, K. J., B. SONNE, P. A. FARRELL, B. TRONIER, and H. GALBO. Effect of physical exercise on sensitivity and responsiveness to insulin in humans. *Am. J. Physiol.* 254 (*Endocrinol. Metab.* 17): E248–E259, 1988.

222. MILLER, T. R., S. J. GROSSMAN, K. B. SCHECTMAN, D. R. BIELLO, P. A. LUDBROOK, and A. A. EHSANI. Left ventricular diastolic filling and its association with age. *Am. J. Cardiol.* 58: 531–535, 1986.
223. MONTAGNANI, C. F., B. ARENA, and N. MUFFULLI. Estradiol and progesterone during exercise in healthy untrained women. *Med. Sci. Sports Exerc.* 24: 764–768, 1992.
224. NAJJAR, M. F., and M. ROWLAND. Anthropometric reference data and prevalence of overweight. In: *Vital and Health Statistics. Series 11: Data from the National Health Survey,* 1987, vol. 238, p. 1–73.
225. NARIMYA, S., C. B. DOLKAS, C. E. MONDON, C. SIMS, D. W. WRIGHT, and G. M. REAVEN. Insulin resistance in older rats. *Am. J. Physiol.* 246 (*Endocrinol. Metab.* 9): E397–E404, 1984.
226. NELSON, M. E., C. N. MEREDITH, B. DAWSON-HUGHES, and W. J. EVANS. Hormone and bone mineral status in endurance-trained and sedentary postmenopausal women. *J. Clin. Endocrinol. Metab.* 66: 927–933, 1988.
227. NISHIMURA, H., H. KUZUYA, M. OKAMOTO, T. YOSHIMASA, K. YAMADA, T. IDA, T. KAKEHI, and H. IMURA. Change of insulin action with aging in conscious rats determined by euglycemic clamp. *Am. J. Physiol.* 254 (*Endocrinol. Metab.* 17): E92–E98, 1988.
228. NOTELOVITZ, M., D. MARTIN, R. TESAR, F. Y. KHAN, C. PROBART, C. FIELDS, and L. MCKENZIE. Estrogen therapy and variable-resistance weight training increase bone mineral in surgically menopausal women. *J. Bone Min. Res.* 6: 583–590, 1991.
229. NOVAK, L. P. Aging, total body potassium, fat-free mass and cell mass in males and females between ages 18 and 85 years. *J. Gerontol.* 27: 438–443, 1972.
230. O'DEA, K. Marked improvement in carbohydrate and lipid metabolism in diabetic Australian aborigines after temporary reversion to traditional lifestyle. *Diabetes* 33: 296–303, 1984.
231. OGAWA, T., R. J. SPINA, W. H. MARTIN, III, W. M. KOHRT, K. B. SCHECHTMAN, J. O. HOLLOSZY, and A. A. EHSANI. Effects of aging, sex, and physical training on cardiovascular responses to exercise. *Circulation* 86: 494–503, 1992.
232. ORLANDER, J., K.-H. KIESSLING, L. LARSSON, J. KARLSSON, and A. ANIANSSON. Skeletal muscle metabolism and ultrastructure in relation to age in sedentary men. *Acta Physiol. Scand.* 104: 249–261, 1978.
233. ORWOLL, E. S., J. FERAR, S. K. OVIATT, M. R. MCCLUNG, and K. HUNTINGTON. The relationship of swimming exercise to bone mass in men and women. *Arch. Intern. Med.* 149: 2197–2200, 1989.
234. OSBORNE, G., L. A. WOLFE, G. W. BURGGRAF, and R. NORMAN. Relationships between cardiac dimensions, anthropometric characteristics and maximal aerobic power (VO_{2max}) in young men. *Int. J. Sports Med.* 13: 219–224, 1992.
235. OSCAI, L. B., and J. O. HOLLOSZY. Effects of weight changes produced by exercise, food restriction, or overeating on body composition. *J. Clin. Invest.* 48: 2124–2128, 1969.
236. OSCAI, L. B., P. A. MOLÉ, and J. O. HOLLOSZY. Effects of exercise on cardiac weight and mitochondria in male and female rats. *Am. J. Physiol.* 220: 1944–1948, 1971.
237. OSCAI, L. B., P. A. MOLÉ, L. M. KRUSACK, and J. O. HOLLOSZY. Detailed body composition analysis in female rats subjected to a program of swimming. *J. Nutr.* 103: 412–418, 1973.
238. OVEREND, T. J., D. A. CUNNINGHAM, J. F. KRAMER, M. S. LEFCOE, and D. H. PATERSON. Knee extensor and knee flexor strength: cross-sectional area ratios in young and elderly men. *J. Gerontol.* 47: M204–M210, 1992.
239. PACINI, G., A. VALERIO, F. BECCARO, R. NOSADINI, C. COBELLI, and G. CREPALDI. Insulin sensitivity and beta-cell responsivity are not decreased in older subjects with normal OGTT. *J. Am. Geriatr. Soc.* 36: 217–323, 1988.
240. PARÉ, P. D. The effect of chronic environment stress on premature aging in the rat. *J. Gerontol.* 20: 78–84, 1965.
241. PARIZKOVA, J., E. EISELT, S. SPRYNAROVA, and M. WACHTLOVA. Body composition, aerobic capacity, and density of muscle capillaries in young and old men. *J. Appl. Physiol.* 31: 323–325, 1971.
242. PAY, H. E., A. E. HARDMAN, G. J. JONES, and A. HUDSON. The acute effects of low-intensity exercise on plasma lipids in endurance-trained and untrained young adults. *Eur. J. Appl. Physiol.* 64: 182–186, 1992.
243. PEARL, R. *The Rate of Living,* New York: Knopf, 1928.
244. PHILLIPS, S. K., S. A. BRUCE, D. NEWTON, and R. C. WOLEDGE. The weakness of old age is not due to failure of muscle activation. *J. Gerontol.* 47: M45–M49, 1992.
245. PIERSON, R. M., J. WANG, S. B. HEYMSFIELD, M. RUSSELL-AULET, M. MAZARIEGOS, M. TIERNEY, R. SMITH, J. C. THORNTON, J. KEHAYIAS, D. A. WEBER, and F. A. DILMANIAN. Measuring body fat: calibrating the rulers. Intermethod comparisons in 389 normal Caucasian subjects. *Am. J. Physiol.* 261 ((*Endocrinol. Metab.* 24): E103–E108, 1991.
246. PLOUG, T., B. M. STALLKNECHT, O. PEDERSEN, B. B. KAHN, T. OHKUWA, J. VINTEN, and H. GALBO. Effect of endurance training on glucose transport capacity and glucose transporter expression in rat skeletal muscle. *Am. J. Physiol.* 259 (*Endocrinol. Metab.* 22): E778–E786, 1990.
247. POEHLMAN, E. T., E. M. BERKE, J. R. JOSEPH, A. W. GARDNER, S. M. KATZMAN-ROOKS, and M. I. GORAN. Influence of aerobic capacity, body composition, and thyroid hormones on the age-related decline in resting metabolic rate. *Metabolism* 41: 915–921, 1992.
248. POEHLMAN, E. T., T. L. MCAULIFFE, D. R. VAN HOUTEN, and E. DANFORTH. Influence of age and endurance training on metabolic rate and hormones in healthy men. *Am. J. Physiol.* 259 (*Endocrinol. Metab.* 22): E66–E72, 1990.
249. POEHLMAN, E. T., C. L. MELBY, and S. F. BADYLAK. Relation of age and physical exercise status on metabolic rate in younger and older healthy men. *J. Gerontol.* 46: B54–B58, 1991.
250. POEHLMAN, E. T., C. L. MELBY, S. F. BADYLAK, and J. CALLES. Aerobic fitness and resting energy expenditure in young adult males. *Metabolism* 38: 85–90, 1989.
251. POLLOCK, M. L., C. FOSTER, D. KNAPP, J. L. ROD, and D. H. SCHMIDT. Effect of age and training on aerobic capacity and body composition of master athletes. *J. Appl. Physiol.* 62: 625–731, 1987.
252. POLLOCK, M. L., H. S. MILLER, and J. WILMORE. Physiological characteristics of champion American track athletes 40 to 75 years of age. *J. Gerontol.* 29: 645–649, 1974.
253. PROBART, C. K., M. NOTELOVITZ, D. MARTIN, F. Y. KHAN, and C. FIELDS. The effect of moderate aerobic exercise on physical fitness among women 70 years and older. *Maturitas* 14: 49–56, 1991.
254. PROFANT, G. R., R. G. EARLY, K. L. NILSON, F. KUSUMI, V. HOFER, and R. A. BRUCE. Responses to maximal exercise in healthy middle-aged women. *J. Appl. Physiol.* 33: 595–599, 1972.
255. REAVEN, E., D. WRIGHT, C. E. MONDON, R. SOLOMON, H. HO, and G. REAVEN. Effect of age and diet on insulin secretion and insulin action in the rat. *Diabetes* 32: 175–180, 1983.
256. REAVEN, E. P., G. GOLD, and G. REAVEN. Effect of age on glucose-stimulated insulin release by the beta cell of the rat. *J. Clin. Invest.* 64: 591–599, 1979.
257. REITMAN, J. S., B. VASQUEZ, I. KLIMES, and M. NAUGLESPARAN. Improvement of glucose homeostasis after exercise-training in non-insulin-dependent diabetes. *Diabetes Care* 7: 434–441, 1984.
258. RETZLAFF, E., J. FONTAINE, and W. FURUTA. Effect of daily

exercise on lifespan of albino rats. *Geriatrics* 21: 171–177, 1966.
259. RICE, C. L., D. A. CUNNINGHAM, D. H. PATERSON, and M. S. LEFCOE. Arm and leg composition determined by computed tomography in young and elderly men. *Clin. Physiol.* 9: 207–220, 1988.
260. RICE, C. L., D. A. CUNNINGHAM, D. H. PATERSON, and P. A. RECHNITZER. Strength in an elderly population. *Arch. Phys. Med. Rehab.* 70: 391–397, 1989.
261. RICO, H., M. REVILLA, E. R. HERNANDEZ, L. F. VILLA, M. A. DEL BUERGO, and A. L. ALONSO. Age- and weight-related changes in total body bone mineral in men. *Miner. Electrolyte Metab.* 17: 321–323, 1991.
262. RISSER, W. L., E. J. LEE, A. LEBLANC, H. B. W. POINDEXTER, J. M. H. RISSER, and V. SCHNEIDER. Bone density in eumenorrheic female college athletes. *Med. Sci. Sports Exerc.* 22: 570–574, 1990.
263. RIVERA, A. M., A. E. PELLS, III, S. P. SADY, M. A. SADY, E. M. CULLINANE, and P. D. THOMPSON. Physiological factors associated with the lower maximal oxygen consumption of master runners. *J. Appl. Physiol.* 66: 949–954, 1989.
264. ROBINSON, S. Experimental studies of physical fitness in relation to age. *Arbeitsphysiologie* 10: 251–323, 1938.
265. ROBINSON, S., D. B. DILL, R. D. ROBINSON, S. P. TZANKOFF, and J. A. WAGNER. Physiological aging of champion runners. *J. Appl. Physiol.* 41: 46–51, 1976.
266. ROCKWELL, J. C., A. M. SORENSEN, S. BAKER, D. LEAHEY, J. L. STOCK, J. MICHAELS, and D. T. BARAN. Weight training decreases vertebral bone density in premenopausal women: a prospective study. *J. Clin. Endocrinol. Metab.* 71: 988–993, 1990.
267. RODEHEFFER, R. J., G. GERSTENBLITH, L. C. BECKER, J. L. FLEG, M. L. WEISFELDT, and E. G. LAKATTA. Exercise cardiac output is maintained with advancing age in healthy human subjects: cardiac dilatation and increased stroke volume compensate for a diminished heart rate. *Circulation* 69: 203–213, 1984.
268. RODNICK, K. J., E. J. HENRIKSEN, D. E. JAMES, and J. O. HOLLOSZY. Exercise-training, glucose transporters and glucose transport in rat skeletal muscles. *Am. J. Physiol.* 262 (*Cell Physiol.* 31): C9–C14, 1992.
269. RODNICK, K. J., J. O. HOLLOSZY, C. E. MONDON, and D. E. JAMES. Effects of exercise training on insulin-regulatable glucose transporter protein levels in rat skeletal muscle. *Diabetes* 39: 1425–1429, 1990.
270. ROGERS, M. A., J. M. HAGBERG, W. H. MARTIN, A. A. EHSANI, and J. O. HOLLOSZY. Decline in $\dot{V}O_{2max}$ with aging in master athletes and sedentary men. *J. Appl. Physiol.* 68: 2195–2199, 1990.
271. ROGERS, M. A., D. S. KING, J. M. HAGBERG, A. A. EHSANI, and J. O. HOLLOSZY. Effect of 10 days of inactivity on glucose tolerance in master athletes. *J. Appl. Physiol.* 68: 1833–1837, 1990.
272. ROGERS, M. A., C. YAMAMOTO, J. M. HAGBERG, W. H. MARTIN, III, A. A. EHSANI, and J. O. HOLLOSZY. Effects of 6 d of exercise training on responses to maximal and submaximal exercise in middle-aged men. *Med. Sci. Sports Exerc.* 20: 260–264, 1988.
273. ROGERS, M. A., C. YAMAMOTO, D. S. KING, J. M. HAGBERG, A. A. EHSANI, and J. O. HOLLOSZY. Improvement in glucose tolerance after one week of exercise in patients with mild NIDDM. *Diabetes Care* 11: 613–618, 1988.
274. ROWE, J. W., K. L. MINAKER, J. A. PALLOTTA, and J. S. FLIER. Characterization of the insulin resistance of aging. *J. Clin. Invest.* 71: 1581–1587, 1983.
275. RUBNER, M. *Das Problem der Lebensdauer und seine Beziehungen zur Wachstum und Ernährung,* Munich: Oldenbourg, 1908.

276. SALTIN, B., G. BLOMQUIST, J. H. MITCHELL, R. L. JOHNSON, K. WILDENTHAL, and C. B. CHAPMAN. Response to exercise after bed rest and after training. *Circulation* 38: 1–78, 1968.
277. SARTIN, J. L., M. CHAUDHURI, S. FARINA, and R. C. ADELMAN. Regulation of insulin secretion by glucose during aging. *J. Gerontol.* 41: 30–35, 1986.
278. SATO, Y., A. IGUCHI, and N. SAKAMOTO. Biochemical determination of training effects using insulin clamp technique. *Horm. Metab. Res.* 16: 483–486, 1984.
279. SCHNEIDER, S. H., L. F. AMOROSA, A. K. KACHADORIAN, and N. B. RUDERMAN. Studies of the mechanisms of improved glucose control during regular exercise in type 2 (non-insulin dependent) diabetes. *Diabetologia* 26: 355–360, 1984.
280. SCHOELLER, D. A. Changes in total body water with age. *Am. J. Clin. Nutr.* 50: 1176–1181, 1989.
281. SCHWARTZ, R. S., W. P. SHUMAN, V. LARSON, K. C. CAIN, G. W. FELLINGHAM, J. C. BEARD, S. E. KAHN, J. R. STRATTON, M. D. CERQUEIRA, and I. B. ABRASS. The effect of intensive endurance exercise training on body fat distribution in young and older men. *Metabolism* 40: 545–551, 1991.
282. SEALS, D. R., J. M. HAGBERG, W. K. ALLEN, B. F. HURLEY, G. P. DALSKY, A. A. EHSANI, and J. O. HOLLOSZY. Glucose tolerance in young and older athletes and sedentary men. *J. Appl. Physiol.* 56: 1521–1525, 1984.
283. SEALS, D. R., J. M. HAGBERG, B. F. HURLEY, A. A. EHSANI, and J. O. HOLLOSZY. Endurance training in older men and women 1. Cardiovascular responses to exercise. *J. Appl. Physiol.* 57: 1024–1029, 1984.
284. SEALS, D. R., J. M. HAGBERG, B. F. HURLEY, A. A. EHSANI, and J. O. HOLLOSZY. Effects of endurance training on glucose tolerance and plasma lipids in older men and women. *JAMA* 252: 645–649, 1984.
285. SEIDELL, J. C., A. OOSTERLEE, P. DEURENBERG, J. G. A. J. HAUTVAST, and J. H. J. RUIJS. Abdominal fat depots measured with computed tomography: effects of degree of obesity, sex, and age. *Eur. J. Clin. Invest.* 42: 805–815, 1988.
286. SELYE, H., and G. TUCHWEBER. Stress in relation to aging and disease. In: *Hypothalamus, Pituitary and Aging,* edited by A. V. Everitt and J. A. Burgess. Springfield, IL: Thomas, 1976, p. 553–569.
287. SHIMOKATA, H., D. C. MULLER, J. L. FLEG, J. SORKIN, A. W. ZIEMBA, and R. ANDRES. Age as independent determinant of glucose tolerance. *Diabetes* 40: 44–51, 1991.
288. SHIMOKATA, H., J. D. TOBIN, D. C. MULLER, D. ELAHI, P. J. COON, and R. ANDRES. Studies in the distribution of body fat: I. Effects of age, sex, and obesity. *J. Gerontol.* 44: M66–M73, 1989.
289. SIRI, W. E. Gross composition of the body. In: *Advances in Biological and Medical Physics,* edited by J. H. Lawrence and C. A. Tobias. New York: Academic Press, 1956, p. 4.
290. SLONAKER, J. R. The normal activity of the albino rat from birth to natural death, its rate of growth, and duration of life. *J. Anim. Behav.* 2: 20–42, 1912.
291. SNEAD, D. B., S. J. BIRGE, and W. M. KOHRT. Age-related differences in body composition by hydrodensitometry and dual-energy x-ray absorptiometry. *J. Appl. Physiol.* 74: 770–775, 1993.
292. SNOW-HARTER, C., and R. MARCUS. Exercise, bone mineral density, and osteoporosis. *Exerc. Sports Sci. Rev.* 19: 351–388, 1991.
293. SOUMINEN, H., E. HEIKKINEN, H. LIESEN, D. MICHEL, and W. HOLLMAN. Effects of 8 weeks' endurance training on skeletal muscle metabolism in 56–70-year-old sedentary men. *Eur. J. Appl. Physiol. Occup. Physiol.* 37: 173–180, 1977.
294. SPARROW, D., G. A. BORKAN, S. G. GERZOF, C. WISNIEWSKI, and C. K. SILBERT. Relationship of fat distribution to glucose

tolerance: results of computed tomography in male participants of the Normative Aging Study. *Diabetes* 35: 411–415, 1986.
295. SPINA, R. J., T. OGAWA, W. M. KOHRT, W. H. MARTIN, III, J. O. HOLLOSZY, and A. A. EHSANI. Differences in cardiovascular adaptations to endurance exercise training between older men and women. *J. Appl. Physiol.* 75: 849–855, 1993.
296. SPINA, R. J., T. OGAWA, T. R. MILLER, W. M. KOHRT, and A. A. EHSANI. Effect of exercise training on left ventricular performance in older women free of cardiopulmonary disease. *Am. J. Cardiol.* 71: 99–104, 1993.
297. SPURGEON, H. A., M. F. STEINBACH, and E. G. LAKATTA. Chronic exercise prevents characteristics age-related changes in cardiac contraction. *Am. J. Physiol.* 244 (*Heart Circ. Physiol.* 15): H513–H518, 1983.
298. STALBERG, E., O. BORGES, M. ERICSSON, B. ESSEN-GUSTAVSSON, P. R. W. FAWCETT, L. O. NORDESJO, B. NORDGREN, and R. UHLIN. The quadriceps femoris muscle in 20–70 year old subjects: relationship between knee extension torque, electrophysiological parameters and muscle fiber characteristics. *Muscle Nerve* 12: 382–389, 1989.
299. STARNES, J. W., R. E. BEYER, and D. W. EDINGTON. Myocardial adaptations to endurance exercise in aged rats. *Am. J. Physiol.* 245 (*Heart Circ. Physiol.* 16): H560–H566, 1983.
300. STARNES, J. W., G. CANTU, R. P. FARRAR, and J. P. KEHRER. Skeletal muscle lipid peroxidation in exercised and food-restricted rats during ageing. *J. Appl. Physiol.* 67: 69–75, 1989.
301. STARNES, J. W., E. CHEONG, and F. M. MATSCHINSKY. Hormone secretion by isolated perfused pancreas of aging Fischer 344 rats. *Am. J. Physiol.* 260 (*Endocrinol. Metab.* 23): E59–E66, 1991.
302. STEEN, B. Body composition and aging. *Nutr. Rev.* 46: 45–51, 1988.
303. STEINHAUS, L. A., R. E. DUSTMAN, R. O. RUHLING, R. Y. EMMERSON, S. C. JOHNSON, D. E. SHEARER, R. W. LATIN, J. W. SHIGEOKA, and W. H. BONEKAT. Aerobic capacity of older adults: a training study. *J. Sports Med. Phys. Fitness* 30: 163–172, 1990.
304. STILLMAN, R. J., T. G. LOHMAN, M. H. SLAUGHTER, and B. H. MASSEY. Physical activity and bone mineral content in women aged 30 to 85 years. *Med. Sci. Sports Exerc.* 18: 576–580, 1986.
305. TATE, C. A., G. E. TAFFET, E. K. HUDSON, S. L. BLAYLOCK, R. P. MCBRIDE, and L. H. MICHAEL. Enhanced calcium uptake of cardiac sarcoplasmic reticulum in exercise-trained old rats. *Am. J. Physiol.* 258 (*Heart Circ. Physiol.* 29): H431–H435, 1990.
306. TAYLOR, R., P. RAM, L. R. ZIMMET, L. R. RAPER, and H. RINGROSE. Physical activity and prevalence of diabetes in Melanesian and Indian men in Fiji. *Diabetologia* 27: 578–582, 1984.
307. TERJUNG, R. L., K. M. BALDWIN, W. W. WINDER, and J. O. HOLLOSZY. Glycogen repletion in different types of muscle and in liver after exhausting exercise. *Am. J. Physiol.* 225: 1387–1391, 1974.
308. THOMAS, D. P., R. J. MCCORMICK, S. D. ZIMMERMAN, R. K. VADLAMUDI, and L. E. GOSSELIN. Aging- and training-induced alterations in collagen characteristics of rat left ventricle and papillary muscle. *Am. J. Physiol.* 263 (*Heart Circ. Physiol.* 34): H778–H783, 1992.
309. TROVATI, M., Q. CARTA, F. CARALOT, S. VITALI, C. BANAUDI, P. G. LUCCHINA, F. FIECCHI, G. EMANUELLI, and G. LENTI. Influence of physical training on blood glucose control, glucose tolerance, insulin secretion, and insulin action in non-insulin-dependent diabetic patients. *Diabetes Care* 7: 416–420, 1984.
310. TZANKOFF, S. P., and NORRIS, A. H. Effect of muscle mass decrease on age related BMR changes. *J. Appl. Physiol.* 43: 1001–1006, 1977.
311. VANDERVOORT, A. A., and A. J. MCCOMAS. Contractile changes in opposing muscles of the human ankle joint with aging. *J. Appl. Physiol.* 61: 361–367, 1986.
312. VAN LOAN, M. D., and L. S. KOEHLER. Use of total-body electrical conductivity for the assessment of body composition in middle-aged and elderly individuals. *Am. J. Clin. Nutr.* 51: 548–552, 1990.
313. VOGEL, J. A., J. F. PATTON, R. P. MELLO, and W. L. DANIELS. An analysis of aerobic capacity in a large United States population. *J. Appl. Physiol.* 60: 494–500, 1986.
314. WALFORD, R. L., S. HARRIS, and R. WEINDRUCH. Dietary restriction and aging: historical phases, mechanisms, current directions. *J. Nutr.* 117: 1650–1654, 1987.
315. WALLBERG-HENRIKSSON, H., and J. O. HOLLOSZY. Activation of glucose-transport in diabetic muscle: responses to contraction and insulin. *Am. J. Physiol.* 249 (*Cell Physiol.* 18): C233–C237, 1985.
316. WATSON, P. E., I. D. WATSON, and R. D. BATT. Total body water volumes for adult males and females estimated from simple anthropometric measurements. *Am. J. Clin. Nutr.* 33: 27–39, 1980.
317. WEINDRUCH, R., and R. L. WALFORD. *The Retardation of Aging and Disease by Dietary Restriction.* Springfield, IL: Thomas, 1988.
318. WENDORF, M., and I. D. GOLDFINE. Archaeology of NIDDM: excavation of the "thrifty" genotype. *Diabetes* 40: 161–165, 1991.
319. WEST, K. M. Diabetes in American Indians and other native populations of the new world. *Diabetes* 23: 841–855, 1974.
320. WHITE, T. P., and S. T. DEVOR. Skeletal muscle regeneration and plasticity of grafts. *Exerc. Sports Sci. Rev.* 21: 263–295, 1993.
321. WOMERSLEY, J., J. V. G. A. DURNIN, K. BODDY, and M. MAHAFFY. Influence of muscular development, obesity, and age on the fat-free mass of adults. *J. Appl. Physiol.* 41: 223–229, 1976.
322. WOOD, P. D., M. L. STEFANICK, P. T. WILLIAMS, and W. L. HASKELL. The effects on plasma lipoproteins of a prudent weight-reducing diet, with or without exercise, in overweight men and women. *N. Engl. J. Med.* 325: 461–466, 1991.
323. YARASHESKI, K. E., J. J. ZACHWIEJA, and D. M. BIER. Acute effects of resistance exercise on muscle protein synthesis rate in young and elderly men and women. *Am. J. Physiol.* 265 (*Endocrinol. Metab.* 28): E210–E214, 1993.
324. YOUNG, A., M. STOKES, and M. CROWE. The size and strength of the quadriceps muscles of old and young men. *Clin. Physiol.* 5: 145–154, 1985.
325. YOUNG, J. C., M. CHEN, and J. O. HOLLOSZY. Maintenance of the adaptation of skeletal muscle mitochondria to exercise in old rats. *Med. Sci. Sports Exerc.* 15: 243–246, 1983.
326. YU, B. P., E. J. MASORO, I. MURATA, H. A. BERTRAND, and F. T. LYND. Life span study of SPF Fischer 344 male rats fed ad libitum or restricted diets: longevity, growth, lean body mass and disease. *J. Gerontol.* 37: 130–141, 1982.
327. ZAVARONI, I., E. DALL'AGLIO, F. BRUSCHI, E. BORONA, O. ALPI, A. PEZZAROSSA, and U. BUTTURINI. Effect of age and environmental factors on glucose tolerance and insulin secretion in a worker population. *J. Am. Geriatr. Soc.* 34: 271–275, 1986.

Index

acid-base balance 487
acromegaly 387
adipocytes 126–128, 132, 653–654
  lipolysis 126
adipose tissue 96, 102, 150, 162, 165, 314, 455
  subcutaneous 314
adipose tissue–free weight 150
adiposity 97, 103, 106, 129, 132, 134–135, 651, 654, 657 (also see obesity)
adrenal cortex 128, 355–356, 381–385, 387, 491
  effects of adrenalectomy 383
  glucocorticoids 128, 355–356, 381–384, 387
    circadian rhythms 381
    corticosterone 382
    cortisol 381
    hydrocortisone acetate 384
    plasma corticosterone 382–383
    plasma cortisol 381–382
    plasma free corticosterone 383
    plasma free cortisol 381–382
    prednisolone phosphate 383
    salivary cortisol 381
  mineralocorticoids 381, 384, 387, 491
    acid-hydrolyzable glucuronide conjugate of aldosterone 384
    aldosterone 381, 384, 391
    plasma aldosterone 384
  reticularis 384
  steroids 381–385
adrenal gland, weight 383
adrenocorticotrophic hormone (ACTH) 382, 384
age-associated disease processes 15, 40–41
  age-dependent diseases 15
  age-related diseases 15
age-associated diseases 29–31, 83–86, 164–167
  influence of adiposity 164–167
  risk factors 29–31, 83–84, 86
age-associated physiological changes 14–17
aging 3, 8–9, 13–15, 25, 27–30, 54, 372, 378, 381–382, 385–387, 592, 613–631
  changes during 25
  definition of 3, 13, 25, 54, 592
  individual differences 30
  interventions 613–631
  maturational changes 25
  phenotype 3, 9, 14–15, 372, 378, 381–382, 385–387
  stability during 25, 27–28, 30
  stability of individual differences 29–30
  universality of 8
aging and health 86
aging populations, variance in 30–31
aging studies, design issues 16, 25–29, 31–34, 38, 83–92, 327, 329, 363, 413, 454–455, 486, 488, 649–650

causal inferences 32–33, 83, 86
cross-sectional designs 16, 25–26, 28, 33, 38, 84, 327, 329, 363, 413, 454, 486, 649–650
  cohort effects 84, 650
cross-sequential designs 25, 27
human subjects 83–92
longitudinal designs 16, 25–29, 33–34, 83–86, 90, 327, 329, 363, 413, 455, 488
mathematical modeling 31–32
population based 85
practice effect 27
problem of attrition 28, 84, 89
problem of disease 28–29
sample representativeness 28, 85
secular effects 26–27
subject participation 89–90
subject selection 85
time-sequential designs 25, 27
albumin 180, 185, 195, 395
  serum 395
albumin gene 186, 190
aldolase 217–218, 221
algae 592–593
allergy 312, 561
alpha$_{2u}$-globulin 180, 185–186, 194
Alzheimer's disease 85–89, 325–327, 332–337, 344–349, 352–357, 383, 499, 529
  aborative sprouting neurites 334–335
  amygdala 334
  amyloid 334
  amyloid precursor protein 335, 354
  antibodies recognizing cholinergic neurons 357
  antibodies recognizing microglia 357
  antibrain antibodies 357
  aphasia 334
  apolipoprotein E 335–336
  apolipoprotein E-4 335
  apraxia 334
  association neocortex 334
  basal nucleus of Meynert 334
  beta-amyloid 335–337, 349, 354, 357
  beta-amyloid-induced immune response to microglia 357
  choline acetyltransferase 333–334
  cholinergic projection system 334, 352
  degenerating neurites 334–335
  dopaminergic projections 344
  education, influence of 337
  entorhinal cortex 334
  frontal lobe 334
  glutaminergic projections 334
  hippocampus 334
  immune system 356–357
  interleukin-1 357
  locus ceruleus 334

  memory 334
    delayed recall 334
  neocortical association areas 334
  neuritic plaque biogenesis 357
  neuritic plaques 333–334, 354
  neurofibrillary tangles 332–334, 336, 357
  norepinephrine projections 334
  paired helical filaments 335–336
  parahippocampal areas 334
  perforant pathway 332, 348
  risk factors 336
    head injury 336
    myocardial infarction 336
  selective brain region vulnerability 334
  senile plaques 353
  serotonergic projections 334
  sprouting fibers 354–355
    re-express neonatal factors 355
  tacrine 334
  tau protein 335–336
  therapeutic use of nerve growth factor 352
  visual agnosia 334
amyloidosis 336, 495
androgen receptors 195
androgens 378–381, 384–385, 387, 499, 577, 624–625, 654
  adrenal 381, 384–385, 387, 577, 624–625
  dehydroepiandrosterone (DHEA) 381, 384, 387, 577, 624–625
  plasma dehydroepiandrosterone (DHEA) 384
  plasma dehydroepiandrosterone sulfate 385
  dihydrotestosterone 379, 654
  testicular, Leydig cells 378–379
  testosterone 379–380, 387, 499
    bioavailable 380
    plasma levels 379–380
    sex hormone binding globulin 380
aneuploidy 11
angiogenesis 313
angiotensin 415
animal models for aging studies 37–52, 109–113, 120, 122, 125, 188, 195, 197, 204, 241–242, 346–347, 378–384, 386, 414, 436, 441–442, 452, 541, 634–635, 646, 653–654
  bats 111–112
  birds 112
  Caenorhabditis elegans 48
  carnivores 48
  cats 48
  commonly used species 45–47
  crustaceans 46–47
  Daphnia 110
  diet 41–43
    ad libitum feeding 41
    AIN-76 41
    cancer 41–43
    closed formula 41

animal models for aging studies, diet (*continued*)
  dietary restriction 41
  lymphoma 41–42
  open formula 41
 diversity of 37
 dogs 48, 382, 436
  beagles 436
 Drosophila 37–39, 46–48, 109–110, 113, 195, 197, 204, 383–384
 environmental conditions 41–44
 exercise 44
 frogs 46–47
 genetics 44–45
 gerbils 46–47
 health status 38, 40
 housing 43–44
 husbandry 43–44
 late-life disease patterns 40–41
 longevity characteristics 40
 marsupials 111
 Mastomys 46–48
 mice 39–40, 45, 48, 188, 347, 378–379, 381–383
  $C3B10F_1$ strain 40
  C57BL/6J strain 379, 381, 383
  Cr1:CD-1 (ICR)BR strain 381–382
  DBA/2J strain 383
  MRL/lpr strain 39
  NIA subsidized strains 45
  NZB strain 39
  (NZB × NZW) F_1 strain 39
  senescence accelerated strains 39, 347
  transgenic 48
 microbial status 43–44
  specific pathogen-free (SPF) 44
 mollusks 46–47
 nematodes 195, 204
 nonhuman primates 40, 49, 111, 120, 346, 378–380, 382, 384
  baboons 382, 384
  bonnet macaques 379–380
  chimpanzees 111
  dietary restriction 49
  monkeys 346
  pigtail macaques 49, 379
  rhesus macaques 40, 49, 120, 379
  squirrel monkeys 49
 Peromyscus 45–48, 188
 rabbits 40
 rats 38–39, 44–45, 47–48, 122, 125, 241–242, 378–379, 381–382, 386, 414, 441–442, 452, 541, 634–635, 646, 653–654
  Brown-Norway strain 48, 382
  F-344 strain 38, 47–48, 122, 381–382, 386, 441, 645, 653
  gnotobiotic 541
  hypertensive strains 241–242
  Lobund-Wistar strain 44, 48
  Long-Evans strain 382, 386, 634–635, 646, 653
  nephropathy 42
  NIA subsidized strains 45
  spontaneously hypertensive strains 39, 452
  Sprague-Dawley strain 45, 122, 125, 382, 441–442, 634, 646, 653
  testicular interstitial cell tumors 47
  Wistar strain 125, 441, 634
  Wistar-Kyoto strain 441
 rodents 37, 379
 sheep 46–47
 Syrian hamsters 381–382
antioxidant defenses 113
antioxidant enzymes 222
antioxidant feedings 621–622
apocrine glands 313–314
 androgen stimulation 314
apoptosis 10, 596; *see also* cell death
arteries 165, 235, 272, 414–417, 431, 457
 aorta 165
 arterial impedance 417, 431
  impedance modulus 417
 collagen 415
 elastic fibrils 415
 elastin 415
 interstitial matrix 415
 mechanical properties 414–417
  stiffness 414–417
  volume elasticity 414–415
 pulse wave velocity 415
 reflected pulse waves 415
 rigidity 235, 272
 structure 414–417, 457
  diameter 414
  wall thickness 414
arteriosclerosis and collagen 241
arthritis 383, 641
ascorbate 112
atherosclerosis 57, 138, 165–167, 275, 415, 488, 495, 533, 657
atherosclerotic plaques 385
athletes, endurance trained 655–656
atrial natriuretic factor 491
autocrines 310
autoimmunity 317, 385
autonomic nervous system 421, 428, 433–441, 505, 525–526; *see also* sympathetic nervous system; parasympathetic nervous system

basal metabolic rate (BMR) 98–104, 106, 108, 112
basement membrane 237
beta-carotene 112
bile 518–519, 535–538
 bile salts 518–519, 535
  deconjugation by bacteria 518–519
 cholelithiasis 536
 cholesterol 535–537
 composition 536
 digestive functions 535
  lipids 535
  triglycerides 535
 flow 536
 gallstones 536–538
 immunoglobulins 535
 mucus 535
 sterol vitamins 535
biodiversity 593
biological age 8–9, 17, 31, 249
biomarkers of aging 9, 17, 31, 249–250, 261–262, 599–600, 603, 613
 advanced glycation end-products 261–262
 non-linear dynamics 599–600
 tail tendon breaking time 249
blood 137–138, 218, 319, 355–356, 381, 395, 403, 436, 523
 clotting 319, 395, 523
  vitamin K 523
 glycosylated hemoglobin 137
 hematocrit 381
 leukocytes 355–356
 monocytes 138, 319, 403
 neutrophils 319
 platelets 319, 436
 reticulocytes 218
blood pressure 134, 148, 165, 416–417, 420, 427–428, 431; *also see* hypertension
 aortic 420
 central arterial pulse pressure 416
 diastolic 417, 427–428
 dietary sodium chloride 416
 mean 427–428
 pulse pressure 416
 systolic 416
body cell mass 158
body composition 95, 113, 150, 158–161, 164, 514, 647–652
 measurement 158–161
  bioelectric impedance 160–161
  in vivo neutron activation analysis 158–160
 multicompartment models 649
body density 156, 648–649
body fat 96–97, 129, 132, 149–167, 385–386, 639, 648–652, 654–656; *see also* adipose tissue; adiposity; obesity
 distribution 129, 132, 149, 161–162, 164–167, 651–652, 654–656
  computerized tomography measurement 162
  exercise 652
  magnetic resonance imaging measurement 162
  measurements 161–162, 166
  waist to hip circumference measurement 161–162, 166
 exercise 650
 measurements 150–161, 650
  direct method 150–153
  indirect methods 153–160, 650
body fat–free mass 96–102, 104, 108, 113, 150, 156, 158, 161, 648–652; *see also* lean body mass
 endurance training 650
body height 647–648
body mass index (BMI) 147, 149, 153–155, 165–166, 385
body potassium 648
body surface area 156
body temperature 16, 105–107
 Arrhenius equation 105
 core 106–107
 Q_{10} 106
 set point 106
body water 156, 158–159, 648, 650
 measurement by isotope dilution 156, 158

body weight 164–165, 647–648
  exercise 648
  Metropolitan relative weights 164
bone 98, 160, 185, 319–320, 379, 381, 395–412, 523, 649–651
  cells 396, 401–402
    osteoblast progenitor cells 402
    osteoblasts 396
    osteoclast progenitor cells 401
    osteoclasts 396
    osteocytes 396
  composition 395–396
    calcium phosphate 395
    hydroxyapatite 395
  density 98, 319–320
  formation, vitamin K 523
  formation to resorption coupling 401
  Harvesian system 404
  loss 379, 395, 397–406, 650
    alcohol 405–406
    appendicular 397
    appropriateness of rat model 400–401
    biphosphonate therapy 400
    caffeine 405–406
    cancellous bone 400
    cortical bone 400
    dietary calcium 398, 405
    dietary phosphorus 405
    dietary protein 405
    distal radius 401
    estrogens 399
    exercise 400, 404–405
    hematopoiesis-local factor hypothesis 401–404
    intestinal calcium absorption 399
    mechanical stress 404
    menopause 650
    ovarian hormone actions 398
    ovariectomized premenopausal women 399
    ovariectomized-induced in rats 400–401, 403
    postmenopausal 399–400
    postmenopausal rat model 400–401
    risk factors 404–405
    smoking 405–406
    tamoxifen therapy 400
    trabecular 379
    vertebral 397
    vertebral cancellous bone 401
  mass 160, 185
    dual photon absorptiometry measurement 160
  matrix 395–396
    collagen 395
    fibronectin 396
    matrix-gla-protein 396
    osteocalcin 396
    osteopontin 396
    proteoglycans 396
    sialoprotein 396
  mineral content 650–651
    exercise 651
    physical activity 651
  mineral density 399–400
  morphometric proteins 401
  remodeling 396–397
    "basic multicellular units" (BMUS) 396
    basic structural unit (BSU) 396
    function of 396
  resorption 398, 400
    osteoclastic 400
  turnover 400
bone marrow 312, 401–402, 568–569, 572, 577
  hematopoietic mononuclear cells 401–402
  prothymocytes 569
  stem cells 568
  TRAP-positive multinucleated cells 401–402
brain 138, 325–337, 345–362, 381–383, 385, 496, 498, 604, 621; see also Alzheimer's disease; nervous system; sense organs and sensation
  amygdala 333
  anxiolytics 349
  benzodiazepine receptors Types I and II 351
  "cage" convulsants 349
  cerebral blood flow 330–331
  cerebral metabolism 330–331
  cholecystokinin 350
  choline acetyltransferase 333
  cognition 138, 325–327, 332–333, 337, 345, 349–350, 381–382
    impairment 381–382
    phosphatidylserine effect 349
  compensatory plasticity 345
  cortical atrophy 332
  degenerating terminals repair 355
  dementia 496
  deprenyl 333
  depression 329, 349–351, 498
    benzodiazepines 349–351
    chlorazepate 350
    chlordiazepoxide 350
    diazepam 350
    prazepam 350
  entorhinal cortex 332, 348, 353–355
  extrapyramidal system 333
  frontal cortex 346
  glial cells 333–335, 352, 355–357
    astrocytes 333–335, 352, 355
    microglia 334, 355–357
  hippocampus 327, 332–333, 346–347, 352, 354–357, 383
    dentate gyrus 347, 354–356
    neuron death 383
    neuropeptide Y m-RNA 383
    pro-opiomelanocortin m-RNA 383
    pyramidal cells 383
    reinnervation 356
  hypnotics 349
  injury 351
  intellectual performance 326
  ischemic damage 355
  learning 352
  memory 326, 328–329, 332, 337, 352, 382, 385
    "benign forgetfulness" 326
    episodic 328
    procedural 328
    semantic 328
    spatial 382
    working 329
  1-methyl-4-phenyl, 1,2,3,6, tetrahydropyridine (MPTP) 333, 353, 621
  microtubular system 336
  neocortex 327
  neuritic damage, complement factors 357
  neuritic plaques 332
  neurofibrillary changes 332
  neurons 326, 332, 345–346, 348, 351–353
    axon sprouting 345
    loss 326, 332, 346, 348, 351–353
    regrowth 345
  occipital cortex 346
  parietal cortex 346
  perforant pathway 353
  plasticity 333, 351
  remodeling 358
  repair 358
  reserve 337
  semantic knowledge 327–328
  synaptic reorganization 348
  temporal neocortex 333
  volume 327
  weight 327, 332
  "wisdom" 604
brain stem 332–333, 381; see also nervous system
  basal nucleus of Meynert 332
  locus ceruleus 332
  stria terminalis 381
  striatum 333
  substantia nigra 332–333
brown adipose tissue 104, 107–108, 639
Build Study 147, 154, 164

calcitonin 195, 398–400, 406
  deficiency 406
  hetrogeneity of circulating forms 400
  plasma 399–400
  thyroid source 400
calcium 395–396, 398–399, 405, 521–522
  adaptation to low dietary intake 521
  body 395
  extracellular 395
  homeostasis 395–396, 398, 522
  recommended daily allowance 405
  urinary 399
caloric restriction. See dietary restriction
cancer 57, 85, 113, 161, 165, 188, 309, 316–318, 365, 378–379, 381, 383–384, 495–496, 500, 542–543, 576, 594
  breast carcinoma 379, 384
  colon 542–543
  colorectal 383
  endometrial carcinoma 379
  lung 85, 161
  multiple myeloma 496
  nephrotic syndrome association 495
  prostate carcinoma 381, 500
  skin 309, 316
    basal cell carcinoma 316
    mechanisms 316
    multiple hit theory 316
    squamous cell carcinoma 316

cancer and aging 15
carbohydrate metabolism 119–145, 385, 652–657; *see also* glucose entries
  exercise 652–657
  glucose-6-phosphate dehydrogenase 385
  reduced NADP 385
cardiovascular reserve 428–433
cardiovascular system 165, 378, 383–384, 413–474, 525, 535, 642–644; *see also* arteries; blood pressure; heart
  chemoreceptor reflex 428
  chronic physical conditioning 453–457
    middle-aged people 454
  coronary artery alpha$_1$-adrenergic receptors 436
  disease 165, 378, 383–384
  exercise response 642
  exercise training 643–644
  liver blood flow 535
  peripheral vascular resistance 417, 428, 431
    kidney 417
  postural reflexes 428–429
    baroreceptor sensitivity 428
    response to gradual tilt 428–429
    response to lower body negative pressure 428–429
  splanchnic blood flow 525
    noradrenergic innervation 525
  sympathetic modulation 433–440
  vasodilation, beta-adrenergic mediated 436
  venous responsiveness, alpha$_1$-adrenergic receptor 436
  ventricular-vascular coupling 418, 420–421
    aortic impedance 418
    vascular loading 418
cartilage 270–272, 274, 276
case-control studies 86
catalases 112, 180, 186, 195, 638
catecholamines 128–129, 133, 137, 425, 428
  plasma levels 428
cell culture systems for the study of aging 53–82, 247–248, 542, 605–606
  cell migration 54
  cell physiology 57
  cellular senescense markers 62–64, 68
    acute hyperthermia 68
    cell size 62
    chromosomal changes 63
    cytoplasmic microfilaments 62
    endoplasmic reticulum 62
    Golgi apparatus 62
    lysosomal bodies 62
    morphological alterations 62
    multinucleated cells 62
    nuclear size 62
    nucleolar size 62
    polyploidy 63
    saturation density 62
    tetraploidy 63
    vacuolated cytoplasm 62
  clonal size distribution 57
    donor age 57
  cloning efficiency 57
    diabetes mellitus 57
  cortisol 59
  cortisone 59
  epidermal 57
  fibroblasts 56–57, 67, 542
    phorbol esters 542
    skin 56
    WI-38 57, 67
  human diploid fibroblasts 69
  human liver cells 57
  immortality 53, 68–69
    embryonic stem cells 53
  immortalization 57
  IMR-90 cells 67
  indefinite life span 57
  lysosomal enzymes 57
  molecular senescence markers 62–65, 67–68, 72–73
    alpha (1) procollagen 63
    cathepsin B 65
    Cdc 2 64
    cell contact 62
    c-fos 64
    chromatin structure 64
    cip-1 72
    collagenese 63
    cyc A 64
    cyclin-dependent kinase 72
    cyclin-dependent kinase genes 67
    cyclins 67
    DNA content 63
    elongation factor I alpha 72
    epidermal growth factor (EGF) receptors 65
    extracellular matrix 62, 72
    fibronectin 63, 72
    histones 68
    inhibitors of DNA synthesis 68
    insulin-like growth factor I (IGF-I) 63
    insulin-like growth factor I receptors 63, 72
    P^{21} 73
    pic-1 73
    plasminogen activator inhibitor types 1 and 2 63
    proliferating cell nuclear antigen (PCNA) 68
    protein synthesis 64
    protein turnover 63
    RNA content 63
    RNA synthesis 64
    secretory proteins 62–63
    stromelysin 63
    TIMP-1 63
    waf-1 72
  nutritional requirements 60
  postmitotic population 62
  progeroid syndrome 63
  proliferation 55–59, 65–67, 69
    arachidonic acid metabolism 67
    calcium ions 67
    calcium mobilization 67
    calmodulin 67
    cell generation times 58
    crisis 69
    donor age 56–57
    epidermal growth factor (EGF) 66
    growth factors 65
    insulin-like growth factor-I (IGF-I) 66
    insulin-like growth factor-I receptor 66
    phosphodiesterase activity 67
    phospholipid turnover 67
    platelet-derived growth factor (PDGF) 66
    prostaglandin metabolism 67
    protein kinase A 67
    protein kinase C activation 67
    replication capacities 59
    serum 65
    tyrosine kinase activity 66
  proliferation and differentiation 57, 59
  proliferative life span 53, 57, 60–62, 64–65, 67, 70
    adeno-virus E1A 70
    alpha-tocopherol 65
    c-fos 60
    cumulative population doublings 61
    DNA replication 60
    DNA synthetic capacity 60
    Down syndrome 57
    endothelial cells 53
    fibroblasts 53
    glial cells 53
    glutathione 65
    human papilloma virus (HPV-E7) 70
    Hutchinson-Gilford syndrome 57
    hydrocortisone 60
    keratinocytes 53, 57
    lens cells 53
    monozygotic twins 57
    oxygen tension 65
    P^{53} protein binding activity 70
    phase out 62
    phorbol-12-myristate-13-acetate 60
    plasma membrane 60
    progeroid syndrome 57
    retinoblastoma (RB) protein 67, 70
    simian virus 40 (SV 40) 60
    simian virus 40 large T antigen 67, 70
    stochastic mechanisms 64–65
    vascular smooth muscle cells 53
    Werner syndrome 57
  senescence 605–606
  senescence and collagen 247–248
  senescence genetic mechanisms 68, 71–72
    c-DNA libraries 72
    cell fusion studies 68
    chicken SM22 gene 72
    DNA tumor viruses 68
    Drosophila MP20 gene 72
    EPC-1 (early PDLcDNA-1) 72
    HeLa cells 68
    heterokaryon 68
    human chromosome 1 71
    human chromosome 4 71
    LPC-1 (late PDL cDNA-1) 72
    mitochondrial genes 72
    monoclonal antibody (MAb) 72
    SDI-1 72
    senescence-associated gene (SAG) 72
    WS3–10 gene 72
    selective libraries 72–73
  signal transduction pathways 65–68

cell cycle 56, 63–64, 67–69, 72
  c-myc 64, 67
  DNA polymerase alpha 68
  G_0 phase 64, 68, 72
  G_1 block 63
  G_1 phase 63
  G_2 phase 64, 68
  H-ras 67
  mitosis 56, 64
  nuclear fluorescence 64
  nucleolar association 64
  ornithine decarboxylase 64
  S phase 64, 68
  signal transduction 64
  thymidine kinase 64
cell cycle-dependent genes 64
cell death 55–56, 59, 62, 345; *see also* apoptosis
  intracelluar clocks 56
cell membranes 11
cell proliferation 56
cell transformation 69
cellular senescence 549; *see also* cell culture systems for the study of aging
cellular signal transduction 387, 437–439, 450, 525, 535
  adenylate cyclase activity 437–438
  calcium 525
  cyclic AMP 438–439
  cyclic AMP phosphodiesterase 439
  cyclic AMP-dependent protein kinase 438
  G-proteins 437–438
  intracellular phosphorylation 438–439
  protein kinase activation 438–439
  protein kinase C 450, 525
central nervous system 346, 349, 352, 355–357, 479, 497, 525–526, 529; *see also* brain; nervous system
cerebrospinal fluid 349, 357
cerebrovascular disease 138, 167, 496, 499; *see also* stroke
chaos theory 13, 595
chaotic dynamics 595
chemical senses 363–375
cholesterol 148–149, 165, 167, 385
  plasma 148–149, 165, 167
  hypercholesterolemia 148–149
chondroitin 270
chondroitin sulfate 270, 272, 274–275
chromatin 175, 187–188, 222
chromosomal abnormalities 11
chronological age 249
chylomicrons 518
circadian clocks 600
coelenterates 592
collagen(s) 137, 235–264, 270–271, 274, 313, 315, 319, 381, 395
  chemical properties 236, 251–264, 395
    cross-links 236, 251–264
      glycation-mediated 257
      histidinoalanine 254–255
      lipid peroxidation-mediated 254–256
      lysyl oxidase-mediated 251–254
      Maillard/glycation reactions-mediated 256–264
      nonreducible cross-links 252–253
      pyridinium 395

  pyridinoline 252–253, 395
  reducible cross-links 252
  content of tissues 237–240
  degradation 246–247
  fibrillar 236
  glycosylated hydroxylysines 395
  hydroxyproline 241, 246–247, 381, 395
    urinary excretion 246–247, 381
  nonfibrillar 236
  physical properties 248–250
    solubility 248
    stiffness 249
    tensile strength 248–249
    thermostability 248
  prohydroxylase 313
  synthesis 245–246, 313, 315
  turnover 242–248
    tissue differences 242, 245
  types 237, 242
  vascular 242
collagenase 247, 319
colon 515, 521, 528–532
  calcium absorption 521
    1,25 dihydroxyvitamin D 521
    short-chain fatty acids 521
  cellular function 530–531
    cytochrome P450 531
    sodium absorption 530
  constipation 528, 531
  distal 530
  gastrocolic reflex 530
  goblet cells 531
  hydrogen production 515
  proximal 530
  short-chain fatty acid production 515, 531
  transit 528–529, 531
  fiber 531
component failure death 594
connective tissue 313, 317, 395, 641
coronary heart disease 29–30, 85–87, 162, 165, 167, 413–414, 417–418, 432, 639, 643
cross-sectional studies. *See* aging studies design issues
Cushing's syndrome 384
cytokines 106, 138, 180, 195, 310, 318, 346, 352, 355–357, 386, 401–403, 524, 557–559, 570, 574–576, 578–579, 625; *see also* growth factors
  gamma-interferon 401, 558, 574, 576, 579
  granulocyte/macrophage colony stimulating factor 180, 403
  interleukin-1 106, 138, 310, 352, 355–357, 386, 401, 403, 575
  interleukin-2 180, 195, 386, 524, 557–559, 576, 579, 625
  interleukin-3 180, 352, 355
  interleukin-4 557–558, 570, 579
  interleukin-5 558
  interleukin-6 402–403, 575, 578
  tumor necrosis factor-α 138, 401, 403

decubitus ulcers 309
dehydration 158, 491–492
dementias 325–326, 329, 333–334; *see also* Alzheimer's disease
  memory 333

deprenyl 621–624
  free-radical scavenger enzymes 623–624
dermatan sulfate 270, 274–275
dermatin sulfate 313
diabetes mellitus 106, 113, 119–120, 124, 132–138, 148–149, 162, 164–165, 236, 256, 261, 264–266, 279, 282, 385, 451, 490–491, 495, 526, 655
  hyperosmolar non-ketotic coma 136
  insulin deficient 451
  insulin-dependent 490
  non-insulin-dependent (NIDDM) 120, 124, 133–136, 138, 164–165, 451, 655–657
diatoms 592
diet 132–133, 579
  micronutrients 579
  vitamins 579
dietary restriction 7, 14, 41, 108–109, 112, 194–196, 202–204, 206, 220–222, 236, 249–250, 383, 542–543, 565, 577, 601, 614–621, 635, 637
  age-associated diseases 615–616
  $alpha_{2u}$-globin mRNA 195–196
  bone 616
  carcinogenic insult response 383
  cellular actions 619–621
  cellular membranes 619–620
    lipid peroxidation 620
  DNA repair 620
  free-radical damage 620–621
  free-radical scavenger enzymes 620
  gene expression 194–195, 220, 620
  glucocorticoids 618–619
  growth retardation 614
  immune function 616–617
  insulin 618
  intestinal alkaline phosphatase activity 542
  intestinal disaccharidase activity 542
  life span extension 614
  metabolic rate 618
  oxidative damage 621
  physiological processes 616–619
  protein biosynthesis 202–204, 206, 222
  protein degradation 220–222
  protein metabolism 617–618
  protein turnover 220, 222
1,25 dihydroxyvitamin D, plasma levels 520
disuse atrophy 600, 645, 657–658
DNA 11–12, 65, 72, 113, 175, 187–191, 193, 222, 316, 594
  AP-1 element 191
  cDNA 175
  cross-linking 11
  damage 316
  heat shock element 193
  methylation 11, 72, 188–191, 222
  repair 12, 65, 113, 316, 594
  structure 11
dopa decarboxylase 333
Down's syndrome 237, 335
drug metabolism 527

ear. *See* hearing
eccrine glands 313–314, 317
edema 158

elastin 235, 241, 264–269, 313, 315
  chemical properties 266–268
    amino acids 267
    desmosine 266–267
    fluorescence 268
    isodesmosine 266
    racemization 267
  physical properties 266
  synthesis 268–269
  turnover 268–269
electrolyte homeostasis 491–492
endocrine glands 377–394; see also individual glands and hormones
energy balance 105, 113, 655
  positive 655
energy expenditure 100–104, 108–109, 112–113, 655
  components of 101–104
  twenty-four hour 100–104
energy metabolism 95–118, 385
  caloric utilization 385
energy metabolism and body composition 96–97
energy utilization 104–105
enolase 217
epidemiological studies 33, 85–86
epinephrine 127, 129, 136, 427, 434
  plasma levels 427, 434
erythema 316
esophagus 526–527
  achalasia 527
  Barrett's esophagus 527
  lower esophogeal sphincter 526
  motor function 526
    monometry studies 526
    pH monitoring 527
  sphincters 526
  tertiary contractions 526
  neuropathy 526
  transit 526–527
  upper esophageal sphincter 526
estrogen receptors 406
  intestinal cells 406
  m-RNA 406
estrogens 378–380, 383, 387
  estradiol 378–380, 387
    plasma concentrations 379–380
    plasma levels, males 380
  replacement therapy 379
    all-cause mortality 379
    postmenopausal 379
    potential risks 379
evolutionary biology of aging 13–14, 17, 56, 608
  age-specific fitness 13, 17
  antagonistic pleiotropy 14, 56
  deleterious late-acting genes 14
  force of natural selection 13–14, 17
  group selection 13
evolutionary complexity 593
evolutionary pathways 592
execution-driven processes 596
exercise 99, 103, 107, 132, 167, 245, 331, 384–386, 414, 429–437, 453–458, 479, 633–666
  aerobic 132
  aerobic capacity 429–431, 642–643

aortic impedance 431
arterial impedance 431
arteriovenous oxygen difference 429–430
beta-adrenergic relaxant effect 434
blood pressure 431
  diastolic 431
  systolic 431
capacity 386, 479
dynamic 429–437
dyspnea 431
endurance, skeletal muscle adaptation 645
endurance training 99, 245, 453, 455, 645
  collagen synthesis 245
heart 430–434
  beta-adrenergic blockade 433
  beta-adrenergic modulation 433–434
  cardiac output 430
  ejection fraction 432
  left ventricular end-diastolic volume 431–432
  left ventricular end-systolic volume 431–432
  stroke volume index 432
heart rate 432, 454, 457
  maximal 454, 457
isometric 429
  maximal hand grip 429
isometric training 455–456
longevity 633–639
maximum oxygen consumption (VO_{2max}) 429–430, 433, 454–455, 479
peripheral vascular resistance 431
respiratory factors 479
training 639–644
  aerobic 639
  cardiac output 644
  endurance athletes 639–642
  lean body mass 639
  left ventricular filling 643
  ventricular ejection fraction 643
extracellular fluid 385, 491
  volume 491
extracellular matrix 235–276, 287, 450
extracellular water 96, 650
eye 138, 165, 276, 278–281, 283–288, 329–330; see also lens; vision
  aqueous humor 284
  cataractogenesis 283–284
    antioxidant defenses 283
  cataracts 165, 276, 278–281, 283–288, 329
    hydrogen peroxide 329
  glaucoma 329
  macular degeneration 329
  presbyopia 329
  pupillary constriction 329
  retina 330
  retinopathy 138, 165
  visual acuity 329

fasting 121, 123, 530; see also starvation
fatty acids 165
feeding 530
ferritin 217
fever 106, 355
fiber, dietary 522, 540
fibronectin 270, 396

fibronectin gene 185
fibrotic disease 237
folate 522–523
  dietary 522–523
    digestion by folate conjugase 522
    pteroylpolyglutamate 522
  plasma 523
food intake 385
fractals 13
Framingham Heart Study 147, 164, 167
free radicals 112, 259
  hydroxyl radicals 259
  superoxide radicals 259
fuel mobilization 107
functional assessment 87–89, 372
  cognitive assessment 88–89
  Older Americans Resources and Services Questionnaire 372
  physical function 87–88
fungi 593

gallbladder 535, 537, 539
  calcium mobilization, cholecystokinin-induced 537
  cholecystokinin receptors 537
  contractions 535, 537
    cholecystokinin-induced 535
  intracellular calcium 539
gallbladder disease 165, 539
gastrointestinal tract 123, 505–554; see also colon; esophagus; liver; mouth; pancreas; rectum, small intestine; stomach
  anus 530
  cellular proliferative activity 509, 538–543
    adaptive response 542
    alcohol 540
    cell turnover 540
    colon 542
    duodenum 541
    epidermal growth factor-receptor 542
    epithelial cell generation time 541
    esophagus 540–541
    gastrin-binding sites 541
    ileum 541
    intestinal resection 542
    jejunum 541
    metaphase arrest technique 541
    ornithine decarboxylase 540, 542
    polyamines 542
    postnatal development 540–541
    protein kinase C 542
    refeeding 541–542
    small intestine 541–542
    starvation 541–542
    stem cells 540
    stomach 540–541
    thymidine kinase 540, 542
    tyrosine kinase 542
  fecal incontinence 531–532
  hormones 123, 506–509, 525, 529–530, 532–534, 537–539, 541
    bombesin 532, 539
    cholecystokinin 525, 530, 532, 534, 537, 539
    gastric inhibitory polypeptide 123, 530

gastrin 506–509, 530, 532–533, 539, 541
gastrin family 530
gastrin-cholecystokinin family 538
metenkephalin 530
motilin 525, 529–530, 538–539
neurotensin 538–539
pancreatic polypeptides 538–539
pancreatic polypeptides family 538
peptides 538
secretin 525, 532, 534
secretin family 530
somatostatin 506–507, 509, 525, 538–539
substance P 538
vasointestinal peptide 525, 532, 538
motility 510, 525–532
  Auerbach's plexus 529
  interdigestive migrating myoelectric complex 530
  intestine 510
  longitudinal muscle 529
  Meissner's plexus 529
  myenteric ganglia 529
  myenteric neurons 529
  neuromuscular functioning 529–530
  smooth muscle contractions 525
mucosal morphology 509
steatorrhea 518
transit 528
gene expression 12, 171–212, 220, 222, 310, 450, 563, 567
  transcription 171–195, 220, 567
  transcription factors 186–187, 189–195, 222, 450, 567
    c-fos 191
    c-jun 191, 195
    c-myc 186–187, 189–190, 195
    heat shock transcription factor (HSF) 193
    jun-B 191
    jun-D 191
    SPI 191, 195
    TF III A 194
  translation 171, 195–212, 567
glucagon 121, 127–128, 532, 539
  hyperglucagonemia 539
  secretion 121
glucose clamp procedures 122–123, 126, 132, 652–653
glucose effectiveness 128–129
glucose homeostasis 120–122, 124, 129, 132
glucose metabolism 119, 121–122, 125–129, 132–135, 164
glucose production 121, 125–126
  hepatic 121
glucose tolerance 119–123, 126–127, 129, 132–133, 135, 137–138, 164–165, 451, 652–657
  impaired 119–121, 127, 129, 132–133, 135, 138, 164–165, 451, 653–655, 657
  tests 119, 122–123, 126–127, 129, 132, 135, 653–654, 656–657
    intravenous 119, 126–127, 129, 132, 653
    oral 119, 122–123, 132, 135, 654, 656–657
glucose transport 127–128, 132, 652
  exercise 652
  insulin-mediated 127

glucose transporters 121, 125, 127–128, 132, 135, 652–653
glucose utilization 126–127
glucose-insulin axis 236
glucose-pancreatic interaction 124
glutamine synthetase 220
glutathione 280
glutathione peroxidase 112, 195
glycation 137, 236, 255–257, 260–262, 279
  advanced glycation end-products 137, 260–262
    fluorescence 260–261
    pentosidine 261–262
  glycation and oxidation 258–259
    glucose autoxidation 259
glycemia 236, 313; see also hyperglycemia; hypoglycemia
glycogen 652
  biosynthesis 652
  skeletal muscle concentration 652
glycoproteins 272
glycosaminoglycans 237, 265, 269, 313, 315–316
"glycoxidation" 262
gonadal steroids 378–383
  follicular reserve 378
growth factors 101, 138, 310, 386, 395–396, 401, 490, 540; see also cytokines
  beta$_2$-microglobulin 401
  epidermal growth factor (EGF) 310, 490, 540
  epidermal growth factor receptor 310
  fibroblast growth factors 401
  insulin-like growth factor I (IGF-I) 138, 386, 396, 401, 490
    plasma levels 386
  insulin-like growth factor II (IGF-II) 401
  platelet-derived growth factor (PDGF) 395, 401
  transforming growth factor-β 396, 401
  transforming growth factors 396, 401
growth hormone 13, 128, 377, 385–387
  deconvolutional analysis 386
  insulin-like growth factor-I (IGF-I) 386
  human aging 385–386
  plasma levels 386
  pulsatile secretion 385
  recombinant human 386
  replacement therapy 386–387
    risk of cardiovascular complications 387
    risk of carpal tunnel syndrome 386–387
    risk of hyperglycemia 387
    risk of malignancy 387
  rodent aging 386

hair 310, 313–314
  graying 310, 313–314
hair follicles 313
  androgen action 313
  telogen phase 313
hearing 326, 328–330
  auditory acuity 330
  central perceptual processing 330
  organ of Corti 330
  presbycusis 329–330

heart 213, 215, 217, 386, 414, 417–429, 431–453, 456–458, 639, 642–643
  adenosine levels 439
  alpha-adrenergic stimulation 437
  amyloid protein 418
  arrhythmias, ventricular 450
  atria 450
  atrial natriuretic factor 449
  AV block, chronic 451
  beta-adrenergic desensitization 439–440
  beta-adrenergic receptor number 436
  beta-adrenergic receptor response 436, 438
  beta-adrenergic stimulation 421, 437
    Ca_i transient 437
  Ca^{2+} channel blocker 429
  Ca^{2+} channel current 439
  Ca^{2+} homeostasis 439
  cardiac filling 421–423
    Ca^{2+}-dependent myofilament interaction 421–422
  cardiac output 421, 427–428, 432–433, 639, 642–643
  catecholamine content 436
  cellular RNA 450
  cholinergic receptors 441
  collagen 441
  contractility 424, 643
    beta-adrergic stimulation 643
    "E_{max}" 424
  contraction 420, 439, 442–453, 457
    actin 443
    actomyosin-ATPase activity 448
    alpha-MHC ("V_1")-protein isoform 448–449
    beta-MHC ("V_3")-protein isoform 448–449
    law of La Place 420
    myofibrillar-ATPase activity 448
    myofilament proteins 448–449
    myofilaments 443
    myosin 443
    myosin Ca^{2+}-activated ATPase activity 448
    myosin heavy chain 443
    postextrasystolic potentiation 445
    prolonged 449, 451, 457
    sarcomeres 443
    tropomyosins 443, 450
    troponins 439, 443
  C-protein 439
  coronary blood flow 452–453
  echocardiography, M-mode 418
  ejection fraction 420, 423
  endothelium 450
  excitation-contraction coupling 442–447, 450, 458
    action potential 443–445
    after depolarizations 450
    Ca^{2+} current inactivation rate 445
    calmodulin 447
    cytosolic Ca^{2+} concentration 445–446
    cytosolic Ca^{2+} transient 450
    cytosolic Na^+ concentration 447
    "inward-going rectifier" K^+ current 445
    ionic channel restitution 445
    outwardly directed K^+ current 445

heart, excitation-contraction coupling (*continued*)
  sarcoplasmic reticulum 446–447
  sarcoplasmic reticulum Ca^{2+} recycling 443
  sodium–calcium exchange 443
  sodium–potassium pump 447
  voltage-gated sarcolemmal Ca^{2+} channels 442–443
 failure, chronic 436
 gene expression, regulation 450–451
 G_s-protein 436
 hypertrophy 450, 643
 in vitro studies 443, 445, 453
  cardiac myocyte preparations 443
  cell capacitative area 445
  detergent (Triton X-100) treatment 445
  isolated working heart 453
  papillary muscle preparation 443
  trabeculae preparations 443
  whole-cell patch clamp 445
 left ventricular systolic pressure 423
 lipofuscin 418, 441
 mass 417, 441
 MHC genes 449
 mitochondria 456–457
 muscle 443–449
 myocardial contractile properties 423–426
 myocardial contractile reserve 432, 458
 myocardial function 421–428
  contractile state 421
  inotropic state 421
 myocytes 443–449
 oxidative metabolism 452–453
  free energy of ATP hydrolysis (ΔG_{ATP}) 453
  Krebs cycle 453
 oxygen consumption 452–453
 performance 386
 pre-proenkephalin gene 449
 pressure overload, experimental 449–450
 pump function 421–428
 rate 425–429, 432–435, 440, 453, 457, 643
  acetylcholine 440
  exercise response 643
  isoproterenol infusion 434–435
  resting 426
  vagal modification 440, 453
 rhythm 425–427
  AV node 425
  SA node 425
 sarcoplasmic reticulum 439, 447, 456
  Ca^{2+}-ATPase 447, 456
  Ca^{2+}-ATPase-mRNA 447, 456
  Ca^{2+} pump 439
  calsequestrin-mRNA 447
  phospholamban 447
  spontaneous Ca^{2+} oscillations 447
 stiffness 442
  active 442
  passive 442
 stroke volume 414, 420–421, 432–433
  afterload factor 421
  preload factor 421
 stroke volume index 427
 stroke work index 421, 425
 structure 417–419, 441–442, 457

cardiothoracic ratio 417
left ventricular cavity size 418
left ventricular hypertrophy 441
left ventricular wall thickness 418–419
life style influences 418
myocyte number 442
myocyte size 418, 441–442
subendocardial fibrosis 442
ventricular filling 422
 early filling rate 422
 echo-Doppler measurement 422
 radionuclide measurement 422
ventricular tachycardia 432
volumes 423, 427–429, 431–432
 end-diastolic 427, 431–432
 end-systolic 431–432
 equilibrium-gated cardiac blood-pool scan measurements 429
heat shock gene 68, 186, 193, 195, 222
heat shock protein-70 195
hematopoiesis 401–404
hematopoietic tissue 396
 granulocyte-macrophage series 396
heparan sulfate 270
heparin 270, 313
histones 187
homeodynamic senescence 11
homeodynamics 11, 598–601, 607
 action modes 601
 chaotic dynamics 600
 clamping 600–601, 607
 clocks 598
 constraints 598–599
 degrees of freedom 599
 differentiation 598
 entropy 599
 fluctuations 599–600
 fluctuation spectrum 601
 fractal space 599
 fractal time 599
 holonomic constraints 598
 information 601
 irreversibility 598–599
 isolated systems 598
 kinetic irreversibility 598
 near-periodicity 599
 nonholomonic constraints 599
 open systems 598, 600
 phase space 598
 physical-chemical potentials 600–601
 power spectrum 599
 reductionistic analysis 601
 second law of thermodynamics 598
 self-organizing system 600
 spectral analysis 599
 stability 599
 stochastic fluctuations 600
 thermodynamic engine cycles 598
 thermodynamic irreversibility 599
homeostasis 9–13, 17, 598
homeostatic control systems 12–13
homeotherms 99, 106
hormones 355, 377–394, 535, 538; *see also* individual hormones and endocrine glands
 receptors 538
 replacement therapy 377

horseradish peroxidase 217–218, 220
human subjects. *See* aging studies, design issues
Huntington's disease 349
hyaluronic acid 270–272, 275, 313
hydrogen peroxide 112
hydroxyl radicals 113
hyperadrenergic state 108
hyperadrenocorticism 13
hypercapnia 478
hyperglycemia 121, 123, 129, 132, 135, 137–138, 164, 279, 385, 655
hyperinsulinemia 122, 124, 132–133, 135, 165, 654–656
hyperlipemia 655
hypertension 85, 87, 133–135, 138, 148–149, 165, 417–418, 421–423, 427–433, 450, 488, 495, 498, 655
hypertension and collagen 241–242
hypoglycemia 652
hypophysectomy 624
hypothalamic-pituitary-adrenal axis 383
hypoxia 97, 428, 478

immune system 13, 56, 317–318, 346, 352, 355–357, 381, 510, 524–525, 555–590; *see also* lymphocytes; macrophages
 accessory cells 573–576
 anergy 580
 antibody responses 574, 577
 antibody secretion 56
 anti-CD28 antibodies 574
 antiidiotypic antibodies 573
 autoimmunity 572
  encephalomyelitis 572
  lupus-like syndrome 572
  thyroiditis 572
 autoreactive antibodies 572
 cell-mediated immunity 317–318
 central nervous system 356
 class I histocompatibility complex 556
 delayed-type hypersensitivity 318, 559, 580
 dendritic cells 555, 573–574
  follicular 574
 functional deficiencies 381
 germinal centers 574
 gut-associated 524–525
  lymphoid tissue 524–525
  lamina propria lymphocytes 524
  mesenteric lymphoid cells 524
  mucosal immune response 524
  oral tolerance to antigens 524
  plasma cells within lamina propria 524
 humoral response 318
 immunoglobulin A 524–525, 571
 immunoglobulin D 569
 immunoglobulin G 525, 571
 immunoglobulin M 525, 569–571
 immunoglobulins 357
 infections 579–581
  influenza 581
  polio virus 580
  Leishmania major 579
  tuberculosis 580
 influenza vaccination response 560
 intestine 510

immunoglobulin A secretion 510
immunoglobulins 510
isoprimosine 579
Langerhans' cells 574
Leishmania major infection 579
lymphocyte proliferation, phorbol esters 524
major histocompatibility class II antigens 356
natural killer cells 576, 581
  virally infected cells 576
patch tests 318
radioallergosorbent test 318
response to interleukin-2 559–560
responses 346, 355–357
risk of mortality 580
role of cytokines 357
scrum complement 357
  anaphylotoxins 357
  C1 complement 357
  classical pathway of complement activation 357
  membrane attack complex 357
skin 317–318
  epidermal 318
superantigens 559
tumor rejection 559
vaccination responses 560, 581
vaccines 577–578
immunity and disease 579–581
immunosuppression 13
infectious illness 579
inflammation 259, 314, 316, 318, 355–357, 383
  acute phase response 356–357
  carrageenan-induced 383
  histamine 318
  prostaglandin E_2 318
inflammatory processes 383
insects 593–594
insulin 121–129, 132–135, 138, 165–166, 236, 532, 652–658
  action 122, 124–129, 132–133, 135, 652–654, 656–657
    antilipolytic 127
    antiproteolytic 127
  clearance 123
  C-peptide 122–123
  deficiency 655–656
  plasma 352; see also hyperinsulinemia
  resistance 122–123, 125, 132–135, 138, 165, 653–658
  responsiveness 654
  secretion 121–124, 127, 129, 133–135, 652–653, 655–656
    glucokinase activity 135
  sensitivity 125–126, 128–129, 132–135, 165, 652–656
insulin clamp procedure 127
insulin-mediated glucose utilization 121
insulin-mediated signal transduction 125
insulin receptor 125–126, 135
  tyrosine kinase 125
intracellular water 96, 650
in vitro aging 56; see also cell culture systems for the study of aging

keratan sulfate 270, 272, 274–275
kidney 138, 165, 261, 381, 384, 386, 485–496
  afferent arteriole 487
  blood flow 486–487
  concentration ability 487
  diluting ability 487
  disease 138, 165, 261, 488, 490, 493–496
    acute glomerulonephritis 494
    acute interstitial nephritis 493–494
    acute renal failure 493–494
    acute tubular necrosis 493
    arteriolar nephrosclerosis 495
    chronic renal failure 495–496
    glomerulosclerosis 490
    nephrotic syndrome 494–495
    polycystic renal disease 496
    postural obstruction 494
    primary glomerulopathies 494–495
    pyelonephritis 490
    rat chronic nephropathy 488
    renal artery stenosis 495
    rodent glomerulosclerosis 488
    urinary tract infections 496
  efferent arteriole 487
  filtration fraction 487
  function 386, 485–491
    high protein diet 490
    osmotic diuresis 491
    serum creatinine concentration 486
  glomerular filtration rate 386, 485–486, 489
  glomerular permeability 488
  hydrogen ion excretion 487–488
  morphology 488
    glomerular number 488
    mass 488
    tubular cell number 488
  plasma flow 486–487
    arteriolar constriction 486
  salt balance 384
  tubular reabsorption maxima 487
  tubular secretory maxima 487

laminin 237
lean body mass 96, 150, 158, 381, 385–386; see also body fat-free mass
  estimated from total body potassium 158
lens 236, 276–287; see also eye
  aldose reductase 283, 287
  aminopeptidase 283
  ascorbic acid 283–284
  calpains 283
  catalase 283–284
  cathepsin B 283
  crystallins 236, 276–287
    aging mechanisms 283–285
    conformational changes 279
    cross-linking 281–282
    damage from ascorbic acid 286
    damage from reducing sugars 286
    deamidation 282
    deamination 282
    fluorescence 279–280
    fragmentation 279

glycation 282–283
oxidation 280–281
photooxidative damage 285
racemization 279
solubility 278–279
yellowing 279–280
glucose-6-phosphate dehydrogenase 283
glutathione 283–284, 287
glutathione peroxidase 283
glutathione reductase 283–284, 287
hydrogen peroxide 284
metabolism 277
metal-catalyzed oxidation 284–285
neutral endopeptidase 283
oxidative damage 284
partial pressure of oxygen 287
protein carbonyl groups 284–285
sodium-potassium ATPase 283
superoxide dismutase 283
taurine 287
life expectancy 5
life span 5–6, 38–39, 250, 379, 381, 383, 604, 637
  alcohol 381
  antioxidant enzymes 39
  antioxidants 39
  castration 381
  cephalization factor 39
  DNA repair 39
  main histocompatibility complex 39
  maximum 5–6, 250, 637
  maximum potential 604
  mean 250
  metabolic factor 39
  rodents, ad libitum fed vs. dietary restricted 383
  smoking 381
  species 38–39
  thymectomy 39
life span and metabolic rate 111
life span extension 604, 613
life table 4, 40
lipid metabolism 135, 138
  disorders of 135
lipid peroxidation 113
lipid profiles, plasma 165
lipids 165
  plasma, dyslipidemia 165
lipofuscin 113, 256, 314
lipoproteins 148, 165–167, 195, 381, 518, 524
  apolipoprotein A1 195
  plasma 148, 165–167, 381
    apolipoprotein B 165
    dyslipoproteinemia 148
    high density 165–167
    low density 165–167, 381
    very low density 166–167
  very low density 518
  vitamin A-containing 524
liver 218, 512, 523, 531, 535–538; see also bile; gallbladder
  bile salt secretion 536
  bile salt synthesis 537
  function 531, 535–536, 538
    detoxification 531, 536
    drug clearance 536

liver, function (*continued*)
  drug metabolism 536
  sulfobromophthalein 535, 538
  hepatocyte plasma membranes 536
  lipid peroxidation 512, 536
  membrane fluidity 512
  morphology 535
   size 535
  ornithine decarboxylase 536
  P450 536
  partial hepatectomy 536
  regeneration 536
  reticuloendothelial system 535
  thymidine kinase expression 536
  transplantation 536
  vitamin A stores 523
  vitamin K metabolism 523
longevity 7, 110, 579–581, 604, 633–639
  cold exposure 638
  exercise 633–639
  Gompertzian hazard function 604
  "hormesis" 604
  immunity 579–581
  sex differences 7
longitudinal studies. *See* aging studies design issues
lymphocytes 180, 187, 317–318, 355, 524, 555–574; *see also* immune system
  B cells 318, 524, 555, 559, 569–574
   antibody diversity 572
   antibody secretion 571
   calcium signals 571
   CD5 antigens 570
   development 572–573
   frequency 571
   heavy and light-chain variable region 571
   I_a surface antigens 570
   immunologlobulin loci 573
   memory subset 574
   phosphorylation activity 571
   pre-B cells 572
   response to influenza antigens 571
   response to phosphorylation 571
   response to pneumococcal vaccine 570
   T 15 antiidiotype antibody 571
   V_H gene segment 572
  T cells 187, 317–318, 355, 524, 555–569, 571, 573
   A23187 stimulation 566
   activation 563–568
   calcium influx and efflux 565–566
   calcium ionophore effects 567
   calcium level 563
   calcium pump 566
   calcium signal generation 564–565
   CD3 marker 557
   CD4 marker 557
   CD8 marker 557
   CD25 marker 558
   CD29 marker 558
   CD44 marker 558
   CD45RA marker 558
   CD45RO marker 558
   c-myc protooncogenes 567
   c-myc mRNA 567
   cytotoxic 318, 556–557, 559
   development 568–569
   granulocyte–macrophage colony stimulating factor 562
   helper 318, 556–557
   inositol phosphate metabolism 565
   inositol triphosphate 563–564
   inositol triphosphate generation 565
   interferon-γ production 561–562
   interleukin-2 production 559, 564, 566–567
   interleukin-2 receptors 560, 566
   interleukin-3 production 562
   interleukin-4 production 561
   interleukin-5 production 561
   ionomycin stimulation 564, 566
   membrane potential 567
   memory subset 557–558, 561, 563–565, 573
   naive subset 557–558, 563, 565
   P-glycoprotein 559
   phorbol myristate acetate stimulation 564, 566
   phospholipase C 563
   proliferation 524, 559, 566
   protein kinase C 563, 571
   protein kinases 563–564
   subsets 556–559
   T-cell receptor (TCR) 569
   T-cell receptor (TCR) genes 558
   T-cell receptor (TCR) marker 557
   tyrosine-specific protein kinase 563
   Vβ gene 567
lymphokines. *See* cytokines
lysosomes 211
lysozyme 218

macrophages 138, 319, 355, 555, 573–575; *see also* immune system
Maillard reactions 256, 258
  aminocarbonyl reactions 256
mast cells 313, 315
matter, animate 592
measurement reliability 29–30, 32
melatonin 624
meniscus 274
menopause 165, 378–379, 397
  androgen levels 378
  estradiol levels 378
  progestin levels 378
  vasomotor instability 379
metabolic economy 105
metabolic efficiency 104
metabolic mass 101
metabolic rate 95, 98–105, 107–109, 112–113; *see also* basal metabolic rate
  diet-induced thermogenesis 100, 103–104, 108
  measurement 100
   doubly labeled water 100
   indirect calorimetry 100
  physical activity 100, 103
  postprandial thermogenesis 103
  resting 100–102, 104, 108–109
  tissue 98
  whole body 98–105
   metabolism 97–99, 104, 109, 112
    aerobic 109, 112
    futile cycles 104
   tissues 97–99
    adipose 97
    brain 97
    heart 97
    kidney 97
    skeletal muscle 97
microvascular disease 165
mineral metabolism 395
minerals, total body 159
minimal oxygen consumption 103, 108
mitochondria 11, 95, 99, 104, 109–110, 113, 174, 197, 566
  calcium pool 566
  DNA 95, 99
  genome 11
  membrane surface area 99, 109
  oxidative phosphorylation 104
  structure 11
  volume density 99
mitochondrial content 99, 107
mitochondrial density 109, 113
mitochondrial function 113
mitochondrial metabolism 99
models in science 591–592
monoamine oxidase B 333
morphogenesis 596
  adhesion processes 596
  determination 596
  differentiation 596
  pattern formation 596
mortality 4–8, 379, 384, 592, 594, 603, 606–607, 614
  age-specific 4–8, 603, 606–607, 614
  Gompertz exponential analysis 603, 606–607, 614
  all cause 379, 384
  Gompertzian analysis 5–8
  probability 594
  rate 592
mortality rate doubling time 6–7, 17, 613–614
mouth 363, 506, 526; *see also* salivary glands; swallowing
  "mouthsense" 363
  pharynx 526
mouth-pharynx, Zenker's diverticulum 527
mucopolysaccharides 270
multicellularity 593–594
muscle mass 96, 102; *see also* skeletal muscle
mutagenesis 65

National Health and Nutrition Examination Survey (NHANES) 147–148, 164
nervous system 325–346, 351–357, 381, 623; *see also* autonomic nervous system; brain; brain stem; cental nervous system; neurons; neurotransmission; neurotransmitters; sense organs and sensations
  basal forebrain 352
  central processing 326, 328
  cholinergic system 333, 352

circadian activity rhythms 381
dopaminergic system 353
gait 326, 331–333
growth factors, insulin-like growth factor-1 352
locomotion 381
mobility 331
motor coordination 381
motor function 331–332
motor speed 328
neurotrophic factors 345–346, 351–357
  brain-derived growth factor (BDGF) 352
  fibroblast growth factors 352, 355
  nerve growth factor (NGF) 352, 354–355, 357
  nerve growth factor receptor synthesis 352
  neurotrophin family 352
nigrostriatal dopaminergic system 331, 333, 337, 623
postsynaptic receptors 326
posture 326, 331
presynaptic terminals 326
reaction time 328
sensory systems 326
somatosensory systems 328, 330
  central perceptual processing 330
synapses 327, 332–333
synaptic activity 351
synaptic plasticity 356
timed tasks 326
walking 331
neurodegenerative disease 345, 348–349, 351, 355
neuroendocrine system 13, 107–108, 379
neuromuscular function 431
neurons 346–347, 349, 355, 357
  benzodiazepine binding 349
  calcium influx 346, 349
  calcium-mediated channels 346
  excitotoxicity 346, 349, 355
  long-term potentiation 346, 357
  MK-801 binding 346–347
    glycine effect 347
    zinc effect 347
  N-methyl-D-aspartate binding 346
  plasticity of response 346
  substance P 357
neuropathy 165
neurotransmission 129, 134, 345–352, 428–429, 432–433, 437, 491, 498, 529
  adrenergic receptors 129, 134, 433, 437
    alpha 129, 134
    beta 129, 433, 437
    beta$_1$ 437
    beta$_2$ 437
  alpha-adrenergic 429, 498
  alpha-amino-3 hydroxy-5 methyl-4 isoxazolepropionic acid receptors 346–347
  beta-adrenergic 428–429, 432, 491, 498
  excitatory 345
  excitatory amino acid receptors 348
  gamma-amino butyrate receptors 349–352
    turnover 349
  glutamate receptors 346–349

glutamate system 351
inhibitory 345
kainic acid receptors 346–347
N-methyl-D-aspartate (NMDA) receptors 346–347, 349, 352
  acetylcarnitine effect 349
  phosphatidylserine effects 349
  zinc inhibition 349
non-N-methyl-D-aspartate receptors 346
opiate receptors 529
neurotransmitters 103, 108, 129, 134, 326, 333, 346–349, 351–352, 357, 415, 440, 497, 529, 621
  acetylcholine 357, 497
  catecholamines 415
  dopamine 333, 621
    monoamine oxidase 621
  gamma-aminobutyrate (GABA) 346–347, 351–352
  gamma-aminobutyrate synthesis 349
  glutamate 346, 348–349, 352
  norepinephrine 103, 108, 129, 134, 333
  substance P 529
  vagal 440
nitrogen, total body 159
nonlinear oscillations 595
norepinephrine, plasma 427, 434, 439
"normal aging," concept of 15, 38, 657
nucleosome 187, 194, 222
nutrition, micronutrients 513

obesity 103, 122, 125, 132–133, 135, 138, 148–149, 153, 156, 160–161, 164–167, 385, 637, 653–655, 658; see also adiposity
  android 164
obesity, index 153
olfaction 363, 370–373
  allergic rhinitis 372
  anosmia 370
  hyposmia 370
  loss 372
    cribiform plate damage 372
    head trauma 372
    viral infections 372
    nasal polyposis 372
    National Geographic Survey 371
  normosmia 370
  orthonasal route 363, 370–372
    labeled scale 371
    loss 372
    magnitude matching 371–372
    magnitude scale 371
    odor identification 371
    thresholds 370–371
  orthonasal vs. retronasal route 372–373
  retronasal route 363, 372–373
    dentures effect 373
    loss 373
    magnitude matching 372
    odor identification 372
    saliva production effect 373
    thresholds 372
  sensory-specific satiety 373

testing, Baltimore Longitudinal Study of Aging 372
organismal senescence 594
ornithine decarboxylase 217
osteoarthritis 237, 274, 288, 331
osteomalacia 319
osteoporosis 13, 331, 381, 395, 397–398, 405–406, 520
  cost to society 397
  estrogen therapy 406
  intestinal calcium malabsorption 406
  intestinal resistance to calcium absorption 406
  involutional 397
    postmenopausal 397
    senile 397
    type I 397
    type II 397
  primary 397
  secondary 397
ovalbumin 218, 220
ovarian failure 378–379
ovarian steroids 378–379
  postmenopausal 379
oxidative damage 112
oxygen consumption 106, 108–109, 113, 132, 639–645, 658
  maximum ($\dot{V}O_{2max}$) 106, 108, 132, 639–645, 658
oxygen molecules, reactive 113
oxygen toxicity 638

pancreas 515, 518, 522–523, 532–535, 539
  amylase 533
  cholecystokinin receptors 539
  chymotrypsin 533
  DNA 533
  exocrine secretion 515, 518, 522–523, 532, 534
    amylase 515, 532, 534
    bicarbonate 534
    chymotrypsinogen 532
    folate conjugase 522–523
    lipase 532, 534
    proteolytic enzymes 532
    trypsin 534
    trypsinogen 532
  idiopathic pancreatic exocrine deficiency 533
  Islet of Langerhans 532
  lipase 533–534
  morphology 532–533
    metaplasia 533
    pancreatitis 533
    polyamines 534
    proliferation 533
    protein biosynthesis 533
    proteins 533
    spermidine 534
    stones 533
    trypsinogen 533–534
pancreatic alpha cells 121
pancreatic beta cells 121–123, 132, 135, 137, 653, 656
  glucokinase activity 123

pancreatic polypeptide 532
paracrines 310, 401
parasympathetic nervous system 426, 428, 440–441, 497, 505, 529–530, 532
parathyroid hormone 396, 398–399
  plasma levels 399
Parkinson's disease 331, 333, 349, 496, 499, 527, 621–623
peripheral neuropathy 138
peripheral vascular disease 138
peroxidases 638
peroxisomes 112
phagocytosis 355, 357
  complement facilitation 357
phosphate, plasma 398
physical activity 132, 135, 165–166, 451, 665
physical fitness 106, 132
physical inactivity 642–645
pituitary gland 385–386, 578, 624; see also individual hormones
  adenohypophysis, somatotropes 385
  adenoma 386
plants 593, 602
  callus 602
poikilotherms 99, 106, 109–110
potassium 491
  balance 491
  hyperkalemia 491
primary aging processes, concept of 9–13, 17
progesterone 379
proinsulin 122–123
prokaryotes, anaerobic 593
prolactin 377
proliferation-related pathologies 57
  hyperplastoid cells 57
  neoplastoid cells 57
prostaglandins 396, 403–404, 507–509, 574
  gastroduodenal 508
  gastrointestinal 508
  gastrointestinal synthesis 508
  prostaglandin E 396
  prostaglandin E_2 404
  stomach 507–509
prostate 380–381, 486, 491, 494, 499–500
  benign hyperplasia 380–381, 494, 499–500
    detrusor function 500
    urinary bladder out flow obstruction 499
  benign hypertrophy 486
  prostate-specific antigen 381
proteins 11–12, 65, 104, 112–113, 120, 159, 171, 195–213, 218–221, 236, 385–386, 450, 517
  abnormal 218–220
  biosynthesis 120, 171, 195–212, 385–386, 450
    elongation 206, 211–212
    elongation factor 1α (EF1α) 206, 209, 212
    elongation factor 2 (EF2) 206
    elongation (S1 protein) 209
    eukaryotic initiation factor 2 (eIF-2) 206
    fidelity 204–206
    initiation 206
    skeletal muscle 386
    carbonyls 113
    cross-linking 236
    degradation 171, 211–212, 219–220
      proteosome 212, 219
      ubiquitin 212
    degradation pathways 211, 213
    dietary 517
    error-containing 65
    fragmentation 236
    oxidized 112, 218–220
    partially degraded 65
    post-translational modifications 11, 218, 221
    racemization 236
    total body 159
    turnover 12, 104, 171, 211, 220
proteinuria 488
proteoglycans 235, 237, 261, 269–276, 313
  aggrecan 272–274
  hydration 271
  synthesis 275
  tissue content 271
  turnover 275–276
proteolysis 12
protozoa 593
psychosocial performance 385
pulmonary system 85, 87, 235, 266, 383, 430, 475–481; see also respiratory system
  airway closing volume 477–478
  chronic obstructive lung disease 85, 87, 479–481
  emphysema 266, 480
  flow rates 383, 476–477
    dynamic compression of airways 476
    forced expiratory volume 383, 476–477
    forced vital capacity 476
  function 475
  gas exchange 477–478
    alveolar-arterial oxygen difference 478
    alveolar capillary surface area 478
    alveolar partial pressure of oxygen (PAO_2) 478
    arterial partial pressure of oxygen (PaO_2) 478
    dead space 478
    diffusion capacity 478
  lung volumes 475–476
    functional residual capacity 476
    residual volume 476
    total lung capacity 475
    vital capacity 476
  lungs 235, 477–478
    alveolar ventilation 477
    elasticity 235
    perfusion 477
    ventilation-perfusion dynamics 478
    ventilation-perfusion ratio 477
  mechanics 475–477
    chest wall 475
    lung elastic recoil 475
    respiratory muscles 475
    physiological changes 475
    respiratory muscle reserve 430

Raynaud's phenomenon 526
rectum 530–532
  ampulla sensation 531
  compliance 531–532
  defecation 530
  external sphincter 530
    neuropathic damage 531
  fecal bacteria 531
  function, childbirth damage 532
  internal sphincter 530–531
  manometric studies 531
  sphincters 530
  tissue elasticity 532
regular phenomena 595–596
  approximate entropy 595
  complexity 595
  constraints 595
  coupling constants 595
  execution driven phenomena 596
  intentionality 596
  near periodicity 595
  phase space 595
  programmatic phenomena 595–596
  regularity 595
  spectral analysis 595
  stable modes 595
  symmetry breaking 596
renin activity, plasma 491
renin-aldosterone response 491
renin-angiotensin-aldosterone system 491
replicative senescence 10; see also cell culture models for aging studies
reproduction 377–379
  decreased fertility 379
  estrous cyclicity 379
  implantation 379
  menstrual cyclicity 379
  persistent estrous 379
  prolonged cycles 379
  ovulatory cyclicity 379
respiratory system 475–483, 639, 642; see also pulmonary system
  airway responsiveness 479
  arteriovenous oxygen difference 639, 642
  defense mechanisms 479
    cough mechanisms 479
    laryngeal reflexes 479
  respiratory control 478
    central chemoreceptors 478
    peripheral chemoreceptors 478
  sensations 478–479
ribonuclease A 218
ribosome aggregation 206, 212
ribosomes 204, 206, 210
RNA 11, 171–189, 190–191, 194, 201, 205–209, 220–221
  hnRNA 175, 184
  mRNA 174–187, 191, 194, 201, 206, 221
    post-transcriptional processing 184–187
    post-transcriptional splicing 185
  poly(A^+) RNA 174, 186
  rRNA 174, 190
  synthesis 171–175, 188
  tRNA 174, 205–209
    aminoacylation 206
  turnover 220
RNA polymerases 175, 184, 187, 205, 221

salivary glands 505–506, 515, 524, 526
  parotid 505–506
  saliva 526
  secretions 505–506, 515, 524
    amylase 506, 515
    immunoglobins 524
  sublingual 505
  submandibular 505
scleroderma 495–496
sebaceous glands 313–314
  androgen stimulation 314
senescence 3, 8, 54, 592, 596–598, 601–607
  binary fission 602
  component death 602, 605–606
  connectivity 606
  definition of 3, 54, 592
  degrees of freedom 601
  differentiation 601
  dynamic instability 602
  germ line 602
  homeodynamic instability 602–603
  isolated systems 603
  mathematical models 607
  physical background 596–598, 601–603, 607
    Aristotelian causes 597
    broken symmetry 598
    causality 597
    complexity 596
    complex systems 596
    constraints 598, 601–602, 607
    coupling strengths 597
    entailments 597
    execution driven 598, 602
    heterarchy 597
    hierarchical organization 597
    horizontal integration 597
    marginal stability 597
    nonholonomic constraints 596
    order 597
    order parameters 597
    phase space 597
    re-initialization 598, 602
    resilience 597
    second law of thermodynamics 598, 603
    self-organizing systems 598, 602
    stability 597–598
    vertical integration 597
  program-driven systems 602
  rate 8, 604
  redundancy 606
  soma 602
  specific metabolism 601, 604
  system death 602–603, 604
sense organs and sensations 309, 314, 326, 328–332, 363–366; see also eye; hearing; olfaction; taste
  central perceptual processing 330
  cutaneous senses 314
    Meisner's corpuscles 314
    Merkel's corpuscles 314
    nerves 314
    nerve endings 314
    Pacinian corpuscles 314
    radiant heat 314
    touch 314

vibration 314
intensity 364–366
  category scale 364
  magnitude matching 366
  magnitude scale 364
  perceived 364–366
  tape-pull method 366
itching 309
measurement of sensation 363
pain 309, 314
perception 329–330
perceptual processing 328
proprioception 331
thresholds 364
trigeminal sensation 363
vibration sense 326, 331–332
skeletal muscle 104, 107–108, 125, 127, 132, 151–153, 162, 165, 195, 213, 215, 271, 326, 331, 381, 386, 417, 430–431, 455–456, 479, 486, 639, 644–647, 652–653, 657
  atrophy 195
  decline in maximum oxygen consumption 644–645
  fatigue, glycogen stores 652
  force development 646
  grip strength 331
  mass 386, 417, 430–431, 479, 486, 644–647, 657
    loss of muscle fibers 647
    strength training 646–647
    weight-bearing muscles 646
  metabolism, ^{31}P nuclear magnetic resonance measurements 430
  motor units 645
  myofibrillar protein 195
  strength 326, 331, 386, 430, 645–647, 657
skeleton 395; see also bone
skin 235, 309–324, 522
  achochordons 310
  basement membrane zone 312
  bruises 313
  cherry angioma 310
  cytokines 311, 318
  dermal-epidermal junction 312
  dermal fibroblasts 309, 313–315, 319
  dermis 312–314, 316
    appendageal structures 313
    elastic tissue 313
  dryness 310
  elastic fibers 315
  elasticity 235
  elastosis 315
    "grenz" or border zone 315
  epidermal stem cells 310
  epidermis 310–312
  extrinsic aging 314–317
    cigarette smoking 314, 316
    environment 314
    sunlight 314
  keratinocytes 309–312, 315–316, 318–319
  Langerhans' cells 312, 315, 318
    immune function 312
  laxity 310
  lentigines 310
  melanocytes 309, 311–321

melanin pigment 311
microvasculature 313, 315
photoaging 309, 314–316
  dermatoheliosis 314
  heliodermatitis 314
  microvasculature 315
  pathophysiology 316
  ultraviolet light 316
photocarcinogenesis 312, 316
  physical influence 316
physiology 317–320, 522
  barrier function 317
  percutaneous absorption 317
  stratum-corneum function 317
  transepidermal water loss 317
  vitamin D production 319–320, 522
pilosebaceous units 313
seborrheic keratosis 310, 315
spider nevi 315
sun damage, clinical features 315
superficial varicosities 315
telangiectasia 315
thickness 313
vascular changes 313
wrinkling 310, 313, 315–316
xerosis 315
skin-fold measurements 156–157
slime molds 592–593
small intestine 398, 507–524, 528–529, 534, 537
  absorption 398, 507, 511–524, 534, 537
  active transport 513–514
  amino acids 517
  arginine 517
  bile salts 517
  biotin 522
  calcium 398, 507, 519–523
  capacity 514
  carbohydrate 513–518
  cholesterol 518–519
  copper 519
  1,25 dihydroxyvitamin D 522
  drugs 524
  electrolytes 519
  facilitated difusion 514
  fat 518
  fat-soluble vitamins 513
  fatty acids 519
  folic acid 507, 522–523
  fructose 515
  galactose 515
  glucose 514–516
  glucose transporters 517
  glycine 517
  ileum 517
  iron 507, 519
  jejunum 516–517, 519
  lipids 513, 518–519
  long-chain fatty acids 518
  magnesium 522
  malabsorption 513, 519, 534
  membrane fluidity 514
  methods of study 514–515
  microvillar brush border membranes 514
  monosaccharides 515
  3-O-methylglucose 516

small intestine, absorption (*continued*)
  passive transport 514, 516
  phenylalanine 517
  phosphate 398, 522
  potassium 519
  proline 517
  proteins 514, 517–518
  rate 514
  receptor-mediated 514
  riboflavin 522
  short-chain fatty acids 518
  sodium 519
  surface area 511, 514
  thiamine 522
  triglycerides 514, 518
  tryptophan 517
  unstirred water layer 514, 519
  vitamin A 514, 518–519, 523–524
  vitamin B_{12} 507
  vitamin B_{12} malabsorption 523
  vitamin D 518–519
  vitamin E 518
  vitamin K 523
  water soluble vitamins 513
  xylose 515
  zinc 519
 bacterial overgrowth 514, 529
 brush border membranes 512–517, 519–520
  alkaline phosphatase 512–513
  composition 512
  disaccharidases 513, 515
  fluidity 512
  glucose transport 516
  lactase 513, 515
  lactase deficiency 515
  lipid thermotropic transition 512
  maltase 513
  receptors 517
  sucrase 513
 calbindin 520–521
  1,25 dihydroxyvitamin D influence 520
  vitamin D influence 520
 calbindin mRNA 521
  1,25 dihydroxyvitamin D influence 521
 calcium transport system 520
  basolateral membrane calcium transporters 520
 cellular proliferation 512
 digestion 512–513, 515–518
  carbohydrate 515–518
   sucrose in jejunum 515
   sucrose in ileum 515
 1,25 dihydroxyvitamin D 520, 523
 1,25 dihydroxyvitamin D receptors 521
 duodenal bicarbonate secretion 508–509
 enzymes 512–513
 folate 522
  active receptor-mediated transport 522
  malabsorption 522
 folate conjugase activity 522–523
  duodenum 523
  ileum 523
 folylpolyglutamate hydrolysis 522–523
 glycocalyx 522
 lipid transport 519
 membrane vesicles 516
 microvillus 516
  glucose transport 516
  membrane vesicles 516
 morphology 510–512, 524
  crypts 511
  duodenum 511
  goblet cells 511
  jejunum 511
  ileum 511–512
  mucosal membranes 510
  Paneth cells 510
  Peyer's patches 510, 524
  villi 511
  weight 511
 motor patterns 529
  migrating motor complex 529
 mucosa 513, 515
  glycoproteins 513
  ribosomes 513
 mucus 510
 permeability 513, 517, 519
 protein biosynthesis 513
  mucosa 513
  serosa 513
 transit 528–529
  breath-hydrogen testing 528
smooth muscle 133, 415, 434, 526, 529
 esophageal 526
 intestinal 529
 vascular 133, 415, 434
sodium 491–492
 balance 491
 hypernatremia 491–492
 hyponatremia 492
somatostatin 123, 127, 195, 532
splenocytes 386
 mitogenic response 386
  concanavalin A 386
  pokeweed 386
sponges 592
starvation 109, 510, 540; *see also* fasting
statin 73
steroids, anabolic 381
stomach 506–510, 518, 521–523, 527–529
 achlorhydria 507–508, 521–522, 528
 antral gastrin 509
 atrophic gastritis 506–507, 518
 emptying 527–529
 fiber processing 507
 gastrin receptors 509
 gastrin-binding sites 508
 hypochlorhydria 507
 intrinsic factor 508
 lipase 508, 518
 morphology 506–508
  parietal cells 508
 mucosal energy metabolism 509–510
 pepsin 508
 pepsinogen 508
 secretion 507–510, 523, 529
  acid 507–508, 529
  intrinsic factor 507, 523
  lipase 507
  pepsinogen 507
stress 13, 106–108, 128–129, 355, 383–384, 414, 421, 428, 434, 441, 457
 acute 108
 cold 107, 384
 heat 106
 neurotransmitter elaboration 434
 orthostatic 428, 457
 postural 441
stress and neoplasms 384
stroke 87, 138, 162, 165, 378
"successful aging" 16–17, 325, 363, 373, 397, 485
superoxide 112
superoxide dismutases 65, 112, 180, 186, 195
survival analysis 32
survival curves 4–5
swallowing 506, 526
sweat glands. *See* eccrine glands
symbiosis 593
sympathetic nervous system 103–104, 106–108, 129, 133, 329, 426, 428, 433–440, 498–499, 505, 529–530, 579
syndrome of inappropriate antidiuretic hormone 492
system death 594–595

taste 363, 366–370
 consistency of responses 370
 intensity 367–370
  labeled scales 368–369
  magnitude estimates 367–368
  magnitude matching 369–370
 loss 370
 suprathreshold studies 370
 thresholds 366–367
teeth 506
telomeres 11, 71
tendons 272
terminin 73
testicular steroids 379–381
theories of aging 9–14, 17, 64–65, 95, 110–113, 188, 204–205, 236, 346, 603–608, 618–619, 633, 637–639
 aspect theories 603–604
 centralized clock theory 10
 classification 9–10
 codon-restriction theory 10
 cross-linking theory 236
 decreasing oxygen consumption hormone theory 10
 disposable soma theory 14
 "dysdifferentiation" theory 12, 188
 energy metabolism theories 110–113
 error catastrophe theory 10–11, 65, 204–205
 free-radical damage theory 10, 12, 65, 95, 112–113, 637
 free-radical-glycation theory 10
 genetic programs 9–10, 17
 glucocorticoid cascade hypothesis 10, 12–13, 618–619
 glycation theory 12, 112
 imbalance hypothesis of brain aging 346
 immunologic theory 10
 "intrinsic mutagenesis" theory 11

lifetime metabolic potential 110
metabolic rate theories 12, 95
neuroendocrine-immune theory 10
oxidative damage theory 12
oxygen-radical mitochondrial injury theory 11
rate of living theories 95, 110–112, 603–605, 633, 637–639
reliability theories 604–608
  Gompertz-Makeham law 605–606
  mathematical models 605
somatic mutation theory 10–11, 64–65
  epimutations 65
  methylation 65
  mutational interactions 65
  transposable elements 65
wear and tear theories 10, 14
thermic effect of food 103
thermogenesis 104, 106–107
  nonshivering 107
  shivering 106–107
thermoregulation 100, 105–107, 313–314
  sweating 106
thiamine, dietary deficiency 522
thirst 491–492
thromboembolism 379

thymopoietin 318
thymus 318, 383, 386, 558, 568–569, 578
  hormones 578
  involution 568–569
  weight 383, 386
thyroid gland 107–108, 451
  euthyroid 108
  hormones, metabolism of 108
  hyperthyroidism 108
  hypothyroidism 108, 451
  thyroxine 108, 451
  triiodothyronine 108, 451
transcription. *See* gene expression
translation. *See* gene expression
transplantation 56, 577
triglyceride 165
  plasma 165
tyrosine hydroxylase 180, 333

urinary incontinence 485, 497–499
  established 499
  transient 498
urinary tract 496–500
  detrusor (bladder) 496–498
  urethra 497
"usual aging" 16

vasopressin 381, 491–492
  binding sites 381
  mRNA 381
vision 326, 328–330, 352; *see also* eye
  central perceptual processing 330
  optic nerve 352
vitamin A 317
vitamin B_{12}, dietary 523
vitamin D 319, 398–399, 523
  cholecalciferol 398
  dietary 523
  1,25 dihydroxyvitamin D 319, 398–399
  plasma levels 399
  25 hydroxy-1α-hydroxylase 399
  25 hydroxyvitamin D, plasma level 399
  provitamin D 319
  skin precursor 7 dehydrocholesterol 398
vitamin E (alpha tocopherol) 112, 574
vitamin K 396
  gamma-carboxylated proteins 396

water balance 491–492
wound healing 310, 318–319

yeast (*Saccharomyces cerevisiae*) 73